YOUR GUIDE TO

Fundamentals of Nursing Care

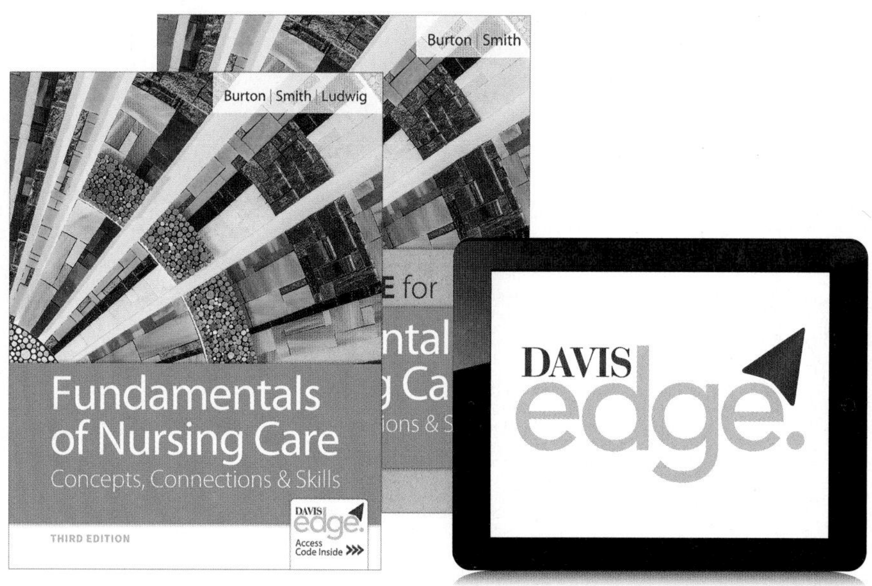

Your journey to success BEGINS HERE!

Your text works together with your Study Guide, online resources, and Davis Edge to make this foundational content easier to master.

Don't miss everything that's waiting online to make learning less stressful... and save you time. Follow the instructions on the inside front cover to use the access code to unlock your resources today.

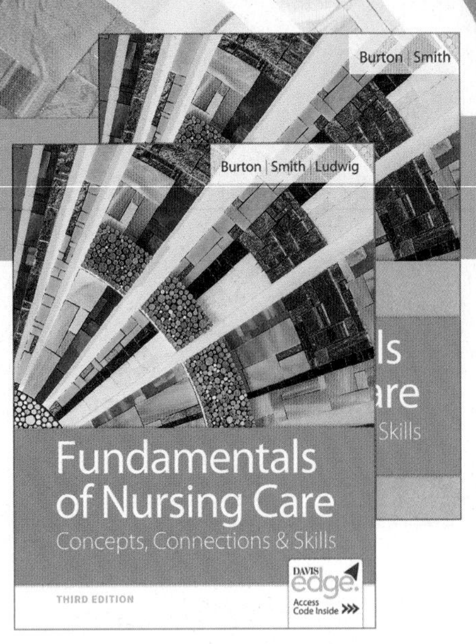

STEP #1

Build a solid foundation.

Knowledge Connection boxes check your understanding of the material you just read.

KNOWLEDGE CONNECTION

What areas will you inspect when assessing a patient with impaired oxygenation? When you palpate, what two evaluations are you making? How can you tell if the patient is becoming hypoxic or hypoxemic?

Step-by-step procedures for over 120 skills make every concept easy to grasp.

Skill 28.3 Assisting With Incentive Spirometry

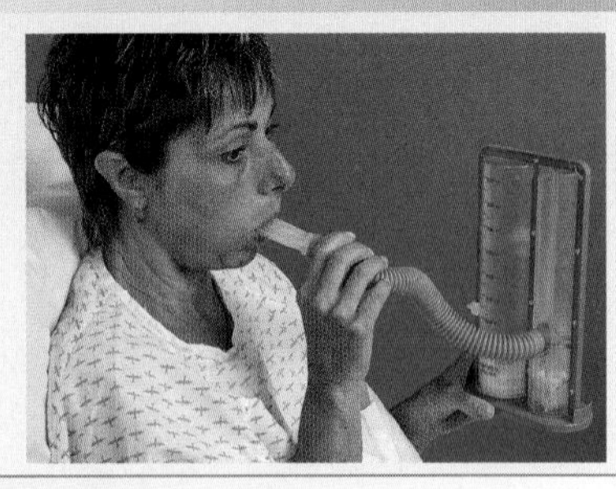

Assessment Steps

1. Verify the health-care provider's order for incentive spirometry. ***Note: Some hospitals do not require a health-care provider's order for this because it is considered a nursing or respiratory therapy order. Always follow your facility's policy.***
2. Determine the patient's pain level, availability, and willingness to perform the procedure. It may be necessary to medicate the patient for pain before beginning the procedure.

Planning Steps

1. Obtain an incentive spirometer.
2. Plan for appropriate time for incentive spirometry; avoid mealtimes.

Implementation Steps

1. Follow the Initial Implementation Steps locat[...] front cover.
2. Assist the patient to an upright position in th[...] chair ***to enlarge the rib cage and allow for m[...] lung expansion.***
3. Splint abdominal or chest incisions with a pill[...] ***pain during deep inhalation and exhalation***
4. Place the mouthpiece of the incentive spirom[...] the patient's lips ***to prevent air from escapin[...] during inhalation.***
5. Instruct the patient to take a deep breath thr[...] mouth, then exhale through the nose. ***This h[...] patient understand that the focus is on deep[...] not exhalation.***

CRITICAL THINKING CONNECTION

Clinical Assignment

You are assigned to care for a hospitalized patient tomorrow in clinical who has a tracheostomy. He was injured in a car accident and was on a ventilator for several weeks. He is breathing on his own now, but he still has the tracheostomy in place. In addition, he has recently developed pneumonia in his right lung. He has a large amount of secretions and requires suctioning every 2 to 3 hours. The tracheostomy will have to be cleaned on your shift and a new inner cannula put in place. He has humidified oxygen at 4 L/min via a tracheostomy collar.

Critical Thinking Questions:

1. Why is a tracheostomy done?
2. How does a tracheostomy work?
3. How will you suction it?
4. How will you clean it and replace the inner cannula?
5. What is a tracheostomy collar?

Post Conference boxes at the end of every chapter provide answers to the questions posed in the Critical Thinking Connections.

POST CONFERENCE

You were really worried when you walked into your patient's room the first morning and saw him with his tracheostomy, sounding all bubbly and coughing frequently. He pointed to the tracheostomy and mouthed the word "suction." Without much time to think, you grabbed a suction catheter and glove kit and set up quickly but without contaminating your sterile field or sterile supplies. You remembered as you suctioned to hold your own breath and not suction for longer than 10 seconds. It was obvious to you that the suctioning procedure tired your patient and made him a little sho[...] of breath. However, once you had suctioned his tracheostomy several times, he could breathe considerably better and mouthed "thank you." After that, you weren't afraid to suction him. His tracheostomy collar stayed in place pretty well, and you were able to replace his inner cannula the first day with your instructor's guidance. By the second day, you were feeling far more confident about all of his care. By the third day of clinicals, you were showing other students how to suction him.

Critical Thinking Connections at the beginning of every chapter help connect what you read to what you will see and do in the clinical setting.

Evidence-Based Practice

Ventilator-Associated Pneumonia in Acute Care Hospitals

Clinical Question

Do patients have a higher risk for ventilator-associated pneumonia (VAP) who receive mechanical ventilation (MV)?

Evidence

Patients who receive MV are at a higher risk for nosocomial pneumonia. VAP is a type of HAI. A patient is at risk for VAP if they are on MV for 13 to 51 per 1,000 ventilator days. A patient is also at risk for developing MRSA while on mechanical ventilation. When the patient must be frequently

Evidence-Based Practice boxes demonstrate the link between research and practice that underlies the best nursing care.

Elder Care Connection

Teaching Elderly Patients

Have a caregiver or family member present during teaching, if possible. Allow plenty of time for teaching so that your elderly patient does not feel rushed. Be alert to cues that the elderly patient does not understand the teaching. He or she may put you off, saying, "I'll do it later" or "I already read it." This may occur because the patient is confused or does not understand but does not want to say so. Be very patient with elderly learners. Use plenty of repetition without getting frustrated.

Geriatric content throughout familiarizes you with this important patient demographic.

STEP #2

Make studying easier.

Study Guide*

Corresponds to your text chapter by chapter to reinforce the "connections" each step of the way with exercises and activities that develop the critical-thinking and problem-solving skills essential to your success. Documentation exercises are included.

eBook

Lets you access your text online anytime, anywhere for study, review, and reference. You can also add notes, highlights, and bookmarks.

Online Resources

Feature Audio Chapter Summaries that help you to prepare for exams and let you study on the go as well as Skills Checklists that ensure you master must-know procedures.

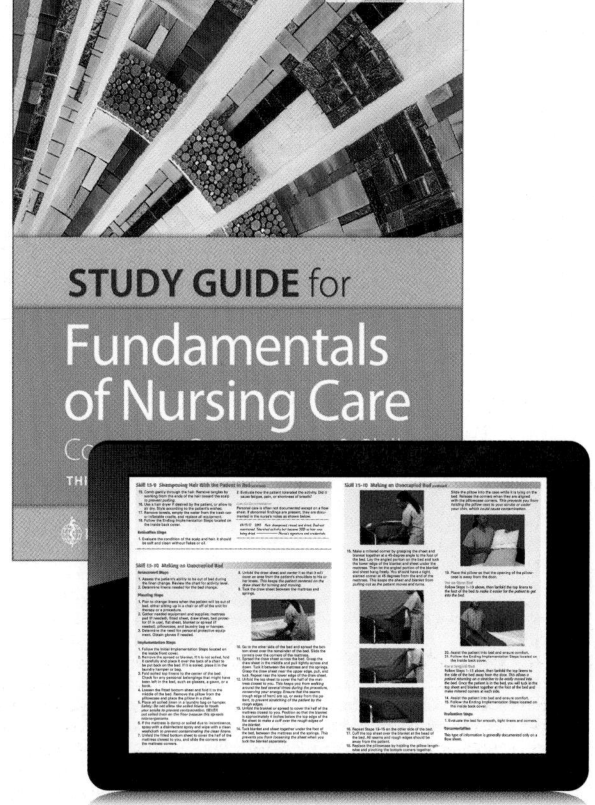

*Purchase separately.

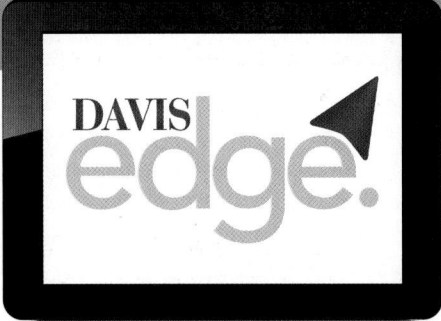

STEP #3

Test Yourself.

Davis Edge is the interactive, online Q&A review platform that provides the practice you need to master course content and to improve your scores on classroom exams. Access it from a laptop, tablet, or mobile device for review and study on the go.

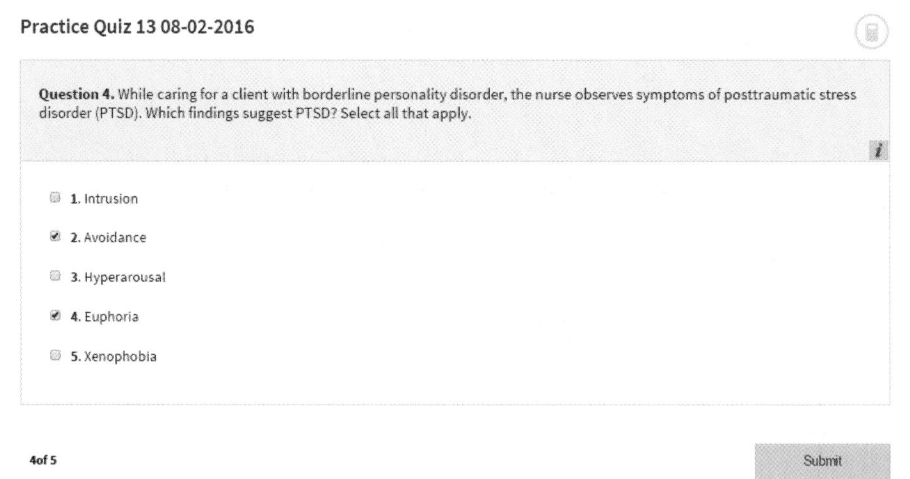

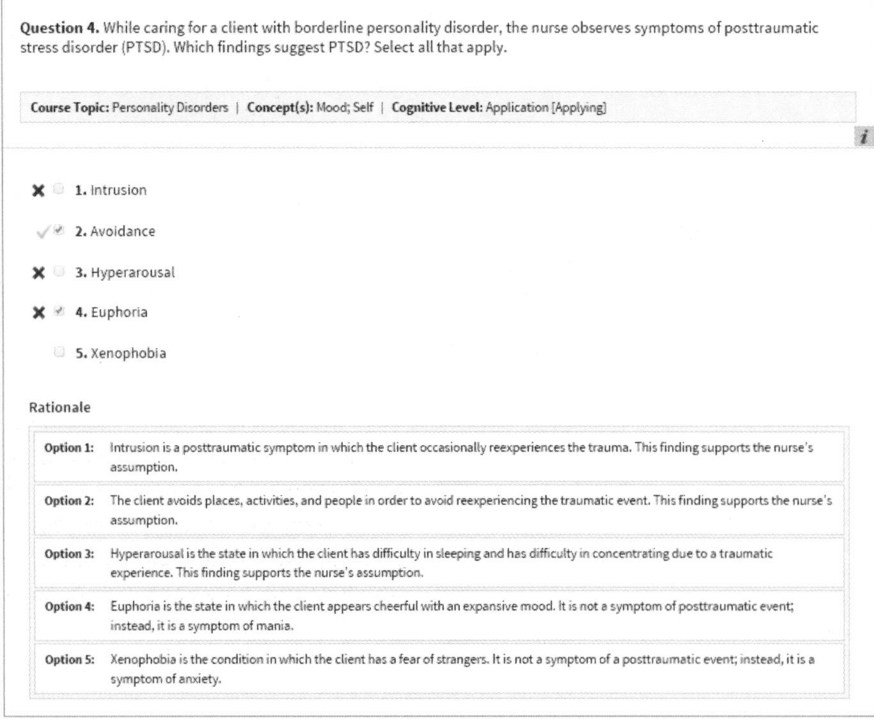

Practice Quiz 13 08-02-2016
Question 4. While caring for a client with borderline personality disorder, the nurse observes symptoms of posttraumatic stress disorder (PTSD). Which findings suggest PTSD? Select all that apply.
1. Intrusion
2. Avoidance
3. Hyperarousal
4. Euphoria
5. Xenophobia
4of 5
Submit

Question 4. While caring for a client with borderline personality disorder, the nurse observes symptoms of posttraumatic stress disorder (PTSD). Which findings suggest PTSD? Select all that apply.
Course Topic: Personality Disorders | Concept(s): Mood; Self | Cognitive Level: Application [Applying]
1. Intrusion
2. Avoidance
3. Hyperarousal
4. Euphoria
5. Xenophobia
Rationale
Option 1: Intrusion is a posttraumatic symptom in which the client occasionally reexperiences the trauma. This finding supports the nurse's assumption.
Option 2: The client avoids places, activities, and people in order to avoid reexperiencing the traumatic event. This finding supports the nurse's assumption.
Option 3: Hyperarousal is the state in which the client has difficulty in sleeping and has difficulty in concentrating due to a traumatic experience. This finding supports the nurse's assumption.
Option 4: Euphoria is the state in which the client appears cheerful with an expansive mood. It is not a symptom of posttraumatic event; instead, it is a symptom of mania.
Option 5: Xenophobia is the condition in which the client has a fear of strangers. It is not a symptom of a posttraumatic event; instead, it is a symptom of anxiety.

NCLEX®-style questions prepare you for the exams you'll encounter throughout your education, including the more difficult alternate-format questions like "select all that apply."

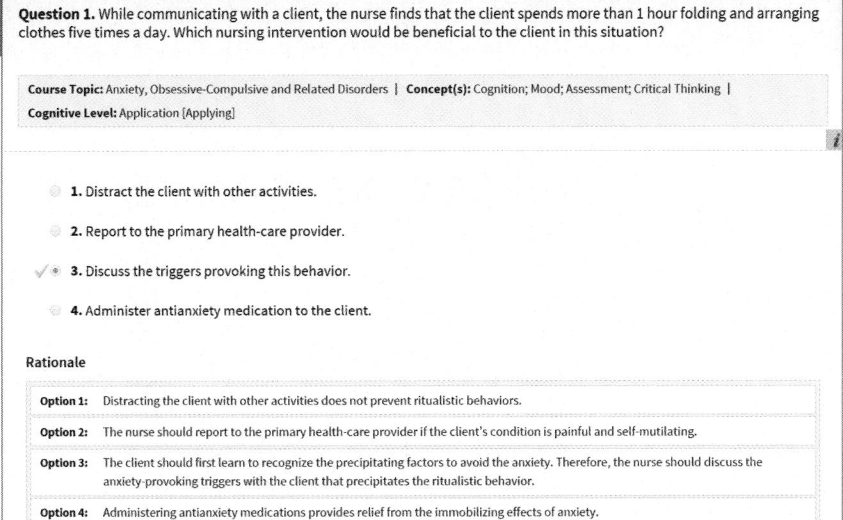

Comprehensive rationales explain why your responses are correct or incorrect. Page-specific references direct you to the relevant content in *Fundamentals of Nursing Care.*

The Success Center offers a snapshot of your progress and identifies your strengths and weaknesses.

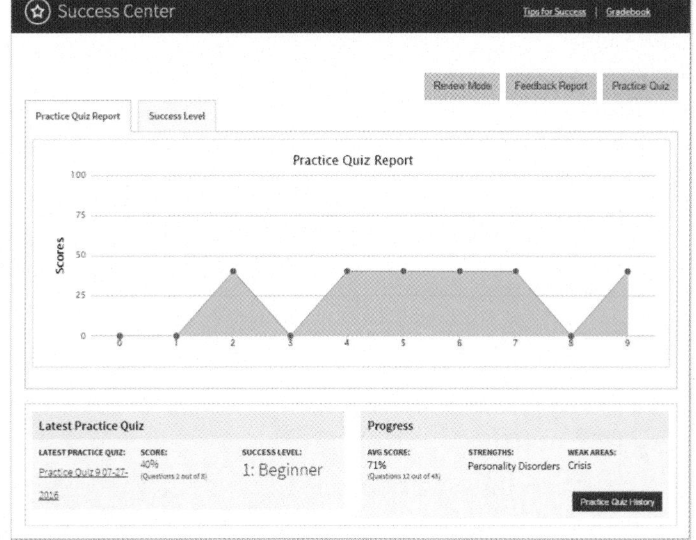

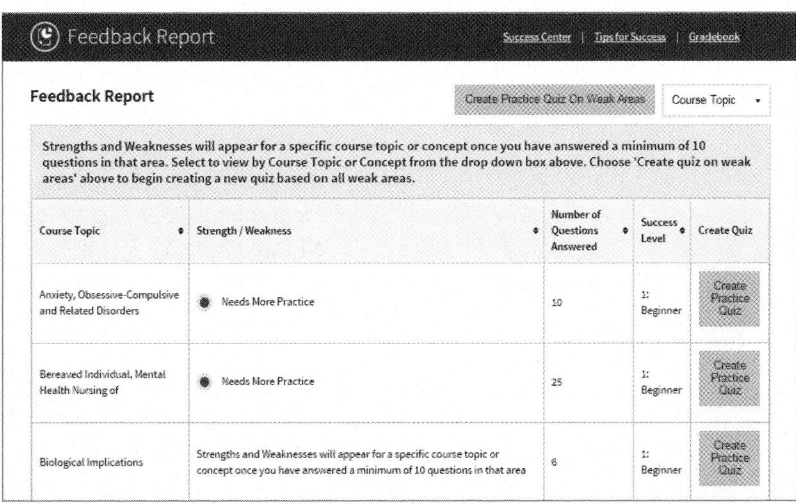

The Feedback Report drills down to show your performance in individual content areas. It's easy to create new practice quizzes that focus on your areas of weakness or to select the topics or concepts you want to study.

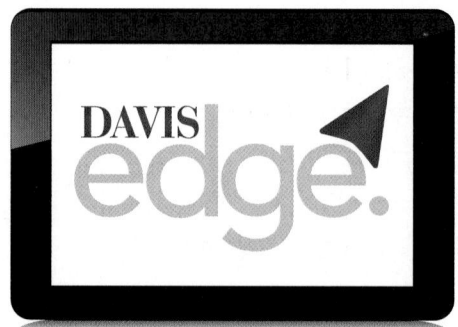

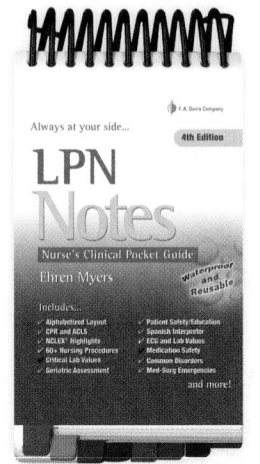

Brief Contents

F. A. Davis Company
1915 Arch Street
Philadelphia, PA 19103
www.fadavis.com

Printed in the United States of America

Last digit indicates print number: 10 9 8 7 6 5 4 3

Publisher, Nursing: Terri Wood Allen
Content Project Manager II: Amy M. Romano
Illustration & Design Manager: Carolyn O'Brien

As new scientific information becomes available through basic and clinical research, recommended treatments and drug therapies undergo changes. The author(s) and publisher have done everything possible to make this book accurate, up to date, and in accord with accepted standards at the time of publication. The author(s), editors, and publisher are not responsible for errors or omissions or for consequences from application of the book, and make no warranty, expressed or implied, in regard to the contents of the book. Any practice described in this book should be applied by the reader in accordance with professional standards of care used in regard to the unique circumstances that may apply in each situation. The reader is advised always to check product information (package inserts) for changes and new information regarding dose and contraindications before administering any drug. Caution is especially urged when using new or infrequently ordered drugs.

Library of Congress Cataloging-in-Publication Data

Names: Burton, Marti, author. | Smith, David W. (Of University of Texas at Arlington), author. | Ludwig, Linda J. May, author.
Title: Fundamentals of nursing care : concepts, connections & skills / Marti A. Burton, David W. Smith, Linda J. May Ludwig.
Description: Third edition. | Philadelphia : F.A. Davis Company, [2019] | Includes bibliographical references and index.
Identifiers: LCCN 2018018864 (print) | LCCN 2018019575 (ebook) | ISBN 9780803689879 | ISBN 9780803669062 (pbk.)
Subjects: | MESH: Nursing Care | Nursing Process | Nurse's Role | Nurse-Patient Relations
Classification: LCC RT41 (ebook) | LCC RT41 (print) | NLM WY 100.1 | DDC 610.73—dc23
LC record available at https://lccn.loc.gov/2018018864

Fundamentals of Nursing Care

Concepts, Connections & Skills

THIRD EDITION

Marti A. Burton, RN, BS
Curriculum Developer and Designer
Former Instructor, Link to Nursing Program
Canadian Valley Technology Center
Yukon, Oklahoma

David W. Smith, MSN, RN
Former LPN/LVN Instructor
North Central Texas College
Gainesville, Texas
Clinical Assistant Professor
University of Texas at Arlington
Arlington, Texas

Linda J. May Ludwig, RN, BS, MEd
Retired Nursing Instructor
Canadian Valley Technology Center
El Reno, Oklahoma

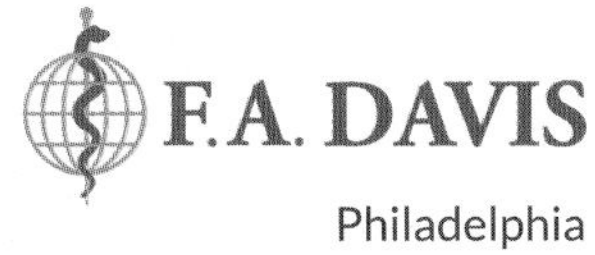

Philadelphia

List of Skills, Nursing Care Plans, and Concept Maps

Skills

Nursing Care Plans

Concept Maps

Dedications

To our past, present, and future nursing students: You are the inspiration for this book. May you each be not just a nurse, but a ***good*** nurse.

To our fellow nursing instructors: You, too, inspired us to write this book. We wanted the book to explain concepts the way you explain them to your students. Our goal was to write the book in a way that the students could easily read and understand in order to make your jobs easier.

To my husband, Barry: You passed away so suddenly and left a giant hole in my heart. Thank you for being a wonderful husband and my best friend for 33 years. I will always love you.

To Kelsea and Gabriel, my precious daughter and son-in-law: I don't know how I could make it without your love and support. I am so thankful that you are with me. You are my rocks and I love you so very much.

To my "sister" Vicky: I so appreciate your support and caring during this year I was writing, and for being there during the hard times.

To honor my parents, my oldest brother, and my soul-mate Barry, who are no longer with us here but who live on in my heart.
Marti A. Burton

To my wonderful wife, Michelle: I want to thank you for encouraging me every day while I wrote and revised this book. I am thankful you came into my life 13 years ago, and I love you.

To my parents, Kenny and Jayleane Smith: You are both my rock and support as you continue to push me every day in life. I love you both.

To my dear friend, Jane Lopes: I want to thank you for giving me an opportunity to teach at North Central Texas College. You guided me to be the best nursing instructor I can be. Thank you for believing and trusting in me.
David W. Smith

Acknowledgments

We want to express our thanks to the following people, without whom this book would have never been completed:

To Terri Allen, Nursing Publisher: We are so grateful for your enthusiastic support of this book and the insight you give us into the publishing process. You have great ideas, and we are so glad to be a part of them.

To Jean Rodenberger, Editor in Chief, Nursing: We are thankful for your support and encouragement as we planned this revision. You have been a great resource for us.

To Amy Romano, Content Project Manager II: We are thankful for all you have done to help us. You have been so enjoyable to work with, and you have great talents for negotiating that we truly appreciate. You have helped this process go so smoothly, and we do appreciate all of your work to make that happen.

To Julie Scardiglia, Developmental Editor: Thank you for your amazing work on all the details that kept the book organized and the revision process smooth. You caught the vision for this third edition and really helped us make the book better than ever. We so appreciated you noticing all those details that we missed and fixing all the little boo-boos along the way.

To Will Welsh, Manager of Content Development: We appreciate your input at the planning meeting and the work that went into making this book better than ever. Thank you for helping us revise certain areas to improve how we say what we say.

To our Photographer, Family, Friends, Students, and Peers: You made all the pictures we originally shot for the book look great.

To Canadian Valley Technology Center: Thank you for supporting this book, from our original photoshoot to the third edition. The school helps us to make the book look good. Thank you again Sharon Mitchell, Business and Industry Supervisor, and Rhonda Reherman, former PN Director, for your support and understanding during all the revisions of this book.

About the Authors

Marti A. Burton, RN, BS
Marti has been an RN for 40 years and taught LPN/LVN students for 25 years. She worked in the areas of medical intensive care and coronary care for several years, as well as a pulmonary nurse specialist. She also has worked in home health, as a field nurse, as a supervisor, and as a quality assurance specialist. She has taught entry-level health-care education to adults and high school students for 30 years. She has been an instructor in several practical nursing programs. She has also taught and directed the Link to Nursing program, and she designs and develops curricula for all the entry-level health-care education programs at Canadian Valley Technology Center. She also does massage therapy part time and serves as a faith community nurse for her congregation in Mustang, Oklahoma.

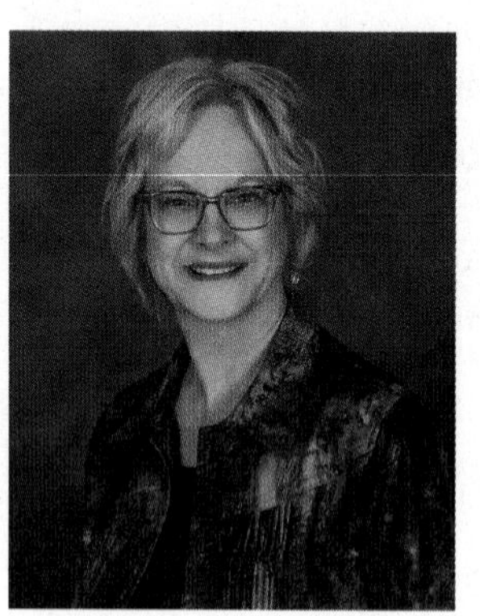

David W. Smith, MSN, RN
David has been an RN for 13 years. He entered the nursing field as a certified nursing assistant at Presbyterian Hospital of Dallas and graduated from North Central Texas College as an LPN/LVN and then New York University as an RN. He worked for over 13 years as a pediatric cardiac nurse at Children's Health in Dallas, Texas. He has worked for North Central Texas College as a curriculum developer, as part of the mentoring program for at-risk students, as an instructor for the ADN and LPN/LVN programs, and in the simulation department. He is an executive board member for the Texas Association of Vocational Nurse Educators. He currently teaches at the University of Texas at Arlington as a pediatric clinical assistant professor.

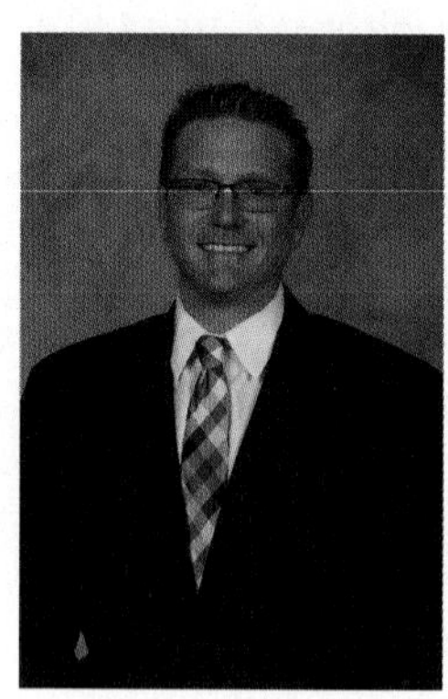

Preface

When we decided to write a nursing textbook, we wanted it to be written to the entry-level student, not about the student. We designed it so that students could truly understand what they are reading without the need for prior nursing experience or knowledge. We wrote it to guide the student in developing simple problem-solving skills and then progressing to critical thinking in real-world nursing. Our aim is to teach students to understand and connect the what, why, and how of safe and effective care.

Themes

We want to help students learn how to truly individualize care by choosing the most appropriate interventions for each patient. We take the students through the steps of the nursing process as it applies to each selected patient and situation. The book's organization and content enable students to make their own connections without requiring an instructor's lecture to do so. Our book incorporates the following themes:

1. **Making the Connection:** In this text, we assist students to see that each feature connects to something the student can relate to or something important the student will need to take into consideration. When students memorize information, it is often only retained in their short-term memory, so it is unavailable when it is needed later. The more a student can relate information to previous learning, such as anatomy or physiology and clinical experiences, the easier it is for them to remember what they have learned. This book uses multiple areas of focus to help make these connections.
2. **Thinking Like a Nurse:** Our book teaches students to identify patient problems and contribute to the development of the care plan. We help students identify what problems a patient is experiencing or may be expected to experience and relate them to nursing interventions. Our book provides students with a solid understanding of how to problem-solve in the clinical arena, holistically view their patients' needs, and apply a working knowledge of nursing fundamentals.
3. **Safety:** We focus students on safe and effective nursing care by using red type to emphasize this content throughout the chapters and in the skills.
4. **Personalizing Care:** We include situations that require students to think about the individual and his or her needs as opposed to a generic one-size-fits-all care plan guide. We want students to take individual patients' preferences and requirements into consideration as they deliver care, rather than caring for all patients with the same diagnosis in the same manner. With this in mind, students are encouraged to understand themselves as cultural beings and to think critically about culture and its relevance to effective nursing care.
5. **Utilizing Real-World Nursing:** Quite often there are gaps in how to take what is in a textbook and apply it to what the student sees during clinical experience. Often, as instructors, we have found ourselves saying, "I know what your book says, but in the real world. . . ." This book is designed to help students learn to prioritize care and manage patients who have more than one illness. We also help students think through ways care might need to be adapted or could be more easily implemented. We emphasize the need for thorough care delivered by a thinking nurse so that students are not tempted to take shortcuts.

Features

This book contains the following special features. The 126 step-by-step skill presentations are found at the end of the chapters to prevent interruption to the flow of the text.

- ***NEW* Elder Care Connection:** Our students and graduates will care for elderly patients regardless of their work settings. Some aspects of elder care are the same as caring for younger adults, but other aspects are not. In this feature, we highlight issues that are specific to caring for the elderly patient.
- ***NEW* Settings Connections:** LPN/LVNs may go to work in long-term care facilities, home health agencies, or medical offices. In this feature, we highlight information that is important to nurses working in those different settings.
- ***NEW* Evidence-Based Practice:** This feature is included in chapters where newer evidence demonstrates a need to change our nursing practice. These boxes pose a clinical question and then provide a brief summary of the research and how it affects the nursing practice of LPN/LVN students. They also point the students to the research so they can read it themselves or find similar research for comparison. This helps our LPN/LVN students think about how they will practice as nurses and how they need to base their practice on the newest and best evidence available.
- ***NEW* Word-Building Footnotes** appear in most chapters to help nursing students master medical terminology.
- ***NEW* Phonetic pronunciations** have also been added to the key terms that begin every chapter.
- **Critical Thinking Connection:** Clinical assignments that nursing students commonly face are featured at the beginning of each chapter. They are designed to put the student in a realistic situation that could occur during clinical experiences. The critical thinking questions in this feature help students connect what is in the chapter to what they will be doing when they care for real patients. At the end of each chapter, we have included a **Post Conference**

exercise that encourages students to reflect the effectiveness of his or her interventions.

- **Knowledge Connection:** These questions occur after sections of text so that students can make certain they have understood the main ideas of the section. This feature is in addition to workbook questions and review questions at the end of each chapter.
- **Anatomy and Physiology Connection:** This feature provides students with the connection between anatomy and physiology and their nursing diagnoses and interventions. It is not designed as a system review but rather is intended to connect the concepts of anatomy and physiology with the critical aspects of nursing fundamentals.
- **Patient Teaching Connection:** This feature outlines the important points to emphasize when talking with patients or explaining their care; its emphasis is on helping students capture teachable moments during patient care.
- **Real-World Connection:** This feature shares stories to explain how errors have led to patient harm, how to improve patient compliance or care, and how situations could play out in the real world. We asked our contributing writers to share stories from their own experiences to illustrate a major concept of the chapter. We also drew from our experiences as staff nurses, instructors, and students to share illustrations that students will remember far beyond the course for which they use this book.
- **Laboratory and Diagnostic Connection:** These features relate elevated or decreased results for one laboratory test or a group of tests to effects in the body or explain the use of specific laboratory or diagnostic tests to help determine diagnoses. The laboratory tests chosen coordinate with the topic of each chapter.
- **Supervision/Delegation Connection:** These features point out aspects of appropriate delegation to nurse assistants and unlicensed assistive personnel, as well as the critical elements that should not be delegated to unlicensed personnel. Additional information included will help students learn to supervise care given by nursing assistants and unlicensed assistive personnel.
- **Skills:** We designed our book to be very comprehensive regarding the skills we present. We wanted this book to be a go-to resource for skills for the entry-level nurse, with nothing important omitted. Our book includes step-by-step procedures with appropriate rationales for 126 skills. In addition, we are passionate about making the book about real-life nursing, so the steps in the skills are reasonable, rational, and understandable to the student.

Ancillaries

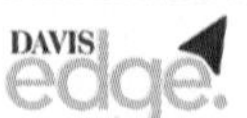

This online assessment platform includes more than 1,600 questions and integrates seamlessly with the textbook and course. Its interactive, question-based format provides the practice students need to build comprehension and improve their scores on classroom exams and the NCLEX® through a series of quizzes that can be personalized to meet individual student needs.

The tool provides real-time analysis of the following:

- Comprehension: How well are students understanding and retaining the content?
- Participation: Are students engaging with their reading and keeping up with their assignments?
- Test-taking skills: Are students adapting to NCLEX-style questions and improving their skills?

Suggestions for implementing Davis Edge into your course are included in the Active Classroom Instructor Guide. By incorporating assignments into a course, instructors are able to monitor engagement, participation, and areas of strengths and weaknesses.

Additional Online Resources for Students

- **Audio Chapter Summaries** for studying "on the go"
- **Skills Checklists**
- **Chapter References**
- An **eBook** of the text

Study Guide

The study guide is designed to assist the student to develop critical thinking skills. The study guide includes application-style questions, matching and multiple-choice questions, true-or-false questions, examples of "blank forms" such as incident reports, head-to-toe assessment flow sheets, graphic sheets, activity flow sheets, intake/output sheets, and progress notes. To assist the student with documentation, there are assignments within the specific study guide chapters that refer the student to the blank form on which the documentation is to be completed.

Instructor Resources on DavisPlus

The online resources for instructors include the following:

- **NCLEX-Style Test Bank**
- ***NEW* Active Classroom Instructor's Guide**, which provides guidance on how to utilize and assign the text and ancillaries throughout the course. Abundant activities to promote an active classroom are included.
- **PowerPoint Slides**
- **Electronic Image Bank**
- **Study Guide Answer Key,** which is posted on the instructor's Davis*Plus* site to allow instructors the option of providing answers to students for self-study, or assigning the Study Guide exercises for grading.
- An **eBook** of the text

BONUS If you use *Davis's Nursing Skills Videos for LPN/LVN*, 3rd edition in your program you can assign the quizzes in Davis Edge to ensure that students have viewed the videos as assigned.

LPN/LVN Connections

F.A. Davis is pleased to introduce **LPN/LVN Connections**, a consistent and recognizable approach to design and content that will make it easier for students and instructors to use multiple F.A. Davis textbooks throughout the LPN/LVN curriculum.

We have increased continuity whenever possible, without erasing the authors' autonomy or changing legacy content that has been popular in past editions. This makes it easier for instructors and students to move through the textbooks and ancillary products while recognizing shared themes and featured content.

Textbook Design, Style & Pedagogy

- All textbook chapters include:
  - Numbered Learning Outcomes
  - Key Terms with phonetic pronunciations listed on the chapter opener and boldfaced where first defined in the chapter
  - Chapter Concepts
  - Bulleted Key Points
  - NCLEX-style Review Questions, with answers right on the page for students' ease of reference
  - Chapter References, located online
- A Reading Level Evaluation is performed during the manuscript development, to ensure readability
- Word-Building Footnotes to help students build understanding of root terminology
- A uniform, space-saving internal design features special heads and colors that are shared across titles for features with similar content, to increase recognition
- Consistent and current terminology and laboratory values across titles; the authors followed *Davis's Comprehensive Handbook of Laboratory & Diagnostic Tests with Nursing Implications* by Van Leeuwen and Bladh for all values

Standardized Student and Faculty Resources

- For Students:
  - *Davis Edge* personalized online quizzing to help master course content and prepare for the NCLEX-PN examination
  - Gratis eBook with purchase of the print text, to allow flexibility in accessing course content
  - Study Guide with perforated pages so that students can hand in assignments if requested; the Answer Key is provided to instructors online, to distribute if desired
- For Instructors:
  - *Davis Edge* pre-set quizzes and classroom management tools, with instructor reserve questions
  - Active Classroom Instructor's Guide (ACIG) provides pre-, during, and post-class suggestions for activities and assignments, focusing on the active classroom
  - eBook
  - NCLEX-style test bank
  - PowerPoint presentations
  - Digital image collection

F.A. Davis LPN/LVN Advisory Board

Paula K. Mundell, MSN, RN
Coordinator, Nursing Program
Delaware Technical Community College
Dover, Delaware

Sonia Rudolph, APRN, FNP-BC
Nursing Division Chair
Jefferson Community & Technical College
Louisville, Kentucky

Patricia Taylor, MSN Ed, RN
Practical Nursing Coordinator
Kapi'olani Community College
University of Hawaii
Honolulu, Hawaii

Contributors

Rita Armstrong, DNP, MSN Ed, RN
Dean of Nursing/Nurse Consultant
Education Affiliates/Fortis College
Baltimore, Maryland
Chapter 5: Documentation

Alene M. Homan, MEd, BSN, RN, CSN, CPN
Practical Nursing Instructor
Clearfield County Career and Technology Center
Clearfield, Pennsylvania
Chapter 32: Care of Elderly Patients

Connie Hunt, MS, RN
LPN Instructor
Indian Capital Technology Center
Stilwell, Oklahoma
Chapter 33: Care of the Surgical Patient

Kathleen Hutchins-Otero, MSN, RN, CNE
Assistant Professor
College of the Mainland
Texas City, Texas
Chapter 30: Bowel Elimination and Care

Thirty Lacy, BSN, RN, CDP
Instructor, Vocational Nursing
Alvin Community College
Alvin, Texas
Chapter 8: Ethnic, Cultural, and Spiritual Aspects of Care

Shirley MacNeill, MSN, RN, CNE
Allied Health Department Chair
Lamar State College Port Arthur
Port Arthur, Texas
Chapter 12: Patient Teaching

Julie Martin, MSN, RN, CHSE
Health Sciences Director of Simulation
North Central Texas College
Gainesville, Texas
Chapter 4: The Nursing Process: Critical Thinking and Decision Making

Patricia A. Perryman, MSN, RN
Dean of Nursing
Fortis College
Grand Prairie, Texas
Chapter 18: Applying Heat and Cold Therapies

Molly M. Showalter, MSN Ed, RN
Vocational Nursing Instructor
Texas Southmost College
Brownsville, Texas
Chapter 9: Growth and Development Throughout the Lifespan

Tetsuya Umebayashi, DNP, MSN, RN
Director of LVN Program
Tarrant County College
Fort Worth, Texas
Chapter 35: Researching and Preparing Medications

Patricia Williams, MSN, RN
Assistant Professor for the Practical Nursing Program
Hagerstown Community College
Hagerstown, Maryland
Chapter 21: Physical Assessment

Reviewers

Janice Ankenmann MSN, CCRN, FNP-C, RN
Nursing Director/Professor
Napa Valley College
Napa, California

Chanda D. Beaty MSN, RN/NP
Nursing Facilitator
Upper Cape Cod Regional Technical School
Bourne, Massachusetts

Gretheline Bolandrina MSN Ed, RN, CRRN
Program Director
Bay Path RVTHS Practical Nursing Program
Charlton, Massachusetts

Karla Cepeda BSN, RN
Nursing Faculty
Kapiolani Community College
Honolulu, Hawaii

Joan Eula Conde MS, RN, AGCNS-BC
Instructor
Kapi'olani Community College
Honolulu, Hawaii

Denise Daffin BSN, RN
Nursing Instructor
Indian Capital Technology Center
Sallisaw, Oklahoma

Denese Davis MEd, BSN, RN
Instructor
Wiregrass Georgia Technical College
Valdosta, Georgia

Mary Davis MSN, RN
Nursing Faculty
Wiregrass Georgia Technical College
Valdosta, Georgia

Deanna Dubay MSN
Nursing Instructor
Davenport University
Midland, Michigan

Shelley Eckvahl MSN, RN
Professor, Nursing
Chaffey College
Rancho Cucamonga, California

Louise S. Frantz MHA, Ed, BSN, RN
Coordinator, Practical Nursing Program
Penn State Berks
Reading, Pennsylvania

Alice Gilbert RN
Director/Instructor
Ukiah Adult School
Ukiah, California

Janis Grimland BSN, RN
Vocational Nursing Program Director
Hill College
Hillsboro, Texas

Kimberly D. Hagerman ADN, RN, BS
PN Instructor
McDowell County CTC School
Welch, West Virginia

Theresa Hallowell BSN, RN
Nursing Instructor
Lincoln Technical Institute
Allentown, Pennsylvania

Robin Hill MSN, RN
Program Coordinator, Practical Nursing Program
Hagerstown Community College
Hagerstown, Maryland

Thomas H. Hodges MN, RN
Director of Nursing
MCI College of Health Science of ECPI University
Greensboro, North Carolina

Pamela B. Hoffeditz MSN, RN
Nurse Educator
Franklin County Career and Technology Center: Practical Nursing Program
Chambersburg, Pennsylvania

Alice Hupp BS, RN
Lead Instructor of Vocational Nursing
North Central Texas College
Gainesville, Texas

Shirley Kelley RN
Instructor
University of Arkansas Pulaski Technical College
North Little Rock, Arkansas

Sheri Kline MSN, BSN, RN
Instructor
Blackstone Valley Regional Vocational Technical Nursing Program
Upton, Massachusetts

Thirty Lacy BSN, RN-CDP
Instructor, Vocational Nursing
Alvin Community College
Alvin, Texas

Cynthia L. Lapp RN, BS
Nursing Instructor
Jefferson-Lewis BOCES
Glenfield, New York

Ronnell R. Leftwich MHS, MA, BSN, RN
Program Chair
Athens Technical College
Elberton, Georgia

Mandi M. Mauck MSN, RN
Instructor, Program Coordinator
Columbus State Community College
Columbus, Ohio

Cinthia dos Santos Mesquita BSN, RN
Faculty
Assabet Valley Practical Nursing Program
Marlborough, Massachusetts

Amanda Perkins MSN, RN
Assistant Professor of Nursing
Vermont Technical College
Randolph, Vermont

Thomas L. Petricini MSN, RN
Nursing Instructor
Sharon Regional Health System
Sharon, Pennsylvania

Helen Rogers-Koon MSN, RN
Instructor, Practical Nursing Program
Central Pennsylvania Institute of Science and Technology
Pleasant Gap, Pennsylvania

Jackie Shrock MSN, MEd, RN
Nursing Faculty
Wayne County Schools Career Center Practical Nursing Program; HS and AE
Smithville, Ohio

Patricia A. Taylor MSN-Ed, RN
Associate Professor, Practical Nursing Program Coordinator
University of Hawaii, Kapi'olani Community College
Honolulu, Hawaii

Sharon Weaver EdS, MSN/Ed, BSN, RN
Instructor of Nursing
Lincoln Technical School
Allentown, Pennsylvania

Lauren Winters BSN, RN
Practical Nursing Faculty
Nunez Community College
Chalmetter, Louisiana

Karen Leslie Znajda MS, RN
Nursing Instructor
Northland Community & Technical College
East Grand Forks, Minnesota

Contents

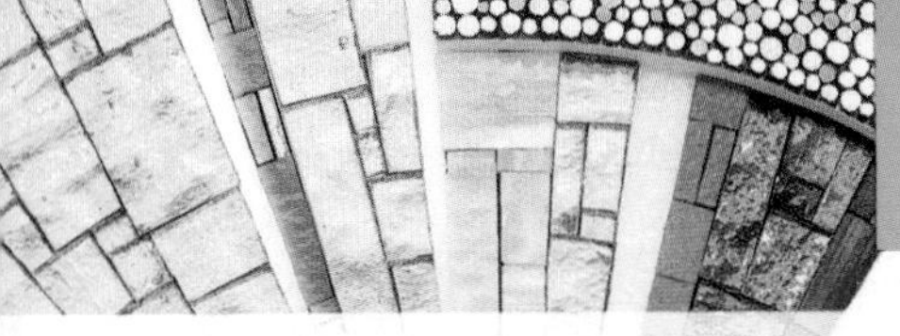

CHAPTER 1
The Vista of Nursing

KEY TERMS

Associate Degree Nurse (a-SOH-see-uht de-GREE NERS)
Baccalaureate Degree Nurse (bak-uh-LAW-ree-uht de-GREE NERS)
Diploma program nurse (dip-LOH-mah PROH-gram NERS)
Evidence-based practice (EV-ih-dents-BAYST PRAK-tiss)
Health Occupations Students of America (HELLTH AHK-yoo-PAY-shunz STOO-dents uv a-MER-ih-kah)
Licensed Practical/Vocational Nurse (LYE-senst PRAK-tih-kuhl/voh-KAY-shun-uhl NERS)
National Association of Licensed Practical Nurses (NASH-nuhl a-SOH-see-AY-shun uv LYE-senst PRAK-tih-kuhl NERS-uhz)
National Council Licensure Examination for Practical Nursing
National Council Licensure Examination for Registered Nursing
Nurse Practice Act (NERS PRAK-tiss AKT)
Quality and Safety Education for Nurses (KWOL-ih-tee and SAYF-tee eh-juh-KAY-shun for NERS-uhz)
Scope of practice (SKOHP uv PRAK-tiss)

CHAPTER CONCEPTS

Professionalism
Evidence-Based Practice
Quality Improvement

LEARNING OUTCOMES

1. Define various terms associated with nursing practice.
2. Trace the providers of nursing care from ancient history until the mid-1800s.
3. Summarize the development of modern nursing.
4. Describe the history of nursing at both the LPN/LVN and RN levels.
5. Differentiate four pathways for entering nursing education.
6. Discuss career ladders and specialization in nursing.
7. Identify commonalities of nurse practice acts in all states.
8. Define scope of practice.
9. Describe four characteristics of nurses.
10. Evaluate professional appearance and behavior.
11. Discuss the purposes of professional organizations you can join as a nursing student.
12. Discuss unprofessional conduct and its consequences.
13. Discuss selected nursing theories and theorists.
14. Explain the impact of nurses on patients' lives.
15. Discuss information found in the Connection features in this chapter.
16. Identify specific safety information.
17. Describe trends in nursing practice, including evidence-based practice and QSEN.

CRITICAL THINKING CONNECTION

Feature Overview

Near the beginning of each chapter in this book, you will read about a specific patient that you could be assigned to care for during a clinical experience. This Critical Thinking Connection will guide you as you read the chapter, helping you think about actions you would need to take and information you would need to consider if you were caring for this patient. The Critical Thinking Connections in each chapter are designed to help you connect what you read in the textbook with what you will actually see and do in the clinical setting.

When you stand at the top of a mountain and look out, you see a vista—an open, unblocked view. When you begin nursing school, it is like standing at the top of that mountain. You may have followed quite a winding path to get where you are now, and you bring many life experiences with you. After suffering through entrance examinations, waiting lists, and preference points, you are finally here—you have started nursing school. But "here" is only the beginning. This is just the first step in your nursing career.

Look out across the vista of nursing and see the possibilities. From here, you can go many places and work in a variety of settings. You may work in a hospital, outpatient surgery center, health-care provider's office, or specialty clinic. Your path might take you to a career in home health care, long-term care, or assisted living. You may choose to continue your education. Some people work while they go on with college to obtain higher degrees in nursing. You may even decide to climb another mountain and become an advanced practice nurse. Sometimes students start out in nursing and then decide to go into other areas of health care, such as physical or occupational therapy, legal nurse consulting, or even medical school. Many possibilities are available in the vista of nursing.

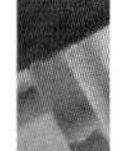

HISTORY OF NURSING—A LOOK AT WHERE WE HAVE BEEN

Through ancient history, nursing care was provided by family members and male priests. Around 1000 AD, after the end of the Dark Ages, the Italian town of Salerno allowed women to attend school to study midwifery. As Christianity spread, care for the sick and poor was considered a valuable endeavor. Convents were then established for training caregivers and providing care for the sick. Deaconesses (religious women who served by helping the poor and sick) administered care similar to today's public health nurses.

In the 1700s to 1800s, very little was known about antisepsis. Hospitals were not clean, nor were they places of hope. Educated women did not pursue nursing because it was considered beneath them. It was left to the poor—the low class, the "Sairey Gamps"—to care for sick people. (Sairey Gamp was a fictional drunken midwife created by Charles Dickens. Her name became synonymous with low-class, poorly qualified health-care workers.) Wealthier people cared for sick family members at home because it was considered a disgrace to send one's family away to a hospital.

Modern nursing began in the mid-1800s. In 1836, the first school of nursing was established in Kaiserworth, Germany, by Pastor Theodore Fliedner. Many women who were educated there were then assigned to various places around the world to teach other women to be nurses. They were referred to as *Kaiserworth deaconesses,* and the most famous of them was Florence Nightingale (Fig. 1.1). Information on women who helped mold modern nursing is given in Table 1.1.

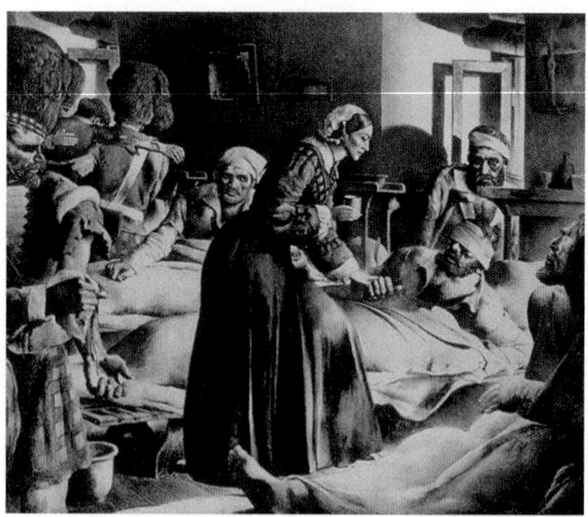

FIGURE 1.1 Florence Nightingale during the Crimean War (from Neeb KC. *Fundamentals of Mental Health Nursing.* 4th ed. Philadelphia, PA: FA Davis; 2014).

In 1897, the Nurses Associated Alumnae of the United States was formed in Baltimore, Maryland, in an effort to oversee training so as to protect patients from incompetent nurses. Soon afterward, the American Society of Superintendents of Training Schools for Nurses was established. This group later became the National League for Nursing Education. Its purpose was to set standards and rules in nursing education, and it continues to fulfill that function today.

In the early 1900s, some states began to pass laws requiring the licensure of nurses. Requirements for entering nursing school also were established. The *American Journal of Nursing* was published for the first time during this era to help keep nurses aware of the newest medical information and the newest information about nursing education.

In 1892, the first training program for practical nurses was established in New York City at the Young Women's Christian Association (YWCA). The next year, the first official school for practical nurses, called the Ballard School, was opened, also through the YWCA. This school was established to help meet the need for educated bedside nurses, recruiting those who "had a special way with the sick." Because many people were cared for at home during this era, these first practical nurses were essentially home health nurses. The training program was 3 months long and focused on homemaking skills as well as skills in caring for the sick.

It was not until 1955 that all states required practical nurses to be licensed. The title licensed practical nurse, or LPN, is used in all states except California and Texas. Those states use the title licensed vocational nurse, or LVN.

KNOWLEDGE CONNECTION

When did modern nursing begin, and who is recognized as its founder? When did states start requiring RN licensure? What type of training did the first practical nurses receive?

Table 1.1
Women Who Molded Nursing History

Person or People	*Role in History*
Clara Barton	Known as the "Angel of the Battlefield" during the U.S. Civil War, she cared for soldiers both from the North and the South. She was the first president of the Red Cross Association, now the American Red Cross.
Dorothea Dix	An activist for better mental health care and the establishment of psychiatric hospitals, she was appointed as the Superintendent of Female Nurses in the Army in 1861, where she organized staff and equipment for Army hospitals. She was not a nurse or a military officer, but a retired teacher.
Florence Nightingale	Seen as the person who established modern nursing, she attended the Kaiserworth School in Germany in 1851 and also studied in Paris under the Sisters of Charity. She is famous for her work giving nursing care during the Crimean War. She also kept records during that time, shared them with the Secretary of War, and influenced war strategy. She was instrumental in the establishment of the Nightingale School in London, England, which became a model for other nursing schools.
Mary Mahoney	The first African American nurse in the United States, she worked tirelessly to improve acceptance for African Americans in nursing. She established an association for this purpose, the National Association for Colored Graduate Nurses, and served as its first president.
Linda Richards	Recognized as the first "trained nurse" in the United States, she graduated from Boston's New England Hospital for Women and Children in 1872. Her system of noting information about her patients at Bellevue Hospital in New York became the foundation for modern nurse's notes. She later went to Japan on a medical mission and established the first school of nursing there.
Isabel Hampton Robb	An activist for nursing labor reform in the late 1800s, she helped usher in 12-hour shifts with meal breaks for nurses, when 24 hours had been standard. She also was instrumental in establishing a 3-year training program for nurses and worked for licensure examinations and nursing registration.
Mary Adelaide Nutting, Lillian Wald, and Annie Goodrich (the "Great Trio")	These three nurses made great strides in nursing education and community health nursing. Nutting graduated in the first nursing class from Johns Hopkins University and established the Nursing and Teachers College at Columbia University, where she was the first professor of nursing. Wald, known as the first visiting nurse, opening the Henry Street Settlement to provide health care to the poor. Goodrich was devoted to establishing nursing as a profession. She received the Distinguished Service Award for developing the Army School of Nursing. She also served as the director of the Visiting Nursing Service at the Henry Street Settlement. In addition, she served as the dean of nursing at Yale University and as president of the American Nurses Association.

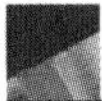

OPTIONS FOR ENTERING NURSING

When you decide to pursue a nursing career, many pathways are open to you (Box 1.1). It is unusual for so many choices to exist when entering a field of study, and often students find those choices confusing. Remember, too, that these options do not have to be selected in any particular order.

Licensed Practical/Vocational Nurse

The **licensed practical/vocational nurse** (LPN/LVN) is the most basic of all the entry-level options for nurses. The educational programs range from 9 months to 1 year for full-time programs and generally 18 months to 2 years for part-time programs. Some college courses may be required before entering LPN/LVN school, but many states have no requirements for previous education except a high school diploma or the equivalent.

When students finish their educational program, they will take the **National Council Licensure Examination for Practical Nursing** (NCLEX-PN) to become licensed. This examination is standardized in all 50 states and is taken by computer at specified locations. Results are mailed to graduates within a short period of time (usually 5–7 days), and the newly licensed LPNs/LVNs can quickly begin to work in health care.

Associate Degree Nurse

The **associate degree nurse** (ADN) is an entry-level educational option for registered nurses. Students in these programs attend a private or community college for a minimum of 2 years to obtain their associate degree in nursing. An associate degree includes some basic general education courses, such as science,

Box 1.1

Nursing Education Levels

A number of entry-level and advanced practice education options are available to those entering the nursing field.

Entry-Level Education

- **Licensed Practical/Vocational Nurse:** 9 to 12 months of education at a technical college or career technology center
- **Registered Nurse, Associate Degree:** 2 to 3 years at a community college or state college
- **Registered Nurse, Diploma Program:** 3 years in a hospital-based program affiliated with a college or university
- **Registered Nurse, Baccalaureate Degree:** 4 years at a college or university

Advanced Practice Education

- **Masters of Science in Nursing (MSN):** 2 or more years in the graduate school of a university; may teach in BSN, ADN, and LPN/LVN programs; may also choose to specialize further in one of these areas:
  - Clinical nurse specialist
  - Nurse practitioner
  - Certified registered nurse anesthetist
  - Nurse midwife
- **Doctorate in Nursing (PhD, DNP):** 2 or more years in a doctoral program at a university; may serve as the dean of nursing for a university program or the director of nursing at a large hospital; may teach in MSN and doctorate programs; and may direct and design formal research programs

math, history, English, and social sciences, at the college level. In addition, these students take three to four semesters of nursing courses. For students who have not attended college previously, it is not uncommon for this educational preparation to take up to 3 years to complete.

When students complete all coursework and graduate, they are eligible to take the **National Council Licensure Examination for Registered Nursing** (NCLEX-RN). Upon successfully passing the examination, the graduate becomes a registered nurse and uses the title "RN" after his or her name.

Diploma Program Nurse

A **diploma program nurse** is educated in a hospital-based nursing education program, of which few remain. Before universities and community colleges were numerous and easily accessed, nursing education was delivered through hospitals. Students worked on the patient units and gained experience while they attended classes. Eventually, hospitals offering such programs affiliated with colleges or universities. The college or university faculty, either at the hospital or at a convenient location, provides general education courses such as the sciences, history, English, and math. The hospital oversees and employs the faculty who teach nursing courses. Diploma programs last about 3 years, often with required summer sessions. Graduates of these programs also take the NCLEX-RN for licensure to become RNs.

Baccalaureate Degree Nurse

The **baccalaureate degree nurse** (BSN) program can also be an entry into nursing. Students who choose this option enter a university to pursue their nursing education. They take all required courses for a 4-year college degree: general education courses as well as four to five semesters of nursing courses. It is not uncommon for students to complete their first 2 years of college before they apply and are admitted to the university's school of nursing to obtain their bachelor of science in nursing (BSN) degree.

Upon completion of all coursework, these students also take the NCLEX-RN. The focus of their nursing education puts more emphasis on management and leadership than the ADN and diploma programs. Therefore, these nurses are more in demand for management positions.

ADVANCING YOUR CAREER

Career ladder options are available to every nurse (Box 1.2). The LPN/LVN may wish to obtain an ADN and become an RN but still focus mostly on direct care. The same nurse may later wish to go to a university for a BSN and then move into a management or leadership opportunity. An ADN may return to school quickly and obtain a BSN or may work several years before doing so. Some nurses choose not to obtain higher degrees and find working as LPNs/LVNs, ADNs, or diploma nurses very rewarding. You are the best judge of what level of education is best for you.

KNOWLEDGE CONNECTION

How many ways can a person become an RN? Which preparation path for RN takes the longest? What is the advantage of a "one-plus-one" program?

Specialization in Nursing

Nursing students often ask about specializing in different areas, such as critical care or pediatrics. In nursing school, you will rotate through many areas of nursing care: medical-surgical floors, surgery and recovery, emergency, mental health, obstetrics, and pediatrics, just to list a few. As a newly graduated entry-level nurse, you may be encouraged to work in a medical-surgical unit for a year to gain experience in nursing and to develop good nursing judgment before obtaining a position in a specialty area. Many metropolitan hospitals limit specialty areas only to RNs. However, in more rural areas, LPNs/LVNs may work in a greater variety of settings. Once you have completed school and passed the NCLEX, you may find one area of work that you prefer above all others.

Scope of Practice

All nurses are responsible for knowing their own **scope of practice;** that is, the limitations and allowances of what they

Box 1.2

Career Ladder in Nursing

Once you become a nurse, you can continue your education in a variety of ways.

- **One-Plus-One Programs:** Offered at community and state colleges. In the first year, the curriculum prepares the student to take the NCLEX-PN. After passing the examination, the student can work as an LPN/LVN while completing the second-year curriculum. The student then takes the NCLEX-RN to be licensed as a registered nurse.
- **PN to ADN Programs:** Offered at community and state colleges. The student is given credit for LPN/LVN education that counts toward requirements for RN education, making the time spent in school shorter to complete coursework to become a registered nurse.
- **PN to BSN, ADN to BSN, and Diploma to BSN Programs:** All previous entry-level nursing education programs are credited toward the course requirements for a baccalaureate degree in nursing, making the time in school shorter.

can do as nurses. In every state, a **Nurse Practice Act (NPA),** or the law governing nurses' actions, exists. This law is written to specifically address each level of nursing. In every state, LPNs/LVNs are required by law to practice under the supervision of an RN or physician, and RNs are required to practice under the supervision of a physician. The Nurse Practice Act in each state establishes the scope of practice for each level of nurse based on educational preparation. The Board of Nursing in each state determines and enforces the contents of the Nurse Practice Act. Other specific allowances or limitations vary from state to state. For example, in some states, LPNs/LVNs are prohibited by the Nurse Practice Act from initiating intravenous (IV) therapy. In other states, LPNs/LVNs are allowed under the law to perform this skill. ***Safety: It is your responsibility to know the content of the Nurse Practice Act in your state regarding your scope of practice and to follow it faithfully.***

KNOWLEDGE CONNECTION

What does "scope of practice" mean? Who determines the nurse's scope of practice? How is the care of an elderly individual different from the care of a younger adult?

BEING A LIFELONG LEARNER

Whatever choice you make for your basic nursing education, you will work hard to achieve your nursing license. You will be expected to learn an enormous amount of information in a relatively short period of time. You will be expected to remember what you learned in previous courses and apply that knowledge to new situations in patient care. Nurses must constantly connect known information while absorbing new information. All nurses, whether LPN/LVN, RN, BSN, or advanced practice, should strive to deliver good nursing care. Although we may have different scopes of practice based on our initial time in school, we all share skills and knowledge, and we all work together to provide excellent patient care. All nurses must continue to learn after they complete their basic nursing education. Whether you choose to do so through formal degree programs or through continuing education, seminars, and short courses, you will need to stay current in the ever-changing field of nursing.

Settings Connection

Feature Overview

As a nurse, you will work with a variety of people in a variety of places. The Settings Connections help you see how what you are learning may apply differently when you work in various practice settings, including home health care, health-care providers' offices, and in long-term care settings.

Medical Office Setting

When you work in a family practice office, for example, you will care for patients of all ages. It is important to remember that very young patients may present different challenges than adults, including difficulty understanding what is happening and expressing their feelings during medical procedures. They have no previous experience to prepare them for illness or treatment, so they often are frightened. It will be your responsibility to help reassure younger patients and explain in terms that they can understand.

Home Health Setting

Your educational program will focus mainly on hospital care. When you care for patients in the home-care setting, there are differences in how care is delivered, with fewer supplies and less equipment available than in a hospital. You have to adapt and sometimes be creative. You are generally alone in the patient's home, with no other health professionals to help you make decisions about care. You must have good nursing judgment to make quick decisions in the home.

Long-Term Care Setting

In the long-term setting, care is delivered in a more home-like environment that is less institutional than a hospital. Residents are surrounded by familiar items from home, and they may participate in activities together. When you work in this setting, you will encourage residents to participate in their care and decision making when possible. Because confusion and agitation can be a problem for some residents, it is essential to use an easy, calming approach when providing care. To help detect health problems in elderly individuals, it is as important to recognize changes in residents' behavior as it is to recognize changes in vital signs. This feature will provide tips to help you care for patients of all ages and in all settings.

Elder Care Connection

Feature Overview

While much of your educational program will focus on adults and adult health problems, the elderly population has additional health issues, such as multiple chronic illnesses, sensory deficits, and multiple prescription medications, that require you to be even more focused in your assessments and interventions. The Elder Care Connections help you be aware of the unique health-care challenges faced by the elderly.

CHARACTERISTICS OF NURSES

If you asked people on the street to choose one word to describe nurses, chances are great that the word you would hear most often is "caring." Other descriptions might include "compassionate," "comforting," and "helpful." According to several Gallup polls, nurses are considered to be honest, ethical, and trustworthy. Although you might not hear this from interviewing random strangers, words such as "technologically savvy," "troubleshooter," "problem solver," "intelligent," and "multitalented" are equally appropriate for describing nurses. In this section, we will discuss four important characteristics—being responsible, honest, caring, and organized.

Being Responsible

The job of nursing requires that you be able to think critically about each patient while carrying out all of their health-care providers' orders and handling unexpected admissions and emergencies that may arise. Nursing is a unique field in which to work because of the amount of responsibility involved. You are responsible for the following:

- Caring for several patients, including their medications and comfort, and seeing that their physical, emotional, and spiritual needs are met
- Helping families understand what is happening to the patient and preparing them for his or her care after discharge
- Noticing changes in the patient's condition and notifying the appropriate health-care professional if negative changes occur

Contrast this with the job of a bank teller, who is responsible for greeting customers; performing requested transactions, such as deposits and withdrawals; cashing checks; and, at the end of the day, balancing his or her drawer with the transaction record. Although handling money certainly is a big responsibility, the responsibilities of a nurse far outweigh those of most other jobs.

Being Honest

Nurses have to be honest—far more honest than the average person. You can put patients at risk for developing infection, illness, or complications when you make an error in medication dosage, sterile technique, or assessment. It is extremely difficult for most of us to admit that we made a mistake. It is even harder to tell your supervising nurse or doctor about an error. And if you make an error while caring for patients, it is possible that no one would ever know unless you admit to it. However, for the sake of protecting patients from possible complications, you must be responsible and honest enough to admit your mistake. In other words, you must be willing and able to put your patients' well-being first, before your pride. Patients place their trust in you and depend on you, so you must be completely honest about anything that could potentially harm them.

Being Caring

Much has been written about nurses and caring. Dr. Jean Watson, a nurse, educator, and theorist, advocates stressing the art of nursing with an emphasis on caring. In this way, nurses respond to patients in a way that confirms their individuality, emotions, and needs. A caring nurse does not treat patients in a "one-approach-fits-all" manner, but rather individualizes care for that particular patient. A caring nurse does not see a patient in terms of a cellular disorder or an illness to be cured. Instead, the caring nurse sees patients as people who have needs for touch and understanding as much as they have needs for IV fluids and antibiotics. In fact, "high-touch" nursing is just as important as "high-tech" nursing (Fig. 1.2).

Being Organized

There is also another side to nursing—the side that integrates information from laboratory values, normal structures

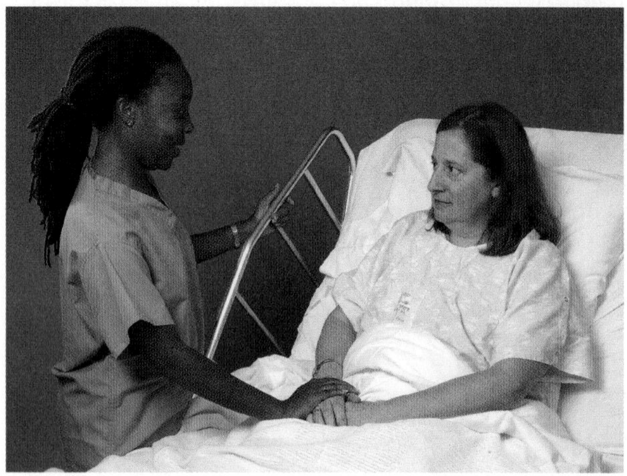

FIGURE 1.2 Caring and listening are some of the skills needed for the art of nursing (from Wilkinson JM, Treas LS. *Fundamentals of Nursing: Theory, Concepts & Applications.* Vol. 1. 2nd ed. Philadelphia, PA: FA Davis; 2011).

and functions, nursing diagnoses, patient needs and problems, supervision and delegation issues, vital sign readings, and medication orders to determine what nursing care to perform for each patient. In addition, the nurse uses highly technical equipment and troubleshooting for problems when alarms sound. It is extremely important that you be able to keep track of all this information about your patients. You also must deal with changing orders from health-care providers and meet the changing needs of your patient.

The only way to accomplish all of this for several patients during one shift is to be very organized. You will learn to make notes on a shift report or other form rather than to trust your memory with important information. You also will learn how to prioritize the care you give your patients so that nothing gets missed. In some ways, when you are striving to be organized and on time with treatments and medications, it is easy to lose sight of the fact that your patients are people who need a human touch rather than a list of tasks to be completed (Box 1.3).

Laboratory and Diagnostic Connection

Feature Overview

Most hospitalized patients undergo frequent laboratory and diagnostic tests that help identify illnesses and evaluate the treatment of disease. Some medications affect balances in the body, so frequent laboratory tests are necessary to detect any potential imbalance. It is your responsibility as a nursing student to check laboratory and diagnostic tests often, to note any abnormal findings, and to notify the appropriate health-care professionals of significant abnormal findings. In future chapters, this Laboratory and Diagnostic Connection feature will provide information to help you learn about different laboratory values and their significance in your patients' care.

KNOWLEDGE CONNECTION

How is nursing different from other jobs? Why is it so important that nurses be honest? Explain how nursing can be both an art and a science.

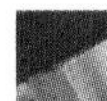

PROFESSIONALISM IN NURSING

Sometimes, beginning nursing students talk about past experiences with nurses that were both positive and negative. A student's motivation to become a nurse may be a desire to emulate a positive nurse role model or the aspiration to be a better nurse than one who was a negative example. As students learn more about nursing, they often discover that a "negative example nurse" simply failed to communicate what was about to happen and why. When you do not communicate well with your patients and their families, you will leave a negative impression about your abilities as a nurse.

Professional Appearance and Behavior

You can be a nurse, or you can be a good nurse. There is a difference. Good nurses communicate well. Before beginning a procedure they tell their patients what will happen and why. Good nurses take responsibility for their own behavior, including mistakes they may have made. Good nurses also see themselves as professionals and act in a corresponding manner. Not everyone views appearance as important, but you are judged as a nurse by how you look and present yourself. If you are not neat and clean, patients may feel that you will not provide meticulous nursing care. If you do not act like a professional, patients may feel that you are not competent to care for them (Box 1.4).

Box 1.3

The Art and Science of Nursing

Nursing is both an art and a science. The art of nursing describes the caring, creativity, communication, and compassion necessary to connect with patients in a meaningful way. The science of nursing describes the analysis and integration of data, the decision-making process, and the technical monitoring of patients. Figure 1.3 shows a nursing instructor teaching with a computerized manikin, one of many high-tech tools for learning about clinical patient care. Good nurses blend both the art and the science into their daily nursing practice.

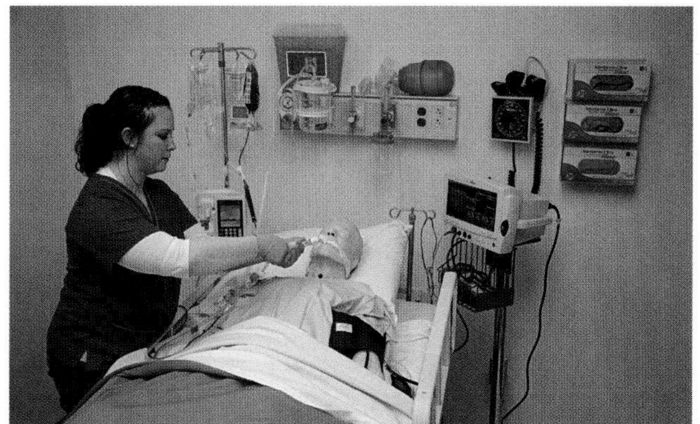

FIGURE 1.3 A nursing instructor using a computerized manikin to teach students about the science of nursing, including managing monitors and equipment.

Box 1.4

Professional Appearance and Behavior

You will be expected to appear and behave in a professional manner during your nursing education and your nursing career.

Personal Hygiene and Appearance

- Shower or bathe and apply deodorant daily.
- Keep hair clean and styled appropriately.
- Wear clean undergarments.
- Wear clean scrubs that fit well, without tears or wrinkles.
- Wear shoes that are clean and in good condition with clean shoelaces.
- Cover any visible tattoos according to school and facility policy.
- Remove studs, barbells, and gauges from piercings as required by facility policy.
- Keep fingernails short and clean; this helps prevent scratching patients or injury to self.

Professional Behavior

- Arrive on time, prepared to work.
- Complete assigned care during your shift. If you are unable to do so, ask for help. If you are caught up on your assignments, offer to help someone who is behind.
- Give thorough care with no shortcuts that compromise patient safety or comfort.
- Take breaks on time and return on time so that others can go at their assigned times.
- Leave the unit only after you have ensured that another nurse is aware that you are gone and will be responsible for your patients while you are gone.
- Assume responsibility for other nurses' patients when they leave the unit.
- Be kind and supportive of other nurses and health-care professionals.
- Avoid criticizing the mistakes of others since you will undoubtedly make mistakes, too.
- Look for the positives in people—patients, family members, coworkers, and supervisors.

Unprofessional Conduct

Professional behavior is so important that the nurse practice acts in many states define unprofessional conduct as a reason to revoke or suspend a nurse's license. Some examples of unprofessional conduct that could result in the loss of your nursing license include:

- Use of drugs or alcohol in a way that could endanger patients
- Diversion of drugs from prescribed patient use to personal use
- Failure to adequately supervise certified nursing assistants and unlicensed assistive personnel
- Failure to adequately care for patients or conform to minimum standards of nursing practice
- Criminal conduct

Professionalism is extremely important in nursing. You represent all nurses each time you care for a patient in any setting, so it is essential that you appear and conduct yourself in a manner that says you are not only a nurse, but that you are a good nurse.

Professional Organizations

Another aspect of professional behavior is participation in professional organizations, both as a student and as a nurse. Professional organizations give you a collective voice that will be heard by those who enact laws and establish policy for health care. In addition, professional organizations provide opportunities for leadership in nursing.

LPN/LVN Student Organizations

While in nursing school, you can belong to the **Health Occupations Students of America** (HOSA) and the **National Association of Licensed Practical Nurses** (NALPN) as a student affiliate.

HOSA is a national organization specifically for students in health occupations educational programs. Membership is open to both high school and adult students, with separate chapters for each group. HOSA holds two state or regional events per school year. In the summer, a national conference is held in a different major city each year. The state or regional events include a fall leadership conference to provide training for chapter officers and the election of state officers. In the spring, a skills competition is held, allowing qualifying students to compete in a variety of contests. Some examples are job-seeking skills, outstanding chapter, CPR/First Aid, and practical nursing skills. For more information about HOSA, look on their Web site (www.hosa.org).

NALPN is the professional organization for LPNs/LVNs. It was established in 1949 by Lillian Custer, and only those with an LPN or LVN license can join. Student affiliation is allowed. NALPN offers updates on legislation affecting LPNs/LVNs, recognition of practical nursing students with a B average or above who are recommended by their instructors and are in the NALPN Student Honor Society, and participation in state events and the national convention. State affiliates often sponsor a Student Day at their annual convention, with topics of interest to students and new LPNs/LVNs. The official publication of NALPN is the journal *Advance for*

LPNs. They also publish *NALPN Extra!* for members. For more information about NALPN, look on their Web site (www.nalpn.org).

Supervision/Delegation Connection

Feature Overview

It will be your responsibility to know the scope of practice not only for yourself, but also for the unlicensed assistive personnel (UAP) and certified nursing assistants (CNAs) that you supervise. If you delegate a task to a CNA or UAP that is not within his or her scope of practice, you put the assistant and yourself in legal jeopardy. In this book, we will include information about appropriate delegation and supervision to help you learn what you can and cannot delegate. We also will include tips for successfully supervising assistants.

KNOWLEDGE CONNECTION

What professional organizations can you join as a nursing student? What can result when a nurse exhibits unprofessional conduct?

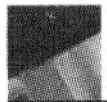

NURSING THEORIES AND THEORISTS

Nursing theories are ideas that a particular nurse or nurse educator has developed to explain how he or she looks at the purpose and focus of nursing. Each theory addresses the theorist's views regarding the person, environment, health, and nursing itself. A variety of nursing theories have been developed over the past 160 years. Table 1.2 presents a brief outline of some of the best-known nurse theorists and the basic premise for their theories. As you might imagine, no one theorist is "right" and the others "wrong." Rather, each theory approaches the overall idea of nursing with a different view. The more you learn about nursing theories, the better you will understand every aspect of being a nurse.

TRENDS IN NURSING PRACTICE

As nursing grows and evolves, improvements in quality and delivery are accomplished. Not all trends are lasting ones, but many stand the test of time. As we look at major trends now, two areas are of great importance: (1) using evidence-based nursing practice and (2) an emphasis on preparing new nurses to improve patient care and the health-care environments in which they work.

Evidence-Based Practice

As a practicing nurse, it is easy to perform skills and care the way you have always done it without questioning whether it is the best practice of nursing. In fact, that is how nursing education worked for a very long time. We passed information from one generation of nurses to the next based on how the instructors learned to practice.

Now, as you are becoming a nurse, there is a better way: to learn the best practices rather than only the tradition of nursing practice. In order to determine best practices, nurses are doing research to test which of our traditional care methods stand the test of evidence. Now nurses use **evidence-based practice** (EBP) as a problem-solving approach to delivering health care. This approach uses the best evidence from nursing research studies and patient care data; it also considers the patient's preferences and values. In other words, research is very important to determine what care is appropriate for certain situations; however, making the care fit a patient's preferences and values is just as important.

EBP is not a new idea. Back in the 1800s, Florence Nightingale searched for evidence that what she was doing for her patients was effective. However, the emphasis on testing and researching our care is becoming more widespread now. Once accurate, scientifically sound data have been collected and demonstrated to prove positive outcomes, they are written into policies and procedures at health-care facilities. It is possible that some information that you learn during your course of nursing studies will be changed in light of evidence once you are working as a nurse.

Evidence-Based Practice

Feature Overview

In some chapters of this book, you will find a box describing evidence-based practice research and outcomes. These boxes will include the clinical question that was researched, the evidence that was found, the implications for nursing practice—in other words, how it affects what you do as a nurse, and the reference where the research was published. You can go to the reference site and read the research for yourself. You can also look up other research on the same or a similar topic.

Quality and Safety Education for Nurses

In order to equip the next generation of nurses to help make needed changes in health care, the Quality and Safety Education for Nurses (QSEN) project was established in 2005. The project focuses on the knowledge, skills, and attitudes (KSAs) needed by nurses to continually improve the quality and safety of patient care. It includes prelicensure KSAs for nursing students and graduate KSAs.

Table 1.2
Selected Nurse Theorists

Theorist	*Date*	*Theory*
Peplau, Hildegard E.	1952	Interpersonal relationships model: interpersonal communication can improve mental health
Henderson, Virginia	1955	14 basic needs addressed by nursing care; definition of nursing; do for the patient what he or she cannot do for himself or herself
Abdellah, Faye G.	1960	21 nursing problems; deliver care to the whole person
Orlando, Ida Jean	1961	Interpersonal process; nursing process theory
Wiedenbach, Ernestine	1964	Purpose of nursing is to support and meet patients' need for help; nursing is a helping art
Levine, Myra	1967	Conservation model, published in 1973; designed to promote adaptation of the person while maintaining wholeness or health
Johnson, Dorothy	1968, 1980	The behavioral system model: incorporates five principles of systems thinking to establish a balance or equilibrium (adaptation) in the person; the patient is a behavioral system consisting of subsystems
Rogers, Martha	1970	The science of unitary human beings focuses on the betterment of humankind through new and innovative modalities; maintaining an environment free of negative energy is important
Orem, Dorothea	1971	The self-care deficit nursing theory explains what nursing care is required when people are not able to care for themselves; the goal is to help client attain total self-care
King, Imogene	1971	First of two theories was the interacting systems framework, designed to explain the organized wholes within which nurses are expected to function: society, groups, and individuals; the first theory led to the theory of goal attainment, which focuses on mutual goal setting between a nurse and patient and the process for meeting the goals
Neuman, Betty	1972	Neuman systems model is based on general systems theory (a nonnursing theory) and reflects the nature of living organisms as open systems
Roy, Sr., Callista	1974	Adaptation model was inspired by the strength and resiliency of children; the model relates to the choices people make as they adapt to illness and wellness
Leininger, Madeleine M.	1978, 1984	Cultural care diversity and universality theory; caring theory
Newman, Margaret	1979	Theory of health as expanding consciousness describes nursing intervention as nonintervention, where the nurse's presence helps patients recognize their own pattern of interacting with the environment
Watson, Jean	1979	Caring theory; nursing is an interpersonal process
Parse, Rosemarie Rizzo	1981	Theory of human becoming focuses on the human-universe-health process and knowledge related to human becoming (or reaching one's potential)
Benner, Patricia, and Wrubel, Judith	1989	Primacy of caring model; caring is central to the model and helps the client cope with stressors of illness

QSEN focuses on six areas for prelicensure KSAs:

1. ***Patient-Centered Care:*** This is a quality focus that emphasizes the patient and their family members as the center of care and as a full partner as nurses provide compassionate and coordinated care. This care is based on respect for the patient's preferences, values, and needs. This may sound rather familiar because it was also discussed in the section on EBP. In Chapter 4, you will learn to develop nursing care plans and to *individualize* them to each patient according to his or her preferences, values, and needs. You will learn how to tailor your care to the values and preferences of another culture in Chapter 8.
2. ***Teamwork and Collaboration:*** This area requires that you function effectively within the nursing team and with other professionals. This involves showing mutual respect, open communication, and shared decision making to achieve quality patient care. In this chapter and in Chapter 2, you will learn about how you fit into the health-care team. In Chapter 6, you will learn about how to communicate in the health-care setting within the health-care team, including how best to communicate during a crisis.
3. ***Evidence-Based Practice:*** This area integrates the best practices proven with research and evidence and the clinical expertise to deliver excellent patient care while still taking into consideration the patient's preferences and values. As discussed earlier in this chapter, EBP is a big part of making sure that you deliver quality care to your patients.
4. ***Quality Improvement:*** This practice requires that you review and evaluate your care and use that data to improve your processes. Nurses must continuously improve the quality and safety of health-care systems based on the results of those reviews and evaluations. Although you may not be directly involved in quality improvement, you may collect data for evaluation or have ideas that could be tested to improve the quality of patient care.
5. ***Safety:*** This area includes ways to prevent risk and harm to patients and health-care workers. This includes not only the systems that are used, but also the safe performance of each individual. Chapter 13 focuses on safety for patients and a safe environment for nurses. In addition, the red print throughout the book is used to emphasize safety issues in each chapter.
6. ***Informatics:*** This area emphasizes the use of technology to communicate, manage data, and prevent errors. As more technology is used to manage health information, the nurse must be knowledgeable about its implementation and use to support EBP. Chapter 5 includes information about electronic health records, and Chapters 35 through 38 discuss information about the technology used in medication administration.

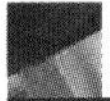

THE IMPACT OF NURSING

Nurses have an amazing opportunity to impact patients' lives every day. People who are ill or recovering from illness or surgery have many needs. They often are unable to perform normal activities and rely on the nursing staff for help with the most basic needs.

Although other health-care professionals come in and out of patients' lives with short-term contact, nurses are the caregivers 24 hours a day, 7 days a week. This gives nurses a number of opportunities to develop relationships with patients. In establishing such relationships, nurses can influence patients in many positive ways. For example, nurses can teach their patients about adopting healthier lifestyles, when and how to take medications, which side effects or complications to watch for, and when to contact their health-care provider.

You will have opportunities to help patients and their families in countless ways throughout your nursing career. Frequently it is the nurse who notices changes and concludes that the patient's condition is worsening. The nurse then contacts the health-care provider regarding the problem. Without an alert, competent nurse, a patient's condition can quickly become dangerous. Often patients never know what could have happened were it not for a thinking nurse. And although not everyone will always say "thank you," you will have the satisfaction of a job well done.

Real-World Connection

Becoming a "Good Nurse"

As one nursing instructor reflected over her 25 years of teaching LPN/LVN students, she said, "I have seen all kinds of students who came from all walks of life be successful in nursing school. The one thing they had in common was the desire to learn and to care for people. My desire was that they not just become nurses, but that they become good nurses, the kind of nurse I would want caring for my family members or me." Her advice to you is, "Do not settle for just being a nurse. Settle for nothing less than being a good nurse, a thinking nurse, one whose presence makes a difference."

• WORD • BUILDING •

collaboration: col – together + labor – work + ation – action

informatics: informat – information + ics – study of

POST CONFERENCE

The Post Conference at the end of each chapter will help you understand how to evaluate the clinical experience of caring for the assigned patient in the Critical Thinking Connection. You will participate in Post Conferences after you care for real patients in the long-term or acute care setting. You will find that you can learn something new from each experience of caring for people. What new things have you learned from reading and studying this chapter?

Key Points

- Many educational opportunities and a variety of practice settings are available to nursing students after graduation.
- Throughout much of history, nursing was provided by religious orders and then by the poor, lower classes.
- Modern nursing originated in the mid-1800s with Florence Nightingale as its founder.
- The standardization of nursing education came into being through the American Society of Superintendents of Training Schools for Nurses (now the National League for Nursing).
- Education for LPNs began in 1892 in New York City through the YWCA.
- The title LPN is used in all states except California and Texas, where the title LVN is used.
- Four entry-level options for nursing education are LPN/LVN, ADN (RN), diploma (RN), and BSN.
- It is your responsibility to know the content of your state's Nurse Practice Act and to follow it faithfully.
- Nurses must be responsible, honest, caring, and organized.
- You represent all nurses to your patients and their families, so it is extremely important to be professional in appearance and behavior.
- There is a difference between being a nurse and being a good nurse.
- Two organizations LPN/LVN students can join while in school are HOSA and NALPN. After graduation, NALPN is the professional organization.
- Unprofessional conduct is described in the nurse practice acts of most states. If you are found guilty of certain conduct, you could lose your license and the legal right to practice as a nurse.
- Nursing theories by selected theorists form the basis for how nurses think about nursing and how they implement care.
- Trends in nursing include using EBP to promote quality care and using the KSAs to improve quality and safety in nursing.
- Think about the kind of nurse you would want to take care of your family or to care for you. Be that kind of nurse.

Review Questions

Select the answer that is most appropriate for each of the following questions. Some questions may have more than one correct answer. Select all that apply.

1. The first role for a woman in health care was that of a:
   1. nun.
   2. midwife.
   3. deaconess.
   4. teacher.

2. The most famous Kaiserworth deaconess was:
   1. Sairey Gamp.
   2. Clara Barton.
   3. Florence Nightingale.
   4. Mary Mahoney.

3. Which is true of a "one-plus-one" program?
   1. One year after a student becomes an ADN, he or she can finish college with a BSN.
   2. One year after working as an RN, the nurse can achieve advanced practice status with 1 more year of college.
   3. One RN and one LPN/LVN work together for 1 year in a hospital setting, and then the LPN/LVN can become an RN after passing the NCLEX.
   4. The first year of a 2-year program prepares the student to take the NCLEX-PN. The student can work as an LPN/LVN while completing the second year of nursing school to become an ADN.

4. The NCLEX is:
   1. an examination to determine entry into a practical/vocational nursing school.
   2. an examination taken to become licensed as a nurse.
   3. a review course to help students do well on their licensure examination.
   4. a national survey of all nurses to determine average age and work settings.

5. An RN student asks a friend who is an LPN/LVN student, "Will you be able to start IVs when you get out of school?" Which is the best response?
   1. "It will depend on the Nurse Practice Act of the state where I work."
   2. "Sure. I'm sure I will learn how to do that in school."
   3. "Maybe. If the hospital where I work allows it."
   4. "No. LPNs/LVNs are never allowed to do that."

6. Which is a description of professional behavior by a nurse?
   1. Taking several breaks when you need to make personal phone calls.
   2. Criticizing another nurse in the break room because of an error made when administering medications.
   3. Requesting assistance if you realize you will not be able to finish your assigned duties on time.
   4. Leaving the patient unit without notifying anyone to run to the gift shop for a few minutes.

7. Which of the following are entry-level nursing programs? Select all that apply.
   1. A minimum of 2 years at a private or community college
   2. Two or more years in graduate school at a university
   3. Nine months to 1 year at a technical college or career technology center
   4. Four-year college degree at a university
   5. Three years in a hospital-based program affiliated with a college or university

ANSWERS 1. 2, 2. 3, 3. 4, 4. 2, 5. 1, 6. 3, 7. 1, 3, 4, 5

Critical Thinking Exercises

Answers available online.

1. What would you do if you, a nursing student, made an error that could harm a patient?

2. How would you respond to the following statement? "Nursing is more science than art in today's world. 'Caring' nurses are equated with subservient handmaidens."

Additional Resources

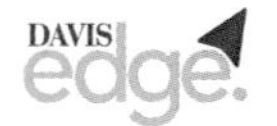

Use the scratch off code on the inside front cover of your book to access online quizzes that will help you to improve your scores on course exams and prepare for the NCLEX-PN®.

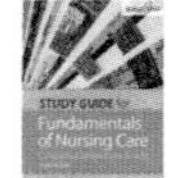

Study Guide

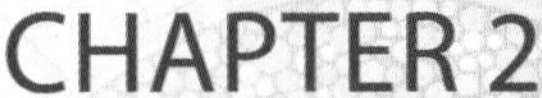

CHAPTER 2
Health-Care Delivery, Settings, and Economics

KEY TERMS

Capitation (KAP-ih-TAY-shun)
Case management (KAYSS MAN-aj-ment)
Client-centered care (KLY-ent SEN-terd KARE)
Diagnosis-related groups (DYE-ag-NOH-siss rih-LAY-ted GROOPS)
Health-care provider (HELLTH KARE proh-VYE-duhr)
Health maintenance organization (HELLTH MAYN-tuh-nanss OR-ga-nih-ZAY-shun)
Home health care (HOHM HELLTH KARE)
Hospice (HOS-pis)
Inpatient (IN-pay-shent)
Managed care (MAN-ajd KARE)
Medicaid (MED-ih-kayd)
Medicare (MED-ih-kare)
Outpatient (OWT-pay-shent)
Point-of-service plan (POYNT-uv-SER-viss PLAN)
Preferred provider organization (PPO) (prih-FERD pro-VYE-duhr OR-ga-nih-ZAY-shun)
Primary care nursing (PRY-mare-ee KARE NER-sing)
Primary care physician (PRY-mare-ee KARE fih-ZIH-shun)
Referral (rih-FER-uhl)
Rehabilitation (REE-ha-BIL-ih-TAY-shun)
Team nursing (TEEM NER-sing)
Third-party payer (THERD-PAR-tee PAY-uhr)

CHAPTER CONCEPTS

Collaboration
Health-Care System
Communication

LEARNING OUTCOMES

1. Define various terms associated with health-care delivery and economics.
2. Discuss health-care collaboration and how it links to patient safety.
3. Identify the two most important factors in health-care delivery and economics.
4. Describe members of the health-care team and their functions.
5. Describe inpatient health-care settings and their services.
6. Describe outpatient health-care settings and their services.
7. Explain two types of rehabilitation services.
8. Distinguish between types of nursing care delivery systems.
9. Contrast Medicare and Medicaid.
10. Describe various types of private health insurance.
11. Discuss information found in the Connection features of the chapter.

CRITICAL THINKING CONNECTION

Clinical Assignment

You have been assigned to care for a 60-year-old female patient diagnosed with colon cancer. She underwent abdominal surgery to remove the tumor, and now she has an infected abdominal wound. Her care plan calls for dressing changes on the wound twice a day and IV antibiotics. She is very anxious to get home so that she can take care of her two young grandchildren of whom she has primary custody. There are no other adults in the home to help care for her.

Critical Thinking Questions:

1. What concerns do you have regarding discharge of this patient?
2. What resources are available to help her?
3. How can the hospital staff help prepare her for discharge?

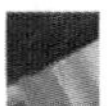

THE HEALTH-CARE TEAM

A patient in a health-care facility sees an amazing number of different workers, all of whom are members of the health-care team. These team members provide medical and mental health services to patients in various settings. They have a common goal of providing quality, cost-efficient care to all patients in order to restore their patients to their optimal level of functioning and wellness.

While caring for patients on a busy day, the last thing on the minds of many nurses is who is paying for each patient's care. Yet some entity is responsible for payment. It is important for you to be cost conscious as a nurse, to conserve supplies when possible, and to avoid any waste. In this chapter we will talk more about who pays for health care and how.

Collaboration of the Health-Care Team

You will work with a variety of team members with different types of training and areas of focus (Table 2.1). Please note that physicians, physician's assistants, and nurse practitioners are referred to in this book as **health-care providers** (HCPs)

Table 2.1
The Health-Care Team

Staff Member	*Description*
Health-Care Providers	
Medical Doctor (MD) Doctor of Osteopathy (DO)	Responsible for diagnosing and treating disease, illness, and injury; ordering diets, tests, medications, treatments, therapies, and procedures; and directing overall care of patients
Physician's Assistant (PA)	Employed by a physician or hospital to work closely with the physician and assist in directing patient care
Nurse Practitioner (NP)	Masters-prepared registered nurse certified in a specific area of practice and identified with advanced practice license who diagnoses illnesses and prescribes medications and treatments
Nursing Staff	
Registered Nurse (RN)	Practices nursing within a defined scope under the direction of a physician; provides direct patient care, manages departments, and supervises other nurses and assistive personnel
Licensed Practical/Vocational Nurse (LPN/LVN)	Practices within a defined scope under the supervision of a physician, dentist, or RN; provides direct patient care and supervises assistive personnel
Unlicensed Assistive Personnel (UAP)	Performs more complicated tasks than the certified nursing assistant, including sterile procedures, in some states
Certified Nursing Assistant (CNA)	Performs patient care duties and assists nursing staff
Therapy Staff	
Respiratory Therapist (RT)	Evaluates, treats, and cares for patients with breathing problems due to heart and lung disease
Respiratory Therapy Technician (RTT)	RTT generally works under the supervision of an RT
Physical Therapist (PT)	Provides services to help improve or restore function and mobility, relieve pain, and prevent or limit permanent physical disabilities for patients suffering from injuries and disease
Physical Therapy Assistant (PTA)	PTA generally works under the supervision of a PT and carries out the PT's orders
Speech and Language Therapist (ST)	Assesses, diagnoses, treats, and helps to prevent disorders related to speech, language, voice, swallowing, and fluency

Continued

Table 2.1
The Health-Care Team—cont'd

Staff Member	*Description*
Occupational Therapist (OT) Certified Occupation Therapy Assistant (COTA)	Assists patients with disabilities to develop, recover, or maintain their skills for daily activities and work
Laboratory Staff Pathologist (MD)	Medical doctor who examines tissue and blood samples to determine the origin or existence of disease
Medical Laboratory Technologist (MLT) Medical Technician (MT)	Examines and analyzes body fluids and tissues, matches blood for transfusions, and tests for blood levels of medications
Phlebotomist	Draws blood specimens from patients for testing
Radiology Staff Radiologist (MD)	Medical doctor who specializes in procedures involving x-rays and radiation therapy; reads radiographs and other radiological films
Radiologic Technologist (Rad Tech)	Operates x-ray machines and other radiological equipment, such as computed tomography (CT) scanners, as well as magnetic resonance imaging (MRI) and ultrasound equipment; assists the radiologist by performing ordered tests to determine diagnoses and treat certain diseases
Ancillary Staff Pharmacist	Pharmacist distributes prescription medications and advises patients and prescribers on the selection, dosages, interactions, and side effects of medications
Pharmacy Technician	Pharmacy technician assists pharmacist by helping to prepare prescribed medications, answering phones, and stocking shelves
Registered Dietitian (RD)	RD plans regular menus and develops special menus to meet the dietary needs of patients, works with health-care providers to meet special dietary needs, and instructs patients on special diets
Dietary Technician	Dietary Technician assists the RD by distributing and picking up selective menus and monitoring patient food intake
Medical Social Worker Public Health Social Worker	Provides psychosocial support to patients, families, or vulnerable populations; advises caregivers; counsels patients; plans for patients' needs after discharge; and arranges for needed care such as home health care
Chaplain	Provides spiritual care for patients in hospitals and hospice settings, meets the spiritual needs of families and patients when diagnosis is terminal or when death occurs, and provides spiritual care for hospital staff

because they all write orders for patient care. It is important that you realize the valuable input of each health-care team member. It takes all of us working together to deliver quality health care to our patients. Communication between members of the health-care team is also extremely important. This is discussed further in Chapter 6.

When health-care workers collaborate with one another, one of the most positive outcomes is improved patient safety. Poor quality care occurs, along with a higher rate of preventable errors, when health-care personnel act alone, or in a "silo."

One program, called Team STEPPS, is available through the Agency for Healthcare Research and Quality (AHRQ). This program uses evidence-based teamwork to improve communication and teamwork skills. This in turn eliminates barriers to quality and safety.

Interprofessional collaboration helps improve the ability of health-care professionals and patients to consider one another's unique perspectives to better address the needs of all patients and their families. No one can do this all alone.

Multidisciplinary Team Conferences

One way to help facilitate communication between professionals caring for the same patients is through multidisciplinary team conferences. These conferences bring together all of the disciplines involved in the patient's care. For example, a patient who has had a stroke and is paralyzed with difficulty swallowing and eating might have a multidisciplinary team that includes the health-care provider, the physical therapist, the occupational therapist, the speech therapist, the dietician, and a representative from the nursing staff. Each discipline has input for the care of the patient to bring about the best outcomes.

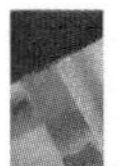

DETERMINING THE DELIVERY OF EFFECTIVE CARE

When the economics of care is a foremost consideration, two factors help guide decisions about patient care: *medical necessity* and the *appropriate level of care*. These factors are important to ensure that patients get the care they need in the correct setting to be cost-effective and promote patient improvement. In order to make these decisions about care, insurers use some form of managed care. **Managed care** has been defined as "any method of financing and organizing the delivery of health care in which costs are contained by controlling the provision of benefits and services."

Medical Necessity

Insurers determine medical necessity by comparing the patient's clinical/medical information against accepted medical review criteria. According to government funding sources, *medical necessity* is defined as services or items reasonable and necessary for the diagnosis or treatment of illness or injury or to improve the functioning of a malformed body member. This means that the services must seem reasonable and necessary to the entity paying for them.

Example of Reasonable and Necessary Services

If a person has health insurance and submits a claim for a face lift, the insurance company would not pay it because a face lift is not needed to diagnose or treat an illness or injury, nor does it improve the functioning of a malformed body part. However, another person could submit a claim for facial reconstruction surgery after a car accident, and that claim would be paid because it is reasonable and necessary to repair the person's facial structures after an injury.

Appropriate Level of Care

Another aspect of paying for health care requires determining an appropriate level of care to meet the patient's needs. In today's health-care environment, there is a continuum of care that the patient may travel in his or her efforts to reach an optimal level of health, function, and wellness. It is important that the patient is cared for at the most cost-effective, yet safe and effective, level. This may be either at an inpatient or outpatient level.

Inpatient Settings

Inpatients stay overnight or longer in a health-care facility. Inpatient care may be provided in an acute medical or mental health-care hospital, a skilled nursing facility in a nursing home or hospital, a long-term acute care hospital, a long-term chronic care facility such as a nursing home or assisted living facility, or a rehabilitation facility.

ACUTE CARE HOSPITAL OR MEDICAL CENTER. An acute care hospital may be the only hospital for many miles, or it may be one of several hospitals in a medical center complex where a number of different specialty hospitals are grouped together and share resources. Acute care hospitals provide emergency care, surgeries, inpatient care, diagnostic testing, and usually some types of outpatient care. Staff is composed of a variety of doctors, nurses, assistants, therapists, laboratory workers, and other medical personnel. Rural hospitals may be smaller, with fewer departments and less staff than their larger city counterparts. Regardless of size or location, when a person is ill or injured, he or she generally seeks care at the closest hospital.

LONG-TERM ACUTE CARE HOSPITAL. A long-term acute care hospital (LTACH) provides a level of care similar to that of an acute care hospital. However, an LTACH focuses on patients with serious medical problems that require intense, special treatment for a long period of time, usually about 20 to 30 days. These patients often transfer from intensive care units in traditional hospitals. It would not be unusual for a patient in an LTACH to need ventilator or other life support medical assistance.

The health-care team in an LTACH is composed of members similar to those in the acute care hospital. A health-care provider visit is required daily.

Example of the Effective Use of This Level of Care

A patient is in intensive care on a ventilator after lung surgery and develops an infection in the chest cavity. The patient is stable on the ventilator and will have to remain on it until the infection is completely cleared, which could be up to a month. It would be extremely expensive for the patient to remain in an acute care hospital during that time. The patient is transferred to an LTACH for continued treatment of the lung infection and ventilator support.

SKILLED NURSING FACILITY. A skilled nursing facility (SNF) may be associated with a hospital or long-term care facility. The SNF provides a less intense level of care than that found in a traditional or long-term acute care hospital. It usually is

• WORD • BUILDING •

ventilator: ventilat – ventilate + or – a thing performing an action

a transitional care setting. Patients may stay in an SNF for a few days or as long as 100 days, but they eventually move to a rehabilitation, nursing home, or home-care setting.

SNF care consists of skilled nursing care and physical, occupational, and speech therapy as needed. Health-care providers usually do not visit daily and are more likely to see patients on a weekly basis. Laboratory, radiology, or surgical services usually are not available at an SNF. An SNF level of care usually is covered by Medicare and most private insurers, but there are certain requirements:

- The patient must have been hospitalized for at least 3 days prior to admission.
- The patient must enter the nursing home within 30 days of a hospitalization.
- There is a 100-day stay maximum per year related to any one hospitalization and diagnosis.
- The patient must be making regular progress as documented by the medical professionals.

Example of the Effective Use of This Level of Care

An elderly man falls at home and suffers a fractured hip. While in the acute care hospital, he has surgery to repair the fracture but does not want to eat after surgery. Eventually a feeding tube is placed, and the patient is fed through the tube. He begins to eat a bit, but not enough to take out the tube. The surgery was successful, but the patient is not strong enough to return home. He is placed in an SNF unit for skilled nursing care. He continues to increase his oral intake and is discharged to his home in 40 days.

REHABILITATION FACILITY. **Rehabilitation,** often shortened to rehab, is a level of care in which the patient can receive intense physical, occupational, and speech therapy services. The rehabilitation facility may be part of a hospital, or it may be a freestanding facility. A physician specialist in physical medicine and rehabilitation oversees the patient's care during his or her stay. Other health-care team members who may participate in patient care include nurses, therapists, therapist assistants, nursing assistants, and technicians. As a rule of thumb, the patient must be capable of participating in at least 3 hours of therapy a day to be admitted to a rehabilitation facility. If the patient becomes ill or has other medical problems while in rehabilitation, he or she may be transferred back to an acute care hospital.

Example of the Effective Use of This Level of Care

A female patient suffers a stroke and has weakness on the left side of her body. She is discharged from the hospital to a rehabilitation facility for 2 months of intensive therapy to regain as much strength and use as possible in her affected side. The therapy sessions are held every morning and afternoon. She is also expected to perform activities such as bathing and grooming with assistance. As her stay lengthens, she is expected to need less assistance.

Another type of rehabilitation facility focuses on treating patients with chemical dependency and mental health issues. Some of these facilities provide medical care in the form of *detoxification,* or the removal of drugs and alcohol from the person's body, which generally takes several days.

If the rehabilitation facility does not provide this type of care, patients have to be admitted to an acute care hospital for the detoxification process as it can lead to a medical emergency. After going through the detoxification process, patients can then be admitted to a rehabilitation facility designed to treat chemical dependency and mental health issues. Most generally, the physician who oversees the patient's care is a psychiatrist who specializes in treating mental or behavioral disorders. The health-care team in this type of rehabilitation setting consists of nurses, nursing assistants, clinical social workers who usually function as therapists or counselors, and psychologists.

Example of the Effective Use of This Level of Care

A young male patient is addicted to the pain medication OxyContin®. He cannot really begin treatment for addiction until the drug is completely out of his body and the withdrawal symptoms are past. He goes through detoxification for the first few days after he stops taking the drug. The health-care staff monitors him closely for physical problems related to withdrawal, such as seizures, sweating, hallucinations, muscle pain, and nausea and vomiting. He then begins individual and group counseling sessions and group activities to deal with the issues that led to his addiction.

RESIDENTIAL CARE FACILITIES. The term *residential care* is used to describe care given in settings where the patients, or residents, stay for long periods of time. Box 2.1 lists examples of residential care facilities and their functions.

KNOWLEDGE CONNECTION

Give an example of a procedure that would be considered medically necessary. List four settings for residential care. List four criteria that a patient must meet to be admitted to an SNF. What is the difference between an acute care hospital and an LTACH?

Outpatient Care

Outpatient care is provided in many settings and is designed to meet the needs of the patient in 1 day and then allow him or her to return home. Care and services provided on an outpatient basis usually are less expensive than care provided on an inpatient basis. Outpatient care is preferred when possible

• WORD • BUILDING •

detoxification: de – removal + toxi – poison + fication – make

Box 2.1
Examples of Residential Care Facilities

A client may live in a variety of residential care settings. Each provides a different level of assistance.

- **Long-term care facilities:** Also called nursing homes or convalescent homes, these facilities are where residents often live for many years. Nursing care is provided around the clock for the residents in these facilities. The residents usually have chronic illnesses or disabilities. Long-term care facilities may also be affiliated with skilled nursing facilities. Therapies are available through the facility or through home health agencies. They are staffed by RNs, LPN/LVNs, and CNAs. In some states, medication aides help administer medications to these residents.
- **Assisted living facilities:** These facilities provide less nursing care than that found in long-term care facilities. They offer 24-hour protective oversight. Residents are assisted with medications and personal care such as bathing and dressing. Meals are provided, and a choice of activities may be available. Therapies and specific nursing care, such as dressing changes, are provided through home health agencies. These facilities are staffed with one or more RNs, one or more LPN/LVNs, and numerous CNAs.
- **Memory care facilities:** These are secure facilities for residents with cognitive issues who are likely to wander or to be unsafe unless they are in a protected environment. Twenty-four hour care is provided by CNAs with specialized training to work with cognitive-impaired clients. An RN or LPN/LVN is usually available on the unit during the daytime hours but may be only on-call in the evenings. In this environment, the residents are provided with personal care, meals, a safe environment, and appropriate activities.
- **Independent living facilities:** These facilities do not provide nursing care. They generally have staff available around the clock to respond to urgent situations by contacting emergency medical services for the residents. Meals usually are available, as well as transportation and activities.

to decrease costs while still providing quality care. A patient may require surgery that can be provided at an outpatient facility, but the appropriate level of care for this patient may be for the surgery to be performed in an inpatient setting because the patient has other health conditions that could influence his or her recovery.

HOSPITAL OUTPATIENT DEPARTMENT. Hospitals offer a wide range of outpatient services. Most larger hospitals or medical centers provide outpatient surgery; cardiac, pulmonary, physical, occupational, and speech therapy/rehabilitation; laboratory, radiation, and diagnostic testing; and mental health services such as intensive outpatient or partial-day treatment. Most hospitals also have a 24-hour observation setting in which patients can receive care and diagnostic testing to determine whether they need to be admitted.

Outpatient surgery is performed in a hospital setting, but the patient is allowed to return home on the same day that the surgical procedure is performed. Outpatient surgery is also referred to as *ambulatory surgery* or *same-day surgery.* It is suited best for healthy people undergoing minor or intermediate procedures. Some outpatient surgeries may require a 24-hour observation stay to make sure the patient does not have any immediate complications after surgery. More than 60% of elective surgical procedures in the United States are currently performed as outpatient surgeries. Health experts expect that this percentage will increase to nearly 75% over the next decade.

Ambulatory surgery centers (ASCs) are freestanding health-care facilities that provide outpatient surgery only. The type of surgeries performed at ASCs may be directed by state regulations.

Example of the Appropriate Use of This Level of Care

A patient has her gallbladder removed via a small abdominal incision called *laparoscopic surgery.* The patient is monitored after she awakens from the anesthetic. The nurse assesses the patient to ensure that she can tolerate liquids and can urinate after surgery. Then the patient is discharged to home with follow-up instructions.

OUTPATIENT MENTAL HEALTH SERVICES. Some hospital mental health outpatient services include intensive outpatient and partial-day treatment programs. Intensive outpatient programs generally provide group counseling and therapy sessions for mental health and chemical dependency illnesses; these sessions generally last 2 to 3 hours per day, two to five times per week. Partial day treatment programs provide group and individual counseling and therapy sessions for mental health and chemical dependency illnesses, lasting approximately 7 to 8 hours per day during the week.

Example of the Appropriate Use of This Level of Care

As a continuation of the treatment for the client addicted to OxyContin® whom we discussed earlier, after detoxification and inpatient treatment, he transitions to partial-day treatment. He comes to the mental health facility every day for 8 hours. As the client improves, he begins a job during the day. He then comes back to the facility 2 nights per week for group therapy sessions.

CARDIAC REHABILITATION. The American Heart Association describes cardiac rehabilitation as a medically supervised program to help patients with cardiac disorders recover quickly and improve their overall physical, mental, and social functioning. The goal is to stabilize, slow, or even reverse the

• **WORD • BUILDING** •
ambulatory: ambulat – move about + ory – relating to

progression of cardiovascular disease. Cardiac rehabilitation programs include the following:

- Counseling so that the patient can understand and manage the disease process
- Exercise programs
- Nutritional counseling
- Risk factor modification
- Counseling on the appropriate use of prescribed medications

The cardiac rehabilitation health-care team consists of cardiologists (physicians who specialize in the diseases and treatments of the heart), nurses, physical/exercise therapists and assistants, and dietitians. Cardiac rehabilitation is provided through an outpatient setting of a hospital or at a freestanding facility.

PULMONARY REHABILITATION. Pulmonary rehabilitation is a program of education and exercise classes that teaches patients about their lungs, how to exercise and perform activities with less shortness of breath, and how to live better with a lung condition. The health-care team for pulmonary rehabilitation includes a pulmonologist (physician who specializes in diseases and treatments of the lungs), nurses, respiratory therapists, and respiratory assistants. Pulmonary rehabilitation is provided through an outpatient setting of a hospital or at a freestanding facility.

AMBULATORY CARE CLINICS. Ambulatory care clinics operate much like a medical office and provide the same type of services. Some may specialize in one type of care, such as urgent care or occupational health care. Ambulatory care clinics may provide a variety of health-care services under one roof. These services may include medical, dental, laboratory, x-ray, psychological, and/or pharmaceutical care.

HEALTH DEPARTMENTS. Health departments are public facilities that provide health-care services. These facilities are funded by county, city, state, and federal governments. Therefore, the cost of care at these facilities is lower than the cost of care at private clinics. In some cases, care is provided at no cost. The services provided are determined by the governing entity but may include immunizations, family planning, maternity education, well-baby clinics, child developmental services, and environmental health.

Health departments are also responsible for the tracking and treatment of certain communicable diseases such as tuberculosis, sexually transmitted diseases, measles, mumps, rubella, hepatitis, flu, and certain viruses.

Example of the Use of This Level of Care

A teenage mother who is pregnant with her second child does not work because of the pregnancy and caring for her 18-month-old son. Her husband has been laid off from his construction job. She is seen at the health department for assistance with food and health care for herself and her child through the Women, Infants, and Children (WIC) health program. She is provided with vouchers to buy healthy food, and her pregnancy is monitored for problems. Her son is provided with the appropriate immunizations and is monitored for normal growth and development.

MEDICAL OFFICE. The medical office setting offers evaluation, assessment, treatment, simple diagnostic testing, and simple surgical treatment. The health-care provider and staff may specialize in one particular area of health care, seeing only patients with specific health conditions. The health-care team in a medical office usually consists of one or more physician, physician's assistants and/or nurse practitioners (health-care providers), an office nurse or medical assistant, and medical office personnel. Administrative medical assistants are responsible for appointments, phone calls, collaboration with health insurance companies, billing, and other duties assigned by the health-care providers.

HOME HEALTH CARE. **Home health care** can be one or many types of health or medical services provided to patients in their homes because they are confined to their homes by an illness or disability. Home health agencies provide care in the form of skilled nursing visits with or without home health aide visits; physical, occupational, and speech therapy; medical social worker visits; infusion therapy; durable medical equipment; and hospice. Home health services must be ordered by a physician and be medically necessary in order to be covered by Medicare and private insurance plans.

Home health care allows people to stay in their homes rather than being forced by medical needs to live in a health-care facility. Home visits for skilled care are a cost-effective way to provide limited care.

Skilled services are those that require a license to be performed, and Medicare requires that a patient need skilled services in order to qualify for home health care. These skilled services may be a need for nursing, therapy, or social work. Skilled nursing visits include performing nursing assessment and evaluation, complicated dressing changes, and the administration of IV medications. Home health aides provide nonskilled services such as assisting with bathing and grooming, housekeeping, transportation, and food preparation and delivery.

Physical, occupational, and speech therapy services can be provided in the home by therapists who make home visits through a home health agency. The patient must be homebound to receive these services; otherwise, the patient could go to an outpatient therapy center for this type of care.

Medical social worker visits can be ordered to assist patients and families with psychosocial support to help them deal with chronic, acute, or terminal illnesses. They also can help patients and their families with financial needs. They may arrange for community services such as Meals on Wheels, public transportation, medication assistance, and legal assistance.

Example of the Effective Use of This Level of Care

An elderly man whose wife died last year recently underwent abdominal surgery to repair a bowel perforation. His abdominal wound has not healed, and he requires dressing changes twice each day. A home health nurse comes each morning and evening to change the dressing, and a home health aide comes 2 days per week to help him take a sponge bath, change his sheets weekly, and prepare a light lunch for him. The social worker has arranged for meals to be delivered through a neighborhood Meals on Wheels program. The patient's wound gradually heals, and he gains strength. He no longer needs home health assistance and goes to the senior center for his noon meal most days.

HOSPICE. Hospice is defined as an interdisciplinary program of palliative care and support services that addresses the physical, spiritual, social, and economic needs of terminally ill patients and their families (Taber's 23e). The appropriate time for hospice care is when the patient is no longer seeking treatment to arrest or cure the disease and is expected to live 6 months or less. The patient is treated with medications and other measures to relieve pain and remain comfortable. This treatment is usually in the home but may also occur in a free-standing hospice building or a hospice wing in a hospital. Hospice services include managing the patient's pain and symptoms, lending emotional support to the patient and family, administering medications, providing medical supplies and equipment, providing caregiver instructions and support, coordinating all health-care services, and providing grief support for surviving loved ones and friends.

The hospice team usually consists of home health aides, a hospice physician, nurses, social workers, a chaplain or clergy, and trained volunteers, and it may include the patient's personal health-care provider. For more information about hospice, see Chapter 10.

KNOWLEDGE CONNECTION

How are inpatient and outpatient settings different? What types of diseases are treated and tracked by health departments? How are home health care and hospice care similar? How are they different?

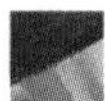

DELIVERY OF NURSING CARE

Whatever the setting or level of care, nurses provide quality care to patients. This requires organization, in-depth knowledge of patient care, and application of that knowledge in a variety of situations.

When you care for patients, you deliver nursing care. This may be accomplished in several different ways. It is important for you to be familiar with these delivery systems to understand your role in each of them. Some systems are well suited to specific settings but would not work as well in others. The most commonly used types of delivery for nursing care include team nursing, client-centered care, primary care nursing, and case management.

Team Nursing

Team nursing uses a team consisting of nurses and certified nursing assistants (CNAs) or unlicensed assistive personnel (UAP) to provide care for a group of patients. This type of delivery system for nursing care is often used in the acute care hospital, rehabilitation setting, and long-term care setting. In team nursing, each member of the team provides nursing care depending on his or her skills, education, and licensure.

For example, a nursing care team in the acute care hospital might consist of a registered nurse (RN), a licensed practical nurse (LPN), and a UAP or CNA, all of whom are responsible for the care of 10 patients. The RN might be responsible for assessing patients, administering some or all of the IV medications, maintaining the IV sites, communicating with health-care providers and obtaining orders, and ensuring that other team members have performed and documented care appropriately. The LPN/LVN might be responsible for administering medications to all of the patients as well as performing any treatments (for example, dressing changes), assessing the patient for any changes from baseline, evaluating pain levels and medicating appropriately, and providing patient teaching. The UAP or CNA might be responsible for helping each patient bathe and dress in a clean gown, changing sheets on the beds, assisting patients to the bathroom, and taking routine vital signs. The job duties are divided by the nursing team's level of knowledge and education. That is not to say that only nursing assistants should help a patient to the bathroom. The needs of the patients must be the first priority of everyone on the team.

A disadvantage of team nursing is that, without excellent communication between team members, care may become fragmented.

Client-Centered Care

Client-centered care empowers the patient to take control of and manage his or her care. This type of system is often seen in a rehabilitation setting. It allows patients to achieve independence within the limits of their disability by permitting them to have a voice in their rehabilitation, schedule, goals, and method of attaining those goals.

Client-centered care in the acute care hospital setting varies. In that setting, the goal is to decrease the number of people who give care to the patient so that there is less chance of miscommunication or error and to provide care as soon as it is needed instead of having to wait for people from different departments to arrive. Health-care workers are cross-trained to perform as many tasks as possible for each patient. For example, in some client-centered care settings, the nurse not only performs the usual nursing care, but also obtains needed blood specimens, runs an *electrocardiogram* (ECG; a tracing of electrical heart activity) when indicated, and may even administer respiratory therapy treatments. In this situation, no phlebotomist comes in to draw blood, no ECG technician is requested if the patient is having chest pain, and no respiratory therapy technician is needed to give a breathing treatment. One disadvantage of this type of care in the acute care hospital is the time and education needed for each staff member to cross-train in all of these areas.

Primary Care Nursing

In **primary care nursing,** one nurse is responsible for all aspects of nursing care for his or her assigned patients. This means that there is no UAP or CNA to take vital signs, no other nurse to call the health-care provider or take orders, and no one else to bathe the patient or change the bed. In this type of nursing, the nurse carries a great deal of responsibility. A secondary nurse is assigned care for the patient when the primary nurse is off duty.

The primary care nursing model is often used in intensive care units. An RN or LPN/LVN provides all aspects of nursing care to one or two critically ill patients. These nurses must be able to work quickly and efficiently in a crisis or under stress. In addition, they must be able to assess the patient carefully, making sure to note any small change in the patient's condition and correctly interpreting its significance. A disadvantage of this type of nursing delivery is that it works best when the number of patients assigned to the nurse is very limited, so it does not work well outside critical care areas.

Case Management

The delivery of nursing care via a **case management** system is associated with a managed care strategy. The nurses providing case management services act simultaneously as coordinators, facilitators, impartial advocates, and educators. These case managers can be found in hospitals, rehabilitation facilities, and home health agencies. They handle workers' compensation claims resulting from severe injury or disability. The process of case management involves seeing each patient as an individual and each situation as unique. The goal of case management is to assist patients who are vulnerable, at risk, or cost-intensive so that their care is coordinated, meets their specific needs, and is cost-effective while still bringing them to optimum health.

Case managers may supervise the care of a group of patients within one facility, such as an acute care hospital or home health agency. In that situation, the case manager ensures that each assigned patient is receiving cost-effective care while reaching the goals of a return to optimal health and function. Case managers may also supervise the care of patients in a wide geographical area who have been injured on the job. These case managers make sure that their patients make it to their scheduled health-care appointments and assist with arranging for retraining if the patient cannot return to his or her previous work situation.

A disadvantage of this type of nursing delivery is that case managers' options may be limited depending on the availability of adequate facilities and funding to move the patient to the optimum facility.

KNOWLEDGE CONNECTION

Give one advantage and one disadvantage for each type of nursing care delivery system. Which system seems the best for providing optimum patient care? Which system seems the most cost-effective?

Supervision/Delegation Connection

The Secret to Good Supervision

RNs and LPNs may function as managers or supervisors. It is important to remember that when you supervise other nurses, you are supervising health-care professionals. Avoid allowing a position of supervision to "go to your head." Put yourself in the place of the people you supervise. Always treat them with respect and avoid being overly critical. Everyone responds well to positive comments about their work. Find positives to praise, and if you must correct another nurse or nursing assistant, be as kind as possible.

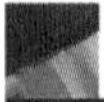

HEALTH-CARE ECONOMICS

In health-care economics, we will discuss how health care is paid for and why that matters to you as a nurse. As this book is being written, our national health-care provisions are in a state of flux. Since 2010, the Affordable Care Act (ACA) has been the law regarding health care. It made some sweeping changes to provide health insurance or Medicaid for what was hoped would be all Americans.

The Affordable Care Act

The ACA has addressed four major issues: cost containment, pre-existing conditions, small business premiums, and lifetime benefit caps. These were helpful to most people who had trouble getting or paying for health insurance in the years previous to the ACA.

Also, under the ACA some services were made available at no cost to the consumer. These included preventative care and vaccinations. In addition, young adults were allowed to stay on their parents' insurance policy until age 26 years to help them pay for the cost of insurance.

• WORD • BUILDING •

electrocardiogram: electro – electricity + cardio – heart + gram – writing

Health-care exchanges were set up for people to purchase insurance if they did not have coverage through their employers. The coverage varied according to the plan they chose, and some people received tax subsidies to help them pay for the cost of their insurance premiums.

The ACA also required that everyone buy health insurance or else pay a special tax. Larger businesses who didn't insure their workers were also required to pay a special tax.

Currently, however, many insurers are leaving the health-care exchanges, and in some counties in the United States there is only one insurer or no insurers available. The enrollees in the ACA insurance plans have been sicker than expected, and providing health care to them has therefore been costlier than expected. This has caused premiums to increase greatly and has caused a number of large insurance companies to stop offering insurance coverage through the exchanges.

There are many ideas about how to fix our nation's health-care cost and coverage issues, but none have yet been signed into law.

Payment of Health-Care Costs

Health-care costs are paid for in one of five ways:

1. Public health insurance (e.g., Medicare and Medicaid)
2. Private health insurance (e.g., Aetna, Blue Cross, United Healthcare, Prudential)
3. Insurance for special populations (e.g., CHAMPVA, TRICARE, Indian Health Service [IHS], Workers' Compensation, and disability insurance)
4. Charitable organizations (e.g., Shriners and the Kaiser family)
5. Self-pay (those who are uninsured)

Public Health Insurance

Public health insurance is funded by the government, either state or federal, or a combination of both. Medicare and Medicaid are forms of public health insurance, as is the IHS.

Medicare

Medicare is the federal government's health insurance program for people older than 65 years. It may be available to those younger than 65 years who have end-stage renal disease and certain other debilitating illnesses. Often private insurers adopt the requirements and payment policies determined by Medicare. It includes four programs, which are described in Box 2.2.

Medicare uses a payment schedule based on **diagnosis-related groups** (DRGs). These classifications of illnesses and diseases are used to determine the amount of money paid by Medicare to the hospital for the care of a patient with that particular illness or disease. For example, a patient might be admitted to the hospital with diabetes. According to the DRGs, Medicare will pay the hospital a certain amount for the care of this diabetic patient, which includes all nursing care, tests, treatments, and teaching. If the patient stays in the hospital longer than the allowed time or it costs the hospital more than the set amount for the patient's care, the payment will still be the set amount of the DRG. If the patient has complicating factors that affect the hospital stay (for example, the patient gets an infection or develops a new problem in addition to diabetes), the hospital can submit bills for the additional problems under a different DRG.

> **Box 2.2**
>
> **Medicare Programs**
>
> Medicare includes several types of programs. Parts A through D each provide a different aspect of care for eligible patients.
>
> - **Part A:** Insurance for hospitalization, hospice, home health, and skilled nursing facility services
> - **Part B:** Supplementary health insurance to help pay participating providers, such as health-care providers, laboratories, x-ray technicians, and home health nurses, and for durable medical equipment
> - **Part C:** Also called Medicare Advantage Plans, which are health insurance plans administered by private insurance companies in place of traditional Medicare
> - **Part D:** Also known as Medicare Prescription Drug Coverage; provides payment for prescribed medications and is run by insurance companies or other private companies approved by Medicare

Medicaid

Medicaid is a federal-state program in which the federal government helps states pay for the health care of those with an income below the poverty level as well as certain other individuals. Because the state is required to set coverage policies and administer the program, the benefits are slightly different in each state. This program offers assistance for poor and medically indigent individuals, pregnant women with an income below the poverty level, children, and certain disabled individuals who meet income-level requirements.

Indian Health Service

The IHS provides government funding for health care for qualified Native American individuals. The IHS may fund hospitals, ambulatory medical and mental health-care clinics, and dental care facilities. It may contract with one or more of the federally recognized tribes to fund health-care services in that tribe's reservation territory. Individuals utilizing these health-care services must meet criteria for a "certificate of degree of Indian blood (CDIB)" in order to be eligible to receive care. A CDIB card is issued when an individual meets the criteria set by the tribe. This card enables the individual to receive health-care services at tribal and IHS facilities.

Private Health Insurance

When a person uses private health insurance, he or she, known as the beneficiary, pays premiums to the insurance company. If people do not have health insurance through their employer, they must purchase it through the Health Exchange. When the beneficiary is cared for by a health-care provider or hospital and the bill is sent to the insurance company, the insurance company is referred to as a third party or a **third-party payer.** Blue Cross Blue Shield, Aetna, United Healthcare, and Prudential are a few of the largest private health insurance companies currently operating in the United States.

Private health insurance companies offer several types of health insurance plans and services. Box 2.3 provides a brief explanation of the most common types. The development of these plans came about as a strategy to help contain the cost of health care by restricting patients' access to only those groups of health-care providers who have contracted to provide specific services at a negotiated price.

Capitation refers to the payment system used by **health maintenance organizations** (HMOs). In this system, **primary care physicians** (PCPs) are paid a set amount per member per month to manage the health care of those members. This PCP is considered the gatekeeper to health services for the individual enrolled in the HMO. For example, a PCP may have 200 patients assigned to him or her. Perhaps the set amount per member is $40. The PCP is paid $8,000 per month to see all the patients who make appointments. If the PCP is unable to successfully treat the patient's condition, he or she makes a **referral** to a specialist. The patient cannot self-refer, and the specialist cannot accept the patient without a referral. In this way, access to more costly care and potentially redundant testing is controlled.

Patient Teaching Connection

Teaching About HMO Regulations

Teach patients enrolled in HMOs the importance of going through their PCPs before accessing care to ensure that the care will be covered. If it is not ordered by their PCP, the insurance company may deny the claim. It is extremely important that patients understand the requirements of their insurance plan. Teach patients that before any procedures, surgeries, and tests are performed, the patient or health-care provider's staff must obtain prior authorization by contacting the insurance company and acquiring approval for the treatment.

Private health insurance is available in different venues. Individuals may participate in group health insurance plans provided by employers. With this type of health insurance, the employer pays a portion or all of the cost of the premium. The company may offer one type of health plan or may offer a variety of plans, and the individual can choose from several types of coverage for different prices. The employer decides what types of policies are available to the employee. The options available to the employer include HMOs, **preferred provider organizations** (PPOs), and **point-of-service plans** (POS plans).

The company may also define and fund its own benefits and have a health insurance company administer the benefits according to the employer's defined requirements. The employer generally negotiates with the health insurance company to utilize their HMO, PPO, or POS networks to provide health-care services to their members.

Underinsured patients are those that have purchased some form of medical insurance, but it pays a relatively small portion of their medical expenses. Some people on the lowest level of the health exchanges have insurance, but it only pays 60% of their costs and has a high deductible. For example, if a person had an acute and severe illness, such as an infection in the lining of the heart, he or she may be in an intensive care unit for a week or longer. With a high deductible of $10,000 plus 40% of the total cost of the hospitalization, which could amount to $80,000 or more, the patient would owe around $42,000. This patient will have difficulty paying such a bill. In this case, the patient would have been underinsured for the situation.

Box 2.3
Common Types of Health Insurance Programs

Health insurance programs fall under several main categories:

- **Health Maintenance Organization:** A cost-containment program featuring a primary care physician as the gatekeeper to eliminate unnecessary testing and procedures. This is a capitated system that requires the insured person to remain within the network.
- **Preferred Provider Organization:** In this type of plan, a group of health-care providers contract with a health insurance company to provide services to a specific group of patients on a discounted basis.
- **Point-of-Service Plan:** This plan is similar to a Health Maintenance Organization in that a primary care physician still serves as a gatekeeper, but it is not capitated. Insured people can seek care from health-care providers who are both in and out of the network. The patient pays a part of the bill (usually 20%–30%), and the insurance company pays the remainder.

Health Insurance Plans for Specific Populations

Some health insurance plans are designed to serve only a specific group of people. TRICARE is an insurance plan for active and retired military service members and their families, and CHAMPVA provides free health benefits for veterans of military service. Workers' Compensation insurance provides for people who are injured on the job. It pays for medical costs and some living costs while the person is unable to work. Disability insurance is designed specifically for those who cannot work because of some type of temporary or permanent disability.

Charitable Organizations

There are also local, state, and national charitable organizations that provide free health-care services to individuals. These organizations may be funded by religious denominations, private individuals, or national or community organizations such as the Catholic and Jewish health systems, Shriners, the Kaiser family, and the Robert Wood Johnson Foundation, just to name a few.

Self-Pay (Uninsured Patients)

Although it has been the goal of the ACA that all people in the United States will have health insurance, there are still some who do not have it and must pay for their health care on their own. They may prefer to pay the nominal fine compared with the cost of health insurance, or they may be unable to afford the least expensive insurance on the exchange. Many health-care providers will offer discounts to those who must pay for their own care, and most will require a payment plan to pay a fixed amount monthly on the bill.

Some physicians are opting for a self-pay option called *concierge medicine.* The patient pays a yearly fee, often $2,000 or $3,000, to have full access to their physician. In return for that fee, the physician is available by phone 24 hours per day, 7 days per week. The patient is seen quickly when the need arises. The patient also pays a visit fee to the physician, which varies according to what is done and may be covered by insurance. This type of care often can prevent the need for hospitalization by allowing early intervention in an acute illness or complication of a chronic illness.

KNOWLEDGE CONNECTION

What are the differences between Medicare and Medicaid? List three types of private health insurance. What populations are covered by TRICARE and CHAMPVA?

POST CONFERENCE

During your post conference with your clinical group, a discussion about your patient's situation ensues. She wants and needs to be at home, yet she also needs IV antibiotics and dressing changes. Although everyone understands her desire to go home right away to care for her young grandchildren, it is hard to understand why she doesn't want to stay in the hospital for the needed treatment so that she can get well completely. You explain that you have no idea how to help her with this situation, but that you are learning a great deal from the RN in charge of her care. He has brought in the hospital social worker to help the patient apply for state help. He has also talked to her doctor about arranging for home health care to do the dressing changes, IV antibiotics, and assessments. The physician has agreed, and the RN has scheduled everything. The patient will therefore be discharged today, and the home health nurse will see her this evening.

Key Points

- The ACA was designed to eliminate many problems in the current health-care system. It does away with lifetime limits and the denial of coverage based on pre-existing conditions. It allows young people to stay on their parents' policy until age 26 and provides some preventative care without cost to the consumer.
- One of the most positive outcomes of health-care workers collaborating with one another is improved patient safety. Team STEPPS is a program that uses evidence-based teamwork to improve communication and teamwork skills, which will, in turn, help to improve quality care and patient safety. When we work alone and do not collaborate well with other health-care team members, we increase the risk of preventable errors.
- The two most important factors in determining payment for health-care delivery are medical necessity and appropriate level of care.
- The health-care team is made up of a number of professionals and assistants, including medical, nursing, therapeutic, laboratory, radiology, and ancillary staff. It is impossible to provide thorough health care without the help of everyone on the team.
- A variety of inpatient and outpatient settings exist to provide health care. It is important for patients to obtain needed care in the most appropriate setting to deliver cost-effective health care.
- Nursing care is delivered in a variety of ways. Some commonly used delivery systems are team nursing, client-centered care, primary care nursing, and case management.
- Health care is costly, and the costs may be paid in numerous ways. These include public and private health insurance, insurance for special populations, charitable organizations, and self-pay.
- Public health insurance is funded by the federal government, the state government, or a combination of both. It includes Medicare, Medicaid, and the IHS.
- Private health insurance companies, also known as third-party payers, include HMOs, PPOs, POS plans, and variations of these services.
- HMOs pay PCPs by a capitation system. The PCP is the gatekeeper for referrals to other health-care professionals such as specialists and therapists.

- PPOs and POS plans rely on previously negotiated discount agreements between the insurance companies and the health-care providers, including specialists.
- Many situations exist that prevent Americans from being able to afford health-care insurance, and this is of great concern to those both inside and outside the health-care system.

Review Questions

Select the answer that is most appropriate for each of the following questions. Some questions may have more than one correct answer. Select all that apply.

1. Which of the following would NOT be considered medically necessary by an insurance company?
   1. Surgery to remove an infected gallbladder
   2. Breast implants to increase breast size
   3. Breast implants after breast cancer surgery
   4. Botox injections to decrease facial wrinkles
   5. Skin grafts to repair a spider bite injury

2. If an elderly person needed help with meals, medications, and personal care but did not need continuous nursing care, which inpatient setting would be the most appropriate level of care?
   1. A skilled nursing facility
   2. A long-term acute care hospital
   3. An assisted living facility
   4. A long-term care facility

3. Which member of the therapy staff would be consulted if a patient had difficulty swallowing?
   1. Speech therapist
   2. Physical therapist
   3. Occupational therapist
   4. Respiratory therapist

4. A cost-efficient way to provide care to people who are confined to their homes because of illness or disability is the use of:
   1. the hospital outpatient department.
   2. a skilled nursing facility.
   3. the health department.
   4. home health care.

5. A patient who is terminally ill with cancer is no longer being treated with radiation or *chemotherapy* (cancer-attacking medication). The most appropriate level of care for this patient would be:
   1. home health care.
   2. hospice.
   3. a skilled nursing facility.
   4. a long-term care acute hospital.

6. You are working on a large medical unit with 30 patients who require medications, therapies, dressing changes, and pain management. Nursing staff for the day shift consists of two RNs, three LPNs, and three CNAs. Which type of nursing care delivery would you expect to work best on this unit?
   1. Team nursing
   2. Client-centered care
   3. Primary care nursing
   4. Case management

7. Payment to hospitals for the care of Medicare patients is based on:
   1. a specified amount per member per month.
   2. the actual costs of all supplies, equipment, tests, and nursing care.
   3. DRGs.
   4. a previously negotiated discount rate.

8. Eligibility for the HIS is:
   1. based on having a CDIB.
   2. available to all people with at least 25% Indian blood.
   3. set by each tribe.
   4. determined by presenting a family genealogy.
   5. determined by blood type.

ANSWERS 1. 2, 4, 2. 4, 3. 1, 4. 4, 5. 2, 6. 1, 7. 3, 8. 1, 3

Critical Thinking Exercises

Answers available online.

1. If a patient with HMO coverage wants to see a specialist for a skin condition, what must the patient do *first*?
2. How would you respond to the following statement made by a fellow nursing student? "With the Affordable Care Act, there is no reason now for people not to have health insurance."

Additional Resources

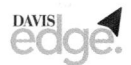

Use the scratch off code on the inside front cover of your book to access online quizzes that will help you to improve your scores on course exams and prepare for the NCLEX-PN®.

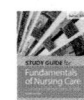

Study Guide

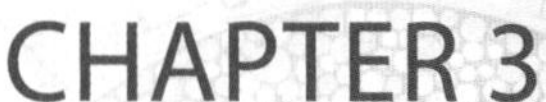

CHAPTER 3
Ethics, Law, and Delegation in Nursing

Donna Walls

KEY TERMS

Abandonment (a-BAN-don-ment)
Advance directive (ad-VANS dur-EK-tiv)
Advocate (AD-vuh-kut)
Assault (a-SOLT)
Battery (BAT-uh-ree)
Centers for Disease Control and Prevention (SEN-tuhrs for di-ZEEZ kon-TROHL and prih-VEN-shun)
Emancipated minor (ih-MAN-sih-PAY-ted MYE-nor)
Empathy (EM-path-ee)
Ethics (ETH-iks)
Good Samaritan Law (GOOD sa-MAR-ih-tuhn LAW)
Health Insurance Portability and Accountability Act (HELLTH in-SHOR-ents POR-ta-BIL-ih-tee and a-KOWN-ta-BIL-ih-tee AKT)
Incident report (IN-sih-dent rih-PORT)
Informed consent (in-FORMD kon-SENT)
Malpractice (mal-PRAK-tiss)
Negligence (NEG-lih-jenss)
Precedent (PREH-seh-dent)
Standard of care (STAN-derd uv KARE)
Value (VAL-yoo)

CHAPTER CONCEPTS

Professionalism
Ethics
Legal

LEARNING OUTCOMES

1. Define various terms associated with nursing ethics and law.
2. Discuss the need to identify your own values and ethics in order to provide ethical care for patients.
3. Identify ways to provide ethical nursing care.
4. Explain what it means to advocate for the patient and why it is important.
5. Describe types of laws that affect nurses and their practice.
6. Explain how the following statutory laws affect nurses: the Health Insurance Portability and Accountability Act, the Health Information Technology for Economic and Clinical Health Act, nurse practice acts, and licensing laws.
7. Identify two situations that must be reported under the mandatory reporting statutory law.
8. Describe five areas of civil law (torts) that affect nurses.
9. Discuss four legal documents and the licensed practical/vocational nurse's responsibilities regarding each of them.
10. Explain the five rights of delegation and how they apply to licensed practical/vocational nurses.
11. Describe the professional responsibilities of nurses and nursing students.
12. Discuss information found in the Connection features in this chapter.
13. Identify specific safety information.

CRITICAL THINKING CONNECTION

Clinical Assignment

You are assigned to care for an 86-year-old patient who had a massive stroke 2 weeks ago. He is totally unresponsive and has been since the stroke occurred. His family must decide whether to put in a feeding tube. The family does not have an advance directive or durable power of attorney but says their father had spoken of his wishes in the past.

Critical Thinking Questions:

1. What are your own feelings about the ethical aspects of this situation?
2. How will you support the family in whatever they decide?
3. What are the two valid sides of this ethical dilemma?
4. How might an ethics committee in the hospital be helpful regarding this situation?

The goal of your nursing care should be to improve the quality of the patient's living and dying. As you strive to determine how to best accomplish this goal, there are many laws and regulatory guidelines that will help you determine what you can, cannot, should, and should not do. In this chapter, we will discuss not only ethical guidelines, but laws that govern your nursing practice, as well as your responsibilities in delegation and receiving delegation from others.

In addition to legal and regulatory boundaries, the codes of professional ethics and personal ethics will help guide you in your nursing practice. *Professional ethics* are published formal statements indicating a profession's expectations for its members. The National Association of Licensed Practical Nurses code of ethics for licensed practical nurses (LPNs) can be found at http://nalpn.org/wp-content/uploads/2016/02/NALPN-Practice-Standards.pdf.

One principle that can provide overall guidance during your career is the following: ***Safety: Never do anything that you know is not in the patient's best interest.*** This requires you to evaluate your own moral and ethical codes. But such self-evaluation does not happen overnight. It requires inquiry, thought, analysis, and time to identify the moral and ethical codes that dictate who you are and how you relate to others. We encourage you to initiate this process now as you begin your nursing education.

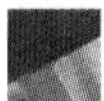

ETHICAL ISSUES IN NURSING

As a nurse, you will face many ethical dilemmas regarding honesty; organ transplantation issues; informed consent; child and elder abuse; surrogacy issues; honoring advance directives; and other life-and-death decisions such as abortion, assisted suicide, euthanasia, do-not-attempt-resuscitation (DNAR) orders, and the withdrawal of artificial nutrition or ventilators. The more technology provides for artificial ways to preserve life, the more situations may arise that require ethical decisions. In this chapter, we will focus on how to provide ethical care for patients, how to advocate for patients, and how to respond when orders or decisions are made to no longer support life or to refrain from resuscitation if breathing or a heartbeat stops. In addition, we will discuss examples of how to report unethical behavior by others.

Identifying Your Own Values and Ethics

Before you can comfortably make decisions in your nursing practice, you must determine your own values and ethics. A **value** is related to your belief of something's worth and may differ from the values of others around you. Your values are learned from your life experiences and determine who you are. Your **ethics** are made up of the values that influence your decisions and behavior. They are partially determined by what you believe is morally right and wrong as well as other principles, including the following:

- The patient's welfare is our primary concern.
- Individuals have the right to make choices, even when those choices may not be in their best interest.

An *ethical dilemma* is a situation in which a decision must be made between two opposing alternatives when there is not an exact right or wrong answer. Ethical decisions are not made with one's emotions or feelings but are based on principles and logical reasoning. As you prepare to enter nursing, a profession rich with ethical dilemmas, you will need to examine your feelings about life, death, health, disease, spirituality, and religion.

Also reflect on each of your patients' expectations. For example, patients will expect to be provided the highest quality medical care conceivable in a safe environment. They will expect their treatment options to be explained in terms that they can understand. Patients will want to be included in the decision making regarding their own care. It is our responsibility to strive to deliver care reflective of the care we would personally desire for ourselves and our loved ones.

Providing Ethical Patient Care

Patients have the right to be treated with respect, dignity, honesty, and compassion. In addition, the nurse is the patient's advocate. To **advocate** for a patient means to stand up for that which is in the patient's best interest, as opposed to that which is in the best interest of the health-care provider, hospital, or staff.

- Treat patients with respect, including honoring the patient's feelings, beliefs, opinions, and decisions whether or not you agree with them.
- Maintain a patient's dignity by allowing and honoring the patient's self-respect.
- Treat a patient with dignity, which may mean allowing the patient to refuse an aspect of care that he or she does not want, such as a particular medication or procedure.
- Care for patients with honesty, being completely truthful about the patient's condition, test results, treatment options, and potential for recovery. Honesty also means acknowledging when you make a mistake and reporting any type of illegal, incompetent, or impaired medical or nursing practices that you may come across.
- Provide compassion by delivering nursing care with a gentle and caring attitude.

A good rule for ethical patient care is to treat every patient as you would want to be treated yourself or as you would want important people in your life to be treated. This may mean that you have to report inappropriate or unethical behavior of your coworkers if you observe it (Box 3.1).

Advocating for the Patient

It is paramount to remember your number one role: you are to serve as the patient's advocate. In the acute care setting, nurses care for the patient 24 hours a day, 7 days per week. In longer-term care settings, nurses may care for the same patients over a period of months or years. As an advocate for

• **WORD** • **BUILDING** •
advocate: ad – to + vocate – call

Box 3.1

Reporting Unethical Behavior

The authority to which you report unethical behavior differs from state to state, so you must be familiar with your own state laws. Most unethical behaviors are reported to your immediate supervisor and the Board of Nursing.

Examples of unethical behaviors that you should report include the following:

- Impairment of a nurse by alcohol, prescription or illegal drugs, or severe fatigue
- Diverting drugs by taking a patient's medications, such as narcotics, for personal use but charting them as administered to the patient
- Abuse or mistreatment of patients, both known and suspected
- Fraudulent documentation
- Practicing without a license
- Incompetence
- Failure to follow the health-care provider's orders
- Failure to perform a necessary action
- Practice outside the individual's scope of practice

patients, you will stand up for them when they cannot stand up for themselves. You will be sure that they are cared for when they cannot care for themselves. You will do these things without imposing your own values on patients. *You must stand with the patient, you must stand for the patient, and you must stand by the patient, always ensuring that everything is done in the patient's best interest.*

When a patient is admitted to a hospital, he or she is given a copy of the American Hospital Association's brochure, titled "Patient Care Partnership" (PCP). This replaces the "Patient Bill of Rights" used in the past. The PCP discusses the expectations, rights, and responsibilities of the patient during their hospital stay. Each item in the PCP is a way of advocating for the patient and includes such things as a clean and safe environment, protection of privacy, and help with billing and discharge from the hospital.

To be not just a nurse, but a good nurse, you will need to develop empathy for patients and families as well as coworkers. **Empathy** is the awareness of and insight into the feelings, emotions, and behavior of another person and their meaning and significance. It is different from *sympathy,* which is usually not objective and involves such a strong feeling of closeness that something that affects one affects the other (Taber's 23e).

KNOWLEDGE CONNECTION

Explain what it means to serve as the patient's advocate. Discuss the importance of advocating for the patient.

Do-Not-Attempt-Resuscitation Orders

Another area that is ethically difficult in some situations is the order not to resuscitate a patient if he or she stops breathing or the patient's heart stops beating. According to the law, you must initiate cardiopulmonary resuscitation unless there is a written order not do so, called a DNAR order.

In certain situations, such as when a patient is in the terminal stages of a disease and is not expected to live much longer, the health-care provider may write a DNAR order in the patient's chart. This order may be the result of a living will or a verbal request made by the patient to the physician. If the patient is unable to request it, the family may ask the health-care provider to write such an order.

When a DNAR order is in the health record, you, as the nurse, will provide comfort and care to the patient just as you would any patient. If the patient stops breathing or the heartbeat ceases, you will remain with the patient and quietly be present during the dying process. You will also provide emotional support to the family during this time.

Ethics Committees

To help make decisions that are difficult and may present ethical dilemmas involving patients and their care, most hospitals have an ethics committee to provide assistance. The committee members may serve the hospital by developing its policies and procedures for handling ethical issues such as DNARs and organ transplantation. When there is a decision to be made concerning ending life support or artificial nutrition, it may be reviewed by the ethics committee. The committee generally focuses on the patient and his or her rights. Disagreeing family members may request that the ethics committee be consulted when difficult decisions must be made.

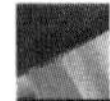

LEGAL ISSUES IN NURSING

The world of nursing that you are entering is not exempt from the increasing frequency of lawsuits, which is reflective of the rest of society. While working as a nurse, you will constantly be responsible for making decisions that can impact the lives of your patients. It is of the utmost importance that you understand the state and federal laws, rules, and regulations that regulate your nursing practice. These laws and ethics define the boundaries in which nurses may work and still be protected.

There are many legal terms that you may hear in your practice as a nurse. Table 3.1 provides a list of commonly used legal terms and their definitions.

One of the most important things you can do is to treat all patients with respect and dignity. It is also very important for you to develop a trusting relationship with each patient. When trust exists, the patient believes that you are doing your best for him or her. When you have this kind of relationship, the patient is less likely to sue you, even if mistakes are made. Be careful to maintain good relationships with your patients and to be proactive regarding their needs.

• WORD • BUILDING •

empathy: em – in + pathy – feeling

sympathy: sym – with + pathy – feeling

Table 3.1
Common Legal Terminology

Term	*Definition*
Abandonment of patient	To desert or forsake a patient in your charge; to leave a patient in your charge without appropriate nursing replacement; wrongful termination of care
Advance directive	A written statement indicating a patient's wishes regarding future medical care in the event the patient becomes unable to voice his or her decisions; it may give consent for certain aspects of care as well as refusal of specific care
Appeal	To challenge the decision of a court to a higher court, where the decision will be either confirmed or reversed
Assault	To purposely threaten physical harm to an individual
Battery	To touch an individual without consent
Civil law	The individual or personal rights guaranteed by federal law, such as the Constitution and the Bill of Rights
Competency	The legal qualification to make one's own decisions
Consent	To give permission for, to agree to; the consent generally must be written
Controlled substances	Drugs regulated by laws; drugs that have potential for abuse, such as narcotics
Criminal law	Laws that protect the public or society
Damages	Money awarded to a plaintiff upon proving injury by the defendant
Defendant	The one accused of breaking criminal or civil law
Durable medical power of attorney	Legal written designation making another person responsible for one's medical decisions
Emancipated minor	Legal consideration of one younger than age 18 years as an adult because he or she lives alone and is self-supporting, has joined the military, is married, or is a parent
Liability	One's responsibility for his or her own actions, such as acts of negligence
Libel	False written statements about another that are made publicly known, with intent to harm
Malpractice	Injury, loss, or damage to a patient because of failure to provide a reasonable standard of care or demonstrate a reasonable level of skill
Negligence	Failure to provide certain care that another person of the same education and locale would generally provide under the same circumstances
Plaintiff	The one accusing another of criminal or civil law violation
Statute	A written law
Tort	A violation of a civil law; involves a wrong against an individual or his or her property

KNOWLEDGE CONNECTION
Why is treating patients with dignity and respect important? Why is trust a key to preventing lawsuits?

Types of Laws

Laws vary according to where they originate (federal, state, or local government) and how they are enforced. In this chapter, we will briefly discuss types of laws and then discuss in more details laws that affect your nursing practice.

- *Constitutional law* is in place to protect our constitutional rights. An example is the U.S. Bill of Rights.
- *Statutory laws* may be federal, state, or local laws and are sometimes called *statutes.* Examples include the *nurse practice acts* (NPAs) that are passed by each state. Statutory laws are discussed in more detail later in this chapter.
- *Case* or *judicial laws* are written in response to specific legal questions brought before the courts. Once the question is decided by the courts, it is used as a **precedent** to judge similar cases in the future.
- *Criminal laws* protect the public or society as a whole. An example of criminal law is a nurse found guilty of murder who intentionally injected a patient with a lethal dose of medication.
- *Civil laws* protect an individual's personal rights, which include most health-care issues.

Statutory Laws Affecting Nurses

As you begin your journey as a nurse, it is important that you recognize that your nursing practice and license are subject to federal laws. Even though you are not yet licensed, as a nursing student you are held to the same standards as a licensed nurse. You are responsible to meet all federal and state requirements while *competently* performing *only* those skills for which you have been trained.

HEALTH INSURANCE PORTABILITY AND ACCOUNTABILITY ACT OF 1996. Better known as the privacy protector, the Health Insurance Portability and Accountability Act (HIPAA) was implemented by regulations of the U.S. Department of Health and Human Services in 1996. It provides for confidential maintenance of protected health information. HIPAA includes the Privacy Rule and the Security Rule.

Privacy Rule. The privacy rule establishes national standards designed to protect the individual's health information. It applies to insurance plans, billing clearinghouses, and electronic transactions in health care. It requires appropriate safeguards to personal health information, including who can and cannot have access to it without the patient's authorization. Examples of such safeguards that affect nurses include the following:

- You may not tell a person making a telephone inquiry that a person is a patient in the hospital unless you have permission to do so.

Box 3.2
Use of Social Media and Confidentiality

The use of social media, such as Facebook, Twitter, YouTube, Instagram, and Snapchat, is a common practice for many people. You must clearly understand the ethical and legal aspects of its use related to nursing and confidentiality. Health-care employers, nursing schools, state Board of Nurses, and the National Council of State Boards of Nursing have policies regarding social media use. It is your responsibility to know these policies and to strictly follow their guidelines. You must not discuss your patients on social media, even if you do not use the patient's name or location. You are responsible for maintaining patient confidentiality at all times and in all situations, not just at your job or in your clinical experiences. ***Safety: You can be required to appear before the Board of Nursing if you use social media in a way that violates your state NPA and rules.***

- You may not give a visitor or family member information about a patient's condition unless you have permission to do so. ***Safety: Always check the patient record to see who is approved to receive health information about the patient.***
- Patient information can only be discussed in areas where privacy is ensured.
- The only health-care providers who have a right to access the patient record are those workers directly involved in the care of that patient.
- Avoid discussing patient information in all public places—both in health-care facilities and other public places, such as restaurants and stores—such as hallways, cafeterias, vending machine areas, and elevators.
- Keep any notes that you make face down to prevent them from being read by unauthorized persons.
- Shred all report and shift notes before leaving the clinical/work site.

The Privacy Rule also ensures that patients have the right to view and amend their own health record, as well as obtain a copy of the entire medical record on request. This is discussed further in Chapter 5. Patient confidentiality safeguards also apply to social media use (see Box 3.2).

Security Rule. The Security Rule establishes national standards for protecting electronic health records (EHRs). It also protects health information that is created, received, used, and maintained by a covered entity. This rule requires reasonable safeguards to ensure the confidentiality and security of protected health information. The following are examples of safeguards that affect nurses:

- Computers with electronic health records on them cannot be left visible to the public.
- All computers must be password protected. ***Safety: Never share your password with anyone.***

• WORD • BUILDING •
judicial: judicialis – related to judges and law courts
precedent: pre – before + cedent – going

- Change your password often as required by the facility where you work.
- Only those health-care providers who are caring for the patient can access the EHR of that patient.

Safety: As a student, it is your responsibility to closely follow your nursing school's and clinical sites' policies and regulations regarding the confidentiality of patient information.

HEALTH INFORMATION TECHNOLOGY FOR ECONOMIC AND CLINICAL HEALTH ACT. In 2009, a federal statute was enacted known as the Health Information Technology for Economic and Clinical Health (HITECH) Act. This was designed to stimulate the adoption of EHR and its supporting technology as part of the stimulus bill. It established grants for training personnel to support new health information technology. It also established penalties for those health-care providers not using EHR by 2015. The HITECH Act includes a breach notification rule that requires health-care businesses to notify individuals in writing when the individual's private health information is known to have unauthorized access. This could happen if the company's computer system is hacked.

KNOWLEDGE CONNECTION

What may you write about your clinical assigned patient on Facebook? How is the HIPAA Privacy Rule different from the Security Rule? What are the implications of each for nurses? What is the purpose of the breach notification rule?

Laboratory and Diagnostic Connection

Confidentiality of Test Results

All test results must be treated with confidentiality. You cannot discuss any kind of test results with family members or partners of the patient, even if the results could affect them. For example, if a patient tests positive for sexually transmitted diseases, including HIV and AIDS, the health-care professional cannot share that information without the patient's permission to do so. Discussing such results without obtaining the patient's permission is a violation of HIPAA.

Real-World Connection

How Easy Is It to Accidently Breach HIPAA Laws?

A licensed nurse was finishing up a long and difficult shift. The weather was icy, and the forecast was for even more ice. As the nurse was giving a report to the oncoming shift, her husband called her on her cell phone. Due to the weather, cell connections had been difficult to maintain. She asked her husband to hold and laid down her cell phone, then continued to give the rest of her report. She was later called in by the facility's privacy officer and disciplined for violating HIPAA and patient confidentiality.

As you can see, you can violate confidentiality without intending to do so. A breach of confidentiality such as this could easily have resulted in a civil lawsuit, monetary fine, and termination from employment. A written disciplinary action was placed in the nurse's personnel file. Luckily, there were no lawsuits or fines, and the nurse was not fired from her job...this time.

NURSE PRACTICE ACTS. Each state has in place an NPA that defines the scope of nursing within its state. States differ in the groups of people who are governed by their NPA. For example, California has two separate practice acts, one for registered nurses (RNs) and one for licensed vocational nurses (LVNs), which are the same as LPNs in other states except for Texas, which also has LVNs instead of LPNs. Oklahoma's NPA covers LPNs, RNs, advanced-practice RNs, and authorized unlicensed assistive personnel (UAP). Ohio's NPA includes RNs, LPNs, dialysis technicians, certified medication assistants, and community health workers.

Boards of Nursing. In each state, the state agency designated to administer and enforce the NPA is the Board of Nursing. This board has the authority to:

- License nurses
- Take disciplinary measures against nurses who fail to follow the NPA
- Regulate the practice of nursing as well as nursing education

The primary purpose of NPAs is to protect the public's health, safety, and welfare. The scope of practice sets legal boundaries for nursing care. Both nurses and students are expected to stay within these boundaries. Examples of such boundaries include practicing under the supervision of specified licensed professionals. LPNs/LVNs must be supervised by RNs, health-care providers, or dentists. Other boundaries include professional behavior and relationships with patients. (See the list of unprofessional conduct examples in Chapter 1.) If a student does not follow these boundaries while in school, the student may not be allowed to take the National Council Licensure Examination (NCLEX).

In addition, the National Council of State Boards of Nursing (NCSBN) is a nonprofit organization that is made up of the boards of nursing from all 50 states, the District of Columbia, and 4 U.S. territories. They work together to provide standardization of nursing excellence and protect the public health, safety, and welfare. Student nurses are held to the same legal standards as licensed nurses. Every student nurse and licensed nurse has a moral, ethical, professional, and legal responsibility to follow his or her own state's NPA. To find your state's Board of Nursing contact information, go to https://www.ncsbn.org/index.htm and select your state. To find your state's

NPA, go to https://www.ncsbn.org/npa.htm and scroll to your state. These are the rules you will live by as a student nurse and a licensed nurse.

Licensure

Each state requires nurses, both LPNs/LVNs and RNs, to become licensed in order to practice nursing. To be licensed you will be required to take and pass the NCLEX-PN. RN candidates take the NCLEX-RN.

After successfully completing your nursing education program, you will apply to the National Council of the State Boards of Nursing to take the licensing exam. You will be required to pay a fee when you submit your application.

Once you have passed the NCLEX, you are eligible to apply for licensure in any of the 50 states. Each state has its own procedures to follow for initial licensure application. Under the nursing license compact agreement, 25 states allow nurses to practice in their states if they are licensed in other states without having to be processed and licensed again. This is especially helpful to nurses who may live near the border of one state and work in another state and for traveling nurses. ***Safety: Follow your state's requirements to obtain and keep your nursing license. Never assume that you are safe to practice in another state without confirming it.***

MANDATORY REPORTING LAWS. Most states have laws requiring the reporting of certain situations to the proper authorities, particularly communicable diseases and abuse. Such laws are called statutes and help to protect the public and track outbreaks or occurrences of disease. The **Centers for Disease Control and Prevention** (CDC) is a federal agency that supports health promotion and the prevention of disease. They also help health-care professionals be prepared to respond to outbreaks of diseases and illnesses.

CHILD ABUSE MUST ALSO BE REPORTED. All 50 states require that you report to authorities even suspected child abuse, including physical, sexual, and emotional/verbal abuse, as well as abuse by neglect. In addition, many states require that you report suspected domestic violence or partner abuse. (See Box 3.3 for signs of different types of abuse.) Reports can be made to local law officials or directly to specific state agencies such as Child Protective Services. It is also important to report the abuse of disabled individuals and those older than 60 years regardless of whether it is mandated by statute. (See Chapter 32 for a discussion of elder abuse.) Most states also have statutes that mandate reporting to the police situations such as gunshot or stab wounds, rapes, and sexual assaults.

KNOWLEDGE CONNECTION

List two categories of individuals for whom you must report suspected abuse. Identify four types of patient injuries mandated by state statutes to be reported.

Box 3.3

Common Signs of Abuse

Physical Abuse

- Bruises, burns, and fractures that are unexplained or do not match the given explanation
- Long-sleeved clothes worn to cover injuries even on a hot day

Sexual Abuse

- Inappropriate sexual behavior and knowledge for the child's age
- Sexually transmitted diseases and/or pregnancy under the age of 14
- Acting out sexually with other children
- Pain for a child in sitting or walking

Emotional Abuse

- Being withdrawn and fearful
- Depression
- Vague pains, such as stomachaches and headaches, with no medical basis
- Avoiding social situations such as going to school
- Delayed emotional development

Neglect

- Poor hygiene, lack of appropriate clothing, and clothes that do not fit
- Hoarding food and excessive hunger
- Poor attendance records at school
- Unsupervised play or play in an unsafe environment

Domestic Abuse/Partner Abuse

- Unexplained injuries or injuries that do not match the given explanation
- Being fearful and withdrawn
- Trying to make peace with or excuses for partner's behavior
- Being embarrassed or belittled by a partner in front of others
- Being verbally abused and/or controlled by a partner

Sources: Adapted from Mayo Clinic Staff. Signs of Child Abuse. Mayoclinic.org. http://www.mayoclinic.org/diseases-conditions/child-abuse/basics/symptoms/con-20033789. Accessed May 26, 2017; NCADV. Signs of an Abusive Partner. Ncadv.org. http://www.ncadv.org/learn-more/what-is-domestic-violence/abusive-partner-signs. Accessed May 26, 2017; Stanford Medicine. Signs and Symptoms of Abuse/Neglect. Stanford.edu. http://childabuse.stanford.edu/screening/signs.html. Accessed May 17, 2017; Office of Women's Health. Violence Against Women. Womenshealth.gov. https://www.womenshealth.gov/violence-against-women/. Accessed May 26, 2017.

Civil Laws Affecting Nurses

Civil law is applicable when two or more private parties seek resolution to a dispute. The most common area of civil law that affects the nurses is *tort law,* which deals with claims of injury or harm due to someone else's actions. The following five areas of tort law cover most aspects of nursing care.

MALPRACTICE. Malpractice occurs when the nurse's action fails to meet professional standards of care and injures a patient. For example, a nurse incorrectly reads an order to insert a retention catheter on a postoperative patient. Instead of performing an in-and-out catheter, the nurse inserts a urinary retention catheter and does so incorrectly: The balloon is inflated in the urethra instead of the bladder, and it causes permanent damage to the patient's urinary tract. In this situation, the nurse is liable in a court for damages to that patient.

NEGLIGENCE. If a nurse does something that a reasonable prudent person would not do, or fails to do something that a reasonable prudent person would do, it is called **negligence.** An example of negligence is a nurse who does not notice that a patient's vital signs are falling into an unsafe range. The nurse does not report this to the health-care provider, so no corrective action is taken. Eventually the patient becomes comatose due to low blood pressure. The nurse is liable for failure to monitor the patient and failure to communicate the change in the patient's vital signs to the health-care provider.

FALSE IMPRISONMENT. A competent patient has the right to leave a health-care facility even if it may prove harmful to his or her health and even if the health-care provider feels the patient should remain for medical treatment. Intentionally preventing a patient from leaving a facility or restricting his or her movement within the facility is considered false imprisonment.

When a health-care provider believes that a person is a threat to himself or herself or others, the patient can be admitted to a psychiatric facility involuntarily for a limited time, usually 72 hours. This is done with a court order and is not considered false imprisonment.

If a patient who is not under a court order expresses the desire to leave a health-care facility, you are responsible for explaining to the patient why it is important for him or her to remain under the health-care provider's care. If the patient still refuses to stay, he or she will be required to sign the facility's Leaving Against Medical Advice (AMA) form according to the facility's policy (Fig. 3.1). ***Safety: Never attempt to physically prevent the patient from leaving.***

Protective Restraint Devices

In the health-care facility, some other types of false imprisonment could include the use of restraint devices, which might include bed rails, tied sheets, wrist or ankle restraints, and vest or halter restraints. Even medications to make a patient less combative can be considered false imprisonment depending on how they are administered.

Restraint devices can only be used if the patient presents a clear danger to either self or others and other methods of protecting the patient from injury have already been attempted. If other methods fail to provide adequate safety, the health-care provider must be notified, and then he or she will write an order for a protective restraint. You will learn more about the safe use of restraints and restraint alternatives in Chapter 13.

ASSAULT AND BATTERY. To threaten a patient with harm or to show intent to touch him or her without permission is considered **assault**. An example of this is a nurse who threatens a patient by saying, "If you do not start eating better, I will put a tube down your nose and feed you through it."

Intentional and wrongful physical contact without consent that causes injury or offensive touching is termed **battery.** An example of battery would be a nurse that becomes angry and shakes a patient. A less obvious example of battery would be obtaining a blood sample without the patient's consent.

SEXUAL HARASSMENT. Sexual harassment is a form of discrimination that violates the Civil Rights Act of 1964. Sexual harassment has become a real threat to male and female nurses alike. Harassment can be defined as continued unwanted or annoying actions. Sexual harassment is harassment that includes unwelcome sexual advances, comments of a sexual nature, or offensive remarks about a person's sex.

Some examples of types of behaviors that could be considered sexual harassment include the following:

- Touching or rubbing against another person
- Physically standing within another's "personal space"
- Telling or playing jokes on another that are sexual in nature or carry a sexual innuendo
- Engaging in personal conversations regarding reproductive organs or sexual activity that can be overheard by someone who is offended by the context
- Having wandering eyes or facial expressions that make the recipient uncomfortable
- Stalking

This is another situation in which being proactive is superior to just reacting. It is better to prevent situations that may be misconstrued as sexual harassment rather than trying to defend yourself after you have offended someone. Some other areas of potential liability for the nurse may be found in Box 3.4.

KNOWLEDGE CONNECTION

Name five areas of tort law that apply to the nurse. Explain the differences among them.

CIVIL PROTECTION FOR NURSES. Most states have a law called the **Good Samaritan Law** that provides legal protection to the voluntary caregiver at sites of accidents and emergencies. It serves to protect a citizen, nurse, or other health-care provider from legal liability if they choose to stop and render aid to someone in an emergency situation, such as an automobile accident. It does not apply to staff in health-care facilities or to individuals who are employed as emergency response workers.

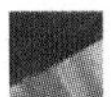

LEGAL DOCUMENTS

The patient's entire medical record is considered a legal document and must be handled accordingly. In addition, some

• **WORD • BUILDING •**
negligence: neglegentia – carelessness

Leaving Before Medical Evaluation – Treatment Completed: ♦ LWBS ♦ Elopement ♦ AMA

Complete applicable section (1 or 2) only

Left Without Notification to Staff (LWBS or ELOPEMENT)

The patient has: ☐ **LWBS** ☐ **Eloped**

No answer when called: 1. Time: ________ Signature: ______________________________

2. Time: ________ Signature: ______________________________

3. Time: ________ Signature: ______________________________

Searched ☐ Emergency Room ☐ Hospital Room ☐ Patient waiting areas ☐ Cafeteria ☐ Parking area

☐ Additional actions taken: ______________________ ☐ MD Notified:(as needed)

X____

Nurse or EDT Signature

LWBS—Left Without Being Seen by a physician or nurse.

Elopement - An ER Patient who leaves after a physician or nurse initiates triage / initial Medical Screening Exam. Or an inpatient or outpatient leaving with out authorization and or notification of their departure.

Leaving Against Medical Advice (AMA) *To be completed by physician or nurse*

☐ **This patient is leaving AMA despite being encouraged to stay for further examination and treatment**

☐ The patient has been advised of the risks of leaving and benefits of remaining at Kingfisher Regional Hospital for further examination and treatment. The risks and benefits include:

☐ Potential threat to life, limb, and/or safety; including death or permanent disability.
☐ Other: (specific to presenting complaint) ______________________________
☐ MD Notified: ______________________ Time:______________________

• Reason(s) for leaving: ____

____

Patient Acknowledgment

You have been advised to stay for further examination and treatment. Please follow up with your provider. Return to an Emergency Department if your symptoms persist or worsen.

I am voluntarily leaving or I am voluntarily taking ______________________ from the facility without a written discharge order from Dr. ______________________. I have been advised of the risk(s) involved, and against the advice and consent of the patient's doctor and / or healthcare providers.

I hereby release the physicians, hospital, and it's employees and agents from all responsibility for any ill effects that may result from my refusal of further medical examination and/or treatment for myself or the person I am taking from the facility.

x______________________________
Physician or Nurse Signature

x______________________________
Patient Signature or authorized representative
☐ *Patient refused to sign*

FIGURE 3.1 Leaving Against Medical Advice form. This form includes a section to be used when the patient leaves without the staff's knowledge. There is also a section for leaving against medical advice. (Courtesy of Kingfisher Regional Hospital, Kingfisher, OK.)

Box 3.4

Common Reasons for Lawsuits Against LPN/LVNs

While LPN/LVNs are sued less frequently than RNs and Nurse Practitioners, it is still a very real possibility. It is important for you to learn your scope of practice and responsibilities as an LPN/LVN to prevent making errors that could lead to lawsuits.

Most Common Reasons

- **Medication-related errors**—this can be administering medications by the wrong route, to the wrong patient, at the wrong time, administering medications that should not have been given, or failure to administer medications at all.
- **Treatment and care-related errors**—this can include failure to provide care, giving incorrect care, misinterpreting order for treatments, or ignoring the need for care.
- **Patient abuse-related errors**—this can include depriving patients of their rights, abusing patients physically, verbally, sexually, or emotionally, or simply ignoring patients' needs.

Less Common Reasons

- **Conduct-related errors**—this could include unprofessional behaviors with patients or patients' families, diversion of patient medications, or inappropriate behavior in the workplace.
- **Assessment-related errors**—this could include failure to do a complete assessment, thereby missing injuries or illness, or failing to report your assessment findings to the health care provider for further treatment and care.
- **Scope of practice-related errors**—this most often is the result of an LPN/LVN acting outside his or her scope of practice and performing tasks that he or she was not educated to perform.
- **Documentation-related errors**—this could include documenting on the wrong chart, documenting opinions rather than facts, and most often, failure to document what occurred and care that was given.

Sources: Nurse Professional Liability Exposures: 2015 Claim Report Update available at www.nso.com/Learning/Artifacts/Claim-Reports/Nurse-Professional-Liability-Exposures-2015-Claim; Gower, T. Top reasons nurses get sued. *OR Management News,* Sept 17, 2018. Available at www.ormanagement.net/Feature/Article/09-18/Top-Reasons-Nurses-Get-Sued/52732

Nurse and Medical Malpractice Case Study with Risk Management Strategies Presented by NSO and CNA, available at www.nso.com/Learning/Artifacts/Legal-Cases/nurse-and-medical-malpractice-case-study-with-risk.

information contained in the record is important legal documents separate from the EHR.

Patient Health Record

A medical record is kept on each patient who enters into any aspect of the health-care system. It provides data about the patient's health status and problems as well as the medical and nursing care provided to that patient. The medical record is also used for communication among health-care providers regarding a specific patient. It serves as a source of information about the patient's condition, test results, care provided, and effectiveness of care, among other things.

The medical record does not belong to the patient but is the property of the hospital or of the physician in a medical office setting. The patient has the right to access it and to request copies of the record as guaranteed by HIPAA. The EHR may not be copied for students to use in their care planning or written assignments. Any data that students obtain must be noted in a way that does not identify the actual patient. ***Safety: Do not write the patient's name and identifying numbers on any of your paperwork that will be taken outside the facility.***

In the United States, government hospitals are even stricter about patient privacy. Any notes that are written while caring for the patient must be shredded before you leave the facility. Most agencies provide a shredder for this purpose.

When you make entries in the patient EHR, keep in mind that it is a legal document and can be used as evidence in a court of law. Make your entries in a timely manner, being accurate and pertinent. Keep all entries objective and factual, without adding your opinions or assumptions. (See Box 3.5 for more information about legal aspects of the patient health record.)

Box 3.5

Legal Aspects of Documentation

The standard accepted in a court of law is "if it's not charted, it wasn't done." Never document something that you did not actually do, do not document anything before it is actually done, and never document anything less than the full truth. To document under any of these circumstances constitutes fraud.

Do not leave medical records visible on any computer screen. Charts and items such as laboratory reports must be secured in a manner that will not be conducive to the public casually glancing over or reading them. All patient information is considered confidential. Failure to handle charts appropriately breaches HIPAA.

KNOWLEDGE CONNECTION

Who may legally access a patient's chart? To whom does the chart belong?

Informed Consent

Informed consent is a voluntary agreement made by a well-advised, mentally competent patient to be treated by a health-care provider or institution. If the patient is a minor or unconscious, a legal representative will sign the consent form. The patient or representative should have a clear understanding of the procedure or process to be performed, along with its accompanying risks and possible outcomes.

It is the responsibility of the person performing the procedure to explain the procedure using terminology that the patient can understand. The health-care provider may delegate obtaining the patient's signature on the consent form to the nurse; however, it is still the legal responsibility of the physician to explain the procedure and risks to the patient and to be sure that the patient understands. The patient must voluntarily give consent without any pressure to do so. If informed

• **WORD • BUILDING •**

delegate: de – down + legate – deputize emancipated: e – out + mancip – slavery + ated – action

consent in not obtained for a procedure or surgery, a charge of assault and battery could be brought in court. ***Safety: Consent forms must never be signed after the patient has received mind-altering medications or has consumed alcohol.***

All persons who sign the consent form must be at least 18 years old and *competent,* both mentally and legally fit. The only legal way for an individual younger than 18 years to sign his or her own consent form is if the individual is an emancipated minor.

The following signatures are required on the informed consent form:

- The health-care provider
- The patient or custodial parent or legal guardian (stepparents cannot sign in most states)
- A witness

Nurses may only sign a consent form as a witness to the patient's signature. Your primary role is to make certain that informed consent has been obtained. If the patient tells you that he or she does not understand what is to be done or changes his or her mind about having a procedure after signing the consent form, it is your duty to inform the health-care provider.

The only time that medical treatment may be provided without written consent is when a life-threatening emergency exists. The law then allows for what is termed *implied consent.* The emergency may also allow parental permission to be given via the telephone, but this must be witnessed by two individuals who heard the permission granted over the phone.

KNOWLEDGE CONNECTION

What are the components of informed consent? Whose responsibility is it to inform the patient of the procedures for which consent is sought and of the risks of those procedures?

Advance Directives

Advance directives are written documents that provide guidelines for making medical decisions in the event a person becomes incapacitated and is unable to make his or her wishes known. All states recognize two types of advance directives: proxy directive, such as power of attorney, and instructional, such as a living will. However, from state to state, there are considerable differences in restrictions, interpretation, and the scope of decision making that may be included.

A proxy directive designates the individual legally responsible for making medical decisions once the person is unable to make decisions. Once a proxy has been appointed, a living will is required for the proxy to know what types of care the person does or does not desire. The proxy will also know when to apply the decisions the patient has made in advance of the incapacitating illness.

Federal law requires hospitals, nursing homes, and home health agencies to ask each patient when admitted if he or she has a living will or other advance directive. This must be documented in the patient's medical record. The patient should provide the facility with a copy of the directive so that it may be scanned into the medical record and used if needed.

Incident Reports

Incident reports may also be known as *unusual occurrence reports* or *variance reports.* They are to be completed in the event of an unusual occurrence or an accident. For example, if a patient falls out of bed or a visitor faints in the hallway, an incident report is filled out. The report should include what happened, who was involved, who witnessed it, and any treatment provided. Most agencies have their own incident report form to use for patient or visitor incidents and one to use if an incident occurs to an employee (Fig. 3.2).

When accidents or unusual occurrences happen to a patient, it is documented in the EHR. All information about the incident is factual and objective, without impressions, assumptions, or conclusions. An incident report is also completed according to agency policy and includes a record of notifying of the supervisor and other appropriate personnel. The existence of an incident report is not mentioned in the patient's medical record. Quality assurance committees or risk management committees review all incident reports to improve quality of care and reduce risk.

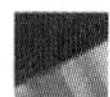

PROFESSIONAL RESPONSIBILITIES

Even as a nursing student, you are responsible for acting in a professional manner. The same will be true when you are a licensed nurse. Some key areas of professional responsibility include being accountable for your actions, securing professional liability insurance, establishing professional boundaries, achieving competence, and following standards of care.

Being Accountable

As a nurse, you are held to a certain level of professional accountability. This means that you are responsible for your own actions. You must take actions to ensure that you are providing safe care for your patients. Such actions include the following:

- Assuring that when you accept a patient assignment or delegation of a task, the assignment or task is within your level of education, training, experience, and ability.
- Refusing to take extra shifts if you are so fatigued that you are not a safe practitioner.
- Staying on the job and caring for patients until someone else can take over their care. This is known in nursing as continuity of care. If you leave or walk away from patient assignments without replacement by another nurse, you are guilty of abandonment. **Abandonment** is defined as the premature cessation of the professional care nurse-patient relationship without adequate notice or the patient's permission.

Even though you are a student nurse, this does not relieve you of accountability. You are expected to know and follow

• **WORD • BUILDING •**
variance: variantia – difference

INCIDENT REPORT EXAMPLE

Incident Date: ____________ Incident Time: ____________ Department: ____________

Injured Person's Name: ____

Injured Person is a:

- ☐ Patient
- ☐ Visitor
- ☐ Employee

Physician's Name if a Patient: ________________________________

Name of Employee Reporting the Incident: ________________________

Details of the Incident:

____

____

Details of the Injury:

____

____

Physician Notified? ____________ New Orders? ____________________

Contributing Factors to the Event:

- ☐ Unsafe environment
- ☐ Failure to follow policies and procedures
- ☐ Incomplete or inaccurate documentation, including MAR
- ☐ Problem with equipment
- ☐ Other (Explain below)

____

____

Signature: ______________________ Date: ________ Department ________

FIGURE 3.2 This Incident Report form can be used for patients, visitors, and employee incidents.

your scope of practice and your school's policies and procedures regarding clinical experiences. In addition, you are accountable for performing only the skills that you have been taught to do. During clinical experiences, you will be expected to report changes in your patient's condition to your instructor or staff nurse immediately.

Even as a student, it is important to know that if you do make an error that harms a patient, you have financial protection for yourself in case of a lawsuit.

Securing Professional Liability Insurance

You will be required to carry professional liability insurance as a nurse and also as a student. While you may have some coverage under a facility's group liability insurance, it is best to know that you have your own coverage in case it is needed.

The cost varies from state to state, but $1 million of coverage can generally be purchased for $200 or less per year.

> ### Supervision/Delegation Connection
> **Responsibility of Patient Advocacy**
>
> Patient advocacy is something that you may NEVER delegate to another individual. It is your primary responsibility to fill this role for your patient.

Establishing Professional Boundaries

It is important to make a distinction between advocacy and becoming personally involved with a patient. When you are in intense situations of life and death and when you care deeply about giving good nursing care, sometimes the situation becomes very emotional. It is important to step back and not allow yourself to become inappropriately involved with your patients or their families. Examples of inappropriate involvement include the following:

- Seeing a patient socially or dating a patient while he or she is still your patient. An example of this is a student nurse who was attracted to a patient she was caring for and went after clinical to hang out with him in his hospital room.
- Any physical or sexual relationship with a patient or the patient's family. An example of this is a nurse who helps code an older male who has had a massive heart attack. The patient's son is very grateful to the nurse and becomes infatuated with her. They are found in a compromising situation in an empty hospital room the next day.
- Taking money or gifts from a patient or handling a patient's finances for them. An example of this is a private duty nurse who takes over paying a patient's bills and the other caregivers who came to the home. The access to the elderly patient's bank account becomes a temptation to the nurse, who embezzles money from the patient.

Delegating Tasks in Nursing

According to the American Nurses' Association and the National Council of State Boards of Nursing, in their Joint Statement on Delegation, delegation is defined as "the process for a nurse to direct another person to perform nursing tasks and activities." This is distinguished from an assignment, because that is the distribution of work that each staff member is responsible for during a given work period.

In delegating, a nurse must determine if the tasks are appropriate for the other person to perform. For the task to be appropriate, the delegatee, who is the person to whom a task is delegated, must have the knowledge and skills to perform the task and it must be within his or her scope of practice. You must know your state's NPA before delegating tasks because different states have different laws.

The National Council of State Boards of Nursing established the five rights of delegation in 1997:

1. The right task: The delegatee can perform the task according to the facility's policies and procedures and has had training to do so.
2. Under the right circumstances: The patient must be stable. If the patient's condition changes, the delegatee must inform the licensed nurse who can then reassess the situation.
3. To the right person: The delegatee has the knowledge and skills to perform the task.
4. With the right directions and communication: Each situation is unique, and the licensed nurse must communicate clear instructions. The delegatee must understand and agree to accept the delegated activity.
5. Under the right supervision and evaluation: The licensed nurse must provide appropriate monitoring, evaluation, intervention as needed, and feedback.

It is important to know that some activities cannot be delegated. Nurses cannot delegate nursing judgment, critical decision making, or care for an unstable patient unless this is within the delegatee's scope of practice in the NPA for that state.

Achieving Competence

Another professional responsibility that you have is to perform all that you have learned in school in a competent manner, which means you are able to perform them successfully and efficiently as a nurse. This comes with practice and experience, which is why your clinical experiences are so important.

You must always know when you need further guidance. The LPN/LVN must know when to solicit advice or assistance from the RN or health-care provider. The RN must know when to solicit guidance or assistance from a supervisor or health-care provider. ***Safety: Do not perform a skill or procedure that you have not been trained to do or that you are not sure should be done. Always ask for help or guidance in such situations.***

Following Standards of Care

If your nursing actions are judged in a court of law, they will be judged according to **standards of care.** These are statements of actions that are consistent with minimum safe professional conduct under specific conditions. You may also hear them called *standards of performance* or *clinical guidelines*. They can be found in nursing textbooks, nursing journals, on the Web sites of nursing accreditation, regulatory agencies and nursing associations, or in facility policy and procedure manuals.

Regardless of where they are found, standards of care represent the level of skill and nursing care that another nurse in the same area of the country, with the same educational level, would perform in the same situation. In court or hearings before the nursing board, your actions are judged by whether or not you followed these standards of care. An example is the *Standards of Practice and Educational Competencies of Graduates of Practical/Vocational Nursing Programs* published by the National Association for Practical Nurse Education and Service, Inc. (NAPNES), which can be found in Box 3.6.

Continuing Your Education

Even when you are a licensed nurse, you are not finished learning. Continuing education helps you maintain, improve, expand, and enhance your nursing knowledge. Because nursing is dynamic or ever-changing, continuing education is necessary to stay abreast of these changes. Many states require a specified number of hours of continuing education each year in order to renew your nursing license. However, even if your state does not have a mandatory continuing education requirement, you will want to take steps to ensure that your skills, training, and knowledge remain current. Between the time you began your education and the day you graduate, there will be many significant discoveries that will affect your practice. The only way to be a good nurse is to continue your education as a nurse.

Box 3.6

NAPNES Standards of Practice and Educational Competencies of Graduates of Practical/Vocational Nursing Programs

Professional Behaviors

Professional behaviors, within the scope of nursing practice for a LPN/LVN, are characterized by adherence to standards of care, accountability for one's own actions and behaviors, and the use of legal and ethical principles in nursing practice. Professionalism includes a commitment to nursing and a concern for others demonstrated by an attitude of caring. Professionalism also involves participation in lifelong self-development activities to enhance and maintain current knowledge and skills for continuing competency in the practice of nursing for the LPN/LVN, as well as individual, group, community, and societal endeavors to improve health care.

Upon completion of the LPN/LVN program, the graduate will display the following program outcome: demonstrate the professional behaviors of accountability and professionalism according to the legal and ethical standards for a competent LPN/LVN.

The following competencies demonstrate that this outcome has been attained:

- Complies with the ethical, legal, and regulatory frameworks of nursing and the scope of practice as outlined in the LPN/LVN NPA of the specific state in which licensed
- Utilizes educational opportunities for lifelong learning and maintenance of competence
- Identifies personal capabilities and considers career mobility options
- Identifies own LPN/LVN strengths and limitations for the purpose of improving nursing performance
- Demonstrates accountability for nursing care provided by self and/or directed to others
- Functions as an advocate for the health-care consumer, maintaining confidentiality as required
- Identifies the impact of economic, political, social, cultural, spiritual, and demographic forces on the role of the LPN/LVN in the delivery of health care
- Serves as a positive role model within health-care settings and the community
- Participates as a member of an LPN/LVN organization

Source: National Association for Practical Nurse Education and Service. *Standards of Practice and Educational Competencies of Graduates of Practical/Vocational Nursing Programs*. Springfield, OH: NAPNES; 2007.

This does not necessarily mean you must go on to earn additional degrees, although we encourage you to continue your formal education. However, it does mean that you must continue to learn and stay current so that you are competent to practice safe nursing. The following are some ways to remain current:

- Subscribing to and reading nursing journals regularly
- Attending educational seminars and workshops
- Attending employer training opportunities and in-service education offerings
- Researching nursing topics and health-related issues in both current textbooks and professional Web sites
- Taking individual courses and workshops online or at a college or university
- Taking continuing education courses in professional journals or online
- Staying up to date with the published Board of Nursing meeting reports
- Joining and participating in your professional organizations

We cannot overemphasize the importance of being a lifelong learner when you are a nurse. There will constantly be new medications, new treatments, new trends and issues, and new evidence-based practice determinations to learn about. You will never be completely finished learning new things. A nurse who does not continue to learn becomes a danger to his or her patients, so it's a benefit both to you and your patients to keep learning.

KNOWLEDGE CONNECTION

What are five things you can do to maintain current knowledge and practice? Why is lifelong learning necessary for nurses?

POST CONFERENCE

After you began caring for the patient described in the Critical Thinking Connection, you were notified that the decision was made to not insert a feeding tube. The family finally agreed that this decision was what their father would have wanted. While it makes you a little sad, you also understand the family's feelings. You can be empathetic to their situation. You find it easy to be supportive of them as they make this difficult decision.

Key Points

- Values and ethics are different but related, and they influence your decision making as a nurse.
- Providing ethical patient care requires you to treat your patients with respect, dignity, honesty, and compassion.
- When you advocate for your patients, you will stand for them, stand by them, stand with them, and always act in their best interest.
- It is important for you, as the patient's advocate, to report unethical behavior that could cause harm to patients.
- Types of laws that affect nurses include constitutional, statutory, case or judicial, criminal, and civil.
- HIPAA requires confidentiality of patient information through the Privacy Rule and the Security Rule. Both protect patients' health information from being seen or accessed by anyone other than those giving care or those given permission by the patient.
- The HITECH act helped move the nation toward EHRs. It also put in place the *breach notification rule.*
- NPAs and licensure laws ensure that the scope of practice for each level of nursing is clearly established in each state. Licensure laws ensure that all nurses pass the appropriate NCLEX exam and follow other requirements in each state.
- Mandatory reporting laws require that nurses report certain communicable diseases to the CDC and suspected or actual child abuse to the proper authorities.
- Areas of civil law (torts) that affect nurses include malpractice, negligence, false imprisonment, assault and battery, and sexual harassment. The Good Samaritan Law protects nurses who volunteer to assist in an accident from legal liability.
- The five rights of delegation include the right task, under the right circumstances, to the right person, with the right directions and communication, and under the right supervision and evaluation.
- Legal documents that LPN/LVNs have responsibilities for include the patient's health record, informed consent, advance directives, and incident reports.
- Professional responsibilities of nurses and nursing students include accountability, securing professional liability insurance, following standards of care, establishing professional boundaries, being competent, and continuing your education.

Review Questions

Select the answer that is most appropriate for each of the following questions. Some questions may have more than one correct answer. Select all that apply.

1. You are suspicious that a coworker might be diverting drugs from patients for her own personal use. Which of the following are the least appropriate actions to take?
   1. Accuse her of being a drug addict
   2. Ask your best friend with whom you work what she thinks about it
   3. Report your suspicions to your supervisor
   4. Ignore the situation because it is none of your business
   5. Wait until you can catch her yourself before reporting it

2. Which of the following can be considered restraint devices?
   1. Bed rails
   2. Belts
   3. Tied sheets
   4. Sedatives
   5. Wrist restraints
   6. Vest restraints

3. Who is responsible for serving as the primary advocate for the patient?
   1. The nurse
   2. The health-care provider
   3. The nurse supervisor
   4. The hospital
   5. The laboratory technician

4. Violation(s) of HIPAA include:
   1. failure to comply with mandatory reporting of suspected child abuse.
   2. documenting inaccurate information in your nurse's notes.
   3. discussing the patient's condition in the hospital dining room.
   4. filling out an incident report.
   5. leaving a patient's EHR visible on a computer screen that visitors can see.
   6. a nursing student tells her neighbor about a mutual friend hospitalized for treatment of a sexually transmitted disease.

5. You need to have a patient sign informed consent for a procedure that the doctor has explained. The patient is a 17-year-old female who is married and has a child. Her mother is also in the room. Who should sign the form?
   1. The patient's mother if the patient lives with her
   2. Only the patient's father can sign the form
   3. The patient
   4. Whichever parent is the custodial parent

6. An LPN plans to delegate the task of getting an informed consent form signed to a CNA. Which of the five rights of delegation would be violated by this decision, if any?
   1. Right task
   2. Right circumstances
   3. Right person
   4. Right directions and communication
   5. Right supervision and evaluation

7. An LVN is being sued for malpractice. He testifies that he did turn the patient every 2 hours and did not observe any signs of pressure injuries during the shifts he worked. There is no documentation of this in the patient's medical record. This is an example of:
   1. the NPA being violated.
   2. rules for documentation not being followed.
   3. an advance directive not being followed.
   4. HIPAA laws being violated.

8. A nursing student posted a comment about her clinical experience on Facebook. She did not use the patient's or the nurse's names but described them both in negative terms. This was
   1. acceptable because no names were used.
   2. unacceptable because it can be considered slander.
   3. unacceptable because it violates confidentiality.
   4. acceptable because the location of the patient was not revealed.

ANSWERS 1. 1, 2, 4, 5, 2. 1, 2, 3, 4, 5, 6. 3. 1, 4. 3, 5, 6. 5. 3, 6. 1, 3, 7. 2, 8. 3

Critical Thinking Exercises

Answers available online.

1. Your patient, who has already signed the informed consent for a surgical procedure, indicates to you that he does not understand the risks of the procedure or exactly what will occur during the procedure. What should you do as the patient's advocate?

2. During the night, Jim Jones, a 46-year-old male, was admitted with alcohol intoxication and cirrhosis of the liver. His liver enzyme and bilirubin levels are elevated. He is severely distended and has multiple bruises covering much of his extremities and lower abdomen. The health-care provider has ordered Mr. Jones to have nothing by mouth (NPO) and IV fluids to infuse at 100 mL/hr. Mr. Jones repeatedly asks for breakfast, stating he is going to "starve to death" if not fed. After explaining to the patient why he is NPO, Mr. Jones tells you to get his clothes for him and that he is going home. What are your responsibilities as his nurse?

Additional Resources

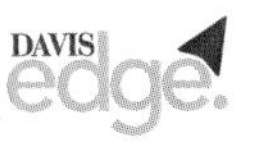

Use the scratch off code on the inside front cover of your book to access online quizzes that will help you to improve your scores on course exams and prepare for the NCLEX-PN®.

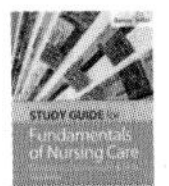

Study Guide

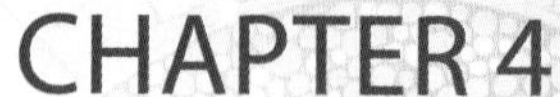

CHAPTER 4
The Nursing Process: Critical Thinking and Decision Making

KEY TERMS

Care plan (KARE PLAN)
Collaborative intervention (ko-LAB-o-ra-tiv IN-ter-VEN-shun)
Critical thinking (KRIT-ih-kuhl THING-king)
Defining characteristic (dih-FYE-ning KAR-ik-ter-RIS-tik)
Dependent intervention (dih-PEN-dent IN-ter-VEN-shun)
Direct patient care (dih-REKT PAY-shent KARE)
Expected outcome (eks-PEK-ted OWT-kum)
Independent intervention (IN-dih-PEN-dent IN-ter-VEN-shun)
Indirect patient care (IN-dih-rekt PAY-shent KARE)
Nursing diagnosis (NER-sing DYE-ag-NOH-siss)
Nursing goal (NER-sing gohl)
Nursing process (NER-sing PRAH-sess)
Objective data (ob-JEK-tiv DAY-tah)
Primary data (PRY-mare-ee DAY-tah)
Rapport (rah-POR)
Secondary data (SEK-un-DARE-ee DAY-tah)
Subjective data (sub-JEK-tiv DAY-tah)
Validate (VAL-ih-DAYT)

CHAPTER CONCEPTS

Patient-Centered Care
Informatics

LEARNING OUTCOMES

1. Define various terms associated with the nursing process and decision making.
2. Discuss ways in which critical thinking is used in nursing.
3. Enumerate the steps of the nursing process.
4. Contrast subjective and objective data.
5. Explain how to conduct a nursing interview.
6. List techniques used to gather data during a physical assessment.
7. Describe how Maslow's hierarchy of human needs is used to prioritize nursing diagnoses.
8. Explain how NANDA-I nursing diagnoses are listed.
9. Compare one-part, two-part, and three-part nursing diagnoses.
10. Differentiate between long-term and short-term goals.
11. Explain how to write correct outcomes statements.
12. Compare types of nursing interventions.
13. Explain the importance of individualized nursing interventions.
14. Enumerate the initial intervention steps.
15. List types of nursing care plans.
16. Explain the process for writing a student care plan.
17. Discuss the use of concept maps to plan care.
18. Discuss information found in the Connection features in this chapter.
19. Explain safety issues related to the nursing process and decision making.

CRITICAL THINKING CONNECTION

Clinical Assignment

You have been assigned to care for a 68-year-old male patient with congestive heart failure, diabetes, and emphysema. He has had two significant heart attacks (myocardial infarctions) in the past 6 years. You are also assigned to write your first student plan of care concerning this patient. You are supposed to arrive for your first day of clinical with a list of probable and possible nursing diagnoses and appropriate nursing interventions and a patient goal for each.

CRITICAL THINKING CONNECTION—cont'd

Critical Thinking Questions:

1. Where will you find this information?
2. How can your instructor expect you to figure out nursing diagnoses before you even see the patient or talk with him?
3. How does knowing the patient's medical diagnoses help you determine possible nursing diagnoses?

It can feel confusing to be asked to come prepared to care for a patient whom you know nothing about, yet every day nurses care for patients who are newly admitted to their units. The nurse knows nothing about the patient, other than perhaps a working medical diagnosis, yet he or she must find out the pertinent information about the patient and develop an appropriate plan of care in an hour or less. In this chapter, you will learn about the steps of the **nursing process,** a decision making framework used by all nurses to determine the needs of their patients and to decide how to care for them. You will learn how to obtain pertinent information from various sources so that you make correct decisions about your patients' care. You also will learn how to organize the information in a care plan that other nurses can follow so that patient care is both consistent and appropriate during their hospital stay. A **care plan** is a documented plan for giving patient care and includes the health-care provider's orders, nursing diagnoses, and nursing orders.

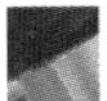

DECISION MAKING IN NURSING

How do nurses know what to do for patients, particularly patients with multiple problems who are very ill? Do they just perform the orders left by the physicians, nurse practitioners, and physician assistants? How do they know when or if it is necessary to call the health-care provider?

Critical Thinking Skills

One way nurses make such decisions is by the use of critical thinking. Many definitions exist for this term, but to keep it simple and clear, **critical thinking** is using skillful reasoning and logical thought to determine the merits of a belief or action. To think critically, you must think about *how* you think so that you can improve your ability to make sound decisions about patients and their care.

Nurses who use critical thinking avoid jumping to conclusions about patients or patient care. They also avoid making decisions based on assumptions. They **validate,** or ensure the correctness of, the information they obtain. It is sometimes tempting to simply "do what you are told" or to "just follow orders" rather than to think critically about your nursing practice. However, you must learn to think purposefully, using reasoning and logical thought, to determine whether your actions are appropriate for the optimal care of your patient. The following example depicts a nurse who uses critical thinking when caring for patients.

> *A nurse receives an order from the health-care provider for an antibiotic to be administered IV to a patient who has developed pneumonia. The nurse remembers that the patient has an allergy to another medication in the same family of antibiotics and validates that memory by checking the patient's allergies in the chart. The nurse further validates the information by asking the patient to relate again the name of the medication and the type of reaction that occurred in a previous hospitalization, ensuring that it is entered in the chart. The nurse then notifies the health-care provider of the potential for the patient to have a reaction to the ordered antibiotic.*

This thinking nurse is not working on "automatic pilot" and simply carrying out the health-care provider's orders. The nurse has prioritized the patient's health and well-being and has prevented a potentially severe medication reaction.

You will use critical thinking skills many, many times during a shift when you work as a nurse. Your job now is to learn to think in a way that perhaps is different than you are accustomed to and to practice that thinking at every opportunity. In addition to learning to think critically, you must learn to make nursing decisions using a framework for decision making known as the *nursing process*.

Real-World Connection

Critical Thinking in Patient Care

An elderly woman was admitted to the hospital due to shortness of breath. Eventually she required mechanical ventilation because she could not breathe well on her own. A tracheostomy was performed to prevent problems of a long-term ventilator run. After some time and treatment, she was weaned from the ventilator. The weaning process was rocky, however, because she kept experiencing severe respiratory distress after a few hours of breathing on her own and would have to go back on the ventilator.

This continued for over a week. Some of the nurses thought that she was just anxious, and others felt that she had simply become dependent on the ventilator and would never be able to breathe on her own for more than a short time.

One of her nurses and her respiratory therapist decided to think critically about this case. They shared the observation that shortly after receiving the breathing treatment with medication to open her airways, the patient would experience distress every time and have to go back on the ventilator. One of them wondered aloud, "Could she be allergic to the medication, causing it to have the opposite effect?"

It was not easy, but the nurse approached the pulmonologist about discontinuing the medication in the breathing treatments. He was quite skeptical but eventually agreed. The patient stopped relapsing ... until the medication was reordered a week and a half later. The pulmonologist again discontinued the medication, and the patient's chart was marked with a red allergy tag.

If these two staff members had not been willing to think outside the box and think critically, this patient would have remained on the ventilator when it was not necessary.

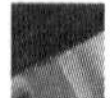

THE NURSING PROCESS

As early as the 1950s, nurses were attempting to define and explain their function. They are not simply the handmaidens of physicians or task-oriented assistants who are unable to think critically. Nurses see the whole patient and all of the patient's problems and needs, and they work to meet those needs. One way nursing function can be defined is by the use of the five steps of the nursing process: assessment, diagnosis, planning, implementation, and evaluation.

Steps of the Nursing Process

Remember that the nursing process is a framework for decision making. By following these five steps, nurses determine actions to take and the effectiveness of those actions. An easy way to remember the first letter of each step is to use the mnemonic ADPIE:

- ***A*ssessment** is the gathering of information through signs and symptoms, patient history, and both subjective and objective findings. Just as a health-care provider gathers information by performing a physical examination and a patient history, the nurse gathers information about the patient through asking questions (interviewing), performing a head-to-toe assessment, and reviewing laboratory and diagnostic tests.
- ***D*iagnosis** is the formulation of nursing diagnoses through an analysis of the assessment information that you have gathered. **Nursing diagnoses** are related to the needs or problems a patient is experiencing. These are completely different from medical diagnoses and are selected based on definitions and defining characteristics.
- ***P*lanning** is the process of determining priorities and what nursing actions should be performed to help resolve or manage each patient problem. In addition, the nurse determines expected outcomes for the patient to meet for the nursing diagnosis to be resolved, as well as a realistic time frame for that to occur. The nurse then decides on appropriate interventions to resolve each patient problem or nursing diagnosis.
- ***I*mplementation** is the process of taking actions to resolve the patient's problems (i.e., the nursing diagnoses). These actions are also called *interventions.* When the nurse performs these interventions, it is called *implementation.* The nurse implements the plan to help resolve the patient's problems.
- ***E*valuation** is performed when the nurse reflects on the interventions he or she has performed and decides if they have brought the patient closer to achieving the goals and outcomes set in the planning step. If not, the nurse then revises and changes the interventions and perhaps the goals to better fit the needs of the patient.

Although it looks like this process is performed in a step-by-step sequence, flexibility in the order of the steps is often necessary to best meet the patient's needs. The steps may overlap, and the nurse may move among the steps as he or she makes decisions about patient care. Figure 4.1 presents an example of the overlapping aspects of the nursing process. Box 4.1 looks at the steps of the nursing process from a non-nursing perspective.

Roles of Registered Nurses and Licensed Practical/Vocational Nurses in the Nursing Process

According to the American Nurses Association (ANA) Standards of Practice for registered nurses (RNs), all the steps of the nursing process, from assessment through evaluation, are the responsibility of the RN. This includes outcome identification in addition to planning. The National Federation of Licensed Practical Nurses (NFLPN) Nursing Practice Standards for the licensed practical/vocational nurse (LPN/LVN) identify assessment and nursing diagnosis as the responsibilities of the RN, while the LPN/LVN participates directly in the remaining steps of planning, intervention, and evaluation. This does not mean that the LPN/LVN cannot perform assessment skills, but it does mean that the findings of the LPN/LVN are shared with and sometimes confirmed by the RN. The same is true of formulating a nursing diagnosis. The LPN/LVN contributes greatly to the development of the nursing diagnosis. All data and information gathered by all nurses are considered when the nursing diagnoses are identified and prioritized.

All members of the health-care team contribute to providing quality patient care for patients (Fig. 4.2). No one, from the housekeeping staff to the director of nursing, is less valuable than anyone else when it comes to providing care for patients.

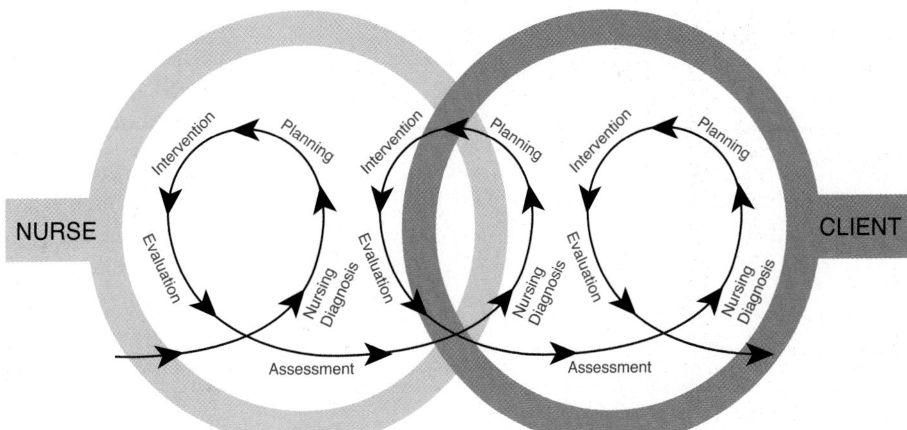

FIGURE 4.1 The interconnected steps of the nursing process and how the nurse continuously uses this decision making process (from Doenges M, Moorhouse MF. *Application of Nursing Process and Nursing Diagnosis*. 6th ed. Philadelphia, PA: FA Davis; 2013).

Box 4.1

The Nursing Process From a Nonnursing Perspective

As you look at the steps of the nursing process, you may realize that you use a similar method for making many decisions in your life. You gather information, analyze the information, develop a plan, execute the plan, and then decide how well it worked. Based on your evaluation, you may modify or change your plan. This way of making decisions is not really new to you, but using it to make nursing decisions may feel different.

Let's look at a nonnursing example of this decision making process: You are at a family gathering when you hear your son, Charlie, crying in the backyard. You can tell that he is hurt, so you rush out to see what has happened.

Assessment

You see Charlie standing next to the slide with blood coming from his left knee. As you look closer, you see a "goose egg" forming above his left eye, and you notice that his lower lip is swollen and bleeding. You ask your niece, "What happened?" She tells you that as Charlie was going down the slide, he flew over the side and hit his head and face on the pole of the swing set. You ask Charlie, "How did you fall off of the slide?" He replies through his tears that his tennis shoe caught against the side of the slide, stopping him and causing him to fall over the side. Then you notice that he is holding onto his left wrist, so you ask him if it hurts. He nods, still crying, and says that it hurts a whole lot.

All of the above is the assessment phase of the nursing process. You gather information by asking questions, observe Charlie's injuries, and ask about additional injuries that you might not be able to see at first glance.

Diagnosis

You begin the diagnosis portion of the nursing process when, after assessment, you begin to analyze the information you have gathered and determine the problems that Charlie is experiencing. In this case, you wonder if his wrist could be fractured. You must decide if you need to take him to the urgent care center for x-rays.

Planning

Now you have to decide what you will do to resolve the problems. This is the planning phase. Can you clean and bandage all the injuries yourself, or do you need to take him to the doctor or hospital? You know that you need to clean his knee and lip so they do not get infected. You also think that you had better check his teeth to be sure that he has not broken or loosened a permanent tooth. You plan to put some ice on the goose egg to keep it from getting any bigger.

Implementation

Next, you put your plan into action. You gently wash his knee and lip. You inspect his lower teeth for damage, but find none. You apply antibiotic ointment to his knee and cover it with a bandage to keep out dirt that could cause infection. You make an ice pack and place it on the goose egg over his left eye to help prevent further swelling.

While doing that, you check his eye for bruising or damage, but it seems uninjured. You notice that Charlie is not moving his left wrist during the time you are working on him. He keeps it close to his body with his elbow bent. You ask Charlie if he can move his hand without pain. He replies that it feels better not to move it. When you look closer, you can see a lump just above his wrist. Now you decide that you need to take him to the urgent care center for x-rays and help him into the car.

Evaluation

After performing your care (the planned interventions), you think that all of Charlie's problems are resolved. Now it is time to re-evaluate because you have now gathered more information about Charlie's wrist injury. The additional information helps you determine that Charlie needs to see a health-care provider for further testing.

After his wrist is x-rayed, the health-care provider determines that Charlie has fractured his wrist, and she applies a cast. She also checks his other injuries, validating your findings that nothing else is serious. You have taken the right steps to get Charlie the help he needs, and now he will heal with time.

As you can see, you make similar decisions all the time. The nursing process is simply a way to help you make good, sound nursing decisions while caring for patients.

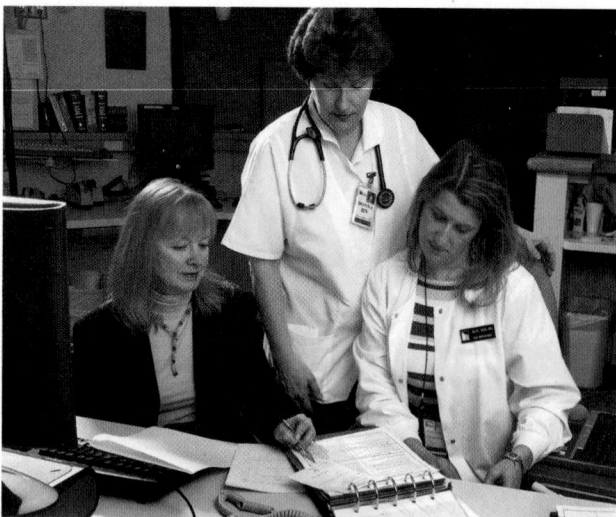

FIGURE 4.2 These nursing team members are collaborating on the care plan for a patient (from Williams LS, Hopper PD. *Understanding Medical-Surgical Nursing*. 5th ed. Philadelphia, PA: FA Davis; 2015).

Supervision/Delegation Connection

Collaboration, Not Delegation, in Care Planning

You cannot delegate nursing decisions or care planning. Those activities are strictly the role of the licensed nurse. However, it is absolutely necessary that all members of the health-care team share observations and information about patients so that the best possible care can be provided. Everyone must work together in collaboration to develop a thorough care plan.

KNOWLEDGE CONNECTION

What is the difference between the role of the RN and the role of the LPN/LVN in the nursing process? What does ADPIE stand for?

Performing the Steps of the Nursing Process

Although you now may realize that you use decision making processes in your daily life and that you also use critical thinking to decide what is important even in nonnursing settings, you may be confused about how to actually use the nursing process to make nursing decisions.

We will discuss each step in detail so that you can see how you, as a nursing student now and as a licensed nurse later, will gather information to determine patient needs, then decide what actions to take to meet those needs, and finally evaluate the effectiveness of each action.

Assessment

As discussed earlier, there are three components to the assessment of patients when gathering information about their problems and needs:

- Interviewing, which involves asking questions, listening, and using both verbal and nonverbal communication skills
- Performing a focused body system assessment to determine deviations from normal in the patient's physical condition (Chapter 21 gives you a complete guide to performing a physical assessment)
- Reviewing the results of laboratory and diagnostic tests to determine problems and needs caused by abnormal findings

SUBJECTIVE AND OBJECTIVE FINDINGS. When you gather information regarding a patient, your data will fall into one of two categories: objective or subjective. **Objective data** are those things that you can observe through your senses of hearing, sight, smell, and touch. Examples of objective data include "pale, cool, moist skin" and "dark brown, formed bowel movement." Box 4.2 shows how senses are used to gather objective data. Information that is known only to the patient and family members is **subjective data.** Although some clues to these symptoms may be observable, only the patient knows exactly what he or she is feeling. Examples of subjective data include nausea, pain, anxiety, fear, depression, and discouragement. It is very important that you report and document objective data. If you are relaying subjective data, they must be attributed to the patient; for example, you would say that *the patient* states that she has a headache. The objective data that support this might include the fact that she is pale and holding her head in her hands. More information about documenting and reporting subjective and objective data can be found in Chapter 5.

Notice that objective data provide a description of what you see, hear, smell, and touch, but they do not involve drawing conclusions or inferences. If a patient is crying, your objective data are that the patient's eyes are red and that she is wiping away tears. If you draw a conclusion or an inference, you might assume that the patient is sad, depressed, or discouraged. However, you must validate your assumptions before acting on them. The patient may be crying because she or he feels happiness or relief about the results of a diagnostic test.

INTERVIEWING. When you enter a patient's room or area to perform a nursing interview, it is important to first establish **rapport,** creating a relationship of mutual trust and understanding. You can do this by introducing yourself and explaining your role in the patient's care. For example, you would say, "I am John Smith and I will be your nurse until 7 p.m." To avoid asking the patient the same questions he or she has already answered, review all the available information about the patient first. Then you can ask the patient to validate that information. Another way to establish rapport is to tell the patient the purpose of the interview and the approximate length of time it will take. Sometimes nurses take a few moments to ask some general questions and make small talk before beginning the interview, allowing the patient to relax with them.

Box 4.2

Use of Senses to Obtain Objective Data

Objective data are limited to that which you can detect with your five senses. Because we no longer need to rely on our sense of taste, we only document that which we can see, hear, smell, or feel.

Use of Vision

- Make direct observations of the patient's physical characteristics, facial expressions, actions, or behavior.
- Make direct observations of the characteristics of eliminated bodily fluids, such as blood, urine, emesis, feces, or drainage.
- Read results of laboratory, x-ray, or diagnostic reports.
- Read reports and documentation within the patient's current or past medical records.
- Read results and detect the function of equipment, such as sphygmomanometer, thermometer, pulse oximeter, various monitors, oxygen or suction flowmeters, or fingerstick blood sugar equipment.
- Observe the measured volume of urine or drainage in a graduated container, the volume of fluid remaining in the IV bag, and/or the amount of liquid drunk from a cup with graduated markings.
- Read textbooks, medical journals, and multimedia devices used to research medical diagnoses and treatments.

Use of Hearing

- Note patient-made sounds heard with the naked ear, such as belching, passing flatus, crying, moaning, snoring, spoken words of the patient or family, and laughter.
- Note sounds heard during auscultation.

Use of Smell

- Detect patient body- or bodily fluid–related odors, such as foul, fetid, sweet, fruity, acidic, ammonia-like, sulfurous, fresh, or musty.

Use of Touch

- Assess pulse rate.
- Palpate for edema, firmness or softness, nodules, papules, taut skin, masses, or mushy tissue.
- Detect the temperature of the patient's skin.
- Detect the moisture of the patient's skin.
- Detect the texture of skin, hair, or nails.
- Measure the strength of muscular contractions.

For example, the nurse might ask if the woman with the patient is his wife and then ask if they have children. Another nurse might comment about the weather or ask whether the patient is from the immediate area or an outlying one.

Once rapport is starting to be established, you will begin the nursing interview. While you begin your interactions with patients based on an admitting medical diagnosis, you are gathering evidence about patient problems that will be the foundation of your nursing care. The medical diagnosis is the disease or illness diagnosed by the physician. For example, the patient may be admitted with a diagnosis of appendicitis, pneumonia, or thrombophlebitis, all of which describe physical conditions. Nurses are concerned with how medical diagnoses affect patients' abilities to care for themselves and their families, as well as how the diagnoses affect the patients' lives.

During the interview, you will often obtain information from more than one source. When the patient provides information, it is considered **primary data.** When you obtain information from family members, friends, and the patient's chart, it is considered **secondary data.**

When interviewing your patients, avoid simply asking questions on a form and obtaining minimal answers. Rather, listen carefully to the answers and ask for additional information as it is appropriate. This requires you to think of and ask questions that may not appear on your nursing interview form. In many situations, patients do not volunteer important information simply because they do not realize it is important. If this happens, you may find out valuable facts that are crucial to providing appropriate nursing care much later than you needed to know about them. When questioned at that time, the patient will tell you, "No one asked me about that before."

Most facilities use an admission form that requires a nursing history to be performed as well as a head-to-toe assessment. Figure 4.3 shows an example of a hospital admission form. Such a form cues you to questioning the patient and completing a full assessment. However, it is appropriate to ask for additional information that is not specifically on the form if you identify other problems as you talk with the patient. For example, if the admission form asks about previous hospitalizations and the patient responds by listing two recent surgeries, it is appropriate to ask, "What about when you were a child, or a young adult? Were you ever hospitalized then?"

In addition to asking for further information, be alert to how the patient responds to questions. Notice the words the patient uses or if he or she hesitates before answering. Box 4.3 lists ways to respond to different nuances of patient responses in order to obtain the most complete information from the patient.

Sometimes patients want to give more detail than is necessary for you to obtain pertinent information. For example, a patient may spend a great deal of time describing what was happening before he fell and injured his back. You must listen carefully to extract what is important, but if the interview is taking an extended amount of time, it is appropriate to find a polite way to redirect the patient to the subject at hand. Some ways to do this include saying,

- "Can you tell me more about the pain you have been experiencing?"

CODE NA - NOT APPLICABLE UTA - UNABLE TO ACQUIRE 0 - OTHER (SPECIFY IN NOTES)

COGNITIVE - PERCEPTUAL PATTERN

MENTAL STATUS ☐ ALERT ☐ RECEPTIVE APHASIA ☐ UNRESPONSIVE ☐ COMBATIVE

☐ POOR HISTORIAN ☐ ORIENTED – ☐ PERSON ☐ PLACE ☐ TIME ☐ CONFUSED – ☐ TOTAL ☐ INTERMITTENT ☐ NIGHTTIME

CHANGE IN MEMORY ☐ NO ☐ YES SPECIFY ______

HEARING ☐ WNL ☐ IMPAIRED ☐ RIGHT ☐ MILD ☐ MODERATE ☐ SEVERE ☐ PROFOUND

☐ LEFT ☐ MILD ☐ MODERATE ☐ SEVERE ☐ PROFOUND

☐ HEARING AID – ☐ RIGHT ☐ LEFT ☐ TINNITUS

VISION ☐ WNL ☐ CORRECTIVE LENSES ☐ BLIND – ☐ RIGHT ☐ LEFT ☐ CATARACT – ☐ RIGHT ☐ LEFT

☐ BLURRED

☐ DOUBLE ☐ ARTIFICIAL EYE – ☐ RIGHT ☐ LEFT ☐ OTHER ______

☐ GLAUCOMA

SPEECH ☐ WNL ☐ SLURRED ☐ GARBLED ☐ EXPRESSIVE APHASIA ☐ LANGUAGE BARRIER (EXPLAIN)

SPOKEN LANGUAGE ______ INTERPRETER ☐ NO ☐ YES ______ (NAME)

EYES	R	L	PUPILS	R	L
CLEAR	☐	☐	REACTIVE	☐	☐
DRAINING	☐	☐	NONREACTIVE	☐	☐
REDDENED	☐	☐	☐ EQUAL ☐ UNEQUAL		
OTHER ______	☐	☐			

(CIRCLE NUMBER)

RIGHT SIZE (mm) 1 2 3 4 5 6 7 8

LEFT SIZE (mm) 1 2 3 4 5 6 7 8

MOUTH

GUMS/MUCOUS MEMBRANES ☐ WNL ☐ MOIST ☐ DRY ☐ LESIONS ☐ OTHER ______

TEETH ☐ WNL ☐ CAPPED ☐ ORTHODONTIA ☐ DENTURES ☐ EDENTULOUS ☐ OTHER ______

RESPIRATORY ☐ WNL ☐ SHALLOW ☐ RAPID ☐ LABORED ☐ OTHER

COUGH ☐ NO ☐ YES ☐ DRY ☐ MOIST ☐ PRODUCTIVE (DESCRIBE):

AUSCULTATION COMMENTS

LEFT LUNG ☐ CL ☐ ABNORMAL ______

RIGHT LUNG ☐ CL ☐ ABNORMAL ______

CIRCULATORY

APICAL HEART RATE ☐ REG. ☐ IRREG. ☐ PACEMAKER

NUMBNESS ☐ NO ☐ YES WHERE ______

SYNCOPE ☐ NO ☐ YES WHEN ______

ANEMIA ☐ NO ☐ YES ______

EDEMA ☐ NO ☐ YES WHERE ______

PAIN / ANGINA ☐ NO ☐ YES WHERE ______

LEG CRAMPS ☐ NO ☐ YES WHEN ______

H / A ☐ NO ☐ YES WHERE ______

COMMENTS:

ABDOMEN ☐ SOFT ☐ FIRM ☐ FLAT ☐ DISTENDED

BOWEL SOUNDS ☐ PRESENT ☐ ABSENT

COMMENTS:

SKIN EXTREMITIES COLOR ☐ WNL ☐ PALE ☐ CYANOTIC ☐ GRAY ☐ JAUNDICED ☐ FLUSHED

TEMP. ☐ WARM ☐ COOL MOISTURE ☐ DRY ☐ DIAPHORETIC

TURGOR ☐ WNL ☐ POOR AMPUTATION (SPECIFY)

INTEGRITY ☐ INTACT ☐ NO SPECIFY AND LOCATE ON DIAGRAM ON RIGHT

LESIONS ☐ NO ☐ YES ______

BRUISES ☐ NO ☐ YES ______

REDDENED ☐ NO ☐ YES ______

PRURITIS ☐ NO ☐ YES ______

EDEMA ☐ NO ☐ YES ______

OTHER ☐ NO ☐ YES ______

RIGHT PEDAL PULSE ☐ STRONG ☐ WEAK ☐ NON-PALPABLE

LEFT PEDAL PULSE ☐ STRONG ☐ WEAK ☐ NON-PALPABLE

RN SIGNATURE ______ DATE ______ TIME ______

FIGURE 4.3 Sample assessment portion of an admission form: Parts 1 and 2. (Courtesy of Kingfisher Regional Hospital, Kingfisher, OK.)

DISCOMFORT/PAIN ☐ NONE ☐ ACUTE ☐ CHRONIC

DESCRIPTION/LOCATION ______

RATING CODE CIRCLE ONE NUMBER ➧ 0 1 2 3 4 5 6 7 8 9 10

NONE MINIMAL ——→ MODERATE ——→ SEVERE

PAIN MANAGEMENT AT HOME:

MUSCULOSKELETAL RANGE OF MOTION ☐ FULL ☐ LIMITED SPECIFY: ______

HAND GRASPS ☐ EQUAL | ☐ LEFT ☐ STRONG ☐ WEAK ☐ PARALYSIS | ☐ RIGHT ☐ STRONG ☐ WEAK ☐ PARALYSIS

LEG MUSCLES ☐ EQUAL | ☐ LEFT ☐ STRONG ☐ WEAK ☐ PARALYSIS | ☐ RIGHT ☐ STRONG ☐ WEAK ☐ PARALYSIS

BALANCE AND GAIT ☐ STEADY ☐ UNSTEADY ☐ BEDFAST

☐ CONTRACTURES

COMMENTS:

NUTRITION TYPE OF DIET: ______

APPETITE: ☐ GOOD ☐ FAIR ☐ POOR AVERAGE FLUID INTAKE: ______

TYPICAL DAILY FOOD INTAKE: NUMBER OF MEALS: ______ SUPPLEMENTS ______ AMOUNT OF WEIGHT LOSS/GAIN: ______

NAUSEA / VOMITING ☐ NO ☐ YES HEARTBURN ☐ NO ☐ YES

DYSPHAGIA ☐ NO ☐ YES ☐ SOLIDS ☐ LIQUIDS ABD. PAIN / CRAMPING ☐ NO ☐ YES

COMMENTS:

ELIMINATION BOWEL PROBLEM: ☐ NO ☐ YES DATE OF LAST BM: ______ LAXATIVE / DIETARY CONTROL: ☐ NO ☐ YES

DIARRHEA: ☐ NO ☐ YES CONSTIPATION: ☐ NO ☐ YES BOWEL INCONTINENCE: ☐ NO ☐ YES

URINARY FREQUENCY: ☐ NO ☐ YES URINARY PAIN, BURNING, HESITANCY: ☐ NO ☐ YES URINARY RETENTION: ☐ NO ☐ YES

CATHETER / OSTOMY: ☐ NO ☐ YES LAST CHANGED ______ URINARY INCONTINENCE: ☐ NO ☐ YES

COMMENTS:

REPRODUCTIVE ☐ N/A DATE OF LAST MENSTRUAL PERIOD: ______ LAST PAP SMEAR: ______ MENOPAUSE: ☐ NO ☐ YES

BREAST: SELF EXAM ☐ NO ☐ YES ☐ NA MENSES: ☐ NO ☐ YES ______

PROSTATE PROBLEMS: ☐ NO ☐ YES ☐ NA ______

COMMENTS:

ACTIVITY/EXERCISE PATTERN

1. MOBILITY STATUS: ☐ AMBULATORY ☐ AMBULATORY WITH ASSIST ☐ BEDREST ☐ TRANSFER WITH ASSISTANCE
2. ASSISTIVE DEVICES: ☐ NONE ☐ CANE ☐ WHEELCHAIR ☐ WALKER ☐ CRUTCHES ☐ PROSTHESIS

☐ NO PROBLEM ☐ CONTRACTURES ☐ JOINT STIFFNESS ☐ MUSCLE STIFFNESS ☐ FRACTURES ☐ PARALYSIS ☐ ARTHRITIS

☐ PROSTHESIS ☐ PAIN ☐ WEAKNESS ☐ OTHER

COMMENTS: ______

COPING - STRESS TOLERANCE/SELF-PERCEPTION/SELF-CONCEPT PATTERN

DO YOU OR YOUR FAMILY HAVE ANY CONCERNS ABOUT YOUR HOSPITALIZATION OR ILLNESS?

☐ NO ☐ YES COMMENTS:

DO YOU FEEL: ☐ CALM ☐ ANXIOUS ☐ FEARFUL ☐ HOPELESS ☐ POWERLESS ☐ OTHER

COMMENTS:

HAVE YOU HAD A MAJOR LOSS OR CHANGE IN YOUR LIFE IN THE PAST YEAR? ☐ NO ☐ YES

COMMENTS:

SUPPORT PERSON(S): ☐ MOTHER ☐ FATHER ☐ SISTER ☐ BROTHER ☐ GUARDIAN ☐ OTHER

NAME(S):

SAFETY EVALUATION: SCORE 1 FOR EACH CRITERIA MARKED

☐ CONFUSION/DISORIENTATION ☐ BOWEL/BLADDER INCONTINENCE/NOCTURIA | ☐ MINIMAL RISK FALL PRECAUTIONS - 1 OR 2 SELECTED

☐ HX OF FALLS ☐ VERTIGO | ☐ HIGH RISK FALL PRECAUTIONS - 3 OR MORE SELECTED

☐ REQUIRES ASSIST TO AMBULATE

ADDITIONAL COMMENTS ______

RN SIGNATURE ______ DATE ______ TIME ______

KRH DISK #3

FIGURE 4.3—cont'd

Box 4.3

Responses to Nuances in Patient Interviews

During the patient interview, a patient may respond to your questioning in a number of ways. The patient may be open, honest, and talkative or quiet, evasive, and vague. It is up to you to get the appropriate responses from your patient. Below are some possible tips to utilize when interviewing a patient.

Patient Response: Patient hesitates before answering a question.

Nurse's Response: Give the patient time because he or she may be thinking through an answer. If the patient continues to hesitate, you may need to reword the question.

Patient Response: Patient responds with a vague answer, using phrases such as "not exactly," "sort of," "maybe," or "you could call it that" in reply.

Nurse's Response: Ask the patient to provide more detail or to be more specific. Ask the patient to be precise and accurate so that you can get a clear picture of what it is he or she is describing.

Patient Response: Patient looks away or acts uncomfortable when you ask a question.

Nurse's Response: Apologize if the question seems intrusive and explain that the information is necessary for you to completely comprehend how the illness is affecting his or her life and relationships.

- "Now, let's get back to what happened after you fell."
- "After that happened, what did you do to relieve the pain?"

You will use many techniques for interviewing and extracting pertinent information from your patients. Chapter 6 explains how to use open-ended questions when talking with patients. It includes phrases to avoid because they can shut down communication.

PHYSICAL ASSESSMENT. Physicians, physician's assistants, and nurse practitioners often perform extremely in-depth physical assessments to detect signs and symptoms that contribute to formulating medical diagnoses. Nurses in the acute care setting, both RNs and LPNs/LVNs, perform thorough physical assessments to collect additional data used in formulating nursing diagnoses according to facility policy and the state Nurse Practice Act (NPA).

In general, the RN is responsible for performing a complete assessment when the patient is admitted to a nursing unit in the hospital. The RN will establish the nursing diagnoses and goals for a patient during their hospital stay. However, in many settings, the LPN/LVN may do all or part of the assessment, which is then confirmed by the RN. ***Safety: Always follow facility policy and practice within the scope established by your state's NPA.*** Nurses gather data about how the patient's body is functioning using the following techniques:

- *Inspection,* which is the visual examination of the patient's body for rashes; breaks in the skin; and normal appearance of the eyes, ears, nose, mouth, limbs, and genitals
- *Palpation,* which is touching or feeling the torso and limbs for pulses, abnormal lumps, temperature, moisture, and vibrations
- *Auscultation,* or listening for abnormal sounds in the lungs, heart, or bowels
- *Percussion,* or using tapping movements to detect abnormalities of the internal organs

Physical assessment usually is performed in a head-to-toe pattern to avoid omitting any important data. Many hospital admission forms include a head-to-toe assessment guide for the nurse to follow. However, you are responsible for obtaining thorough data whether or not it is found on an assessment form. Performing a physical assessment is discussed in detail in Chapter 21.

Laboratory and Diagnostic Connection

How Laboratory and Diagnostic Results Affect Patient Care

Sometimes nurses think that analyzing laboratory and diagnostic test results is strictly in the realm of the health-care provider. Although the health-care provider will review the results of laboratory and diagnostic tests, it is important for nurses to examine them as well. As you learn more about abnormal results of such tests, you will understand how they affect a patient's nursing care. For example, if you have a patient whose white blood cell count is very low, you know he or she is at high risk for developing an infection because white blood cells are responsible for fighting invading pathogens. That information is important when you think about how to care for your patient and how to protect him or her from potential infections.

Nursing Diagnosis

The formulation of **nursing diagnoses** is a uniquely nursing function. Physicians, physician assistants, and nurse practitioners all focus on medical diagnoses based on signs, symptoms, laboratory findings, and test results, but nurses focus on the needs of patients. As discussed in the previous section, a medical diagnosis is a label for a disease, illness, or injury, such as coronary artery disease, pneumonia, or hematoma. A nursing diagnosis, however, is a label or statement for a problem that a patient is experiencing as a result of his or her medical diagnoses. This type of diagnosis is treated by the nurse using interventions to improve the patient's ability to function as normally as possible.

PRIORITIZING DIAGNOSES. Nursing diagnoses address physical, psychosocial, and environmental needs of patients, with some of them being a higher priority than others. For example, the nursing diagnosis "Ineffective airway clearance" would be considered a higher nursing priority than "Chronic low self-esteem." Both diagnoses are important, but the first is critical to the patient's ability to breathe. How do nurses decide which diagnoses are the most important?

Maslow's Hierarchy of Human Needs. One helpful tool for determining priority is Maslow's hierarchy of human needs. This pyramid identifies human needs in an ascending order of importance. The first level is composed of physiological needs, those things a human being needs to survive. The next level addresses safety and security needs, those things a human being needs to remain alive and protected. The third level includes the need for love and belonging, such as meaningful relationships. The next level is the need for self-esteem and feelings of self-worth. This is followed by the level that addresses cognitive needs for learning and exploring. The sixth level is composed of aesthetic needs for beauty and order. The seventh level addresses the need for self-actualization, which is the need for reaching one's own growth potential, and the highest level is that of transcendence, or the need to help others reach their highest potential. Figure 4.4 shows Maslow's hierarchy of human needs depicted as ascending steps.

According to Abraham Maslow, who was an American psychologist, humans must meet their physiological needs first, before needs on higher steps can be addressed. For example, a homeless person is focused on finding food and shelter in a safe area and would not be interested in joining a self-help group until his or her basic needs have been met. Nurses, therefore, must address the physiological needs of survival first with their patients and then the needs related to relationship issues in the love and belonging tier.

An example of this in the hospital setting is a patient who has recently undergone an abdominal surgery that is causing him or her to be in pain and to not sleep well. This patient would not be ready or able to learn how to perform a dressing change on his or her abdominal wound until the basic physiological needs of pain relief and rest have been met.

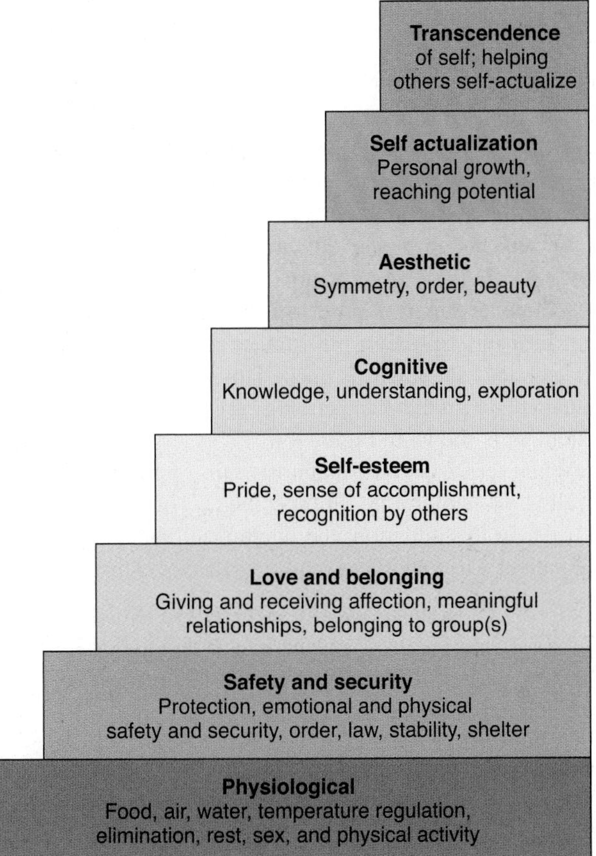

FIGURE 4.4 Maslow's hierarchy of human needs moves upward from survival needs to transcendence (from Wilkinson JM, Treas LS. *Fundamentals of Nursing: Theory, Concepts & Applications*. Vol. 1. 3rd ed. Philadelphia, PA: FA Davis; 2016. Adapted from Maslow A. *The Farther Reaches of Human Nature*. New York, NY: Viking Press; 1971; and Maslow A, Lowery R, eds. *Toward a Psychology of Being*. 3rd ed. New York, NY: Wiley & Sons; 1998).

Patient Teaching Connection

Meeting Patient Needs First

It is important to remember what you have learned about Maslow's hierarchy when you prepare to teach patients. If a patient is uncomfortable, is in pain, needs to go to the bathroom, is too cold or hot, feels nauseated or hungry, or is feverish, these things are barriers to learning and need to be alleviated and/or removed before teaching should occur. You need to be alert to cues that the patient is not ready or able to learn because of lower level needs that have not been met. Do your best to determine what the problem is, take care of the physiological and safety needs first, and then begin your patient teaching.

SELECTING NURSING DIAGNOSES. Although formulation of nursing diagnoses is identified by the ANA and NALPN as an RN function, all nurses, both LPN/LVNs and RNs, collaborate and contribute to the development of the care plan. NANDA-I, which stands for North American Nursing Diagnosis Association International, is responsible for creating and maintaining an approved list of nursing diagnoses to be used throughout most countries, including the United States and Canada. By establishing and revising this list, nursing diagnoses are standardized for use by nurses everywhere and lend themselves more easily to computerized documentation than individually developed diagnoses.

NANDA-I Lists. Most lists are written to make the diagnoses easy to find. The main topic is listed first, followed by modifiers such as "risk for," "readiness for enhanced," "acute," "chronic," "family," "impaired," "disturbed," and "deficient." Nursing diagnoses on care plans are written as they would logically be read, not the way it appears on the list. For example, on the list, one nursing diagnosis reads "Infection, risk for." This makes it easy to find within the list when infection

• WORD • BUILDING •

taxonomic: taxo – arrangement + nomic – relating to distribution

is a potential problem. However, on the care plan, it would appear in the logical form of "risk for infection."

The NANDA-I diagnosis list, titled Taxonomy II, is published every 2 years. The nursing diagnoses are updated based on evidence-based practice. Lists should be available for 2018 to 2020 and 2021 to 2023. They are divided into 13 domains for organizational purposes.

DETERMINING NURSING DIAGNOSES. All data collected in the assessment step of the nursing process are analyzed to determine the correct nursing diagnoses by the RN. It is not simply a matter of choosing a diagnostic label from the list. Rather, the RN must understand the definition of the nursing diagnosis as well as the **defining characteristics,** or signs and symptoms, exhibited by the patient. The following example will help you understand the selection of a nursing diagnosis:

> *A male patient has been admitted with the medical diagnosis of pneumonia. The nursing assessment reveals that he is short of breath at rest, has a weak cough, and is unable to bring up mucus that can be heard in his lungs and throat. He complains of chest discomfort and has a temperature of 101.8°F (38.8°C), pulse of 112 beats per minute (bpm), respirations at 22 per minute, and blood pressure of 128/84 mm Hg. His pulse oximetry reading is 94% at rest. When the nurse listens to his lungs, she hears crackles and wheezes. The patient breathes easiest when he is sitting upright in bed. He is very weak and is unable to get out of bed without assistance. When he attempts to walk to the bathroom, he becomes short of breath and his pulse increases to 128. His laboratory test results show normal oxygen levels in the blood when he is resting.*

Several nursing diagnoses, particularly some related to breathing, ventilation, and gas exchange, look like they might apply to this patient. So how does the RN determine which is appropriate? The nurse must use the definition of the diagnosis and the defining characteristics found in the nursing diagnoses manuals that are derived from the NANDA-I approved lists of approved nursing diagnoses. In this situation, the nurse narrows the possible diagnoses about the patient's respiratory problems down to two possibilities: "Impaired gas exchange" or "Ineffective airway clearance."

The RN rules out "Impaired gas exchange" because that diagnosis is used when the patient's oxygen level is low or the carbon dioxide level is high. Although this may be the case in a patient with a similar diagnosis, from the information the nurse has collected, the patient's oxygen level is now within normal limits. When the nurse looks at the definition and defining characteristics for "Ineffective airway clearance," the patient's symptoms match several of the defining characteristics as well as the definition. This diagnosis fits because it is used when the patient is unable to cough mucus up and out of the airway to keep the airway clear. Looking further, this patient matches several of the defining characteristics for this diagnosis, including crackles and wheezes in the lungs, needing to sit upright to breathe easily, and the inability to bring up mucus from his throat and airways.

As the RN continues to review the assessment data, other clusters of data become evident, such as the patient's weakness and inability to tolerate getting out of bed. The nurse chooses the nursing diagnosis "Activity intolerance." The nurse confirms that the patient fits this diagnosis because of his weakness and inability to ambulate to the bathroom due to shortness of breath and an increased pulse rate.

WRITING NURSING DIAGNOSES. Up to this point, we have discussed only one part of the nursing diagnosis: the first part, also referred to as the diagnostic label or diagnostic concept. This is the portion of the nursing diagnosis that is identified through definitions and defining characteristics, and it is the core of the diagnosis.

A complete nursing diagnosis may be a one-part, two-part, or three-part statement. The three-part statements are often called PES statements. This stands for problem, etiology, and signs and symptoms:

- The *problem* is the diagnostic concept or label based on the patients' needs.
- The *etiology* refers to the causative factor(s) and is connected to the diagnostic label by the words "related to."
- The *signs and symptoms* include the data collected and the evidence used to support the diagnostic label. They are linked to the statement with the words "as evidenced by."

Using the diagnostic concepts selected for our patient in the previous section, the complete three-part nursing diagnosis statements are shown in Figure 4.5.

In some circumstances, all three parts of the statement will not apply. In that case, a two-part statement may be a better fit. When the nursing diagnosis is one that expresses the risk for a problem, a possible problem, or certain actual problems, the two-part statement is used. This is referred to as a PE statement, or problem and etiology only. An example of a PE statement is shown in Figure 4.6.

When the NANDA-I diagnosis falls into the category of "wellness," "syndrome," or "specified," a one-part statement is used. In this situation, the diagnostic label clearly states the patient's need without requiring further elaboration:

- A *wellness* diagnosis usually includes the phrase, "readiness for enhanced ..., " which means that the patient is willing to improve his or her lack of hope, knowledge, coping, or other needs.
- A syndrome is a label for a group of signs and symptoms, so *syndrome* diagnoses already refer to defining characteristics and do not need further elaboration. Examples of syndrome diagnoses include "Post-trauma syndrome," "Rape-trauma syndrome," and "Frail elderly syndrome."

• WORD • BUILDING •

etiology: etio – cause + logy – study of

syndrome: syn – together + drome – run

Ineffective airway clearance	related to	secretions in the airways	as evidenced by	abnormal lung sounds, orthopnea, and dyspnea
Problem		Etiology (cause)		Signs and symptoms (evidence)

Activity intolerance	related to	generalized weakness	as evidenced by	dyspnea on exertion, and elevated heart rate with activity
Problem		Etiology (cause)		Signs and symptoms (evidence)

FIGURE 4.5 Three-part nursing diagnosis statement samples.

- *Specified* diagnoses are those that clearly apply to one defined patient need so that any more description would only be redundant. An example of a specified diagnosis is "Latex allergy response." There is no need to say "related to allergy to latex" because it is the only cause of that response.

Sometimes the available nursing diagnoses do not really fit the situation with a patient. Rather than using a diagnosis that is not completely accurate, the RN may use his or her own words to describe the patient's problem. It is more important to communicate effectively with the nursing staff regarding the patient's problems than to use official NANDA-I language.

Once you have been given the appropriate nursing diagnoses for the patient, you are ready for the next step of the process: planning.

KNOWLEDGE CONNECTION

List three ways to obtain assessment data. How do nurses decide which nursing diagnoses have the highest priority?

Planning

The planning step of the nursing process involves several areas: setting long-term and short-term goals, planning outcomes for each nursing diagnosis, and planning the interventions you will use in the implementation step.

LONG-TERM AND SHORT-TERM GOALS. A **nursing goal** is the overall direction in which one must progress to improve a problem. Long-term goals are not expected to be met before the patient is discharged from the hospital. It may be an ongoing process of improvement or a gradual change in circumstances. Short-term goals are expected to be met by the time of discharge or transfer to another level of care. They may be met in a brief teaching session. Some facilities and schools do not include these broad long- and short-term goals. They use expected outcomes only.

EXPECTED OUTCOMES. While goal statements are general, outcomes are specific. **Expected outcomes** are statements of measurable action for the patient within a specific time frame and in response to nursing interventions. According to the ANA Standards of Practice, expected outcomes are to be developed by the RN. Again, the LPN/LVN contributes information and provides input in the development of expected outcomes.

Just as NANDA-I creates and revises standardized nursing diagnoses, a similar classification and standardization process is underway for nursing expected outcomes. The Nursing Outcomes Classification (NOC), originally developed at the University of Iowa College of Nursing, currently contains a list of 500 nursing expected outcomes designed to coordinate with established NANDA-I diagnoses. For example, an expected outcomes label to go with the nursing diagnosis "Activity intolerance" could be *Endurance* or *Mobility*. Standardization of the terminology of expected outcomes is helpful for computer documentation and electronic medical records.

An expected outcomes statement is often the exact opposite of the problem or diagnostic label. For example, if the nursing diagnosis for a patient is "Self-care deficit related to weakness and pain after surgery," the outcome statement might be *Patient will shower with standby assistance by the second postoperative day.* However, once you are clear on the difference between nursing diagnoses and outcome statements, you will realize that these two components of the nursing process work hand in hand to help deliver only the best in patient care.

Outcomes statements should include the following information:

- **A realistic, specific action to be taken by the patient (not the nurse):** To be specific, the expected outcome must state precisely what is to be accomplished. To be realistic, the expected outcome must be something the patient is capable of doing. For example, *Patient will ambulate 30 feet in the hallway with walker* tells where and with what assistance the patient will perform the activity.
- **An action that the patient is willing and able to perform:** To be an action that the patient is willing and able to perform, the expected outcome must be something the patient wants to do and will cooperate in achieving. For example, the nurse may think that a good action for the patient is to ambulate in the hallway, but if the patient is too short of breath or in pain, he or she will be unable to meet the expected outcome.
- **An action that is measurable:** To be measurable, it is necessary to use verbs that can be evaluated. In the previous example, we can evaluate whether the patient was able to ambulate 30 feet.

Risk for poisoning	related to risk factor of	confusion
Problem		Etiology

FIGURE 4.6 Sample of a PE statement.

- **A definite time frame for the action to have been accomplished:** To include a definite time frame, the expected outcome could be *Patient will ambulate 30 feet in the hallway with walker before discharge from hospital.*

Because expected outcomes are often required before a patient can be discharged from the hospital, they are sometimes referred to as *discharge criteria.* Long-term goals may require follow-up by health-care providers such as physicians, nurse practitioners, physician assistants, home health-care staff, and physical and occupational therapists.

When you are given outcomes and goals, you will also participate in planning the nursing interventions that will be used to improve the patient's health status and meet his or her health-care needs. We will discuss the selection of interventions in the next step of the nursing process, implementation.

Implementation

Nursing actions, or interventions, are sometimes referred to as *nursing orders.* Just as the physician makes a medical diagnosis and writes physician's orders to improve the patient's condition, nurses formulate nursing diagnoses and write nursing orders to resolve the patient's problems. To a beginning nursing student, this may seem totally overwhelming. However, learning which nursing actions to take and the reasons behind each action will help you become a better nurse. Just as every skill prepares you to give needed care to patients, understanding how nursing diagnoses work helps you know when such care is indicated. You will become so familiar with nursing actions that when you hear a nursing diagnosis, you will automatically begin thinking of nursing interventions for it.

In the same University of Iowa College of Nursing project that is standardizing and classifying nursing outcomes (NOC), a group is also working to do the same for nursing interventions. The standardized language for nursing interventions is found in the Nursing Interventions Classification (NIC).

TYPES OF NURSING INTERVENTIONS. Nurses must work together, as well as with other health-care professionals, to accomplish established goals and outcomes. Nursing interventions may involve direct or indirect patient care. **Direct patient care** is performed when the nurse interacts directly with the patient. It includes activities such as bathing, teaching, listening, and administering medications. **Indirect patient care** is performed when the nurse provides assistance in a setting other than with the patient. Examples of indirect care include documenting care, participating in care conferences, talking with the health-care provider, and receiving new health-care provider's orders.

Nursing interventions can also be classified as independent, dependent, or collaborative. When nurses determine that interventions are needed, they may be able to provide the intervention without consulting anyone else. These are **independent interventions** because a physician's order is not required to perform them. An example of this type of intervention is when the nurse assesses a patient's urine and notices that it is dark yellow and concentrated and that the amount is lower than normal. The nurse decides to put the patient on intake and output measurement because the patient has a risk for imbalanced fluid volume. This nursing action does not require a physician's order but instead is a nursing order, and it is a way to obtain more data about the patient's possible problems.

Some nursing interventions do require a health-care provider's order before they can be performed; these are referred to as **dependent interventions.** For example, if a patient was complaining of constipation, the nurse would assess the date of the last bowel movement and assess the abdomen. The nurse would use independent interventions to help promote peristalsis, such as increasing fluid intake, encouraging high-fiber foods, and assisting with ambulation, if allowed. The nurse also would administer laxatives or stool softeners as ordered by the physician. If the patient still was unable to have a bowel movement and further orders were needed, the nurse would call the health-care provider to obtain an order to administer an enema to the patient. *Nurses always need an order from a health-care provider for administering or changing a patient's diet, activity level, medications, IV therapy, treatments, diagnostic tests, and discharge.*

Collaborative Nursing Interventions. **Collaborative interventions** are those that involve working with other health-care professionals in the hospital setting, such as therapists, social services workers, and dietitians. An example of this is when the nurse caring for a resident in a long-term care facility learns that hospice has been called in to see the resident. The hospice nurse provides certain types of care to the resident related to his or her terminal diagnosis. The nurse employed by the long-term care facility also provides care to the resident, including medications and treatments. The two nurses work together to provide the best possible care to this terminally ill resident.

Individualized Nursing Interventions. In the world of computer lists and preprinted actions for nursing diagnoses, it is tempting to simply select nursing orders from a list of possible interventions without taking into account what is most appropriate for your particular patient and without considering the patient's likes or needs. However, such "cookie-cutter care" is dangerous because you can miss cues about a patient's unique problems that can lead to adverse effects for the patient, including a life-threatening situation.

Individualized care for patients ensures better nursing care. Your patient is not just a diagnosis or the person in Room 537, but a person with individual responses to being ill and who is in a hospital clinic, hospice, or home care setting. It is important to remember that no two patients are the same. Even though some patients share the same diagnoses, their care should reflect their individual needs. Box 4.4 provides an example of how to provide individualized nursing care.

Sometimes a nursing order is to carry out the health-care provider's order. For example, a patient complains of a moderate headache, which he or she attributes to not sleeping well. The nursing orders include administering a back and neck rub, keeping the patient's room quiet, and dimming the lights. The nurse also administers 400 mg of ibuprofen,

Box 4.4

Providing Individualized Nursing Care

You are caring for a female patient who has a nursing diagnosis of "Deficient fluid volume." The short-term goal is for the patient to increase her oral fluid intake to 1,500 mL/d. What will your nursing interventions be? You want the patient to drink, so you offer her iced tea between meals. However, she says she does not like it. How do you ensure that you and the other nursing staff know what fluids to provide to this patient and how often to do so?

First, ask the patient which fluids she likes. She responds that she likes fruit juices and that she prefers grape juice, orange juice, and lemonade, as well as coffee with cream.

Next, you divide up the 1,500 mL of fluid so that she consumes it throughout the day and not all at once. You determine that the day shift fluid goal is 750 mL, the evening shift fluid goal is 500 mL, and the goal for the night shift is 250 mL.

You now write the following nursing orders:

- Offer 8 ounces of fruit juice every 2 hours, especially grape juice, orange juice, and lemonade.
- Record intake and output every shift to detect improvements in fluid balance.
- Offer coffee with cream with meals and between meals. Inform the dietary department of the patient's dislike for tea.
- Encourage water intake from the bedside water pitcher for additional fluid intake.
- Assess mucous membranes, tongue, and skin turgor every shift to evaluate signs of dehydration.

If you looked at a standard care plan without individualization, it might list nursing interventions such as these:

- Encourage fluid intake.
- Record intake and output.
- Assess for signs and symptoms of dehydration.

You can see the difference in the details of nursing care for this patient. In addition, other nursing staff will know specifically how to improve this patient's fluid status, and no one will bring fluids that the patient does not like to drink. As a bonus, the patient does not have to tell each nursing staff member which fluids she prefers.

which is ordered by the health-care provider for relief of mild to moderate pain. The nursing orders and the medical orders combine to improve the patient's health status. We are all working in collaboration toward the same goal.

INITIAL IMPLEMENTATION STEPS. Nursing students learning to perform interventions soon discover that the initial steps for each intervention are very similar. Before you begin any intervention, you must be sure that you know how to perform it. ***Safety: Never perform any skill or intervention that you have not been taught how to do or you feel unsafe in attempting to perform.*** In some situations, you will have the opportunity to observe a skill being performed before you learn how to do it yourself because you have not yet reached that area of your curriculum. In that case, you must be an observer only; you cannot try to perform a skill or intervention with a staff nurse attempting to "talk you through it." It is dangerous for the patient, and you put yourself in a position of liability in such a situation.

The initial steps of most nursing interventions include the following:

- Checking the health-care provider's order. ***Safety: Always review the order before executing it rather than simply going by what someone tells you is ordered.*** Be sure the order is appropriate for this patient and nothing has changed to contraindicate it.
- Referring to facility procedures unless you already know them.
- Gathering needed equipment and supplies. Check to ensure that a consent form has been signed, if needed.
- Washing your hands. Follow facility policies and CDC guidelines for hand hygiene.
- Obtaining assistance if needed.
- Identifying your patient using two methods of identification according to facility policies. In the hospital, all patients wear armbands for identification purposes. In addition, you ask the patient his or her name and birthdate. You read the armband and ask the patient to state his or her name and birthdate. ***Safety: Always ensure that you are providing ordered care to the correct patient.***
- Introducing yourself to the patient if you have not previously done so. Include your name and title, such as "I'm Jane Johnson, a student nurse."
- Explaining the procedure to the patient, using words the patient understands. Include information about what the patient will do, what he will feel, and what he is expected to do.
- Providing privacy by closing doors and window blinds and, if needed, asking visitors to step out briefly. Wash your hands or use hand sanitizer according to facility policies (see Chapter 14).
- Using standard precautions (see Chapter 14). Use good body mechanics. ***Safety: Raise the bed to a comfortable working height to prevent injury to your back and lower the near side rail.***
- Making any assessments needed to ensure that the patient still requires the procedure and is able to tolerate it.
- Continuing to observe the patient during the procedure to be aware of pain, discomfort, or any other problems.

These initial implementation steps and the following ending implementation steps are also listed inside the back cover of this book for quick reference when you are performing nursing interventions.

ENDING IMPLEMENTATION STEPS. When you complete a procedure, you need to evaluate the patient's response and the effectiveness of the procedure, if applicable. In addition, there are things you must do to restore the patient to a comfortable situation and tidy the room. The ending steps of most nursing interventions include the following:

- Evaluating the patient's response to the procedure
- Ensuring that the patient is safe and comfortable, in proper body alignment, and with clean linens and a call light within reach

- ***Safety: Lower the bed to its lowest height to reduce risk of falls. Raise the bed rails as appropriate and according to facility policies.***
- Performing hand hygiene
- Asking the patient if he or she needs anything and informing him or her when you plan to return
- Leaving the room door open or closed according to the patient's preference
- Documenting your interventions and their effectiveness according to facility policies
- Properly disposing of used supplies, personal protective equipment, and trash, as well as returning equipment to the proper location

As a nurse you will be caring for more than one patient at a time, so you must learn to plan your shift in such a way that you implement all nursing and health-care provider's orders for all of your patients in a timely manner. In addition, you must document all the nursing interventions that you perform. Chapter 5 offers more information about organizing and documenting your nursing care.

During the implementation stage, it can feel like you are running around all day checking tasks off of a list. Sometimes you can lose your focus and forget why you are performing these interventions, and you can forget to add the human touch to the technology. Never lose sight of the individual patients that you care for. Step back to evaluate what is and what is not working and whether goals are being accomplished. This is the next and last step in the nursing process—evaluation.

Evaluation

As you look at your patient's nursing diagnoses and desired outcomes, you will evaluate whether your nursing interventions brought about the desired outcomes. Evaluate the following factors:

- Are the nursing diagnoses correct?
- Have you established realistic, reachable goals?
- Have you determined the correct priorities for your nursing diagnoses?
- Have you selected and implemented the correct interventions?
- Has the patient's condition changed?

Box 4.5 illustrates the process of evaluating nursing care.

KNOWLEDGE CONNECTION

What is the difference between short-term goals and expected outcomes? Give an example of an independent nursing intervention. Give an example of a dependent nursing intervention.

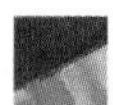

NURSING CARE PLANS

Care plans are documented on various forms, depending on the type of facility and the policies of that facility. In hospitals, a detailed care plan of some type generally is included

Box 4.5

Evaluating Your Nursing Care

You are caring for a patient whose nursing diagnosis is "Activity intolerance related to generalized weakness as evidenced by shortness of breath and increased heart rate when ambulating to the bathroom." The expected outcome is, *Patient will ambulate to the bathroom with minimal assistance by the third hospital day.* Your interventions include gradually increasing activity to increase strength. Your nursing orders are the following:

- Get the patient to sit in a chair for 30 minutes three times per day, increasing the time by 30 minutes each day.
- Encourage protein-rich foods to help promote healing and strength.
- Assist the patient to ambulate from the bed to the chair and back two times before sitting up, starting on the second day.

Now it is time to evaluate this approach. On the third hospital day the patient is stronger but now complains of left calf pain when taking steps. You must go back to the assessment step of the nursing process. When you assess the leg, you find that the calf is warm, red, and swollen. You notify the physician, who orders tests that confirm the presence of thrombophlebitis in the saphenous vein of the left leg. The physician orders bedrest for the patient to prevent a pulmonary embolus.

Now your nursing diagnosis changes to "Impaired physical mobility, level 4, related to impaired leg circulation as evidenced by redness, pain, and swelling of the left calf." Your nursing interventions change to:

- Maintaining bedrest
- Elevating the leg to reduce swelling
- Maintaining moist heat on the leg as ordered by the physician
- Assessing for changes in the leg, such as decreased swelling, decreased redness and warmth, and decreased pain
- Assessing for symptoms of a pulmonary embolus, such as chest pain and dyspnea
- Administering anticoagulants as ordered by the physician

The expected outcome changes to *Restored physical mobility when blood clot has resolved.* As you go through the evaluation process, you realize that everything has changed and nothing from your original plan applies now.

Your nursing day will be filled with similar scenarios when you care for patients. One hallmark of a good nurse is that he or she is ready to make changes and use a fresh approach when necessary.

in the patient's chart. In addition, a short summary of specific care may be written on the Kardex. (See Chapter 5 for more information about the Kardex.)

Types of Care Plans

A care plan is often used as a basis for documentation, as in the problem-oriented medical record. (See Chapter 5 for more information about documentation.) A detailed care plan may be documented in a variety of ways.

Computerized Care Plans

In most hospitals, computerized care plans are the standard. The RN highlights or checks appropriate nursing diagnoses on the computer screen and then selects corresponding goals and nursing interventions listed for that diagnosis. The care plan is saved in the computer and may not be printed out. It is available to all nursing staff with computer passwords. The use of standardized language for nursing diagnoses (NANDA-I), outcomes (NOC), and interventions (NIC) is essential for the computerized care plan to be consistent from facility to facility. ***Safety: Always turn off or shut down the computer monitor screen so that other people cannot see the patient's private information.***

Standardized Care Plans

Standardized care plans are preprinted documents with typical nursing diagnoses and corresponding nursing intervention choices to coordinate with a particular medical diagnosis. For example, a standardized care plan for a patient with pneumonia might include choices of the following nursing diagnoses:

- Ineffective airway clearance
- Impaired gas exchange
- Activity intolerance

The nurse checks the nursing diagnoses that match the assessment data and then selects from the listed interventions those that are appropriate for this patient. Many standardized care plans provide the opportunity to individualize further by writing details or dates in blank spaces. An advantage to these standardized care plans is that they help you remember most of the interventions for a specific diagnosis, preventing oversight.

Multidisciplinary Care Plans

Another type of care plan frequently used in hospitals is a collaborative or multidisciplinary plan of care. This type of care plan includes choices of different nursing diagnoses with options the nurse may select in order to individualize the patient's care (Fig. 4.7). In addition, the multidisciplinary care plan contains similar areas for respiratory therapists, social services workers, physical therapists, and dietitians to document their plans and the patient's response in the electronic health record. One major advantage of this type of care plan is that all health-care professionals involved in the patient's care are working together and communicating with one another. (See the Evidence-Based Practice box, "Making Care Plans More Relevant.")

Evidence-Based Practice

Making Care Plans More Relevant

Clinical Question

Could care plans be more relevant to patient care and contribute to collaborative care?

Evidence

At White Plains Hospital in White Plains, New York, the nursing staff felt that current care plans were designed for nurses only and had way too many nursing diagnoses and patient problems to be effective. After research using surveys and EHR review, they determined that a different approach was needed. They developed care plans that were disease specific and interdisciplinary in nature. They included only the patient problems that were preventing them from moving on to the next level of care.

Implications for Nursing Practice

After performing this research, these nurses found that this type of care plan improved communication between departments and helped them develop a cohesive and collaborative team. Their research after implementing the evidence-based care plans showed improved efficient quality of patient care. Prior to implementing the change in the design and use of care plans, only 60% of patients had a care plan developed. Afterwards, 95% of patients had care plans because they were useful tools in helping patients improve.

Source: You can read more about this study at http://www.himss.org/reinventing-care-plan-wheel-our-process-implementing-evidence-based-care-plans

Critical Pathways

Critical pathways, also called clinical pathways, are similar to standardized care plans except that they are based on the progression expected for each day the patient is in the hospital. Certain nursing interventions are provided each day, and they change as the patient improves and requires less comprehensive nursing care. The critical pathway uses the average length of stay for a particular medical diagnosis as the basis for the progression of care. When a patient has more than one major medical diagnosis, it becomes more difficult to use critical pathways. Figure 4.8 shows an example of a critical pathway.

Student Care Plans

For many years in nursing education, student care plans have been used to help students make connections between the patient's medical diagnoses, medications, laboratory and diagnostic tests, assessment data, nursing diagnoses, nursing orders or interventions, and evaluations. It is true that once you are out of school you will no longer complete these detailed care plans because of time constraints. However, while you are a student, these care plans are excellent tools for sharpening your critical thinking skills and your nursing decision making. In fact, it is one major way that you learn to think like a nurse. Figure 4.9 shows an example of a student care plan.

PREPARING TO CARE FOR PATIENTS PRIOR TO CLINICAL EXPERIENCE. As a student, you may be required to prepare for your clinical experiences by completing a portion of your care plan form before you actually care for your patients. This gives you background and sparks ideas about the types of problems and assessment data that you may find when you care for the patient. For example, suppose your instructor gives you the following information about the patient:

- George Marquez, a 54-year-old male patient with medical diagnosis of coronary artery disease
- Admitted after experiencing radiating chest pain to left arm and jaw while bicycling with his son
- Scheduled for an arteriogram at 1 p.m. tomorrow
- Nothing by mouth (NPO) after midnight
- Healthy heart diet
- Vital signs every 4 hours
- Bedrest with bathroom privileges
- IV line in left arm
- Intake and output
- *Telemetry* (a remote heart monitoring device)

Your instructor tells you that he has arranged for you to accompany Mr. Marquez to the catheterization laboratory and to observe the arteriogram procedure tomorrow. He also tells you that the patient is very anxious about the procedure and

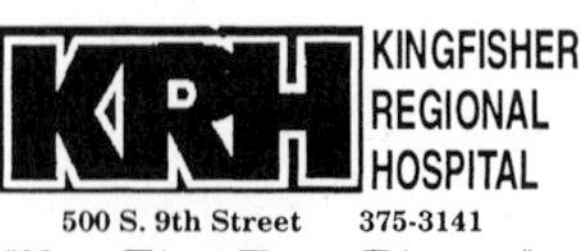

"Your Home Team Advantage"

MULTIDISCIPLINARY PLAN OF CARE

Page 1

PHYSICAL MEDICINE AND REHABILITATION

INITIAL EVAL. DATE	INITIAL EVAL. INITIALS	PATIENT PROBLEMS	EXPECTED OUTCOMES / GOALS	INTERVENTIONS / APPROACHES	RESOLVED DATE	RESOLVED INITIALS
		☐ Activity Intolerance ☐ Pain 2° ____ ☐ Decreased Strength ☐ Decreased Endurance ☐ Decreased ROM ____	☐ Increased Activity Tolerance ☐ Decreases Pain ☐ Increase Strength ☐ Increase Endurance ☐ Increase ROM ____	☐ Therapy: ☐ Hot Packs ☐ Ultrasound ☐ Massage ☐ Tens ☐ Therapeutic Exercise ☐ Progressive Gait Training ☐ Other ____		
		☐ Impaired Physical Mobility ☐ Bed mobility ____ ☐ Transfers ____ ☐ Ambulation ____ ☐ Balance ____ ☐ Decreased Safety Awareness	☐ Bed mobility ____ ☐ Transfers ____ ☐ Ambulation ____ ☐ Balance ____ ☐ Improve Safety Awareness	☐ Bed mobility Training ☐ Transfers Training ☐ Progressive Gait Training ☐ Balance Training ☐ Safety Awareness ☐ Precautions ☐ Written Instructions - Precautions		
		☐ Wound	☐ Wound Cleansed ☐ Increased Circulation ☐ Healing Promoted ☐ Reduced Potential for Infection	☐ Whirlpool ☐ With Additive ____ ☐ Without Additive ☐ With Debridement ☐ Sterile Dressing ☐ Dry ☐ Dry with Topical Ointment ☐ Wet/Dry with Saline With Packing ____ Other ____		

Therapy, Evaluation. Treatment Flow Sheets and Progress Notes can be found in the Physical Therapy section of the patient's current medical record.

Additional Comments: ____

FOOD & NUTRITION

INITIAL EVAL. DATE	INITIAL EVAL. INITIALS	PATIENT PROBLEMS	EXPECTED OUTCOMES / GOALS	INTERVENTIONS / APPROACHES	RESOLVED DATE	RESOLVED INITIALS
		Actual / potential nutrition risk factors identified: ☐ Patient requires enteral and/or parenteral support ____ ☐ Knowledge deficit related to ____ ☐ Dental status ☐ Protein/Energy Depletion ☐ Cultural Influence ☐ Other:	Maintain / improve nutritional status as evidenced by ☐ Weight maintenance or gain ☐ Improved PO intake > 75% meals ☐ Lab Values: ____ ☐ Improved: ____ ☐ Patient/Significant Other able to demonstrate comprehension of diet modification. ☐ Other:	☐ Provide supplement and/or snack ____ ☐ Provide consultation/recommendation ____ ☐ Provide education/counseling ____ ☐ Monitor tolerance/response to: Meals ____ Supplements ____ Snacks ____ Enteral feedings ____ Parenteral nutrition ____ ☐ Calorie counts ____ ☐ Monitor weight/lab values ____ ☐ Other ____ ☐ Refer to Pt. Nutrition Evaluation found in patient's Medical Record		

Additional Comments: ____

FIGURE 4.7 Sample of a multidisciplinary care plan that combines a standardized nursing care plan with those of other disciplines. (Courtesy of Kingfisher Regional Hospital, Kingfisher, OK.)

RESPIRATORY MULTIDISCIPLINARY PLAN OF CARE (Continued)

RESPIRATORY

INITIAL EVAL.		PATIENT PROBLEMS	EXPECTED OUTCOMES / GOALS	INTERVENTIONS / APPROACHES	RESOLVED	
DATE	INITIALS				DATE	INITIALS
		☐ Impaired Gas Exchange ☐ Dyspnea related to: __________ ☐ Ineffective airway clearance related to: ________ ☐ Secretions: ________ ☐ Knowledge deficit related to: __________ __________ __________ ☐ Other:	☐ Improved Oxygenation ☐ Establish effective respiratory pattern ☐ Reduce potential for atelectasis ☐ Diminished or absence of rales ☐ Mobilize secretions ☐ Patient / significant other able to demonstrate: ☐ ABG's within normal limit ______ ☐ Respiratory rate normal ______ ☐ Other:	☐ Assess respiratory function __________ ☐ Monitor: Breath Sounds ______ ABG ____ Oximeter ____ CXR ____ Other ____ ☐ Oxygen ________ ☐ HHN / MDI ________ ☐ IPPB ________ ☐ Incentive Spirometry ________ ☐ Aerosol Therapy ________ ☐ CP&PD ________ ☐ Bronchodilator ________ ☐ Suction ________ ☐ Other:		

Additional Comments: ______________________________

DISCHARGE PLANNING / SOCIAL SERVICES

INITIAL EVAL.		PATIENT PROBLEMS	EXPECTED OUTCOMES / GOALS	INTERVENTIONS / APPROACHES	RESOLVED	
DATE	INITIALS				DATE	INITIALS
		☐ Concern: patient's ability to return to premorbid living arrangements related to: ☐ Living alone ☐ Has disabling illness ☐ Not alert / disoriented ☐ Has no identified family / significant other ☐ Depressed / anxious ☐ Suspected abuse / neglect ☐ Conservatorship ☐ Other ________ ☐ Cultural Influences ☐ Agitated / Combative / Suicidal ☐ Hallucinations / Delusions	☐ Patient / significant other will be aware of appropriate D/C arrangements as evidenced by verbalizing what services are being arranged ☐ Increased awareness of adjustments needed to cope with disabling illness ☐ Financial assessment will result in referral to eligible programs ☐ Other:	Arrange for: ☐ Home Health ________ ☐ Attendant care ________ ☐ Rehab ________ ☐ SNF / Sub-acute ________ ☐ Board & care ________ ☐ Durable medical equipment ______ ☐ Counseling / support group referrals ____ __________ ☐ Transportation ________ ☐ Nutrition program ________ ☐ SSI ____ ☐ IHSS ______ ☐ Medicaid ________ ☐ Educ. re: Advanced Directive ______ ☐ Initiated short-term counseling ______ ☐ Other:		

Additional Comments: ______________________________

FIGURE 4.7—cont'd

Continued

MULTIDISCIPLINARY PLAN OF CARE (Continued)

Page 3

NURSING CARE PLAN

INITIAL EVAL.			PATIENT PROBLEMS	EXPECTED OUTCOMES / GOALS	INTERVENTIONS / APPROACHES	RESOLVED	
DATE	INITIALS					DATE	INITIALS
		1	Knowledge deficit related to: ______ ______ ______	☐ Patient / family will verbalize and/or demonstrate understanding of education during hospitalization: ______ ______	☐ Initiate Education Profile ☐ Other: ______ ______ ______		
		2	Anxiety ☐ Potential ☐ Actual related to: ☐ Hospitalization ☐ Perceived threat to self concept or health status ☐ Perceived threat to significant other ☐ Other:	☐ Patient / family will verbalize decreased feeling of anxiety during hospitalization ☐ Other:	☐ Assess level of anxiety ______ ☐ Encourage patient / family to verbalize feelings ______ ☐ Give information regarding: test, disease process / surgery as patient is ready to learn ______ ☐ Answer questions appropriately and concisely ______ ☐ Encourage patient input into plan of care ______ ☐ Offer appropriate reassurance and support ______ ☐ Pastoral care referral ______ ☐ Social services referral ______ ☐ Other:		
		3	Alteration in Respiratory Status related to: ☐ Infection ☐ Loss of functioning lung tissue ☐ Post-op status ☐ Other:	☐ Patient will obtain adequate ventilation during hospitalization ☐ Other:	Monitor: ☐ CXR's ______ ☐ Respiratory status ______ ☐ Character of sputum ______ ☐ ABG's / Labs ______ ☐ O2 as ordered: ______ ☐ Respiratory therapy: ______ ☐ Assess Home Health needs ______ ☐ Other:		
		4	Alteration in Cardiac Status related to: ☐ Hemodynamic instability ☐ Potential ☐ Actual ☐ Dysrhythmia ☐ Hypo / hypertension ☐ Pulmonary congestion ☐ Edema ☐ Cardiac output, diminished ☐ Other:	Patient will exhibit, within potential: ☐ Hemodynamic stability ______ ☐ Rhythm stability ☐ Blood pressure stability ☐ Fluid and electrolyte balance ______ ______ ☐ Other:	Monitor: ☐ Cardiac rhythms ______ ☐ Vital signs per protocols ______ ☐ Invasive lines ______ ☐ Medications ______ ☐ Fluid balance / I&O ______ ☐ Daily weight - type of scale ______ ☐ Lab values per protocols ______ ☐ Test results (EKG, CXR, ECHO) ______ ☐ Cardiac teaching (diet, meds, activity, etc.) ☐ Other:		
		5	Alteration in Comfort related to: ☐ Illness / surgery ☐ Nausea / vomiting ☐ Pain ☐ Itching ☐ Other:	☐ Patient will verbalize and/or demonstrate relief of discomfort 30-60 minutes p intervention using pain scale 1-10 ______ ______ ☐ Other:	☐ Assess for discomfort and relief pos: intervention ______ ☐ PRN meds as ordered ______ ☐ Provide comfort measures ______ ☐ Position changes ______ Teach pain relief options ______ ☐ Breathing ☐ Relaxation exercises ☐ Other: ☐ Other:		
		6	Alteration in Bowel Elimination related to: ☐ Diarrhea ☐ Constipation ☐ Ileus ☐ Neurogenic bowel ☐ Other:	☐ Patient will ______ pattern of bowel elimination ☐ Patient demonstrate management ☐ Other:	☐ Assess and monitor causative factors ______ ☐ Increase fluids / bulk ☐ PRN meds as ordered ______ ☐ Monitor bowel sounds q ______ ☐ Bowel program ______ ☐ Other:		
		7	Alteration in Urinary Elimination related to: ☐ Incontinence ☐ Retention ☐ Neurogenic bladder ☐ Other:	☐ Patient will ______ pattern of urinary elimination ☐ Patient / family will demonstrate management ______ ______ ☐ Other:	☐ Assess and monitor causative factors ______ ☐ Assess and monitor signs and symptions ______ ☐ Offer bedpan / urinal q ______ ☐ Comfort measures ______ ☐ Catheter ______ ☐ Teach patient / family ______ ☐ Other:		

FIGURE 4.7—cont'd

Estimated Length of Stay: 7 Days – Variations from Designated Pathway Should Be Documented in Progress Notes						
Nursing Diagnoses and Categories of Care	Time Dimension	Goals and/or Actions	Time Dimension	Goals and/or Actions	Time Dimension	Discharge Outcome
Risk for injury related to CNS agitation					Day 7	Client shows no evidence of injury obtained during ETOH withdrawal
Referrals	Day 1	Psychiatrist Assess need for: Neurologist Cardiologist Internist			Day 7	Discharge with follow-up appointments as required.
Diagnostic studies	Day 1	Blood alcohol level Drug screen (urine and blood) Chemistry Profile Urinalysis Chest x-ray ECG	Day 4	Repeat of selected diagnostic studies as necessary.		
Additional assessments	Day 1 Day 1–5 Ongoing Ongoing	VS q4h I&O Restraints p.r.n. Assess withdrawal symptoms: tremors, nausea/ vomiting; tachycardia, sweating, high blood pressure, seizures, insomnia, hallucinations	Day 2–3 Day 6 Day 4	VS q8h if stable SC I&O Marked decrease in objective withdrawal symptoms	Day 4–7 Day 7	VS b.i.d.; remain stable Discharge; absence of objective withdrawal symptoms
Medications	Day 1 Day 2 Day 1–6 Day 1–6	*Librium 200 mg in divided doses Librium 160 mg in divided doses Librium p.r.n. Maalox ac & hs *NOTE: some physicians may elect to use Serax or Tegretol in the detoxification process	Day 3 Day 4	Librium 120 mg in divided doses Librium 80 mg in divided doses	Day 5 Day 6 Day 7	Librium 40 mg DC Librium Discharge; no withdrawal symptoms
Client education			Day 5	Discuss goals of AA and need for outpatient therapy	Day 7	Discharge with information regarding AA attendance or outpatient treatment

FIGURE 4.8 Sample of a critical pathway showing the progression of nursing care for a patient with alcohol withdrawal (from Townsend M. *Psychiatric Mental Health Nursing.* 8th ed. Philadelphia, PA: FA Davis; 2014).

about what the doctors might find. He mentions that, as Mr. Marquez had chest pain ambulating to the bathroom on two different occasions, it looks like he probably has significant blockage in his coronary arteries.

Step 1: Research. With this information, you are ready to do some further research. Before you care for Mr. Marquez the next day, you need to know more about his likely problems and potential problems. What are the signs and symptoms of this condition? Which diagnostic tests do you expect? What is the usual treatment? You will learn more about diseases, diagnosis, and treatment in the medical-surgical portion of your nursing education. Early in school, you will need to research medical diagnoses in your medical-surgical textbook.

You learn that the common signs and symptoms of coronary artery disease are chest pain with or without radiation to other areas, chest pressure or discomfort, elevated blood pressure, dyspnea with exertion, and possibly an irregular heartbeat. Tests include *coronary arteriography,* which is taking an x-ray after the injection of contrast media into the coronary arteries to detect blockages or narrowing that could lead to a myocardial infarction, or heart attack. The treatment is diet and lifestyle modifications, medications to dilate the coronary arteries (for example, nitroglycerin), medications to lower blood pressure, and possible stent placement or coronary artery bypass grafts if the blockages are severe. A *stent* is a device inserted into a blood vessel to keep it open, allowing blood to flow evenly through it.

Level IV Master Clinical Written Assignment (100 pts)

Admitting Diagnosis:	Admission Date:	Age:	M/F	Admitting Dr.	Student:
	Surgical Procedure (if applicable) & Date		Diet:		Instructor:
			Secondary Diagnosis:		
	History of Presenting Illness: (Get from patient interview & reading the History & Physical in the chart.)		Social History:		
			Past Medical History:		
Allergies:					

Nursing Care to be Provided

Activity:	Fluid Balance: (I & O, Encourage Fluids, Fluid Restriction, etc.)
Safety:	
Vital Sign Frequency:	Treatments (dressings changes, irrigations, FSBS, etc.):
Hygiene & Type Bath:	
Respiratory Therapy:	
Physical Therapy:	

(Worth 5 pts.)

Drug/Dose/ Route	Frequency/ Time	Classification	Why is Patient on This Drug? BE SPECIFIC	What assessment or lab result must be monitored prior to administering this drug?	Was Patient on this drug at home?

(Disease Research worth 5 pts.)

Diagnosis: ______________________

Disease Research of Admitting Diagnosis: *(Describe the processes/changes within the body that result in the signs and symptoms of the disease.)* **5 pts.**

FIGURE 4.9 A student care plan for a student near graduation from an LPN/LVN program. (Courtesy of Canadian Valley Technology Center, El Reno, OK.)

Diagnostic Studies: Level IV Master List routine lab tests/procedures for your patient, the results and possible significance of each. Worth 15 pts.					
Lab Test/X-ray/ Procedure	Normal Value	Admit Results & Date	Day 1 Results & Date	Day 2 Results & Date	Significance
WBC					
RBC					
HGB					
HCT					
PLT					
Glucose					
BUN					
Creatinine					
Sodium					
Potassium					
Chloride					

Lab Test/X-ray/ Procedure	Normal Values	Admit Results & Date	Day 1 Results & Date	Day 2 Results & Date	Significance
Urinalysis:					
Color/ Appearance					
Specific Gravity					
Urine PH					
Protein					
Glucose					
Ketone					
Bilirubin					
Blood					
Nitrate					
Bacteria					
UA WBC					

FIGURE 4.9—cont'd

Because you will be accompanying the patient when the arteriogram is obtained, you research what will be done during the procedure and what the patient can expect after the procedure. You learn that if stents are necessary, they will be placed during the procedure. If the blockages cannot be treated with stents because of their location, the patient may have to undergo open-heart surgery for coronary artery bypass grafts.

Now you know more about what to expect in the care of this patient. But how do you turn all of that medical information into nursing care? You must use the nursing process.

Step 2: Possible Nursing Diagnoses. Even though you cannot perform an assessment on your patient now, you are beginning to have ideas about the possible problems that your patient might have. For student care plans, it is often suggested that only three or four nursing diagnoses be required so that the student can concentrate on learning specifics of those diagnoses. In this case, you can narrow down the possibilities to these diagnoses:

- Acute pain related to decreased oxygen to the heart muscle
- Activity intolerance related to decreased ability of the heart to respond to increased demand as evidenced by pain and dyspnea when ambulating
- Deficient knowledge about pending coronary arteriography

Step 3: Expected Outcomes. Expected outcomes for each nursing diagnosis could be similar to the following:

- Patient will rate chest pain at a 0 to 2 before discharge.
- Patient will ambulate 30 feet in the hallway without chest pain before discharge.
- Patient will verbalize what to expect during and after the coronary arteriography by noon tomorrow.

Step 4: Develop Your Interventions. You now need to determine what you will do for this patient. How will you help relieve his chest pain if it occurs? What do you need to monitor about his chest pain? You can find out more about managing pain in Chapter 19.

What, if anything, do you need to know about his telemetry unit? Are you supposed to do anything with it while you are caring for Mr. Marquez? What will you do with it while the arteriogram is being obtained? Chapter 25 has information about caring for patients on telemetry.

What will you do about his activity problems? How will you get him to the bathroom? What could you do instead? How can you help keep him from getting weak even though he is on bedrest with bathroom privileges? Chapter 16 contains information about moving and positioning patients.

What about his lack of knowledge leading to anxiety about the coronary arteriography? You need to teach him what to expect during the procedure and afterward. You have looked up the information, but how do you teach it to him? Chapter 12 contains information on patient teaching.

As you go through this book and learn to care for patients, you will use information from different chapters for different situations because every patient is a unique individual. That is why it is so important for you to learn what is in this book, allowing you to think on your feet as you provide nursing care for a variety of patients.

CARING FOR THE PATIENT DURING CLINICAL EXPERIENCE.
Step 5: Meet and Assess the Patient. It is the morning of your clinical experience and you have met Mr. Marquez. He is pale and a bit shaky, and you wonder if he is nervous. He was glad to hear that you will be with him for the arteriogram procedure. As you perform your assessment, you obtain the following data:

- His father died suddenly at age 60 years with what was presumed to be a heart attack.
- He verbalizes concern that he "might end up like my dad."
- He verbalizes concern over "what they will find when they look at my heart. I don't want to have open-heart surgery."
- His blood pressure is 160/90, his temperature is 99°F (38.2°C), his pulse is 94 and irregular, and his respirations are 20.
- His skin is pale and moist.
- He has had no more chest pain since the nitroglycerin patch was put on last night; he is able to walk to the bathroom without pain, but he does still have dyspnea with exertion.
- He owns his own business and is frequently on the telephone with his employees while in the hospital.
- He states that he does not want to know what they are going to do today; he just wants them "to do it and get it over with."
- He has a history of smoking a pack of cigarettes per day since he was 16 years old.

Step 6: Evaluate Your Nursing Diagnoses. Now that you have assessed your patient, do you need to make any changes to the nursing diagnoses that you developed last night? Or are they still the priorities in his care? Does another diagnosis need to take priority over these?

As you look at the diagnoses you formulated last night, they still seem to be appropriate. Although Mr. Marquez is no longer having chest pain when he ambulates to the bathroom, he has the potential for chest pain at any time, so it is appropriate to leave it as a priority diagnosis.

Step 7: Implement Your Interventions. Now you will implement the interventions that you developed last night as you asked yourself all those questions about taking care of Mr. Marquez. The Nursing Care Plan on page 68 shows the nursing diagnoses with related interventions.

Step 8: Evaluate Your Care Plan. Now you are finishing up your clinical day. You have completed everything that you had planned to accomplish. Mr. Marquez made it through the coronary arteriography and had two stents placed. He knew what to expect afterward because you had prepared him, so he was able to cooperate fully. He is scheduled for discharge tomorrow and already feels better than he did before the stents were placed.

Before he is discharged, he will need additional teaching about health promotion, such as diet and lifestyle choices, including smoking cessation. Although you will not be taking care of him again, you know the plans for this teaching are already underway. The Nursing Care Plan on page 68 shows the evaluations of your nursing interventions for Mr. Marquez.

You can see that you definitely used the nursing process while developing your care plan. You also realize that you did not follow the exact order in which you learned it. When you are preparing for clinical experiences ("clinicals") the evening before, you must adapt the process to fit your circumstances. It is very important for you to be prepared to care for your patients when you arrive for clinicals each day, and now you have a guide for how to prepare.

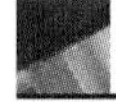

CONCEPT MAPS

Concept maps, also known as "mind maps," can be used to diagram and connect data about any subject. They also can be used to organize and plan nursing care, in effect making them a care plan as well. When you use a concept map to plan care, you still use the nursing process as your basis for decision making.

Concept maps can help you see relationships between nursing diagnoses and assessment data. They also can help you make connections between interventions and diagnoses, even though those are on a separate piece of paper. Sometimes you are not sure what to do with information. Should it be a nursing diagnosis or not? Where might it fit? You can put it on your concept map with a question mark and then see where it fits later. Visual learners often enjoy using concept maps.

Steps for Concept Mapping of a Care Plan

You will follow the steps of the nursing process as you plan care for your patient, but you will also follow steps for concept mapping:

Step 1: In the middle of a blank sheet of paper, write the reason the patient is hospitalized or seeking medical care. (See Fig. 4.10 for an example of a concept map.) This is usually the medical diagnosis, but not always.

Step 2: Using rectangles, write the nursing diagnoses/patient problems around the reason for hospitalization, leaving room to write in additional information. Connect the nursing diagnoses to the patient with a solid line.

Step 3: List supporting information, or evidence, from your assessment and nursing history below each nursing diagnosis (see Fig. 4.10). Write nursing actions or additional information in a triangle beneath the nursing diagnosis or patient problem.

Step 4: Connect nursing diagnoses to other nursing diagnoses with a broken line if there is a relationship. Be prepared to explain your reasons for connecting them.

Step 5: On a separate sheet of paper, make a chart showing the first priority nursing diagnosis at the top and then list the desired outcome beneath the diagnosis. Make two columns beneath the headings (see the Nursing Care Plan).

Step 6: Write the nursing interventions in the left-hand column of the paper beneath the nursing diagnosis. Repeat this for each nursing diagnosis (see the Nursing Care Plan).

Step 7: Write your evaluation information in the right-hand column of the paper beneath the appropriate nursing diagnosis. Evaluate each intervention, nursing diagnosis, and goal and outcome (see the Nursing Care Plan).

This is just one way to create a concept map. You can make them look however you would like. Some students like to use different colors for different things, such as red for medications and green for nursing diagnoses. You can use different shapes to represent different aspects of your map, such as a square for diagnostic tests and a circle for medications. Be sure to follow any guidelines established by your school when you do concept mapping. Some people use very large sheets of paper and include nursing interventions, outcomes, and evaluations in the concept map itself.

Whether you use a traditional care plan, a concept map, or a combination of the two, your main focus is integrating your knowledge and skills to provide the very best, individualized care for your particular patient.

KNOWLEDGE CONNECTION

What types of care plans are available? Why do students write care plans? Which parts of a care plan can be done before your clinical experience and which parts must be done after you have met the patient?

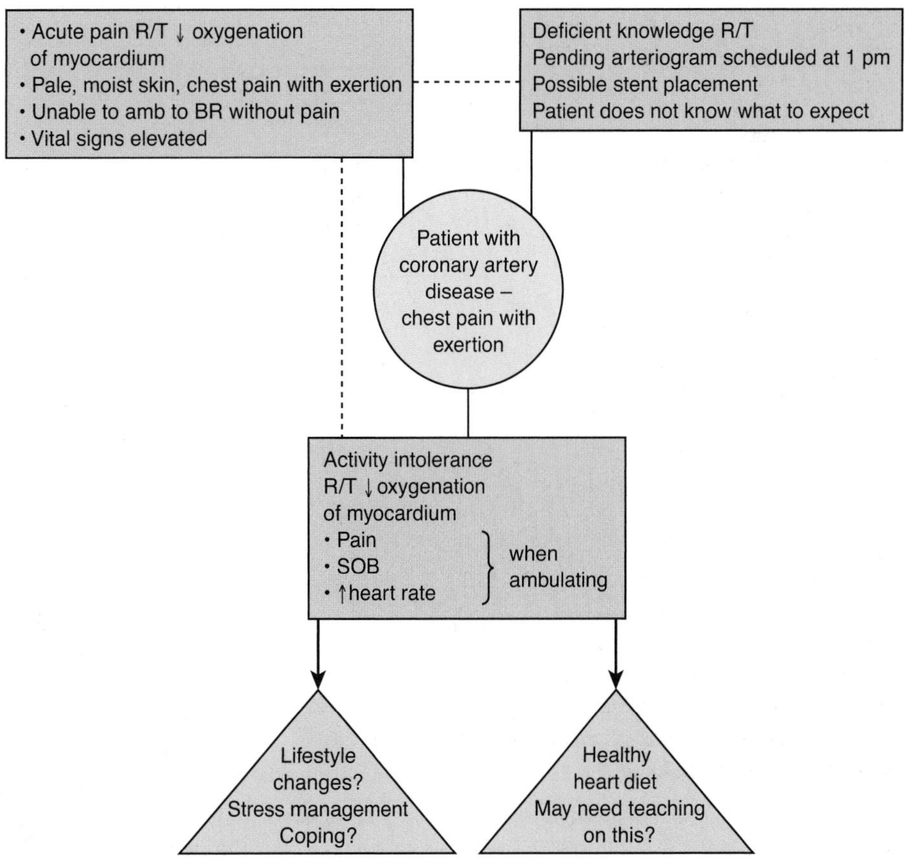

FIGURE 4.10 Sample of a concept map care plan.

Nursing Care Plan Interventions and Evaluation

Nursing Diagnosis: Acute pain r/t decreased oxygenation of the myocardium
Outcome: Patient will rate chest pain as 0 to 1 on a scale of 10 by discharge.

Interventions	Evaluation
Monitor for chest pain episodes. If chest pain occurs, report to nurse immediately and take vital signs. Evaluate effectiveness of nitroglycerin spray in relieving chest pain. Monitor vital signs after use of nitro spray.	Pt had no chest pain during morning prior to arteriography. BP stable at 146/80, P – 92 and irreg, R – 20, T – 98°F.
Maintain telemetry monitoring by ensuring that electrodes and wires are in place.	Telemetry maintained until pt left floor for cath lab.
Notify monitor station before removing telemetry for any reason.	Monitor station notified and telemetry monitor removed.

Nursing Diagnosis: Activity intolerance r/t decreased ability of heart to respond to demands AEB pain and dyspnea when ambulating
Outcome: Patient will ambulate 30 feet in hallway without chest pain before discharge.

Interventions	Evaluation
Assist pt to dangle first and evaluate response before getting up to BR. If pt c/o chest pain, return to bed.	Pt dangles and tol without c/o chest pain.
Ambulate pt to BR slowly, stay close and be prepared to lower to floor if pt becomes weak or loses consciousness.	VS remained stable when dangling at 140/82, P – 94, R – 24. Assisted to BR ×2 without problem. Stopped to rest ×1 when returning to bed. No loss of consciousness.
Consider asking for order for BSC if pt unable to make to the bathroom.	Unnecessary—able to amb to BR.
Monitor VS when pt returns from BR.	VS remain fairly stable. BP – 160/86, P – 98, R – 26 on return from BR.
Provide active ROM exercises for pt to prevent muscle weakness while on bedrest.	Performed active ROM ×2 prior to going to cath lab.

Nursing Diagnosis: Deficient knowledge about coronary arteriography
Outcome: Patient will verbalize what to expect during and after scheduled arteriogram.

Interventions	Evaluation
Allow pt to talk about what he knows about procedure and concerns and fears he may have.	Pt talked about his father's death and his fears that it could happen to him. Acknowledged that his father had ignored health problems, but he was not ignoring his.
Instruct pt on what to expect during arteriogram procedure: • Pt will be awake. • Staff will be dressed in gowns, gloves, masks, goggles. • Puncture will be made into femoral artery and cath will be inserted and passed through to heart. • Pt may feel a warm sensation when contrast medium is injected. • If necessary, stents will be placed in arteries to keep them open.	At first, pt was not interested in hearing this. Said it would make him more nervous, but as time drew closer, he started asking questions, leading to pt teaching. Able to verbalize to me what stents were and what they were for.
Instruct patient on what to expect after arteriogram is performed: • Must lie flat 6 hr afterward. • Cannot bend rt leg at groin for 24 hr. • Staff will check groin frequently for bleeding. • Pt will be attached to heart and BP monitor for 2 hr after procedure.	Pt verbalized what to expect after procedure; very cooperative afterward; kept leg straight and knew what would happen when the staff checked his leg. Pt to be discharged in a.m.

POST CONFERENCE

After being frustrated and upset, you read Chapter 4 and look up your patient's major diagnoses. It is confusing to read about all of those signs and symptoms, tests, and treatments, so you decide to focus on his heart failure. You are actually able to come up with about six nursing diagnoses, and some overlap with his other diagnoses. Your instructor is impressed with your list. You still do not know how to select many interventions, but as the day goes on, you begin to understand better that nearly everything you do for your patient is a nursing intervention.

Key Points

- Nurses make decisions using critical thinking and the nursing process.
- The steps of the nursing process are assessment, diagnosis, planning, intervention, and evaluation. RNs participate in all aspects of the nursing process. LPNs/LVNs contribute to assessment and diagnosis and participate in planning, intervention, and evaluation.
- Assessment includes collecting objective and subjective data through interviewing, physical assessment, and review of laboratory and diagnostic tests.
- Nursing diagnoses are prioritized using Maslow's hierarchy of human needs. Physiological or survival needs must be met before other needs that are of concern to the patient.
- The NANDA-I list contains nursing diagnoses developed and approved by the North American Nursing Diagnoses Association–International. The list is arranged with the primary topic first, followed by modifiers.
- Nursing diagnoses may be one-, two-, or three-part statements. All contain a diagnostic label. Two-part statements also contain an etiology, and three-part statements contain both of these plus defining characteristics exhibited by the patient.
- Expected outcomes are specific measurable actions by the patient within a specific time frame. In care plans, there is an expected outcome for every nursing diagnosis. They are determined by the RN.
- Nursing interventions may be direct or indirect and independent, dependent, or collaborative.
- Nursing care plans provide a communication tool for all nursing staff regarding the care of patients. They may be standardized, computerized, multidisciplinary, or critical pathways.
- Concept maps are alternate ways of making connections between the steps of the nursing process and determining interventions to be performed for each patient.

Review Questions

Select the answer that is most appropriate for each of the following questions. Some questions may have more than one correct answer. Select all that apply.

1. Which of the following are examples of activities in which a nurse would need to use critical thinking?
   1. Prioritizing patient care
   2. Administering medications
   3. Writing nursing orders
   4. Questioning the appropriateness of an order
   5. Starting an IV infusion

2. Which of these is considered subjective data?
   1. The patient is resting on his side.
   2. The patient complains of a headache.
   3. The patient ambulated to the bathroom with assistance.
   4. The patient's mother states that he does not eat well.

3. Given that all of the following are appropriate nursing diagnoses for your patient, which would be the priority?
   1. Ineffective coping
   2. Sedentary lifestyle
   3. Risk for loneliness
   4. Self-care deficit: bathing

4. Which of these nursing diagnoses is correctly written?
   1. Readiness for enhanced knowledge related to problems with diabetes
   2. Risk for injury related to poor balance when walking
   3. Risk for falls as manifested by frequent falls in the past
   4. Anxiety and fear

5. Which are examples of independent nursing interventions?
   1. Placing a patient on intake and output measurement
   2. Assessing the abdomen when a patient is constipated
   3. Encouraging high-fiber foods for a patient who is constipated
   4. Administering an enema to a constipated patient
   5. Administering a laxative and stool softener to a constipated patient

6. Number in order the steps of the nursing process.
   1. Planning
   2. Assessment
   3. Evaluation
   4. Diagnosis
   5. Implementation

7. Which steps of the nursing process does the LPN/LVN directly participate in?
   1. Assessment
   2. Diagnosis
   3. Planning
   4. Implementation
   5. Evaluation

ANSWERS 1. 1, 2, 3, 4, 5. 2. 2, 4. 3. 4. 4. 2. 5. 1, 2, 3. 6. The correct order is 2, 4, 1, 5, 3. 7. 1, 4, 5

Critical Thinking Exercises

Answers available online.

1. A patient is admitted with nausea and vomiting. She has lost a great deal of fluid and is dehydrated. The physician orders IV fluids and NPO. The patient is already very thin. Give two possible nursing diagnoses for this patient, using diagnostic labels only, and etiology if possible.

2. Draw a concept map of the information and nursing diagnoses for the patient in Question 1.

Additional Resources

DAVIS edge **Use the scratch off code on the inside front cover of your book to access online quizzes that will help you to improve your scores on course exams and prepare for the NCLEX-PN®.**

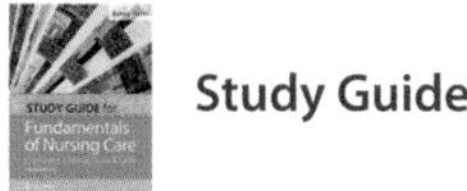

Study Guide

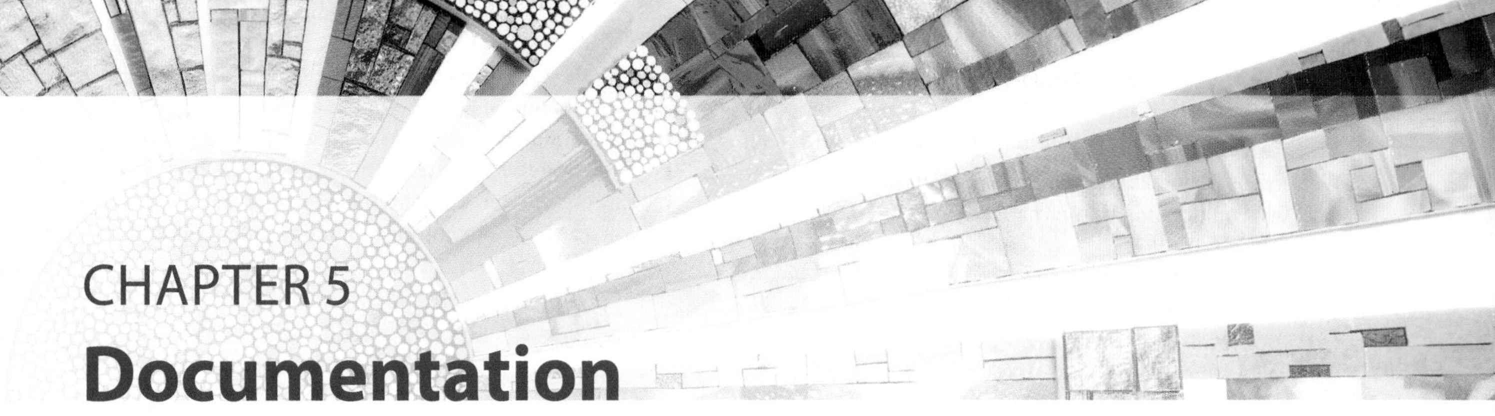

CHAPTER 5

Documentation

Dr. Rita Armstrong

KEY TERMS

Charting by exception (CHART-ing bye ek-SEP-shun)
Documentation (DOK-yoo-men-TAY-shun)
Electronic health record (ee-lek-TRON-ik HELLTH REK-ord)
Focus charting (FOH-kuss CHART-ing)
Kardex (KAR-deks)
Narrative charting (NA-ra-tiv CHART-ing)
PIE charting (PYE CHART-ing)
SOAPIER charting (SOH-pee-uhr CHART-ing)

CHAPTER CONCEPTS

Communication
Informatics
Legal

LEARNING OUTCOMES

1. Define various terms associated with documentation and information systems.
2. Discuss four purposes of written documentation.
3. Discuss confidentiality of patient records.
4. Discuss the appropriate uses of the various documentation forms.
5. Identify guidelines for electronic documentation.
6. Compare source-oriented and problem-oriented documentation systems.
7. List the common sections of a source-oriented documentation system.
8. Discuss various methods of charting patient information, including narrative charting.
9. Explain the use and importance of electronic health records.
10. Describe additional uses for electronic health records other than documentation of patient care.
11. Discuss variations involved in documentation in long-term care and home health care.
12. Identify five documentation mistakes that increase the risk of legal action.
13. Discuss information found in the Connection features in this chapter.
14. Identify specific safety information.

CRITICAL THINKING CONNECTION

Clinical Assignment

You are assigned to take care of a Native American Indian female who is 87 years old. She was admitted with congestive heart failure and to rule out myocardial infarction (a heart attack). You have already sailed through several clinical days and made pretty good grades, but you feel anxious about today because this is the first time that you will be expected to document your nursing care.

Continued

CRITICAL THINKING CONNECTION—cont'd

Critical Thinking Questions:

1. What types of details will you be expected to document?
2. How will you document information in an electronic health record (EHR)?
3. When will you need to chart? How often?
4. The patient's daughter, who is on her HIPAA form, asks to see some information on the EHR about her mother's lab results. What will you do?

Prior to entering nursing school, when you thought of nursing, you probably thought of the physical aspects of providing care to patients, such as administering injections, performing cardiopulmonary resuscitation, or holding the hand of a dying patient—the heroics of nursing. Those are all part of nursing, but nursing also encompasses the routine, daily tasks that every nurse must perform in order to ensure that every patient he or she cares for receives the utmost in care. **Documentation** is the act of recording pertinent medical information in a patient's medical record, which may be handwritten on a paper chart or keyboarded into an electronic medical record (Taber's 23e). When you document, or chart, you will record a patient's progress and treatment during an illness, outpatient procedure, office visit, home health visit, or hospitalization. It is one of the most important tasks you will perform on a daily basis. Any written account of patient care will be maintained in a chart or an **electronic health record** (EHR) to serve as a permanent medical record.

Because the patient's chart is a record of patient care you have delivered, it is imperative that you are as skilled in documentation as you are in assessing vital signs or drawing a blood sample. In this chapter, we will cover the purposes and guidelines pertaining to documentation, explain the various documentation formats that you may see, and explain related legal concerns.

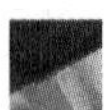

PURPOSES OF DOCUMENTATION

The process of providing ongoing medical and nursing care that meets the patients' needs requires that a large quantity of data be shared among all health-care providers involved with a patient's individualized plan of care. Pertinent data about the patient's condition, the health-care provider's orders, diagnostic results, procedures, treatment, and medications, as well as the effectiveness of each, are recorded within written, typed, or computer-generated documentation. This documentation constitutes the patient's *chart,* otherwise known as the *medical record.* Written documentation serves at least four purposes:

1. To communicate pertinent data that all health-care team members need in order to provide continuity of care
2. To provide a permanent record of medical diagnoses, nursing diagnoses, the plan of care, the care provided, and the patient's response to that care
3. To serve as a record of accountability for quality assurance, accreditation, and reimbursement purposes
4. To serve as a legal record for both the patient and the health-care provider

KNOWLEDGE CONNECTION

Explain what documentation is. Relate the four purposes of documentation.

Continuity of Care

In the health-care setting, nurses provide continuous care for a patient 24 hours a day. Physicians, physical therapists, respiratory therapists, dietitians, laboratory personnel, and other members of the health-care team provide care at intervals, sometimes on a daily basis, but not as continuously as the nurse. It is the nurse's responsibility to document an ongoing account of all pertinent patient data 24 hours a day. This documentation helps to provide physicians and other members of the health-care team with a more complete picture of each patient's individual problems, treatments, and responses to treatment.

For patient care to be effective, it must be delivered and evaluated continuously, systematically, and smoothly from one hour to the next, including through the staffing changes between shifts. This cannot be accomplished without communication of the patient's current condition, changes that have transpired, care that has been delivered and its effectiveness, and medications that have been administered and their effectiveness, as well as the care that is to be delivered in the oncoming hours. Although some of these data can be provided through a verbal shift report, it is impossible to tell the next nurse everything that is contained within the patient's chart. The written documentation serves as a source of information that can be utilized to make decisions regarding care to be given (Fig. 5.1). You will learn more about the verbal shift report in Chapter 6.

KNOWLEDGE CONNECTION

What is meant by *continuity of care?* Why is it so important?

Permanent Record of Care

Another purpose of documentation is to produce a permanent record of the patient's condition, diagnoses, results of diagnostic

• WORD • BUILDING •

diagnostic: dia – through + gnostic – knowledge

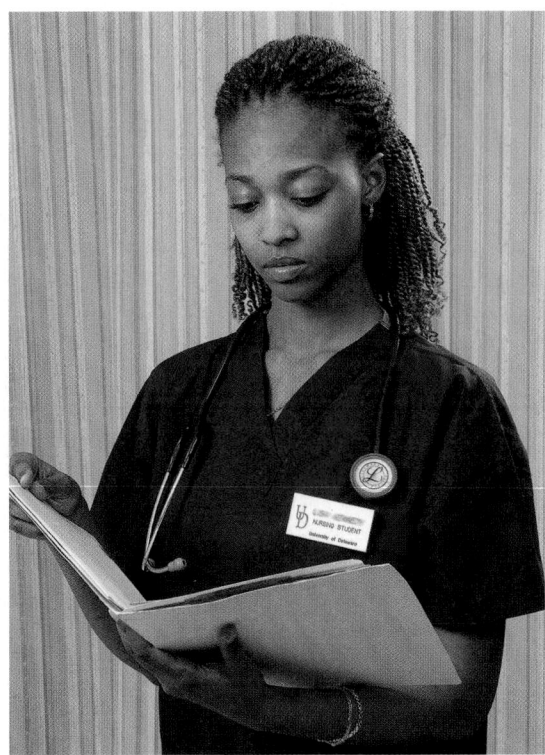

FIGURE 5.1 A nurse gathers data from the patient's medical record (from Wilkinson JM, Treas LS. *Fundamentals of Nursing: Theory, Concepts & Applications.* Vol. 1. 2nd ed. Philadelphia, PA: FA Davis; 2011).

tests and procedures that were performed, and all medical and interdisciplinary care that was provided, as well as the patient's outcome. This record supplies a permanent source of medical history that can be used for reference when the patient requires additional health care in the future. It allows for future comparison of physical assessments, illnesses, injuries, or diagnostic test results with those previously recorded; it also allows for detection of any changes that may have occurred in the interval. It is not uncommon for medical records from past decades to shed light on present-day medical problems.

Accountability

Medical records, or charts, are utilized by facility quality assurance committees as they monitor the quality of care being delivered in their institution. Records help facilities to detect problems, less-than-desirable outcomes, or areas of weakness in their delivery systems so that improvements can be made. Statistics such as rates of hospital-acquired infections, mortality rates, success rates of specific procedures, and number of incidents and accidents serve as defining factors of a medical facility's reputation. This motivates continual internal assessment and evaluation of the care that is delivered.

Government and other accrediting agencies, such as The Joint Commission, also audit medical records to verify facility compliance in meeting established health-care standards. The Joint Commission sets the standards by which the quality of health care is measured both nationally and internationally. It seeks to improve the safety and quality of the care that health-care organizations provide to the public. Standards are written for different types of facilities, such as critical access hospitals, long-term care facilities, home health care, and outpatient surgery offices. To be accredited by The Joint Commission, a facility must practice in a manner that meets The Joint Commission's standards. This is determined by a team of reviewers who visit the facility to assess its policies, procedures, and actual performance and ensure that the standards are met.

Reimbursement by insurance companies and other third-party payers is generally dependent on documentation of specific data in the medical record, making correct documentation an issue of financial survival for medical institutions. Researchers also utilize data from medical records in their experimental work and development.

KNOWLEDGE CONNECTION

Explain what The Joint Commission has to do with documentation. How do quality assurance committees utilize documentation? Describe why insurance companies would have a need for documentation.

Legal Record

The documentation in the permanent record serves as a legal record for both the patient and health-care providers. It can be used in a court of law by the patient to prove that malpractice or negligence occurred, but it also can be used by health-care providers to defend or disprove claims of malpractice or negligence—that is, *if* adequate documentation was performed. ***Safety: From a legal standpoint, it is best to assume that if it wasn't charted, it wasn't done.*** Although that may not always be the case, in many courts that will be the standard, which is why it is so imperative to document thoroughly all patient care and pertinent data.

Not Charted, Not Done

The phrase "Not charted, not done" is interpreted to mean that if something is not documented, then it was not done or did not occur. This can apply to an assessment finding, a change in a patient's condition or situation, or a nursing intervention that you performed, as well as many other things. The concept of "not charted, not done" has been treated as a literal truth in medical negligence and malpractice cases for many years. Quality assurance committees, accrediting agency examiners, attorneys, and nurses continue to function according to this idea, believing that if something is not charted, then it was not done...period. However, this is inherently false if the documentation method is **charting by exception** (explained in more detail later in this chapter), which limits charting to only *abnormal* findings, situations, conditions, or results. Anything falling within the realm of normal would not be charted, making it difficult to prove that you did something.

The phrase "not charted, not done" is not limited to just this particular method of documentation; it may be applied to all documentation methods. It also may be used against you when you simply forget to chart something that is, or later turns out to be, pertinent. This requires you to always chart with a clear understanding of the following: Documentation that is lacking in full detail serves to support even false claims of negligence or malpractice.

Lawsuits often are not filed until years after the precipitating event, possibly long after the patient or event has been forgotten by the medical personnel who delivered care at that time. In some states, events occurring during labor and delivery can be called into evidence for a very long time—until the baby that was delivered is 21 years of age. The longer the interval is between occurrence and legal involvement, the more important the things you documented will be because they will serve as the record of what actually happened. This record is considered much more credible than any one individual's memory. Therefore, documentation is recognized as written evidence.

If you should ever find yourself involved in a malpractice suit brought by one of your patients, especially one whom you do not remember, you will find it comforting to discover that you were careful to document objectively, accurately, and thoroughly. However, if you discovered charting omissions, misspellings, phrases that do not make sense, unapproved abbreviations, illegible handwriting, or any number of unwise shortcuts within your documentation, you would likely find it distressing and worrisome. If you document inaccurate or incomplete descriptions of patient care, or document care that you did not provide, you will be legally responsible for falsifying medical records.

KNOWLEDGE CONNECTION

Explain how documentation is pertinent during a lawsuit. What types of errors could possibly make you, the nurse, "look bad"?

Whose Medical Record Is It?

As you learned in Chapter 3, the original written or computerized medical record, even though it is about the patient, is the property of the hospital or facility. In a physician-owned medical office, the record is the property of the physician. *However, all the information within the chart belongs to the patient.* The patient is guaranteed by the Health Insurance Portability and Accountability Act (HIPAA) the right to view and obtain a copy of the medical record, but the patient does not have the right to take the original chart copy itself. HIPAA ensures the patient's right not only to view and copy his or her own medical record, but also to amend his or her own health information. HIPAA also requires hospitals and medical sites to disclose to each patient, in writing, the way the patient's health data will be used and to ask the patient to specify who can obtain the patient's personal health data. As a result, hospitals have become more careful regarding who may view the chart, and most require that the patient sign a document indicating who may view the medical record or obtain verbal reports about his or her condition or tests and surgery reports.

You are responsible to know your facility's policy and procedure regarding this issue. For EHRs, the Health Information Technology for Economic and Clinical Health Act (HITECH) works to extend the HIPAA regulations for patient privacy and disclosure of personal health information (PHI). HITECH also established requirements for notifications if privacy has been breached, which require a more specific explanation of disclosures of PHI in addition to HIPAA's regulations. ***Safety: Never allow anyone to access the chart until you have verified the facility's policy and ensured that the patient has granted consent in writing.***

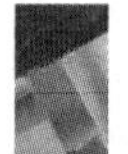

CONFIDENTIALITY OF DOCUMENTATION

As you learned in Chapter 3, federal and state laws govern confidentiality of patients' medical data. HIPAA requires that medical data be maintained in a confidential manner at all times. This applies to the patient's chart, results of diagnostic procedures and consultations, and any notes you might write regarding the patient's health status. **Confidentiality** is the maintenance of privacy by not sharing with a third party privileged or entrusted information (Taber's 23e). Confidentiality is violated when personal information is provided to another person without a patient's permission or knowledge. This can lead to litigation and cause a person unnecessary and unwarranted hardship. For example, two nurses standing in an elevator discussing with each other a patient's condition with other people present in the elevator is a breach of patient confidentiality. ***Safety: Remember that you cannot confirm that an individual is a patient in your facility without specific permission from the patient.*** Therefore, all medical records must be protected and maintained in such a manner that no unauthorized individuals have access to them, only the health-care providers that are directly involved in the patient's care. ***Safety: Take care to avoid leaving patient care notes, laboratory results, medication administration records (MARs), and patient charts lying open and accessible to other facility employees and the public.*** Before you are allowed to send medical records even to another physician to whom the patient is being referred, the patient must sign a written consent. ***Safety: Any handwritten notes or copies of confidential patient information should be shredded once their purpose has been fulfilled.*** Most nurses' stations have a paper shredder to aid you in keeping records private.

Faxing of medical information has become a common occurrence and brings with it another opportunity to breach confidentiality laws. ***Safety: Just before you fax the medical record, telephone the intended recipient to inform him or her of the impending confidential fax.*** This helps to ensure that the intended recipient is present to receive the fax in an effort to prevent it from lying unattended when it is received.

> **KNOWLEDGE CONNECTION**
> To whom does the original patient medical record belong? Explain the rights of the patient regarding his or her medical record. What should you do prior to faxing a medical record?

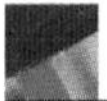

USES OF DOCUMENTATION FORMS

You will need to be familiar with various documentation forms. One piece of documentation you will use is known as an *incident report* or *variance report.* When accidents, incidents, mistakes, or anything out of the ordinary occurs, you will be required to file a written report. There are also various forms in the patient's chart that you must complete every shift. If you work in a hospital or long-term care facility, at the beginning of your shift you will receive a report from the off-going nurse about each of your assigned patients. The shift report will be discussed more thoroughly in Chapter 6, but the written notes that you should make during the shift report will be included in this chapter as a form of written documentation.

Report Form

Because your work shift will begin with an initial patient report, we will begin with the form on which you will document reported information. Most facilities have a standard report form on which to document the report you receive at the beginning of your shift. An example is shown in Figure 5.2. With an EHR in place, however, this form may be replaced by a report printout that contains the information about each patient. The notes that you take during the shift report should be detailed and all-inclusive so that they can serve as your template for scheduled duties for the coming shift if this is not provided on a printout. This form will need specific areas to document the following:

- Room number; patient name, age, and gender; and attending physician
- Date of admission and diagnoses
- Frequency of vital signs and activity orders
- Type of diet ordered, nothing-by-mouth (NPO) status, fluid restrictions, IV, or intake and output (I&O) totals
- Any diagnostics to be done and pertinent results of recent tests
- Personal care that may be needed
- All nursing care to be delivered

You will also need room to make additional notes throughout the shift as things occur. Nurses commonly refer to these notes as their "pocket-brains." Few nurses are able to accurately remember all the necessary details that should be documented and reported to the oncoming shift without some form of pocket-brains. Some nurses prefer to create a self-designed format that works best for them. Figure 5.3 shows a sample of one nurse's pocket-brain. It was designed so that only a glance was required to identify the blank lines and the times of the tasks that were to be performed. One could be made for each patient during a shift; this one, which was handwritten, could be modified when additional nursing care was in order. If you make your own, figure out what works best for you and be certain to use the same order or format for each set of patient data and draw blank lines for marking each task completed. You probably will want to save time and use computer technology to create your pocket-brain.

Safety: The ideal method to ensure documentation accuracy is to consistently chart immediately after care is provided, after assessment data are obtained, and after any event or occurrence that has the potential to affect the patient. However, the reality of documentation is that it is not always possible to chart immediately. The very patient about whom you need to document something may require other aspects of care before you can get to the chart. Other patients may have needs that are higher priority than charting. You simply get busy. However, no matter how busy you get, there are certain things that you can do to increase the accuracy of your documentation.

One thing you can do is to write a quick note on your pocket-brain right at the bedside or just outside the patient's room door, providing yourself with specific times and data that can be transcribed onto the chart as soon as possible. One might argue that to write something down and then be forced to copy or rewrite it on the chart provides another chance for error. This is true; but it also is true that, for most of us, it is safer to write notes as things happen, along with the exact time of occurrence, than to assume that we will remember everything we need to chart at some point later in the shift. We may remember what happened and think that we know the correct time it occurred. However, there are nurses who can testify to the hard lessons learned because of poor memory. It should be understood that our memories are fallible when we are trying to keep track of dozens of facts about multiple patients, especially when you throw in one or two episodes of adrenaline rush due to emergent situations. Excessive stimuli decrease the average individual's ability to recall details. A patient's improvement, even the patient's life, may be dependent on the accuracy of your documentation.

Accuracy of the time at which things occur and tasks are performed can be momentous in regard to legal action as well. It would be difficult, if not impossible, to explain from the witness chair how Patient X could have been "Lying quietly with eyes closed. Respirations even and regular at

Nursing Report

Room	Name	Dr	Diag.	Age/Sex	V. Signs	IV/Rate	FSBS	Diet	Guaiac	Tele	Tests/Notes
101		A G K M S			4 8 12		Da Bid Qid		Emesis 1 2 3 Stool 1 2 3		
102		A G K M S			4 8 12		Da Bid Qid		Emesis 1 2 3 Stool 1 2 3		
103		A G K M S			4 8 12		Da Bid Qid		Emesis 1 2 3 Stool 1 2 3		
104		A G K M S			4 8 12		Da Bid Qid		Emesis 1 2 3 Stool 1 2 3		
105		A G K M S			4 8 12		Da Bid Qid		Emesis 1 2 3 Stool 1 2 3		
107		A G K M S			4 8 12		Da Bid Qid		Emesis 1 2 3 Stool 1 2 3		
108		A G K M S			4 8 12		Da Bid Qid		Emesis 1 2 3 Stool 1 2 3		
109		A G K M S			4 8 12		Da Bid Qid		Emesis 1 2 3 Stool 1 2 3		
110		A G K M S			4 8 12		Da Bid Qid		Emesis 1 2 3 Stool 1 2 3		
111		A G K M S			4 8 12		Da Bid Qid		Emesis 1 2 3 Stool 1 2 3		
112		A G K M S			4 8 12		Da Bid Qid		Emesis 1 2 3 Stool 1 2 3		
114		A G K M S			4 8 12		Da Bid Qid		Emesis 1 2 3 Stool 1 2 3		
115		A G K M S			4 8 12		Da Bid Qid		Emesis 1 2 3 Stool 1 2 3		
116		A G K M S			4 8 12		Da Bid Qid		Emesis 1 2 3 Stool 1 2 3		
117		A G K M S			4 8 12		Da Bid Qid		Emesis 1 2 3 Stool 1 2 3		

FIGURE 5.2 A sample of a facility report form. (Courtesy of Kingfisher Regional Hospital, Kingfisher, OK.)

Rm 201	Matt Hau 54 y/o/m Dr. Evans Adm. MM/DD/YYYY
	Dx: MI Allergic: PCN
	Ordered Tests: EKG today Meds @ ~~7:30, 9,~~ 11:30, 2:00.
	IV Rt wrist, 18g, 1/2 NS @ 60 mL/hr per pump: new bag @___
	Bedrest w/ BRP ✓ Turn q 2 hrs: 8 ✓ 10 ✓ 12___ 2___
	VS @ 8 146/88 98-88irr-18 12___
	O^2 @ 4 L/M per NC con't ✓ SpO_2 @ 8 96% 12___
	Reg diet: B 75 % L___% Foley ✓
	Bedbath @ 10:30 mouth & skin care q4hr 9 ✓ 1___
	I-___mL O-___mL BMs X 1 lg soft brown

FIGURE 5.3 An example of handwritten "pocket-brains."

19/min" at 7:30 p.m., when Patient X was actually in the imaging department having magnetic resonance imaging performed from 7:10 p.m. until 7:55 p.m. It is vital that you vigilantly document things at the correct time they were done and as soon as possible after the event or task.

> **KNOWLEDGE CONNECTION**
> What is a report form? Explain the various types of data that you will document on the report form.

Incident Reports

Another type of documentation that is not part of the patient's medical record is the incident report, also known as the variance report. This report is used to document out-of-the-ordinary things that happen in a facility. The incident or occurrence may or may not actually involve a patient. Occurrences that should be documented on an incident or variance report form include the following:

- Medication error
- Patient injury
- Visitor injury
- Employee injury
- Condition constituting a safety hazard, such as an unsafe staffing situation or failure to repair reported broken or damaged equipment
- Failure of appropriate health-care provider response to an emergency
- Failure to perform ordered care
- Loss of patient's personal belongings, prosthetic or assistive devices, home medications, or secured valuables
- Lack of availability of vital patient care supplies or equipment

Some nurses feel that completion of an incident report is punitive, but that is far from the truth. In fact, the report is designed to better protect the facility, you, and the patient when something unusual occurs by providing accurate facts regarding the incident or occurrence. When completing an incident or variance report, be objective, documenting only what you were able to detect with your senses—what you saw, heard, smelled, or were able to feel with your hands. Avoid interpreting what you saw or heard, such as "Heard the patient fall from the chair to the floor." Keep it completely objective: "Heard loud crashing sound." Rather than write that the "patient fell out of bed," document only objective data such as "found patient lying face down on the floor beside the bed" and "patient reports he fell out of bed while trying to reach his telephone." ***Safety: Never document assumptions or drawn conclusions.***

Incident forms will include not only the incident but also the action taken and any care provided after the occurrence. They will have a section in which you will list any witnesses who observed the occurrence, the physician who was notified and any orders received, the signature of the employee involved or who discovered the variance, and the supervisor's signature. (See the sample incident report form in Chapter 3, Fig. 3.2.) These reports are kept separate from patient records, and they are reviewed and analyzed by facility committees according to policy and procedure. The incident or variance report provides an accurate record of what happened for use if legal action results. Most importantly, however, it helps to identify unsafe conditions or situations for which a change in the facility's policy and procedure may prevent or at least reduce the risk for repeated occurrences.

> **KNOWLEDGE CONNECTION**
> Explain why incident or variance reports are not filed with the patient's medical record. List at least five types of occurrences for which an incident or variance report should be completed.

Care Plans

Another form of written documentation is the plan of care developed for each patient, which was covered in depth in Chapter 4. The care plan serves to communicate the patient's problems, what interventions are to be performed for each problem, and the effectiveness of each intervention. Revisions and modifications to the plan of care are made and documented within the plan as the patient's changing condition warrants, providing a current plan of action for health-care providers to follow each day.

Patient Chart or Medical Record

The most lengthy and encompassing form of written documentation is the patient's chart or medical record. In long-term care facilities, you may see paper charts. However, all hospitals are now required to use EHRs. More information about documenting in a paper chart is found in the section about documenting in long-term care. For computerized documentation, be sure to follow these guidelines:

- **Avoid taking charting shortcuts.** It is tempting at times when using electronic charting to "copy and paste" either your own or another nurse's note. Your intention is to make any changes necessary to update the note without having to write the entire thing. This is, however, absolutely forbidden. This type of shortcut will look very bad in a court and says that if you will take shortcuts when documenting care, you might very well take shortcuts when providing care.

Also, avoid leaving blank spaces in the EHR, just as you would in a paper record. Use "N/A," "denies," or "not observed" to complete lines rather than leave them blank.

- **Use only approved abbreviations.** It is your responsibility to know which abbreviations and symbols may be used in your documentation and which ones may not be used. Most facilities have their own list of approved abbreviations and symbols that may be used in documentation. The Joint Commission issues National Patient Safety Goals. The commission requires that each facility have a documented standardized list of abbreviations, symbols, dose designations, and acronyms that are *not* to be used anywhere in the facility. The facility's list must include each of the items on The Joint Commission's official "Do Not Use" list (Table 5.1). Box 5.1 provides a list of commonly used health-care abbreviations.
- **Be accurate.** Make certain that all pertinent data are recorded. Be factual. Be specific. Avoid using judgmental language. Do not document your opinions, assumptions, interpretations, or self-drawn conclusions. Refrain from using subjective terms such as *strange, well, average, normal, bad, poor, odd,* or *good* because they are vague and mean different things to different people. If you want

Table 5.1
The Joint Commission's "Do Not Use" Abbreviations

Official "Do Not Use" List[1]		
Do Not Use	***Potential Problem***	***Use Instead***
U (unit)	Mistaken for "0" (zero), the number "4" (four), or "cc"	Write "unit"
IU (International Unit)	Mistaken for IV (intravenous) or the number 10 (ten)	Write "International Unit"
Q.D., QD, q.d., qd (daily) Q.O.D., QOD, q.o.d., qod (every other day)	Mistaken for each other Period after the Q mistaken for "I" and the "O" mistaken for "I"	Write "daily" Write "every other day"
Trailing zero (X.0 mg)* Lack of leading zero (.X mg)	Decimal point is missed	Write X mg Write 0.X mg
MS MSO_4 and $MgSO_4$	Can mean morphine sulfate or magnesium sulfate Confused for one another	Write "morphine sulfate" Write "magnesium sulfate"
Additional Abbreviations, Acronyms, and Symbols[2]		
> (greater than) < (less than)	Misinterpreted as the number "7" (seven) or the letter "L" Confused for one another	Write "greater than" Write "less than"
Abbreviations for drug names	Misinterpreted because of similar abbreviations for multiple drugs	Write drug names in full
Apothecary units	Unfamiliar to many practitioners Confused with metric units	Use metric units
@	Mistaken for the number "2" (two)	Write "at"
cc	Mistaken for U (units) when poorly written	Write "mL" or "milliliters"
µg	Mistaken for mg (milligrams) resulting in 1,000-fold overdose	Write "mcg" or "micrograms"

[1]Applies to all orders and all medication-related documentation that is handwritten (including free-text computer entry) or on preprinted forms.

[2]For possible future inclusion in the official "Do Not Use" List.

*Exception: A "trailing zero" may be used only where required to demonstrate the level of precision of the value being reported, such as for laboratory results, imaging studies that report size of lesions, or catheter/tube sizes. It may not be used in medication orders or other medication-related documentation.

Box 5.1
Commonly Used Health-Care Abbreviations

Abbreviations	Meaning
½NS	0.45% sodium chloride
¼NS	0.22% sodium chloride
⅓NS	0.33% sodium chloride
3%NS	3% sodium chloride
ā	before
AAO×4	awake, alert, and oriented times four spheres
abd	abdomen
ac	before meals
ADL	activities of daily living
ad lib	as patient desires
AEB	as evidenced by
AKA	above-the-knee amputation
amb	ambulate, ambulatory
amp	ampule
amt	amount
ASAP	as soon as possible
ax	axillary
BE	barium enema
bid	twice per day
BKA	below-the-knee amputation
BM	bowel movement
BMR	basal metabolic rate
BP	blood pressure
bpm	beats per minute
BR	bedrest
BRP	bathroom privileges
BSC	bedside commode
c̄	with
ca	cancer
cal	calories
cath	catheter
CBC	complete blood count
CCU	coronary care unit; critical care unit
chem.	chemistry
CHF	congestive heart failure
cm	centimeter
C/O, c/o	complained of
CO_2	carbon dioxide
CPR	cardiopulmonary resuscitation
CVA	cerebrovascular accident, stroke
CXR	chest x-ray
D5 ½NS	dextrose 5% in 0.45% sodium chloride
D5RL	dextrose 5% in lactated Ringer's solution
D5W	dextrose 5% in water
D&C	dilation and curettage
DM	diabetes mellitus
Dp Br	deep breathe
dsg or drsg	dressing
Dx	diagnosis
ECG or EKG	electrocardiogram
EEG	electroencephalogram
EENT	eyes, ears, nose, throat
ER	emergency room
ETOH	alcohol
F	female
Fr	French (diameter size measurement)
FSB	fasting blood sugar
FSBS	finger stick blood sugar
ft	foot or feet
fx	fracture
g	gram
GI	gastrointestinal
gr	grain
gtt(s)	drop/drops
GU	genitourinary
GYN	gynecology
HA	headache
Hct	hematocrit
Hgb	hemoglobin
h/o	history of
hob	head of bed
HOH	hard of hearing
H&P	history and physical
hr	hour
ht	height
HTN	hypertension
hyper	above or high
hypo	below or low
ICU	intensive care unit
ID	intradermal
IDDM	insulin-dependent diabetes mellitus
IM	intramuscular
Inj	injection
I&O	intake and output
IV	intravenous
IVP	intravenous push
IVPB	intravenous piggyback
L	liter
lb	pound
liq	liquids
LLE	left lower extremity
LLL	left lower lobe
LLQ	left lower quadrant
LMP	last menstrual period
LOC	level of consciousness
LUE	left upper extremity
LUL	left upper lobe
LUQ	left upper quadrant
med	medication
mg	milligram
mL	milliliter
MN	midnight
NAS	no added salt
NG	nasogastric
NGT	nasogastric tube
NKA	no known allergies
NKDA	no known drug allergies
noc	night
NPO	nothing by mouth
NS	0.9% sodium chloride
N/V/D	nausea, vomiting, diarrhea
O	oral

Continued

Box 5.1

Commonly Used Health-Care Abbreviations—cont'd

Abbreviations	Meaning	Abbreviations	Meaning
O_2	oxygen	RLQ	right lower quadrant
OB	obstetrics	RML	right middle lobe
OOB	out of bed	R/O	rule out
OR	operating room	Rt	right
ortho	orthopedics	RUE	right upper extremity
os	mouth or opening	RUL	right upper lobe
OT	occupational therapy	RUQ	right upper quadrant
OTC	over the counter	Rx	prescription
oz	ounce	$\bar{s}$	without
P	pulse	SCD	sequential compression device
$\bar{p}$	after	SOB	shortness of breath
pc	after meals	SpO_2	percentage of hemoglobin saturated with oxygen
PCA	patient-controlled analgesia		
PEARL	pupils equal and reactive to light	SSE	soapsuds enema
PEARLA	pupils equal and reactive to light and accommodation	stat	immediately
		STD	sexually transmitted disease
PERLA	pupils equally reactive to light and accommodation	T	temperature
		TB	tuberculosis
PERRLA	pupils equally round and reactive to light and accommodation	tid	three times per day
		TO	telephone order
PO	by mouth	TPR	temperature, pulse, respirations
PPP	peripheral pulses palpated	Tx	treatment
prn	as needed	UA	urinalysis
PT	physical therapy	VO	verbal order
q	every	VS	vital signs
qid	four times per day	WBC	white blood cell count
R	rectal	W/C	wheelchair
R	respirations	WDI	warm, dry intact
RLE	right lower extremity	WNL	within normal limits
RLL	right lower lobe	wt	weight

to chart that you think the patient is acting "strangely," describe only what you see or hear that makes you think the behavior is "strange." If you think a patient tolerated the clear liquid diet "well," think of the reasons why you think the patient tolerated it well. Was it because the patient did not experience nausea or vomiting after consumption of the first liquids allowed following being NPO? Whatever caused you to think the patient tolerated it "well" is what you should chart.

- **Be objective.** ***Safety: Do not allow your perspective or your personal feelings and emotions to be expressed in your documentation. Chart only those objective data that you can detect with your senses.***
  - What you can see, read, or observe with your eyes
  - What you can smell with your olfactory sense
  - What you can feel using your sense of touch
  - What you can hear with your ears with or without a stethoscope, which includes subjective data that the patient, family, or significant other may tell you

Refer back to Chapter 4, Box 4.2, for a description of different types of objective data. Table 5.2 lists the differences between subjective and objective entries. The only subjective data that you will chart will be things that the patient, family, or significant other tells you. When you chart direct quotations of the patient, you should use his or her *exact* words and place them in quotation marks. Correct examples of charting what the patient told you might include the following:

- States *"I have vomited everything I have eaten and drunk since yesterday."*
- Supine, holding lower abdomen with both hands. Moaning. States *"The pain is getting worse. I don't know if I can stand it or not."*

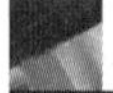

TYPES OF MEDICAL RECORDS

Each facility designates the type of system that is used to organize patient medical records. There are two basic formats: source-oriented records and problem-oriented records. Both systems may be utilized for handwritten medical records, known as hard copies, or for computerized records, which will be discussed later in this chapter.

Table 5.2
Subjective Versus Objective Entries

*Subjective Entry**	*Objective Entry*
Ate *well* and tolerated it well.	Ate 80% full liquid diet unassisted. Tolerated without nausea or vomiting.
Ate *most* of lunch. Tolerated *well.*	Fed 90% clear liquid diet by wife, who stated he swallowed easily without choking or strangling.
Worried & nervous about impending surgery. Instructed about procedure.	Sitting in chair at bedside. Tapping fingertips on arm of chair. Bouncing left leg repeatedly. Inquired if he had any questions or concerns about his surgery tomorrow. Responded by asking several questions about surgery. Sat beside him for 15–20 min: answered questions, marked surgical sites on RUQ abdomen, & explained what to expect preop & postop. Laparoscopic Cholecystectomy Patient Teaching Brochure reviewed verbally with patient & left at bedside. Encouraged to read it and ask any questions that come to mind. States he already understands better and does not feel as nervous as he did but will call if he has more questions. Posture more relaxed. No longer tapping fingers or bouncing left leg.
Wound *worse* today.	Wound measures larger than on 6-1-15. Now 2 cm × 2.5 cm. Wound bed bright red. Now draining green purulent drainage.
Had a *good* night.	1200 Left lateral position. Eyes closed. Resp reg & even. 0115 Supine. Eyes closed. Resp reg & even. 0320 Snoring softly. 0530 Assisted to bedside commode. Voided 350 mL clear, yellow urine. Assisted back to bed. 0615 Supine. Eyes closed. Resp reg & even.

**Note:* Words in *italics* are subjective terms.

Source-Oriented Records

Source-oriented medical records are organized according to the source or type of data, using specific forms for each, with each section designated by a labeled tab. The various health-care providers and staff members will enter their data under the corresponding tab. For example, the physician will write treatment orders in the *Physician's Orders* section and notes about how the patient is doing in the *Physician's Progress Notes* section. A physical therapist would document his or her notes about rehabilitation strength training in the *Rehabilitation Therapy* section. However, while most other disciplines will make entries in only one or two sections, as a nurse you will document in multiple sections of the chart.

Typical Sections of the Source-Oriented Medical Record

Table 5.3 presents a list of the typical sections found in a source-oriented medical record. Note that the sections marked with asterisks are the various areas in which you, the nurse, will document. Most of these section labels are somewhat self-explanatory as to the type of information that is located there, making it easy to locate specific data such as a new physician's order or the results of the chest x-ray, which is an advantage of this system. However, because several members of other disciplines also may be caring for the patient, there may be information related to a patient problem spread out in several different sections of the medical record. If you have to scan the entire record in search of all of the data, it can be a time-consuming task, which is a distinct disadvantage. For example, a patient with diabetes admitted for treatment of pneumonia most likely will be receiving care or services from one or more physicians and nurses, as well as from respiratory therapy, radiology, the pharmacy, the laboratory, dietary services, and possibly physical therapy. When searching for information about the patient's gas exchange and whether it is improving, you would have to look in several sections of the record to locate all the data regarding the patient's gas exchange. Look at the following:

- **Nurse's notes** for latest assessment of breath sounds, characteristics of respirations, amount and color of sputum production, response to medications, and frequency of use and effectiveness of supplemental oxygen
- **Health-care provider's progress notes** for latest report of improvement or decline in the patient's condition
- **Vital signs** for temperature, pulse, and respiratory rate trends, as well as oxygen saturation levels
- **Rehabilitation therapy** for the number of respiratory therapy treatments given and their effectiveness

• WORD • BUILDING •
rehabilitation: re – again + habilitat – make able + ion – action

Table 5.3
Sections of the Source-Oriented Medical Record

Sections	*Type Information*
Admission Record *You may assist with record completion in certain circumstances.	*Demographic data,* including patient name, age, address, telephone number, and religious preference; next of kin and contact information; and occupation and employer's name and address *Personal identification data,* including birth date, Social Security number, and photo ID; insurance data; permission to treat and permission to disclose patient medical data to insurance company and specified individuals; hospital identification number; and admitting medical diagnoses
Advance Directive	Each patient must be asked if he or she has an advance directive such as a living will; any instructions regarding the extent to which the patient wishes to be provided medical care
*Surgical and Procedure Consents	Any signed consent forms for surgery or invasive procedures
Physician's Orders *You may write verbal orders.	Orders for treatments, medications, diet, procedures, care to be performed, activity level to be allowed
*Graphic Data	Vital sign graph, I&O record, weights
*Care Flow Sheet	Form on which check marks or brief entries are made regarding percentage diet consumed, type of bath, activity level, ROM exercise, repositioning intervals, number of bowel movements, Foley care, oral care, use of assistive devices, and safety measures such as raised bed rails, height of bed, and activation of bed brakes
*Care Plan	Plan of care identifying specific prioritized patient problems, interventions for them, and effectiveness of interventions; may include interdisciplinary contributions in addition to nursing's contributions
*Nurse's Notes	Chronological record of patient problems and condition along with the nursing care provided and the effectiveness of interventions
Laboratory Results	Results of laboratory tests run on blood or other body fluids or tissues
X-Ray (or Radiological) Results	Results of x-rays
Consultation Reports	Reports by consulting physicians
History and Physical	Physician's initial assessment of body systems on admission; includes medical diagnoses, past illnesses and surgeries, patient complaints and reason for seeking medical care, and medications patient has been taking at home
Surgical Reports *You will complete postanesthesia notes	Reports of all surgeries performed during this hospitalization, explanation of anesthesia administered, description of actual surgical procedure, and post anesthesia or recovery room record
Rehabilitation Therapy	Any physical, respiratory, occupational, or speech therapy administered along with patient's response and progress
*Medication Administration Record	Lists of administered medications, dosages, route, date, time, and nurse who administered each; only the records for previous days are kept in the chart; the current day's record is kept in a separate medication administration book
Physician's Progress Notes	Physician's notes regarding patient progress and responses to treatment
*Discharge Planning	Data from social services, case managers, home health-care agencies, and discharge planners

**Note:* Sections marked with asterisks are the various areas in which the nurse will document.

- **MAR** for the number of as-needed (prn) doses of cough medication that was required in the last 24 hours and which antibiotic has been administered
- **Laboratory results** for the latest white blood cell count, hemoglobin level, and sputum culture and sensitivity results
- **X-ray results** for latest chest x-ray results

Problem-Oriented Records

Problem-oriented records differ from source-oriented records in that they are organized around the patient's individual problems rather than where the data came from, as in the source-oriented system.

Sections of the Problem-Oriented Medical Record

The problem-oriented medical record will have four primary sections:

1. Database
2. Problem list
3. Plan of care
4. Progress notes

Additional forms, such as a flow sheet or discharge summary sheet, may be used according to the facility's policy. Table 5.4 provides an explanation of data to be included in each of these sections of the problem-oriented medical record.

The primary advantage of problem-oriented record-keeping is that it encourages collaboration between all the disciplines providing care to the patient. All the health-care providers contribute to the same database, problem list, plan of care, and progress notes. Working together, a plan of care is determined, listing the patient problems and potential patient problems chronologically as they are identified. Another advantage is that the list of patient problems is kept at the front of the chart, where it is easily accessed without thumbing through the entire chart. The fact that all health-care providers write their progress notes chronologically in the same *progress notes* section allows for quick retrieval of all entries of the involved disciplines regarding the patient's responses to treatments.

KNOWLEDGE CONNECTION

List the common sections of a source-oriented chart. Describe types of data that might be found within those sections. What are the four sections of a problem-oriented chart?

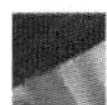

DATA TO DOCUMENT

The types of data that you will be expected to document will vary depending on the facility in which you are working. In an acute care hospital setting, you would chart data for the following categories:

- Physical and emotional assessment
- Nutrition
- Hygiene
- Activity level
- Physician's visits

Table 5.4
Sections of Problem-Oriented Medical Record

Section	*Type Data*
Database	*Demographic data,* including patient name, age, address, telephone number, religious preference; next of kin and contact information; and occupation and employer's name and address *Personal identification data,* including birth date, Social Security number, photo ID; insurance data; permission to treat and permission to disclose patient medical data to insurance company and specified individuals; hospital identification number; and admitting medical diagnoses *Assessments,* including physician's history and physical and nursing's initial assessment Results of diagnostic tests, including laboratory tests and x-rays *Patient's current condition*
Problem list	Derived from the information in the database, a chronological (but not prioritized) list of potential and actual patient problems is developed; updated as problems resolve or worsen, or new problems appear; problems are numbered and kept at front of chart; these numbers are used to reference the specific problem when making an entry in the plan of care or progress notes
Plan of care	For each listed problem: physician's orders, nursing orders and plan of care, and interdisciplinary interventions are listed, including diagnostics, therapeutic plan, and teaching
Progress notes	Organized according to problem list; all disciplines chart on the same progress notes, numbering each entry to correspond with the problem list

- Elimination (both bowel and bladder)
- All nursing care and interventions, including
  - Patient teaching
  - Discharge planning
- Patient's response to each intervention
- All patient complaints
- Safety issues
- Laboratory tests, x-rays, or other diagnostic tests that were done

Box 5.2 lists specific information to be charted for each category.

KNOWLEDGE CONNECTION

Explain what types of daily activities should be documented in the medical record. List at least 2 examples of data that might be found in each of the 11 categories listed.

Box 5.2

Specific Data to Be Charted by Category

Assessment

- Initial shift assessment done at the beginning of your shift to be used as a baseline.
- Any abnormal assessment findings that must be reassessed later in the shift.

Nutrition

- Type of diet.
- How much the patient eats, such as 25%, 50%, 85%, or 100%. If 50% or less, include an assessment of why the patient ate such a small amount. Was there nausea or pain? Did the patient simply not like what was served? Was he or she simply *anorexic* (not hungry)? Did someone bring the patient a burger from the local drive-in?
- How was the diet tolerated: was there nausea, vomiting, indigestion, reflux, gas, or belching? Did the patient have difficulty swallowing? It is important to document if the patient required any assistance to eat.
- Did the patient consume any snacks during the shift? If so, what and how much?
- Is the patient drinking adequate fluids? Is the patient on I&O? Was the patient instructed to record I&O?

Hygiene

- What type of bath was given: bed bath, partial sponge bath, tub bath, or shower?
- Did the patient require assistance, or was he or she able to bathe himself or herself?
- Was mouth care provided by you or performed by the patient? How often?
- Was a back rub performed?
- Was hair care, nail care, shaving, or skin care done?
- What was the patient's response to the hygiene? Did he or she state it made him or her feel better? Or did it make him or her more short of breath?
- Was the patient's skin clean, fresh, and intact? Were any lesions or other problems noted?

Activity Level

- Is the patient on bedrest? Is he or she ambulatory without assistance or with assistance? If assistance is required, how many people are needed to ambulate the patient? Or can the patient only be gotten up for BRP or to sit in a chair?
- Were range-of-motion exercises performed? Active or passive? To which extremities and how often?
- Was the patient logrolled? Or gotten up with the Hoyer lift? How did he or she tolerate the activity? Did the patient become short of breath? Did the pulse rate go from 66 to 110? Did the knees begin to buckle, or did the patient become unsteady?

Physician Visits

- Did a physician see or examine the patient on your shift? If so, who?
- Did the physician remove clips from an incision? Were new orders written?
- Did you have to telephone or communicate data to a physician? If so, what information was reported and what orders were received?

Elimination

- Is the patient continent or incontinent of bowel and/or bladder?
- When was the patient's last bowel movement? Voiding?
- What is the color, clarity, and amount (if on I&O) of urine?
- Did the patient have any complaints, such as burning or frequency?
- If there is a Foley catheter, additional information must be noted as well: Is the catheter patent, is the catheter secured to the leg, and what is the total urine output for the shift?
- What was the color, amount, and consistency of bowel movements? Are there patient complaints of gas *(flatulence)* or cramping?

Note: If there was no BM during your shift, a note indicating no BM should be made at the end of the shift. This makes it easier to track whether the patient has a bowel movement at least every 3 days.

Nursing Care (Implementation Step of Nursing Process)

Any care that you administer must be objectively documented, such as:

- Assisting to turn, cough, and deep breathe
- Changing an IV rate
- Inserting a Foley catheter
- Emptying a Jackson-Pratt drain
- Performing a back rub
- Providing mouth care or skin care
- Administering any one-time meds or prn meds
- Initiating an IV infusion
- Converting an IV line to a PRN lock
- Instilling a PEG tube feeding

Includes patient teaching and discharge planning, such as foot care or insulin administration for a diabetic patient, the use

Box 5.2

Specific Data to Be Charted by Category—cont'd

of patient-controlled analgesia (PCA), wound or incision care, and how to change a dressing.

Patient's Response to Interventions (Evaluation Step of Nursing Process)

How did the patient respond to your intervention, whether it was an assessment of vital signs or the insertion of a Foley catheter? For example, take the intervention of vital signs assessment. What was the patient's response? His pulse was 88, regular and distinct. His temp was 102.4°F. His BP was 138/76. These are his body's physical responses to assessing these areas.

What might be an evaluation of insertion of a Foley catheter? It could be, "550 mL cloudy, amber urine returned—states she feels much better now" or "only 75 mL clear, light yellow urine returned."

If you turn, cough, and deep breathe a patient, the response might be something like "good cough effort, productive of large amount greenish-yellow sputum" or maybe "poor cough effort, cough is nonproductive, only performs coughing & deep breathing exercises when encouraged by nurse."

If you elevate the head of the bed to ease dyspnea, what might be a response from the patient? A couple of possibilities are, "respirations less labored when head of bed is elevated" or "color pink, respiratory rate 27/min, no complaints of shortness of breath."

There is always a patient response to each intervention we perform, and we must chart them.

Safety Issues

These include the bed in a low position, the status of bed rails, suction machine available at bedside, call light within reach, and use of Hoyer lift with three assistants. Also includes such patient instructions to call for assistance before getting out of bed because of possible unsteadiness due to medication, use of shower chair for taking a shower, and numerous other interventions taken to keep the patient from harm.

Laboratory and Diagnostic Testing

Document when a patient is taken to another department for tests or treatments. Include how the patient was transported: did he or she walk, ride in a wheelchair, or go on a gurney? For example: "to radiology via W/C for a CXR." "Returned from MRI via gurney."

All Patient Complaints

This includes any complaints, such as pain, nausea, dizziness, anxiety, fear, tingling, or itching, or that he or she does not like the ordered diet.

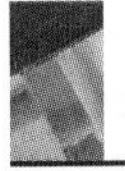

METHODS OF RECORDING PATIENT INFORMATION

While each EHR system has its own method for accessing an area for narrative charting, most routine documentation is done in a "select and click" format.

When additional documentation is required, such as deviations from normal that need to be explained, each facility may have its own preferred method for recording that information. Table 5.5 shows some methods used in paper charting that may be employed in EHR for more detail about a patient's care.

Laboratory and Diagnostic Connection

Your Laboratory and Diagnostic Documentation Responsibilities

Even though you do not normally write the results of very many laboratory and diagnostic tests, you are responsible for monitoring the results of those tests ordered for your assigned patients and documenting whether or not you:

- Notified the physician of the results
- Explained the results to the patient
- Took any other action related to the test results

Because of this responsibility, you must be able to identify when results fall outside the normal range, making the result abnormal. You also must be able to differentiate when an abnormally high or low result has reached the *critical value level*. Your responsibility is not limited to monitoring and reporting results to the physician, however; you must be able to discern when a test result requires that you intervene, such as withholding a medication or treatment, even before you notify the physician. The documentation of performance of appropriate interventions and physician notification is important to protect you legally.

Narrative Charting

It is very important for all nurses to know how to perform narrative charting. **Narrative charting** tells the story of a patient's experiences during their hospital stay. It is written in chronological order and relates the patient's health status from admission through all changes in condition, up to and including their discharge status. It provides a continual description of the patient's condition, complaints, and problems; assessment findings of all systems, activities, treatments, and nursing care provided; and the evaluations of effectiveness for each nursing intervention. It provides more details than most charting styles and a better time line of the patient's changing condition,

• WORD • BUILDING •

chronological: chrono – time + logic – reason + al – related to

Table 5.5
Methods of Charting

Method	*Description*
SOAP/SOAPIER	Can be used with source-oriented or problem-oriented records. Stands for Subjective data, Objective data, Assessment data, Plan/Intervention, Evaluation, and Revision
PIE	Addresses patient's problems and what is done to solve them. Seen mostly in nurse's notes. Stands for Problem, Intervention, and Evaluation
Focus	Focused on patient and less structured than PIE. A common type is DAR, which stands for data, action, and response
Narrative	No set formula is followed; rather, the health-care professional writes a detailed account of the care the patient receives and events that occur in chronological order Most thorough but most time-consuming type of documentation
Charting by Exception	Notes written by health-care providers that focus only on abnormal findings; normal findings are not charted, and checklists are used for routine care Works best with EHR

especially during life-threatening emergencies such as cardiac and respiratory arrests.

Imagine you are working a 12-hour shift from 7:00 a.m. to 7:00 p.m. in a facility that uses the narrative charting style. After you have completed and documented the initial shift assessment, your next couple of entries might look something like the following example. Note that facilities use military time to decrease confusion between a.m. and p.m.:

06/23/22 0755 C/O RUQ abdomen pain at 6 on scale of 0–10. Still NPO. IV 1/2NS 100 mL infusing per pump in Lt. dorsal hand. Site without erythema or edema. C/O dry mouth. Mucous membranes pink, intact, dry. ——————————————— Nurse's signature and credentials

06/23/22 0805 Demerol 100 mg IM administered Rt. ventral gluteal. Mouth care & lip moisturizer provided. Instructed to call for assistance before getting up. R/T drug may cause drowsiness or dizziness. 2 rails up. Bed in low, locked position. Call light within reach. ——————————————— Nurse's signature and credentials

06/23/22 0845 Dr. Taylor here. New orders received to begin clear liquids & ambulate 4 times per day. ——————————————— Nurse's signature and credentials

Box 5.3 presents an example of narrative charting for a typical 8-hour day shift.

Patient Teaching Connection

Documenting Patient Teaching

You will find that you need to perform patient teaching in most types of nursing. It is important to document the teaching needs of the patient, the specific information that was taught, the methods utilized to teach the information, and the effectiveness of your teaching. For example, did you assess the patient's learning needs? Did he or she know pieces of the necessary information, or did you need to teach everything about the subject? Was the patient literate and able to read English? (This is pertinent, especially if English is a second language for the patient.) Did the patient have sensory deficits that required the use of specific teaching methods? Did you ask the patient how he or she preferred to learn, or was there one style of teaching format that worked better than others? What methods did you use to teach the information? Did you use only verbal explanation as your method of teaching, or did you also use pamphlets or charts? Did you use a video or other multimedia method? Did you actually demonstrate the skill or process being taught? Exactly what facts did you teach? For example, what did you teach the patient about "good nutrition for diabetics"? Did you determine the effectiveness of your teaching? How did you evaluate the patient's or family's understanding of the information taught?

Note: Some state nurse practice acts require licensed practical nurses (LPNs)/licensed vocational nurses (LVNs) to use an established teaching plan, or a plan that has been approved by a registered nurse (RN), to perform patient teaching. Complex patient teaching subjects are to be taught by the RN.

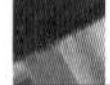

ELECTRONIC HEALTH RECORDS

A law signed by President Barack Obama mandated that the health-care industry participate in the development of computerized patient records that could be utilized by all health-care facilities by 2016. To see an example of computerized/electronic documentation, refer to Figure 5.4.

Box 5.3

An Example of Narrative Documentation for a "Typical Day"

This is the verbal shift report you received at 0615 when you came on duty:

Luddy Julius, a 54-year-old male, a patient of Dr. Evans, was admitted at 0120 with a diagnosis of bacterial pneumonia and a secondary diagnosis of dehydration. He has a history of hypertension and gastroesophageal reflux disease. He presented in the ER with severe shortness of breath and stated that he had been coughing up quite a bit of thick yellow sputum for 3 days. He also stated he had been vomiting and unable to keep anything down for the past 24 hours and that he last urinated approximately 9 hours prior to admission. Admission vital signs were BP 102/58, temperature 102.6°F, pulse 105, respirations 33, and oxygen saturation 87%. Mucous membranes were pale and dry, and his lips were cracking. His skin was flushed, hot, and dry. Breath sounds were diminished in both lower lobes and almost nonexistent in the right lower lobe. Crackles were heard in the left upper lobe and both crackles and inspiratory wheezes in the right upper and middle lobes. He was dyspneic and using accessory respiratory muscles. We applied oxygen 6 liters per minute via nasal cannula and oxygen saturation was up to 90% by 0155. Respiratory therapy gave him a handheld nebulizer treatment with DuoNeb. His dyspnea improved, respiratory rate went down to 25. I started an IV of 1,000 mL of 0.45% normal saline with 20 mEq of potassium chloride in his left forearm with a 20-gauge intracath. It's infusing at 125 mL/hr via IV pump. At 0210, I gave him guaifenesin with codeine cough syrup 10 mL orally for his cough and Tylenol 650 mg orally for fever. At 0545 his temperature was 101.8°F and respirations 26. At 0615 his eyes were closed and respirations were regular but shallow at 25 per minute. He still has had no urinary output. His breath sounds were the same except with slightly less wheezing in the right upper and middle lobes, still minimal breath sounds in the right base.

The narrative documentation for the day shift might look something like this:

0720 BP - 136/74, T - 102.6°F, P - 92, R - 32, SpO_2 - 92% on O_2 4 L/min per NC
Productive cough with yellow sputum at intervals. States he slept couple hrs after cough med. Tylenol 650 mg administered PO for fever. ---------- M. Monett, RN

0745 AAO × 4, PEARL, skin pale, hot, dry, & nonelastic. Cool wet cloth applied to forehead. Conjunctiva pink. Mucous membranes pale & dry, lips cracking. Mouth care performed. Speech clear & appropriate. No neck vein distention. Slightly dyspneic, using accessory respiratory muscles. C/O SOB but states it has improved since admission. Elevated HOB 30 degrees. Lungs auscultated, coarse crackles in all lobes except RML & RLL, where there are no breath sounds. O_2 at 4 L/min per NC. SpO_2 92%. Deep breathed & coughed × 10; productive of lg amt thick yellow sputum. Apical-radial pulse strong & equal at 92. Emptied urinal of 180 mL cloudy amber urine. States last BM was yesterday morning. Abdomen is flat, soft, and nontender to palpation. Active bowel sounds in all 4 quadrants. IV 1,000 mL 1/2NS with 20 mEq KCl infusing Lt. forearm at 125 mL/hr per pump, site free of erythema, edema, & no c/o tenderness at site. PPP strong & equal bilaterally × 4 extremities. Extremities pink & warm with brisk cap refill × 4, no edema. Strong hand grips bilaterally. Strong plantar & dorsal flexion bilaterally. No limitations of ROM detected. Call light within reach. Bed left in low position. Instructed to drink a glass of fluid every hour to help with rehydration and fever. Explained how to record I&O. Verbalized understanding. Requested a soft drink, provided. ------------------ J. Ludwig, RN

0815 Ate 45% ADA diet without N/V. Drank soft drink, juice, & coffee. -------------- M. Monett, RN

0835 Dr. Imagod here to see pt. No new orders.---------- -------------- M. Monett, RN

0850 Assisted to bathroom, voided 120 mL cloudy, amber urine. A little weak and unsteady. Back to bed with 1 assist. Drank 240 mL. ------------ M. Monett, RN

0930 C/O fatigue & not feeling good enough to take shower. Bed bath, mouth & skin care given. States feels "lots better after bath." Encouraged to drink. Requested coffee, provided & drank 150 mL. ----------- M. Monett, RN

1010 To radiology via W/C for CXR. ------------------- --------- M. Monett, RN

1025 Returned from x-ray via W/C. No change in respiratory status. ---------------- J. Ludwig, RN

1135 BP - 152/82, T - 101.4°F, P - 91, R - 23. C/O chest discomfort R/T coughing, 5 on scale of 0-10. Ibuprofen 400 mg given PO. Drinking fluids without N/V. ------------------ -------- M. Monett, RN

1225 States pain at 2. T - 100.6°F. Assisted to chair. Dp Br × 10, with good effort & productive of yellow sputum. IV site unchanged. ------------- M. Monett, RN

1245 Ate only a few bites reg diet. Drank 500 mL fluids. States is just "not hungry." No complaints of nausea. IV site without erythema or edema. ------- M. Monett, RN

1420 Assisted to bathroom, voided 180 mL clear, dark amber urine. Became dyspneic, R - 31 and slightly irreg. Assisted back to bed. O_2 reapplied at 4 L/min per NC. O_2 sats 89%. After 4-5 min, O_2 sats 92%, T - 100.6°F, P - 87 reg & strong, R - 29 shallow, states dyspnea better. Skin & mucous membranes pale. ------------- M. Monett, RN

1450 Eyes closed, resp shallow & reg. IV site unchanged from 1245. In total - 1,700 mL (IV - 950 mL, Oral - 750 mL); out - 490 mL. Wife at bedside. Rails up × 2. Bed low position. ----------------- M. Monett, RN

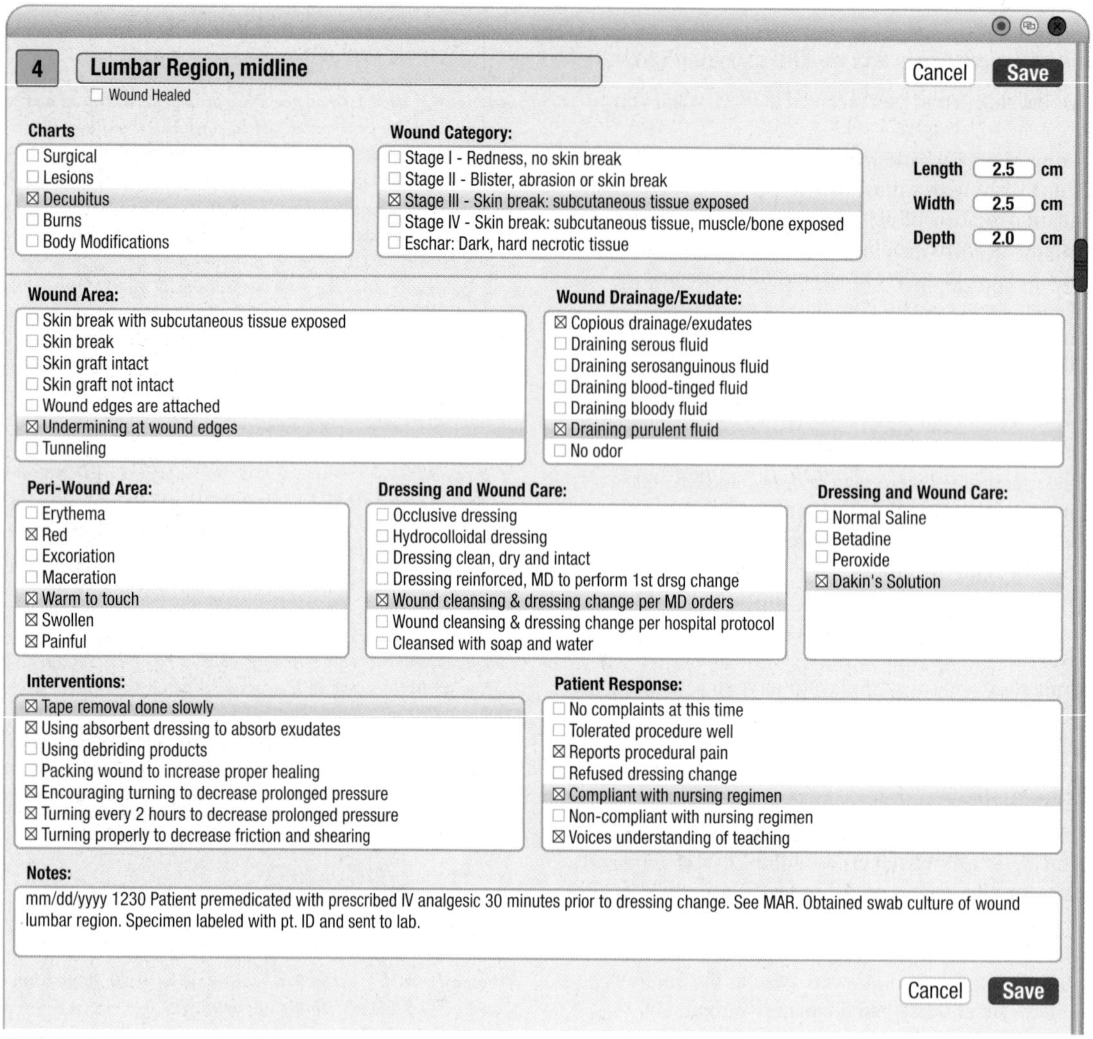

4 Lumbar Region, midline

☐ Wound Healed

Cancel Save

Charts
☐ Surgical
☐ Lesions
☒ Decubitus
☐ Burns
☐ Body Modifications

Wound Category:
☐ Stage I - Redness, no skin break
☐ Stage II - Blister, abrasion or skin break
☒ Stage III - Skin break: subcutaneous tissue exposed
☐ Stage IV - Skin break: subcutaneous tissue, muscle/bone exposed
☐ Eschar: Dark, hard necrotic tissue

Length 2.5 cm
Width 2.5 cm
Depth 2.0 cm

Wound Area:
☐ Skin break with subcutaneous tissue exposed
☐ Skin break
☐ Skin graft intact
☐ Skin graft not intact
☐ Wound edges are attached
☒ Undermining at wound edges
☐ Tunneling

Wound Drainage/Exudate:
☒ Copious drainage/exudates
☐ Draining serous fluid
☐ Draining serosanguinous fluid
☐ Draining blood-tinged fluid
☐ Draining bloody fluid
☒ Draining purulent fluid
☐ No odor

Peri-Wound Area:
☐ Erythema
☒ Red
☐ Excoriation
☐ Maceration
☒ Warm to touch
☒ Swollen
☒ Painful

Dressing and Wound Care:
☐ Occlusive dressing
☐ Hydrocolloidal dressing
☐ Dressing clean, dry and intact
☐ Dressing reinforced, MD to perform 1st drsg change
☒ Wound cleansing & dressing change per MD orders
☐ Wound cleansing & dressing change per hospital protocol
☐ Cleansed with soap and water

Dressing and Wound Care:
☐ Normal Saline
☐ Betadine
☐ Peroxide
☒ Dakin's Solution

Interventions:
☒ Tape removal done slowly
☒ Using absorbent dressing to absorb exudates
☐ Using debriding products
☐ Packing wound to increase proper healing
☒ Encouraging turning to decrease prolonged pressure
☒ Turning every 2 hours to decrease prolonged pressure
☒ Turning properly to decrease friction and shearing

Patient Response:
☐ No complaints at this time
☐ Tolerated procedure well
☒ Reports procedural pain
☐ Refused dressing change
☒ Compliant with nursing regimen
☐ Non-compliant with nursing regimen
☒ Voices understanding of teaching

Notes:
mm/dd/yyyy 1230 Patient premedicated with prescribed IV analgesic 30 minutes prior to dressing change. See MAR. Obtained swab culture of wound lumbar region. Specimen labeled with pt. ID and sent to lab.

Cancel Save

FIGURE 5.4 An example of electronic documentation.

What Is an Electronic Health Record?

An EHR is defined as a record of an individual's lifetime health information and is easily updated and transferable. EHRs are used to document patients' interactions with the health-care system, as well as to record tests, appointments and medications, signs and symptoms, diseases, immunizations, and allergies. The nurse's documentation in an EHR can significantly improve the quality of patient care by reducing errors, emphasizing a patient's needs and problems, and providing communication for all health-care staff caring for a patient.

Protecting Confidentiality of EHR

When you are planning or providing care for patients, electronic access to software tools for patient care plans, medication administration, and patient teaching is beneficial. The information you need to care for your patient is available at your fingertips.

To access EHR you will need a user ID and a password assigned to you by your facility. A patient's health record is password protected so that it cannot be viewed by unauthorized staff. It is your responsibility to keep both your user ID and password in a safe place so it cannot be used by others. If you allow another nurse to use your ID and password, you could be guilty of violating confidentiality. You could be subject to civil and criminal penalties, and you could also be fired from your facility. Computer systems can be hacked into illegally, which puts patient information at risk for unauthorized access. Security and confidentiality of medical records are a major concern. Secure passwords must be changed at regular intervals. As a student, you may be given a password, and, if so, you must guard your password closely. ***Safety: Never allow any other individual to see or use your password to access patient records for any reason.*** As with all medical records, you must remember that a nurse only has access to those records of patients for whom the nurse is caring. A computer password does not give you permission to access the records of other patients for whom you are not providing care. This applies to the medical records of your friends and family members as well.

Learning to Use EHR

Interacting with employees via email, documenting the change in a patient's condition in an EHR nurse's note, and completing a health assessment on the computer are common tasks of nurses. Some nurses, however, are not as confident using technology as others and may avoid thorough documentation for that reason. Unfortunately, this can cause inconsistency in the quality of patient care and can pose major problems within the department, not to mention potential harm to the patients. As with documenting on paper, the misuse of electronic medical records, medication records, and nursing documentation (i.e., assessments and care plans) can have an adverse effect on the outcome of the patient's care. Now that EHRs have expanded to clinics, physician offices, nursing homes, laboratories, and pharmacies, there needs to be further research conducted to identify what necessary updates and enhancements are needed for facilities to provide higher-quality health care.

Most facilities using computerized charting have computer stations at various locations in each patient hall as well as at the nurse's station. Other facilities may use bedside terminals (Fig. 5.5). This enables entries to be made right at the bedside, which is a great advantage and helps to reduce documentation errors and omissions. Other examples of computerized charting can be found in Figures 5.6 and 5.7.

When you have completed documenting on a patient's EHR, you must remember to log out. Otherwise, another person can change or add documentation to the patient's health record under your name. ***Safety: Always log out as soon as you have completed your documentation to prevent the chance of others documenting under your name.***

Additional Uses for EHR

In addition to being a record of the patient's health needs and care, EHRs help contribute to the development of evidence-based practice. The records can be a source of research to determine causes or contributing factors regarding adverse events, such as medication errors or falls.

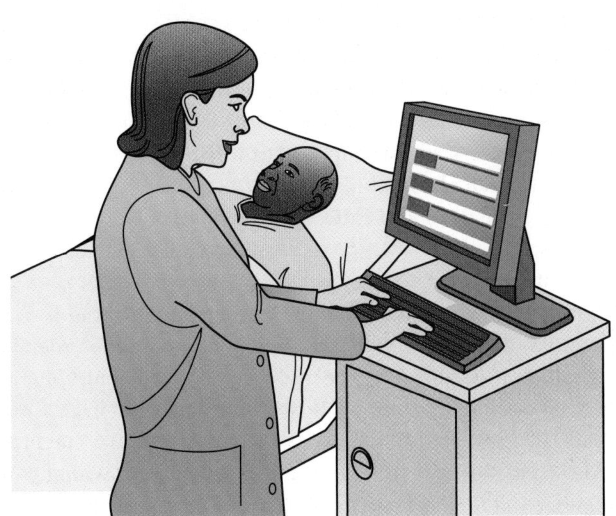

FIGURE 5.5 Point-of-access computing: A bedside terminal.

For example, information collected about the incidence of falls on a nursing unit might show a pattern of falls occurring mostly at night and on the weekends when the staff-to-patient ratio is the lowest. The staff of the nursing unit could then meet to review the findings and brainstorm ways to improve outcomes for patients by decreasing falls. In this example, the staff might determine that having one more CNA on the 7 p.m. to 7 a.m. shift on weekends would help decrease the incidence of falls. After approval to increase staff, the incidence of falls does decrease significantly. The staff on the nursing unit thus demonstrate a difference in positive patient outcomes using EHR to research and institute evidence-based practices.

EHRs also provide a way for the health-care community to collect and share information and to identify needs based on trends seen in electronic health records. For example, collecting data and information about patient illnesses and care can lead to more effective care, a better use of evidence-based practices, and identifying the need for staff continuing education.

KNOWLEDGE CONNECTION

Explain what an EHR is and how it is used. How is confidentiality of information in an EHR protected? What are other uses for EHRs in addition to documenting patient care? How can nurses stay current regarding EHRs?

Continuing Education

The field of nursing changes frequently and so does health-care technology. Nurses at all levels of training and education are expected to be able to both input patient information into and retrieve patient information from the EHR. All health-care providers, including nurses, should participate in annual training in order to keep up with advances in health-care technology.

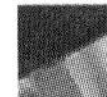

LONG-TERM CARE DOCUMENTATION

Because long-term care facilities are not yet required by law to use EHR exclusively, many continue to use paper charts while some are moving slowly toward electronic formats.

In long-term care, documentation frequency is different than in acute care. What to document and how to document it remain similar in both settings. Some aspects of documentation and communication without computers include the use of a Kardex, paper charts, and handwritten documentation. In addition, the assessment for long-term care differs dramatically from acute care.

Kardexes

Some long-term care facilities use a **Kardex,** which contains written data and is used for quick reference about each resident's care. The Kardex page lists all the care that should be provided for that specific resident. It places the physician's orders and the nursing orders for each resident on a single

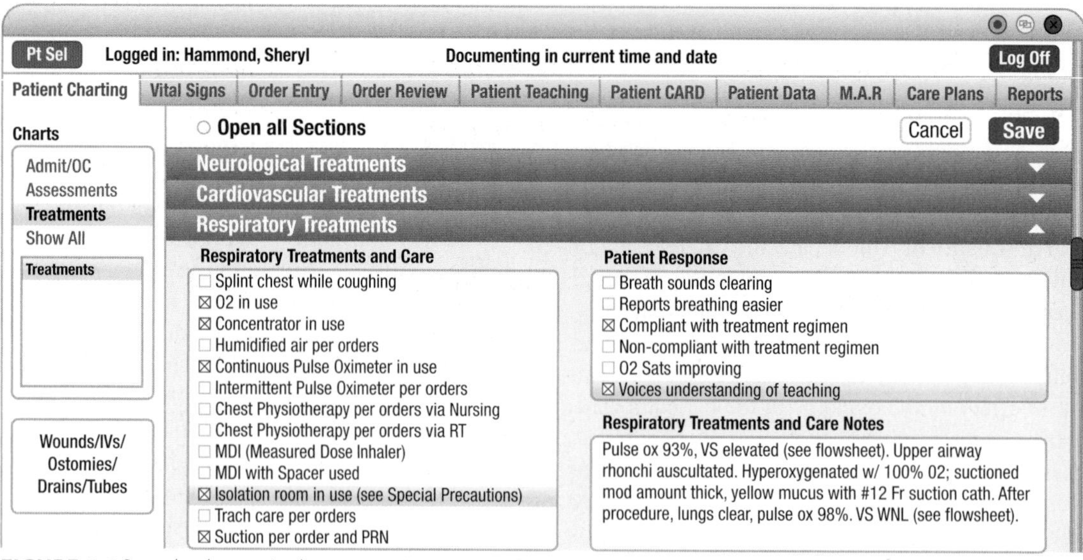

FIGURE 5.6 Sample electronic documentation.

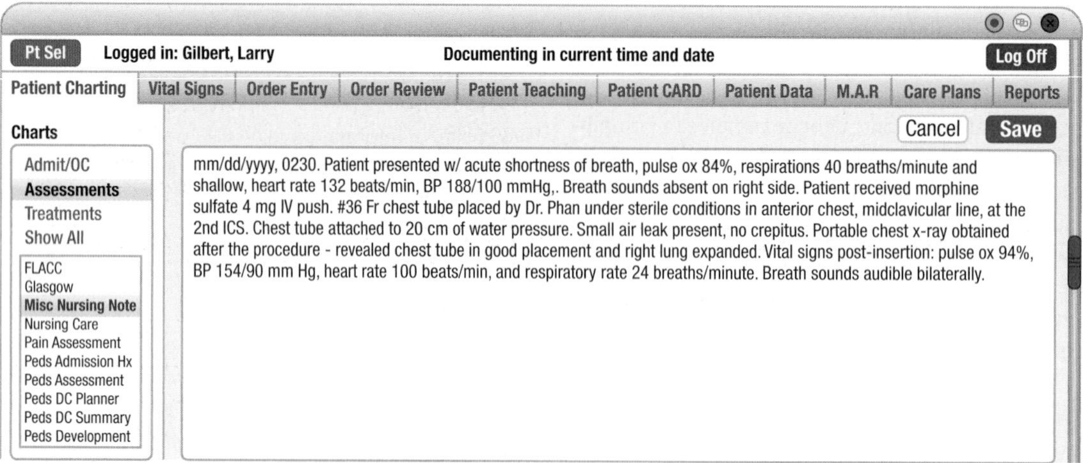

FIGURE 5.7 Sample electronic documentation.

page where it can be retrieved or referred to quickly without having to go through an entire patient chart or medical record. Basic patient data and all physician's and nursing orders are noted along with the date ordered (Fig. 5.8).

> **KNOWLEDGE CONNECTION**
> Describe what is meant by a Kardex form.

Guidelines for Paper Documentation

There are various guidelines that should direct your documentation in an effort to produce a more accurate, objective, complete, and reliable record of the patient's changing condition, the nursing care you provided, and the effectiveness of that care. If you are in a long-term setting with paper charts in use, follow these guidelines for documenting in a paper chart.

- **Use black or blue ink.** Avoid using pencil, erasable ink, or colored inks such as purple, red, or green.
- **Write neatly and legibly.** If your cursive writing is not legible, print your notes. If you always remember that the chart is a *legal* document, it may help motivate you to keep it readable.
- **Sign each entry.** Always sign each entry with your first initial, last name, and credentials according to the facility's policy. A registered nurse signs RN and a licensed practical or vocational nurse signs LPN or LVN. Your signature must be legible.
- **Include the date and time with each entry.** Remember, facilities use military time to decrease confusion between a.m. and p.m. (Fig. 5.9).
- **Follow chronological order.** Documentation should begin at the start of your shift and continue in the order in which it occurs. Use specific times for each entry. Avoid documenting in blocks of time, such as "from 0830 to 1230."
- **Make entries in a timely manner.** ***Safety: Document all assessment findings and the care provided as soon as possible after the occurrence. If you are unable to document on***

DOCTOR'S ORDERS

Activity *MM/DD/YYYY increase activity daily*

- ☐ Bedrest
- ☒ BRP
- ☐ Dangle
- ☒ Ambulate *T/D*
- ☐ Up in Chair
- ☐ Up ad lib
- ☒ TCDpBr q2º
- ☐ BSC only

DATE	ORDER
MM/DD/YYYY	*TED*
MM/DD/YYYY	*Chg. abd drsg daily*
MM/DD/YYYY	*DC foley in AM*

PROSTHESIS
X Dentures
X Hearing Aide
__ Contact Lens
X Glasses
__ Limb ______
__ Eye ______ Rt. ______ Lt.

HOME MEDICATIONS
X None with Pt. (Home)
__ In Room With Pt.
__ In Pharmacy
__ In Drug Cart

BATH/HYGIENE
X Bed X Complete
__ Tub __ Assist
__ Shower __ Self
__ Sizt X Mouth Care
______ X Skin Care

BLADDER/BOWEL
__ Independent
X Foley
__ Straight Cath.
__ Incontinent
__ BSC
__ Ostomy ______

SMOKER
☐ Yes ☒ No

DIET

Date	Type
MM/DD/YYYY	*NPO*
MM/DD/YYYY	*Full liq*

☒ Assist ☒ Set up
☐ Self ☐ Feed

FLUIDS
X I/O
__ Force Fluids
__ Restrict Fluids
7–3 ______
3–11 ______
11–7 ______

SAFETY PRECAUTIONS
X Siderails *x2*
__ Night Only
X Constant
__ Restraints
__ PRN
__ Constant
__ Smoking Precautions

IV #	SOLUTION	SIZE	ADDITIVE	RATE
2	*D5½ NS*	*1000 mL*	*20 mEq KCL*	*125 mL/hr*
3	*D5½ NS*	*1000 mL*	*ø*	*80 mL/hr*

IV - Lt forearm MM/DD/YYYY 10pm
Restarted Rt hand MM/DD/YYYY 4pm

ORDERED LAB & X-RAYS

Date	Test
MM/DD/YYYY	*CBC, UA, CXR,*
	EKG, Chem 21,
	PT, PTT
MM/DD/YYYY	*CBC today*
	Lytes in AM

ATTENTION
MM/DD/YYYY Exp lap in AM
Pre-op teaching tonight

ALLERGIES *PCN, Compazine*

Patient Classification Number ______
Room # *1126* Name *Ruth Weaver*

ADM. DX. *MM/DD/YYYY abd pain & N/V unknown etiology MM/DD/YYYY appendicitis*

ADM. TIME *9:15 pm*
ADM. DATE *MM/DD/YYYY*
DOCTOR *Keast*
AGE *73*

FIGURE 5.8 A sample Kardex page. (Courtesy of Kingfisher Regional Hospital, Kingfisher, OK.)

the chart immediately, write a note on your pocket-brain, including the time and pertinent details. Then transcribe the information to the patient's chart as soon as you are able. Otherwise, another staff member may make an entry before yours, making your out-of-sequence entry a late entry. Never chart something before it is done because that is fraudulent.

- **Be succinct.** Make entries brief, concise, and to the point. It is not necessary to use complete and grammatically correct sentences when documenting. The accepted standard is to omit unnecessary words that are not pertinent to the clarity of the entry, such as "the" or "a." Because the chart is written about the patient, it is not necessary to use the word "patient." Table 5.6 lists examples of succinct documentation.
- **Use punctuation.** Begin the first word of each phrase with an uppercase letter and use punctuation, usually a period, at the end of each phrase. Avoid using exclamation

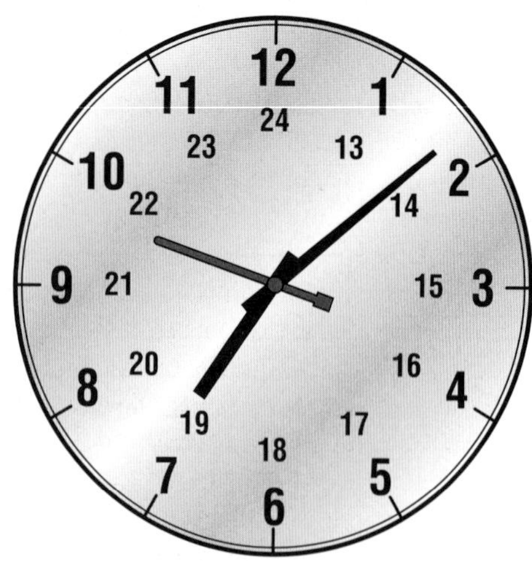

FIGURE 5.9 Many health-care facilities use the 24-hour clock. (Courtesy of Kingfisher Regional Hospital, Kingfisher, OK.)

marks or question marks because they tend to imply emotion or doubt, which can make the entry appear subjective.

- **Do not leave blank lines.** ***Safety: Avoid leaving a blank line, or even a blank portion of a line.*** Blank lines serve as an invitation for another individual to write something in the middle of your charting that could be attributed to you. If you do not fill the line completely, draw a single straight line through the middle of the space, extending from the last word to your signature. Then sign your name and credentials (Fig. 5.10). If your charting completely fills the line, leaving no room for your signature, avoid crowding your signature at the end or in the margin. Simply draw a single straight line through the middle of the space on the next line, leaving room for your signature and credentials.
- **Use continued notes.** When there is not enough room to complete your entry on a page, it must be continued on the next page. Stop writing on the last line at a point that leaves room for you to write "(continued)______Nurse's signature and credentials" (Fig. 5.11).
- **Correct mistaken entries.** If you make an incorrect entry, mark a single horizontal line through the incorrect word or phrase. Write "mistaken entry" and your initials just above the incorrect words (Fig. 5.12). Then proceed with the correct entry. ***Safety: Never use correction fluid or correction tape to totally blank out the mistaken entry. Avoid using markers or making multiple ink marks in an effort to blacken the incorrect entry so that it cannot be read because this may raise suspicion regarding the entry. Also avoid trying to "write over" incorrect letters.*** This only serves to make documentation sloppy and difficult to read.
- **Keep the medical record intact.** The medical record must be kept intact. ***Safety: Never delete any part of the chart.*** Even if a page of your nurse's notes becomes saturated with the soda you were drinking, do not discard the page after you recopy it. If a portion of page 2 or the page in its entirety is so damaged that it is not legible, requiring that you rewrite the data, keep the damaged page in the chart. Make a notation on the damaged page indicating the portion of the page that will be rewritten and make reference to the recopied page

Table 5.6 Examples of Succinct Charting

When charting, remember that it is not necessary to use complete sentences as long as the correct meaning is conveyed.

Lengthy Entry	*Succinct Entry*
"The patient got up to the bathroom to urinate and was able to go on her own without any help. She voided into the specimen pan. I measured 450 mL of real light yellow urine that does not have any sediment or particles in it. Then she walked from the bathroom back to bed."	"Ambulated unassisted to bathroom. Voided 450 mL clear, pale yellow urine. Back to bed."
"Upon entering the room, I found the patient just lying there. I spoke to him, but he did not answer me and did not open his eyes. He was pale and did not have as much color as he did this morning. His skin felt real moist and also cooler than it did at the beginning of the shift. He did not respond to me touching him, either. Then I used pressure on one of his nailbeds on each hand, and he moaned softly. But he did not open his eyes at all. I took his blood pressure and got 84/46. I took his apical pulse and got 116. It was also irregular and quite hard to hear both the S_1 and the S_2...."	"Lying supine. Eyes closed. Responds only to pain stimuli: moans when pressure applied to nailbed. Pale, cool, & clammy. BP – 84/46. AP – 116 muffled & irregular. R – 9 shallow & irregular...."

William, Mayson #91208 Rm. # 804 BD 6-4-61 Admit MM/DD/YYYY		Mission Nursing Center
Date	Time	Nurse's Notes
MM/DD/YYYY	1330	C/O indigestion & mild nausea after eating
		pizza brought by wife. Requests antacid.
		Mylanta 30 mL given p.o. Instructed to call if
	1420	no relief within 30 min. -----J. Hammond, LPN
		States nausea completely relieved &
		indigestion improving. ----------J. Hammond, LPN

FIGURE 5.10 Sample documentation: leave no blank lines.

First Page:

MM/DD/YYYY	1720	Dyspneic. Coughing decreasing. Skin cool, dry,
		pale. No cyanosis. BP-136/88 P-102 Irr. R-29
		Shallow & regular. SpO^2 90%. Breath
		sounds---(continued)------------J. Hammond, LPN

Second Page:

William, Mayson #91208 Rm. # 804 BD 6-4-61 Admit MM/DD/YYYY		Mission Nursing Center
Date	Time	Nurse's Notes
MM/DD/YYYY	1720	(continued) - auscultated: rales in LUL, LLL,
		RUL, rhonchi RML & RLL. HOB elevated
		to 45°. O^2 at 4 L/min applied via NC. Dr.
		Holsted notified of condition per phone. New
		orders received. ----------------J. Hammond, LPN

FIGURE 5.11 Sample documentation: continued note.

(e.g., "Recopied to page 3"). Then, on the new blank page, write "Recopied from page 2" and include the current date and time and your signature. Recopy the notes word-for-word from the damaged sheet and sign it. Leave both pages in the record to prevent doubt or suspicion regarding the recopied page.

KNOWLEDGE CONNECTION

Explain why it is important that all entries are legible and why you must sign each entry.

Why are date, time, chronological order, and documenting in a timely manner such a high priority? Why do you think it is important to start each phrase with an uppercase letter and place a period at the end of the phrase?

Long-Term Care Admission Documentation and Required Assessments

The U.S. government regulates the documentation that is required in long-term care facilities, and those requirements vary according to the level of care required by the resident. Upon admission to the facility, in order to meet Medicare and Medicaid requirements for certification and reimbursement, the facility must complete an admission assessment document for each resident that is many pages in length.

Once the admission paperwork has been completed, there are differences in the amount and type of documentation that is performed on a more regular basis. When one considers the documentation that is needed and required in a long-term facility, it is important to remember that a long-term care facility is considered to be each individual's place of residence—his or her home, whether temporary or permanent. Rather than charting continually through each 24-hour day as with hospital documentation, an update regarding the patient's condition is only required to be documented once a week, or more often if problems or changes in condition occur. This update is known as the *weekly summary*. If a resident becomes acutely ill or suffers an accident or injury, documentation steps up to a daily recording of vital signs and assessments until it is determined that the resident has no need for continued daily monitoring.

KNOWLEDGE CONNECTION

Explain how long-term care documentation differs from acute care documentation.

The Minimum Data Set for Resident Assessment and Care Screening

A federal law known as the Omnibus Budget Reconciliation Act (OBRA) mandates that an extensive assessment form called the *Minimum Data Set (MDS) for Resident Assessment and Care Screening* must be completed for each resident within 4 days of admission to the facility and updated every 3 months. The form consists of many assessments that must be made. A partial list of required assessments includes the following:

- Demographics
- Identification and background patterns
- Customary routines of the patient, including cycle of daily events, eating patterns, activities of daily living patterns, and level of involvement (with others)
- Communication and hearing patterns

• WORD • BUILDING •

demographics: demo – people + graphics – writing

Mistaken entry-LL
"Phenergan 50 mg IM Z-track method administered Lt. ~~dorsogluteal~~ ventral gluteal."
L. Ludwig, RN

FIGURE 5.12 Sample documentation: mistaken entry.

- Cognitive patterns
- Vision patterns
- Psychosocial well-being
- Mood and behavior patterns
- Physical functioning and structural-related problems
- Continence of bowel and bladder
- Health conditions
- Disease diagnoses
- Medications the patient is taking

The entire government form may also be viewed and downloaded from the Internet at http://www.cms.gov/Medicare/Quality-Initiatives-Patient-Assessment-Instruments/NursingHomeQualityInits/downloads/MDS20MDSAllforms.pdf.

Weekly Assessment Data

Because the long-term care facility is the home of the resident, some additional data are collected and documented in the weekly assessments mentioned above, along with the typical data found in a more traditional acute care assessment. This will include the following information:

- **Use of all prostheses,** such as glasses, dentures, hearing aids, and prosthetic limbs
- **Activity level,** whether the resident is bedridden or ambulatory, as well as the level of assistance that is required to perform the activity
- **Elimination control and habits,** whether the resident is continent or incontinent and if bowel training is performed
- **Nutrition versus malnutrition,** such as type of diet, percentage routinely consumed, type and frequency of supplemental nutrition, and weight records
- **Ability to communicate** and, if the resident is unable to speak, the method utilized to communicate
- **Visitors and support system,** whether the resident has regular visitors or rarely receives guests, as well as whether there is a strong support system for the resident
- **Social activities,** such as the types in which the resident participates and the frequency of participation
- **Ability to perform activities of daily living,** including hygiene, dressing, and nutrition and fluid intake

Medication Administration Records

Medication administration is charted each time medications are given, just as it is documented in the hospital. However, there is not a separate MAR for each day as there is in acute care. On the MAR used in long-term care, administration of each drug is documented for the entire month on a single page. This must be done to decrease paper volume of charts that may extend over months and even years.

> **KNOWLEDGE CONNECTION**
> Describe the types of data that should be included in weekly summaries in a long-term care facility. How is the long-term care MAR different from the MARs found in hospitals?

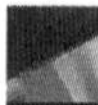

HOME HEALTH DOCUMENTATION

Most home health agencies use EHRs now. Each home health nurse carries a laptop computer and makes nurse's notes while in the home. Home health-care documentation is governed by the federal government agency known as the Centers for Medicare and Medicaid Services (CMS). Certain criteria must be met to admit a patient to home health care, just as in long-term care; documentation of these data is part of the certification process. The admission forms must be extensive to provide adequate data to verify that the patient meets certification requirements. One example of an admission form is the *Outcome and Assessment Information Set,* known as *OASIS.* Figure 5.13 shows the first page of a five-page admission form used by one agency. A copy of a complete OASIS form can be found at www.cms.hhs.gov/oasis/. These admission forms are on the laptop computer that a nurse uses.

You must be an RN to perform this initial visit and assessment, as well as to complete the OASIS form. Either RNs or LPN/LVNs may make subsequent visits. Each time you make a patient visit as a home health nurse, you will be expected to complete the organization's specified home health skilled nursing note form to document the visit. It is important to show in your documentation that the patient is making progress toward specific goals. This documentation is regulated and audited by both the state health department and Medicare.

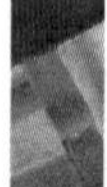

FIVE DOCUMENTATION MISTAKES THAT CARRY INCREASED RISK OF MALPRACTICE

You will want to avoid all documentation mistakes, particularly those for which the very nature of the mistake carries increased risk for being sued for malpractice or negligence. This would include failure to document:

- Assessment findings
- Medications administered
- Pertinent health history
- Physician's orders

Documenting on the wrong chart or MAR also carries increased risk of a lawsuit.

Failure to Document Assessment Findings

It is your responsibility to be competent in assessment and to determine if the findings indicate a change in the patient's condition. Because nurses are the only health-care

• **WORD • BUILDING** •

prostheses: pros – in addition + theses – placed

malnutrition: mal – bad + nutri – feeding + tion – action

<table>
<tr><th colspan="8">PARKVIEW HOSPITAL HOME HEALTH ADMISSION</th></tr>
<tr><td colspan="3">HH #:</td><td colspan="2">☐ New ☐ Readmit</td><td colspan="3">Patient Name:</td></tr>
<tr><td>Sex:
☐ M ☐ F</td><td>Date of Birth</td><td>Age</td><td>Marital Status
S M D W</td><td colspan="2">Race:
☐ White ☐ Black
☐ Hispanic ☐ Other</td><td colspan="2">Social Security Number:</td></tr>
<tr><td colspan="3">Street Address</td><td>City</td><td>State</td><td>Zip</td><td colspan="2">County</td></tr>
<tr><td colspan="8">Mailing Address</td></tr>
<tr><td colspan="2">Medicare</td><td colspan="2">Medicaid</td><td colspan="2">Insurance</td><td colspan="2">Private Pay</td></tr>
<tr><td colspan="3">Pt. Phone #:</td><td colspan="3">Emergency Contact:</td><td colspan="2">Phone #:</td></tr>
<tr><td colspan="3">SOC Date:</td><td colspan="5">Certification Period:</td></tr>
<tr><td colspan="8">Admit Source: ☐ Physician ☐ Emergency Room ☐ HMO ☐ Court/Law Enforcement ☐ Hospital ☐ Clinic ☐ SNF ☐ Not Available ☐ Other Facility</td></tr>
<tr><td colspan="4">Primary Physician:</td><td colspan="2">Date Last Seen:</td><td colspan="2">UPIN #:</td></tr>
<tr><td colspan="6">Address:</td><td colspan="2">Phone:</td></tr>
<tr><td colspan="4">Secondary Physician:</td><td colspan="2">Date Last Seen:</td><td colspan="2">UPIN #:</td></tr>
<tr><td colspan="6">Address:</td><td colspan="2">Phone:</td></tr>
<tr><td colspan="5">Pharmacy Name:</td><td colspan="3">Phone #:</td></tr>
<tr><td colspan="8">Travel Directions:</td></tr>
<tr><td colspan="8"></td></tr>
<tr><td colspan="8">Caregiver(s) in Home:</td></tr>
<tr><td colspan="8">Diagnosis:</td></tr>
<tr><td colspan="8">Start of Care Orders: ☐ SN ☐ Aide ☐ PT ☐ OT ☐ ST ☐ MSW</td></tr>
<tr><td colspan="4">Rehab/SNF:</td><td>Adm. Date:</td><td colspan="2">Disch. Date:</td><td></td></tr>
<tr><td colspan="4">Hospital:</td><td>Adm. Date:</td><td colspan="2">Disch. Date:</td><td>Surgery
☐ Yes ☐ No</td></tr>
<tr><td colspan="6">Referred By:</td><td colspan="2">Phone #:</td></tr>
<tr><td colspan="5">Nurse Receiving Verbal Order:</td><td colspan="3">Referral Date:</td></tr>
<tr><td colspan="8">Team Leader:</td></tr>
<tr><td colspan="5">Initial Nurse:</td><td colspan="3">Date:</td></tr>
</table>

FIGURE 5.13 Portion of a home health OASIS admission form. (Courtesy of Parkview Hospital Home Health, El Reno, OK.)

providers who provide patient care 24 hours per day, 7 days per week, it is most likely that it will be a nurse who is first present when there is a change in the patient's condition. Failure to identify and document even what may initially appear to be a minor change in condition may put the patient in jeopardy.

Some facilities have a policy stating that only the floor supervisors are to call problems in to physicians, meaning that problems must be reported to the supervisor when they are identified. If you are working under this type of policy and discover pertinent abnormal assessment findings, you may immediately go to your supervisor and report the findings, assuming that the supervisor will contact the physician and take care of the reported data. Avoid this line of thinking and method of performing. Even if the supervisor is responsible for notifying the physician, he or she is *not* responsible for documenting your assessment findings. You are responsible for documenting not only your abnormal assessment findings but also the actions you took to address any actual or potential problems related to those abnormal findings. Never depend on another individual to document your assessments or care. Be diligent to document all assessment findings.

Failure to Document Medications Administered

Follow your facility's policy for administering and documenting medications. Always record the drug name, dosage, and route of administration and the correct time of administration as soon as possible. Failure to document administration of a medication carries the potential for another mistake to be made. If another nurse sees no documentation that the medication was given, he or she may give it again, thinking this to be the correct course of action for the patient and also thinking that he or she is doing you a favor as well. The patient has then received an extra dose, the significance of which is affected by several factors: the type of drug that was given, the safe dosage range, the patient's age, the patient's liver and kidney functions, and the patient's response to the medication.

Failure to Document Pertinent Health History

This could include failure to document things such as the patient's allergies to a medication, food, or latex; a diagnosis of hemophilia; or a previous methicillin-resistant *Staphylococcus aureus* (MRSA) infection. An allergy that is not documented presents an opportunity for an allergic reaction to examination gloves or to a medication administered IV, both of which carry the potential to be life-threatening. The safety measures that should be used when caring for a patient with hemophilia may be overlooked if staff are unaware of the diagnosis, endangering the patient. A patient with a history of previous MRSA infection is at risk for a repeat MRSA infection following surgical procedures. A physician probably would want to order a *prophylactic,* or preventive, dose of vancomycin or another antibiotic effective against MRSA to be administered prior to a scheduled surgery. However, if the history of MRSA is not documented, it may be overlooked, which again endangers the patient.

Documenting on the Wrong Chart or MAR

It can be easy to mistake one electronic chart for another of a patient with a similar name and document about the wrong patient. Patients can have the same last name, and sometimes even the same first and last names, making it difficult to differentiate between their charts and MARs. Always check the electronic chart for the patient's full name, birth date, physician, and other identifiers as necessary before documenting in or following the orders located in either the chart or MAR.

Real-World Connection

How Many Can There Be?

During a clinical day at a government hospital, one student nurse had a patient by the name of William Hershell May (not the patient's real name). All medical records were computerized, and the student was required, after entering her multiple pass codes, to type in the name of the patient for whom she needed to view the chart. She typed in "William May," and a medical record came up on the screen. The instructor was standing not far behind the student when she began to scan through the chart. The instructor stepped close enough to read over the student's shoulder, when a particular diagnosis caught his attention. The instructor asked the student if this was, indeed, the chart of her patient. The student replied that it was and began once again to flip through the various sections of the record. Immediately, the instructor noted another piece of information that did not make sense compared with the information he knew about the student's patient, so he asked the student to show him the room number on record in this particular chart. It was not the room number that the student had been going to during her nursing care, so the instructor requested that she pull up the Social Security number listed in the chart. She compared it to the last four numbers that they had been checking against on the MAR and they were not the same; the student was in the wrong chart.

When the instructor backtracked the steps the student had taken to pull up the chart, the instructor showed her that there was more than one patient with the same first and last names. The biggest surprise for the student came when she saw that the nurse had pulled up not only two patients with the name William May but a total of seven patients named William May, two of whom also had "H" for the middle initial. Only two of the seven patients were currently in the hospital; the other five records were from previous admissions. The student was grateful that she had not had time to carry out any physician's orders from the wrong chart.

Failure to Accurately Document Physician's Orders

Once the physician writes an order for any type of treatment, test, procedure, medication, or interval frequency of any aspect of nursing assessment or monitoring, the orders go through a process known as *noting* or *transcribing* the order. This refers to the process of documentation that is required to ensure that the proper health-care providers are notified of the order. This may include documentation in the Kardex in long-term care; making computer entries; written or electronic notification to the pharmacy, dietary services, or physical, occupational, or respiratory therapy; scheduling of procedures or appointments; and various other forms of documentation. If the required documentation is not completed, physician-ordered diagnostics, treatments, and care will not be delivered. Because the physician's orders are the foundation of patient care, your accuracy in transcribing them serves as the scaffolding for delivery of patient care.

You will learn how to perform this skill at a later point in your education, probably after you begin attending clinicals. However, we mention it here because it is a vital area of documentation. Failure to accurately transcribe physician's orders can have harmful consequences and carries the potential to even be life threatening for your patients. In Chapter 6, we will address how to decrease the risk of error while documenting verbal or telephone physician's orders. An example of a consequence that could occur as a result of failure to note a physician's order is shown in Box 5.4.

KNOWLEDGE CONNECTION

Explain the five types of documentation mistakes that carry increased risk for malpractice.

Supervision/Delegation Connection

Must "You" Document Everything?

Although most documentation must be completed by you, the licensed nurse, there are some portions that may be performed by a certified nursing assistant (CNA) or unlicensed assistive personnel (UAP) who has been instructed in the proper manner to document the data. In a hospital, the completion of forms such as the vital signs graphic sheet or a portion of the nursing care checklist or flow chart may be assigned to UAP. As previously noted, a unit clerk or ward clerk may transcribe physician's orders, but you still are responsible to ensure that all required documentation for each order has been correctly completed. You also are responsible for signing the physician's order sheet, complete with date, time, and signature with credentials.

In long-term care, it is common to assign the CNA to document on designated records the following data:

- Date and type of bath given
- I&O shift totals
- Number of times resident is incontinent
- Number of bowel movements
- Percentage and type of nutritional supplements consumed

All other documentation remains your responsibility.

Box 5.4
The Importance of Accurate Order Transcription

The following scenario highlights why it is so vital to accurately follow all physician orders:

The physician's order "NPO at midnight for EGD (esophagogastroduodenoscopy) in a.m." is overlooked by the nurse when the orders are being entered in the computer, so the dietary department did not receive the order. A breakfast tray is available for the patient the next morning and is served by the dietary aide. The patient eats because the tray was served. A technician from the procedure room brings a wheelchair and takes the patient back for the EGD. The patient receives conscious sedation. As the physician begins to insert the scope into the patient's throat, she vomits a moderate amount of undigested food. The procedure was canceled at that point and rescheduled for another day. Luckily the patient did not aspirate and was fine.

This documentation oversight could have resulted in the patient aspirating and developing respiratory complications, all because one nurse missed one physician's order.

POST CONFERENCE

Your clinical shift is almost over and you are giving the end-of-shift report to your instructor. You have a smile on your face because you are very pleased with your performance and the documentation that you had worried about so much. After determining which type of documentation was used in the facility, you also reviewed your fundamentals textbook and then discussed it with your instructor before you began to chart. It all began to "come back" as you reviewed and talked with your instructor. You did quite well with that first day's charting; in fact, your instructor had only a couple of minor recommendations for ways to improve it the next time you get to document. You leave clinicals *almost* looking forward to the next opportunity.

Key Points

- Purposes of documentation include continuity of care; a permanent record of a patient's medical experiences; a record of accountability for quality assurance, accreditation, and reimbursement; and a legal record for both the patient and the health-care providers.
- HIPAA guarantees confidentiality of the patient's medical record.
- Forms used in documentation may include a nursing report or printout, incident reports, care plans, and the patient's medical record.
- Guidelines for electronic documentation include avoiding shortcuts, such as copy and paste; using only approved abbreviations; and being accurate and objective.
- There are two types of medical records: source-oriented and problem-oriented records, and each is organized differently.
- A variety of methods for recording patient information exist. With the use of EHR, charting by exception is often used. All nurses need to know how to record patient information using narrative charting since it is used in a variety of settings.
- EHR use is required by law for hospitals but not for long-term care facilities. However, some facilities are changing over to the use of EHRs.
- When working in an EHR, it is important to never share your password.
- In addition to the documentation of patient care, an EHR provides a way to pool collected data and information, provides evidence for evidence-based practice, and helps identify needs for staff continuing education.
- If you are using paper documentation in long-term care, many rules apply on how nurses' notes are to be written and corrected. Be sure you know and follow all these rules.
- Long-term care documentation frequency and emphasis are very different from acute care documentation. Home health-care documentation is also different from acute and long-term care.
- When using electronic documentation, do not share your user ID and password with anyone.

Review Questions

Select the answer that is most appropriate for each of the following questions. Some questions may have more than one correct answer. Select all that apply.

1. Which of the following phrases are written objectively?
   1. "Ate 45% full-liquid diet. Did not act very hungry and acted like she should not have drunk all that she did."
   2. "Complaining of really severe pain and wants something for it."
   3. "Ambulated unassisted the length of hallway without complaints of fatigue or shortness of breath."
   4. "Does not feel good today. Angry and depressed."
   5. "Makes good eye contact, smiling. States feels 'much better today than yesterday.'"

2. When you use an EHR, you may enter information in which of the following ways?
   1. Hand-held computer
   2. Computer at a computer station in the hallway
   3. Computer at the nurses' station
   4. Bedside terminal in the patient's room
   5. Your personal laptop wherever it is convenient

3. Which of the following times during a 7 a.m. to 7 p.m. shift would be appropriate to document on a patient's chart?
   1. As soon as possible after an occurrence or event
   2. Once at the beginning of the shift, again about midway through the shift, and the last time at the end of the shift
   3. Before the physician makes morning rounds at 10:15 a.m.
   4. Following the performance of physical assessments
   5. Not until all your patient care has been completed for the shift
   6. At least every 2 hours

4. Which of the following entries are good examples of succinct charting?
   1. "Bed bath was given and teeth brushed. Hair was shampooed and tangles combed out. Soaked fingernails in warm soapy water for 20 minutes, then filed them and cleaned them using an orange stick. Legs were shaved and lotion applied to all pressure points and areas of dry skin. Gave her a back rub."
   2. "Sacral wound measures 2 × 4 cm with 1-cm depth. Wound bed pale and dry, with 1-cm black eschar center circumferenced by 0.5-cm dark erythema. No granulation noted. Moderate amount foul-smelling green purulent drainage."
   3. "Patient is having moderate amount of cramping in her abdomen. It seems to be from her uterus. When I inquired, the patient said it is time for her to start her menses. The patient also said she usually does not experience premenstrual cramping."
   4. "BP – 124/72, T – 98.8°F orally, P – 64 strong & reg, R – 17 reg & even."

5. What type of documentation would you, as a nurse, be responsible for performing in the section marked *Physician's Orders?*
   1. The patient's plan of care to be followed
   2. The vital signs taken during your shift along with the I&O totals
   3. Transcription date, time, and your initials
   4. When you noted the orders
   5. Verbal order given to you by the physician
   6. Nursing orders

6. In a source-oriented medical record, which of these would be found in the *Nurse's Notes* section?
   1. Nurse's assessment data
   2. HCP's assessment data
   3. Patient's response to initiation of IV therapy
   4. Patient's living will
   5. Report of chest x-ray results
   6. Patient's complains of incisional pain

7. Which document would be found in the Advanced Directive section of a source-oriented medical record?
   1. Signed surgical consent
   2. Living will
   3. Discharge plans
   4. Treatment plan for the diagnosis

8. Which setting(s) may use Kardexes and paper charts?
   1. Inpatient hospitals
   2. Outpatient surgery centers
   3. Home health care
   4. Long-term care

9. When working in long-term care, the nurse is required to document assessment data on a resident how often?
   1. Every 2 hours
   2. Every 24 hours
   3. Every week
   4. Every month

ANSWERS 1. 3, 5, 2. 1, 2, 3, 4, 3. 1, 3, 4, 5, 4. 2, 4, 5. 3, 4, 5, 6. 1, 3, 6, 7. 2, 8. 4, 9. 3

Critical Thinking Exercises

Answers available online.

1. Using the narrative charting method, document the following data in the most complete, organized, and succinct manner you can:
   It is 2:00 p.m. and about 30 minutes ago you started an IV of 1,000 mL D5W in the patient in Room 1212. It took you only one attempt to access the patient's vein. You set the pump to infuse the D5W at 80 mL each hour. You left the bed in the low and locked position when you were done starting the IV and put the two rails up. You explained to the patient that when she needed to get up to the bathroom, she should not go until she calls you and you have arrived to help her. You told her that it would be too hard for her to handle the tall IV pole with the heavy pump attached to it by herself. The patient told you that she already needed to call for assistance any time she got up, so she certainly would need help now with the new IV.

2. Chart data below using the narrative charting method. The patient in Room 231 does not feel as good now (11:15 a.m.) as she did when you assessed her at the beginning of your shift. She says she aches all over and feels restless. You came on at 7:00 a.m. and completed her assessment at 7:40 a.m. Her temperature is currently 102.4°F orally, and her pulse is 104, strong but irregular. You notice she is flushed over her face and neck. You decide to administer a prn medication, Tylenol 650 mg by mouth because she has not had any in over 12 hours. When you touch her arm, you detect that it is hot and dry. You help to relieve discomfort by applying a cool cloth to her forehead and neck. Later, around 12:55 p.m., you return to her room. She is no longer flushed. Her temperature is 100.2°F, and her pulse is 84, regular and strong. Her eyes are closed and she is snoring softly, but she wakes up when you speak her name. She tells you that she is not restless anymore. Now her skin is warm and slightly damp. She also says that the aching is beginning to improve.

Additional Resources

DAVIS edge Use the scratch off code on the inside front cover of your book to access online quizzes that will help you to improve your scores on course exams and prepare for the NCLEX-PN®.

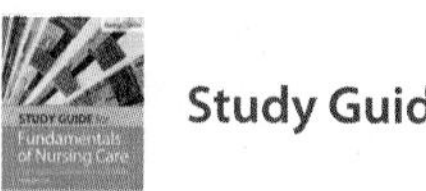

Study Guide

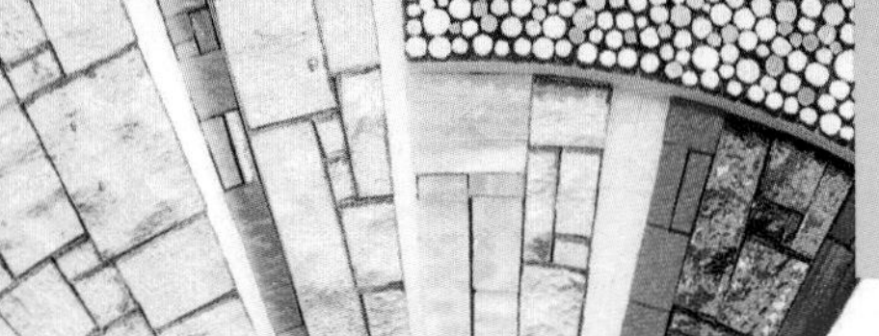

CHAPTER 6
Communication and Relationships

KEY TERMS

Active listening (AK-tiv LISS-uh-ning)
Aphasia (ah-FAY-zee-ah)
Body language (BAH-dee LANG-gwij)
Communication process (kuhm-YOO-ni-KAY-shun PRAH-sess)
Congruent (KON-groo-ent)
Connotative meaning (ko-NOH-tuh-tiv MEE-ning)
Denotative meaning (dee-NOH-tuh-tiv MEE-ning)
Feedback (FEED-bak)
Nonverbal communication (non-VER-buhl kuhm-YOO-ni-KAY-shun)
Proxemics (prok-SEE-miks)
Shared meaning (SHAIRD MEE-ning)
Therapeutic communication (thair-uh-PYOO-tik kuhm-YOO-ni-KAY-shun)
Verbal communication (VER-buhl kuhm-YOO-ni-KAY-shun)

CHAPTER CONCEPTS

Communication
Patient-Centered Care
Culture
Sensory Perception

LEARNING OUTCOMES

1. Define various terms associated with communication and relationships.
2. Describe the communication process.
3. Enumerate types of communication.
4. Discuss the factors that influence communication.
5. Explain personal space and touch preferences within selected cultures.
6. Describe active listening.
7. Classify styles of communication.
8. Explain the DESC method of communication.
9. Differentiate between therapeutic communication techniques and communication barriers.
10. Describe how to communicate to manage conflict effectively.
11. Discuss effective methods of communicating with the health-care team.
12. Discuss the nurse–patient relationship, including the importance of trust and empathy.
13. Describe the interview process, including ways to prevent bias regarding sexual preferences and information.
14. Identify effective communication techniques for patients with special needs.
15. Discuss information found in the Connection features in this chapter.

CRITICAL THINKING CONNECTION

Clinical Assignment

You have been assigned to care for a 54-year-old male patient with heart disease who has undergone coronary artery bypass surgery. In the report, you are told that he is very quiet and does not talk much with anyone. He is not married and has few visitors. You already feel uncomfortable about caring for him because you don't know what to say or how to get him to talk to you.

Continued

CRITICAL THINKING CONNECTION—cont'd

Critical Thinking Questions:

1. What actions can you take while caring for this patient to communicate effectively?
2. Should you ask him lots of questions, or is that prying?
3. Should you just perform his care in silence if that is the way he wants it?
4. How can you draw him out?
5. Does it even matter whether he talks or not as long as you do a good job taking care of him?

You may be wondering whether communication is truly important in nursing. It is. Effective communication is the foundation of nurse–patient relationships: It helps establish the proper transfer of health-care information, is essential in proper documentation practices, and is a key element when reporting information to other members of the health-care team—all vital components of building relationships and carrying out professional responsibilities of caring for others. Yet, despite its importance, surveys tell us that nurses often feel unprepared for the wide range of communication skills that are necessary in clinical situations. Even in the best of circumstances, communication can be challenging. When the situation is stressful, such as when a patient becomes critically ill, effective communication becomes even more challenging.

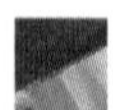

THE COMMUNICATION PROCESS

Think of communication much like a gift exchange; you give a gift to a person and he or she gives you one in return. Likewise, the **communication process** is an exchange of information, feelings, needs, and preferences between two people. When people are face to face, communication is not a passive one-sided event, like watching the news on television. It is not as simple as informing or telling. Rather, it is an active process that involves informing, or *sending,* and *receiving,* which includes listening, observing, processing, and comprehending in a reciprocal fashion. In face-to-face interactions, both parties will send and receive messages simultaneously by interpreting both the words spoken and the tone, as well as the body language and inflection of the voice. To complete the communication process, the receiver will send **feedback,** or a return message, that indicates the message has been received, processed, and comprehended.

The goal of communication is to establish a mutual understanding of the meaning of a message, known as **shared meaning,** that indicates the message was communicated as intended. Figure 6.1 shows the receiver and sender in the communication process.

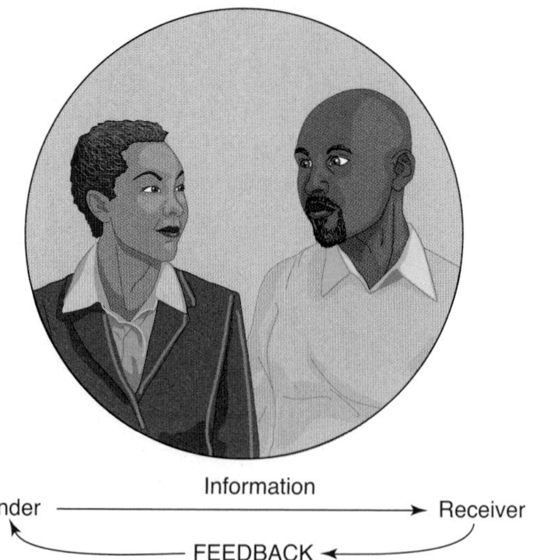

FIGURE 6.1 A sender and receiver participating in the communication process and offering feedback (adapted from Wilkinson JM, Treas LS. *Fundamentals of Nursing: Theory, Concepts & Applications.* Vol. 1. 3rd ed. Philadelphia, PA: FA Davis; 2016).

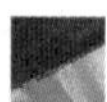

TYPES OF COMMUNICATION

The communication process consists of verbal and nonverbal language. **Verbal communication** is a conscious use of words, either spoken or written. An individual's choice of words may be dependent on age, education, developmental level, and culture. Verbal communication is more direct than nonverbal communication and is often used to give or receive specific information. Feelings can be expressed verbally by a speaker through changes in pitch, pace, and tone of voice.

Nonverbal communication is conveyed by **body language—**facial expressions, posture, body position, behavior, gestures, touch, and general appearance. Nonverbal communication is less conscious and more indirect than verbal communication; consequently, it often conveys more of what a person feels, thinks, and means than what is stated in words. It requires observation and forming a valid, or a true or intended, interpretation of the language. Verbal and nonverbal language should be **congruent,** or in agreement, to effectively meet the goal of shared meaning in communication.

Real-World Connection

Communicating With a Smile

One thing students can do to improve the nurse–patient relationship is to smile. Smiling has a positive effect, not only for those receiving the smile but also for the person giving it. Smiling signals that you are friendly and approachable and that you are enjoying what you are doing. Young children, elderly individuals, and those with dementia respond especially well to smiling; it is a positive way of making a connection with them.

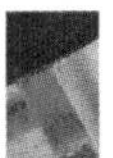

FACTORS THAT AFFECT COMMUNICATION

Personal space, body position, language, culture, attitude, and emotions all contribute to the way people communicate. These are some of the factors that help to establish the norms of the communication process in a given situation.

Personal Space

The distance, or personal space, people place between themselves and others is called **proxemics.** It reflects feelings and attitudes and affects communication. Four personal space–distance zones have been identified for use in the United States:

- *Intimate:* Ranging from physical contact to 18 inches
- *Casual-personal:* 18 inches to 4 feet
- *Social-consultative:* 4 to 12 feet
- *Public:* 12 feet if possible

People who have a negative attitude toward a situation or who view a speaker as unfriendly will maintain a more distant position than someone with a more positive outlook. Generally, the more that people are acquainted with each other, the less personal space they place between themselves. Nurses are an exception.

You most likely will not be closely acquainted with those you care for, yet often you must be in close physical contact with them to provide effective care. Part of your job when caring for individuals within an intimate space range is to communicate to them that you respect that you are invading their personal space but that the closeness is necessary in order to help them at that moment.

Patients from different cultures may have different comfort levels for touch and personal space. Be sure to communicate with the patient about his or her preferences. More information about cultural aspects of nursing care can be found in Chapter 8.

Body Position

A person's body position will communicate messages in several ways. For example, when a nurse stands over and peers down at a seated patient, it may demonstrate the desire of the nurse to maintain some distance physically or appear to have a position of authority. This quite rightly may be perceived by the patient as indicating that the nurse is not really concerned and does not care to listen. Slumping body posture may indicate disinterest or boredom. Folded arms may indicate a resistance to hearing a message. To demonstrate a willingness to communicate effectively with your patients, you need to communicate at eye level with the other person, lean slightly forward, and maintain an open body posture.

Language

Language or words convey our ideas to others when we communicate. Our choice of language is a factor in the success of the shared meaning of the message. Often there are misunderstandings in communication because of language choices. Nurses in particular need to ensure they use language that is clear; is unequivocal, meaning that the words have one meaning; and is free of bias.

You should avoid the use of medical jargon when communicating with patients to promote better understanding. Tailor your language to the patient's stage of development. When communicating with a person who speaks a language other than English, you may point to an object or use a picture board to communicate basic ideas. Arrange for an interpreter who speaks and understands the language in which your patient is communicating to prevent any misunderstandings.

Settings Connection: Medical Office

Communicating Across Developmental Stages

Language is part of a person's psychosocial and intellectual development, which occurs in varying stages over a lifetime. Knowledge of a patient's stage of development allows the nurse to tailor communication appropriately. Nurses care for patients in many stages of development from childhood to elderly patients, as well as mentally challenged patients, and you cannot take a cookie-cutter approach to communication. Adapt your communication strategies to coincide with the patient's stage of development. As a nurse, you will need to be aware of developmental stages and work within them to establish effective, patient-centered communication, including patient teaching.

Culture

Culture consists of the shared values, beliefs, and practices of the majority within a group of people. It includes the attitudes, roles, behaviors, and religious or spiritual practices accepted by the group.

• **WORD • BUILDING •**

proxemics: prox – nearness + emics – study of

Culture influences communication to a great extent. To be sensitive to an individual's culture you must recognize and respect the accepted patterns of communication in that culture. For example, a person is showing cultural sensitivity when he or she refrains from using language that would be deemed offensive or disrespectful by another culture when interacting with a person of that culture.

The most obvious cultural difference among people is language or verbal communication. If a patient does not speak and understand English and the nurse does not fluently speak the language that the patient is using, an interpreter who is familiar with health-care practices can help to translate so that misunderstandings and mishaps in treatment do not occur. Most health-care facilities maintain a registry of employee interpreters or community agencies that provide interpreting services, and telephonic interpreting devices are available in most areas of the country.

As a nurse, you should also be aware that there are cultural variances in nonverbal communication patterns in your patients. Nonverbal communication, such as eye contact, personal space, the use of touch, and the meaning of gestures, may have varying significance in different cultures. Because these factors have a direct effect on communication meaning and will affect the quality of the care experience, observe your patients' nonverbal language to see what the cultural norms are for them and act based on those observations.

Attitude

Your choice of language and nonverbal behavior will be influenced by attitude. By definition, attitude is the manner, disposition, feeling, or position toward a person or thing. It is also defined as the position or posture of the body that is appropriate to or expressive of an action or feeling. An accepting, nonjudgmental attitude toward your patients and their situation is expressed by attentive language and open, focused nonverbal communication.

If you have a negative attitude toward your patient or situation, you may express it by disinterested verbal language, a stern expression, and a closed body stance and by maintaining a greater distance of personal space. As a nurse, you must be conscious of the attitude you display in your professional role and how communication of that attitude will affect your relationships with your patients and coworkers.

Emotion

Language has the ability to stir powerful feelings known as emotions. Language can inspire, give hope, and convey caring, but it also can generate negative feelings such as antagonism, fear, and prejudice. Problems occur when speakers use terms that seem objective but unknowingly hold an emotional bias.

Many words have two layers of meaning. The **denotative meaning** is the literal meaning, absent any interpretation. The **connotative meaning** refers to the emotional associations that can be attached to the word. Connotative language, whether used consciously or unconsciously, has the potential to shape a listener's attitude. Some words hold such strong emotional associations, like a trigger, that they may set off a storm of intense emotional reactions—good or bad. Words such as "love," "cancer," and "death" are emotionally charged words; they can elicit emotional responses that distract the listener because of past experiences, resulting in a message that is distorted and altered.

> **KNOWLEDGE CONNECTION**
> List the three components of the communication process. Explain how body position and attitude are different and how they are similar in the ways they affect communication.

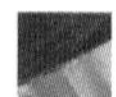

ACTIVE LISTENING

Active listening techniques use all the senses to interpret verbal and nonverbal messages. In active listening, attention is paid to what the speaker is saying but also to what the speaker is not saying. The mind focuses on the interaction and detects feelings as well as the spoken words. It takes real practice for the mind to tune out other intrusions and distractions, focus on the speaker, and then wait for the entire message to be delivered before interpreting what is said. With experience, you will be able to observe and interpret sensory stimuli to form a perception of what your patient may be feeling physically and emotionally but is not verbalizing. Certain facial expressions, body postures, and movements can indicate what the patient is feeling.

To complete the process of active listening, you respond to the content heard in the message, share your perceptions, and state as feedback what you, as the listener, understood was said by the speaker. When you practice active listening as a nurse, you demonstrate to your patients that you are interested in their feelings, concerns, and needs. This interest helps build the foundation of a trusting relationship between nurse and patient that is critical to providing quality care. An example of this would be when a patient says, "I am so tired of all these treatments. They don't seem to do much good, anyway." As an active listener, the nurse would respond by confirming that he or she understood what was stated and what was meant. A possible response might be, "It sounds as though you are getting discouraged about the treatments. It must be difficult to go through the radiation and not know if it is really helping." This gives the patient the opportunity to confirm the nurse's perceptions and discuss the patient's feelings further or to correct any misperceptions the nurse may have.

Elder Care Connection

Communicating With Older Adults

Older adults formed their values and beliefs at a time when society was very different than it is today. Their outlook may be different from that of a younger person. It is important for caregivers to bridge the generational gap with effective, therapeutic communication.

Active listening with all the senses is a necessary part of the process because older adults may have several physical changes that will alter their ability to perceive messages or communicate their needs. For example, an older adult may have hearing or vision impairments, chronic pain, or dementia. Although hearing and vision are the main senses we use in communication, the other senses of touch, smell, and taste may also play a part when communicating with the older adult. Make sure you have the older adult's attention before speaking. Try to minimize environmental distractions such as a loud television.

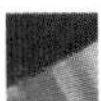

STYLES OF COMMUNICATION

Individuals develop a style or way of communicating that is based on their personality and self-concept. The three common types of style are passive or avoidant, aggressive, and assertive.

The *passive* or *avoidant* behavior style is characterized by the desire to avoid confrontation and the inability to share feelings or needs with others. Individuals with this behavior style have trouble asking for help and allow others to take advantage of them, resulting in feelings of anger, emotional pain, and anxiety.

The *aggressive* behavior style is characterized by putting one's own needs, rights, and feelings before those of others. Individuals with this behavior style exhibit a superior attitude; they try to humiliate others and communicate in an angry, hostile way that does not acknowledge the feelings of others.

The *assertive* behavior style is characterized by standing up for one's self without violating the basic rights of others. Individuals with this behavior style show respect for others, express their own feelings in an honest and direct way, and act in a consistent manner that enhances self-worth.

Assertive communication is the most effective communication style for nurses to practice. An assertive style provides self-esteem and self-confidence and allows the nurse to care for others with a higher degree of commitment and respect. Unfortunately, many nurses do not consistently act or communicate in an assertive manner. Box 6.1 provides an explanation of the Describe, Explain, State, Consequences (DESC) method used to promote assertive communication.

Box 6.1 DESC Method

A communication method, abbreviated as **DESC,** helps promote assertive communication. The four letters are used as a template to help the communicator to practice assertive communication.

- **D**escribe the behavior. Focus on what is observed or heard without a personal attack. Discuss the behavior, not the person.
- **E**xplain the impact of the behavior. Do not minimize the impact of the behavior.
- **S**tate the desired outcome. When you describe what you need from the other person, he or she does not have to guess and may be more likely to make changes.

The first three elements of the DESC method may be sufficient to get the person to change behavior, but if not, then you must initiate the fourth step:

- **C**onsequences should grab the person's attention. You will need to restate your position and then ask the person something, such as "What else do I need to do to get your attention?" or make the statement, "If you continue what you are doing, you and I will need to meet with the supervisor to resolve this." For most people, this will be the most difficult step to implement because nobody likes to go out of their comfort zone.

Learning a New Communication Style

The style in which you communicate is a learned behavior, and it has surely been reinforced over time. We all were taught to "be nice" as children, but some adults take advantage of the nice behavior of others. Also, childhood experiences may have started a pattern of negative messages about self-worth. Additional comments or experiences while working in nursing may reinforce those negative messages of self-worth, especially if a nurse is fearful of repercussions from acting assertively.

It can be difficult to change behavior. It requires time, practice, and a conscious decision to change. To honor your own needs and to fulfill your responsibilities to your profession and patients, you will have to stick up for yourself in an assertive manner. Part of this is learning to avoid ambiguous language. Phrases such as "Do you think you could...," "Sort of," and "Maybe try..." are nonassertive and rarely get a person to change behavior. The ability to practice assertiveness can depend on a number of variables, including a high-stress work environment, self-esteem issues, and the behavior of others. Practice using the DESC method when it is appropriate until you gain confidence in communicating in that middle ground between passivity and aggression.

KNOWLEDGE CONNECTION

Which style of communication do you use most often at school? At home? How can you change that style if it is not effective?

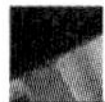 THERAPEUTIC COMMUNICATION

Therapeutic communication is patient-centered communication. The goal of therapeutic communication is to promote a greater understanding of a patient's needs, concerns, and feelings. When practicing therapeutic communication, the nurse helps patients explore their own thoughts and feelings, encourages expression of them, and avoids barriers to communication.

There are a variety of techniques a nurse can use to enhance therapeutic communication in a nurse-patient interaction. Over time you probably will become comfortable with a few of the techniques, but it is a good idea to become familiar with all the techniques and to try new ones periodically so that you do not overuse certain techniques and come across as insincere. Also, be aware that some techniques, such as silence and reflecting, should be used in small doses because they may slow down communication. A list of therapeutic communication techniques and examples is found in Box 6.2.

Barriers to Therapeutic Communication

Many factors can contribute to unsuccessful communication. A sender may send a confusing or incomplete message. A message may become distorted or misunderstood, or it may not be received at all.

Factors that lead to unsuccessful communication are called blocks or barriers to communication. Everyone uses communication barriers from time to time, whether consciously or unconsciously. People may change the subject when they discuss uncomfortable topics, use clichés when they are unsure how to respond, or voice defensive comments when faced with a complaint. Nonverbal barriers to communication include looking distracted, turning away, or intimidating patients by standing over them when they are seated. Nurses should avoid using barriers when communicating with patients and learn ways to promote effective, therapeutic interactions. Other examples of barriers to communication include:

- *Asking questions that can be answered with a "yes" or "no" response:* "Do you feel better after talking to the doctor?"
- *Giving false reassurance:* "Don't worry, everything will be alright."
- *Asking too many personal, probing questions:* "Why do you think that?"
- *Giving advice:* "I think you should…" or "If I were you…"
- *Belittling a patient's feelings:* "There are other patients who need more help than you."
- *Expressing disapproval:* "I would never decide against chemotherapy."

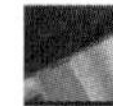 COMMUNICATION IN A CRISIS

In a crisis situation, things can happen suddenly and without warning, demanding that the nurse react quickly to ensure a good outcome for the patient. An important part of ensuring a good outcome in a crisis situation is the ability of the nurse to use effective communication tools to help manage the crisis. In such a situation, the nurse must use focused communication with language that is very clear and concise. A good communication tool to utilize in a crisis is called ISBARR (Introduction, Situation, Background, Assessment, Recommendation-Readback).

By following the ISBARR guide, your communication will systematically be focused on the crisis situation, and use

Box 6.2

Therapeutic Communication Techniques

Practice using these therapeutic communication techniques with your friends and family as well as with your patients. You may be surprised at what you learn.

- **Providing General Leads:** Encourages initiation or elaboration of a conversation. Some examples would be:
  - "I see what you are saying. Then what happened?"
  - "Tell me what treatment plan Dr. Smith talked to you about yesterday."
- **Using Silence:** Utilizes pauses or silence for up to several minutes without verbalizing. An example would be sitting quietly and waiting for the patient to explore thoughts and feelings.
- **Offering Self:** Shows concern and willingness to help. An example would be, "What can I do to help you?"
- **Using Open-Ended Questions or Statements:** Encourages elaboration and discourages answering questions with one or two words. An example would be "Tell me more about…."
- **Using Restatement (Validation):** Restates in different words the heart of what a patient said. Encourages further communication. Also conveys to the patient that you were actively listening. An example would be: *Patient:* "My daughter made me so mad yesterday!" *Nurse:* "Your daughter upset you yesterday?"
- **Seeking Clarification:** Helps to verify that the message sent was what was intended. This is necessary if the communication has detoured into many topics. An example would be, "Are you saying…?"
- **Giving Information:** Provides relevant information. An example would be, "You will need to report to the x-ray department at 8:00 a.m."
- **Using Reflection:** Reflects the same words back to the patient. This encourages verbalization of feelings. An example would be: *Patient:* "I'm so anxious about what my tests will show." *Nurse:* "You are anxious about your test results?"
- **Looking at Alternatives:** Helps patients explore options when making decisions about their care. An example would be, "Have you thought about…?"
- **Summarizing:** Sums up the important points. An example would be, "It looks like you've covered everything…."

of ISBARR can be adopted when you communicate with fellow staff nurses, supervisors, and health-care providers. Along with focused communication, your tone of voice should convey urgency but not panic. Likewise, your nonverbal behavior should display confidence and control, especially in front of your patients and their family members. Having others observe you communicating in a focused, controlled manner will help them cope with the crisis.

An example of using ISBARR could be when a patient was accidentally given the wrong medication and the doctor must be notified. It is hard to admit that you have made an error that should not have happened. Using ISBARR, you will give the doctor a clear picture of the situation using concise explanations:

- **I** (Introduction): "Dr. Jacob, this is Sharon Smith, LPN, at Sunnyview Acute Care Hospital. I am calling about your patient, Alan Jones."
- **S** (Situation): "Mr. Alan Jones was given Mr. Alex Jones's medication in error at 9 a.m."
- **B** (Background): "Mr. Alan Jones received 1,000 mg of metformin and a 100-mg Januvia tablet as well as an 81-mg aspirin that were not prescribed for him."
- **A** (Assessment): "I did a finger stick blood sugar on Mr. Alan Jones at 9:45 a.m. when I realized the error. It was 84 mg/dL. I gave him a glass of orange juice to drink. He is alert, oriented, and says he does not feel weak. His skin is warm and dry."
- **R** (Recommendation): "To prevent such an error from happening again, we have flagged both Mr. Alan Jones' and Mr. Alex Jones's medication administration records with a similar name alert, as well adding an alert to the computer and the medication armband. Would you like us to keep checking his finger stick blood sugars and, if so, at what intervals?"
- **R** (Readback): "Repeating that order, we will check his finger stick blood sugars every 4 hours until tomorrow at noon. We will report to you if his blood sugar falls below 80 and will give the patient 6 ounces of skim milk if his blood sugar is found to be below 80. Thank you, Dr. Jacob."

The ISBARR method of communicating can also be used to ensure that all patient information is covered during a shift report. It is a good format to follow to prevent overlooking important patient data when handing over patients to the next shift.

Anger or Hostility in Communication

Anger is a strong emotion that researchers say is often a cover-up for what a person is really thinking and feeling. Anger can be a signal or a message that we are being hurt, our rights are being violated, our needs are not being met, we are giving too much of ourselves, or we are not doing enough for ourselves. When we experience feelings of frustration, disappointment, or powerlessness, anger is never far behind.

There are two sides to anger. One side is guilt, which is directed inward at something we did or did not do. The other side is resentment, which is directed outward at others for what they did or did not do. Both guilt and resentment build up over time. If there is no change in the situation or no resolution to the problem, a person may become consumed in the negativity of anger and end up harming relationships and hindering personal growth.

Anger expressed as hostility in communication can present in several forms, including screaming, sarcasm, rudeness, belittling comments or jokes, and direct personal insults. Conflict is a by-product of anger projected outward toward others. Conflict is common in health care because it is a highly emotional and people-oriented business. Patients are sick, confused, and frightened. Family members may feel helpless, sad, or guilty. Staff members are stressed by the daily physical and emotional demands of their work. As a result, conflicts may arise between patients and staff, families and staff, or members of the health-care team. Conflict affects the quality of care and must not be allowed to continue unchecked! Box 6.3 presents tips for resolving conflict.

KNOWLEDGE CONNECTION

Which therapeutic communication techniques come the most naturally to you? Which should you be careful not to overuse? Which barriers do you use most often?

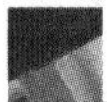

HUMOR IN COMMUNICATION

Humor has a place in health care. It often helps to create an atmosphere that is relaxed and sociable. Research tells us that patients value informal, humorous social interaction because it allows them to step out of their sick role, helps establish rapport and trust, and passes the time, all while helping to relieve anxiety and tension. One study indicated that nurses who used humor appeared more approachable to the patients. Humor also makes anger more tolerable and can work to diffuse pent-up guilt and resentment if used appropriately.

Although humor has its place, it is not appropriate when dealing with highly emotional or difficult issues. In addition, not all people who are ill may appreciate frivolous conversation or joking. When it comes to humor, you should be observant and take your cue from the patient before initiating humorous encounters or backing off from them.

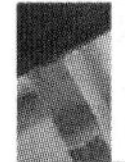

COMMUNICATION WITH THE HEALTH-CARE TEAM

Not only will you communicate with patients and families, you also will communicate frequently with other members of the health-care team. Whether you are communicating with your supervisor or coworker, it is important to approach the situation well prepared so that a clear message is given in a respectful, professional way.

Box 6.3

Tips on Resolving Conflict

Conflict is very uncomfortable for most people. Some may try to avoid it or ignore it because they are unsure of what to do or say. These tips will help you positively confront and resolve conflicts.

- Speak privately with the other person. Remain polite and professional and thank him or her for taking the time to meet with you.
- When speaking, remain focused on the specific area of conflict. Do not focus on how you feel about the other person or how you think he or she should have acted.
- Be specific about what you perceive the problem to be. Express your feelings but do not be accusatory. Use "I" instead of "you" in your statements. This will allow you to take responsibility for your emotions and allow the other person to explain his or her side of the story. For example, it is preferable for you to say "I am bothered by the comments you made the other day" instead of "You hurt my feelings the other day with your comments."
- Be prepared to hear how the other person feels toward you or the problem.
- Apologize for any misunderstandings.
- Ask the other person for ideas on how to resolve the conflict.
- It may be necessary to "agree to disagree." Try to focus on what you have in common, but you can civilly disagree on certain issues. Learning to respect another's beliefs and opinions is part of becoming a professional.

If you cannot satisfactorily resolve a conflict on your own, involve your supervisor.

Upward Communication

The terms *upward communication* and *downward communication* refer to your placement on an organizational chart. Upward communication is the interaction with those in authority over you and is formal by nature. You will need to learn and utilize the channels of communication within your organization. If you are a team member, you will share information with your team leader. The team leader will share information with the unit manager, who in turn will report information to a supervisor, and so on up the chain of command. When you begin working, you will realize there are many layers of nursing between the bedside nurse and the nurses who have major decision making responsibility for the entire facility. Those many layers can affect information flow. Box 6.4 offers tips for talking with your supervisor.

In grade school you probably played the whisper game, in which someone whispers a message to the next person and each person in turn repeats the message down the line. Oftentimes, when the message reaches the end of the line it is unrecognizable as the original message. Likewise, messages can get distorted when they travel through many people in an upward flow of communication. When communicating with supervisors, experts say it is important to state your needs clearly, explain the rationale for your requests, and suggest the benefits to others and not just to you. Also, it is important for you to listen objectively to your supervisor's response because there may be good reasons for granting or not granting your request.

Communicating With Health-Care Providers

When the need arises, you may have to telephone a health-care provider at his or her home or office. You may need to call a health-care provider to clarify orders or to report on a change of a patient's condition. You also may need to call a health-care provider if a patient has a special request or concern that cannot wait for regular rounds. You may even have to contact a health-care provider who is on call for the primary health-care provider. The way you communicate in all these circumstances is crucial to the continuity of care and safety of the patient.

TELEPHONE AND VERBAL HEALTH-CARE PROVIDER'S ORDERS. Communicating face to face with someone can sometimes be difficult. It is important to make certain that the sender's delivered message is received, interpreted, and understood by the receiver in the way intended by the sender. Getting your message delivered correctly or receiving the

Box 6.4

Tips for Talking With Your Supervisor

It is important to communicate effectively when you need to talk with your supervisor about a problem.

- Keep your supervisor informed.
- If a problem develops, make an appointment to talk it over. Have specific information available, especially written documentation. Focus on problem-solving, not just problems.
- Show that you have important information to share and hold a sense of responsibility.
- Be careful which words you choose. Avoid blaming others, exaggeration, and overly dramatic expressions.
- Do not talk to your supervisor when you are angry and do not respond with anger. Use "I" statements and explain what you are thinking.
- If you want to present a new idea, give your supervisor a written proposal and then meet to discuss it.
- Accept feedback and learn from it.
- Never go above or around your supervisor. Always communicate directly with your supervisor before you go up the chain of command.

exact message that was intended becomes even tougher when the communication occurs over the telephone. Over the telephone, you cannot see the individual's eyes, facial expression, or body language, all of which contribute significantly to delivery of the true intended message. The other disadvantage of verbal communication is the lack of the sender's written word to use for clarification as needed.

When you need to telephone a health-care provider regarding a patient's condition, be prepared by having access to the patient's electronic health record (EHR) and paper and a pen to write down any orders the health-care provider gives to you. It is a good idea to also have a pad or paper in case the health-care provider gives you verbal orders on a different patient than the one about whom you are phoning.

Certain guidelines should be followed when contacting a health-care provider. Before calling the health-care provider, make sure you prepare the following:

- A quick assessment of the patient, reviewing the chart for history and background information
- A concise statement of the problem and why you are calling, making sure you have a list of all points you want to cover
- Current data, such as vital signs, laboratory results, diagnostic tests, surgeries, medications received, and allergies

Also try to anticipate what information the health-care provider may need to make a sound decision.

When you call a health-care provider, first identify yourself and then state where you are calling from, the name of the patient you are calling about, and the reason you are calling. Have the chart handy to refer to if necessary. Do not give your personal opinion unless asked to do so.

Box 6.5

Required Data for a Telephone or Verbal Order

When you take a telephone or verbal order, it is very important that you have complete and correct information.

- Include all of the following:
  - Patient's first and last name
  - Date order received
  - Time order received
  - What needs to be done
  - When it should be done
- Indication whether order is a:
  - Telephone order (T.O.)
  - Verbal order (V.O.)
- Provide the following information:
  - Your name and credentials
  - Name of health-care provider giving the order
  - Documentation that the order was read back to the prescriber for verification and validation

Sample Telephone Order Documentation

12/17/22 0815 Change IV fluids to LR 1,000 mL @ 80 mL/hour. ____________ T.O. Dr. Arthur/B. Huntley, RN: order read back for verification and validated

Note: In the patient's EHR, enter the order as above and then search for and select the health-care provider's name from the list. Click "sign" or whatever the EHR provides to indicate that the order is signed. There is a box to check to indicate that the order was read back to the prescriber for verification.

Writing Health-Care Provider's Orders

Write the orders as the health-care provider says them and always read them back to the health-care provider, who should then verify that they are correct. Because it is easy to hear something different than what was actually said, this is a necessary step that should always be carried out. One of The Joint Commission's 2017 National Patient Safety Goals *is to improve staff communication,* so it is very important to ensure that you have correct orders when taking them from a health-care provider. Be certain that the health-care provider allows you time to ask any questions you may have regarding his or her orders and to read back the orders as you wrote them for verification. The ideal method for taking telephone orders is to have a second nurse listen on an extension to further verify what is said and to co-sign the telephone order; however, this is not easily accomplished when you are busy or working shorthanded.

Refer to Box 6.5 for a list of data to include when writing a telephone or verbal order and an example of a correctly written telephone order.

All of these guidelines will take on greater importance if you need to call a health-care provider during the middle of the night. Anticipate that you have awakened the health-care provider and that you should give him or her a moment to wake up and be able to listen attentively to your call. You will want to follow all the guidelines listed above and be especially concerned with clarifying information or orders that do not seem to be correct or are out of the ordinary. If you need to call a health-care provider who is on call and probably does not know the patient, be prepared to give more background information to present a clear, concise profile of the patient.

Downward Communication

Nurses provide direction to and supervise other licensed and unlicensed assistive personnel. Communicating with those you supervise is called downward communication. When supervising, it is important to keep in mind that those you supervise have needs for satisfaction and self-esteem. Your method of supervision and communication should respect those needs. Even nurses who may have many years of experience may be still working on developing effective communication skills. New and inexperienced assistive personnel may need guidance to enhance their communication.

This focus on communication is especially important as the trend in health care is to employ a culturally diverse workforce and provide services to a culturally diverse population. Supervising nurses frequently use several types of downward communication techniques:

- *Job Instruction:* What to do or how to do it. The instruction should include information about deadlines for job completion or other expectations about when to give any feedback of information.
- *Job Rationale:* Explanations about how one task relates to other tasks.
- *Practices and Procedures:* Information about what needs to be done, how it needs to be done according to the facility's policies and procedures, and possible benefits.
- *Feedback:* Information about how effectively a person is performing and outcomes or verification of instruction before a task is initiated, as well as during or after completion of a task.
- *Role Modeling:* Communicating in such a way that you demonstrate to assistive personnel how to interact effectively and appropriately regarding the needs and care of your patients.

Shift-to-Shift Reporting

Ineffective communication is a major cause of medical errors. Hand-off or shift-to-shift reporting can be an area of patient care that is vulnerable to ineffective communication. The *shift report* is the communication of the patient's condition and required nursing care by the off-going nurse to the oncoming nurse, which is a necessary step in preparation for the oncoming nurse to receive the patient into his or her care. The problem of ineffective communication has prompted experts to recommend standardizing the reporting process to make it more relevant and patient centered. The focus of end-of-shift reporting should be to pass along detailed, accurate, current information about the patient and changes in orders or plan of care, including changes that have already occurred and anticipated changes.

Shift Report

Each day when you report to work, especially if you work in a hospital, you will find that you need to know not only which patients you will be providing care for but also what type of care you must provide. Many methods of shift-to-shift reporting have been tried, but most of the time it has been decided that face-to-face reporting is the safest and most effective manner in which to communicate the information (Fig. 6.2). When you are the oncoming nurse, face-to-face reporting provides you with the opportunity not only to listen to the data reported to you by the off-going nurse, but also to ask questions. No one has a perfect memory, especially at the end of a work shift. When the oncoming nurse is given the opportunity to ask questions and clarify what the off-going nurse just said, the shift report becomes a safer and more effective communication tool. The Joint Commission requires that the oncoming shift must have the opportunity to ask questions and receive responses from the off-going shift regarding the care of the patient. The Commission highly recommends a bedside report, in which nursing staff go to each room together and the patient is introduced to the oncoming shift person who will be caring for them. In addition, questions can be asked and answered about the equipment, supplies, and other needs of the patient. Be careful during the bedside report not to violate the Health Insurance Portability and Accountability Act (HIPAA) when discussing the patient's diagnoses and condition.

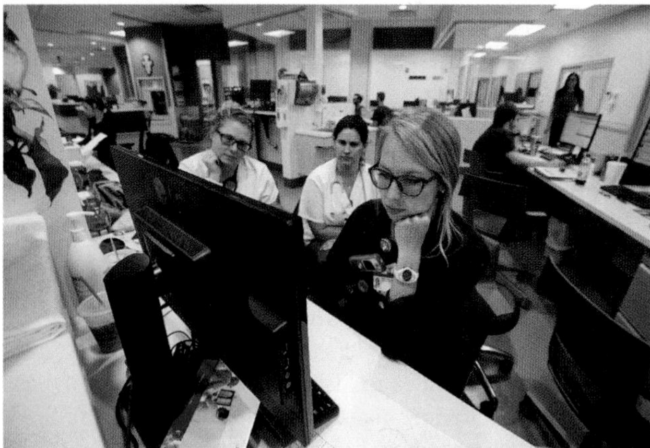

FIGURE 6.2 This nurse is finishing her shift and giving the end-of-shift report to the oncoming nurses. (Courtesy of Texas A&M University.)

CONFIDENTIALITY OF THE SHIFT REPORT. Confidentiality as mandated by HIPAA includes discussion of a patient's condition, such as during a shift report. Such discussions about patients must be conducted where privacy is ensured, not in the hallway or in the cafeteria where others may overhear.

DATA TO INCLUDE IN A SHIFT REPORT. There is certain information that you must always include in your shift report, and there are times when it constitutes a tremendous amount of data, bringing up the issue of length of time spent in reporting. By the end of your shift, you will generally desire to report off and leave on time. Employers have a vested interest in you getting off duty in a timely manner to reduce overtime expenses. This requires you to be succinct while being thorough. If you select some sort of sequence or order in which to present each patient's report and use it consistently while you are learning how to give an end-of-shift report, you will develop a sequence that will become routine without having to think hard about it. Table 6.1 presents a list of specific items that should be included in a shift report. Box 6.6 provides an example of one nurse's shift report.

As soon as you begin the clinical portion of your training, start to develop your own format and order in which you present the information in your report. It will be helpful to use written documents to cue you about things you need to report rather than relying totally on your memory. (See Chapter 5 for information about pocket-brains.)

Table 6.1
Items to Include in the Shift Report

Basic Patient Data Room number Patient name Patient age Patient gender Health-care provider Admitting diagnoses Other diagnoses Allergies Frequency of vital signs Diet order Activity order Type bath Bowel/bladder status Any complaints	**Special safety issues such as:** Fall risk Aspiration risk Confusion Paralysis Tracheostomy Inability to communicate **Sensory deficits such as:** Blindness Deafness	**Assistive equipment such as:** Hearing aid Cane Walker **Prosthetic devices such as:** Eye Arm Leg
Scheduled Procedures Laboratory tests X-rays Radiology procedures Other diagnostic procedures Surgery	***Pertinent Diagnostic Results*** Normal results Abnormal results	
Abnormal Assessment Findings All findings outside of normal range Any changes in patient condition		
Interdisciplinary Therapies Ordered		
Respiratory therapy Speech therapy	Occupational therapy Dietary consult	Physical therapy
Various Ordered Treatments		
Suction Antibiotic therapy	Dressing change Intravenous access	Wound care Telemetry monitoring

Box 6.6
Sample Shift Report

Nurses communicate with one another about patients all the time. Here is an example of a complete and detailed shift report between a nurse who is completing one shift and the nurse who will be relieving him.

Off-going nurse: "In Room 1237 is Melissa Summers, a 37-year-old female patient of Dr. Holsted who was admitted this morning with an acute exacerbation of asthma. She also has diabetes mellitus type 2 that is under good control with diet and Januvia. She's allergic to penicillin, sulfa, and latex. On admit she was very hypoxic, pale with circumoral cyanosis, SpO_2 was 85%, respirations 44 shallow, irregular, and gasping, hardly able to speak. She improved rapidly with application of O_2, nebulizer treatment with DuoNeb, and an IV of aminophylline. Her vital signs with SpO_2 are ordered every 4 hrs. SpO_2 was 90% with O_2 at 4 L/min per NC an hour ago. She had 100.4°F oral temp and respiratory rate of 29 half an hour ago. Other vitals are within normal limits. She still has wheezes throughout all five lobes but has no complaints of dyspnea at this time. Color is pale but no cyanosis. She's on a regular diet, up ad lib unless shortness of breath increases, and can take a shower using a shower chair and someone not in bathroom with her but in the room on stand-by in case she becomes dyspneic. She has voided and had a BM this shift. Drinks lots of fluids without prompting. Her chest x-ray showed some infiltrate starting in both lower lobes, and another chest x-ray is ordered for in the morning. Doc started her on ampicillin IVPB every 6 hours."

Oncoming nurse: "Did they do a WBC on her?"

Off-going nurse: "Oh, yeah. It was 16,500, and he wants it repeated in the morning."

SHALL WE CHAT? The end-of-shift report is not a time for social conversation among coworkers. It is easy to fall into that trap, but it is important to remember that extraneous conversation is distracting and increases the risk of forgetting a piece of pertinent information that may affect the patient's care or condition. Be sure to save any conversation that is not patient centered for another time, such as when you are on break. This will save everyone time and decrease unnecessary time spent in shift reporting.

Written Communication

Nurses communicate not only with the spoken word, but also with written language that is read by other members of the health-care team. A good deal of communication that occurs in health care is in written form, and nurses in particular should develop the ability to write effectively. Written communication includes care plans, progress notes, emails, reports, and assignments.

Before you begin writing, know your audience, which is the person or group of people who will be reading what you write. It is important to know the audience because that will help define what writing style to use. You would use a more formal style for upward communication, making sure you utilize proper titles, format, grammar, punctuation, and spelling. You could use an informal style, more conversational, among your peers or those you may be supervising. In any case, do not let anything that you have written be sent out without first proofreading the material and making revisions if necessary.

Identify the purpose before you begin writing. Knowing the purpose will enable you to organize your thoughts around the "why" of your writing. Write what you mean. Choose words that are clear, specific, and concise. Use technical words appropriately, when the reader will understand the meaning. Keep sentences simple, with one idea per sentence. Your reader should not have to guess what you are trying to say. A reader should be able to follow your thoughts easily without being diverted by unnecessary language. Finally, what you write will make a lasting impression and strongly influence how you are evaluated. People will make judgments about your credibility for a long time after you have written the words.

A quick tip for written communication is KISS: **K**eep **I**t **S**hort and **S**imple!

> **KNOWLEDGE CONNECTION**
> Give an example of downward communication. How can you be certain you have correctly heard the orders a health-care provider is giving you over the telephone? Why is accuracy in communication between shifts so important?

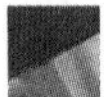

THE NURSE–PATIENT RELATIONSHIP

It is extremely important for nurses and patients to develop *rapport,* or a relationship with mutual trust and understanding. It is your responsibility to take the lead in establishing the relationship with a patient, and it must be one that is based on trust.

Establishing Trust

When individuals become ill, they lose a measure of control of their environment and must rely on others to care for them until they recover. For nurses to be able to give care to patients, they must quickly establish a relationship with them. At the heart of the relationship is trust. You will establish a trusting relationship with your patients by what and how you communicate with them. Your nonverbal communication should convey that you are knowledgeable about their physical care needs and that you are confident and competent when providing care. Your nonverbal behavior also should communicate that you are approachable and ready to listen. When you keep patient medical information confidential and do not discuss patients with friends and coworkers, you are also establishing trust.

Patients will look to you to provide emotional support, encouragement, and understanding. Fear of the unknown is emotionally upsetting to patients and may interfere with their treatment and recovery. When patients understand what is happening and have someone to trust, it helps empower them to face the emotional and physical demands of illness and allows them to participate more fully in their care.

You can provide emotional understanding and support by communicating empathy to your patients. *Empathy* is the ability to intellectually, not emotionally, identify with or experience the feelings, thoughts, or attitudes of others. You can understand and respect what a patient is experiencing without taking on the burden of experiencing it yourself. When you communicate empathetically, the patient knows that you acknowledge and respect his or her feelings and that it is safe to express these feelings to you.

As a nurse, you must keep some emotional distance and not allow the patient's problems to become your problems. You need that distance to think and act on behalf of the patient. Being empathetic will help you conserve your own emotional reserves so that you can be available to all who need your care.

Patient-Centered Communication

Patient-centered communication has been defined as communication that encourages and empowers patients to participate in their care. It is an essential component to establishing a positive nurse–patient relationship. There are several ways a nurse conveys patient-centered communication as opposed to task-centered communication. One method is by demonstrating accessibility and readiness to listen through the use of attentive nonverbal behaviors. Attentiveness or attending behavior is considered a patient-centered form of communication, and it does require the nurse to display genuineness,

• WORD • BUILDING •
empathy: em – in + pathy – feeling

warmth, and empathy. The nurse's behavior and communication must be perceived as real or genuine to the patient.

Verbal communication, such as language used and tone of voice, has also been identified as an important component of patient-centered communication. A friendly tone of voice will signal to patients that you have a genuine interest in and a willingness to listen to them.

Researchers say spending long periods of time with patients does not necessarily mean that a positive nurse–patient relationship will occur. What determines whether a positive relationship develops is not the quantity but the quality of the time spent and communication practiced.

Nurses often blame being short-staffed or "not having the time" during a work shift for not practicing patient-centered communication. Focusing only on the task side of care is like putting blinders on and forgetting about the person beneath those tasks. When nurses are solely task centered, they may be very efficient in performing tasks but may avoid therapeutic, patient-centered communication, which encourages and empowers patients to become partners in their care.

When you communicate with patients in a patient-centered way, you will keep the focus of the conversation on the patient, not on yourself. Even if patients ask you about your personal life, try to answer as briefly as possible and turn the focus back on the patient. For example, if the patient asks, "Are you married? Do you have children?" You could answer by saying, "Yes, I am, and I have two kids. What about you? How long have you been married? Where do your children live?"

Communication During a Patient Interview

An interview is a more formal way of communicating. It is planned communication with a purpose. An interview is used to get or give information. Because this is a planned event, you will need to consider certain factors that will influence the interview. For instance, time, place, seating arrangement, and distance are some factors that will affect the interview. Also, the format of the interview should contain three major stages: the opening, body, and closing.

- The *opening* of an interview includes introducing yourself, explaining the purpose of the interview, and establishing rapport with the patient. For example, you might say, "My name is Jane Jones, and I am going to be talking with you about the problems you have been having due to your heart condition."
- The *body* of the interview is the main part during which you will ask questions and obtain answers from the patient. It accomplishes the purpose of the interview.
- The *closing* of the interview occurs as you complete all the questions, offer the patient a chance to ask any questions he or she might have, and thank him or her for participating. It might include information about what will happen next. For example, you might say, "Dr. Jacobs will be in to see you shortly, and she will order any tests needed to determine your diagnosis."

Interviewing is used extensively in the nursing process. Interviews can be conducted face to face or over the telephone. In all cases, the nurse uses two main types of interviewing techniques. The *directive interview* is structured and conducted to find out specific information. Close-ended questions are used to request specific data from a patient; they usually require a "yes" or "no" or a short response of specific, factual information. Close-ended questions begin with one of the following words:

- Who
- What
- When
- Where
- How
- Do
- Is

The patient gives information or answers questions without going into detail. The directive interview is used when time is limited or during an emergency.

Open-ended questions are used in the *nondirective interview*. The patient has much more input in the nondirective interview and is able to explore thoughts and feelings. An open-ended question states the broad topic that will be discussed and invites the patient to elaborate on responses. Open-ended questions are good questions for beginning an interview, changing topics, and drawing out attitudes. You will use close-ended questions as an interview progresses to obtain specific data, such as a health history. Nurses will use a combination of open- and close-ended questions during an interview to obtain needed information.

Using Nonverbal Communication During an Interview

Nonverbal communication is another important consideration during an interview. Verbal communication can be easily manipulated by interview participants to create a selected impression. Nonverbal language can rarely be manipulated and most often reveals what is really going on with the interview participant. Body language should be observed for unstated feelings or behaviors. Also, be aware of your own body language and how it influences the effectiveness of the interview process.

Because so much of the information a patient provides to you must be entered into a computer for an EHR, it is easy to focus your eyes solely on the computer screen as you ask your patient questions and enter the answers. This is very depersonalizing for the patient and does not convey interest or caring to them. Be especially careful to position the computer screen so that you can look at patients as you ask questions and make eye contact as they answer. Then enter the information into the EHR.

The interview is an opportunity to assess an individual's health literacy. *Health literacy* is defined as the ability of an individual to obtain, process, and understand basic health information and services to make appropriate health decisions.

Low health literacy has been linked to increased rates of hospitalizations, outpatient visits, and health-care costs, as well as noncompliance with instructions about chronic disease conditions. During an interview, the nurse must assess the patient's health literacy and communicate information in a way and language the patient will understand so that he or she can become an active participant in his or her care.

Avoiding Bias During an Interview

In The Joint Commission's safety and quality advisory regarding implicit bias in health care, they have pointed out that all patients are not always treated equally. This can occur as a result of racial, ethnic, or gender bias. It is important that we, as nurses, speak for those who cannot or do not advocate for themselves.

Some individuals are going to be less likely than others to speak up, ask questions, or seek treatment. In addition, bias toward the lesbian, gay, bisexual, and transgender (LGBT) community often keeps these patients from being open with their health-care provider and nurses. Sometimes these patients do not fit in a box on a form.

When discussing a sexual history with a patient, be sure to be open and relaxed. Avoid making any negative facial reactions, even if the patient's lifestyle is very different from your own. When working with a transgendered patient, it is extremely important to be sensitive while still obtaining factual information that you need. When a transgendered patient is admitted, he or she may not want to be called by their legal name if it does not match their chosen gender. Ask the patient how he or she would like to be addressed or what name he or she would like to be called. Then use the gender-appropriate pronouns for the chosen gender. Avoid asking about sex change surgery unless it is necessary for the patient's care. Remember that HIPAA applies to everyone regardless of lifestyle.

It is also important to advocate for the LGBT community and their health needs. It is important to discuss sexually transmitted infections, HIV, AIDS, and depression because there are high incidences of all of these in the LGBT community. Routine screenings such as mammograms and Pap smears are important for every woman regardless of their sexual preference. The same is true for prostate exams for gay, bisexual, and transgender men.

> **KNOWLEDGE CONNECTION**
>
> How can you establish trust with a patient? When is it appropriate to use close-ended questions in an interview? What is meant by health literacy? How can you best discuss sexual history with a transgendered patient?

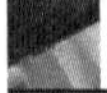

SPECIAL COMMUNICATION NEEDS

When you are working with patients with special needs, you will have to alter how you communicate with them to accommodate those needs. The following are effective communication techniques to use with patients with special sensory needs.

People Who Are Deaf or Hard of Hearing

When patients are hard of hearing, you must make an extra effort to be understood. Communication with patients who are deaf requires that you position yourself in front of them so that they can see your lips. Other strategies for communicating with patients with a hearing deficit include the following:

- Find out how the person communicates best—verbalizing, writing, lip reading, or signing
- Refrain from using an intercom and developing an alternative way of communicating
- Get the person's attention before starting to communicate
- Face the person
- Speak clearly with adequate volume without shouting or mumbling
- Ask for clarification and feedback to make sure you have been understood
- Speak to the patient, not the interpreter, if one is present
- Verify that the patient's hearing aid is inserted and working properly, if appropriate, and make sure batteries are checked frequently
- Eliminate background noise, such as turning down the volume on the television or other distractions

If the person reads lips, use the following strategies:

- Speak in a normal way and not in an overly exaggerated manner
- Use short, simple sentences
- Do not block the view of your face with your hands
- Do not chew gum
- Make sure the lighting is good

Other tips include the following:

- When someone asks, "What did you say?," avoid answering with comments such as "Never mind" or "Nothing." These comments are insulting and demeaning because they communicate that the person is not worthy of the effort of repeating yourself.
- Engage hard-of-hearing or deaf persons in one-on-one communication whenever possible because they may struggle in large groups or when there are two or more speakers.
- Do not show impatience or exasperation when communicating because this may cause the hearing-impaired person to shut down and back off from expressing needs.

People Who Have Speech and Language Impairments

Many people have difficulty with speech or language due to conditions such as deafness, cerebral palsy, cerebral vascular accident (CVA), head injury, multiple sclerosis, and ventilator dependency. Chances are you will encounter patients who

Box 6.7

Types of Aphasia

Patients who are unable to speak may have one or more types of aphasia.

Expressive aphasia (Broca's aphasia) is a disturbance in speech planning and speech production. Persons with expressive aphasia cannot produce fluent speech. Their speech has been described as "halting." Expressive aphasia presents as:

- Single-word responses; inability to produce spontaneous conversation
- Slow, monotone utterances
- Inappropriate words
- Hearing, reading abilities are intact

Receptive aphasia (Wernicke's aphasia) is a deficit in auditory comprehension or in receiving information. The patient can hear but cannot understand what is said, may be slow to respond, or may understand only a portion of what is said. Receptive aphasia presents as:

- Abnormal language
- Impaired reading and writing skill because the person does not understand what is supposed to be accomplished
- Speech sounds with normal rhythm, rate, and fluency

Global aphasia (expressive and receptive) is a deficit of planning, production, and comprehension of language. Patients with global aphasia can speak and understand only a few words. Global aphasia presents as:

- Meaningless speech sounds
- Possibly *perseveration,* or the repetition of one word or thought

Communication with patients with aphasia is difficult. Patients with severe impairments may have to learn to read body language and gestures to communicate.

Box 6.8

Communication Techniques for Patients With Aphasia

It is possible to communicate with patients who are unable to speak or are unable to speak clearly. To do so, use these techniques:

- Make sure you have the patient's attention by touching him or her if necessary and addressing him or her by name.
- Speak slowly.
- Use short sentences.
- Repeat what you said.
- Use gestures, demonstration, and facial expression if necessary.
- Speak in a normal tone of voice.
- Be respectful. The patient's social awareness and sensitivities are not impaired.
- Ask yes-or-no questions and write messages to help the patient understand.
- Listen carefully.
- Allow the patient to speak without interruption.
- Try to make the patient a "partner" in the communication.

Make no issue of the use of swear words or excessive jargon. A speech-language pathologist can make recommendations to deal with those behaviors.

have some form of a speech or language problem, and you must have some understanding of how to best work with these individuals.

Two of the most important functions involving communication are language and speech. Language includes writing, listening, and reading skills. It also includes receiving information. Speech is the process by which language is communicated through sound. In combination, speech and language, as well as nonverbal methods of communication, are the mechanisms through which humans share thoughts, feelings, and information.

Aphasia is the inability to speak or understand language. A patient may have trouble processing language output, known as expressive aphasia, or may have difficulty understanding speech, known as receptive aphasia. Box 6.7 presents an explanation of different types of aphasias. Caregivers should not assume that a patient comprehends communication until the patient's actions indicate an understanding. A speech-language pathologist will evaluate the patient for the type and level of impairment.

It will be your responsibility as the nurse to understand what speech and language deficits your patients may experience and to develop an appropriate plan of care for mutual understanding. You must encourage your patients to communicate to the best of their abilities. Box 6.8 lists some techniques to use when working with patients who have aphasia. Other ways to help communicate with individuals who have aphasia are to use picture boards, write on paper, or utilize a computer or a telecommunication device for the deaf.

People Who Have Vision Impairments

When you care for people who have vision impairments, it is important to remember that they cannot always see you clearly when you enter the room. Always identify yourself because it may be difficult for the patient to recognize your

• WORD • BUILDING •

aphasia: a – not + phasia – speak

voice. Speak naturally—there is no need to raise your voice. Use body language the same way you would with a sighted patient as this makes your tone sound more natural. Be sure to introduce the patient to anyone else who is in the room and avoid speaking to others as though the patient is not there. Before leaving the room, tell the patient that you are going to leave and ask if there is anything needed before you go. Avoid just slipping quietly out the door because the patient will not know that you are gone. Before providing care, touch the patient gently on the arm to signal that you are close.

Anatomy and Physiology Connection

The Nervous System's Role in Communication

The brain and nervous system directly affect our ability to communicate. Activities that precede, initiate, or support communication are controlled by the brain and nervous system. A variety of communication problems occur when there is a brain or nervous system malfunction. Parkinson's disease, CVA (also known as "brain attack" or stroke), and trauma cause damage to the brain and nervous system and often affect a person's ability to engage in the communication process.

The cerebral cortex of the brain has several areas that control voluntary muscle movement, sensory perception, and sensory interpretation—all of which are necessary in the communication process. The left frontal lobe contains Broca's motor speech area, which controls the movements involved in speaking. The left temporal and parietal lobes hold speech areas that are involved in thoughts that precede speech. The parietal lobes contain the general sensory areas where sensations such as touch are felt and interpreted. The occipital lobes contain visual areas that receive impulses from the eyes that allow us to "see" and interpret what is being seen. Deep within the cerebral hemispheres, gray matter called the basal ganglia regulates the use of accessory movements, such as gestures, when communicating.

Patients on Mechanical Ventilation

Attempting to communicate with patients who are intubated via an endotracheal tube and who cannot speak poses challenges for the nurse and causes high levels of patient anxiety and stress. Without the ability to speak, patients are unable to express thoughts, feelings, desires, and needs in the usual manner. The following are some guidelines to enhance communication when caring for the mechanically dependent patient:

- Place the patient in a comfortable position to communicate; this is usually with the patient sitting and positioned upright. Provide adequate pain relief if needed. Assess communication methods to determine what works best.
- Make sure the call light is within easy reach, and instruct the patient on how to use it. Reassure the patient that someone will come when the call light is activated.
- If the patient uses a hearing aid or glasses, make sure they are on or in place and in good working order. If the patient does not speak English, make sure a translator is available.
- Assess the patient for the ability to communicate by writing. Provide a tablet or a magic slate. Do not place an IV line in the patient's writing arm if possible.
- Instruct the patient on other ways he or she can call for attention, such as tapping the over-the-bed table or side rail or using a bell or a clicking device.
- Evaluate the patient's ability to communicate without talking. Mouthing words may not be possible for every patient to master. Communicate with the patient by asking yes-or-no questions and asking him or her to blink the eyes a certain number of times or to shake or nod his or her head for a response.
- If available, use a portable text-to-speech communication device or a communication board.
- Encourage communication and reassure the patient often. If the patient is unresponsive, use therapeutic touch and stroke the patient to convey a sense of security. Continue to communicate with the patient using simple, conversational language and explain what you are doing. Instruct family members and visitors to do the same.
- Be sure to document your communication assessment and the communication strategies you have developed. Also, ensure that successful communication strategies are passed along in the shift report so that all staff may be able to communicate successfully with the patient and the patient may benefit from the continuity of care.

Remember, being intubated is a highly stressful event for the responsive patient. Try to alleviate some of the stress by developing effective communication strategies with the patient and making them part of the care plan.

Patients Who Are Unresponsive

In a critical care environment, where the patients are very ill or need close observation, the nurse must be intensely focused on tasks related to their many physical needs. This often places communication with patients as a lower priority.

There is a strong relationship between patient responsiveness and the amount of verbal communication made by nurses. When patients are unconscious or connected to a ventilator, it is difficult for the nurse, especially the nurse with little clinical experience, to engage in effective nurse-patient communication. Conversation is one-way—with no verbal response from the patient. Consequently, nurses who are working with sedated or unconscious patients will often "undervalue" the importance of talking with them. Inadequate nurse-patient communication in these instances has been shown to increase stress, anxiety, and social isolation for the patient.

Communication content with the unconscious patient often is more "informative" rather than conversational, meaning nurses will explain what tasks they will be performing or if a medical procedure is to be carried out. Informative language is important, but conversational language also is important because it conveys to the patient that you are taking the time to attend to the psychosocial needs that all humans require, as well as their physical needs.

Most sedated or unconscious patients still can hear and comprehend verbal communication, and they respond emotionally to it. Do not speak about other patients while caring for a sedated or unconscious patient. It is a HIPAA violation. In addition, the patient may misinterpret and become distressed. Patients perceive nurses who do not make communication a high priority to be uninterested, unskilled, and not professional.

POST CONFERENCE

As you evaluate the care you gave your patient during post conference, you share that at first it was difficult to talk to him and you found yourself chattering about inane things. Then, every time you asked him a question, he would respond just with a "yes" or "no." That is when you remembered to use open-ended questions. When you asked your patient open-ended questions, he responded better. You learned a little bit about his family. Eventually, you became a bit more comfortable with silence in the room. When his sister came to visit, she was very talkative and told you that her brother "never says more than two words to anybody." Hearing that made you smile because you knew that, by using silence, asking open-ended questions, and establishing rapport, you were able to communicate well with this patient.

Key Points

- Communication is a reciprocal process that occurs simultaneously between two parties. It involves sending and receiving messages to arrive at a shared meaning.
- Communication occurs in two ways, verbal and nonverbal.
- Personal space, body position, language, culture, attitude, and emotions are factors that contribute to the way people communicate.
- Different cultures have different preferences and norms for personal space and touch. For example, people in Canada, the United States, and Great Britain require the most personal space, while people from the Middle East require the least personal space.
- Active listening techniques use all the senses to interpret verbal and nonverbal messages. The mind focuses on the interaction and listens for feelings as well as spoken words.
- The DESC method is used to help promote assertive communication. ***D*** stands for "describe the behavior," ***E*** stands for "explain the impact of the behavior," ***S*** stands for "state the desired outcome," and ***C*** stands for "consequences" of not complying.
- Therapeutic communication is patient-centered communication. The goal is to promote a greater understanding of a patient's needs, concerns, and feelings. There are defined techniques that promote therapeutic communication, such as empathy, and barriers we all use to block communication.
- Anger and/or hostility can lead to conflict. Conflict will affect the quality of care and must be managed.
- Nurses and patients need to build a relationship based on mutual trust. Patients will not share information with someone that they do not trust or someone that they do not think cares about them. When you can intellectually identify with the patient, you show empathy, which will help promote trust.
- Hand-off or end-of-shift reporting is an area of communication vulnerable to ineffective communication that increases the chances of medical errors.
- The interview is formal, planned communication designed to give or obtain information. It is very important to be aware of implicit bias during an interview and take steps to prevent it.
- The very young and elderly individuals have specialized communication needs that must be recognized and individualized.

Review Questions

Select the answer that is most appropriate for each of the following questions. Some questions may have more than one correct answer. Select all that apply.

1. What is the term that indicates that a message was communicated as intended?
   1. Sending
   2. Receiving
   3. Comprehending
   4. Shared meaning

2. Factors that affect communication include:
   1. personal space.
   2. culture.
   3. attitude.
   4. emotions.

3. Active listening involves:
   1. looking at a chart while the patient is speaking.
   2. pausing before speaking.
   3. checking your watch often during conversation.
   4. nodding your head in agreement.

4. An example of nonverbal communication that is congruent to the verbal statement by the patient "I'm having a lot of back pain" would be:
   1. smiling.
   2. reading a magazine.
   3. looking up at the ceiling.
   4. grimacing and rubbing his back.

5. An assertive behavior style includes:
   1. standing up for one's own self.
   2. putting one's own needs, rights, and feelings before others.
   3. showing respect for others.
   4. acting in a consistent manner that enhances self-worth.

6. You promote trust with a patient by:
   1. allowing family members to visit whenever they want.
   2. keeping medical information confidential.
   3. talking with her at length about her life.
   4. being sure to carry through when you say you will do something.

7. When communicating with people who are hard of hearing:
   1. set the intercom on high.
   2. speak in an exaggerated way.
   3. find out how the person communicates best.
   4. if the person uses an interpreter, speak to the interpreter.

8. Open-ended questions are good types of questions to use in what situations?
   1. Introducing broad topics during an interview
   2. Beginning an interview
   3. Changing topics in an interview
   4. Asking a patient about his or her feelings

ANSWERS 1. 4, 2. 1, 2, 3, 4, 3. 2, 4, 4. 4, 5. 1, 3, 4, 6. 2, 4, 7. 3, 8. 1, 2, 3, 4

Critical Thinking Exercise

Answers available online.

1. You are caring for Mrs. Etta Jones, a 79-year-old female who suffered a CVA 2 years ago that left her with an aphasic disorder. Mrs. Jones suffers from expressive aphasia and utters the word "yes" for all responses. What communication techniques would you use to ensure that Mrs. Jones' needs are being met and that she is being supported emotionally?

Additional Resources

Use the scratch off code on the inside front cover of your book to access online quizzes that will help you to improve your scores on course exams and prepare for the NCLEX-PN®.

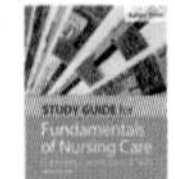

Study Guide

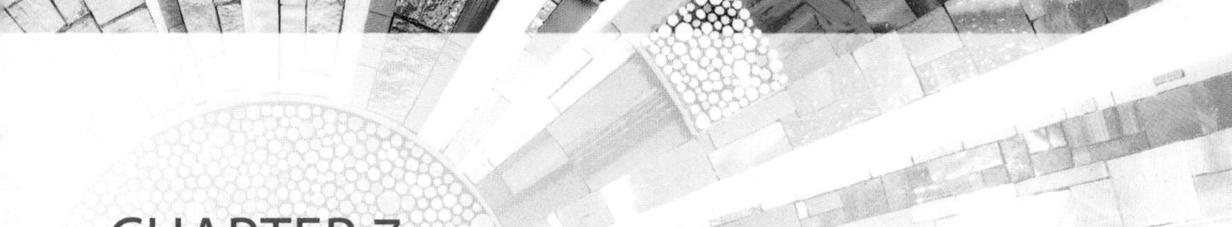

CHAPTER 7
Promoting Health and Wellness

KEY TERMS

Acute illness (ah-KEWT ILL-ness)
Adaptation (ad-ap-TAY-shun)
Chronic illness (KRAH-nik ILL-ness)
Continuum (kon-TI-new-uhm)
Coping strategies (KOH-ping STRA-tuh-jeez)
Dependency phase (dih-PEN-den-see FAYZ)
Exacerbation (egg-sass-sir-BAY-shun)
Fight-or-flight response (FIGHT OR FLIGHT ree-SPONS)
Health literacy (HELLTH LIT-er-ah-see)
Healthy People 2020
Prodromal phase (proh-DROHM-uhl FAYZ)
Recovery phase (ree-KUV-uh-ree FAYZ)
Remission (ree-MISH-un)
Risk factor (RISK FAK-ter)
Seeking help phase (SEE-king HELP FAYZ)
Stress (STRESS)
Symptomatic phase (SIMP-toh-MAT-ic FAYZ)

CHAPTER CONCEPTS

Stress
Health Promotion

LEARNING OUTCOMES

1. Define various terms related to health promotion and wellness.
2. Explain the wellness-illness continuum.
3. Describe two theories of wellness and illness.
4. Discuss different types and phases of illness.
5. Identify the 4 overarching goals and 12 leading health indicators of Healthy People 2020.
6. Explain health literacy.
7. Identify risk factors for selected illnesses.
8. Explain the theory of stress and adaptation.
9. Describe the symptoms of stress.
10. Describe the body's reactions during the "fight-or-flight" response.
11. Categorize coping strategies in response to stress.
12. Describe defense mechanisms and their use.
13. Discuss information found in the Connection features in this chapter.

CRITICAL THINKING CONNECTION

Clinical Assignment

You are caring for a 45-year-old woman who is a very healthy, long-distance runner. She has been diagnosed with gallstones and is scheduled for a *cholecystectomy,* the surgical removal of the gallbladder. She seems very anxious and tells you that she has never really been ill before. In fact, she tells you that she doesn't understand how she could get gallstones because she is such a healthy eater. She has many questions for you about her postoperative recovery; she asks you, "Will I be well again after this surgery? Can I run again right away and eat my normal diet? I hate being sick. This was never supposed to happen to me."

Critical Thinking Questions:

1. How does your patient view illness?
2. How does your patient view wellness?
3. How does lifestyle influence her diagnosis, if at all?
4. How will you promote wellness with this patient?

In our society, the idea of wellness covers a wide spectrum. Getting plenty of exercise, eating healthy foods, avoiding unhealthy activities, and perhaps taking dietary supplements may mean wellness to some people. To others, the quality of exercise is stressed above all else, such as 30 minutes of cardiovascular exercise and 30 minutes of weight training, followed by 15 minutes of walking on the treadmill to cool down. Still others focus more on the types of food and intake, with only a nod to exercise: They might eat raw fruits and whole grains in the morning, lean protein and raw vegetables at lunch, and cooked vegetables with lean protein and whole grains for dinner, with snacks of nuts and dried fruits.

So, what is wellness? Is it what you eat or do not eat? Is it dependent on exercise? Or is it more than all of these things?

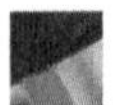

THEORIES OF WELLNESS AND ILLNESS

To some individuals, a person is well when he or she is without a diagnosed illness. However, does that mean that a person who has a well-controlled condition that is ongoing, such as hypertension, cannot be considered well? As nurses, we may see people with critical illnesses every day and, as a result, lose our perspective. We may think that anyone who is not in an intensive care unit is not actually ill. What about people whose lifestyle has been less than perfect? What about those who are overweight, do not exercise, eat unhealthy foods, or smoke tobacco? Are they guaranteed to become ill? Do they even deserve their illness because they were not actively trying to prevent it?

These questions are difficult to answer because illness means different things to different people. One popular definition of illness states that illness causes changes in a person's functioning, whether it be physical, mental, spiritual, or emotional. Some people have illnesses that affect their ability to function even though they appear perfectly normal, making it difficult for others to sympathize. Other people are visibly ill, such as the person who is very thin, weak, and pale and the person who becomes short of breath with the slightest exertion.

The Wellness-Illness Continuum

Most of us are not completely well or completely ill at any given time. Rather, we move up and down along a **continuum,** or scale, with exceptional wellness at the top and severe illness at the bottom. Figure 7.1 shows such a continuum. Even within a day, a person may move up or down on this continuum. For example, you may wake up with a sore throat and nasal congestion and you might consider yourself at 5 on the continuum. By afternoon, you are feeling better and may move up the scale to 7.

It is important to remember that physical health is not the only issue that is involved when discussing wellness and illness. A person may be well physically but may be depressed or have other mental conditions that would prevent him or her from being considered healthy. However, if a mental illness is being treated and managed well, the person moves closer to the exceptional wellness end of the scale.

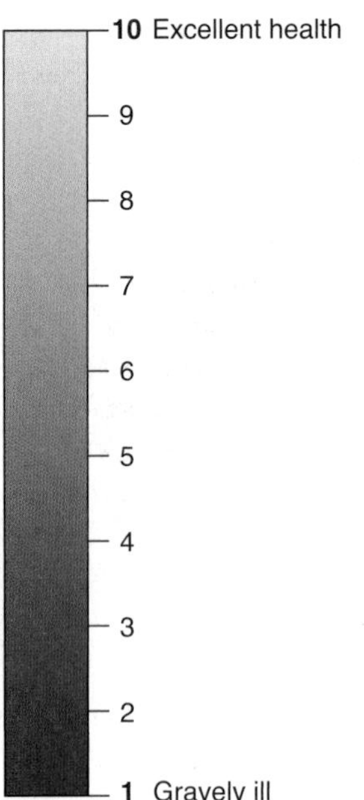

FIGURE 7.1 The wellness-illness continuum (from Wilkinson JM, Treas LS. *Fundamentals of Nursing: Theory, Concepts & Applications.* Vol. 1. 3rd ed. Philadelphia, PA: FA Davis; 2016).

Dunn's Theory of High-Level Wellness

In 1959, H. L. Dunn developed a theory about achieving high-level wellness. In his theory, there is not only a continuum of health and wellness, referred to as the Health Axis, but also a vertical axis to represent the person's environment. In this theory, there are four quadrants to describe a person's condition based on the influences of wellness or illness and a favorable or unfavorable environment.

On the environmental axis of the grid, one end of the continuum is labeled "Very Unfavorable Environment," while the opposite end of the continuum is labeled "Very Favorable Environment." On the health axis, one end of the continuum is labeled "Peak Wellness," while the opposite end is labeled "Death." The four quadrants of the grid include:

- ***Protected Poor Health:*** This occurs when the environment is favorable but health is not.
- ***Poor Health:*** This occurs when both health and environment are not favorable.
- ***Emergent High-Level Wellness:*** This occurs when the environment is not favorable, but health is favorable.
- ***High-Level Wellness:*** This occurs when both the environment and health are favorable.

If a person with an ongoing health condition such as severe congestive heart failure is in a favorable environment with family, caregivers, needed medications, appropriate diet, and regular health-care provider visits, on Dunn's grid this person would be identified as having "protected poor health."

• WORD • BUILDING •

hypertension: hyper – excessive + tension – stretching

It is easy to see that a person with an illness such as tuberculosis who is homeless would be considered to have "poor health" on this grid.

Fitzpatrick's Rhythm Model

A nursing theory that deals with health and wellness is Dr. Joyce Fitzpatrick's rhythm model. One of the major concepts of Fitzpatrick's theory is that of wellness-illness. Nursing is rooted in the promotion of wellness practices, the attentive treatment of those who are acutely or chronically ill or dying, and the restorative care of people during convalescence and rehabilitation. In this model, health is a dynamic state that results from the interaction of a person and his or her environment. A person's state of health can vary from wellness to illness, disease, or dysfunction, and it changes continuously throughout the person's life span.

> **KNOWLEDGE CONNECTION**
> Where do you place yourself on the wellness-illness continuum today? Where would you have placed yourself yesterday? What are the reasons for your choice?

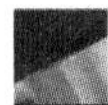

PROMOTING WELLNESS

Concern regarding the overall health of our citizens has led the U.S. government to establish an initiative for moving us all toward wellness and living long, healthy lives. The current version of this initiative is known as Healthy People 2020.

Healthy People 2020

Healthy People provides science-based health goals and objectives to improve national health and prevent disease. The goals and objectives are revised every 10 years. Through the Office of Disease Prevention and Health Promotions, part of the Department of Health and Human Services, **Healthy People 2020** continues to work toward improving the prevention of disease and promoting health in the United States. The overarching goals of this program are as follows:

- Attain high-quality, longer lives free of preventable disease, disability, injury, and premature death
- Achieve health equity, eliminate disparities, and improve the health of all groups
- Create social and physical environments that promote good health for all
- Promote quality of life, healthy development, and healthy behaviors across all life stages

The current 10-year promotion, Healthy People 2020, includes 12 leading health indicators (LHIs) that are the highest-priority health issues that serve as measures of our nation's health. The Web site, www.healthypeople.gov/2020/leading-health-indicators/2020-LHI-Topics, includes actions that can be taken to address each of the objectives. (See Box 7.1 for a list of these LHIs.)

Health Literacy

When health-care professionals explain to patients how to prepare for a test, how to take medications, or any number of other instructions, they assume the patients understand, especially if they ask no questions. The truth is that sometimes patients do not actually understand, resulting in illnesses or complications that could have been prevented. In an effort to address this communication gap, the concept of health literacy was developed. **Health literacy** refers to the ability of individuals to understand basic health information and to use that information to make good decisions about their health. Assessing health literacy is so important that it has been referred to as the "newest vital sign."

The idea behind the concept is that health-care professionals should assess patients for their ability to comprehend health-care information and to use it to make decisions. Several tools are available to measure health literacy, but one very popular tool uses an ice cream label to assess the patient's ability to use numbers, make calculations, identify potentially harmful ingredients, and make informed decisions before taking action.

The patient is given a specific ice cream label to refer to during the assessment. The health-care professional then asks the patient six questions and scores the answers according to a score sheet. The questions are always asked orally. Examples of such questions include the following:

- If you ate the entire container of ice cream, how many calories would you eat?
- If you usually eat 2,500 calories in a day, what percentage of your daily calories will you be eating if you eat one serving?

Box 7.1

Healthy People 2020 Leading Health Indicators

The 12 LHIs included in the Healthy People 2020 initiative are:

- Access to health services
- Clinical preventive services
- Environmental quality
- Injury and violence
- Maternal, infant, and child health
- Mental health
- Nutrition, physical activity, and obesity
- Oral health
- Reproductive and sexual health
- Social determinants
- Substance abuse
- Tobacco

Source: Office of Disease Prevention and Health Promotion. Leading Health Indicators. Available at: www.healthypeople.gov/2020/Leading-Health-Indicators. Accessed May 2, 2017.

- Pretend that you are allergic to the following substances: penicillin, peanuts, latex gloves, and bee stings. Is it safe for you to eat this ice cream?

You may not be surprised to learn that only 12% of the population has a proficient health literacy score according to the National Assessment of Adult Literacy. Research has shown that people who have low health literacy are at higher risk for poor health regardless of other factors such as educational level and age. ***Safety: It is extremely important for health-care professionals to ensure that patients understand the information they receive.***

> **KNOWLEDGE CONNECTION**
> Which of the 12 Leading Health Indicators do you see as most important? Why? Why is it important for nurses to assess a patient's health literacy?

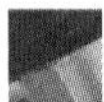 ILLNESS

Despite efforts to promote wellness and decrease risky behaviors, people do become ill. Illness is not always due to the person's lack of effort to remain healthy. Some people do nothing to achieve a healthy lifestyle, engage in a number of risky behaviors, and are diagnosed with an illness, as expected. At other times, people work very hard at being healthy and are shocked when they develop a sudden severe illness. Although cause and effect regarding lifestyle choices and illness have been proven to exist, sometimes illness occurs without previous risk factors. Therefore, it is important that you do not "blame the victim" when you care for patients who have been diagnosed with an illness or disease.

Just as it is difficult to know what caused an illness or why it happened to a particular person, it also is difficult to predict each person's response to illness. Some people seem to take even devastating diagnoses in stride, while others seem to panic over a diagnosis of a relatively minor, easily treated disorder.

Types of Illness

To some people, illness is defined as "not being able to do what I want to do." To others, illness could be defined as "any pain or discomfort because it means my body is not functioning normally." It is difficult to determine a single definition of illness because several types of illness exist, and people perceive illness differently.

An **acute illness** strikes suddenly and lasts for a limited time. An example of an acute illness would be food poisoning: You become very ill a few hours after ingesting contaminated food. You experience severe symptoms of nausea, vomiting, and diarrhea for 24 to 48 hours. Once your body rids itself of the offensive contaminants, you begin to feel better. Acute illness also can occur in situations in which hospitalization is required. For example, a patient is admitted with acute appendicitis and has an emergency *appendectomy,* or removal of the appendix. After surgery, the incision gradually heals and the patient eventually returns to normal activities.

A **chronic illness** is one that lasts for 6 months or longer and is characterized by intensifying or improving symptoms. Chronic illness may require treatment and medications or limitation of a person's activities. An example of a chronic illness would be chronic obstructive pulmonary disease (COPD). People with COPD often are dependent on supplemental oxygen and have a low energy reserve because of the effort required to breathe, thus limiting activities in which they are able to participate.

Chronic illness is characterized by periods of either minimal symptoms or a complete absence of symptoms, called **remissions,** and periods of worsening symptoms, called **exacerbations.** Rheumatoid arthritis is an example of a chronic illness with periods of remission when joint pain lessens and mobility improves and periods of exacerbation when the opposite occurs.

Phases of Illness

Before a person develops symptoms of a specific illness, he or she may simply "not feel good," with generalized body aches and fatigue. This is referred to as the **prodromal phase** of illness.

As observable symptoms develop—for example, a sore throat and congestion or a rash with a fever—the person enters the **symptomatic phase.** At this point, he or she makes a choice to wait and see if the symptoms resolve, treat himself or herself with over-the-counter products or home remedies, or seek advice from friends and relatives.

Next comes the **seeking help phase.** The majority of people in Western society seek help from a medical professional, such as a physician, physician assistant, or nurse practitioner. However, some people may seek help from healers rather than physicians. Some seek out herbalists or other alternative practitioners (see Chapter 11 for additional information on alternative medicine).

Once a person has sought help, he or she must decide to follow the advice or recommended treatment or to seek help elsewhere. In this **dependency phase,** a person relies on others for help in diagnosis and treatment. In many cases, the individual not only must depend on others for medical care, but he or she also may be forced to rely on others to perform his or her work or family duties. Different people react in different ways to the dependent role. As the nurse, you are often the one whom patients must depend on during this phase of illness. Many patients adapt to this dependent role without difficulty, realizing it is a short-term situation; other patients react by becoming angry, fearful, or overly dependent; and still others may become manipulative.

• WORD • BUILDING •
remission: re – back + mission – send
exacerbation: ex – induce + acerbation – aggravation
prodromal: pro – before + dromal – running

The final phase is the **recovery phase,** when the person is slowly able to resume independence and regain his or her health. It should be noted that people with a chronic illness often remain in the dependency phase because complete recovery is not possible.

> **KNOWLEDGE CONNECTION**
> Contrast acute and chronic illness. Contrast exacerbation and remission. List the five phases of illness.

Risk Factors for Illness

Researchers have identified **risk factors** for some illnesses. These are physiological, psychological, or genetic elements that contribute to the development of an illness or disease. Another type of risk factor is environmental elements, such as exposure to a chemical hazard that could lead to illness. Some risk factors can be modified or changed by alterations in lifestyle and nutrition. Other risk factors are nonmodifiable, such as heredity, age, and gender. People who have risk factors for illnesses such as diabetes, heart disease, stroke, and cancer may be able to decrease their risk of developing the illness by modifying their diet and exercise routine, as well as managing their blood pressure and blood sugar. Table 7.1 lists modifiable risk factors for selected illnesses. ***Safety: An increasingly common modifiable risk factor for many illnesses is overwhelming stress and a lifestyle that lacks balance among work, play, and rest.***

Cancer can have some familial tendencies (be passed down in families), which is a nonmodifiable risk factor. The American Cancer Society has identified seven warning signs of cancer; these are listed in Box 7.2. ***Safety: Knowledge of these warning signs can contribute to early detection and diagnosis.***

Table 7.1
Modifiable Risk Factors for Selected Diseases

Risk Factor	*Diseases*
Obesity	Diabetes, heart disease, breast cancer, colon cancer
Diet high in trans-fatty acids, cholesterol, and triglycerides	Diabetes, stroke, heart disease
Hypertension	Stroke, heart disease, kidney disease
Smoking	Heart disease, bronchitis, COPD, stroke, lung cancer, and other types of cancer

Box 7.2
The Seven Warning Signs of Cancer

The first letter of each sign indicating that a condition may be cancerous together spell out the word CAUTION.

- **C**hange in bowel or bladder habits
- **A** sore that does not heal
- **U**nusual bleeding or discharge from any body orifice
- **T**hickening or a lump in the breast or elsewhere
- **I**ndigestion or difficulty in swallowing
- **O**bvious change in a wart or mole
- **N**agging cough or hoarseness

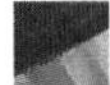

STRESS AND ADAPTATION

According to Hans Selye, who developed the response-based model of stress, **stress** is identified as a nonspecific response of the body to any demand made on it. Any stress-inducing event is referred to as a *stressor;* it can include a physical, emotional, pleasant, or unpleasant occurrence. How these stresses of daily life affect an individual depends largely on the individual's ability to adapt. **Adaptation** is the ability to positively adjust to changes that occur in an individual's world. If one does not adapt to changes, the physiological and psychological responses can be harmful. Ongoing stress not only can result in illness and injury, but also can lead to death if it is not relieved.

> **Anatomy and Physiology Connection**
>
> **The Fight-or-Flight Response**
>
> When your brain perceives a threat to your well-being, it sends messages to the body to prepare to either *stay and fight* or *run away.* This innate protective response saved our ancestors from wild animals and other predators and is known as the **fight-or-flight response.** Your brain engages the sympathetic nervous system, which stimulates the endocrine glands to pump cortisol, adrenaline, and other hormones into the bloodstream, enabling you to hit harder, jump higher, see farther, and think or run faster. These hormones cause the bronchial airways to dilate and the respiratory rate to rise, which both help to increase oxygen intake. The hormones also cause the heart rate to increase, blood vessels in the skin to constrict, and central blood vessels to dilate in an effort to deliver more oxygen-rich blood to the brain, heart, and muscles needed for the fight-or-flight response. Glycogen is converted to glucose to provide additional fuel and energy. The pupils of the eyes dilate to allow better vision. The sense of hearing is heightened to detect warning sounds. Salivary glands decrease their secretions and peristalsis slows in the digestive tract to prevent the need for bowel elimination during this "emergency" or high-stress time.

Arm and leg muscles tense in preparation for running or physical fighting. When the threat is removed, the parasympathetic nervous system dominates and reverses these responses.

Selye's theory of stress and illness probably has been demonstrated at some time in your life when you were in a situation of ongoing, unrelieved stress and then developed an illness. When we are stressed, our body responds with the fight-or-flight response described in the Anatomy and Physiology Connection. This is referred to as the *alarm phase.* If the stressor is removed in a relatively short period of time, our bodies return to normal. However, if the stressor continues in our life and we do not find positive ways of relieving it, our bodies get stuck in that fight-or-flight response, producing high levels of cortisol and other stress hormones. The body works hard trying to resist the threats of stress and to keep working efficiently to prevent illness. Selye calls this the *resistance phase,* and it can continue for weeks, months, or years. Eventually, our bodies cannot keep up the pace of dealing with stressors and fighting off illness. This is the *exhaustion phase,* when the body's resources are depleted and we are most vulnerable to physical and psychological disease. Selye titled this the *general adaptation syndrome* (GAS) because it describes the body's attempts to adapt to the stressors we encounter.

Stress can be considered either negative or positive, but the body cannot tell the difference between the two. Negative stress has the potential to cause harm. Examples would be physical illness, disease, or death of a family member. Positive stress involves events that, although anticipated, still may be viewed as stressful. Examples would include an upcoming marriage, job change, or graduation.

People use different ways of coping to manage their stressors. The possible outcomes of stress and ways of coping are changing the stressor, adapting to the stressor by changing thoughts and behaviors related to it, or avoiding the stressor. If the stressor—or in many cases a variety of stressors—remains in place without the person adapting to it, the stressor eventually causes illness or even death.

When a person is dealing with several stressors at one time or a stressor that lasts for a long time, it is much more difficult for him or her to adapt. Your response to stressors depends on several factors:

- How do you view the stressor? Do you see it as something major or something that can be adapted to with increased time and energy?
- What is your current health status? Do you already have a chronic illness such as diabetes or hypertension? Are you constantly in a state of exhaustion with few energy reserves?
- What are your support systems? Do you have friends and family who can help you with the details of life so that you can use your energy to adapt to the stressor? Do you have people to listen to you when you need to talk about your stressors?
- What other factors are at play? Your age, life stage, and life experiences can influence your ability to adapt to your stressors.

The outcome of stress is that either you adapt to it or you develop a disease or illness. Our bodies use various feedback mechanisms to maintain *homeostasis,* or balance in the internal environment of the body. These are physiological responses and include GAS. The process of making changes, physical or psychological, in response to stress is adaptation.

The psychological response to stressors includes feelings, thoughts, and behaviors. Common responses are fear and anxiety. Anxiety is a vague, uneasy feeling that is not centered on a specific source, and it is emotional in nature. Fear is an identified danger or threat with a real or imagined source, and it is cognitive in nature. One way we manage our fears and anxieties is by using *defense mechanisms,* which are unconscious reactions to decrease the stress. They help decrease tension caused by various stressors in our lives. Table 7.2 lists the types of defense mechanisms and examples of each.

Effects of Stress on Illness

When stress is continuous, it causes the sympathetic nervous system to go into "overdrive." Constricted blood vessels and an increased heart rate can lead to hypertension and heart disease. Vasodilation in the brain may contribute to migraine headaches. Illness and hospitalization also are stressors that can worsen some conditions, such as diabetes. In fact, research has shown that simply being admitted to the hospital will increase most individuals' blood glucose levels even though they do not have diabetes. Stress also can cause exacerbations in patients with some chronic disorders, such as systemic lupus erythematosus, multiple sclerosis, fibromyalgia, arthritis, and asthma.

When a family member has a major illness, it inflicts stress on the healthy members of the family because of concerns over the cost of health care, the care the patient is receiving, and fear of the ultimate outcome. It is vital that nurses be aware of all the stressors that both the patient and family members are facing.

Recognizing the Symptoms of Stress

How many times have you heard a coworker or fellow student say, "I am so stressed out"? It is a common phrase, and it sounds as if we all know when we are stressed. However, that is not always the case. Some people do not realize that they are experiencing severe stress overload until they are very ill or have caused damage to relationships. Box 7.3 lists some common symptoms of stress.

Stress Management

Coping strategies, the actions people utilize to combat stress, vary from person to person. It is important to note that both positive and negative coping strategies exist. Negative strategies cause harm to yourself or others—for example, drinking

Table 7.2
Defense Mechanisms

Mechanism	*Description*	*Examples*	*Overuse Can Lead To*
Avoidance	Unconsciously staying away from events or situations that might open feelings of aggression or anxiety	"I can't go to the class reunion tonight. I'm just so tired. I have to sleep."	May become socially isolated
Compensation	Making up for something we perceive as an inadequacy by developing some other desirable trait	The small boy who wants to be a basketball center instead becomes an honor roll student. The physically unattractive person who wants to model instead becomes a famous designer.	Use of drugs or alcohol to feel confident in social situations
Conversion reaction	Anxiety is channeled into physical symptoms. (*Note:* Often, the symptoms disappear soon after the threat is over.)	Nausea develops the night before a major examination, causing the person to miss the examination. Nausea may disappear soon after the scheduled test is finished.	Anxiety not dealt with can lead to actual physical disorders, such as gastric ulcers, and possibly some cancers.
Denial	Unconscious refusal to see reality. Usually the first defense learned and used. Is not consciously lying.	The alcoholic states, "I can quit any time I want to."	Repression, dissociative disorders
Displacement (transference)	Transferring anger and hostility to another person or object that is perceived to be less powerful: the "kick-the-dog syndrome"	Parent loses job without notice; goes home and verbally abuses spouse, who unjustly punishes child, who hits the dog	Loss of friends and relationships Confusion in communication
Dissociation	Painful events or situations are separated or dissociated from the conscious mind. Patients will often say, "I had an out-of-body experience" or "it happened to someone else, but it was as though it happened to me."	Patient who had been sexually abused as a child describes the situation as if it happened to a friend or a sibling. Police visit parent to inform parent of death of child in car accident. Parent tells police, "That's impossible. My child is upstairs asleep. You must have the wrong house."	One of the dissociative disorders, such as multiple personality disorder
Identification	A person takes on the ideas or personality traits of someone that he or she fears or respects.	Children playing like they are firefighters, police officers, cowboys, or mothers.	Assumes mannerisms, wears clothing, and arranges hair and appearance to match those of the other person.

Continued

Table 7.2 Defense Mechanisms—cont'd

Mechanism	*Description*	*Examples*	*Overuse Can Lead To*
Intellectualization	Separates self from uncomfortable emotions by focusing on facts and logic. When her husband dies, the wife relieves her pain by saying, "It's better this way because he was suffering so much."	After a breakup, a person focuses on obtaining a scholarship with good grades rather than feel the emotions of rejection and loss.	Allows facts and logic to take the place of feeling emotions over time. Similar to Mr. Spock on *Star Trek*.
Isolation	Emotion that is separated from the original feeling.	"I wasn't really angry; just a little upset."	Avoids dealing with true feeling Can increase stress
Minimization	Not acknowledging or accepting the significance of one's own behavior, making it seem less important.	A person thinks it doesn't matter how much he drinks as long as he doesn't drink and drive.	No motivation to change behavior, so it can become more unhealthy or antisocial with no consequences.
Projection (scapegoating)	Blaming others A mental or verbal "finger-pointing" at another for the problem	"I didn't get the promotion because you don't like me." "I'm overweight because you make me nervous."	Finds faults in everything and everyone Fails to learn to take personal responsibility May develop into delusional tendencies
Rationalization	Use of a logical-sounding excuse to cover up true thoughts and feelings The most frequently used defense mechanism	"I did not make a medication error; I followed the health-care provider's order." "I failed the test because the teacher wrote bad questions."	Self-deception
Reaction formation (overcompensation)	Similar to compensation, except the person usually develops the *exact opposite* trait	The small boy who wants to be a basketball center instead becomes an honor roll student. The physically unattractive person who wants to model speaks out for eliminating beauty pageants.	Failure to resolve internal conflicts
Regression	Emotionally returning to an earlier time in life when there was far less stress Commonly seen in patients while hospitalized (*Note:* Everyone does not go back to the same developmental age. This is highly individualized.)	Children who are toilet trained begin to wet themselves. Adults may start crying and have a "temper tantrum."	May interfere with perception of reality May interfere with progression and development of personality
Repression (stuffing)	An unconscious "burying" or "forgetting" mechanism Excludes or withholds from our consciousness events or situations that are unbearable; a step deeper than "denial"	Having no memory of a traumatic event, such as sexual abuse	Flashbacks, posttraumatic stress disorder, amnesia

Table 7.2
Defense Mechanisms—cont'd

Mechanism	*Description*	*Examples*	*Overuse Can Lead To*
Restitution (undoing)	Making amends for a behavior one thinks is unacceptable Making an attempt at reducing guilt	Giving a treat to a child who is being punished for a wrongdoing. The person who sees someone lose a wallet with a large amount of cash does not return the wallet but puts extra money in the collection plate at the next church service.	May send double messages. Relieves the "doer" of the responsibility of being honest in the situation
Sublimation	Unacceptable traits or characteristics are diverted into acceptable traits or characteristics.	Burglar teaches home safety classes. Person who is potentially physically abusive becomes a professional sports figure. People who choose to not have children run a day-care center.	The "socially accepted" behavior might actually reinforce the negative tendencies, and the person may still show signs of the undesirable behavior or trait.

Source: Adapted from Wilkinson JM, Treas LS. *Fundamentals of Nursing: Theory, Concepts & Applications.* Vol. 1. 3rd ed. Philadelphia, PA: FA Davis; 2016:250-251; Table 12-1. *Wilkinson's table notes the following source:* Adapted from Neeb K. *Fundamentals of Mental Health Nursing.* 3rd ed. Philadelphia: FA Davis; 2006.

Box 7.3
Symptoms of Stress

When you are experiencing stress, you may have a few or a number of these symptoms:
- Frequent feelings of anger, helplessness, or hopelessness
- Headaches, back pain, and insomnia
- Hiding real feelings from family and friends
- Hurting loved ones with words or physical harm
- Constant worry, memory loss, and trouble thinking clearly
- Panic attacks with rapid heart rate, shortness of breath, and dizziness
- Isolation from friends and family
- Inability to make decisions
- Overuse of alcohol, drugs, or food to feel better

too much or kicking the cat. Positive strategies include those that are good for body, mind, and spirit. Examples of positive coping strategies for the body include the following:

- Eating regular meals with lower levels of fat and sugar
- Exercising regularly
- Sleeping an adequate number of hours every night
- Using deep-breathing exercises to relax and relieve stress
- Listening to your body and giving it what it needs, such as extra rest when you are ill

Examples of positive coping strategies for the mind and spirit include:

- Saying "no" to people when necessary, preventing yourself from taking on more responsibility than you can handle
- Taking time out to relax and have fun with family and friends
- Laughing
- Reducing excesses in your life; getting rid of clutter both in activities and in possessions
- Talking about your feelings with people you trust
- Asking for help when you need it
- Participating in worship services or spending time with nature
- Taking a "mental vacation" from time to time. Close your eyes and picture a beautiful, relaxing place. Imagine yourself there. What are you doing? What do you see? What do you hear? What do you smell?
- Keeping a journal, either of daily life or of stressful events and your response to them

Stress is a fact in our daily lives. It is not going to go away. We get to choose how we will respond to it. If you choose to use positive coping strategies, your life will not be ruled by stress.

• WORD • BUILDING •
dissociation: dis – opposite of + sociation – ally with

Patient Teaching Connection

Patient Teaching to Decrease Stress

Hospitalization is a huge stressor. Your patients may need assistance from you to help cope with the experience. To help patients manage the stress of hospitalization, encourage them to:

- Ask questions if they are unsure about a treatment, medication, or diagnosis. Be sure to explain what to expect before performing any procedure or treatment.
- Discuss their feelings with you or another health-care professional if they are distressed about their diagnosis or care. Listen to the patient's concerns and provide reassurance when it is appropriate to do so.
- Ask for assistance if they are unable to sleep. Provide a back massage, warm drink, or other comfort measures to help the patient relax.
- Laugh at a funny story or movie. Use humor therapy when appropriate. Laughter increases endorphins and decreases residual effects of the fight-or-flight response.

KNOWLEDGE CONNECTION

Describe the effects of the fight-or-flight response on the body. Which disease is listed as a result of all risk factors? How does stress affect a person who is hospitalized?

POST CONFERENCE

At post conference, you report on your clinical experiences: Once you were able to calm your patient and understand her concerns, you began to forge a strong nurse-patient relationship. You were able to explain to her what happens in gallbladder disease. You complimented her on her healthy lifestyle and established rapport. You put her mind at ease about what would happen after she recovered from her surgery, and you cared for her postoperatively. You explained her activity orders for discharge: She should not lift anything over 5 pounds in weight for 2 weeks, and then she could return to her usual activities. You explored her feelings about wellness and illness, explained the continuum concept, and helped relieve her anxiety both before and after surgery.

Key Points

- Most people are not completely well or completely ill at any given time; instead we move up and down a continuum.
- The goals of Healthy People 2020 are to increase the quality and years of a healthy life and to eliminate health disparities.
- It is necessary to assess a patient's health literacy in order to address the communication gap that often occurs between the health-care provider giving instructions and the patient being able to understand those instructions.
- Illness can be acute or chronic and can mean different things to different people.
- The five phases of illness are prodromal, symptomatic, seeking help, dependency, and recovery.
- Illness risk factors are modifiable or nonmodifiable. Modifiable factors include exercise, diet, and lifestyle choices. Nonmodifiable risk factors include heredity, age, and gender.
- Stress can be negative or positive, but the body cannot tell the difference and reacts in the same way to both.
- Stress causes a physiological reaction in the body called the fight-or-flight response.
- Frequent or unrelieved stress can lead to increased risk for illnesses.
- Defense mechanisms are ways we manage our fears and anxieties; they are unconscious reactions to decrease our stress.
- Positive strategies for coping with ongoing stress include limiting your obligations and responsibilities, spending time with people you enjoy, laughing, talking about your feelings, and asking for help when you need it.

Review Questions

Select the answer that is most appropriate for each of the following questions. Some questions may have more than one correct answer. Select all that apply.

1. Acute diseases would include which of the following?
   1. Influenza
   2. Measles
   3. Hypertension
   4. Bacterial pneumonia

2. An individual has been to his health-care provider for complaints of back pain and was informed that he has a bulging vertebral disk. He must now decide whether he wants to see a chiropractor for treatment, obtain a second opinion, or follow the instructions of this health-care provider. This individual is in which of the phases of illness?
   1. Prodromal phase
   2. Dependency phase
   3. Seeking help phase
   4. Recovery phase

3. Which of the following could be classified as stressors?
   1. Getting married
   2. Receiving a promotion at work
   3. Losing a loved one
   4. Having a much-wanted baby

4. You are working with a 28-year-old patient who drinks heavily and smokes two packs of cigarettes per day for stress relief. He tells you that his job is stressful because he works with "stupid people" and that his relationship with his girlfriend is often tumultuous. He says he has only hit her "once or twice" but says that they yell at one another often. He is overweight by about 40 pounds and mostly eats fast food. Which of the LHIs would you consider to be concerns for this patient?
   1. Access to health services
   2. Injury and violence
   3. Mental health
   4. Nutrition, physical fitness, and obesity
   5. Oral health
   6. Substance abuse
   7. Tobacco

5. A patient who has been diagnosed with rheumatoid arthritis tells you that she has not had any joint pain or swelling for 3 months. She is hoping it has "gone away for good." What is probably happening with this patient?
   1. She is probably right and the acute phase of the illness is over.
   2. Because this is a chronic illness, she is probably in a remission for now.
   3. She is now in the prodromal phase of illness and no longer in the symptomatic phase.
   4. She is in the recovery phase of illness and will no longer experience those symptoms.

6. Which are included in determining a person's health literacy?
   1. Assess the patient's ability to comprehend health-care information and use it to make decisions.
   2. Use a specific tool, such as an ice cream label, to assess the ability to use numbers and make calculations.
   3. Ask the patient to determine if it would be safe to eat the ice cream if he or she were allergic to certain substances.
   4. Ask the patient to read and define a list of common medical terms used to explain illnesses and treatments.

7. Which are modifiable risk factors for diseases?
   1. Smoking
   2. Diet high in fat
   3. Genetic makeup
   4. Age and gender

8. A patient is extremely stressed and decides to decrease some of her responsibilities outside of her family and job. She resigns from being PTA president and from being a Scout leader, as well as saying "no" to some church and social obligations. This is an example of using:
   1. negative coping strategies.
   2. minimization.
   3. dissociation.
   4. positive coping strategies.

ANSWERS 1. 1, 2, 4. 2. 2. 3. 1, 2, 3, 4. 4. 3, 4, 6, 7. 5. 2. 6. 1, 2, 3. 7. 1, 2. 8. 4

Critical Thinking Exercises

Answers available online.

1. Compare the physiological changes that may occur in the two following situations. Are they the same? If not, how are they different?
   Situation #1: During the night you are home alone. You hear the breaking of glass at the patio entrance door and fear it is an intruder. Your body initiates the fight-or-flight response.
   Situation #2: The physician has just told your patient some devastating news: She has advanced cervical cancer.

Additional Resources

DAVIS edge. **Use the scratch off code on the inside front cover of your book to access online quizzes that will help you to improve your scores on course exams and prepare for the NCLEX-PN®.**

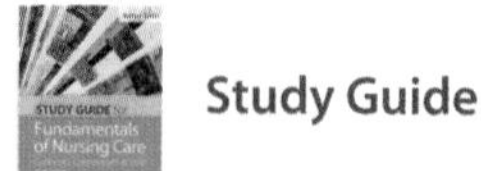

Study Guide

CHAPTER 8

Ethnic, Cultural, and Spiritual Aspects of Care

Thirty Lacy

KEY TERMS

Cultural awareness (KUL-chur-uhl uh-WAIR-ness)
Cultural competence (KUL-chur-uhl KOM-puh-tents)
Cultural diversity (KUL-chur-uhl dih-VER-sih-tee)
Cultural sensitivity (KUL-chur-uhl sen-sih-TIV-ih-tee)
Culture (KUL-chur)
Discrimination (dis-KRIM-ih-NAY-shun)
Ethnicity (eth-NIH-sih-tee)
Prejudice (PREJ-uh-diss)
Religion (rih-LIH-juhn)
Spiritual care (SPIH-rih-choo-ahl KARE)
Spirituality (SPIH-rih-choo-AL-ih-tee)
Stereotyping (STER-ee-oh-tye-ping)
Transcultural nursing (trans-KUL-chur-uhl NER-sing)

CHAPTER CONCEPTS

Culture
Spirituality
Communication

LEARNING OUTCOMES

1. Define various terms associated with ethnic, cultural, and spiritual nursing.
2. Explain why it is important to be aware of ethnic, cultural, and spiritual differences.
3. Compare cultural awareness to cultural sensitivity.
4. Describe some of the ways in which ethnic, cultural, and spiritual differences can affect nursing care.
5. Discuss at least five barriers to health care and how they prevent or lead to inappropriate health care.
6. Contrast the major religions and how they can affect health care of the patient.
7. Relate spiritual distress to possible signs or symptoms indicative of such.
8. Identify nursing interventions that you can use to meet the ethnic, cultural, and spiritual needs of your patients.
9. Discuss information found in the Connection features in this chapter.

CRITICAL THINKING CONNECTION

Clinical Assignment

You are a female student nurse assigned to care for Mr. Habib, a male patient who is Muslim. He is recovering from surgery for prostate cancer and has a suprapubic incision. He is from Iran and has some difficulty speaking English. You know very little about the Muslim faith. You have been told that his wife is always at the bedside, and she seems very nice. One nurse tells you that she cared for the patient yesterday and that he has "something on a string around his neck."

Critical Thinking Questions:

1. How would you familiarize yourself with Muslim beliefs as they affect health care?
2. As a female, what questions might you ask the patient about the care you plan on providing?
3. How would you best meet his spiritual and cultural needs while you care for him?

We all are different in numerous ways. We may be different in the way we believe, think, speak, act, or live, but we are all individuals who deserve to be treated with respect and dignity regardless of our ancestry, beliefs, or way of life. As a nurse, you will find it not only beneficial but necessary to broaden your awareness of the differences that may be found in others. This chapter discusses nursing care issues relating to the cultural and spiritual differences of the most common diverse populations.

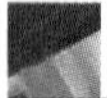

ETHNICITY AND CULTURE

Ethnicity is the categorization of a group of people by a distinctive trait, such as the line of genealogy or ancestry, race, or nationality. **Culture** might be defined as the way of life that distinguishes a particular group of people from other groups. It is the whole of the learned behaviors of individuals within a specific group. It includes the beliefs; values; symbols; art; music; morals; laws; customs; experiences; attitudes; religions; roles; concepts of space, time, and the universe; belongings; communications; races; and ethnicities of an individual or group. Additional aspects included in the definition of culture are traditions, holidays, and specific celebrations and practices. These are addressed in the discussion of beliefs, religions, and spirituality later in this chapter.

Ethnicity and Culture in America

International migration to the United States has dramatically increased over the last 3 decades; this influx has contributed to the country's population explosion and heightened diversity. The Census Bureau report of 2015 indicated that minority groups, including Hispanics, African Americans, Asian Americans, and other people of color, comprised 56% of the population of the United States—and trends continue to show a steady increase in diversity (Fig. 8.1).

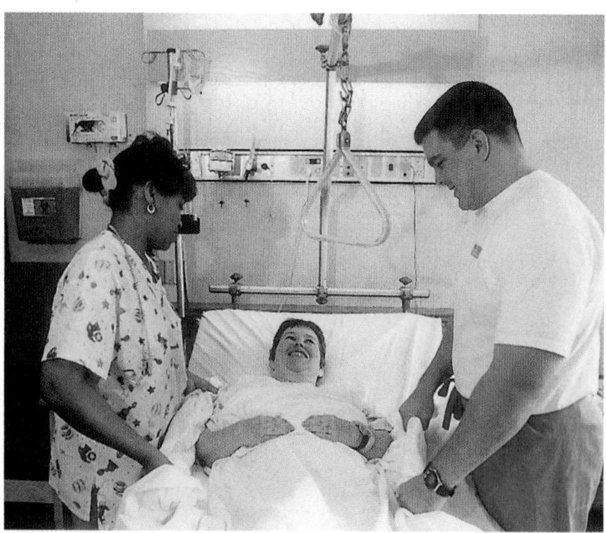

FIGURE 8.1 Nurses commonly care for patients of different cultures than their own (from Williams LS, Hopper PD. *Understanding Medical-Surgical Nursing.* 5th ed. Philadelphia, PA: FA Davis; 2015).

The emergence of these various cultural populations, with their many different beliefs and practices, continues to have an impact on the care that nurses provide. The Joint Commission, the primary evaluation and accreditation agency for health-care facilities, has established that all patients have the right to receive medical care that is considerate of their culture, religion, and spirituality.

Therefore, as America becomes more diverse, nurses and other health-care professionals need to become culturally competent caregivers by increasing their knowledge of the various religious and spiritual beliefs held by people of different cultures. **Cultural competence** requires that the nurse makes a commitment to consider the cultural background of each patient and to provide appropriate care specific to that individual.

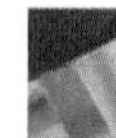

TRANSCULTURAL NURSING AND CULTURAL COMPETENCE

Transcultural nursing is care that crosses cultural boundaries or combines the elements of more than one culture. As America has grown in cultural diversity, the issues of transcultural nursing have increased in importance. Today, health-care providers are being mandated to provide transcultural care by professional and governmental agencies. However, before the nurse can provide care that addresses the culture of the patient, there are several aspects of transculturalism that must be understood, including cultural diversity and cultural awareness.

Cultural Diversity

Cultural diversity is defined as the differences between groups of people in a certain geographical area, such as a city, state, or country; a specific place, such as a church or factory; or a conceptual community, such as the medical community. It is a way of identifying the group through the differences found between groups of people. Factors that determine the cultural diversity of a group might include the different ethnic groups, races, languages spoken, and religions within the larger group. Anything that is specific to the group that distinguishes the group from all other groups of people defines the culture of the group.

An example of cultural diversity found in a hospital would be the different ethnic groups represented among the hospital's employees, as a hospital might employ American, Mexican, Iranian, and Chinese doctors and nurses. Within each of these ethnic groups, a number of races may be represented, including Caucasian, Latino, and Asian (Fig. 8.2).

• WORD • BUILDING •

ethnicity: ethnic – nation + ity – suffix to form abstract noun

competence: competere – to be fit and proper

transculturalism: trans – across + cultural – relating to culture + ism – theory of

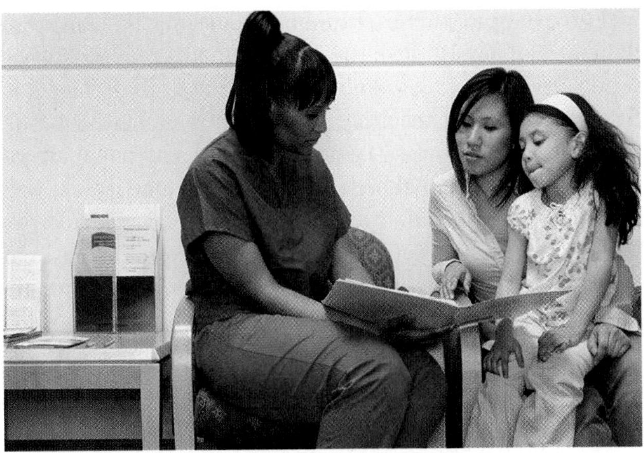

FIGURE 8.2 Diversity of ethnic backgrounds and cultures is common within the nursing profession (Imagine ID: 72421026; from City Hospital 2 CD on www.punchstock.com).

This group of doctors and nurses would speak English as well as their native languages.

Cultural Awareness

Transcultural nursing addresses the following:

- Cultural differences among patients
- Cultural differences among health-care providers
- Culture of the individual nurse

The knowledge of various cultural beliefs and values is known as **cultural awareness.** Patients are different. Their beliefs are different. Their responses to illness and wellness are different depending on their cultural backgrounds—and even patients from the same cultural group may have differences in their health-care beliefs and practices. Being culturally aware requires that you be culturally sensitive. **Cultural sensitivity** means that you provide care to the patient and show respect for and incorporate the patient's specific cultural beliefs and values into your nursing care. Cultural sensitivity also requires that you recognize and respect the accepted patterns of communication. When patients feel that you are being culturally insensitive by ignoring their beliefs, values, and communication patterns, they may delay or reject needed health-care services.

Cultural Competence

Culturally competent care occurs when the nurse provides care to the whole patient, incorporating within that care the cultural context of the patient's beliefs and values. The nurse does not have to have expert knowledge of every culture or cultural group to be culturally competent. However, the culturally competent nurse chooses to be aware of the cultural differences and to become familiar with aspects of the patient's culture that impact and influence the patient's health and care. The nurse strives to understand anything that might influence the patient's health, including the patient's:

- Perceptions
- Expectations
- Behavior
- Decision-making processes

The nurse will work at identifying those cultural factors that will empower the patient to reach his or her full health potential. The culturally competent nurse conveys caring to the patient by showing respect for his or her beliefs and ideas and not assuming that the nurse knows what the patient is thinking or feeling. Providing care that is culturally competent will build trust between the nurse and the patient and promote cooperation.

KNOWLEDGE CONNECTION

What does The Joint Commission say about patients from various cultures, religions, and spiritualities? List some of the factors or differences that might indicate cultural diversity. Describe the difference between cultural awareness and cultural sensitivity.

Real-World Connection

Meeting Rachael's Spiritual Needs

Rachael was a patient with terminal cancer in the community hospital where she had worked as a nursing assistant for many years. The nurse caring for Rachael had carefully planned her delivery of care to include all hygiene, treatments, and medications that were ordered. Shortly after she began her shift, she headed to Rachael's room to perform her initial assessment and begin the delivery of her planned care. As she was completing her initial assessment, there was a knock on the door. Several family members and others had arrived and asked to see the patient. The nurse explained that she was busy giving nursing care, and she asked if they could come back in about an hour. One of the family members took the nurse aside and explained that these were members from Rachael's church who believed that the laying on of hands and anointing of Rachael's body with oil could possibly cure her cancer. The ritual would last approximately an hour to an hour and a half. Even though it would interrupt the schedule of care that she had planned for the patient, the nurse knew that Rachael was a woman of strong faith and religious beliefs. Feeling that Rachael's spiritual needs were just as important as—maybe more important than—her physical needs, she told the family and church friends to take all the time they needed and to call her if they needed any assistance. The ritual took about 90 minutes, and the nurse had to reprioritize her planned schedule, but she knew that she had done the right thing by allowing Rachael's spiritual needs to be met.

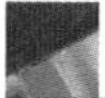

HOW CULTURE AFFECTS HEALTH CARE

Beliefs about illness can impact a patient's health, as shown in Table 8.1. Other cultural beliefs that affect health care include beliefs about food. For instance, patients who practice Hinduism may refrain from eating beef and pork, while pork is prohibited in a Jewish diet but beef is not. Diet restrictions can even impact the medications a patient may take; for example, a Hindu patient may refuse to take medication that is packaged in a capsule because the capsule might be made from gelatin substances derived from beef or pork.

Often tea and coffee are served in the hospital with meal trays. However, it is important to be aware that some cultures and religions prohibit caffeine intake, so decaffeinated beverages would be preferred for these patients.

It is also important to be aware of the different beliefs about illness and wellness that may impact a patient's health and prognosis. Several cultures believe that health is the balance of the internal and external environments of the individual, incorporating the whole of the person, including his or her physical, mental, social, and spiritual components. Some believe that the imbalance of these environments is the cause of illness. Traditional Chinese medicine is based on this belief.

The patient may believe that illness is caused by an imbalance between inanimate forces. Members of certain cultures believe that illness is due to an imbalance between "hot" and "cold." As a result, a member of these cultures may only drink or eat hot foods when ill in an effort to restore balance and health. Because of fears that cold temperatures can cause illness, members of some cultures make efforts to stay warm at all times. For example, a patient holding this belief might refuse to use an ice pack to treat an injured ankle; another patient who is ill may refuse to shampoo her hair because of fear of developing a headache or catching a cold.

According to traditional Chinese medicinal practices, illness is caused when there is an imbalance of the energy forms known as yin (cold) and yang (hot). In this belief system, the terms *hot* and *cold* do not refer to actual temperatures but serve as descriptors of these energy forms, which exist not only in the individual's body but also in foods, actions, and behaviors. India's practice of Ayurvedic medicine, which uses herbs, nutrition, cleansings, acupressure, massage, and yoga, is based on similar beliefs.

It is important for nurses to understand that other cultures are different than their own and that part of our job is to provide care that is culturally sensitive. At the same time, we realize that just because a patient comes from a particular culture, he or she may not embrace the same beliefs and traditions as others of that culture. It is necessary to discuss cultural expectations in a sensitive way.

For example, nurses cannot assume that because the patient is of Jewish descent, he or she will require kosher foods. The only way to know the patient's requirements is to ask if there are specific food restrictions that he or she would like us to honor. It is the same with any patient from any culture. Avoid making assumptions that the patient will or will not react certain ways based on their ethnic, cultural, or religious background. It is always appropriate to ask, in a sensitive manner, how the patient wishes for the nursing staff to provide care in a culturally appropriate way.

KNOWLEDGE CONNECTION
What are the beliefs of traditional Chinese medicine?

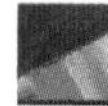

DEATH AND DYING

Although members of a specific culture normally follow the beliefs of their culture, individuals also develop their own beliefs that may or may not be consistent with the practices or religion of their identified culture. Therefore, it is very important that the nurse provide care that is both culturally based and specific to the individual.

One of the common areas in which a patient's beliefs may differ with those of his or her culture is that of death and dying. There are many cultural aspects related to death and dying. It may be viewed as controlled by a supernatural force or purely as a scientifically based phenomenon. The individual, on the other hand, may hold the opposite view.

While members of some cultures prefer to die at home, others feel more comfortable in a controlled environment such as a hospital or hospice unit. Some cultures approve of life support, while others do not permit mechanical means of prolonging life. Some feel that it is important to pray for the person's healing and recovery, while others believe that a person receives his or her just reward and that it is wrong to pray for relief of his or her suffering.

Some cultures have specific persons who care for the body after death, and only those individuals are to touch or prepare the body for burial. Others have no specific regulations or rites related to the care of the body, and the nurses will prepare the body for transfer to the funeral home, where the body will be prepared for burial.

Some cultures promote the presence of the family or of the family and friends, while others prefer that the dying patient be given time alone for reflection and repentance. More expressive cultures may exhibit loud moaning and chanting during the last hours of the patient's life as a means of providing comfort to the patient and family members. Other cultures may prefer a more quiet and peaceful environment. Some desire the continued presence of a spiritual leader,

Table 8.1
Beliefs About Illness

Principles of Beliefs	*Basic Tenets of the Beliefs*	*Examples*
Scientifically Based Beliefs, Biomedical		
Based on scientific research leading to best practices	If it can be proven scientifically, then it is accepted as truth and law. If it cannot be proven scientifically by research, it is an unfounded belief and myth.	Brushing teeth prevents tooth decay. Hand washing prevents the spread of disease. Immunization prevents disease.
Naturalistically or Holistically Based Beliefs		
A healthy state is one of balance and harmony. Examples include beliefs in yin and yang, or "hot" and "cold."	The balance between yin and yang is what maintains and restores health. Yin and yang are compared to the sympathetic and parasympathetic nervous systems and the way they maintain balance in the body. Balance is maintained between hot and cold in order to maintain health. Some cultures believe that certain conditions are cold if they are manifested by vasoconstriction and decreased metabolism. Hot conditions or diseases are manifested by a high metabolic rate and vasodilation. The goal of treatment is to restore balance.	Cold diseases or states: menstrual cramps, rhinitis, colic Hot diseases or states: hypertension, diabetes mellitus, pregnancy
Religiously Based Beliefs		
Called *magico-religious,* the principle of these beliefs is that disease is caused by supernatural forces and health can be restored by supernatural forces.	Although many religions believe in prayer and the laying on of hands for healing, magico-religious beliefs indicate there is an added realm, the realm of magic. Magic can heal the illness as well as be the cause of illness. Others who practice magico-religion believe that illness is caused by some sinful act or by an actual demon spirit who is working against the individual. These patients may also believe that God is punishing them for sinful behaviors or lack of faith.	Depression is thought by some to be the result of sins. There is belief in the "evil eye," which is a term that means a look or an eye that can cast spells on individuals. Amulets, talismans, and rites are used to chase away bad spirits. Many herbs are used to heal.
Folk Healing		
Beliefs in practitioners of specific alternative therapies	There are practitioners who promote the treatment and healing of disease who are not licensed as health-care providers or nurses or recognized by any certifying organization of higher learning. Many people seek assistance from herbalists, spiritualists, naturalists, and more. Other alternative practitioners provide therapeutic touch, iridology, naturopathic medicine, and reflexology.	The patient seeks a reflexologist, who performs massage of the sole of the foot to relieve the pain of a migraine headache.

while others prefer the spiritual leader to come and anoint or pray for them and then leave.

KNOWLEDGE CONNECTION

What are some different beliefs about where the patient dies? What are some different cultural beliefs about caring for the body after death? What are some different cultural beliefs about the environment around the patient who is close to death?

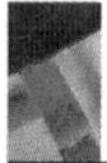

DELIVERING CULTURALLY SENSITIVE CARE

When caring for patients from culturally diverse backgrounds, it is important to incorporate culturally sensitive care that conveys an attitude of caring. It is important to treat the patient with respect. It is not enough to go through the motions of providing care without communicating with the patient, even if the communication is difficult. Actively listening to the patient's expressions, permitting him or her time to express concerns, providing prompts when the words cannot be found, and providing presence all give the patient a sense of being cared for and respected.

Culturally sensitive caring requires awareness of the patient's actions as the nurse performs the care. The nonverbal response becomes most important when there is a language barrier that may prevent the patient from expressing himself or herself. If the care is cold or disrespectful, the patient may become resistive or have changes in his or her physical condition. If the patient becomes fearful or anxious, he or she may have changes in vital signs, such as an elevated heart rate and respiratory rate, an increase in blood pressure, or possibly development of a panic attack. If the patient feels he or she is being attacked or feels totally out of control of the situation, the patient may refuse care, become combative, or leave without the needed health care. In an effort to prevent these problems from arising, try the following approaches:

- Allow the patient time to get his or her thoughts together.
- Use an interpreter if needed. If an interpreter is needed but one is not available, use prompts such as pictures or vocabulary cue cards.
- Be aware of the patient's nonverbal body language. It may alert the nurse to escalating tension and the need for a calm and quiet approach.
- Be aware that hand gestures mean different things in different cultures. For example, the "okay" sign used by many people in the United States may mean consciousness or deliberation to individuals in India.
- Understand that the patient may be able to speak English but that it may be broken or difficult to understand.

BARRIERS TO HEALTH CARE

Several barriers to health care are specific to the individual. Some of the issues that may lead to lack of care or to the provision of inappropriate care include the following:

- Economics
- Education
- Geography
- Language
- Stereotyping
- Prejudice and discrimination
- Misunderstandings

Economics

For many, health care is obtained through individual insurance plans or private pay. Others obtain health care through public programs such as Medicaid, Medicare, and state programs. However, patients who are not insured or are underinsured may not be able to afford health care and may wait until their condition or illness becomes life-threatening before seeking care.

You may find yourself caring for indigent and homeless patients. Although others may look at such individuals as dirty or unpleasant, it is important that you see them as fellow humans deserving of dignity and respect.

Education

Research studies have shown that the higher a person's level of education, the more health care is obtained. The opposite also is true. Sometimes, even though families may be able to financially afford health care, individuals with a low education level tend to seek less medical help than those with higher educational levels. The education and literacy levels of a patient also play a role in dictating how to provide patient teaching (see Chapter 12).

Geography

A patient's geographical area may have an impact on his or her ability to obtain health care. Many rural areas have limited access to health-care providers and facilities, such as clinics or hospitals. Many low-income areas of larger cities have limited health-care providers and facilities as well. Minority groups make up a greater percentage of low-income populations in the United States, leading to decreased access to needed health care for those populations.

Language

A member of a minority group who speaks his or her native language but is not fluent in the common language of the population majority where he or she resides is at a distinct disadvantage. There are often cultural particularities that should be taken into account when communicating with families. For example, in some cultures, the patriarch of the family may be

• WORD • BUILDING •

discrimination: discrimin – distinguish between + ation – action

assigned a special role in decision making. In addition, language barriers, along with fears of possible discrimination, can lead to feelings of powerlessness. This language barrier can make it difficult for an individual to gain access to health care. For example, in the United States, minority group members for whom English is a second language sometimes find it difficult to determine where to go for various types of medical care. Even after the individual has successfully accessed the correct type of health-care facility or health-care provider, if the health-care provider and the nurse do not speak the patient's native language, it can result in miscommunication, misunderstandings, increased anxiety, and frustration for both the patient and the caregiver. The caregiver may be unable to obtain information, or he or she may obtain incorrect information, leading to the provision of improper care and the planning of inappropriate treatment. Sometimes the patient will nod his or her head and indicate that he or she understands what you have said when this is not actually true. Therefore, it is extremely important to use an interpreter when a language barrier exists.

The interpreter should be a trained interpreter and not be a family member or a small child because of the nature of the information that potentially needs to be communicated. The possibility exists that the patient may be afraid to provide truthful information or be embarrassed to speak of the health-care concern in the presence of the family member. With the increased emphasis on confidentiality and transcultural care, the government mandates that trained interpreters are available across the country. In addition, some health-care facilities use computer programs to help translate patient information from their native language (refer to Chapter 6). An example of a language barrier is noted in the story found in Box 8.1.

While understanding that language barriers make communication more difficult, it is important to keep in mind that a patient's limitations with the English language do not reflect limitations in the patient's intelligence. No matter which type of communication method you use, remember to deliver it in a respectful manner and avoid "talking down" to the patient.

It is useful to learn and use key words in the patient's language whenever possible. If an interpreter is not available, ask a family member or do research on the Internet to learn the appropriate terms for words such as "pain," "nausea," "hungry," "urinate," "medication," "feel good," "feel bad," "Can I help you?," and "thank you." This demonstrates respect for the patient and helps to build rapport.

Stereotyping

Stereotyping may prevent individuals from seeking or obtaining the health care they need. **Stereotyping** can be defined in different ways, but essentially it means that a person or group is looked at by another person or group through preconceived ideas and fixed impressions; it can also be defined as ideas or beliefs that lead to prejudice and possibly mistreatment. These preconceived ideas may be based solely on a person's physical characteristics. Stereotyping can occur when a health-care provider identifies a patient according to his or her understanding of the ethnic group or race to which the patient belongs and not as an individual with unique qualities and characteristics.

Most individuals are guilty of stereotyping at one time or another. Work to evaluate your own perceptions and beliefs regarding different ethnic groups or races. Remember that individuals within the same ethnic group or race may have different beliefs or behaviors. A culturally sensitive nurse must avoid categorizing patients simply by their looks, ethnic groups, race, language, or beliefs. Taking the time to assess a patient's cultural preferences can decrease stereotyping and help you provide effective care.

Prejudice and Discrimination

Prejudice is based on a preconceived idea about an individual solely based on physical appearance or a characteristic of his or her social or cultural group prior to determining or examining the facts related to the individual. **Prejudice** is a determination or judgment about a person or group based on irrational suspicion or hatred of a particular group, race, sexual orientation, or religion. **Discrimination,** like prejudice, is a type of unfair treatment of one or more persons or groups. The discrimination is usually due to misguided and unfounded beliefs about the race, ethnicity, age, gender, sexual orientation, or religion of the person or group. When a patient feels that he or she is being discriminated against, he or she will be

Box 8.1

Breaking the Language Barrier: A Case Study

Read the following case study about Anna and note how the simple act of taking time to ensure effective communication makes a difference in Anna's acquisition of medical care.

Anna, who only speaks Spanish, needed medical care and came to the free clinic looking for help. She arrived by herself, carrying a small notebook that had a phone number in it. On arrival at the clinic, her distress was notable by her crying. The caregivers at the clinic could not speak Spanish, and there was no interpreter available. Although the nurse practitioner did not speak Spanish, she was able to convey a sense of patience and caring, which helped to calm Anna. Anna indicated that the nurse should call the phone number written in her notebook, which the nurse did, reaching an individual who spoke both English and Spanish. The interpreter would speak to Anna, then to the nurse, and then again to Anna. Although it took a while and required much work at communication, Anna was able to obtain the care that was needed for her diabetes. The interpreter offered to write a chart of Spanish words and the English equivalents for Anna to bring to future visits. Using this method, Anna came to the clinic several times over the next few months, each time with the chart and the name and phone number of the interpreter who would be available that day. She was able to obtain the medical care she needed to get her blood sugar levels under control again.

reluctant to seek further assistance from the nurse, other health-care provider, or profession.

Before a nurse can be successful in exhibiting sensitivity to those of different cultures, the nurse must examine and identify his or her own prejudices. Many individuals do not realize that they are prejudiced until they actively assess their feelings and beliefs. It is not necessary for a nurse to agree with differing beliefs, but it is paramount that the nurse be able to accept the patient's differences and deliver respectful nursing care in spite of the differences.

Even as you are trying to deliver culturally sensitive care, you may observe other staff members engaging in behaviors that demonstrate racial bias or cultural insensitivity. It is your responsibility to intervene in an appropriate manner on behalf of your patient's rights. That may require you to take the staff member aside and tactfully explain that the observed actions or words could be perceived by the patient as being insensitive and insulting, biased, or even discriminating. Relate the specific cultural beliefs held by the patient so that the staff member will understand why his or her actions or words could have been offensive to the patient. If the staff member continues to persist in behaviors that are culturally insensitive, it is your responsibility as your patient's advocate to report the problem to your supervisor so that resolution can be attained.

Misunderstanding

Misunderstanding is a barrier that is caused by a mistake of meaning or intention. When a misunderstanding arises between a patient and their health-care provider, the patient may fear further encounters with the health-care system. A fear of making mistakes or retaliation may prevent the patient from seeking appropriate medication or diagnosis. Thus, it is important that the nurse verifies a patient's understanding during all communication and patient teaching. You might ask the patient to tell you in his or her own words what he or she understood you to say. Avoid simply asking, "Do you understand?" Out of respect, many patients will automatically answer with a yes whether or not they actually understand what you are saying.

KNOWLEDGE CONNECTION

Name at least five barriers to health care. Describe at least one way to overcome each of the five barriers. What are your own prejudices that you need to overcome?

Settings Connection: Home Health

Respect the Beliefs of Others

When providing home health care to an individual of another culture, it is important to seek information regarding customs, expectations, acceptable behaviors, and courtesies that are unique to their culture. Providing nursing care in the patient's home is likely to involve even more adaptation in services than would be necessary in a hospital. For example, you may have to remove your shoes before entering the home, abstain from wearing pants (if you are a female nurse), avoid touching the patient's prayer rug, or move the patient's bed so that it faces north. Some cultures may expect you to avoid prolonged eye contact, even when speaking directly to a person from that culture. Remember to show respect for the patient's beliefs, just as you would those of your own mother, father, or child.

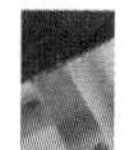

RELIGION, SPIRITUALITY, AND CREATIVITY

Humans are more than just the physical. They are made up of a body, mind, and spirit. The body is the physical, biological part of the person—as a nurse, you will learn about the physical body through the study of anatomy and physiology, as well as the discussion of medical-surgical nursing. The mind is that part of the person that learns, thinks, communicates, makes decisions, and feels, while the spirit is the essence of the person, the vital force or energy, that is distinct from physical matter. Some people believe the soul and spirit to be interchangeable. In this textbook, the soul and the spirit are defined as being the essence of the person.

Religion, spirituality, and creativity are aspects of culture that provide the basis for the development of beliefs, values, morals, and ethical standards. **Religion** is the formal structured system of beliefs, values, rituals, and practices of a person or group, usually based on the teachings of a god or other spiritual leader. It is a belief in a higher power or supernatural being that the members of a religion revere and honor. A religion may incorporate a set of rituals that contribute to the worship of the higher power. For some people, religion may be based on a cause or principle that is sought after with fervent passion rather than on the teachings of or belief in a higher power. Religions often have specific holidays or celebrate specific times of the year.

Some religions can affect health-care choices because of treatment restrictions. For example, Jehovah's Witnesses traditionally do not believe they should receive blood transfusions or have blood products administered to them.

Some cultures incorporate several different religions, while other cultures are known for one major religion. Some religions are monotheistic, believing in one god, while others are polytheistic, believing in multiple gods. Some cultures reject religion of any type, promoting the atheistic belief that there is no god. Regardless of the belief system, most believe there is a sense of humans that is beyond the tangible—a spirit, a sense of creativity, an essence of the supernatural that motivates, stimulates, and gives a sense of purpose and meaning to life. That intangibility is called spirituality.

Spirituality is the descriptive term that explains the spirit and the relationship of the spirit to the body, mind, and environment, including the patient's relationship to others. It is the spirituality of the person that gives meaning and purpose to life, making it the most important aspect of an individual. Although spirituality usually incorporates religion, spirituality and religion may mean two very different things to a patient. For many, spirituality refers to the individual's expression (or living testimony) of his or her religious beliefs and represents the meaning of life, which includes a sense of involvement with the transcendent outside institutional boundaries. Others may believe that spirituality is completely separate from any formal religion and is simply the expression of who the individual is and how that individual relates to things of this world, such as nature.

Research studies have found relationships between a patient's religious beliefs and practices, such as prayer, and his or her health. Findings indicate that expression of spirituality contributes to a healthier lifestyle; people who regularly participate in religious services tend to have a lower frequency of unhealthy behaviors and stronger support systems. In addition, research studies have found improved emotional well-being in patients who claim to be religious. The health benefits of religion appear to be numerous. Religion can give meaning and purpose to the patient's life, empower the patient, and give the patient a sense of control. Religious beliefs also tend to give hope and motivate people toward a better outcome.

KNOWLEDGE CONNECTION

What are three health benefits generally found in patients with strong spiritual or religious beliefs or religious affiliation?

Spiritual Care

Spiritual care begins with an understanding of the differences between spirituality and religion, as well as an understanding of one's own spirituality, beliefs, and values. The nurse who provides spiritual care must understand his or her own purpose and goals related to providing spiritual care to the patient. The relationship of body, mind, and spirit is so closely interactive that an alteration in the body affects the mind and spirit, an alteration in the mind affects the body and spirit, and an alteration in the spirit affects the mind and body. An example of this interaction may be seen in the case study in Box 8.2.

Spiritual care addresses the possible effects of illness on the patient's belief system and spirituality. When a person faces the complications of illness, trauma, or any medical condition, he or she may begin to question his or her faith. The patient may believe that he or she is being punished by God, or the patient may accept a negative outcome, feeling that he or she deserves to be ill. The nurse caring for the patient described in Box 8.2 had a choice to provide holistic care, which provides care to the whole person, including the body, mind, and spirit, or to ignore the spirit of the patient. Any spiritual stress that can be relieved will enhance the patient's physical health as well. It may be extremely helpful to a patient to notify their clergy or spiritual advisor about their condition or hospitalization, but first the patient's permission must be obtained.

Spiritual distress can occur at any time during a patient's life experiences. It may be seen during times of heavy financial stress, during major life changes such as divorce or death of a loved one, and during one's own illness or injury, especially if the illness is terminal. One example

Box 8.2
Spiritual Distress: A Case Study

In this case study about Mr. Govi, note how fear and other effects of spiritual distress can cause or increase physical signs and symptoms of illness.

Mr. Govi is a 42-year-old male who is generally pleasant and self-assured. He is well educated and holds a doctorate in political science. He attended church regularly during his childhood and early adulthood. He has not been attending church or living as he believes he should for some time now. His lack of spirituality has been on his mind and has begun to bother him. Today he began to feel short of breath and had pain in his chest. After an hour or so, he decided that he was having a heart attack. His wife phoned for an ambulance to take him to the local emergency room. In the ambulance, his pain was a 7 on a 0-to-10 scale, his heart rate was 90 bpm, and his respirations were 24 breaths per minute. On arrival in the emergency room, he rated his pain as an 8, his heart rate was 96, and his respiratory rate was 24.

While the nurse connected Mr. Govi to a heart monitor and applied oxygen, his chest pain increased to a 9, his pulse rate increased to 110, and his respiratory rate increased to 29. He became so distressed that he was having trouble thinking clearly. He felt weak and had a strong sense of doom, which produced a sense of fear that stimulated the sympathetic nervous system, causing the adrenal cortex to release adrenaline. It further raised the heart rate and blood pressure, increasing the workload of the heart and the need for oxygen. The nurse applied oxygen. While the nurse was gathering information from the patient, Mr. Govi made the following statement, "I think I'm having a heart attack. God is probably punishing me!"

Eventually a heart attack was ruled out, and Mr. Govi was diagnosed with gastroesophageal reflux and treated with the appropriate medication. During his hospitalization, the nurse obtained permission from Mr. Govi to telephone his minister, requesting that he visit Mr. Govi.

At the time of his admission, Mr. Govi's data had included changes in his body and mind, as well as a feeling of abandonment or punishment by God. Physical changes in the body can be brought on by spiritual distress or emotional distress. When this distress is not addressed, it may lead to worsening spiritual distress, which can continue to feed and worsen the patient's health status.

might be discontinuation of religious beliefs or practices under which the individual was reared. The individual may stop participating in the formal rites or rituals of his or her religion or worship, such as no longer attending church services or failing to pray on a regular basis. He or she may even have a questioning of or a total loss of faith, such as may occur with the death of a child. Others experience spiritual distress when their belief and value systems are challenged by disease, injury, or even nonmedical issues. Sometimes the patient may believe that because he or she made a mistake or a bad choice, illness or intense suffering is a form of discipline by a higher being. The patient may even refuse to seek wellness if he or she believes that the illness or death is deserved.

When the nurse identifies a patient as having spiritual distress, the nurse should respond with compassion and not be judgmental or biased. It is important to realize that anyone can develop spiritual distress. Once the nurse identifies spiritual distress in a patient, the goals or outcomes of their spiritual care should be directed toward restoring the patient's comfort and relationship with himself or herself, others, and/or God. These goals are specific to a patient and to the symptoms of his or her spiritual distress. An example of a goal is "the patient will express a feeling of hope for the future."

First, the nurse must determine the patient's current level of spiritual health by assessing for symptoms of distress. If it is determined that the patient has spiritual distress, you can then determine the appropriate nursing care to provide. Nursing interventions will nearly always include the following:

- Offering presence, which means to give the patient time and attention
- Providing opportunities for the patient to express his or her feelings
- Using therapeutic communication techniques (see Chapter 6) to promote the expression of feelings
- Contacting the religious or spiritual advisor of the patient's choice (only with the patient's permission)
- Providing for religious rituals as the patient desires, such as the practice of communion or the opportunity to pray

When providing spiritual care, nurses must set aside their own beliefs to meet the needs of the patient. The nurse must show respect for the patient's cultural and religious beliefs and practices. Integral to spiritual care is having an open mind and using active listening to determine what the patient needs in terms of spiritual care. As with all nursing care, the nurse must be nonjudgmental and unbiased.

KNOWLEDGE CONNECTION

List at least three interventions that might be appropriate when spiritual distress is identified.

POST CONFERENCE

At the end of your clinical day, you are tired but pleased with the outcome of your care for your patient, Mr. Habib. You have learned a great deal through this experience and look forward to sharing it with the other students. By asking questions and interacting, you learned that the item around his neck was an amulet that contained a portion of the Koran, the Muslim holy book. He asked you to keep it dry and not remove it. Mr. Habib was nice but very quiet. His wife would murmur information to you from time to time. Because he had a suprapubic incision, you asked Mr. Habib if he would prefer that a male student or nurse assess his incision. He nodded, so you got a male student to assess the incision. When you removed the cover from his lunch tray, both you and the Habibs were distressed to learn that his green beans had been seasoned with bacon bits. You quickly offered to get him a new tray, and both he and his wife thanked you repeatedly for doing so.

Key Points

- Every nurse will encounter multicultural patients and staff in the health-care environments in which he or she works.
- The Joint Commission has established that patients have the right to considerate cultural, religious, and spiritual care.
- Culture is defined as the way of life of a group of people that distinguishes the members of one group or category of people from another.
- Religious beliefs, values, and the concept of spirituality are important cultural concepts.
- Cultural sensitivity means that the nurse who provides care to the patient shows respect for and incorporates the patient's specific cultural beliefs and values.
- Cultural beliefs may affect health both negatively and positively.
- Nurses need to be aware of the patient's beliefs about prayer, suffering, death, and dying.
- Certain cultures and religions require that only members of their culture be allowed to touch the body of the deceased patient.

- Some cultures believe that it is wrong to pray for healing and recovery.
- In order to provide culturally sensitive care to a patient and his or her family members, the nurse must maintain a nonjudgmental attitude.
- Expression of spirituality is a healthy activity.
- Religion is the formal structured system of beliefs, values, rituals, and practices of a group based on the teachings of a spiritual leader who is revered and honored.
- The relationship of the body, mind, and spirit are so closely interactive that an alteration in any one of them may affect both of the other two realms.

Review Questions

Select the answer that is most appropriate for each of the following questions. Some questions may have more than one correct answer. Select all that apply.

1. It is important to understand that as individual members of various ethnic, cultural, and religious groups, we all are different and:
   1. we should learn to agree with all the differences in these groups.
   2. we must stick to our own beliefs and avoid accepting those different from our own.
   3. we deserve to be treated with respect and dignity.
   4. yet we still need the exact same care.

2. Which of the following organizations has/have worked to promote the patient's right to culturally competent care in U.S. hospitals?
   1. U.S. government
   2. Bureau of Immigration
   3. The Joint Commission
   4. American Association of Medical Workers
   5. Patient Rights Committee

3. Nursing care that involves or combines the elements of more than one culture is called which of the following names?
   1. Home care
   2. Acute care
   3. Hospice care
   4. Transcultural care
   5. Immigrant care

4. A patient has expressed the feeling that God has caused his illness. Which of the following would be most important for the nurse to consider when responding to the patient's feelings?
   1. The nurse must not be judgmental or biased and should respond with compassion.
   2. The nurse should be comfortable with his or her own religious beliefs and background.
   3. The patient has the right to his feelings, so no response is necessary.
   4. The patient can rely on the family to give direction and support.
   5. The patient's religious clergy should be contacted and a visit arranged.

5. A bedridden patient has a different cultural background and speaks a different primary language than the nurse. In order to provide culturally sensitive care to this patient, the nurse should do which of the following?
   1. Allow the patient time to get his or her thoughts together.
   2. Allow the patient's family member to interpret during conversations.
   3. Ask the patient to speak in his best English.
   4. Be aware of the patient's nonverbal body language.

6. The nurse is assisting a patient of the Jewish culture and faith in planning meals for the day. Which of the following might be a concern for the patient?
   1. Chopped steak
   2. Green beans with bacon
   3. Grilled chicken breast
   4. Pork chops
   5. Spinach

7. A nurse is admitting a 74-year-old Chinese patient to the hospital who says that he practices traditional Chinese medicine. The nurse understands that traditional Chinese medicine is based on which of these?
   1. Balancing Yin (cold) and Yang (hot)
   2. Using acupressure to relieve illness and pain
   3. Using Ayurvedic medicine to treat illness and disease
   4. Unblocking chi in the energy meridians

8. A female nurse is admitting a 24-year-old male Hindu patient to the hospital. The nurse understands that in order to be culturally competent when caring for this patient, she needs to understand anything that might influence his health, including:
   1. perceptions.
   2. behavior.
   3. expectations.
   4. barriers to health care.
   5. the decision making process.

ANSWERS 1. 3, 2. 3, 3. 4, 4. 1, 5. 1, 4, 6. 2, 4, 7. 1,
8. 1, 2, 3, 5

Critical Thinking Exercises

Answers available online.

1. How does a patient's education level affect their health care?

2. Mr. Lambert is admitted with a kidney stone and is in severe pain. Ms. Radania, an African American practical nurse, enters his room to obtain his vital signs and give him his pain medicine. Mr. Lambert becomes very upset and tells her to leave. "I am not going to be touched by the likes of you," he screams. Describe the types of barriers to health care that are demonstrated in this situation. What could the practical nurse do that might improve the situation?

3. A patient who is near the end of life has many family members in the waiting room and in his room. Many are moaning and sobbing loudly. How can the nurse deliver culturally sensitive care to this family?

Additional Resources

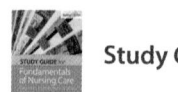

DAVIS edge. **Use the scratch off code on the inside front cover of your book to access online quizzes that will help you to improve your scores on course exams and prepare for the NCLEX-PN®.**

Study Guide

CHAPTER 9

Growth and Development Throughout the Life Span

Molly Showaler

KEY TERMS

Ambivalent (am-BIH-va-lent)
Attachment (a-TACH-ment)
Cephalocaudal (SEF-ah-loh-KAW-duhl)
Cognitive development (KOG-nih-tiv de-VEL-up-ment)
Development (de-VEL-up-ment)
Fontanel (FON-tah-NEL)
Growth (GROHTH)
Menarche (meh-NAR-kee)
Moral development (MO-ruhl de-VEL-up-ment)
Physical development (FIZ-ih-kuhl de-VEL-up-ment)
Proximodistal (PROK-si-moh-DISS-tuhl)
Psychosocial development (SYE-koh-SOH-shul de-VEL-up-ment)
Puberty (PYOO-ber-tee)
Reflex (REE-fleks)
Regression (rih-GRESH-uhn)
Spiritual development (SPIH-rih-choo-ahl de-VEL-up-ment)

CHAPTER CONCEPTS

Patient-Centered Care
Grief and Loss

LEARNING OUTCOMES

1. Define various terms associated with the growth and development of humans.
2. Differentiate between the principles of growth and development.
3. Identify factors that affect growth and development.
4. Describe the stages of physiological development through the life span.
5. Describe the psychological development through the life span according to Erikson.
6. Describe moral development from toddler to adult according to Kohlberg.
7. Explain cognitive development through the life span according to Piaget.
8. Identify the stages of child development.
9. Describe spiritual development from toddler to older adult according to Fowler.
10. Identify specific health concerns for safety issues at each developmental stage.
11. Describe health promotion activities for the nurse to utilize at each developmental stage.
12. Explain nursing implications for each developmental stage.
13. Discuss information found in the Connection features of this chapter.
14. Identify specific safety information.

CRITICAL THINKING CONNECTION

Clinical Assignment

You are assigned to care for José, a 16-year-old male with a newly diagnosed heart condition that was discovered after he collapsed on the basketball court. The family is very concerned, and someone is always with him. He has a 19-year-old sister with an infant son and a younger brother who is 12 years old. His parents are in their late 40s. His 62-year-old grandmother is often at the bedside. All of them have many questions for you. You notice the infant appears underweight and fretful. The grandmother seems fragile and very pale.

Continued

CRITICAL THINKING CONNECTION—cont'd

Critical Thinking Questions:

1. What are the developmental needs of an adolescent?
2. Describe the nursing and health-care issues when caring for an adolescent.
3. What are major aspects of nursing care for an adolescent?

Often you will care not only for a patient, but for his or her family as well. Family members are concerned about the person who is ill, but they may also have health issues. It is not unusual for family members to ask nurses questions about their own health as well as about the care and health of the ill person. When responding to family concerns, it is important to remember the developmental needs and milestones of each age group. This chapter will help you learn how to meet the developmental needs of patients and their families.

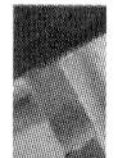

CONCEPTS OF GROWTH AND DEVELOPMENT

Human beings are in a constant state of change from the moment of conception to death. Some of these changes are easily seen, and others, although not visible, are occurring throughout the life span. These changes influence the health and nursing care needs of the individual. When nurses have an understanding of growth and development, they can plan and implement the most appropriate nursing care for each patient at his or her level of development.

Growth is the term for the physical changes that occur in the size of human beings. During growth, the trunk of the body and extremities get longer and heavier. Bones become denser, and teeth erupt. Deciduous teeth appear first, then later fall out and are replaced by permanent teeth. Patterns of growth are similar for all people, but growth rates vary during different stages of development.

Development refers to the increase in complexity of skills performed by a person. Development also refers to the behavioral aspect of growth and includes walking, talking, and meeting psychological benchmarks. Development is more difficult to measure than growth. Several theories about different aspects of development have evolved over time. In this chapter, we will discuss some of the more well-known theories of human development.

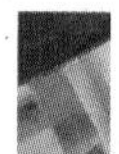

PRINCIPLES OF GROWTH AND DEVELOPMENT

Growth occurs in an orderly and predictable pattern, progressing from the head downward. This is referred to as a **cephalocaudal** pattern. Growth also occurs from the center of the body outward. This is referred to as a **proximodistal** pattern. Infants and children are evaluated by their growth and development patterns to determine developmental delays. Table 9.1 presents principles of growth and development and examples of each.

Factors That Influence Growth and Development

Many factors can influence growth and development. These factors can be loosely divided into biological and hereditary factors, environmental factors, and social factors. It is very important to realize how all of these factors can influence the growth and development of each individual.

- *Biological and hereditary factors* include the presence of physical or mental impairments that may delay or prevent a person from completing developmental tasks or growth benchmarks. Illnesses, whether genetic or due to other causes, also can delay progress through developmental stages. An example of a physical impairment is a child who was born with cerebral palsy who cannot walk. An example of a mental impairment is the child who experienced *anoxia,* or lack of oxygen, at birth and suffers brain damage. An example of an illness that delays progress through developmental stages is the child born with a heart valve disorder who cannot exert himself or herself physically until the valve has been replaced. After that, the child quickly catches up with developmental expectations.
- *Environmental factors* include nutritional concerns and exposure to pollution and chemicals. Exposure to chemicals and heavy metals such as lead can affect the brain, leading to developmental delays. Pollution in the air can lead to respiratory illnesses such as asthma, decreasing physical development because of the inability to tolerate physical activity. Some children do not have nutritionally balanced food available to them, and this decreases their rate of development and growth. An example of this is the child who is given only cow's milk long after solid foods should have been introduced.
- *Social factors* are varied but include expectations, violence and abuse, resources and support systems, and parental influence. When infants are exposed to violence and abuse by caregivers, they are unable to develop healthy trust in those they innately turn to for help. This then affects their ability to complete future developmental tasks. Expectations of behavior and abilities in young children may vary according to the culture. For example, the age at which a child in the United States is expected to be toilet trained and speaking

• WORD • BUILDING •

cephalocaudal: cephalo – head + caudal – tail

proximodistal: proximo – nearest + distal – most distant

Table 9.1
Principles of Growth and Development

Principle	*Example*
Growth and development follow an orderly, predictable pattern.	All children learn to sit before they walk.
Growth follows a cephalocaudal pattern.	Growth begins at the head and progresses to the chest and trunk; then, during the second year, the legs begin to grow rapidly.
Development starts in a proximodistal pattern.	The center of the body develops first, moving outward. Infants hold up their heads, then develop fine motor skills.
Simple skills are learned independently, then become part of complex skills.	Drinking from a cup requires hand-eye coordination, grasping, and hand-mouth coordination.
Development becomes more specific over time.	Infants react with their whole body when expressing pain or happiness. Toddlers react with tears or laughter.
Certain stages of growth and development are more critical than others.	The first trimester in pregnancy is when the fetus is most susceptible to the influence of drugs, chemicals, and viruses that can cause congenital abnormalities.
Growth and development occur at an uneven pace.	There is slower physical growth in school-age children. In adolescence, there is rapid growth of legs and arms.

may be very different from what is expected in another culture.

Theories of Development

Theories are used to describe and organize the growth and development experienced by all human beings. Because you will care for patients of all ages, it is important for you to know appropriate expectations of physical, psychosocial, cognitive, moral, and spiritual development when caring for your patients. In addition, you must tailor your care and patient teaching to the level of your patient. And, as always, *safety must be a primary concern as you care for patients of any age.*

Physical development refers to the physical size and functioning of a person. Influences on physical development include genetics, nutrition, and function of the endocrine and central nervous systems. Table 9.1 provides a summary of the patterns of physical development.

Psychosocial development occurs throughout our lives in distinct stages, according to Erik Erikson, a psychoanalyst who pioneered this area of study. Each stage of psychosocial development requires that specific tasks be mastered. The stages and tasks for psychosocial development are described in Table 9.2.

Cognitive development refers to how we learn. Jean Piaget, a Swiss psychologist and theorist, studied his own children to help him understand how learning takes place as a person develops. Piaget believed that cognitive development occurred from birth to adolescence in an orderly sequence of four stages. Based on this theory, we can see how human beings can adapt behaviors to the demands of a constantly changing environment. Piaget did not differentiate between cognitive development of the adolescent and the adult in his theories. Box 9.1 presents Piaget's four stages of cognitive development.

Moral development is the ability to think at higher levels and develop a value system that differentiates right from wrong. The theory of moral development was established by Lawrence Kohlberg, an American psychologist. He acknowledged that not all people reach all stages of moral development. This is not truly a developmental theory, because progression through the stages may not be age related. All his research was based on males. He studied 84 boys over a period of 20 years to develop his theory. His theory is based on three categories:

1. **Preconventional level:** stages 1 and 2
2. **Conventional level:** stages 3 and 4
3. **Postconventional level:** stages 5 and 6

Box 9.2 gives more information about each of these stages.

Kohlberg is not without his detractors, however. Sharply critical of his work is Carol Gilligan, one of his former students. She feels that the moral development of females is not

• WORD • BUILDING •
psychosocial: psycho – mind + social – related to society

Table 9.2
Erikson's Stages of Psychosocial Development

Stage	*Age*	*Task*	*Nursing Implication*
Trust vs. Mistrust	Birth to 18 months	Learn to trust others	Provide consistent, affectionate care
Autonomy vs. Shame/Doubt	18 months to 3 years	Learn self-control and the ability to express oneself and cooperate	Increase independence by providing praise and encouragement
Initiative vs. Guilt	3 to 5 years	Initiate activities and influence environment	Encourage creativity, answer questions; do not threaten or label behavior as "bad"
Industry vs. Inferiority	5 to 12 years	Develop sense of social skills and self-esteem	Keep realistic expectations for behavior and recognize accomplishments
Identity vs. Role Confusion	12 to 18 years	Seek sense of self and plan according to one's abilities	Assist with planning for future and help with decision making
Intimacy vs. Isolation	18 to 40 years	Develop intimate relationships and choose a career	Avoid criticizing relationships; teach how to establish realistic goals
Generativity vs. Stagnation	40 to 65 years	Become a productive member of society and establish a family	Recognize accomplishments and provide emotional support
Integrity vs. Despair	65+ years	Accept worth, uniqueness, and death	Review accomplishments made by the person

Box 9.1
Piaget's Four Stages of Cognitive Development

Piaget divided his theory of cognitive development into four stages:

- **Stage 1, Sensorimotor:** from birth to 2 years; concept of cause and effect develops; learning through senses and use of body movement and language
- **Stage 2, Preoperational:** from 2 to 7 years; relates objects and events to self; begins to use symbolism; imagination develops
- **Stage 3, Concrete operational:** from 7 to 11 years; concrete problem-solving and inductive reasoning develops
- **Stage 4, Formal operational:** 11 years and older; develops ability to analytically solve problems and engage in abstract reasoning

exactly the same as that of males. Her theory of moral development also has three stages:

1. **Preconventional:** focused on self
2. **Conventional:** interest and concern for others
3. **Postconventional:** focused on social responsibility for self and others

The **spiritual development** theory has been described by James Fowler, an American developmental psychologist. He defines faith as a universal concern that is a process of developing trust. Fowler developed his six stages of spiritual development using information from Piaget and Kohlberg (Table 9.3).

KNOWLEDGE CONNECTION
Explain how knowledge of normal growth and development is important when assessing patients. Which theories of development are based on ages, and which are not?

Settings Connection: Medical Office

Promoting Human Growth and Development
Nurses in a clinic or office setting need insight into human growth and development. Understanding the path of development, including the problems and needs of the various age groups, will allow the nurse to utilize knowledge and provide care that is developmentally appropriate to each age group. Healthy People 2020 has identified a life span goal to "promote healthy development and healthy behaviors across every stage of life." Nurses have the ability to help achieve this goal within the clinic or office setting by advocating for individual improvements in health for all clients.

Box 9.2

Kohlberg's Stages of Moral Development

Kohlberg's stages of moral development include three levels and six stages.

Preconventional Level

Ages 1 to 9 or 10; focuses on avoiding punishment and gaining rewards

Stage 1. Punishment and Obedience Orientation
In this stage, to do right means not being punished, while doing wrong means punishment. The child obeys authority to avoid punishment. An example is the child who tells on herself to avoid being punished when the wrong is found out.

Stage 2. Individualism and Relativism
In this stage, the child no longer views one person as the authority and sees shades of right and wrong. The child focuses on what is fair rather than what might be best for a larger group, such as the family. An example is the child who wants a cat even though other family members are allergic to cat hair. The child sees the situation as completely unfair to him.

Conventional Level

Early adolescence; focuses on conforming to avoid disapproval with respect for authority of law and order

Stage 3. Seeking Strong Interpersonal Relationships
In this stage, the young adolescent focuses on being good and helping others, not just to follow the rules but to feel good about his or her motives. An example is a 13-year-old who helps an elderly neighbor with yard work without being paid to do so.

Stage 4. Law-and-Order Orientation
In this stage, the young adolescent follows laws for the greater good and because of respect for authority. An example of this stage is an adolescent who participates in scouting or other civic clubs.

Postconventional Level

Post adolescence; focuses on behaving according to internal codes and beliefs

Stage 5. Social Rules and Legal Orientation
In this stage, the adult's behavior is motivated by the desire to follow internal values and moral principles. For example, the adult will stop at a red light even though no one is watching and there is no other traffic.

Stage 6. Universal Ethical Principles
In this stage, the adult has concern for human rights and dignity and desires an impartial interpretation of justice. Examples of this stage would include those people who work for justice and human rights throughout the world, such as Mother Teresa.

Table 9.3

Fowler's Stages of Spiritual Development

Stage	*Age*	*Description*
Undifferentiated	0 to 3 years	No concept of self or environment
Intuitive-projective	4 to 6 years	Imitates parents' behaviors about religion
Mythic-literal	7 to 12 years	Symbolism and stories explain religion and morals
Synthetic-conventional	13 to 17 years	While forming own identity, questions values and religious beliefs
Individuating-reflexive	18 to young adult	Referred to as the "demythologizing stage" due to leaving home and developing one's own beliefs
Paradoxical-consolidative	30 years and older	Able to understand different views about faith; more interested in what is true than in what he or she might believe
Universalizing	Adult	Love and justice become tangible as he or she acts on beliefs about the importance of loving and caring for those who are unlovely

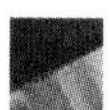

STAGES OF CHILD DEVELOPMENT

In order to study the development of all aspects of children and adults as they grow, categories or stages of development have been identified. As you may have noticed, different theorists use different categories and age groupings. For the purposes of this textbook, we will use the following categories:

- **Infants:** birth to 1 year of age
- **Toddlers:** 1 to 3 years of age
- **Preschoolers:** 3 to 5 years of age
- **School-age children:** 5 to 12 years of age
- **Adolescents:** 12 to 19 years of age
- **Early adults:** 19 to 40 years of age
- **Middle adults:** 40 to 65 years of age
- **Older adults:** 65 years and older

Infants

Infants (birth through 1 year of age) are gradually becoming more aware of the world around them. In addition to the survival skills of eating, sleeping, digesting, and breathing, infants are busy exploring what they can see and touch, including the faces of caregivers.

Physical Development

The first year of life is packed with physical growth and development. It is easy to see the cephalocaudal pattern of development in infants. First, they can hold up their heads at about 2 months of age, can sit up with help at around 6 months of age, and pull up to stand at nearly 1 year of age.

The principle of proximal-to-distal development is also observable in infants. Shortly after birth, they can grasp your finger by reflex. They can wave their arms and legs at approximately 3 months of age, and by 7 months they can reach for and pick up a toy using a pincer grasp.

Infants grow at a rapid rate, doubling their birth weight by 6 months of age and tripling it by 1 year. So the newborn who weighed 7 pounds 8 ounces at birth can be expected to weigh approximately 22.5 pounds when he or she is 1 year old. An infant's length increases at about 1 inch per month during the first year of life. An average length at birth is 18 to 20 inches, so an average height for a 1-year-old child would be 30 to 32 inches.

Newborns possess several reflexes to help them survive. **Reflexes** are automatic responses by the central nervous system and include the following:

- **Rooting reflex:** When a baby's cheek is gently touched, the infant will turn toward the stimulus and open his or her mouth to find milk (Fig. 9.1).
- **Sucking reflex:** When a nipple or finger is placed in a newborn's mouth, the baby begins to suck to obtain nourishment (Fig. 9.2).
- **Startle (Moro) reflex:** When a baby is moved suddenly or jarred in some way, he or she extends their limbs outward and then pulls them toward the trunk of their body to protect themselves from injury (Fig. 9.3).

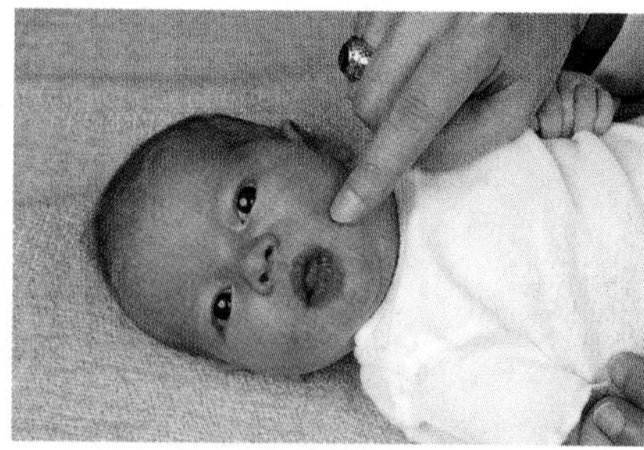

FIGURE 9.1 Rooting reflex (from Dillon PM. *Nursing Health Assessment: A Critical Thinking Case Studies Approach.* 3rd ed. Philadelphia, PA: FA Davis; 2016).

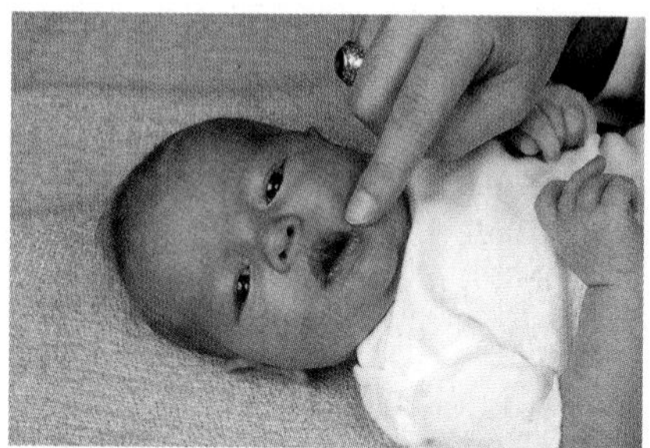

FIGURE 9.2 Sucking reflex (from Dillon PM. *Nursing Health Assessment: A Critical Thinking Case Studies Approach.* 3rd ed. Philadelphia, PA: FA Davis; 2016).

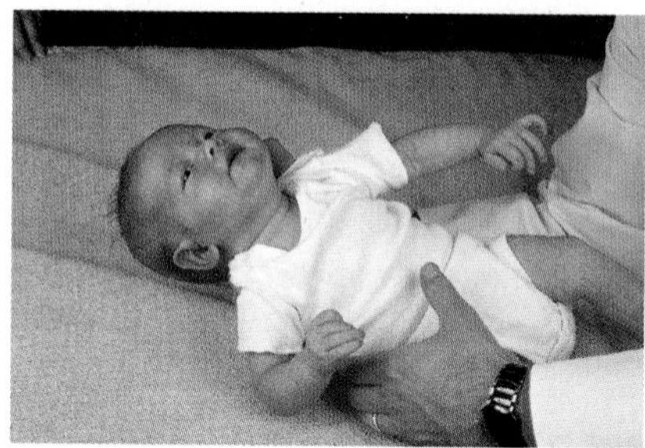

FIGURE 9.3 Moro reflex (from Dillon PM. *Nursing Health Assessment: A Critical Thinking Case Studies Approach.* 3rd ed. Philadelphia, PA: FA Davis; 2016).

- **Babinski's reflex:** When the sole of the foot on a newborn is stroked, the normal response is fanning of the toes while the great toe pulls upward (Fig. 9.4).

These reflexes slowly disappear as the child develops, all decreasing or disappearing by 6 months of age.

Each body system grows and develops more fully during an infant's first year of life. Head circumference is measured to determine brain growth and to detect any signs of problems with cerebrospinal fluid production. Indications of normal growth patterns are that the head circumference will be 2 ½ times the birth circumference by 1 year of age.

Fontanels are the spaces between the bones of the skull that are not yet fused together, sometimes called the *soft spots.* The brain is not protected by bone in these areas during

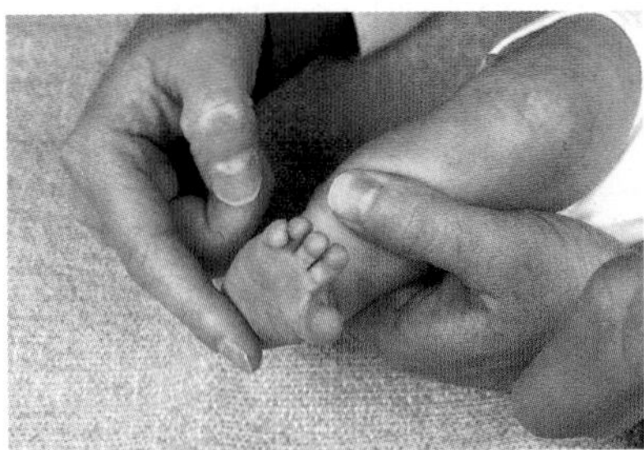

FIGURE 9.4 Babinski's reflex (from Dillon PM. *Nursing Health Assessment: A Critical Thinking Case Studies Approach.* 3rd ed. Philadelphia, PA: FA Davis; 2016).

the first year of life. The posterior fontanel, a triangular-shaped soft area found on the top of the head toward the back, closes first, at about the age of 4 months. The anterior fontanel, a diamond-shaped soft area found on the top of the head toward the forehead, closes last, at about 1 to 1 ½ years of age. Fontanels allow for rapid brain growth during the first year of life. Once the bones of the skull fuse together, there is no longer room for rapid growth.

Psychosocial Development

According to Erikson, the developmental task of the infant is developing trust. In normal situations, mother and baby bond shortly after the birth. The mother looks into the baby's eyes, checks his or her fingers and toes, talks to the newborn, and holds the baby close (Fig. 9.5).

In some situations, the baby is placed in a special care nursery and must remain there for some time. The mother should be encouraged to visit the baby, talking to and holding her newborn as often as allowed to promote mother-baby bonding, also called **attachment.**

If infants' needs for security, food, cleanliness, and love are met, they develop trust in their caregivers. When caregivers do not meet an infant's basic needs, the infant cannot develop trust, and normal psychosocial development is negatively affected.

Cognitive Development

Cognitive development in the infant occurs through sensorimotor experiences. (See Box 9.1 for Piaget's theory of cognitive development.) For learning to occur, the infant must be allowed to have both sensory experiences, such as touching, tasting, seeing, and hearing, and motor experiences, such as moving, rolling, crawling, cruising, and walking. It is a common sight for an infant to pick up any item and then immediately put it in his or her mouth. This is the way the infant learns—through the sensations of touch and taste. Parents have to be vigilant to prevent unsafe items from going into the infant's mouth.

As newborns, infants respond to the environment through reflex action. As they grow older, they respond to repeated sensory and motor experiences by learning through repeated outcomes.

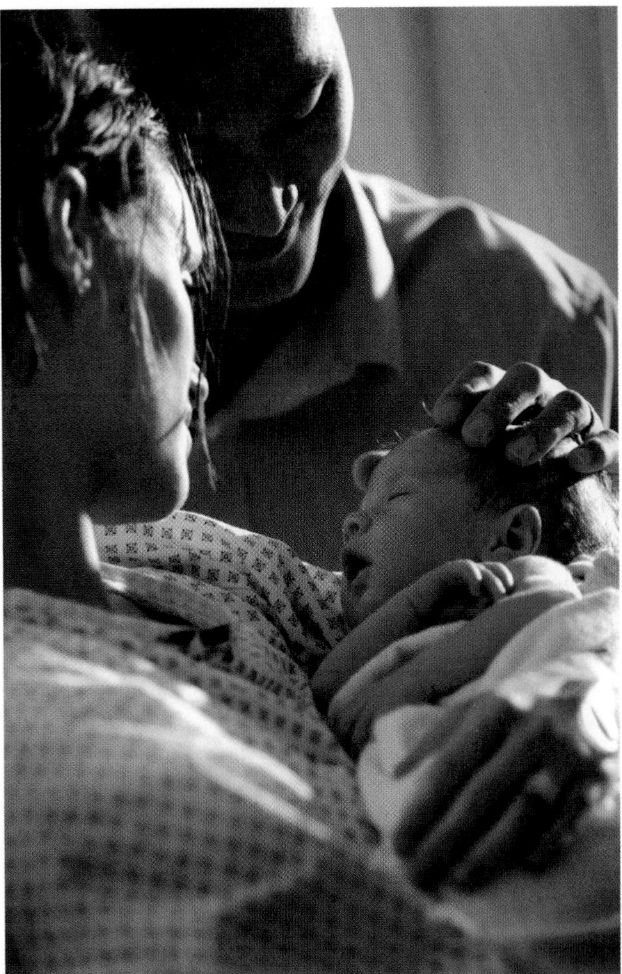

FIGURE 9.5 A new mother bonds closely with her baby (from Wilkinson JM, Treas LS. *Fundamentals of Nursing: Theory, Concepts & Applications.* Vol. 1. 2nd ed. Philadelphia, PA: FA Davis; 2011).

Moral Development

Infants do not possess a sense of right and wrong. They learn through gentle reprimand what behaviors are considered "right" and "wrong." At this age, they do not try to please others, but they respond to the positive feelings of love and affection.

Toddlers

A toddler is a child from 1 to 3 years of age. During this time, the child develops voluntary behaviors and gains control over certain motor skills. The family of the toddler is important in the development of the skills of the child, from toilet training to language development.

Physical Development

Toddlers gain 4 to 6 pounds per year, and their height increases at a rate of approximately 3 inches per year. At age 2, a child is generally about one-half of his or her adult height. So, an infant who is 18 inches long at birth and grows about 12 inches in the first year—or an average of 1 inch per month, as we have seen is normal during the first year of life—would be about 30 inches tall at 1 year of age. By age 2, if the child grew another 3 inches, he or she would be 33 inches tall. Assuming that is half of his or her adult height, the child would reach 66 inches, or approximately 5 feet 6 inches, as an adult.

By 2 ½ years of age, the toddler will have all 20 deciduous teeth. It is important that the child learn to brush his or her teeth or that the parents do so to prevent dental problems in later childhood.

As toddlers' muscles develop and mature, they begin to master additional skills. They learn to control sphincter muscles to master toilet training. Generally, toddlers develop anal sphincter muscle control first and then master bowel control. They develop urinary sphincter control during the daytime before they can stay dry during the night. Accidents and missed cues are common and do not indicate willful disobedience on the part of the child (Fig. 9.6).

Psychosocial Development

Erikson's developmental task for toddlers is autonomy versus shame and doubt. Toddlers struggle to establish their sense of self. Perhaps that is why they like the word "no" so much, because it gives them a sense of control over their daily activities. Toddlers need the opportunity to make decisions with limited choices. Too many choices will be overwhelming for a young child. For example, you might ask a toddler if he or she would like chocolate or vanilla ice cream; listing 14 flavors and asking a toddler to choose just 1 would be too overwhelming. It is important that toddlers be able to make choices without the parent questioning the decision. This helps them develop autonomy.

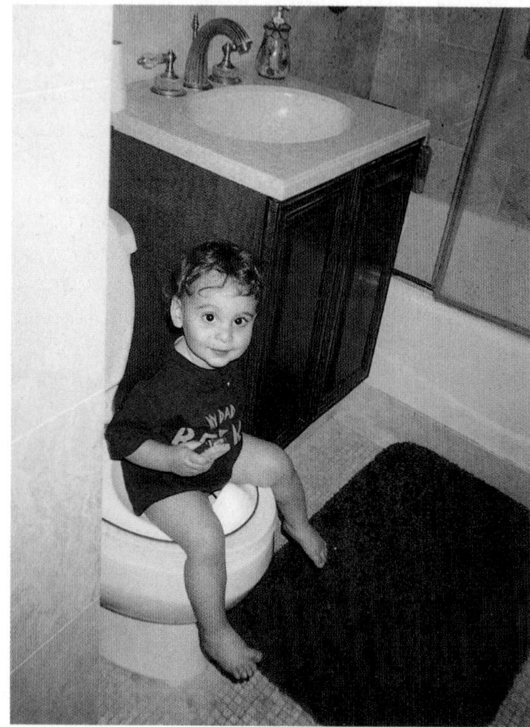

FIGURE 9.6 This toddler is mastering sphincter control and body cues to become toilet trained (from Polan E, Taylor D. *Journey Across the Life Span: Human Development and Health Promotion.* 5th ed. Philadelphia, PA: FA Davis; 2015).

Another way to help toddlers master this developmental task is to allow them to perform and practice skills such as dressing themselves. Even though it would be easier and faster for a caregiver to do this, the child needs to be encouraged to accomplish these skills and to be praised for doing so. If a toddler puts his or her shirt on backward or his or her shoes on the wrong feet, he or she should receive gentle guidance rather than be shamed or ridiculed.

Toddlers are famous for throwing "temper tantrums" when they do not get their way or get their needs and wants met immediately. These tantrums are due to the child's frustration at not being in control. When such tantrums occur, it is best to remove the toddler to a quiet place away from the situation. For example, a toddler may have a temper tantrum in a store, demanding a toy that the parent has refused to purchase. If the parent picks up the child and removes him or her from the toy aisle, going to the restroom or the car, and speaks in a calm, controlled voice, the child will calm down. Then the parent can set firm limits with the child. It can be a challenge to remain calm and in control in such a situation. If the parent gives in and purchases the toy just to keep the child quiet, the child has learned to manipulate the parent using temper tantrums.

Cognitive Development

Piaget describes the cognitive development of a toddler and preschooler as being in the preoperational stage. The child at this age uses trial and error to master new skills and to achieve learning. During this stage of cognitive development, the child is the center of his or her world, or is *egocentric.* Toddlers have no concept of the needs or feelings of others. Their behavior is impulsive, with no thought of how it will affect others.

Toddlers are also developing the concept of object permanence, meaning that they are learning that objects do not disappear when they can no longer be seen. When you play games such as peek-a-boo with toddlers, you are helping them learn this concept.

At this age, the child is also learning by imitation, watching a parent, caregiver, or older sibling and then imitating what they do. Toddlers like to pretend to cook, vacuum, and work with tools.

Moral and Spiritual Development

Again, toddlers imitate parents and caregivers in developing their moral values. As they learn right and wrong from parents and it is reinforced by family and caregivers, toddlers become more secure knowing the limits of acceptable behavior. It is important for parents and caregivers to model the moral behavior they expect from the toddler. For example, if a toddler uses the curse words he or she hears the parents use and then is punished for it, he or she does not understand the expected moral behavior.

At this age, toddlers begin to learn the spiritual beliefs of their parents and caregivers. For example, they may begin to say grace before eating a meal or hear stories that illustrate the family's spiritual beliefs.

KNOWLEDGE CONNECTION

Explain the location and function of the fontanels. How can attachment occur if an infant is in a special care nursery? How tall will a child be as an adult if he is 35 inches tall at age 2? What are two ways to help the toddler develop autonomy?

Preschoolers

The preschool age group is from 3 to 5 years old. This is a time of rapid growth for psychological and cognitive development. The actual physiological growth of the child is not as rapid during these years as in the toddler years.

Physical Development

Lengthening of the trunk and body occurs during the preschool years. The child starts looking taller. Preschoolers gain about 5 to 7 pounds per year and grow 2 ½ to 3 inches per year. They begin to lose some baby fat and look more slender, with extremities that grow quickly and may appear out of proportion with the rest of the body. They are steadier on their feet, with better balance and body control than toddlers. Deciduous teeth have all grown in, so preschoolers must be encouraged to brush often and well, as well as to choose healthy snacks rather than eating mostly sugary foods.

Four- and five-year-olds can dress themselves without difficulty but may still need help tying their shoes. They can handle utensils well and can make their own sandwiches with supervision. They have mastered toilet training but may need reminders to wash their hands and wipe correctly.

Four-year-olds can climb and jump but may overestimate their abilities, so they need to be supervised closely. Five-year-olds can begin more complicated physical activities such as skating and playing sports.

Psychosocial Development

According to Erikson, the major development issue for preschoolers is initiative versus guilt. Children at this age need to be allowed to pretend, role play, explore their identity in the world, and develop a sense of independence. They learn from parents and other adults about roles and initiative. Children in preschool often learn from adults in various positions, such as nurses, doctors, teachers, police, firefighters, and others who serve as role models.

Children at this age should be encouraged to explore within a safe environment. An example of this is allowing a preschooler to be independent within a limited area in a playground under the watchful eye of a caregiver. The child can explore and try new things with a caregiver nearby to ensure safety.

Cognitive Development

As discussed earlier, Piaget's stage for both toddlers and preschoolers is the preoperational stage. However, preschoolers have advanced to the point of being able to take turns, share toys, and obey rules. Preschoolers can respond to only one aspect of a stimulus, rather than being able to understand the whole situation. For example, if a preschooler sees an adult dressed in a mouse costume, complete with a mask covering the face, the preschooler is afraid, believing this is really a giant mouse. A child of this age cannot interpret the situation as an adult dressed up to look like a mouse.

At this stage, preschoolers can grasp concepts based on their previous experiences rather than on their ability to formally reason. An example of this might be when a preschooler hears a parent arrange for a babysitter and becomes upset because it means his or her parents are going to leave for the evening.

Moral and Spiritual Development

The preconventional stage of moral development encompasses the preschool age. At this stage, children learn moral development from the adults in their lives. Examples set by parents and caregivers are imitated and lay the foundation for further moral growth. Preschoolers make moral decisions based on anticipated punishment for bad behavior.

This is the age when many children begin some type of church school or training. Preschoolers understand the concept of being kind and have the same beliefs as their parents. They have vivid imaginations and may misunderstand some spiritual concepts without support and explanation from their parents.

School-Age Children

At the ages of 5 to 12, the child begins to spend a significant part of each day at school away from family. There is less dependence on parents for activities on a daily basis. Children begin to spend time in school- and sports-related activities. Their social groups expand, and their understanding of the world deepens beyond the immediate family.

Physical Development

Children at this age have slow, steady growth of about 2 to 3 inches per year. They gain approximately 4 ½ to 6 ½ pounds per year. Limbs grow steadily at this age, which can cause "growing pains," especially at night. These pains are due to the stretching of muscles and ligaments in the arms and the legs. As school-age children enter puberty, they experience a growth spurt.

Young school-age children, primarily 6- and 7-year-olds, begin losing their baby teeth and replacing them with permanent teeth. When the permanent teeth come in, they may look big in the child's face until more growth occurs. During the school-age years, dental care is very important to detect and correct alignment problems and dental decay.

Psychosocial Development

School-age children have Erikson's developmental task of industry versus inferiority. They are industrious in various ways: schoolwork, sports, and developing new skills. They may have unrealistic expectations of their abilities and become easily frustrated when they do not perform as well as they thought they would. For example, a 10-year-old may be selected to participate in a spelling bee, so he studies hard and expects to take first place. He may then be devastated by misspelling a word in the third round. His parents and caregivers need to be encouraging and positive about how well he did to make it to the spelling bee rather than emphasizing his loss.

Children in this age group often enjoy sports and identify with a specific team. They also like learning and mastering new skills needed to improve in a sport, ride a bike, swim, and skate (Fig. 9.7). As they get older, school-age children learn skills needed to complete more complex tasks and projects. They need recognition and appropriate praise for their accomplishments.

At this age, children become more social and identify with peer groups. Friendships become very important to them, and family becomes less important. They value their privacy, keep locked diaries in secret places, and become extremely distressed if their belongings are disturbed.

It is common for school-age children to be fearful. Younger children (ages 7 and 8) may be afraid of ghosts and being alone at night. Older children (ages 8 and 9) may be afraid that their parents will die or get a divorce, and 10- and 11-year-olds may be fearful of "bad guys" or of developing a life-threatening illness.

Cognitive Development

According to Piaget, young school-age children, up to age 7, are making the transition to concrete operational thought. By age 7, for example, the child no longer believes that an adult dressed in a mouse suit is a giant mouse. Now he or she knows it is just a person in a costume. Younger school-age children begin to understand cause and effect, and older children master this concept. For example, a 7-year-old may tease a dog several times to see what will happen, but an 11-year-old knows that teasing a dog most likely will result in the dog growling and possibly snapping at him or her.

At this stage, children spend a great deal of time in school, which may or may not be a comfortable place for the child. Issues such as bullying, relating to teachers and other children, and being successful in school influence the comfort level of each child. Parents need to be aware of school problems and be ready to act to help the child if needed.

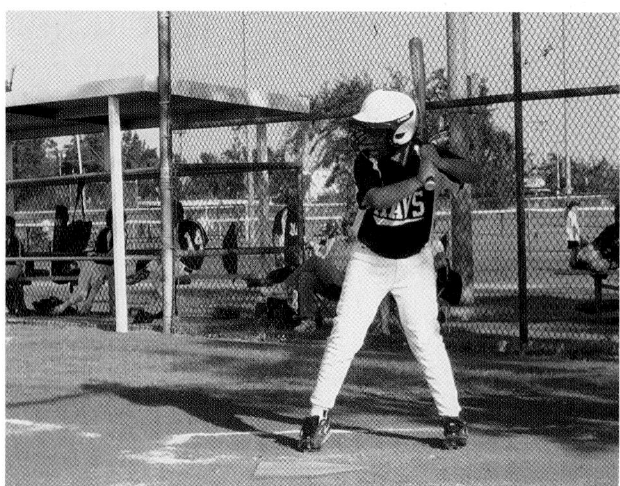

FIGURE 9.7 This school-age child is improving his skills at baseball.

Moral and Spiritual Development

School-age children are moving to the conventional level of Kohlberg's stages. They are learning what it means to be thought of as a good person. By age 11 or 12, children begin to think of others and how to be fair, even if it means sacrificing something they want. Kohlberg refers to concern for others as *reciprocity*. Children at this age are beginning to learn how to regulate their own behavior to win the trust and loyalty of others. Moral beliefs are still based on the teaching of their parents and the behavior they model.

School-age children understand the concept of a god and begin to understand spiritual symbolism in stories with guidance from their parents and religious teachers. They are learning to separate accepted spiritual facts from the fiction of their imagination.

During the years from 12 to 19, teens undergo the change from childhood to adulthood. Both physiological changes and psychosocial adjustments occur. This time of transition is often as challenging for the parents as it is for the adolescent.

Physical Development

At the beginning of adolescence, there is a period of rapid growth referred to as a growth spurt. Boys grow 4 to 12 inches during the adolescent period, and girls grow 2 to 8 inches. Their weight increases in accordance with their height increase. Boys gain from 15 to 65 pounds during these years, and girls gain 15 to 55 pounds.

Puberty, the onset of the development of sexual characteristics and functions, occurs between the ages of 11 and 14. Females develop breasts and experience **menarche,** or the beginning of menstrual periods. Males develop facial hair, and their voices deepen due to the enlargement of their vocal cords and larynx. The penis grows in length and diameter. In both sexes, pubic and axillary hair appears, and hormone production increases.

After puberty, growth slows. Girls reach their adult height by 17 years of age, but boys continue to grow until they reach 18 to 20 years of age. Four more teeth erupt, the third molars or *wisdom teeth,* by about the age of 25. Often there is no room for these teeth, and they have to be surgically removed.

Psychosocial Development

For adolescents, Erikson's developmental task is identity versus role confusion. The teen begins establishing his or her own identity apart from parents and family. It is important that teens test their values, compare them to those of others, and then decide what they truly value and believe. In addition, older teens

• WORD • BUILDING •
menarche: men – month + arche – beginning

are facing the need to make decisions about their future. Will they continue with school or go to work? What kind of degree or career should they pursue?

Adolescents do want guidance and advice from their parents, but at the same time they want to be independent and make their own decisions. This is a time of conflict even in the best of situations. Wise parents expect older adolescents to pull away, to be somewhat critical of them, and to feel **ambivalent,** or to have opposing feelings, about their parents.

Some social issues facing adolescents today include sexually transmitted diseases, teen pregnancy, date rape, and substance abuse. As a nurse, you may be the person a teen turns to for information and help regarding these issues. They often do not want to go to their parents for assistance. Be open and matter of fact. Avoid acting shocked that the teen is involved in these kinds of situations. Provide factual information, answer questions, and be supportive as teens take positive steps to handle these issues.

Cognitive Development

According to Piaget, adolescents are shifting from concrete operational thinking to formal operational thinking. This means that teens are beginning to think logically with problem-solving skills. One example is being able to understand and apply the scientific process to problem-solving. Adolescents can begin to predict outcomes: if this happens, that will result.

In addition to this higher level of thinking, teens begin to have a wider view of the world. They may become interested in politics, environmental issues, and social justice. As their interests increase, adolescents learn about issues with global significance and ways that they can impact their world. You can see that cognitive development of the adolescent closely ties to moral development.

Moral and Spiritual Development

In this transition stage of moral development, teens believe they can make a difference in the world and wish to right the wrongs they see. No longer do they do the right thing simply to avoid punishment. Now they may question the moral rightness of some of their parents' beliefs and examples. They want to try out their own moral code at this age, sometimes without thoroughly thinking about the long-term results of their moral decisions.

This same type of questioning goes on in spiritual development as well. Teens begin to compare what they have always believed with the beliefs of other faiths. They may feel they find more similarities than differences. Adolescents may now be open to spiritual ideas that they have previously opposed. Often they are attracted to less formal worship settings rather than more traditional ones.

KNOWLEDGE CONNECTION

At what age do girls reach their adult height? At what age do boys reach their adult height? Give an example of ambivalent feelings a teen might have about his or her parents.

Laboratory and Diagnostic Connection

Approaches to Procedures for Different Developmental Stages

Although there are no laboratory or diagnostic tests for stages of growth and development, there are often common reactions of children to these procedures. It is very important to keep the age and stage of the child in mind when tests are ordered. Infants need to be held and comforted during and after such procedures. If a parent or family member is not available, you will want to provide this comfort. The same is true of toddlers and preschoolers. They are old enough to anticipate pain when they see a needle for drawing blood or feel anxiety when they are separated from a parent. They may react in a panic. Speak to this age child in a calm, reassuring voice. Try to distract the child with a toy or book if possible. Again, be available to comfort the child if no one else can do so.

School-age children and adolescents may regress when they see a needle or if they have to be separated from a parent or caregiver for tests. At this age, it is important to give a brief explanation of what they will see, hear, and feel. Be honest about whether the procedure may hurt, but reassure them about what it feels like and that the discomfort will be brief.

Adults may be apprehensive about tests and blood draws as well, especially if they have had traumatic experiences in the past. It is important to remain calm and reassuring with adult patients, too. You can distract them during a blood draw by asking questions about their lives and hobbies to keep their minds focused on other things. Answer questions about procedures and explain the purpose for what is being done.

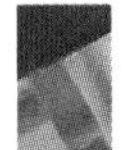

HEALTH CONCERNS FOR INFANTS, CHILDREN, AND ADOLESCENTS

In addition to knowledge of normal growth and development patterns, it is important for you to be aware of safety issues for children of all ages. You may care for children who have been injured in avoidable accidents and need to do patient teaching with the family regarding ways to promote safety in the future. In addition, you may have the opportunity to answer questions from parents about ways to keep their children healthy. You may care for children in a hospital setting, so it is important to adapt your care to meet their needs.

Infants and Toddlers

It is part of your role as a nurse to promote safety and teach family members how to provide for the needs of infants and toddlers. It is also your responsibility to keep infants and toddlers safe while they are in your care.

Safety

When caring for infants and toddlers, it is extremely important to keep the following safety concerns in mind:

- **Prevent Falls.** Never leave an infant alone on an elevated surface. The danger of the infant rolling off and falling is too great. Examples include changing tables or high cribs with the side rails left down. ***Safety: In these situations, keep one hand on the infant at all times. Toddlers like to climb, so keep side rails up and observe the child closely to prevent falls.***
- **Prevent Choking.** Children at these ages tend to put everything in their mouths as a means of exploration. Choking is an ever-present concern. ***Safety: Never leave small objects within reach of infants and toddlers.***
- Nurses must use extra care not to accidentally leave needle covers, IV caps, or other small objects in the infant's or toddler's bed.
- **Prevent Drowning.** Infants and toddlers can drown in as few as 2 inches of water. ***Safety: Never leave an infant or toddler alone in a bathtub.*** Infants can be slippery when wet, so keep a firm grip on infants to prevent them from slipping beneath the surface of the water. Toddlers should never be left unsupervised around bathtubs or swimming pools, even small child-sized pools.

Health Teaching

In addition to teaching parents about safety, you may also teach about health issues. Proper nutrition is essential for young children and can be confusing for parents who may hear conflicting advice from older generations versus current medical thinking. Support parents of infants in following the health-care provider's (HCP's) guidelines for how long to stay on formula or breast milk alone, and when to begin adding cereals and other baby foods.

Toddlers are often finicky eaters, refusing all foods except certain preferred ones for several days in a row. Parents are often very disturbed by this. Encourage parents to provide a variety of healthy finger foods for the toddler to choose from. Examples include small pieces of fruits such as banana, cheese pieces, pieces of cooked vegetables, and small sandwich pieces of peanut butter on bread. Avoid foods that could cause a toddler to choke easily, such as slices of hot dog. The child will usually choose enough foods to stay healthy.

Discipline is often a concern for parents of toddlers during those "terrible twos." Support parents in their choices for discipline, if possible. Provide gentle guidance with suggestions for options to try if you are asked for input. If "time-out" is used, a good guideline is to keep the toddler in the time-out location for 1 minute per year of age.

Parents must have realistic expectations of what an infant or toddler can accomplish. When parents and caregivers expect children to behave in a manner that only an older child could master, the parents may become frustrated. If this frustration mounts, it can lead to child abuse. When caregivers expect behavior that the toddler is incapable of performing, the caregiver may end up harming the child. Many times a caregiver who abuses an infant states that it is because "he just wouldn't stop crying."

Nursing Implications for Hospitalized Infants and Toddlers

Children of this age will want a parent or caregiver with them at all times. If that is not possible, you will need to offer comfort by holding and cuddling the infant or toddler. Remember the importance of meeting the needs of an infant so that he or she will develop trust appropriately. When a hospitalized infant cries and no parent or caregiver is with him or her, be sure that you meet the infant's needs.

Toddlers may respond well when you can take time to play with them. Build rapport by singing a child's song or reading a book to the toddler while you are in the room to perform routine care such as administering medications.

> **KNOWLEDGE CONNECTION**
>
> How long should a 3-year-old be expected to sit in "time-out" when disciplined? What precautions will help prevent an infant from drowning?

Preschoolers and School-Age Children

Preschoolers are unaware of unsafe situations and must be supervised closely while at play. School-age children may see themselves as invincible and dismiss potential for harm.

Safety

Safety issues for this age group include focusing on "stranger danger," playground safety, and water safety.

STRANGER DANGER. Preschoolers must be taught to avoid talking to or trusting strangers. At this age, they believe what they are told and will often talk to anyone, sharing all kinds of information. It is important to teach this safety concept without making the preschooler fearful of everyone all the time. Be sure the preschooler knows it is acceptable to talk to a policeman or fireman to get help.

School-age children need information about how to escape if abduction is attempted. This knowledge gives them confidence that they could handle such a situation. Several programs are available that provide this type of information.

PLAYGROUND SAFETY. Preschoolers may not think through the consequences of their actions and therefore are at risk for playground accidents. For example, they may walk in front of a swing while another child is swinging and be hit. Supervision is necessary to prevent them from attempting unsafe tricks, such as jumping from the top of a slide.

School-age children are very active and are beginning to participate in sports. They must understand safety rules to prevent injury. They are less fearful than when they were younger and want to try out new skills without practicing them first. ***Safety: Safety equipment is required and must be***

used in team sports, cycling, skateboarding, and other activities with potential for injury.

WATER SAFETY. Preschoolers need to learn to swim to prevent accidental drowning. They still should not be left alone in water that is deeper than they are tall.

School-age children may participate in water sports and should be aware of safety rules to protect themselves and others in the water.

Health Teaching

Preschoolers need to have a bedtime routine that involves hygiene, such as brushing teeth and hair, dressing themselves, and some talking time at bedtime, such as with a bedtime story. They are often fearful of real or imagined things, such as a monster under the bed, and require repeated reassurance. Parents and caregivers need to be understanding and avoid impatience or belittling the preschooler.

School-age children need to have health screenings for common problems such as vision impairment, scoliosis, and hearing problems. It is important for them to be active and get exercise each day. Performance in school should be evaluated to help with early detection of learning disabilities or attention problems.

Nursing Implications for Hospitalized Preschoolers and School-Age Children

When you care for preschoolers in a hospital setting, allow them to keep an object such as a blanket or stuffed animal with them for security (Fig. 9.8). A parent or caregiver should be encouraged to stay with the preschooler. To explain medical procedures to a preschooler, show him or her a stuffed animal or doll with a sling or cast to help explain what will happen. Allow the child to act out the procedure with the doll. Use words young children can understand. Remember that children at this age have many fears, so do all you can to help alleviate them. Use a nightlight to help alleviate fear of the dark.

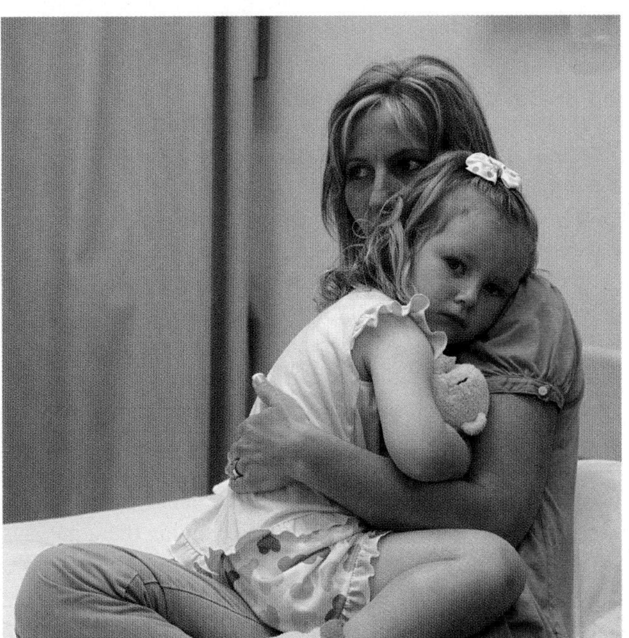

FIGURE 9.8 A preschooler clings to her stuffed animal and her mother for security.

School-age children have a variety of needs due to the wide age range. Younger children, ages 6 to 8, may need frequent reassurance about what is being done because they have many fears about physical injury and bodily harm. Show them what to expect during procedures using a set of dolls created for the purpose. For example, use a set with a doctor doll, a nurse doll, and a patient doll, and then have the child tell you what will happen to be sure he or she understands.

Be honest if the child asks, "Will it hurt?" by replying openly, "It may sting for just a few seconds" or "We will give you medicine to make the hurt go away." Answer questions with enough information to satisfy the child but without overwhelming him or her with information. **Regression,** or returning to earlier behaviors, may occur in school-age children when they feel insecure and threatened by treatments. You may see an 8- or 10-year-old crying, clinging to his or her parent, or having a temper tantrum. Remember to consider the illness and treatment from the child's view to understand the reaction.

> **KNOWLEDGE CONNECTION**
> Why might a preschooler be at risk for injuries on the playground? At what developmental stage do children need routine health screenings? Give an example of regression in a hospitalized school-age child.

Adolescents

Teens tend to exhibit risk-taking behaviors in cars, motorcycles, and all-terrain vehicles. They often feel invincible and ignore safety rules, such as diving into water without knowing how deep it is. The part of the brain controlling judgment is not yet fully developed.

Safety

To help teens prevent accidents and injuries, caution them about the following safety issues:

- **Experimentation.** Teens may be willing to experiment with alcohol, tobacco, street drugs, and prescription drugs of others as a way to demonstrate their independence. All of these activities put them at risk for life-threatening consequences.
- **Internet social networking.** Adolescents often meet others over the Internet. Many times they are simply meeting teens who live in other places when they strike up online friendships. However, the possibility that they are communicating with predators cannot be ruled out. It is extremely important that adolescents not arrange to leave home to

meet someone they have communicated with in this venue, especially if no one knows where they are going or why.
- **Firearms.** Even adolescents who have grown up around firearms for hunting and sport can be at risk for injury or death due to accidental or malicious shootings. Adolescents need to know how to handle firearms if those are kept in the home and how to check that the "safety" is on before handling them. Alcohol and drug use with firearms is a lethal combination.

Health Teaching

Although older adolescents often feel that they are very knowledgeable about most aspects of life, they may be operating on misinformation or partial information. It is important that they have complete and accurate information about topics such as sexually transmitted disease, birth control, and pregnancy. Teens may be hesitant to ask for information or be embarrassed about what they do not know. Give teens accurate, factual information in a nonjudgmental way.

Teens are often extremely distressed by the death of another teen, again because they tend to believe that they are indestructible and the death of a peer contradicts that belief. Teens are easily influenced by others and their experiences. "Epidemics" of teen suicides have occurred when hopelessness or despair seems to be contagious. Be supportive and caring when an adolescent experiences the suicide of a friend or even a mere acquaintance, and allow him or her to verbalize feelings without judging.

Nursing Implications for Hospitalized Adolescents

It is important to allow hospitalized adolescents to have some control over their schedules and environment. Keep in mind that the peer group is the most important to a teen, so the visitors they want to see will be other adolescents. Respect the teen's wishes to either have a parent present or not during examinations and procedures. Treat adolescents with respect and dignity. Avoid saying things that sound like you may be talking down to them. Ask what the adolescent patient knows about his or her illness before beginning any patient teaching.

KNOWLEDGE CONNECTION

Why are teens likely to take risks? What are two things to consider when giving care to a hospitalized adolescent?

Supervision/Delegation Connection

Delegating the Care of Infants and Children

As a licensed nurse, you are responsible for all care given to patients who are assigned to you. You also are responsible for the supervision of unlicensed personnel whenever care or tasks are assigned to them. When delegating care of children to unlicensed personnel, you are responsible to ensure that the care provided is appropriate for the age of the patient. Ensure that the unlicensed health-care provider is aware of any special actions and concerns for various age groups. For example, an infant should never be left unattended on a changing table.

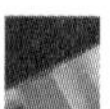

STAGES OF ADULT DEVELOPMENT

Adults continue to develop, experiencing physical, psychosocial, cognitive, moral, and spiritual changes as they age. Adulthood is typically divided into three stages: young adult, middle adult, and older adult.

Young Adults

During this stage, between 19 and 40 years of age, people are often referred to as being "in the prime of their lives." This is due to the maturation of all body systems, the establishment of a career, and the search for meaningful relationships.

Physical Development

Body systems are fully developed and functioning at their optimal level, so many young adults often have no concern for their health. Yet during this time some may begin to experience an increase in cholesterol levels. Women between the ages of 15 and 44 are considered to be at the optimal age for childbearing. People in this age range are often in their best physical condition. The muscles are functioning at the greatest efficiency and coordination is at its peak, giving the young adult an advantage in sports and exercise.

Psychosocial Development

During young adulthood, intimate relationships develop. According to Erikson, the developmental task for this age group is establishing intimacy versus feelings of isolation. Young adults engage in productive work and begin to assume new roles as a husband or wife, and sometimes as parents. Figure 9.9 shows a young couple embarking on these new roles.

Emotional intimacy with family and friends is also a part of this developmental task. They must use introspection to know themselves and to be able to establish healthy relationships with others. Without this, adults of this age group become isolated and self-absorbed, leading to superficial relationships.

Cognitive Development

Young adults become less egocentric, valuing the input and opinions of others. They are able to reason and realistically problem-solve by drawing on experience and researching information. In the first part of young adulthood, they may have completed their basic schooling; however, in the later part of this stage, young adults may continue their education to

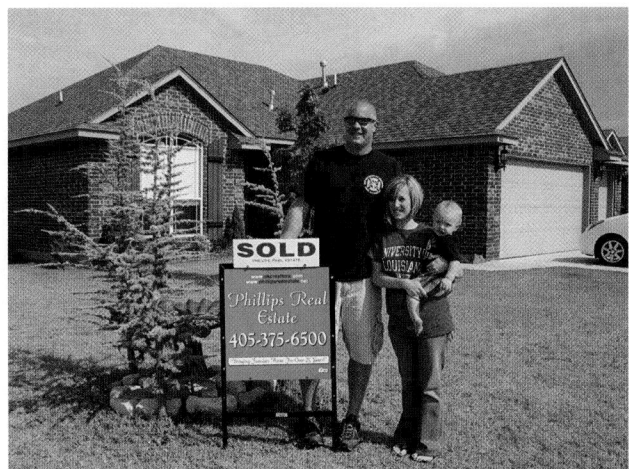

FIGURE 9.9 This young couple is taking on new roles, both as parents and as homeowners.

obtain advanced degrees or certifications to be able to move up the career ladder.

Moral and Spiritual Development

Each adult develops a value system that is based on his or her beliefs and principles. This is how they define right and wrong. Young adults are able to see things within the context of setting rather than always in moral absolutes. This is the postconventional stage of moral development according to Kohlberg. An example of this type of thinking is the young adult believing that injuring another person is wrong, but that knocking an intruder unconscious is not wrong because the person is protecting his or her family and possessions.

Young adults benefit from a spiritual support system that is based on their beliefs. During this time, they may return to the faith of their childhood, especially when they start their own family. They may feel a need to bring up their children with the faith of their family and roots.

Patient Teaching Connection

Teaching About Child Safety

Young adults starting families may need instruction on child safety. Teach parents of toddlers the importance of safety to prevent accidental deaths. You can do this in two ways: teach parents about the developmental stage of the toddler and about the causes of accidents so they can work to maintain their child's safety.

Motor vehicle accidents are one cause of injury and death among toddlers. Encourage parents to use car seats correctly. Teach them about the importance of vigilance when driving in areas where toddlers may be playing. It is very difficult to see a small child when you are backing up or pulling into a driveway. In addition, a child this age may dart out in front of a car without realizing it is dangerous.

Middle Adults

During the middle adult years, which are the years between 40 and 65 years of age, adults are concerned with being productive in both family life and work. Their accomplishments in these areas contribute to feelings of success and satisfaction.

Physical Development

During middle adulthood, the capacity for physical exertion decreases somewhat. It still is important for adults to engage in physical exercise to maintain cardiovascular health because the blood vessels lose some of their elasticity and blood pressure may elevate. During the late middle years, they may notice a decrease in the sensations of heat and cold. Gastrointestinal motility slows, which may cause constipation. There is loss of skin elasticity and subcutaneous tissue, which can lead to wrinkles. Hair begins to lose pigment and turn gray. There is a slight decrease in muscle tone and bone density. It is during middle age that women experience decreased production of estrogen and progesterone, resulting in menopause. Men have a decrease in testosterone, resulting in a decrease in viable sperm.

Psychosocial Development

Erikson's stage of development for this group is generativity versus stagnation. *Generativity* means serving the community, doing meaningful work, and influencing the family in a positive way. Middle adults who are comfortable with their successes generally feel good about themselves and their lives. They may volunteer and become active in the community. During this time, roles change within the family. Middle adults can find themselves caring for their aging parents as well as their adolescent children. For this reason they are often referred to as the "sandwich generation." At this age, they may experience the "empty nest syndrome" because their children leave home. However, they also may help raise their grandchildren. If they do not see themselves as achieving goals, they may stagnate and focus only on themselves.

Cognitive Development

Middle-age adults reflect on the past and anticipate the future. They are able to learn new things, but their reaction time is slower. They need more time to learn complex tasks, but they are very accurate once the task is mastered.

Moral and Spiritual Development

Middle adults may reassess their values and beliefs. It may become important to help others live out their beliefs. Laws are obeyed because they protect the rights and welfare of others. According to Kohlberg, this is the postconventional stage of moral development.

Faith is a source of comfort as adults of this age seek meaning in their life experiences. They may find it easier to deal with illness and death in a framework of the significance of life.

Older Adults

Aging is a process that begins at birth and continues throughout the life span. Encourage older adults, those adults ages 65 years and older, to adopt a healthy lifestyle. It is important to understand that the changes brought about by aging are not indicative of disease.

Physical Development

Older adults experience a variety of changes in their physical condition due to the process of aging. They lose 1 cm of height with each decade of life after age 30, with more rapid height loss after age 70. The nose and ears continue to grow longer because they are made of cartilage and not bone. Table 9.4 describes changes that occur in each body system due to aging.

Psychosocial Development

As older adults reflect on their lives, it is important that they feel a sense of accomplishment. Erikson described this developmental task as integrity versus despair. As older adults think back over their lives, an activity known as *reminiscence,* they often experience feelings of satisfaction and worth. However, if they feel that their life has had little meaning, they tend toward despair. At this stage, older adults have wisdom to share with younger people and may focus on helping others and engaging in meaningful activities.

Cognitive Development

There is no decline in the older person's IQ. Reaction time slows and short-term memory recall decreases, but long-term memory remains unchanged. Older adults can still learn new things, but it requires more time and repeated practice to master a new skill than when they were younger (Fig. 9.10).

Moral and Spiritual Development

Older adults base moral decisions on their own principles and beliefs. They can respect the values of others even though

Table 9.4
Physical Changes in the Older Adult

System	*Changes*
Respiratory	The lung capacity is decreased due to the muscles of the respiratory system being less flexible and to changes in the skeletal structure of the rib cage. There is a decrease in the effectiveness of the cough reflex.
Cardiovascular	The heart requires more time to recover after intense activity, and there is a decrease in cardiac output. The blood vessels have loss of elasticity, which can lead to hypertension.
Urinary	There is a decrease in the ability to filter waste from the blood. Bladder capacity decreases, and due to decrease of muscle tone there is difficulty emptying the bladder completely and stress incontinence.
Gastrointestinal	The taste buds decrease in number. Choking and gag reflex decrease. Peristalsis of the gastrointestinal tract decreases. Liver function diminishes, and the gallbladder is slower to empty.
Musculoskeletal	Muscles decrease in mass and tone. There is decrease in bone density. Degeneration of joints occurs due to "wear and tear" from use.
Neurological	The blood flow and oxygen use in the brain decrease. There are fewer neurons in the brain. Increased time is required to perform tasks that require speed, coordination, fine motor skills, and balance. Sleep disturbances occur. Short-term memory may decrease.
Sensory	The lens of the eye becomes less able to focus and the pupil does not accommodate as easily. There is less lacrimal gland secretion. In the ears, there is a decrease in flexibility of the pinna, and the number of neurons in the cochlea decreases.
Endocrine	The response of the endocrine organs to their target hormones decreases with age. The basal metabolic rate decreases gradually. The body cells become less sensitive to the effects of insulin, causing an increased incidence of diabetes mellitus in older adults. Production of the sex hormones, estrogen and testosterone, decreases.
Reproductive	With the decrease of estrogen, the pelvic organs decrease in size and elasticity. Breast tissue decreases. There is still a need for sexual intimacy and companionship for both men and women. In men, testosterone production decreases. There is a diminished size of the testicles. Sperm count decreases, and the prostate gland may enlarge.

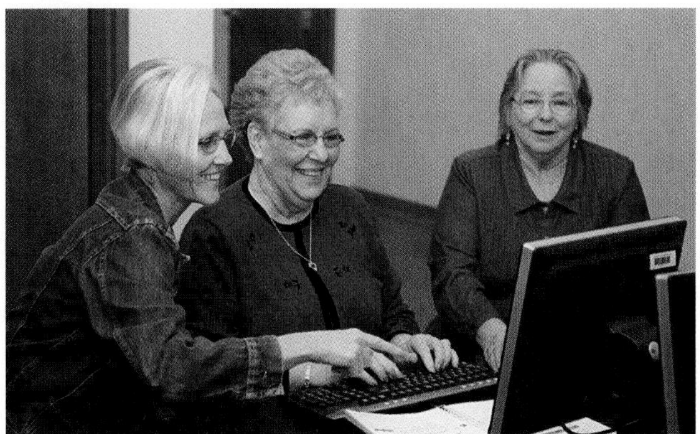

FIGURE 9.10 These older people are learning new skills using the computer.

they differ. Older adults may feel more freedom to act on their beliefs.

As people age, they begin to see their friends and family members die. Older adults may experience the loss of many friends over the last years of their lives. Their spiritual beliefs often help them deal with the grief of losing friends and loved ones.

Health Concerns for Young, Middle, and Older Adults

When you care for adults, it is important to remember the challenges that they face in their own development. Although we are unlikely to see a young adult as having the same concerns as an older adult, we often neglect to consider the issues of safety, health teaching, and nursing implications for adults.

Safety

When you care for young adults, keep in mind that they may have concerns for their children while they are not at home to assume their usual roles. It is important for young adults to provide a safe environment in the home, which includes fire safety. Families need to have a plan for how they will escape and where they will meet in case of fire. The adults need to be sure there are working smoke detectors in the home. It is also important for them to model safe behavior for their children during play and recreational activities.

Middle adults may have more concerns about workplace safety. They know that they should follow all safety guidelines, but sometimes they neglect to do so, even when serious injury can occur. Other injuries at this life stage may result from overexertion when they have not been very active. Damage to muscles and connective tissue may occur when middle adults take on a strenuous project even though they are not used to performing that kind of work.

Older adults are most at risk for injury from falls. This may be due to poor balance, poor vision, or some type of illness. They have very fragile skin that tears easily, leaving them at risk for infections. Adults in this age group may be abused by caregivers. ***Safety: Always be alert for signs of abuse and report them immediately.*** Such signs include unexplained bruises, unexplained fractures or old fractures that appear on x-rays that were never treated, burns that do not match the explanation of how they happened, and an overall fearful attitude by the older adult toward a caregiver.

Health Teaching

Encourage young adults to have yearly physical examinations and screenings for tuberculosis and other diseases. Teach breast self-examination to women and testicular self-examination to men. Encourage regular exercise for cardiovascular health and healthy lifestyle choices, such as staying at a healthy weight, making wise food choices, not smoking, and avoiding excessive alcohol use.

Monitor blood pressure and cholesterol levels of middle-age adults to detect and treat cardiovascular problems early. Encourage them to have vision screenings for *presbyopia* (farsightedness that develops with aging), cataracts, and glaucoma. Early treatment of some eye disorders can prevent serious vision problems later. Encourage regular mammograms to detect breast cancer and regular blood tests to detect prostate cancer. Middle-age adults need to be screened regularly for the development of diabetes.

Many older adults have chronic illnesses that must be monitored, such as diabetes, heart disease, and lung disease. Encourage them to see their health-care professionals on a regular basis for this. They need to obtain influenza vaccines each year and the pneumonia vaccine as well. Some older adults experience confusion, dementia, or Alzheimer's disease. This is not a normal part of aging but a disease process. It is important that they be diagnosed and followed closely to prevent possible injuries or dangers. Adults at this age have decreased kidney and liver function, which can lead to medication toxicity. They need to have blood work done on a regular basis to determine whether toxicity may be occurring.

Nursing Implications for Hospitalized Adults

When younger adults are hospitalized, you must meet their physical needs, but you also need to realize that anxiety over finances, work, and care of their children can influence their recovery. Serious health issues are not as common in young adults, so hospitalization may cause great anxiety. Injury and accidents with lasting disability can devastate the entire family. Be very aware of the concerns and anxieties of young adult patients that you care for, keeping in mind their life stage and responsibilities.

Middle adults may have concerns about the care of elderly parents while they are hospitalized. They may experience a great deal of stress due to their inability to meet family responsibilities in addition to missing work. As a nurse, you can listen to their concerns and be a sounding board as they problem-solve about their situation. Encourage them to ask for help from other family members and friends when they are unable to meet those family responsibilities. Sometimes church members or other community groups are available to help so that the patient's stress can be relieved and he or she can concentrate on getting well.

When older adults are hospitalized, they may be confused by the change in their environment and routine. They need reassurance frequently. If they are very confused, you can help them remember what is happening by reorienting them to their location, the date, and the time when you are with them. (See Chapter 32 for more information on caring for elderly patients.) While they are hospitalized, it is very important for you to keep them safe. Prevent falls by using bed and chair alarms and other alternatives to restraints. Protect older adults from injury by keeping the area around the bed free of clutter and equipment so that they will not trip when they get out of bed. (See Chapter 13 for more information on safety.)

As a nurse who will be caring for patients of all ages, it is important to be knowledgeable about normal growth and development so that you can assess patients of all ages and plan the most appropriate care for them.

Although death can occur at any age, nurses often care for older patients who are close to death or who die in the hospital. (See Chapter 10 for more information on caring for patients at the end of life.)

Settings Connection: Home Health and Long-Term Care

Patient Populations

Home health care and long-term care have typically been associated with the older adult. In the past a major function of home health care was to help elders remain at home. Today, with shortened hospital stays, home health care is needed by patients of all ages to assist them with care they still need after they are discharged from the hospital. Home health care provides things such as dressing changes, IV medications, and care of drainage tubes.

This change from the past is also true of long-term care facilities. Today young and middle-age adults often stay in nursing facilities after they are discharged from a hospital. They may be there to recuperate from surgeries, injuries, or illnesses that require additional care even though they can no longer remain in the hospital.

Real-World Connection

A School Nurse Supervisor's Experience

While working in a large school district in the southwestern part of the United States as a school nurse supervisor, I was responsible for ensuring that children with complex nursing needs at the school were provided with appropriate care and for training the school nurses and staff.

My biggest challenge was when I was asked to evaluate a 3-year-old female who was a quadriplegic, was ventilator dependent, and had a pacemaker. My job was to determine the care needed by this child so that she could attend preschool 3 ½ hours a day. Assessing the nursing needs of this child was challenging because she continued to say "NO" to any question I asked her. She had been in the hospital for over a year, and her parents were very concerned about her entry into school. They needed detailed explanations about how her needs would be met at school. I arranged for the parents to visit the school and spend time in the classroom to increase their confidence that their child would be safe. A nurse was hired and trained specifically on the nursing needs of this child, as well as spending time interacting and playing with the child to establish a relationship and trust. The first day the child attended school, her parents spent time in the classroom. The time that I took to establish a relationship with this child and her parents, as well as the special training for the nurse and school staff, helped this child have a successful school experience for many years.

POST CONFERENCE

In post conference, you have a lot to share. You feel good about the care you have provided. Even though José is 16, he was terrified about having a heart problem. You recognized his moodiness as fear and feeling out of control. You were able to establish a rapport with him, and he talked openly to you about his concerns. What would happen to his planned basketball career? Would he live a long life or a short one? The doctor answered all his questions. He is going to have to take medications, but he should be able to live a long and healthy life, including playing basketball.

His sister asked you a question about her baby, and that gave you the opportunity to teach her a bit about infant nutrition. His grandmother felt ill, and you were able to encourage her to see her HCP. His 12-year-old brother was crying in the hallway because he was afraid José would die, so you were able to reassure and comfort him. And now you understand better how a nurse responds to the needs of the whole family at varying stages of the life span.

Key Points

- Growth of the body includes lengthening of the trunk and extremities and other physical changes in size.
- Development refers to the increasing skills and behavioral changes such as walking, talking, and meeting milestones in abilities.
- A variety of factors can delay or prevent growth and development. These include biological and hereditary factors, environmental factors, and social factors.
- Physical development occurs in an orderly, predictable fashion from the head down and the center of the body out. This is known as a cephalocaudal and proximodistal pattern.
- Psychosocial development requires the completion of specific tasks in each stage of life in order to move successfully to the next stage. This is based on the theory of Erik Erikson.
- Cognitive development involves the progression of learning throughout life, from learning cause and effect at an early age, to concrete problem-solving during the school years, and to analytical problem-solving as an adult. This is based on the theory of Jean Piaget.
- Moral development refers to establishing a value system, distinguishing right from wrong, and the motivations for moral behavior. Lawrence Kohlberg developed this theory of moral development.
- Spiritual development occurs as children first imitate their parents' beliefs and behaviors, learn about religion through symbolism and stories, and then develop their own beliefs. James Fowler developed this theory of spiritual development.
- Nurses need to know the principles of growth and development to assess patients for needs that relate to them.
- Infants and toddlers go through rapid changes in physical development. Their psychosocial development is geared toward developing trust and autonomy.
- Preschoolers and school-age children develop cognitively very quickly, grasping concepts based on previous experiences and using their imaginations. Morally, they begin learning shades of right and wrong. They learn from their parent's behaviors and through symbolism and stories.
- Adolescents struggle to establish their identity and independence. Cognitively, they are beginning to think logically and are developing problem-solving skills. Moral and spiritual development involves developing their own thoughts and beliefs rather than just accepting those of their parents.
- Adult stages of development include younger, middle, and older adults. The major tasks of these stages are establishing intimacy, generativity, and integrity. Cognitive development remains at the formal operational stage. Moral development focuses on behaving according to their internal codes and beliefs. Spiritual development involves the ability to understand others' views about faith, with tangible forms of love and justice.
- Safety, health teaching, and nursing implications for patients of all ages must be addressed to provide optimum care for the whole person.

Review Questions

Select the answer that is most appropriate for each of the following questions. Some questions may have more than one correct answer. Select all that apply.

1. Growth that progresses from the head downward is known as what type of pattern?
   1. Caudocephalad
   2. Cephalocaudal
   3. Proximodistal
   4. Distoproximal

2. When an infant cries, a caregiver comes to give comfort so that the infant learns that her needs will be met. This is an example of:
   1. the theory of physical development.
   2. Piaget's theory of cognitive development.
   3. Kohlberg's theory of moral development.
   4. Erikson's theory of psychosocial development.

3. You are caring for a 10-year-old child who has had major surgery. When you get ready to change his dressing, he begins to scream at you and even tries to hit and bite you. This is an example of:
   1. lack of cognitive development.
   2. attachment behavior.
   3. regression.
   4. lack of moral development.

4. A 16-year-old girl comes to the clinic where you work. She is diagnosed with a sexually transmitted disease. She tells you she is worried that she might be pregnant. Which is the best response for you to make?
   1. "Would you like to have a pregnancy test and find out for sure?"
   2. "Do your parents know about this?"
   3. "If you are pregnant, I hope you don't plan to keep the baby!"
   4. "You should not be sexually active at your age."

5. Which of the following would be of concern to you when you assess a 3-month-old infant?
   1. Rooting reflex is absent.
   2. Sucking reflex is present.
   3. Posterior fontanel is closed.
   4. Infant does not move arms and legs.
   5. Infant grasps your finger and attempts to put it in his mouth.

6. The nurse understands that Erikson's stage of psychosocial development for a 4-year-old is:
   1. autonomy versus shame and doubt.
   2. initiative versus guilt.
   3. industry versus inferiority.
   4. identity versus role confusion.

7. When a baby's cheek is gently touched, he or she will turn toward the stimulus and open his or her mouth to find milk. This is known as:
   1. the sucking reflex.
   2. the rooting reflex.
   3. the startle (Moro) reflex.
   4. Babinski's reflex.

Identify which factor will cause a delay in growth and development for the following children. Write a B for biological/hereditary factors, an E for environmental factors, and an S for social factors.

8. A child born with spina bifida who is paralyzed from the waist down: _____

9. A child who has been sexually abused and does not behave appropriately around other children: _____

10. A child who was exposed to industrial-strength pesticide and suffered brain damage as a result: _____

ANSWERS 1. 2, 2. 4, 3. 3, 4. 1, 5. 1, 3, 4, 6. 2, 7. 2, 8. B, 9. S, 10. E

Critical Thinking Exercises

Answers available online.

1. You are caring for a hospitalized 2-year-old. The toddler has a temper tantrum when you bring in his evening medications. Why is this happening? What will you do?

2. A 45-year-old woman is admitted to the hospital with extremely elevated blood pressure. She seems anxious, and you hear her on the phone telling her 17-year-old son to go check on his grandparents. You can tell the conversation did not go well. How can you help meet this patient's needs? What will you say?

Additional Resources

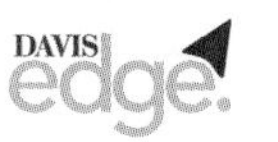

Use the scratch off code on the inside front cover of your book to access online quizzes that will help you to improve your scores on course exams and prepare for the NCLEX-PN®.

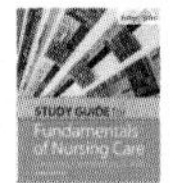

Study Guide

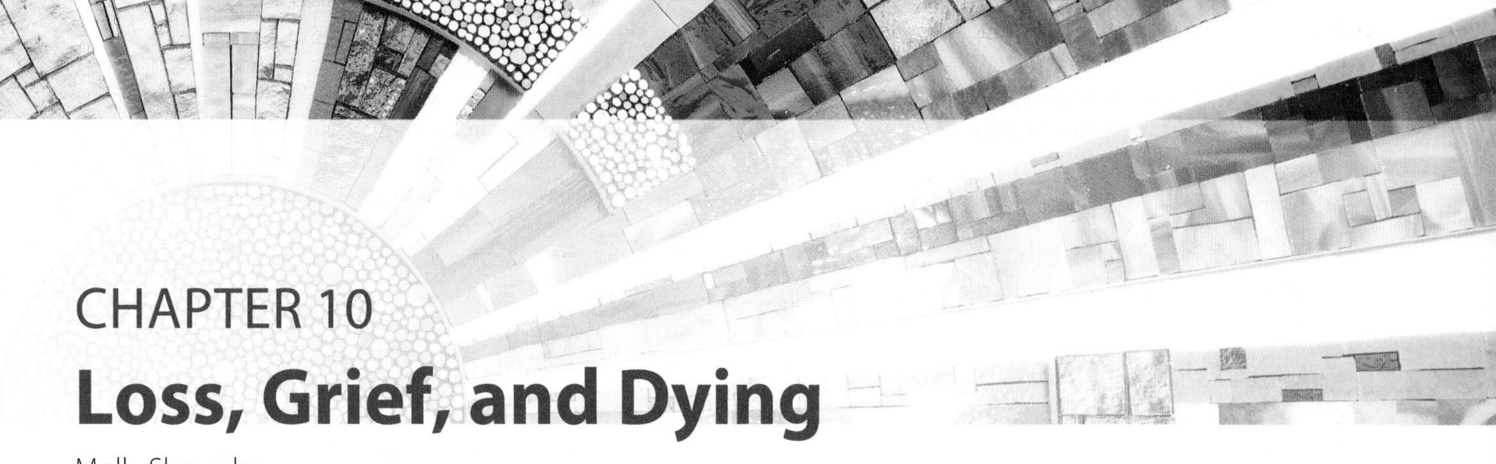

CHAPTER 10
Loss, Grief, and Dying

Molly Showaler

KEY TERMS

Apnea (APP-nee-ah)
Circumoral cyanosis (SIR-kum-OR-uhl SIGH-uh-NOH-siss)
Comorbidity (KOH-mor-BID-i-tee)
Do-not-attempt-resuscitation order (DOO NOT ah-TEMPT ree-SUSS-ih-TAY-shun OR-der)
Durable power of attorney (DYOO-ruh-buhl POW-ur uv uh-TUR-nee)
Euthanasia (yoo-thuh-NAY-zee-ah)
Grief (GREEF)
Living will (LIV-ing WIL)
Palliative care (PAL-ee-ah-tiv KARE)
Postmortem care (pohst-MOR-tuhm KARE)
Respite (RESS-pit)
Role reversal (ROHL ri-VERS-uhl)

CHAPTER CONCEPTS

Grief and Loss
Comfort
Patient-Centered Care

LEARNING OUTCOMES

1. Define various terms associated with loss, death, and grief.
2. Discuss the nurse's role in medicating terminally ill patients.
3. Explain the differences among curative care, palliative care, and hospice care.
4. Discuss durable power of attorney and living wills.
5. Discuss do-not-attempt-resuscitation orders, including the roles of the nurse and health-care provider, and the performance of cardiopulmonary resuscitation.
6. Explain the traditional five stages of grief.
7. Compare religious and cultural differences in death and dying.
8. List at least seven signs and symptoms frequently present in end-stage disease.
9. Contrast the psychological, physical, and emotional changes commonly noted in patients preparing for death.
10. Identify appropriate nursing care for terminally ill patients in specific scenarios.
11. Describe at least four beneficial effects of dehydration at the end of life.
12. Identify comments the patient might make indicating that he or she desires to discuss his or her terminal condition.
13. Discuss information found in the Connection features in this chapter.
14. Identify specific safety information.
15. Answer questions about the skill in this chapter.

SKILL

10.1 Postmortem Care

CRITICAL THINKING CONNECTION

Clinical Assignment

You have been assigned to care for a 68-year-old woman with lung cancer that has *metastasized* (spread) to the brain. Your instructor pulls you aside when you arrive at clinical to explain that your patient is now actively dying. You ask for a different patient, but your instructor tells you that this patient needs your care, even if she is

Continued

CRITICAL THINKING CONNECTION—cont'd

dying. You are terrified. You have never seen anyone die before, and you don't know what to expect.

Critical Thinking Questions:

1. Should you talk to this patient as you would other patients, or should you be silent because she is dying?
2. What if you are in the room with her when she dies? Should you call for help?
3. What will you do after she dies?
4. What will you say to her family, or should you say anything at all?
5. What if you say the wrong thing?

Throughout your nursing career, many medical treatment decisions will become routine. Your patient will be sick. The health-care provider will examine the patient, perform diagnostic studies and laboratory tests, and then prescribe treatment. The treatment plan will be followed, and usually your patient will get better.

However, as your patients become increasingly elderly and subsequently, more ill, medical decisions and treatments can become more complex. Factors such as **comorbidity** (having multiple diseases), dependence on others, and terminal illness can change the range of treatment choices open to them. As chronic illness takes a terminal trajectory, some medical treatments offer little benefit; others can even present potential harm.

In Chapter 3, we discussed the importance of ethics and patients' rights in the general field of nursing. In this chapter, we will provide you with an even deeper look at ethics and patients' rights: those of patients for whom there is no hope of a cure, those who have suffered great losses, and those who are grieving death. In preparation for these eventualities, we will guide you in determining what this means to you the nurse and how to better use the gift you are given when you have the opportunity to assist your patients and their families who are experiencing loss, grief, and even dying.

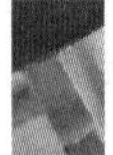

DEALING WITH THE TERMINAL PATIENT

As your patients face difficult life situations, you must be prepared with skill and understanding to help them face serious illness, loss, and death. You must be able to provide them information and referrals to the resources that they will need to make the best decisions. In order to do this well, you will need to think through your own feelings on these issues. What are your attitudes toward aging, chronic illness, cancer, and the losses they represent? How do you feel about withholding treatment that may prolong life but not improve the quality of that life? Providing or withholding artificial nutrition and hydration can be controversial, even for health-care providers. Naturally, these choices can be confusing and even frightening for patients and their families. Fearful patients may consider suicide or assisted suicide, or even ask you about **euthanasia** (the deliberate ending of a terminally ill patient's life). Do not allow this to frighten you. Professionals involved with end-of-life care feel strongly that

- when fear is relieved,
- when pain is managed,
- when the needs for reconciliation with loved ones are met, and
- when spiritual needs are met,

Then patients can approach loss and death without fear and with a sense of peace. When your patient understands that his or her pain and discomforts will be managed, that he or she will be honored, and his or her dignity will be maintained, the issues of assisted suicide and euthanasia often become "nonissues." *However, it is important to note that, in Oregon, it is legal for the health-care provider to write a mentally competent, terminally ill patient a prescription for a lethal dose of a Schedule II drug with which to commit suicide once the patient has asked twice.*

Respect for human dignity is the fundamental principle when making your ethical decisions for practice. When you care for all patients, you are called on to honor their values and beliefs, even if those values are not the same as your own. Although you do not agree, you are still expected to honor the patient's choices and see him or her as a person worthy of respect. When caring for patients who are dying, you will provide support to the patient, family, and significant others. You are expected to support the values and beliefs that the patient has exhibited in life even though they may be different from your own.

Medicating the Dying Patient

It is your responsibility to do everything you can to prevent a patient from needlessly suffering. Explain to the patient that it is his or her right to die with both dignity and comfort. Reinforce that this is one of our goals for the patient's care.

One difficulty in achieving comfort in a terminally ill patient may be getting the patient to take adequate pain medication. Some patients needlessly worry that the use of pain medications will result in addiction. Teach the patient that addiction is not a concern during the terminal stages of illness and that this is not something the patient has to worry about. Teach the patient that pain is easier to control if it is medicated before it becomes severe. Explain that the longer the patient waits to ask for pain medication, the longer it will take for the medication to ease the pain. Encourage the patient to request pain medications as soon as he or she feels the need, explaining that it is not necessary to try to *tough it out.* There are no benefits in suffering.

• WORD • BUILDING •

comorbidity: co – with + morbidity – sickness
euthanasia: eu – good + thanasia – death

Depending on the cultural beliefs of the patient, use of pain medication may not be acceptable. For example, some cultures are very traditional and expect pain to be suffered stoically. However, it is important to note that *not all* individual members of all cultures abide by the traditional beliefs of their culture, so all care must be individualized to the patient.

To do anything to a patient with the purpose of ending his or her life is not an acceptable action, and does not fall within the realm of ethical nursing care, even if the nurse feels that he or she would be helping the patient or relieving the patient's suffering. In other words, it is not acceptable to assist a patient in suicide or to knowingly administer an unsafe dosage of medication that will most likely kill the patient, which is known as **euthanasia.** However, this does not relieve your responsibility to help provide as much comfort as possible and relieve fear and anxiety as death comes near. Although most narcotic pain medications lower blood pressure and slow respirations, it is important that you remember that the disease process is what is killing the patient, not the normal doses of pain medication. Even so, if the patient already has low blood pressure and slower-than-normal respirations, you may have concerns about whether to give the pain medication. If you do have this concern, it must be overcome. If the patient has a do-not-attempt-resuscitation (DNAR) order, your first concern should be to relieve the patient's pain and dyspnea…even if it could hasten respiratory or cardiac arrest.

Real-World Connection

To Give the Medication or Not?

A young registered nurse (RN) had been providing nursing care for several months to a 32-year-old female patient in the terminal stages of breast cancer, with bone and brain metastases. She has a DNAR order. One morning as the nurse came on duty, she found the patient nonresponsive to verbal stimulus but moaning in response to even gentle *tactile* (touch) stimulus. The patient was pale, clammy, restless, and dyspneic, with labored respirations at 10 to 12 per minute. Her Foley drainage bag was still empty, as it had been throughout the previous shift.

Several family members sat quietly next to the bed, at times holding the patient's hand, stroking her brow, and whispering softly to her. One of the family members whispered to the nurse, "Please don't let her hurt. We just want her to be comfortable." The patient had been receiving small doses of morphine sulfate IV at 1-hour intervals, as needed, with good pain relief. The nurse administered the next dose of morphine, and the patient's respirations eased, her restlessness calmed, and the moaning stopped. But within 30 minutes, the patient once again was restless, dyspneic with respirations 10 per minute, and moaning. So the nurse phoned the health-care provider and asked if the morphine could be given more frequently than every hour. The physician gave the order to give the medication as often as every 30 minutes if needed to keep the patient comfortable.

The nurse administered the morphine, which once again seemed to calm the patient's restlessness and ease her respiratory distress. But within 20 to 25 minutes, the patient was having severe dyspnea, respirations were 8 per minute, her heart rate was irregular, and she was moaning continually with each breath. As the nurse administered the next dose of morphine, when about half of the dose was delivered, the patient's respirations dropped to 2 to 3 per minute and then ceased.

Without completing the administration of the morphine, the nurse got her stethoscope and auscultated for heart sounds and breath sounds. A few weak, irregular heartbeats were detected. As the nurse continued to listen with her stethoscope, her tears fell onto the patient's chest as the patient's heart sounds faded away completely.

It is time to do a little reflection before you go on. Have you examined your own feelings regarding terminal illness, dying, and death? How do your personal ethics impact your nursing practice in the areas of assisted suicide and euthanasia? What is your definition of death with dignity? For you, what would represent a dignified death?

KNOWLEDGE CONNECTION

When you make your ethical decisions during nursing practice, what is the fundamental principle you must remember? Why should you honor patients' values and beliefs even when they are not the same as your values and beliefs? Explain what euthanasia is and how it differs from assisted suicide.

Palliative Care and Hospice Care

You may think of nursing as *curative* or healing, and many aspects of nursing do fall within this realm. *Curative care* is that in which medications, treatments, and various therapies are provided with the intent of healing or curing a patient's illness. However, there are aspects of nursing care, known as palliative care and hospice care, which do not heal or cure the disease process; both are areas of growing specialty within the medical community. Hospice and palliative care offer a compassionate and humane approach to end-of-life care that maintains a patient's autonomy and dignity when he or she is facing what can be a very frightening time for the patient and his or her family. Figure 10.1 depicts a model that illustrates the connections among curative care, palliative care, and hospice care.

Palliative care, or comfort care, is health-care provider directed but is not intended to cure the patient's disease. A patient

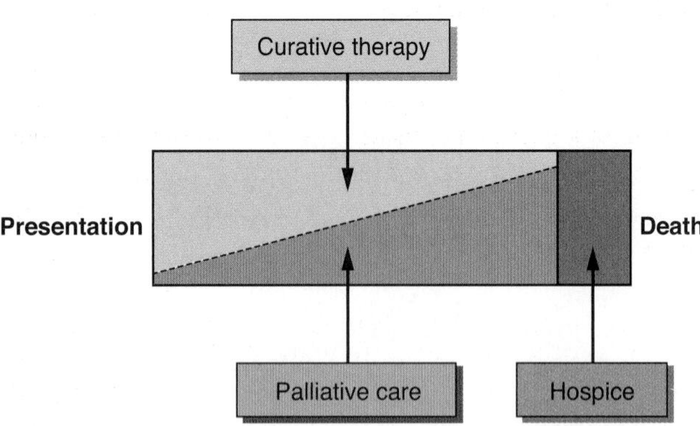

FIGURE 10.1 The simultaneous care model (from Emanuel LL, von Gunten CF, Ferris FD [Eds.]. *The Education for Physicians on End-of-Life Care [EPEC] Curriculum.* Chicago, IL: The EPEC Project; 1999. Copyright 1999. Robert Wood Johnson Foundation. Used with permission from the Robert Wood Johnson Foundation.).

can be admitted to palliative care at any stage of an illness whether terminal or not. It incorporates medication administration, nursing care, and other therapies that are performed to alleviate uncomfortable symptoms such as pain, nausea and vomiting, and dyspnea but have no effect on the disease process itself. Although this type of care may include advanced, aggressive interventions such as chemotherapy, surgery, and radiation, it is important to understand that these therapies are not performed as lifesaving measures. For example, even though a patient may have cancer that is too advanced to be curable, surgery may be performed to debulk a large tumor to provide pain relief and alleviate other distressing symptoms. Whether at home, in acute care hospitals, or in long-term care facilities, patients who receive palliative care services *may* have a life expectancy of more than 6 months.

Hospice care is designed and available for patients in the later stages of terminal illness and does not commonly include measures meant to cure or stop the natural process of dying. Once a patient is referred to hospice care by a health-care provider, a team of hospice professionals will administer care to the patient. Around-the-clock care in a nursing home or home setting is typical; however, a patient may be admitted to a hospital. Admitting a hospice patient to the hospital setting is not the norm. Generally, hospice patients are thought to be in their final 6 months of life, and, as with palliative care, the focus is more on comfort than on cure. Patient and family wishes are followed as the primary direction for care. The primary functions of the interdisciplinary hospice team include the following:

- Relieving patient pain and discomfort
- Lessening patient and family fears and anxiety
- Actively including the patient and family in both patient care and decision making
- Providing both the patient and the family emotional support through the various stages of the grieving process
- Providing respite for the caregivers

The family caregivers may be staying with the patient 24 hours a day, 7 days a week, which is extremely emotionally and physically draining. This increased emotional and physical stress will affect individuals differently, and they will each cope in various ways. You may see increased tension and arguments between family members. You may receive abrupt or curt responses when interacting with them. Remember that these are more than likely just their responses to the increased stress levels and are not directed at you personally. Encourage the family members to take care of themselves during this strenuous and difficult time. Use layman's terminology when explaining things to them. Repeat explanations and answers to questions in a patient manner, even if you have already told them once. Remember that they probably feel overwhelmed and tired, have trouble concentrating, and have little or no energy to deal with things while they are grieving.

Providing **respite** means to make arrangements for provision of care in order that the family members may have a time to get away, rest, and rejuvenate without the strain and worry of continual caregiving. Even a period as brief as 3 to 4 hours can provide temporary relief for the family members. Encourage them to go home for rest or sleep. Remind them that they can call for updates about the patient's condition while they are away. Suggest that they take short walks and breaks several times a day, to allow time to reenergize and clear their mind. A walk outside the facility in the fresh air is important and should be done at least once or twice each day, especially if they are staying with the patient 24 hours a day, 7 days a week. As the team member at the bedside, you are often the coordinator of this team, playing the role of teacher, advocate, and manager to promote best practices for your patient. This is one of those times when you can have a profound impact on a life. By providing holistic patient-centered care and support and by demonstrating your confidence, knowledge, and skills, you can help bring not only physical comfort, but also peace and a sense of life's quality to your patient at the end of his or her life.

KNOWLEDGE CONNECTION

Explain what is meant by palliative care and hospice care. How do they differ from acute care nursing? What is meant by respite care?

Living Until They Die

Preparing for the eventuality of one's own death is not an easy task for most people in our society. But, given the time to consider the subject, most can tell you what they do ***not*** want at the time of their death:

- They do not want to die in pain.
- They do not want to die alone.
- They do not want to be a burden to their family.

Often included in this thought of "not wanting to be a burden" is the statement that they "would not want to be kept on machines" in a hopeless situation. Some will even go so far as to say that they would like to die at home, surrounded by the things and the people they love. A good nurse will assist patients to keep their fears from becoming reality during the dying process.

End-of-Life Documentation

Getting your patient to consider addressing end-of-life decisions is the first step. Once the decisions are made, however, some documentation is needed in order for there to be the assurance that these wishes will be carried out. When a competent individual documents these wishes ahead of time, it is known as an *advance directive* (Fig. 10.2). It can be accomplished with either a living will or a durable power of attorney (DPA).

Living Will

A **living will** is a written document prepared by a mentally competent patient, indicating which procedures and measures the patient does or does not want should an end-of-life condition or disability occur. It may include surgeries, medications, intubation, ventilation, or other extraordinary life-sustaining measures. Many living wills also include instructions on whether or not to provide IV fluids or artificial methods of feeding, such as feeding tubes, if the patient becomes unable to eat and drink normally.

Durable Power of Attorney

While many people have wills in place so that their estates can be administered quickly and efficiently when they die, most individuals never think about who would make decisions for them should they become disabled or lose the ability to make health-related decisions.

A legal court document that grants the authority to make health-care decisions and act as a health-care proxy for the patient should the patient become disabled is known as a **durable power of attorney.** This power is usually bestowed on someone the patient trusts, such as a relative, a friend, or even a trusted financial institution such as the patient's bank. This process does not require an attorney. It simply requires a form with instructions that can be obtained from many hospice agencies or online. The completed document is then signed by the individual, his or her selected representative, who serves as the durable power of attorney, and two nonrelative witnesses to verify the signatures. Then the signatures are verified by a notary public. The form can be very short and simple or very lengthy and complicated, based on the individual's desires included in the document. The nurse may witness the signatures if asked to do so. Without a durable power of attorney, health-care decisions may be left to the legal hierarchy of family relationships, which usually is as follows:

- Legal guardian with health-care decision making authority
- Spouse
- Adult children of patient
- Parents of patient
- Adult siblings of patient

However, when there are no legal instructions dictating how to handle these situations, it can be left to the state courts to appoint a guardian to make these decisions, and the court may not select the person that the patient or family would choose. This can prove to be time-consuming, expensive, and stressful for the patient's loved ones.

Do-Not-Attempt-Resuscitation Order

A **do-not-attempt-resuscitation order** (DNAR) is an order written by the patient's health-care provider meaning that, should the patient's heart and respirations cease, no cardiopulmonary resuscitation (CPR) or other "heroic" efforts to restart the heart and breathing should be performed—a serious and obviously life-ending measure with which you may or may not agree. However, it is your responsibility to know whether or not each of your assigned patients has an AND or DNAR order and to respond accordingly…whether or not you personally agree. If there is no DNAR order, you must initiate CPR. If there is a DNAR order, you may not perform CPR. Some settings recommend replacing DNAR with the acronym AND (allow natural death). The word *death* in the acronym provides the intent of the health-care provider's order. Further reading will focus on using the DNAR acronym. *Follow hospital protocol when determining the use of AND or DNAR.*

HISTORY OF DNAR ORDERS. During the 1960s, researchers developed the techniques involved in CPR as a means of rescuing victims of sudden death when a person's heart or breathing stops. Originally, CPR was intended for use in situations such as drowning or electrical shock, or when an otherwise healthy person experienced complications of a heart attack, such as ventricular fibrillation. Early guidelines stated that there were certain cases when CPR should not be used. Researchers at the time felt it was clearly a violation of a person's right to die with dignity when resuscitation was attempted in cases of terminal, irreversible illness. Today, however, CPR has become the standard-of-care procedure for all patients in hospitals and nursing homes who experience respiratory or cardiac arrest unless there are specific health-care provider's orders stating "Do Not Attempt Resuscitation."

FOLLOWING A DNAR ORDER. In conditions such as advanced metastatic cancer, end-stage acquired immunodeficiency syndrome (AIDS), or renal failure, attempts at CPR frequently are futile. When CPR is successful in restoring breathing and circulation in a patient in an advanced stage of terminal disease, the patient is often revived only to suffer further pain and fear until death finally provides relief of suffering. Because the chain of events puts the start of CPR into motion, your patient could be placed on a ventilator even though he or she might not have wanted it. For many, this risk of prolonged survival "on machines" is a very serious burden. These rather grim thoughts should cause us to look at the ethical and compassionate considerations of performing such procedures on those who have life-limiting illness.

Oklahoma Advance Directive for Health Care

If I am incapable of making an informed decision regarding my health care, I direct my health care providers to follow my instructions below.

I. Living Will

If my attending physician and another physician determine that I am no longer able to make decisions regarding my health care, I direct my attending physician and other health care providers, pursuant to the Oklahoma Advance Directive Act, to follow my instructions as set forth below:

(1) If I have a terminal condition, that is, an incurable and irreversible condition that even with the administration of life-sustaining treatment will, in the opinion of the attending physician and another physician, result in death within six (6) months:

(Initial only one option)

_____ I direct that my life not be extended by life-sustaining treatment, except that if I am unable to take food and water by mouth, I wish to receive artificially administered nutrition and hydration.

_____ I direct that my life not be extended by life-sustaining treatment, including artificially administered nutrition and hydration.

_____ I direct that I be given life-sustaining treatment and, if I am unable to take food and water by mouth, I wish to receive artificially administered nutrition and hydration.

(Initial only if applicable)

_____ See my more specific instructions in paragraph (4) below.

(2) If I am persistently unconscious, that is, I have an irreversible condition, as determined by the attending physician and another physician, in which thought and awareness of self and environment are absent:

(Initial only one option)

_____ I direct that my life not be extended by life-sustaining treatment, except that if I am unable to take food and water by mouth, I wish to receive artificially administered nutrition and hydration.

_____ I direct that my life not be extended by life-sustaining treatment, including artificially administered nutrition and hydration.

_____ I direct that I be given life-sustaining treatment and, if I am unable to take food and water by mouth, I wish to receive artificially administered nutrition and hydration.

(Initial only if applicable)

_____ See my more specific instructions in paragraph (4) below.

(3) If I have an end-stage condition, that is, a condition caused by injury, disease, or illness, which results in severe and permanent deterioration indicated by incompetency and complete physical dependency for which treatment of the irreversible condition would be medically ineffective:

(Initial only one option)

_____ I direct that my life not be extended by life-sustaining treatment, except that if I am unable to take food and water by mouth, I wish to receive artificially administered nutrition and hydration.

_____ I direct that my life not be extended by life-sustaining treatment, including artificially administered nutrition and hydration.

_____ I direct that I be given life-sustaining treatment and, if I am unable to take food and water by mouth, I wish to receive artificially administered nutrition and hydration.

(Initial only if applicable)

_____ See my more specific instructions in paragraph (4) below.

FIGURE 10.2 The Oklahoma Advance Directive for Health Care. (Oklahoma's Advance Directive for Health Care. Public domain.)

(4) OTHER. Here you may:

(a) describe other conditions in which you would want life-sustaining treatment or artificially administered nutrition and hydration provided, withheld, or withdrawn,

(b) give more specific instructions about your wishes concerning life-sustaining treatment or artificially administered nutrition and hydration if you have a terminal condition, are persistently unconscious, or have an end-stage condition, or

(c) do both of these:

____

____

_____
Initial

II. My Appointment of My Health Care Proxy

If my attending physician and another physician determine that I am no longer able to make decisions regarding my health care, I direct my attending physician and other health care providers pursuant to the Oklahoma Advance Directive Act to follow the instructions of ____________________________, whom I appoint as my health care proxy. If my health care proxy is unable or unwilling to serve, I appoint ____________________________ as my alternate health care proxy with the same authority. My health care proxy is authorized to make whatever health care decisions I could make if I were able, except that decisions regarding life-sustaining treatment and artificially administered nutrition and hydration can be made by my health care proxy or alternate health care proxy only as I have indicated in the foregoing sections.

If I fail to designate a health care proxy in this section, I am deliberately declining to designate a health care proxy.

III. Anatomical Gifts

Pursuant to the provisions of the Uniform Anatomical Gift Act, I direct that at the time of my death my entire body or designated body organs or body parts be donated for purposes of:

(Initial all that apply)

_____ Transplantation therapy

_____ Advancement of medical science, research, or education

_____ Advancement of dental science, research, or education

Death means either irreversible cessation of circulatory and respiratory functions or irreversible cessation of all functions of the entire brain, including the brain stem. If I initial the "yes" line below, I specifically donate:

_____ My entire body

or

_____ The following body organs or parts:

_____ lungs _____ liver

_____ pancreas _____ heart

_____ kidneys _____ brain

_____ skin _____ bones/marrow

_____ blood/fluids _____ tissue

_____ arteries _____ eyes/cornea/lens

FIGURE 10.2—cont'd

Continued

IV. General Provisions

a. I understand that I must be eighteen (18) years of age or older to execute this form.

b. I understand that my witnesses must be eighteen (18) years of age or older and shall not be related to me and shall not inherit from me.

c. I understand that if I have been diagnosed as pregnant and that diagnosis is known to my attending physician, I will be provided with life-sustaining treatment and artificially administered hydration and nutrition unless I have, in my own words, specifically authorized that during a course of pregnancy, life-sustaining treatment and/or artificially administered hydration and/or nutrition shall be withheld or withdrawn.

d. In the absence of my ability to give directions regarding the use of life-sustaining procedures, it is my intention that this advance directive shall be honored by my family and physicians as the final expression of my legal right to choose or refuse medical or surgical treatment including, but not limited to, the administration of life sustaining procedures, and I accept the consequences of such choice or refusal.

e. This advance directive shall be in effect until it is revoked.

f. I understand that I may revoke this advance directive at any time.

g. I understand and agree that if I have any prior directives, and if I sign this advance directive, my prior directives are revoked.

h. I understand the full importance of this advance directive and I am emotionally and mentally competent to make this advance directive.

i. I understand that my physician(s) shall make all decisions based upon his or her best judgment applying with ordinary care and diligence the knowledge and skill that is possessed and used by members of the physician's profession in good standing engaged in the same field of practice at that time, measured by national standards.

Signed this _____ day of _______________, 20___.

____
Signature

____
City of

____
County, Oklahoma

____
Date of birth (Optional for identification purposes)

This advance directive was signed in my presence.

_______________________________	_______________________________
Signature of Witness	Signature of Witness
_______________________________, OK	_______________________________, OK
Residence	Residence

FIGURE 10.2—cont'd

When caring for the patient with a life-limiting illness, it is important for you to remember that it is your responsibility to be an advocate for the delivery of dignified and humane care. Withholding CPR is medically justified when it is judged to be of no medical benefit. When fully informed of the potential benefits and risks of performing CPR, many patients choose the DNAR option. ***You should always explain to your patient that having a DNAR order does not mean that he or she will be neglected in any way. Ensure the patient that care will still be provided and his or her comfort will remain a priority.***

DOCUMENTING A DNAR ORDER. A DNAR order can be documented in three ways:

1. The patient may sign a DNAR form.
2. The patient's health-care proxy can sign the form.
3. The health-care provider can write a DNAR order on the patient's chart if he or she feels the clinical situation

warrants. However, the physician does not generally write the order without consulting with the patient and family.

KNOWLEDGE CONNECTION

When should a person execute a durable power of attorney? What preferences does an advance directive establish? When is CPR indicated, and when is it not?

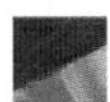

FACING LOSS

As human beings, we face different kinds of loss throughout the course of our lives. Despite the belief of many of us that things will never change and that situations and relationships will be consistent, change happens all of the time—and change usually means loss of one kind or another. Even something as minor as a little surgical scar can represent the loss of body image, so imagine the loss experienced with an amputation of a body part or limb. Consider the loss of one's usual daily routine and freedom when twice-a-day insulin injections become necessary. Once a person has had cancer, even if cured, he or she is forever a "cancer survivor." Once a person is a cancer survivor, his or her sense of security and wellness is forever lost.

Illness and death bring all sorts of loss into a family: not only the loss of that person, but also the loss of all of his or her roles within the family. Many lose parents to Alzheimer's disease long before the parent actually dies. Children, even adult children, feel the loss of a parent comforter, mentor, and advisor. **Role reversal** occurs when the children who are used to being cared for suddenly become the caregivers for their parents. Spouses lose lovers and companions. Losing the breadwinner of the family may bring financial insecurity to the remaining spouse. Even if the surviving spouse is left financially secure, if he or she has not been the one managing the family finances, this new role may be overwhelming. When the family cheerleader and encourager dies, a spark of joy is extinguished for the entire family unit, and with this loss comes grief and mourning as well as a change in their individual family roles. **Grief** is the mental and emotional distress and suffering that one experiences with death and loss, and it is expressed in various ways by each individual. It is important to avoid being judgmental about the way an individual expresses his or her grief. Just because you do not completely understand the person's reaction does not relieve you of your responsibility to be accepting, compassionate, and willing to listen and support the grieving family member or friend. The grieving individual may be extremely tired and worn out by the time the death actually occurs, which can exacerbate the individual's grief. It is your job to encourage the individual to express her grief. Avoid telling the individual that she "must be strong." This discourages the individual from grieving and expressing how she really feels and makes her feel that she should put on a strong front, even when she does not feel that way. Encourage the family members to express their grief and emotions openly with the patient, as well as with you, the nurse. Sharing it with the patient allows the patient a listening ear and another opportunity to talk about his or her fears.

Children and Grief

Many families attempt to shelter children from death, dying, and grieving when a family member is dying, with the intent of *protecting* the child from the unpleasantness of death. However, children are able to detect when something is wrong as they sense changes in the parents or older family members, relatives, and friends. This makes it important to deal openly and honestly with each child, explaining the illness and impending death. The details of the explanation should be based on the child's developmental stage and ability to understand. The younger the child, the more simplified the explanation should be. Without this openness, the child is not prepared for losses to be experienced later in life.

Discuss with the parents (or caregivers) that the child should be encouraged to ask questions and to express his or her feelings openly, rather than try to sidestep the subject. Expect the child to "act out" more often or to act younger than his or her actual age. This is known as *regression* and is commonly seen in children dealing with the illness and death of a close family member. The child needs reassurance that he or she is not to blame for the illness and death.

Five Traditional Stages of Grief

Five emotional and psychological responses have been identified as being common in patients facing the ordeal of coping with loss and grief. Dr. Elisabeth Kübler-Ross was the first to document these findings in her groundbreaking book *On Death and Dying* in 1969. Although there are some differing opinions today on exactly how our patients and their families deal with loss, Kübler-Ross's five stages still provide a method of understanding how people cope with the prospect of dying as part of their life-threatening illness (Table 10.1).

It is also important to realize that there is no script for grief. Those who have experienced loss cannot expect to feel emotions in a particular order or set pattern. People work through and around these stages, sometimes vacillating back and forth and in and out of the various stages. Some experience all five stages, while others experience only a few or just one. Grief is as individual as those who feel it and as varied as the circumstances that surround it.

The actual moment that life is lost to death is always troubling, to say the least. For the patient's loved ones, the separation and loss that accompany death are always sad and often difficult to cope with, let alone accept. However, as the nurse, you have the opportunity to improve the patient's dying experience or journey toward death, to make it as good as is possible, as well as easing the process for the family. This is accomplished by helping the patient and his or her loved ones overcome their fears of the dying

Table 10.1
Kübler-Ross's Five Stages of Grief in Death and Dying

	Stages	*Key Phrases You Might Hear*
Stage 1	Denial	*Not me!* *This isn't happening to me!* *It can't be happening!*
Stage 2	Anger	*Why is this happening to ME?* *Why me? It's not fair!*
Stage 3	Bargaining	*I promise I'll be a better person IF...* *Just let me live to see my children graduate.* *If I could have one more chance.*
Stage 4	Depression	*I don't care anymore.* *I'm so sad; why bother with anything?*
Stage 5	Acceptance	*It's going to be okay.* *I'm ready for whatever comes.*

Source: Kübler-Ross E. *On Death and Dying.* New York, NY: Macmillan; 1969.

process, providing adequate pain relief, performing and teaching interventions to relieve various other discomforts, providing support and understanding, and ensuring that dignity will be maintained.

To minimize some of the natural fears of dying, you will want to provide adequate information regarding the disease process, how it may progress, and that relief of pain and most symptoms is possible. It is helpful to assure the patient that he or she will have full control over his or her own plan of care and degree of pain and symptom control, including the right to refuse any aspect of treatment that may be offered. The holistic needs that must be met include knowing that the patient has control over whether he or she dies at home or in a health-care facility, and who will be allowed to be present as death approaches. It is important to provide for the patient's spiritual needs and any religious rituals that might afford the patient comfort. Encourage the patient to make reconciliation wherever possible and with whomever there is discord. If your patient were dying at this moment, how comforting do you think it would be for the patient to hear the following promise, as stated by Dr. Ira Byock?

> *We will keep you warm and we will keep you dry. We will keep you clean. We will help you with elimination, with your bowels and your bladder function. We will always offer you food and fluid. We will be with you. We will bear witness to your pain and your sorrows, your disappointments and your triumphs; we will listen to the stories of your life and will remember the story of your passing.*
>
> BYOCK I. *DYING WELL: PEACE AND POSSIBILITIES AT THE END OF LIFE.* NEW YORK, NY: RIVERHEAD TRADE; 1997

As a nurse, you can assist the patient to die well by encouraging him or her to live life to the fullest extent rather than just waiting for death and by encouraging the patient to make time to say goodbye to family and friends in his or her own style. Some hospice agencies make it one of their goals to encourage and assist the terminally ill patient to "make wishes come true" as a way of living life to the fullest extent. Examples of ways this might be done include a family reunion, a wedding ceremony, a camping or fishing trip to a favorite lake, a trip to a special seafood restaurant, or a picnic, all things that most dying patients might not attempt or think possible without encouragement.

Patients often seem to be able to exert an uncanny control over the timing of their death. Of course, their primary diagnosis, age, and overall health set a time frame for life expectancy. But a person may either consciously or unconsciously decide to stay alive for a specific event, to complete an important relationship, or to accomplish a special goal. It is a rare gift to your patient for you to recognize this and then offer the opportunity to hear and say the things that will help the patient to experience a peaceful death. Dr. Byock suggested that there are five things that need to be said as we approach the end of our lives:

1. "Forgive me."
2. "I forgive you."
3. "Thank you."
4. "I love you."
5. "Good-bye" and giving the patient permission to go.

These five brief statements represent reconciliation and closure, not only with family and friends, but often with the patient's concept of God and the spiritual. They may be viewed as peacemaking activities and are sometimes expressed in religious tones or seen as a spiritual experience. As human beings, most of us seek or look for eternal significance. Those with that faith often need the support of those around them to find the peace that their faith offers them.

Your job, as the nurse, is to encourage and give your patient and his or her family the space, privacy, and time to explore their experiences and feelings about these issues. You may need to gently let them know these are tasks that they might want to address.

It is critical that you remember that these tasks are very individual, very different for each person. As a nurse, you must be careful *not* to define these experiences for your patients, but let them find their own way. Each person's age, life experiences, and religious background will guide him or her through his or her own unique journey at the end of life. Your own faith and confidence, and especially your presence—just being there if there is no family or friend prepared to do this—are a gift to your patient.

KNOWLEDGE CONNECTION
How can being a cancer survivor represent a loss? How would you outline the stages of grief? Write your own list of things that you feel would help to make your own death a *good death.* What thoughts would you want to impart and to whom? What religious or cultural difference in your patient might cause you the most conflict in caring for him or her?

Culture and Religion

As a nurse, you must be aware that there are many different cultural and religious beliefs regarding death and dying. However, it is also important to understand that an individual being a member of a particular culture or religion does not always ensure that he or she adheres to the traditional death and dying beliefs of that culture or religion. Therefore, it is your responsibility to provide end-of-life care that is specific to the individual.

While members of some cultures prefer to die at home, others feel more comfortable in a controlled environment such as a hospital or hospice unit. Some cultures approve of life support; others do not permit mechanical means of prolonging life.

Some cultures promote the presence of the family and/or friends, while others prefer that the dying patient be given time alone for reflection and repentance. More expressive cultures may exhibit loud moaning and chanting during the last hours of the patient's life as a means of providing comfort to the patient and family members. Other cultures may prefer a more quiet and peaceful environment. Some desire the continued presence of a spiritual leader, while others prefer the spiritual leader to come and anoint or pray for them and then leave.

While some patients may fear death, others may feel that there are things much worse than death. Patient care should be directed toward collecting information about the patient's beliefs and fears; misconceptions should be addressed during patient teaching.

KNOWLEDGE CONNECTION
Describe some beliefs regarding death and dying among different cultural and religious groups.

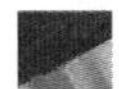

THE DYING PROCESS

Any description of the dying process must be considered as a very flexible list of events. Signs and symptoms of the changes that occur in the mind, spirit, and body as a person prepares to die do not always appear in the same order or in the same way. Death comes in its own time and in its own way, and it is as unique as each individual who experiences it. There are certain symptoms that you might expect to see when your patient begins to enter the end stages of his or her disease (Box 10.1).

These signs and symptoms begin to be exhibited with the patient's initial realization that what is happening is real, when the patient begins to have a true grasp of the idea that time is limited and that he or she is dying. One to 3 months before death, as the knowledge becomes real, your patient will likely begin to withdraw, at least for short periods of time. He or she will have less interest in current events, usual social activities, and sometimes even family members. This withdrawing is a turning in to one's self and can be a time of self-evaluation, life review, or spiritual exploration. It is very unique to each person and may occur in differing sequences or time lines. Box 10.2 presents an example of a typical calendar of events in the dying process.

Psychological and Emotional Changes

As a patient get closer to death, it is common for the patient to review his or her life, sifting through memories, coming to terms with the fact that soon he or she will be leaving the physical body and entering into the afterlife. As your patient mentally processes his or her life, more time will be spent in

Box 10.1

Signs and Symptoms of End-Stage Disease

These signs and symptoms are commonly present during end-stage disease. However, not all of them will be experienced by every patient, and some of the signs and symptoms may be present during earlier stages of certain disease processes.

- Anorexia
- Anxiety/fear
- Cachexia
- Confusion/delirium
- Constipation
- Diarrhea
- Dyspnea
- Fatigue
- Nausea and vomiting
- Pain
- Sadness/depression
- Weakness

Box 10.2

Typical Calendar of Signs and Symptoms of the Dying Process

This *calendar* of signs and symptoms of the dying process relates a *typical* timing of events only. It is important to understand that every patient will exhibit very different timing based on an individualized schedule of his or her own body's design.

1 to 3 Months	1 to 2 Weeks	Last Days and Hours
Realization	Increased sleeping	Congestion and death rattle
Withdrawal	Weakness	Decreased urine output
Life review	Less communication with family	Glassy eyes/tearing
Spiritual exploration	Agitation	Edema of feet
	Anorexia	Mottling of feet and legs
	Changes in vital signs	Nonresponsiveness
		Vital signs: decreased blood pressure, weak and thready pulse, slow and shallow respirations

introspection and reflection, or what appears to be daydreaming, with the patient often not even answering when spoken to. Time spent in withdrawal and noncommunicative states may get longer and longer.

As physical strength decreases, your patient may prefer to stay in bed, resting the physical body while the mind and spirit are working on a level that others cannot really see. Your patient will also have less need to communicate with family and friends. The patient may sleep more and more. This increase in sleeping allows the patient to begin the process of emotionally "detaching" from loved ones and the world as we know it. It is hard to be "awake in this world" and "doing business in the next." Help your patient's loved ones understand this because it can be very hurtful to them. Explain to them that external stimulation such as loud noises, bright lights, strong hugs, and face patting can be very distracting and distressing to the patient and that slow, gentle touch and just being there for the patient take on more importance than long, more demanding conversation.

Another change your patient may undergo as death nears is a loss of interest in food. Liquids are generally more accepted than solids by patients who are dying, but even liquids may become too taxing for them to take in. If this happens to a patient who is in your care, remember that it is acceptable for your patient not to eat. Food is the fuel for the functioning body. It is not needed for the tasks the body now faces.

In the final 1 to 2 weeks prior to death, your patient may appear to be asleep much of the time, but he or she is easily awakened with gentle stimuli. However, keep in mind that it is *absolutely not necessary* to verify level of consciousness with a sternal rub or other painful stimuli you might use in assessing an unconscious patient in another situation. Gentle touch or quiet speech, when necessary, is all that is needed to communicate at this time. If your patient does not respond, respect this too.

Mental Changes

Your patient may experience what appears to be confusion and may talk to people about places and events that do not make sense to you or the family. He or she may pick at linens and have exaggerated arm movements. It is not necessary to restrict these activities; just protect the patient from injury on bed rails or equipment. Your patient may seem to be conversing with loved ones who have died before him or her, such as a parent or spouse. Avoid trying to correct or reorient the patient. This may agitate the patient and result in anxiety, restlessness, or erratic behavior.

Physical Changes

Numerous physical changes will be observed over the days and hours prior to death. Again, it is important to remember that not all patients will follow the same pattern, and some changes will not be experienced by all patients.

Vital Signs

When a patient is dying, his or her blood pressure may be lowered. It is vital to remember, however, that the taking of a patient's blood pressure can be somewhat painful to the patient and that, in the dying process, knowing the patient's blood pressure is secondary to the peace that you can offer by not interfering in his or her comfort. Frequent blood pressure assessment is just not necessary when the patient appears to be within days or hours of death.

It is quite noninvasive to check your patient's pulse, however. You can expect to see your patient's pulse increase up to 140 to 150 bpm, especially if he or she is febrile. Then, as the dying process continues, you can also expect to see the patient's pulse decrease. Just prior to death, the pulse rate may slow into the 30s and 40s.

Skin

Diaphoresis (sweating) and clamminess will be noted along with skin color changes as the body begins to fail. Your patient may be flushed if he or she is feverish, or very pale with cyanosis around the mouth, known as **circumoral cyanosis.** Pallor increases very near the time of death.

• WORD • BUILDING •

circumoral cyanosis: circum – around + oral – mouth; cyan – blue + osis – condition

Respiratory Changes

Respiratory changes also occur with approaching death. Your patient's respirations may increase to between 40 and 50 breaths per minute before decreasing to 6 to 8 breaths per minute. The breaths can be puffing or blowing, and there can be periods of **apnea** (no respirations) for 15 to 50 seconds. Breathing may be cyclic in nature, beginning with periods of shallow, slow breaths before respirations become progressively deeper until they peak as very deep breaths. The respirations then begin to progressively become shallower again, ending the cycle with a period of apnea. This breathing pattern is called *Cheyne-Stokes respirations* and is a strong indicator of nearing death. Observation for more than 1 minute is necessary to identify this breathing pattern accurately.

As death nears, fluids may accumulate in the throat and trachea, causing a moist rattling sound. Often referred to as the "death rattle," this sound does not indicate true respiratory distress for the patient, but it can be very distressing to the family. If the fluids are higher in the throat, suctioning will help reduce the distressing sound. But if the fluids are deep in the throat and trachea, suctioning is not the best solution as it tends to interrupt the patient's ability to breathe and stimulates the body to create more secretions, thus re-creating the problem. This symptom can be addressed with positioning and with medications to dry the secretions, such as a scopolamine patch or atropine. If you are able to alleviate this symptom, you will be making it easier on the family members who are present. This provides another opportunity for you to teach, explaining to the family that although the sound may be frightening, it does not indicate that the patient is in distress.

Physical Activity

In the last days and hours prior to death, the signs that have been present in the last few weeks can intensify. Restlessness can increase as your patient becomes more hypoxic. Short periods of restlessness do not necessarily require treatment. However, a condition of terminal restlessness that is severe and is a reflection of a lack of peace on the patient's part can and should be treated.

Fear and unfinished business are two big factors in determining how much resistance your patient may put into meeting death. Pain should be relieved. Hopefully, all emotional and spiritual issues have been resolved at this point, but occasionally you will have a patient who simply cannot find peace and who will require some kind of sedation.

Eyes

Your patient's eyes may remain closed, but they may also remain open or partly open. There is a glassy look to them, and, because of conjunctival dryness and corneal irritation, there may be tearing. This is not the patient crying. It is important that you communicate this to the family.

Circulatory Changes

As death nears, peripheral circulation continues to fail, and hands and feet become cold and cyanotic. As peripheral circulation fails, you may see *mottling* of the skin, or patches of varying colors of pallor and cyanosis in the feet, legs, hands, and dependent areas of the body. Mottling generally begins distally and progresses proximally. Peripheral pulses become difficult to feel. As the urinary sphincters weaken, the patient may be incontinent. Because of decreased renal perfusion, urine output may decrease or cease completely.

Usually, your patient will become nonresponsive sometime prior to death, a situation in which you cannot awaken him or her with speech or touch. Again, remember that painful stimuli are inappropriate at this time. The period of time from nonresponsiveness to actual cessation of vital signs varies widely from person to person.

> **KNOWLEDGE CONNECTION**
>
> How would you differentiate starvation from the malnutrition and dehydration of the dying process? How would you respond to the question, "How long does mother have to live?" How would you respond if your patient told you he had been visited by a deceased relative? Differentiate between restlessness and terminal restlessness.

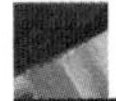

NURSING CARE

Nursing care during the dying process is less about diagnostics, vital signs, and laboratory values and more about caring, touching, teaching the family, and providing presence or simply being there for the patient and family—the fundamentals of nursing that attracted you to the field in the first place (Fig. 10.3). Although great skill, knowledge of the technical aspects of nursing, and understanding of the dying processes are needed, it is the basics of respect for your patient and the maintenance of his or her dignity, even in light of a possible dependence for activities of daily living, that are of the greatest value at this time in your patient's life.

Listening

Listen sensitively and carefully to your patient and to his or her family (Fig. 10.4). Take note of what they say and what they *do not* say. Anticipate needs and fears. This is unfamiliar territory for nearly everyone. Ask about the family and the patient's life, work, and interests. Give the patient your attention and frequent visits, even if for no other reason than to offer caring silence. This presence provides the patient with more opportunity to express his or her fears and concerns because it demonstrates your desire to listen, to support, and to be there any time the patient

• WORD • BUILDING •
apnea: a – without + pnea – breath

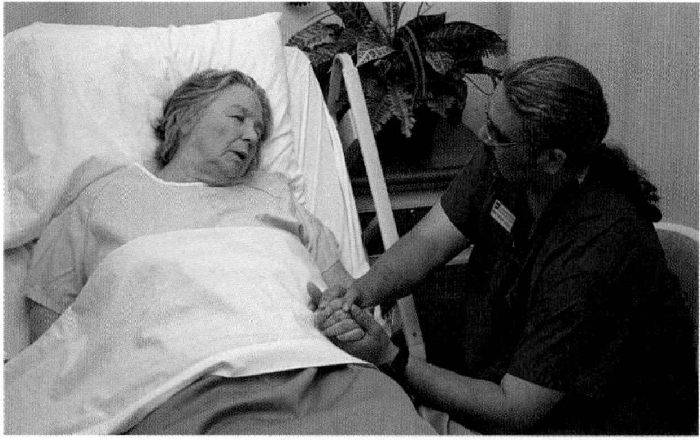

FIGURE 10.3 Sometimes the most important thing you can do for a dying patient is to simply share a little of your time and compassion, just giving your presence.

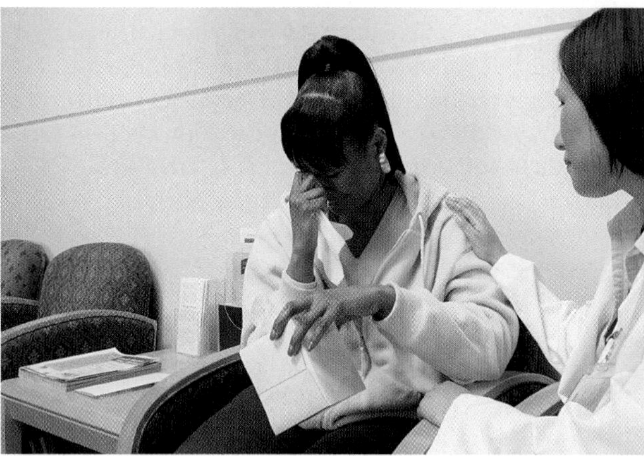

FIGURE 10.4 Encourage your patient and the patient's family members to express emotions and feelings, letting each individual know that these feelings are normal. This will help to build *rapport* (a trusting relationship) with your patient and family members. (City Hospital 2 CD on www.punchstock.com.)

may need you. Hurrying into the room a couple of times per shift and then quickly leaving again tells the patient that you are too busy and just do not have the time for them to talk…so they will not.

Teaching

Using as little medical jargon as possible, gently tell the family what to expect at the level at which they are prepared to hear this information. Two of the most difficult things that families face at this time are nonhealing wounds and poor appetite.

Wounds require adequate circulation and adequate nutrition in order to heal. In the terminal processes, usually neither is present. As with all palliative care, your goals with wounds must generally change from healing to comfort. In the event of a serious pressure ulcer, the best treatment is not usually going to be débridement (removal of dead tissue) because granulation (new tissue growth) is not going to happen in a terminal patient. There is simply not adequate nutrition or body healing processes to heal a severe wound. Keep the area clean, and allow the wound to dry. Allowing a self-sealing eschar (crust or scab) to form over the wound actually helps to control pain and odor.

When the patient is diagnosed with a terminal illness, this is usually the time to throw out all the rules you have learned about nutrition and eating. With rare exceptions, such as renal failure or diabetes, it is usually time to encourage your patient to eat whatever foods he or she thinks sound and look appealing. Generally, you would offer high-protein and high-calorie foods. If your patient wants ice cream and sweets, do your best to accommodate her or his desires. It is not the time to worry about salt or cholesterol intake. Eating three meals a day can be intimidating and nauseating to the patient with *anorexia,* or loss of appetite. Frequent, small snacks can be much more attractive. At a later point in the illness, food will begin to have no appeal at all. Your patient's body will no longer want or need the physical energy that food gives. When that time comes, it is acceptable for your patient to eat as little as he or she wants. This is an extremely difficult time for most families.

When a loved one stops eating, the feelings of fear, anger, frustration, and sadness are often difficult to ease. The sense of loss may be most profound for the family member who had been the food preparer. We nurture by feeding loved ones special holiday meals, therapeutic diets, and their favorite foods. You might hear family members say, "I fix his favorite foods and then he won't eat them," or "He must eat if he is to get his strength back." This can be a terrific source of tension within the family, with the caregiver feeling angry and rejected and the patient feeling hurt and guilty. Helping all understand that the loss of appetite is related to the disease and is something over which the patient has no control may help the family shift the blame from the patient to the disease.

Patient Teaching Connection

Teaching Family Members How to Comfort the Patient

The patient's loved ones may struggle to find ways to help or comfort the individual who is so dear to them. They are often afraid to touch the patient for fear of inflicting pain. Some family members will have a need to physically demonstrate their love and caring. Help the family find nonfood ways of caregiving or nurturing:

- Reading to the patient
- Doing a manicure or pedicure
- Administering gentle massage or soft stroking of feet, hands, or head
- Gently brushing the patient's hair
- Applying moisturizer to the patient's lips
- Singing softly to the patient, especially a song that might hold sweet memories
- Reading aloud favorite Bible scriptures or religious material

- Reminiscing about the good ole' days and telling stories that might hold pleasant memories, allowing the patient to simply listen and drift in and out of recalled happy times
- Viewing old family photographs, especially those that bring particular joy to the patient
- Providing caring silence and simply holding the patient's hand

This is really teaching the family, but patient teaching needs include the family.

The issue of fluid intake has many of the same emotional attachments as does that of eating and feeding solid foods. The parent of an ill child has been encouraged to "give plenty of fluids." As nurses, we have been instructed in the benefits of "forcing fluids" and ensuring adequate fluid intake. And both the medical and lay communities consider dehydration to be a negative state, one that requires correction. ***However, dehydration is a normal part of the physiology of dying and can actually add to the comfort of your dying patient.*** The beneficial effects of dehydration include the following:

- Increased production of endorphins (naturally occurring anesthesia that gives a sense of "well-being" and comfort)
- Decreased urine output, resulting in less incontinence and less need for toileting
- Decreased production of gastric fluids, resulting in less nausea and vomiting
- Decreased pulmonary secretions, resulting in less need for suctioning and less respiratory distress
- Diminished edema and ascites
- Decreased pain perception

Dehydration and the malnutrition that goes along with the dying process are not starvation. Helping your patient's family understand this will be a tremendous gift to the process of providing peace and comfort to all involved.

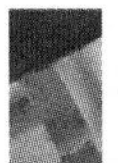

OBSERVATION AND PROVISION OF COMFORT

At the end of life, you will depend *less* on laboratory values and measurements of blood pressures and pulse oximetry readings and *more* on your skills of observation. Observe the patient closely for all aspects of comfort, including:

- **Pain and nausea:** Assess for pain and nausea; do not wait for the patient to find the strength to complain. If these are present, use medications and nonpharmacological methods to relieve them. Box 10.3 lists various nonpharmacological interventions for pain.
- **Gas exchange:** Is the patient dyspneic or cyanotic? If so, provide some oxygen. Is it really important that you know what the peripheral pulse oximetry reading is? No, it really is not.
- **Moisture of mucous membranes:** Are they dry? Then provide oral care. Apply moisturizer to the lips. Dehydration is not uncomfortable for the dying patient if you keep his or her mouth clean and lips moist. If the patient is still taking fluids, offer sips as often as every 30 to 60 minutes or as desired, but do not try to force the patient to drink. The patient may prefer fluids to be room temperature or simply cool rather than ice cold.
- **Emotional or spiritual distress:** If you detect this distress, then address it. Offer to notify a minister or clergy member of the patient's faith or a hospital chaplain if the patient desires.
- **Positioning:** Is the patient restless? Make sure he or she is repositioned frequently, even if only small adjustments are made. It does not take complete side-to-side turning to change a pressure point. Simply placing a small wedge under one hip and one shoulder is often adequate to shift the weight from the previous pressure point to a different area. Apply lotion gently to pressure points and areas of dry skin. The use of an air-fluidized mattress or foam mattress overlay helps to relieve pressure on fragile skin and pressure points over bony prominences. Keep the wrinkles out of the linens under the patient. A very small wrinkle can cause extra pressure on fragile skin.
- **Elimination:** If there is a Foley catheter to drain urine, make certain the catheter is correctly secured to the thigh to avoid tension on the urethra, which is very uncomfortable. If the patient is incontinent, assess frequently and keep both patient and the bed clean and dry to avoid skin excoriation or breakdown. If there is no elimination, gently check for impaction or bladder distention as needed, unless death seems imminent. In this case, lack of output is expected.

Seek help and support from other members of your team as needed for additional ideas and solutions. Offer a symptom

Box 10.3

Nonpharmacological Interventions for Pain

Administration of pain medications is key in providing patient comfort, and these medications should never be ignored or administered sparingly. However, there are many nonmedicinal interventions that have been shown to be as effective as, and sometimes even more effective than, the analgesics themselves. Learn to use all of these interventions, as well as any others you or the patient and family might suggest, to enhance the comfort level of the terminal patient. If one intervention does not work for a patient, try another one, and still another one until you are successful in maximally relieving his or her suffering and distress.

- Distraction
- Heat/cold applications
- Massage
- Meditation/prayer
- Movement and range-of-motion exercises
- Music therapy
- Positioning
- Relaxation and breathing techniques

management plan to the health-care provider. The health-care provider will rarely reject a well-thought-out plan of care with suggestions for solutions rather than just presenting a list of problems. Contact your facility's chaplain or pastoral care department for assistance.

It is important to remember that your first goal at this time is comfort. Withholding narcotic analgesics out of fear of respiratory depression is not appropriate at the end of life. This cannot be emphasized enough. Your patient is dying of his or her disease process. It is natural and normal for respirations to decrease at this time. If narcotics have been part of the patient's medication regimen, dose levels to which he or she has been accustomed will not cause respiratory depression now. Even if narcotics are newly introduced at this time for pain, restlessness, or dyspnea, the small doses prescribed will not compromise your patient's respiratory status. Never withhold comfort medications because you are afraid.

If your patient becomes unresponsive, it is important to remember that research supports the idea that hearing is the last sense to go. It is helpful to discuss this with the family when the time comes, because two things commonly happen:

1. They forget that the patient may be able to hear them and discuss subjects that could be distressing to the patient.
2. They avoid speaking to the patient because they do not know what to say and assume that the patient cannot hear them anyway.

Encourage the patient's family to nurture and comfort the patient even though there does not appear to be a response. You can model these behaviors for the family by continuing to interact with your patient as you would if you knew the patient could hear you, for he or she well might.

KNOWLEDGE CONNECTION

What are the most difficult nursing issues that families face when changing from curative to palliative care? How can you help the family nurture the patient who is too ill to eat? What are the advantages of dehydration in palliative and hospice care?

Symptom Management

Assuring your patient that all symptoms of discomfort can be effectively managed all the way to the point of death addresses one of the greatest fears that people face as the reality of terminal illness descends. It is also one of the most frightening promises you will ever make. However, you can make these promises, and you can make them with confidence:

- Pain can be relieved.
- Nausea can be managed.
- Respiratory distress can be eliminated.

On the rare occasion when symptoms cannot be completely eliminated, they can be brought to a level acceptable to the patient. No one need ever die while suffering in pain or gasping for air.

Box 10.4

Nonpharmacological Interventions for Nausea

As with pain, there are various nonmedicinal interventions that have been successful in alleviating nausea for some patients. Use some or all of these noninvasive, nonpharmacological interventions in addition to medications to prevent or relieve nausea.

- Cool compresses to face and forehead
- Deep breathing
- Meditation/prayer
- Music therapy
- Relaxation techniques
- Small sips of clear liquids at patient's temperature preference

Pain Management

To effectively manage pain, you must first determine what type of pain your patient is experiencing. Accomplish this by asking the patient about the pain and listening closely to his or her answers. Your patient's words will tell you if the pain is visceral, osteogenic, neuropathic, or spastic. Each type of pain must be addressed in very specific ways in order to be effective. Good pain management includes not only medications but also nonpharmacological measures. The different types of pain and pain management will be discussed more completely in Chapter 19. For a list of nonpharmacological interventions for pain, see Box 10.3.

Nausea

Controlling nausea is sometimes one of the greatest challenges of palliative and hospice care. As with pain, you must consider the source of the nausea to begin any effective treatment. Is it opiate induced? Is it caused by neurological problems? Are the symptoms coming from gastrointestinal events? Choices for appropriate medications will be based on these issues. Some examples of nonpharmacological interventions for nausea are listed in Box 10.4.

Dyspnea

Dyspnea may well be one of the most frightening symptoms for your patient. Anyone who has experienced chronic lung disease has experienced air hunger and fears dying while gasping for air. You can be confident when you assure your patient that both pharmacological and nonpharmacological measures are very effective at the end of life to prevent this type of suffering.

Supplemental oxygen, bronchodilators, muscle relaxants, antianxiety agents, and judicious use of morphine all can contribute to your patient's peace and comfort at the end of life.

• WORD • BUILDING •

osteogenic: osteo – bone + genic – production

neuropathic: neuro – nerve + pathic – affected by disease

Morphine reduces the patient's sense of panic that may occur with dyspnea. Use of an electric fan to move the air around the patient often is very comforting to the patient experiencing dyspnea. Box 10.5 lists nonpharmacological treatments of dyspnea.

KNOWLEDGE CONNECTION

What promises can you make to your patient about the care he or she will receive when dying?

Laboratory and Diagnostic Connection

Hypercalcemia

One laboratory result that requires immediate health-care provider contact and possible treatment in hospice care is *hypercalcemia,* an excessively high level of calcium in the blood, usually the result of bony metastasis that is worsened by bedrest. There is a 50% mortality rate if the level is not reduced expediently. It may be evidenced by nausea, vomiting, confusion, constipation, lethargy, decreased deep tendon reflexes, polyuria, and extreme thirst. The common treatment is to increase fluid intake to help dilute the blood level of calcium, using IV fluids if necessary. Furosemide, a common loop diuretic, may be administered to increase urinary excretion of calcium. Calcitonin may also be ordered to lower the blood level by increasing resorption of calcium from blood to bones.

Box 10.5

Nonpharmacological Interventions for Dyspnea

There is nothing more frightening than the feeling that you cannot breathe! Do not hesitate to use every one of these interventions if needed, in addition to use of supplemental oxygen and appropriate medications such as bronchodilators, antianxiety drugs, sedatives, and opioids, which decrease fear and anxiety while providing pain relief. Teach these interventions to the patient and help him or her to optimize a sense of well-being that will help to relieve dyspnea. Take the time for this…it is so very important!

- Fan to move the air
- Meditation/prayer
- Positioning
- Pursed-lip breathing
- Relaxation techniques

Just Be There

Dying patients are experiencing an unfamiliar, but significant, event and usually feel the need to talk about what is happening to them. Although most people do not want to talk about death, your patient will often choose a single person with whom he or she can talk about dying, and it may well be you. Most likely it will not be his or her health-care provider. It is hard for doctors to acknowledge that all of their efforts have still failed and the patient is not going to survive. Death has won and medical science has been defeated. When death is the enemy, defeat is hard to accept.

It is also quite likely that the patient will not choose his or her family for discussion of these things. A dying patient's spouse, children, and even friends feel too much fear and pain, especially at first. It is too risky to talk with someone who does not want to face the grief and separation death will bring, let alone talk about it.

Nevertheless, people need to talk about what they are experiencing. You cannot choose that person for them, nor can you designate yourself as the chosen one, but you should be prepared to be the person with whom the patient feels the most secure and the most comfortable to talk about his or her own death.

Your patient is not likely to just open up and say, "I'm dying and I want to talk to you about it." You will have to listen carefully. The patient may almost talk in code. Statements may be more like, "I don't know what is going on," "I don't think I'm going to make it," "I don't know why God just doesn't take me," or even "I am just so tired." Any of these might be a request for conversation. Listen with a sensitive ear and heart or you might miss the opportunity to give and receive a wonderful gift.

Some of the most meaningful experiences in your nursing career may be sitting at the bedside of your dying patient—not giving great words of wisdom, not having answers to every question, not even talking at all, but just being there, giving presence, providing comforting silence, and helping with your fearlessness and your willingness to just listen. Perhaps you will even shed a tear. That's okay, too. Being willing to feel the patient's feelings and experience his or her emotions is a gift beyond measure.

So often, when you are asked the question, "Why did you choose a career in nursing?," the answer is, "Because I want to help people." Well, here is an opportunity of unbelievable breadth, depth, and height. What greater honor could there be than to be present for the patient when he or she steps out of this world and into the next? As a nurse providing palliative or hospice care, you are there providing help for the patient at a most critical time of life for both the patient and his or her family. You have the opportunity to relieve pain, supply soothing comfort, provide respite, and allay fear, and the rewards for doing so are tremendous. There is not a greater or longer lasting feeling than the self-satisfaction that comes from knowing you helped make the dying process more meaningful, less frightening, and more comfortable for the patient and loved

• WORD • BUILDING •

resorption: resorb – suck in + tion – action

ones. Do not let personal fear cause you to shrink from even one such opportunity that is laid before you.

KNOWLEDGE CONNECTION

What are your gifts to your dying patient? What are his or her gifts to you?

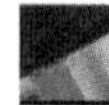

POSTMORTEM CARE

Postmortem care is the care provided after the patient's death. Even after the patient's respirations cease, the heart will sometimes continue to beat irregularly for 2 to 3 minutes. In the hospital or long-term care facility, notify the health-care provider who is responsible for pronouncing death. If the patient is in hospice care, the health-care provider still is notified, but the RN generally makes this pronouncement. Document the time respirations and heartbeat ceased. Incontinence of bowel and bladder generally result with death. Ask the family if they would like to assist with bathing or care. Bathe the body and, if an autopsy is not to be done, remove all tubings such as Foley catheters and IV lines. If there are dressings, leave them intact. Apply a clean gown and linens. Close the patient's eyes and mouth, place the hands across the chest, and elevate the head of the bed slightly. If the patient has dentures, they should be inserted, unless the facility policy states otherwise. A rolled washcloth or small hand towel may be placed under the chin if the mouth will not remain closed. Unless the family prefers to be left alone, remain in the room with the family, providing touch or support as needed. If they do not appear to need your physical touch, just remain unobtrusively in the room. Allow the loved ones as much time as they need. Skill 10.1 provides further information on postmortem care.

Skill 10.1 Postmortem Care

Assessment Steps

1. *Safety: Verify the identification of the patient.*
2. Determine if there are family members and/or clergy that you must notify.
3. Determine whether or not an autopsy is to be performed. Has an autopsy permit been signed?
4. Determine if family members would like to assist in bathing the deceased loved one.

Planning Steps

1. Obtain necessary equipment and clean linens and gown.
2. If there is a roommate present, plan to assist him or her from the room.
3. Close the room door and privacy curtain.
4. Plan to handle the body with all due dignity and respect.
5. Respect cultural beliefs and spiritual practices.

Implementation Steps

1. *Safety: Don clean gloves to protect yourself from body fluids.*
2. Bathe the body to remove all body fluids, including blood, emesis, drainage, urine, or feces. Place a disposable pad under the hips to absorb any further drainage.
   Note: In certain cultures, this step must be omitted. Some religions strictly forbid washing; in others, a special person must perform this task. In cultures in which the family's washing of the body is considered the last service that a family can give a loved one, the family should be given the necessary supplies and left alone in the room with the body.
3. Comb the hair and apply a clean gown and linens as needed.
4. Place the patient in a supine position.
5. Leave or place dentures in the mouth unless facility policy says to remove them. In this case, store in a denture cup and give to the mortician or keep with the body. Be sure to make a note in the chart indicating the disposition of dentures and any other prostheses.
6. Gently close the eyelids. If the eyelids do not close, place a moist compress on the eyelids to moisten for a few minutes and then close the eyes.
7. Gently tie a strip of gauze around the head and underneath the chin if needed to hold the mouth closed.
8. Gently place a pillow under the head and shoulders.
9. Be sure to keep all dressing intact if an autopsy is to be performed. If not, apply clean dressings.
   - ***No autopsy:*** Remove all tubing, such as oxygen, Foley catheter, drains, and nasogastric tube. Remove the IV line and apply a bandage to prevent leakage. Apply clean dressings.
   - ***With autopsy:*** Leave tubes in place, clamp them, cut them off at approximately 6 inches in length, fold over the cut end of the tubing, and tape it closed. Leave the original dressings in place.
10. Place the hands across the deceased's chest to prevent discoloration due to pooling blood.
11. Allow the family to view the deceased patient and to stay as long as they desire. Stay with them to offer emotional support unless they prefer to be alone.
12. When the family leaves, phone the mortuary if the body is to be transported to an independent mortuary.
13. Apply a toe, ankle, or wrist identification band per facility policy.
14. If policy dictates, secure the wrists together and the ankles together to make transport easier.
15. ***If using shroud:*** Place the body in supine position on a flat shroud or sheet. Fold the top and bottom ends of the shroud over the deceased's head and feet. Wrap the two sides of shroud or sheet around the body. Secure the shroud or sheet in place with straps placed around the chest, waist, and ankles. Apply a second identification tag to the ankle strap.
    If no shroud: Cover the body with a clean flat sheet to wait for the mortician.

Skill 10.1 (continued)

16. Transport the body via gurney to the hospital morgue unless the mortician comes to the room to pick up the body.
17. Common courtesy dictates that all patient doors be closed before transporting the deceased down the hallway.

Evaluation Steps

1. Evaluate whether all documentation has been completed per facility policy, including postmortem care; disposition of personal belongings, assistive devices, and valuables; the time that the body was transported; and whether the body was transported to the facility morgue or to an independent mortuary.
2. Make certain that all family members' needs were met and that they have all left the facility.
3. Evaluate whether housekeeping has been notified regarding terminal cleaning of room.

Sample Documentation

03/05/22 0350 Body bathed by wife per her request. Son arrived as wife was completing bath. Informed son and wife to take all the time they needed. Coffee and ice water provided.
——— Nurse's signature and credentials

03/05/22 0420 Personal belongings given to wife. Itemized list signed and placed in chart. No valuables or personal medications in lockup. Orderly assisted wife and son to transport belongings to private car. No further family members present. ———
——— Nurse's signature and credentials

03/05/22 0430 Postmortem care performed. No autopsy to be done. Saint Francis Mortuary notified. ———
——— Nurse's signature and credentials

03/05/22 0520 Body discharged to Saint Francis Mortuary personnel. Both upper and lower dentures were in mouth at time of transport. ———
——— Nurse's signature and credentials

POST CONFERENCE

You share in post conference that this was one of the most amazing days you have had in clinicals. You cared for your patient by keeping her clean and comfortable. You talked to her and her family about her needs and how you would meet them. Her family was so kind to you. They were prepared for her death, but they were not ready to let her go. As her respirations grew slower and more erratic, they gathered around her bed. Each person said a good-bye in his or her own special way, and then she took her last breath. Everything was peaceful and calm. You were glad to help with postmortem care as a final act of reverence and dignity for this special lady.

Key Points

- In order to ensure the right to self-determination, also known as autonomy, the patient should be encouraged to complete an advance directive and durable power of attorney.
- Loss comes in many forms in our lives. All losses are grieved.
- Dying *well* is desirable and possible.
- Although flexible in timing and symptoms, the dying process does have a predictable pathway.
- Nursing care for the dying patient includes observation, listening, teaching, and symptom management.
- All symptoms of suffering can be managed or alleviated.
- It can be one of the nurse's more rewarding roles to facilitate the passing of a life from this world to the next.
- Palliative care, or comfort care, is physician directed but is not intended to cure the patient's disease. It incorporates medication administration, nursing care, and other therapies that are performed to alleviate uncomfortable symptoms but that have no effect on the disease process itself.
- Hospice services are designed and available for patients in the later stages of terminal illness and do not commonly include measures meant to cure or stop the natural process of dying.
- A DNAR is an order written by the patient's health-care provider, meaning that should the patient's heart and respirations cease, no CPR or other "heroic" efforts to restart the heart and breathing should be performed—a serious and obviously life-ending measure with which you may or not agree.
- The five stages of grief in death and dying are the following: (1) denial, (2) anger, (3) bargaining, (4) depression, and (5) acceptance.
- As a nurse, you must be aware that there are many different cultural and religious beliefs regarding death and dying.
- Nonpharmacological interventions for pain include distraction, heat/cold applications, massage, meditation/prayer, range-of-motion exercises, music therapy, positioning, and relaxation and breathing techniques.

Review Questions

Select the answer that is most appropriate for each of the following questions. Some questions may have more than one correct answer. Select all that apply.

1. Your patient can approach loss and death with a sense of peace when which of the following needs are met?
   1. Fear of the unknown is relieved by adequate knowledge.
   2. Pain and other signs and symptoms are effectively managed.
   3. Reconciliation with significant others is accomplished.
   4. The patient receives validation that he or she will die alone.
   5. Spiritual reconciliation is completed.
   6. Estate and financial matters have been settled.

2. Which of the following is not true of hospice care?
   1. It maintains patient autonomy and dignity.
   2. It incorporates therapies to extend the patient's life.
   3. The patient is thought to be in final 6 months of life.
   4. Family wishes are the primary direction for care.
   5. The primary goals are relief of pain, lessening of fear, and provision of caregiver respite.

3. The document that explains the patient's wishes regarding withholding or withdrawing life-sustaining treatments such as artificial nutrition and hydration is the:
   1. durable power of attorney.
   2. power of attorney.
   3. do-not-attempt-resuscitation order.
   4. living will.

4. When your patient states, "It's not fair that my cancer wasn't found sooner!," he is expressing emotions described as:
   1. denial.
   2. anger.
   3. bargaining.
   4. depression.
   5. acceptance.

5. "If I make it through the chemotherapy and radiation, then God will let me live," is an example of:
   1. denial.
   2. anger.
   3. bargaining.
   4. depression.
   5. acceptance.

6. The dying process:
   1. is a flexible list of events.
   2. includes changes that are mostly physical and observable.
   3. includes a time of resting the physical while the mind and spirit are working.
   4. is amazingly similar for most patients.
   5. requires solitude.

7. Of the following symptoms, which is most indicative of imminent death? (Select either 1 or 2 for each of the following choices. You should have six answers when you have completed the question.)

1. Tachycardia	or	2. Bradycardia
1. Circumoral cyanosis	or	2. Peripheral mottling
1. Tachypnea	or	2. Periods of apnea
1. Reaching out to family	or	2. Withdrawal from family
1. Pallor	or	2. Flushing
1. Unresponsiveness	or	2. Agitation

8. When referring to the hospice nurse, the phrase "being there" means:
   1. being with the patient 24 hours a day, 7 days a week.
   2. being honest with patient and family.
   3. being willing to listen.
   4. listening for what the patient/family does not say.
   5. experiencing the emotions elicited during the dying process.
   6. conquering your own fears.

ANSWERS 1. 1, 2, 3, 5, 6. 2. 2, 4. 3. 4. 4. 2. 5. 3. 6. 1, 3. 7. 2, 2, 2, 2, 1, 1. 8. 2, 3, 4, 5, 6

Critical Thinking Exercises

Answers available online.

1. How would you explain the statement that "CPR should not be the *standard of care* for the chronically ill resident of a long-term care facility"?

2. Explain the difference between starvation and the malnutrition/dehydration of the dying process.

Additional Resources

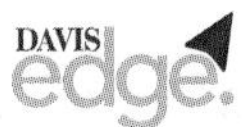

Use the scratch off code on the inside front cover of your book to access online quizzes that will help you to improve your scores on course exams and prepare for the NCLEX-PN®.

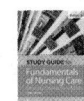

Study Guide

CHAPTER 11

Complementary and Alternative Medicine

KEY TERMS

Acupressure (AK-yoo-PRESH-uhr)
Acupuncture (AK-yoo-PUNGK-chur)
Allopathic medicine (AL-oh-PATH-ik MED-i-sin)
Alternative therapy (awl-TUR-nah-tiv THER-uh-pee)
Chiropractic (KYE-ruh-PRAK-tik)
Complementary therapy (KOM-ple-MEN-tair-ee THER-uh-pee)
Holism (HOH-lizm)
Integrative health care (IN-tuh-gray-tiv HELLTH KARE)
Massage therapy (muh-SAZH THER-uh-pee)
Meridians (me-RID-ee-uhnz)
Yoga (YOH-gah)

CHAPTER CONCEPTS

Health Promotion

LEARNING OUTCOMES

1. Define various terms associated with complementary and alternative medicine.
2. Differentiate between alternative therapy and complementary therapy.
3. Explain the concept of holism and integrative health care.
4. Contrast complementary and alternative medicine/Eastern medicine with Western medicine.
5. Describe the history, use, and effectiveness of chiropractic.
6. Discuss the types and benefits of massage therapy.
7. Explain the use of acupuncture and acupressure.
8. Enumerate six popular herbs and their uses.
9. Describe the purposes and benefits of yoga.
10. Explain how food and lifestyle changes can reverse some diseases.
11. Identify ways nurses can increase communication with patients regarding their use of complementary and alternative medicine.
12. Discuss information found in the Connection features in this chapter.
13. Identify specific safety information.

CRITICAL THINKING CONNECTION

Clinical Assignment

You are assigned to care for a patient hospitalized for a hysterectomy and removal of the ovaries and fallopian tubes. She complains of back pain because she has been lying in a hospital bed for 2 days and nights, but she refuses to take pain medication. She listens to self-hypnosis CDs to help manage her postoperative pain. She tells you that she wants her chiropractor to visit her in the hospital to work on her neck and upper back to relieve her musculoskeletal discomfort. She urges you "not to tell" because her doctor does not believe in chiropractic, herbs, hypnosis, or other alternative therapies.

CRITICAL THINKING CONNECTION—cont'd

Critical Thinking Questions:

1. Does this information need to be passed on to the health-care provider or charge nurse?
2. How will you communicate with this patient in a way that does not convey disapproval?
3. How will you encourage her to share information with you that she withholds from her health-care provider?
4. How will you find out more about the types of complementary and alternative medicines she uses so that you understand what helps her and why?

In a busy nursing unit, you may hear a coworker refer to a patient as "the gall bladder in room 209" or "the MI that went to CCU." This is not an acceptable way to refer to patients in any setting. Patients are people who have many aspects to their lives; being reduced to a medical diagnosis is neither an accurate nor an appropriate way to label them, yet the health-care system in the United States sometimes looks on patients as diseases to be treated or disorders to be repaired. This is partly because of the influence of 19th-century philosopher René Descartes, who championed the idea that the mind and the body are not connected. At that time, medicine was first being pioneered, and the philosophy of Descartes had a huge influence on the way separate treatments were developed for physical illnesses and mental illnesses. Later, other philosophers challenged his ideas and thinking began to change, but such change has been slow to be reflected in Western medicine.

Complementary and alternative medicines (CAMs), some of which originated in Eastern countries such as China and Japan, are at odds with this philosophy. A number of these therapies emphasize **holism**, or the relationships among all living things. Holistic health care, which includes the use of CAM, emphasizes the following:

- The uniqueness of each individual
- The interaction among the mind, body, and spirit
- Multiple factors as causes of illness and disease
- The patient's participation in treatment and healing

For many decades, the Western and Eastern approaches to health care have been in conflict. In the past, if a patient took anything more than a multiple vitamin, the patient might not tell his or her health-care provider for fear of being considered a "health nut." However, over the past 25 years, the use of CAM has become increasingly more mainstream. **Integrative health care** is a term that is used to describe the use of Western medicine and CAM in a coordinated way. Nurses and other health-care practitioners must learn about CAM and how its practices influence and assist traditional medicine. In addition, nurses must remain nonjudgmental about patients' choices to include CAM in their search for health and wellness. This integrative approach is true holistic health care. This chapter will help you understand different types of CAM and why they are helpful. It also will help you adopt a holistic approach to caring for your patients.

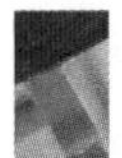

ALTERNATIVE THERAPY VERSUS COMPLEMENTARY THERAPY

Alternative therapy and complementary therapy are technically different. **Alternative therapy** is a therapy used *instead* of conventional treatment, while **complementary therapy** is used along *with* conventional treatment. However, for many people, these two terms have become interchangeable, with a singular definition: treatment or therapies that are *different than* conventional treatment or therapies endorsed and used by the standard medical community.

KNOWLEDGE CONNECTION

How is holistic health care different than your concept of health care? How can you as a nurse help contribute to integrative health care?

The Choice of Complementary and Alternative Therapies

Today's patients, many of whom access health-care information by logging onto the Internet, are more knowledgeable than ever before. The more these patients learn about CAM, the more they become convinced that traditional medicine does not have all the answers; these are the people who eagerly seek out alternative theories and treatments. Other individuals use mainstream medicine but turn to alternative methods for what they believe to be health-enhancing measures. Patients also choose CAM because of issues surrounding the following:

- **Cost:** As traditional medical costs spiral upwards, patients view CAM as a cost-effective option.
- **Access:** In some communities, it is easier to access CAM than traditional medical care.
- **Self-determination:** Patients sometimes feel that the CAM practitioner encourages them to participate more in their own health-care decisions. Some patients may feel that they are not really a participant in their care when consulting conventional medical practitioners.
- **Personal touch:** Some patients feel that CAM practitioners spend more time with them than conventional medical practitioners and are more apt to listen to their concerns. Also, CAM practitioners generally provide more of a hands-on approach. Many types of CAM provide more physical contact and actual touching of the patient, although some do not involve touch.

• WORD • BUILDING •

holism: hol – entire + ism – theory of

KNOWLEDGE CONNECTION
What is the difference between alternative therapy and complementary therapy? List some reasons why people might use CAM.

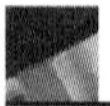

WESTERN MEDICINE

Allopathic medicine is a name used to describe traditional medicine, conventional medicine, or Western medicine. *Allopathic* refers to the treatment of disease by creating an environment that is antagonistic to the disease. The term *Western medicine* is used more commonly and will be used in this chapter to refer to allopathic medicine. One tenet of Western medicine is to prescribe drugs or treatments to kill foreign invaders, such as bacteria or viruses, which have made the body ill. These invaders must be eliminated for a return to health to take place.

Some practitioners of Western medicine tend to see health as the absence of disease, pain, or other symptoms of illness. Symptoms are disagreeable phenomena to be eliminated or suppressed. Prevention, until recently, was not a primary concern, and the mind and body were seen as separate, with no connection of the mind to the body and its function.

This is the type of health care with which most Americans are familiar. You do not seek health care when you feel well, and when you have symptoms of an illness, you go to the doctor, who almost always writes a prescription for you. You then take the medication and hope that soon you are symptom-free, until the cycle repeats itself. For many people, at some point in their lives, an organ or system becomes so diseased that continuous medication is needed to stay symptom-free. And for many, surgery is necessary to repair or remove diseased organs. The Western medicine approach is that the correct medications and surgery will make you well.

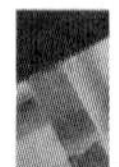

EASTERN AND ALTERNATIVE HEALTH CARE

Eastern medicine is often not what we think of as medicine at all. *Eastern* usually refers to ideas and practices from places such as Asia and India. The awareness and use of bioenergy, also called ch'i, prana, or life force, is extremely important. From this flows a difference in definitions of health, illness, symptoms, and the role of the health-care provider and of health care itself. These differences are often seen in CAM as well.

In Eastern medicine, illness and disease are viewed as a disharmony, imbalance, or defect of energy in the body. Illness is a deviation from normal, healthy function. Symptoms are warning signs that the body is trying to heal itself but needs help; the symptoms are messages or signals about underlying issues of imbalance. The cause of illness is anything that interferes with the balance and movement of bioenergy. Diet, genetic makeup, lifestyle, trauma, negative thoughts, stress, and environmental toxins all are considered possible influences on health.

In Eastern medicine and some CAM, illness progresses in the following manner: An energy imbalance causes functional changes that can initiate a progression of chronic illness preceding pathological changes in tissue.

Personal responsibility is seen as a key to health. According to this philosophy, a person's lifestyle and emotional outlook can help prevent illness; this prevents the viewpoint that people are victims of disease.

A major emphasis in Eastern medicine is the prevention of illness. Humankind is seen as an ecosystem that, when working correctly, functions in harmony. Health-care providers, in turn, are viewed as assistants to help cultivate life and vitality. Mind and body are one, inextricably connected, each affecting the other and overall health.

Mind–Body Connections

Most all CAM have as their basis the belief that the body has the inherent ability to heal itself unless an illness or disease has progressed too far for this self-healing to occur. Also, rather than focusing on symptom relief and removal, CAM practitioners emphasize the need to treat the cause of illness. They also encourage preventive rather than crisis care. A practitioner who follows these tenets and looks at the whole person rather than just the diseased part of the person would be closer to practicing holistic care than the practitioner who practices using a more medical model.

KNOWLEDGE CONNECTION
How does Western medicine view illness and disease? How does Eastern medicine view illness and disease?

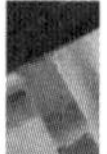

TYPES OF COMPLEMENTARY AND ALTERNATIVE MEDICINE

Many different types of complementary and alternative treatments and medicine exist, some of which are more well known in the United States than others. In this chapter, we will look in-depth at five of the more common practices:

1. Chiropractic
2. Massage therapy
3. Acupuncture and acupressure
4. Herbal supplements
5. Yoga

In addition, we will provide general information about other types of CAM.

• WORD • BUILDING •
allopathic: allo – other + pathic – method of treating disease
chiropractic: chiro – hand + practic – do
acupuncture: acu – needle + puncture
acupressure: acu – needle + pressure

Chiropractic

Writings from China and Greece as long as 4,700 years ago mention spinal manipulation and the maneuvering of the lower extremities to ease low back pain. Hippocrates, who lived from 460 to 357 BC, wrote, "Get knowledge of the spine, for this is the requisite for many diseases."

In the United States, chiropractic was started as an art and science by D. D. Palmer in 1895. Palmer devised the name **chiropractic,** which is a combination of two Greek words meaning "done by hand." It refers to manipulation of the spine to relieve pressure on the nerves. Palmer was well read in the medical journals of the time and had knowledge of the developments that were occurring throughout the world regarding anatomy and physiology. Palmer theorized that the brain and nervous system controlled not only function and movement of the body, but also health or the lack thereof. Statistics show chiropractic to be one of the fastest growing forms of health care in America today in terms of both patients and number of doctors.

The primary tenet of chiropractic is that natural and conservative methods of health care are preferable to invasive treatment and the use of drugs. Another important concept is that the nervous system plays a major role in health and disease. Doctors of chiropractic have a deep respect for the human body's ability to heal itself. They believe that, in many cases, surgery and drugs are not necessary and that once nutrition and other lifestyle factors are improved and the person's nervous system is working at its full potential, the body is designed to correct itself. These doctors devote careful attention to the biomechanics, or movement, of the spine, as well as the anatomy and physiology of the spine and related structures. Additionally, they study the effects of the impulses through the spinal nerves on the musculoskeletal and neurological systems and the role played by the proper function of these systems in the preservation and restoration of health.

Anatomy and Physiology Connection

The Spine, the Nerves, and Correcting Interference

The brain controls the functions of the body through a network of nerves that connect to the spinal cord. These spinal nerves connect with the cord inside the spinal column, where they are protected by the vertebrae, and each spinal nerve passes through openings between the vertebrae cushioned by the intervertebral disks. When pressure is applied to the spinal nerve as it exits the cord, the transmission of messages to and from the brain through that nerve are affected. The organs and muscles that the nerve *innervates* (connects with and passes messages to and from) are at risk for dysfunction due to nerve disturbance. In chiropractic, this is referred to as the *vertebral subluxation complex* (VSC). If the nerve interference is corrected through manipulation of the spine or relaxation of muscle spasm, the messages to and from the brain are restored, and correct function can be reestablished.

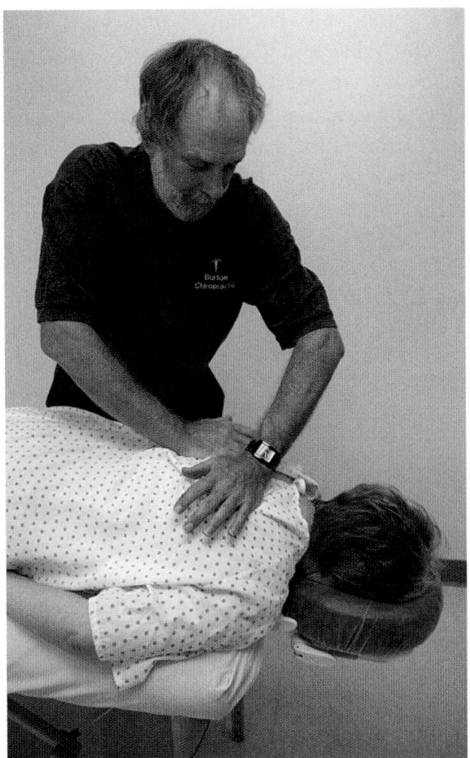

FIGURE 11.1 A chiropractor treating a patient for upper back pain.

Chiropractors regularly treat people with neuromuscular complaints such as headaches, joint pain, and neck and back pain. They also treat people with arthritis, tendonitis, and sprains and strains. Some chiropractors use only hands-on techniques when "adjusting" patients (Fig. 11.1). Others use equipment not unlike that found in physical therapy offices, such as ultrasound equipment, exercise areas, and traction tables.

Chiropractic may not be appropriate for all patients. ***Safety: Patients with certain health conditions such as osteoporosis and cancer and those who have undergone back surgery should share this information with the chiropractic practitioner so that he or she can administer appropriate treatment and avoid causing harm.***

KNOWLEDGE CONNECTION

What is a major tenet of chiropractic philosophy? How do doctors of chiropractic help the body heal itself?

Massage Therapy

Massage has been in use for thousands of years, as confirmed by writings from ancient Rome, Greece, Japan, China, Egypt, and India. **Massage therapy** is the application of stroking,

• WORD • BUILDING •

biomechanics: bio – life + mechanics – science of force and matter

subluxation: sub – less than normal + luxation – dislocation

pressure, friction, and kneading to muscles and other soft tissues to relax muscles and decrease stress (Fig. 11.2).

Massage first became popular in the United States in the mid-1900s, but in recent years it has gained even more in popularity. People seek massage therapy to relieve musculoskeletal pain, decreases stress, relieve depression and anxiety, increase relaxation, and promote an overall sense of well-being. People also seek massage therapy because it feels good. Because of the stress-filled lives of many people, massage therapy has become extremely popular over the past decade.

Many varieties of massage are available. Some of the best known and most popular ones are the following:

- **Swedish:** This type of massage features long, flowing strokes; kneading; vibration; and compression. This is a calming massage shown to help relieve pain and joint stiffness. A variation of this is hot stone massage in which heated stones are placed on different areas of the body to increase circulation to the area with heat. ***Safety: The stones should not be placed directly on the skin; there should be a towel or sheet between the patient's skin and the stones to prevent burns.***
- **Shiatsu:** This is a Japanese-style massage that uses thumb pressure to work along energy meridians, similar to acupressure.
- **Reflexology:** This type of massage uses thumb and fingers to stimulate pressure points on the feet. Practitioners believe that the various internal organs are associated with the different nerve endings on the sole of the foot; it is based on the idea of energy pathways being present in the body.
- **Deep Tissue:** This is a more vigorous, strenuous massage with focused pressure applied to tightened muscle areas and trigger points.
- **Sports:** This type of massage targets muscles and muscle groups that may be strained or injured during sports and vigorous exercise, with a special emphasis on targeting muscle-tendon junctions.

One of the advantages of massage therapy is its ability to relieve muscle tension and stress without using medications that may produce side effects. Another advantage of massage therapy is that it stimulates the circulatory system, which is advantageous to all the body systems. Massage therapy is also known for stimulating the body to produce endorphins. These chemicals, which are developed by the body, are useful in pain relief; they also help to provide a sense of well-being.

Safety: Individuals considering massage who have serious health issues should ask questions of their doctor and massage therapist before proceeding. Some conditions that could contraindicate massage include a history of blood clots in the legs or the lungs, a cancerous tumor that has not been removed, certain heart conditions or irregular heartbeat, certain neck and back surgeries, and severe osteoporosis (with vigorous massage).

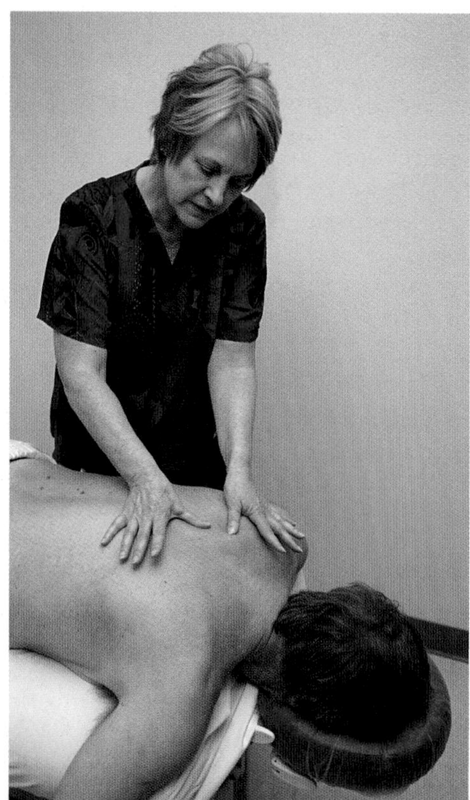

FIGURE 11.2 A massage therapist performing massage.

KNOWLEDGE CONNECTION

What are the benefits of massage therapy? What conditions could contraindicate massage? Describe five common types of massage.

Real-World Connection

Being a Medical and CAM Practitioner

A nurse who is a massage therapist feels that she has the best of both worlds when caring for her clients. As a nurse, she has an hour of uninterrupted time with the client. She can teach about issues that affect the client immediately. For example, she is able to look closely at moles and skin lesions on the client's back and refer him or her to a medical health-care provider if a problem is found. She can teach about the importance of a diet rich in potassium, calcium, and magnesium if the client suffers from muscle cramping. She can explain how the body works and what the client can do to help the body work correctly. As a massage therapist, she can help relax muscle knots, soothe tense muscles, and stretch tight muscles. In addition, she helps the patient relax, rest, and cope with stress. She feels that this is truly integrative health care.

Acupuncture and Acupressure

Acupuncture is the ancient practice of inserting fine needles into carefully selected points located along **meridians,** or energy pathways, in the body. Classic Chinese medicine explains that channels of energy run in regular patterns through the body and over its surface. An obstruction in the movement of energy through these channels backs up energy like a dam backs up water in a river. It is thought that acupuncture stimulates the body's healing ability and corrects dysfunction. The practitioner places needles just below the skin's surface at various points along the meridians and twirls them to help remove the blockage. The existence of these meridians, the cause of disruption of energy through these pathways, and how restoration of energy flow occurs have not been clearly identified.

The National Center for Complementary and Integrative Health, part of the National Institutes of Health (NIH), provides summaries of research of CAM. Their study results have shown that acupuncture is helpful for low back pain, neck pain, migraine and tension headaches, and carpal tunnel syndrome. Studies also show that it reduces chemotherapy-induced nausea and vomiting in cancer patients.

Acupressure is a blend of acupuncture and pressure and is a part of traditional Chinese medicine. All that is said and written about acupuncture is the same for acupressure, except that, rather than applying needles to parts of the body to affect the meridians' flow of energy, pressure is used.

In most states, medical doctors and chiropractors can receive extra training in acupuncture and practice it along with medicine or chiropractic. In addition, in many states an individual can obtain a license to just practice acupuncture without also being a doctor. ***Safety: Patients taking anticoagulant medications (for example, a blood thinner or antiplatelet drugs) should inform the acupuncturist before beginning treatment because bleeding can occur.***

Studies and stories abound in Asian countries about the use of and reliance on acupuncture, although it has not become as popular in the United States. Many hospitals in Asia use acupuncture for most patients before and after surgery. These patients need very little, if any, pain medication. Interest in acupuncture soared in the United States after American visitors to China brought back firsthand reports of patients undergoing major surgery using acupuncture as the sole form of anesthesia.

> **KNOWLEDGE CONNECTION**
>
> What is the explanation for the use of acupuncture to relieve pain or promote anesthesia? For which conditions does the NIH approve the use of acupuncture?

Herbal Supplements

Herbs have been used for at least 5,000 years by the Egyptians, Greeks, and Romans to promote healing and prevent illness. Today, herbs are widely used in Europe and are gaining popularity in the United States. The popularity of herbs in the United States may be due to several factors. One factor is that herbs often have fewer and less severe side effects than prescription medications. Another factor is that people can take a certain amount of control over their own health and try using herbs for conditions that health-care professionals have not been able to successfully treat or for which their prescribed medication has been objectionable in some way. Often people choose to use herbs as a preventative for potential health problems. Some of the more popular herbs, their uses, and cautions are listed in Table 11.1.

Because some herbs can interact with medications and interfere with surgery and its outcomes, it is important that patients tell their health-care providers about their use of herbs. Some people can become very confused about the effective use of herbal supplements; as a result, they take herbs that can interact with one another or cause undesirable outcomes. It is advisable to research herbs thoroughly or depend on the advice of a knowledgeable person such as a nutritionist or an herbalist. ***Safety: Pregnant women should check with their health-care provider before using herbs.***

Yoga

Yoga is considered a mind–body intervention used to decrease the negative effects of stress through the use of breathing exercises, physical postures, and meditation. It originally evolved as a spiritual practice, but in the West it is viewed more narrowly as a form of exercise.

Yoga was first introduced to the United States in the late 1800s, but it has been practiced for more than 5,000 years in the East. Yoga invokes ideas of harmony, health, and balance. It is believed to calm the nervous system and balance the mind, body, and spirit. Practitioners believe yoga prevents diseases and illnesses by keeping the energy meridians open and flowing. Yoga has been used to lower blood pressure; lessen stress; and improve coordination, flexibility, concentration, sleep, and digestion. It also has been recommended by its proponents as supplementary therapy for conditions such as cancer, asthma, diabetes, and irritable bowel syndrome.

As an exercise, yoga has evolved into several subdivisions and variations.

- Hatha yoga is a common and popular form of yoga practiced in the United States. It prepares and conditions the body so that the mind can practice meditation without obstacles. It is slow-paced and gentle, taking the practitioner through basic yoga poses.
- Ashtanga yoga is more fast-paced and intense. It requires the practitioner to change quickly from one pose to another, always following the same order.
- Power yoga follows similar principles to Ashtanga yoga but does not necessarily follow the same set of Ashtanga poses.
- Iyengar yoga emphasizes the use of props such as blocks, straps, and blankets and is concerned with proper body alignment in each pose, as well as holding the poses for long periods of time. This emphasis helps prevent injuries

Table 11.1
Popular Herbs, Their Uses, and Cautions

Herb	*Uses*	*Cautions*
Aloe vera	Used alone and in many products for skin problems; some people drink it for overall health	Using this herb orally has a laxative effect that may cause cramping and diarrhea
Capsaicin	Used in medicated creams and lotions for tenderness and pain of osteoarthritis; some use it for fibromyalgia, diabetic neuropathy, and shingles	Can cause a burning sensation when applied; if severe burning, pain, or blistering occur, seek medical help
Coenzyme Q10	Used to replace naturally occurring coenzyme in the heart, liver, kidney, and pancreas that decreases with aging; may help heart damage due to cancer treatment	Interacts with anticoagulant drugs such as warfarin
Chamomile	May be helpful to treat anxiety, induce sleep, and relieve upset stomach	Belongs to the ragweed family and can cause allergic reaction in those sensitive to ragweed
Cranberry	Some studies show that it reduces recurrent urinary tract infections in pregnant women and in elderly and hospitalized patients	May interact with anticoagulant medications, causing increased bruising and bleeding
Echinacea	Used as an antiviral agent to prevent or eliminate colds, flu, and other infections	Slows metabolism of caffeine, leading to nervousness or jittery feelings
Feverfew	Used as an anti-inflammatory; also used for migraine headaches, fever suppression, and menstrual cramps	Interacts with anticoagulants and antiplatelet medicines, leading to bleeding and bruising
Garlic	Helps reduce total blood cholesterol and low-density lipoproteins (bad cholesterol) over short periods of time (for example, 4-12 weeks)	Interacts with blood thinners, antiplatelet drugs, and HIV antiviral medications
Ginger	Used to help relieve nausea and vomiting of pregnancy in recommended doses for short periods of time (large doses of ginger may be unsafe for a developing baby); may also be used for motion sickness	Interacts with blood thinners
Gingko	Used for memory enhancement and dementia and to help increase blood flow to the brain	Interacts with medicines metabolized by the liver such as omeprazole, donepezil, and fluvastatin; also should not be used with seizure medicines, blood thinners, and diabetic drugs
Ginseng	Used to help lower bad cholesterol and protect the heart; also helps lower blood sugar in type 2 diabetes but not to dangerous levels; may help boost the immune system	May interact with blood thinners, blood pressure medicines, and diabetic medications
Melatonin	Helpful for insomnia, jet lag, and shift-work sleep disorders	May interact with sleeping pills, antihistamines, and opioids; may cause blood sugar to increase and interfere with diabetes medications
Peppermint	Use of peppermint oil combined with caraway oil is helpful in treating heartburn; peppermint oil may improve irritable bowel syndrome and decrease spasms of the gastrointestinal tract before and after endoscopic procedures	Avoid taking with antibiotics or antifungals, iron supplements, and medicines to reduce stomach acid

Table 11.1
Popular Herbs, Their Uses, and Cautions—cont'd

Herb	*Uses*	*Cautions*
Saw palmetto	Used to treat enlarged prostate in men; helps improve the symptom of difficult urination but does not actually shrink the prostate	Do not take with the medication Proscar; can interact with warfarin, estrogens, and birth control pills
Soy	Helps decrease cholesterol and low-density lipoproteins; helps improve acute diarrhea in infants, as in soy formulas; helps decrease menopausal symptoms, such as hot flashes, in some women	Interacts with anticoagulants, antiplatelet medicines, and anti-inflammatory medicines (nonsteroidal); may interact with blood pressure and diabetes medicines
St. John's wort	Used for mild to moderate depression; when used for this purpose, studies have shown it to be at least as effective as some prescription drugs	Interacts with some certain anti-anxiety medications, including diphenhydramine, duloxetine (Cymbalta), and alprozalam (Xanax); should not be taken with valerian or muscle relaxers
Valerian	Used to treat insomnia; helps improve the quality of sleep and helps decrease the amount of time it takes to fall asleep	Interacts with many prescription medications such as muscle relaxers, sleeping medicines, pain medicines, and antidepressants

and assists the body to obtain the maximum benefit from the exercise.

- Bikram yoga, also called "hot yoga," is performed in a studio heated to 105°F with 40% humidity. This is a vigorous yoga done in 90-minute sessions and involves 26 postures. It increases the heart rate and involves vigorous muscle use. This type of yoga can cause heat-related illness.

Yoga usually is performed in classes with sessions conducted several times a week, but it may also be done individually in a studio or at home using a DVD or online instructions.

Additional Forms of Complementary and Alternative Medicine

A large variety of less common types of CAM are available, but these are used by a smaller portion of the general population. Although you may well encounter patients who use one or more of these therapies, you probably will hear more frequently about the types discussed earlier in the chapter. Box 11.1 provides explanations of additional types of CAM.

Lifestyle Changes That Reverse Disease

Another aspect of CAM is the belief that disease can be prevented or even eliminated by adopting a healthy lifestyle and eating whole foods that have not been processed or adulterated. Some studies have been done to validate these ideas.

Terry Shintani, a physician in Hawaii, found that obese patients who also had joint pain issues related to weight as well as diabetes, lost weight and eliminated their diabetes and joint pain by following a diet of nearly unlimited vegetables, certain fruits, and a small amount of fish. Another physician, Dean Ornish, performed research on a way to reverse heart disease without drugs or surgery. This was accomplished by drastically changing the food intake and lifestyle of people with severe coronary artery disease. The subjects in the study actually reversed blockages in their coronary arteries by increasing their activity level and eating a controlled diet rich in vegetables, fruits, and whole grains, with very little meat.

Although both of these physicians have shown how much food and lifestyle changes can truly reverse illness, many others feel that these changes are neither realistic nor attainable for the average American. Some patients would prefer to "take some pills" rather than have to drastically change their lifestyles. This is where Western medicine and CAM differ. While CAM seeks to find ways to avoid drugs and surgery, Western medicine sees no other viable choices.

> **KNOWLEDGE CONNECTION**
> List three herbs and their uses. How can practicing yoga improve health? List four additional types of CAM and their uses. What is your response to the studies showing that food and lifestyle changes can actually reverse diabetes and coronary artery disease?

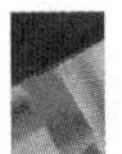

NURSING CARE AND COMPLEMENTARY AND ALTERNATIVE MEDICINE

When you care for patients who use CAM, it is important to respect their preferences and wishes. However, if the CAM modalities can interact negatively with medications or treatments prescribed for them, it is important to be sure your

Box 11.1 Additional Forms of Complementary and Alternative Medicine

There are numerous forms of CAM. Some of the more frequently used forms with their descriptions are listed here:

- **Aromatherapy:** Essential oils with strong fragrances are used to affect a person's mood or health. It has been used for 6,000 years. Some oils may cause irritation if applied directly to the skin. May be added to carrier oil for massage therapy.
- **Meditation:** A discipline in which the mind is focused on an object of thought or awareness. It usually involves turning attention to a single point of reference. Many religions incorporate meditation. Has been practiced for more than 5,000 years. Forms of meditation devoid of religious or mystic content have been developed in the West as a way of promoting physical and mental well-being.
- **Biofeedback:** Use of monitoring devices to help a person become aware of changes in heart rate, blood pressure, and muscle contractions so that they can be controlled using deep breathing and intentional relaxation.
- **Relaxation therapy and imagery:** Uses conscious awareness and visual images to relax muscles, lower respiration, and promote calm. Can ease stress and lower blood pressure.
- **Therapeutic touch or healing touch:** An energy modality that encourages healing. Practitioners place their hands near a patient to detect and manipulate the patient's energy fields, assisting in the natural healing process. Developed in the United States and endorsed by the American Holistic Nurses Association.
- **Homeopathy:** A healing philosophy based on the principle that "like treats like." This is similar to the principles of giving vaccines to stimulate production of antibodies to the disease-causing organism. In this type of approach, the patient is given substances in small amounts that would cause an illness if given in large amounts. They are usually administered in liquid or tablet form to help the body naturally heal.
- **Phytonutrients:** Certain components of plants that are used to promote human health. Fruits, vegetables, grains, legumes, nuts, and teas are rich in phytonutrients, which are thought to protect against many diseases, including cancer.
- **Free radicals and antioxidants:** Oxidation produces free radicals, which begins a process that damages cells and causes aging. Antioxidants are molecules capable of slowing the oxidation of other molecules.
- **Pet therapy or animal-assisted therapy:** Use of animals to help people who are ill. Visits from animals can provide a welcome change from the routine and can help lift depression and loneliness. Research shows that people who have experienced heart attacks and who have pets live longer and that petting a dog lowers blood pressure.
- **Music therapy:** Use of music to promote wellness, manage stress, express feelings, enhance memory, improve communication, and promote physical rehabilitation. Used in many different settings with patients of all ages. Incorporated in therapeutic care of patients with psychiatric disorders, developmental disabilities, speech and hearing impairments, physical disabilities, and neurological impairments.
- **Play therapy:** Used by licensed mental health professionals to communicate with children. The Association for Play Therapy defines this therapy as "the systematic use of a theoretical model to establish an interpersonal process wherein trained play therapists use the therapeutic powers of play to help clients prevent or resolve psychosocial difficulties and achieve optimal growth and development." Usually used with children ages 3 to 11 years to help them express thoughts and feelings.

patients understand this. In most nursing drug handbooks, you will find information about herbs that interact with the medication you are researching. Be sure to ask patients if they are taking any of the herbal supplements listed to prevent potential negative interactions. For example, St. John's wort and ginseng can decrease the effectiveness of warfarin, a blood thinner. Feverfew and Echinacea, among others, can increase bleeding in patients taking warfarin.

When obtaining information for a patient's history, be sure to ask about alternative and complementary therapies. Do so in a nonjudgmental way so that the patient will be comfortable divulging the information to you. Record the information in the patient's nursing history without drawing conclusions. Remember, people use what they can find to help relieve their symptoms.

Patient Teaching Connection

Teaching About CAM and Medical Conditions

Use patient teaching to carefully caution patients about the use of CAM and interactions with their current medications or treatment. For example, a patient recently diagnosed with a compression fracture of the spine states that he goes to a chiropractor once a month. It is important for his chiropractor to know about this diagnosis and the exact location of the compression fracture before the patient is treated again. Instruct the patient to inform his chiropractor that he has a compression fracture of L3.

POST CONFERENCE

After caring for your patient for 2 days, you helped discharge her. It was amazing to see how well she did without traditional pain medication. When one of the nurses said to you, "She's kind of a nut, isn't she?" you found yourself defending your patient and her choices. This experience really opened your eyes to some aspects of CAM that you had never thought about before. While caring for your patient, you encouraged her to tell her doctor about all of her CAM use. He listened thoughtfully and did not judge her negatively for her choices. You also had the opportunity to teach her about some interactions between her natural supplements and her prescription medications that she did not know previously. So, you and your patient both learned from one another.

Key Points

- Holistic health care involves treating patients as people who have many aspects to their lives, not just labeling them regarding their reason for hospitalization.
- CAM is being used increasingly more by our society, so nurses need to be aware and knowledgeable of it.
- Western, or allopathic, medicine bases its approach to disease and illness on the idea that foreign invaders, such as antigens, viruses, and bacteria, cause illness and must be treated with medications or surgery.
- Eastern medicine, and many types of CAM, see disease or illness as a deviation from normal, healthy function and symptoms as warning signs of underlying imbalance. Illness is caused by anything that interferes with the balance and movement of bioenergy, including diet, lifestyle, trauma, environmental toxins, and stress.
- The mind, body, and spirit all are connected and all must be treated. Practitioners of CAM emphasize these connections and believe that the body has the inherent nature to heal itself if given the correct support.
- Chiropractic's primary tenet is that natural and conservative methods of health care are preferable and that the nervous system plays a major role in health and disease. Chiropractors use manual adjustments and other equipment to correct nerve interference.
- Massage therapy involves the use of stroking, pressure, friction, and kneading of muscles and other soft tissues to decrease stress, relieve anxiety and depression, increase relaxation, and promote an overall sense of well-being.
- Acupuncture and acupressure have their roots in Chinese medicine. They involve the use of long, thin, hollow needles inserted beneath the skin (acupuncture) or pressure on acupuncture sites (acupressure) to relieve blockages in the movement of energy through meridians throughout the body.
- Many different herbal supplements are used for a variety of reasons. They can interfere with medications, so question patients about their use of herbal supplements to determine potential interactions.
- Yoga is more than an exercise in Eastern medicine. It invokes harmony, health, and balance; helps calm the nervous system; and balances the mind, body, and spirit.

Review Questions

Select the answer that is most appropriate for each of the following questions. Some questions may have more than one correct answer. Select all that apply.

1. In holistic health care, the emphasis is on the uniqueness of each individual and the interaction among:
   1. health, environment, and disease.
   2. mind, body, and spirit.
   3. herbs, chiropractic, and massage.
   4. Western medicine, allopathic medicine, and CAM.
2. Which is true of alternative medicine and complementary medicine?
   1. They mean the same thing and are simply different than conventional treatment.
   2. They cost more than traditional medicine but may be more effective.
   3. Access to these medicines is limited, so few people can use them.
   4. Alternative medicine is used instead of complementary medicine.
   5. Complementary medicine is used with traditional medicine.
   6. Both 4 and 5.

3. You see a patient while in clinical at a walk-in clinic. This patient has occasional abdominal pain of unknown cause but otherwise is in good health. The doctor suggests blood work and a computed tomography scan of the abdomen to diagnose the cause. The patient says he wants to wait, see his acupuncturist, and give his body the opportunity to heal itself. What is your response?
   1. Tell the patient that he MUST follow through with the doctor's orders.
   2. Express strong disapproval of this plan, both verbally and nonverbally.
   3. Encourage the patient to act quickly and return if the pain persists.
   4. Explain that the body cannot heal itself and requires a doctor's intervention to heal.

4. A patient says he wants to go to a chiropractor to see if it will help his low back pain because medical treatment has been ineffective. How might you respond?
   1. "Some studies have shown chiropractic to be an effective treatment for low back pain."
   2. "You would do better to stick with a real doctor."
   3. "I am not allowed to discuss alternative or complementary medicine with you."
   4. "You need to ask your medical doctor for permission to do that."

5. A person with a tight, sore neck and headaches might use which of these CAM choices for relief?
   1. Echinacea
   2. Chiropractic
   3. Biofeedback
   4. Phytonutrients
   5. Massage therapy
   6. Acupuncture/acupressure
   7. Play therapy
   8. Gingko
   9. Relaxation therapy and imagery

6. Which is accurate regarding the cause and effect of illness according to Eastern medicine and most types of CAM?
   1. Energy imbalance causes chronic illness that leads to functional changes.
   2. Energy imbalance causes changes that can initiate chronic illness preceding pathological changes.
   3. Pathological changes in tissue leads to energy imbalances that precede chronic illnesses.
   4. The mind and body must be in balance or pathological changes will occur.

7. A patient with nausea and vomiting due to chemotherapy for cancer might find relief from which type of CAM?
   1. Yoga
   2. Taking garlic
   3. Massage therapy
   4. Acupuncture

8. Which conditions could cause massage to be contraindicated for a patient?
   1. A history of blood clots
   2. Older than 80 years
   3. Certain heart conditions
   4. Taking medications to lower cholesterol
   5. Osteoporosis

ANSWERS 1. 2, 2. 6, 3. 3, 4. 1, 5. 2, 3, 5, 6, 9, 6. 2, 7. 4, 8. 1, 3, 5

Critical Thinking Exercise

Answers available online.

1. A patient is hospitalized with excessive bleeding after taking the blood thinner warfarin for 2 months. When you ask the patient about the medications she takes, she tells you that she started taking an herbal blend to prevent colds and flu about 6 weeks ago, and she thinks it is helping her. What action will you take and why?

Additional Resources

Use the scratch off code on the inside front cover of your book to access online quizzes that will help you to improve your scores on course exams and prepare for the NCLEX-PN®.

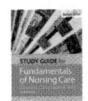

Study Guide

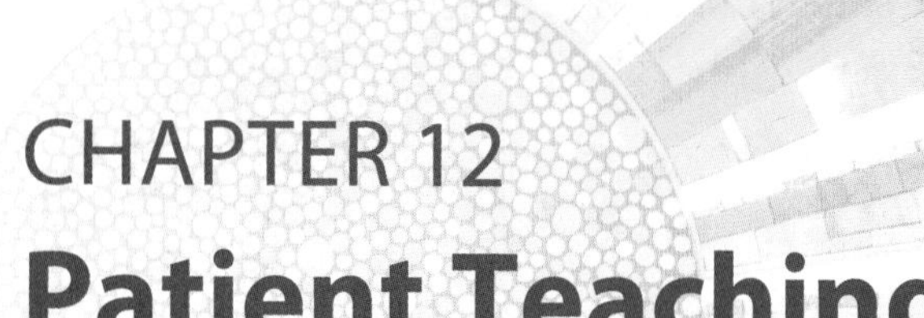

CHAPTER 12

Patient Teaching

Shirley MacNeill

KEY TERMS

Auditory learning (AW-di-tor-ee LER-ning)
Health promotion (HELLTH proh-MOH-shun)
Interpreter (in-TER-pruh-ter)
Kinesthetic learning (KIN-ess-THET-ik LER-ning)
Learning (LER-ning)
Reinforce (REE-in-FORSS)
Teachable moments (TEECH-uh-buhl MOH-ments)
Visual learning (VIZH-yoo-ahl LER-ning)
Wellness strategies (WEL-ness STRA-tuh-jeez)

CHAPTER CONCEPTS

Patient-Centered Care

LEARNING OUTCOMES

1. Define various terms associated with patient teaching.
2. Identify three primary learning styles.
3. Explain ways to address learning styles during patient teaching.
4. Describe factors that affect learning.
5. Discuss information to consider when arranging for an interpreter.
6. Discuss the importance of reinforcement of patient teaching.
7. Identify two primary purposes of patient teaching.
8. Define the concept of teachable moments.
9. Describe how to develop a teaching plan using the nursing process.
10. Discuss ways to implement a teaching plan.
11. Describe three ways to evaluate patient teaching.
12. Explain how to teach patients about Internet resources.
13. Discuss information found in the Connection features in this chapter.

CRITICAL THINKING CONNECTION

Clinical Assignment

You are assigned to care for a 42-year-old female with a new diagnosis of diabetes mellitus. She is overweight and sedentary, eats at restaurants most of the time, and knows very little about diabetes. She is very confused about the lifestyle changes she needs to make. She is scheduled to be discharged today on oral diabetes medication and with a glucometer.

Critical Thinking Questions:

1. How will you find out what she knows about her disease?
2. How does she learn best?
3. When and where will you provide reinforcement for the learning that has already taken place?
4. How will she get additional information and have her questions answered after she goes home?
5. How will you ensure that she knows what medication she is to take, how to take it, and to be alert to side effects?
6. Will she be able to do her own finger stick blood sugar tests twice a day once she is at home or will she need home health care for a short time?

You may think of yourself as a student, not a teacher. Yet you will be a teacher to your patients. Chances are good that you will not stand up in front of a class using a SMART Board, but you will teach all the same. Every time you explain the purpose of a treatment or medication; show a patient how to care for a wound, drain, or tube; or answer a patient's or family member's questions, you will be teaching.

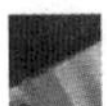

LEARNING

One explanation of **learning** is that when it occurs, behavior changes. True learning is not merely memorizing isolated facts or being able to recite a list of data. True learning is evidenced by applying new information. However, all people do not learn the same way.

Learning Styles

Although many different ideas exist about the ways in which people learn, the most familiar explanation of learning styles is also the first, developed in the 1970s. Known by some as VAK, the identified styles for learning are the following:

- **Visual learning:** learning by seeing, reading, and watching
- **Auditory learning:** learning by hearing and listening
- **Kinesthetic learning:** learning by touching and doing

People can learn in every style, but most people prefer one style when exposed to new information and ideas.

When you teach patients about their care, it is important that you address each style of learning. You may verbally explain information, but you need to provide written information that is appropriate for the patient's reading level as well as providing videos. If you are teaching a task, such as a dressing change, you will need to demonstrate what the patient is to do and then provide an opportunity for the patient to perform the task while you watch. This is referred to as a *return demonstration.*

Factors That Affect Learning

Not only do you need to address all three learning styles when teaching patients, but you also need to consider the following factors that affect learning, including barriers that could delay or impede learning:

- **Environment:** Find a place that is quiet, free of distractions, and offers privacy when you want your patient to learn new information.
- **Comfort:** Your patient will be unable to accomplish learning goals if he or she is in pain, drowsy from medications, too hot or too cold, hungry, or uncomfortable in other ways. Ensure the patient's comfort before you try to begin a teaching session.
- **Readiness:** It is difficult to learn anything if you are not ready to hear the information. Patients may be in the denial phase regarding their diagnosis, or they may feel that they do not need the treatment or medication you are explaining. Patients may believe they already have all of the information needed; establishing what they already know is important. Patients also may simply be too ill to hear and understand your teaching.
- **Language:** Patients cannot learn if the teaching is not provided in a language that they understand. If you do not speak the same language as the patient, arrange for an **interpreter**, or translator, to be present for patient teaching. (Box 12.1 provides information to consider when arranging for an interpreter.) Be sure to look at the patient when you are speaking and not at the interpreter. Another language issue is that of using medical terminology and other terms that the patient may not understand. Be sure you are using general terms and not medical terms when you teach. If medical terms are necessary, be sure to explain the meanings of those terms.
- **Senses:** Patients cannot learn if they have visual or hearing impairments that interfere with their ability to see and hear the information being presented. Position yourself so that the patient can see your lips. Do not sit or stand in front of a window or light that causes a glare. Be sure the patients are wearing glasses or have in hearing aids if they wear them. Use large-print handouts for patients with visual impairments.
- **Cultural or religious beliefs or practices:** It is important to incorporate the patient's specific cultural background and religious beliefs into your teaching for the patient. It is also helpful to ask your patient if there are any family members or other caregivers who may need to be part of the patient's learning.

Box 12.1

Arranging for an Interpreter

When a patient does not speak English, it is necessary to have an interpreter present for patient teaching. Here are some ways to help you choose the best interpreter for the situation:

- Even if the patient can speak and understand some English, arrange for an interpreter who speaks the patient's primary language. During times of illness or crisis, the patient may be less able to speak and understand English.
- Whenever possible, use a professional or certified interpreter rather than a family member. The hospital or other facility will have a list of interpreters available to translate for you. You will need to plan ahead so that you can arrange for an interpreter to be present during patient teaching.
- Arrange for an interpreter who has some understanding of medical terminology so that questions and answers can be translated correctly.
- Try to avoid using young children as interpreters for their parents. This may put the children in a culturally inappropriate situation if taboo areas of the body need to be discussed.
- Some facilities may use a computer and software to provide interpretation from one language to another.

• WORD • BUILDING •

auditory: audit – hearing + ory – relating to

kinesthetic: kin – movement + esthetic – sensation

Repetition

It is not uncommon for patient teaching to be rushed—a last-minute task performed at discharge when the patient is anxious to leave the facility. This is not the ideal time to attempt teaching. For learning to truly take place, information must be introduced, explained, and **reinforced,** or repeated several times. Ideally, you should begin teaching about the disease process, medications, and nursing care as they are introduced in the patient's care, preferably on the day of admission. You may feel that you are boring the patient when you repeat instructions or information, but you probably are not. Although you are familiar with what you are teaching, the information often is completely new to patients. Hearing it repeatedly will help reinforce their learning.

One method of using reinforcement is to introduce the most important concept you want to teach first. Then return to that topic and teach it again last so that the patient will remember it.

> **KNOWLEDGE CONNECTION**
> Name the three learning styles. What should you keep in mind when arranging for an interpreter during patient teaching? What are five factors that affect learning?

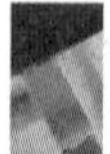

TEACHING ABOUT HEALTH AND ILLNESS

Most information that you teach will focus on the patient's need to know about his or her own health and treatment of illness. Adult learners are motivated to learn in order to solve a problem or meet a need, so you will need to identify issues of care that the patient views as fitting this category. In addition, you will need to establish a realistic expectation of what patients are able to learn in the amount of time available for patient teaching.

Purposes of Patient Teaching

When you provide patient teaching, it will be primarily for two purposes:

1. To instruct patients on health promotion and wellness strategies
2. To explain disease processes, treatments, and care

Instruction regarding **health promotion** includes information about ways to stay healthy. Examples of this teaching include getting regular exercise, making healthy food choices, drinking enough water, and including adequate amounts of fiber, vitamins, and minerals in the diet. When you teach about **wellness strategies**, you will emphasize changing unhealthy practices. Examples of this include stopping smoking, losing weight if appropriate, consuming alcohol and sweets only in moderation, reducing stress, and lowering cholesterol levels.

Before you teach patients about disease processes, you may need to do some research because you want to be sure you are giving correct information to your patients. In the case of our Critical Thinking Connection at the beginning of the chapter, you were assigned to care for a patient with newly diagnosed diabetes. You need to include teaching about insulin and how it works in the body, as well as what happens when the body does not produce enough insulin or cannot use the insulin it does produce. Your teaching should include informing the patient about the signs and symptoms of worsening diabetes, such as unstable blood sugar levels, as well as what to report to the health care provider and when to report it. It is important to explain the potential complications of the disease, including poor circulation, delayed healing, heart disease, kidney disease, *neuropathy* (nerve damage), and *retinopathy* (retinal damage leading to possible blindness).

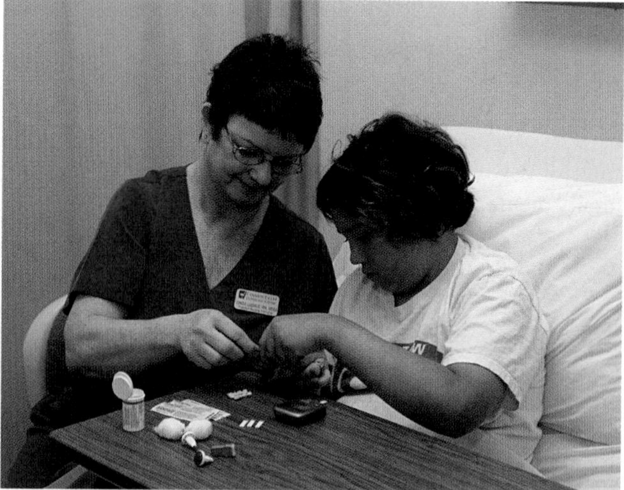

FIGURE 12.1 A nurse is teaching a child about finger stick blood sugar testing.

When you teach patients about treatments, medications, and self-care, you will help them understand how to care for themselves. Patients are more likely to comply with medication orders if they understand the purposes and effects of the medications they have been prescribed. Patients also follow ordered treatments better if they understand the purpose of the treatment and feel comfortable performing it. For example, in the situation of a diabetic patient, you might teach about the effects and side effects of oral medications to treat elevated blood sugar, how to perform a finger stick blood sugar measurement using a glucometer (Fig. 12.1), the signs and symptoms of high and low blood sugar levels, when to report finger stick blood sugar readings to the health-care provider, and how to treat low blood sugar.

As you can see, nurses teach patients repeatedly as teachable moments present themselves throughout care. These **teachable moments** occur when:

- Patients ask you questions about their illness or treatment

• WORD • BUILDING •

neuropathy: neuro – nerve + pathy – disease
retinopathy: retino – retina + pathy – disease

- You hear or observe misinformation or an incorrect procedure and you give correct information
- You point out a cause-and-effect connection to the patient

For example, you might explain to the patient that when he or she bends their wrist, the IV pump starts to beep because the fluid cannot flow freely into the vein. Another teachable moment occurs as you administer medication with a glass of water, when you can stress the importance of drinking a full glass of water with the medication so that it will work better.

As you learn more about providing patient care, you will learn to identify many opportunities for patient teaching. Table 12.1 lists teachable moments in routine care.

KNOWLEDGE CONNECTION

List four topics for patient teaching. What might you teach a patient when serving a meal?

Real-World Connection

The Focus of Patient Teaching

A patient with mild diabetes was brought to the hospital with chest pain. While she was in the emergency room, she had a heart attack. After a stent was placed, she recovered without complications and was sent home. The home health nurse visited the patient at home for follow-up assessment and teaching. She began to discuss diabetes and the patient's diet. The patient told the nurse, "I don't have to be on a diabetic diet. I had a heart attack, so I am on a heart healthy diet now." The patient teaching she received in the hospital focused completely on her cardiac problems, so the patient did not understand that she needed to follow a diabetic diet as well. Remember that patient teaching needs to be focused on all the patient's health issues, not just the primary reason for hospitalization.

Table 12.1
Teachable Moments

During…	*Teach About…*
Bathing and personal care	How to perform skin care and foot care
Daily weights	When weight gain is caused by fluid, not food intake
Ambulation	The benefits of mobility for all body systems
Meals	Intake and output, benefits of water intake, and nutritional needs
Toileting	The benefits of fiber and water intake, intake and output, and signs of constipation and dehydration
Treatments	The purpose of the treatment, expected outcomes, and how to perform the treatment if appropriate
Medication administration	The reasons for the medication(s), possible side effects, and when to report side effects

Teaching Plans

When you have several people with the same teaching needs, it is cost- and time-effective to teach patients in small groups. An example of this is teaching diabetic patients about self-care. When presenting to small groups, you will find it helpful to make a plan for your teaching. You also may use a teaching plan when instructing individual patients, especially when you have a great deal of information to present. Once a patient begins to ask questions in the teaching session, it is easy to lose your train of thought. Using a plan helps to ensure that you do not forget something pertinent.

Developing a Teaching Plan Using the Nursing Process

As you develop a teaching plan, you will use the nursing process to help you make decisions about what to teach and how to teach it. When you develop care plans for patients whom you care for in clinical, do not forget to include teaching as a part of your plan.

ASSESSMENT. To develop a teaching plan, you need to first identify your patient's learning needs. What does the patient already know? What is unclear? What information has yet to be presented? When you take steps to determine what your patient knows, you are assessing your patient's knowledge needs. For example, it is helpful to determine if the patient prefers something visual, such as a video, or prefers to read about the topic before you discuss it.

It is also important to assess the patient's readiness to learn. For example, a patient who was just informed of a serious or life-threatening diagnosis probably is not emotionally ready to learn about treatment or how to take medication. Sometimes a patient may need some time to think about the news just received; other times, the patient may want you sitting quietly nearby. This provides the patient with support while allowing the patient time to develop questions.

NURSING DIAGNOSIS. When you determine what the patient still needs to learn, you are establishing a nursing diagnosis. The two nursing diagnoses that deal with patient teaching are the following:

1. **"Deficient knowledge," with descriptors:** Used when the patient is lacking knowledge about the disease process or management of the disease, including

diagnostic testing, medications, and treatment. Use this nursing diagnosis when planning care according to this example:

"Deficient knowledge about antidiabetic medications related to new diagnosis of diabetes mellitus type II": Indicates that the patient is newly diagnosed with diabetes and has not learned needed information about antidiabetic medications, such as when to take them, what effects are expected, and potential side effects to report if they occur.

2. **"Readiness for enhanced knowledge," with descriptors:** Used when the patient has some basic knowledge about the illness and is ready for further teaching. Use this nursing diagnosis when planning care according to this example:

"Readiness for enhanced knowledge about signs and symptoms of hypoglycemia and hyperglycemia related to new diagnoses of diabetes mellitus type 2": Indicates that the patient is newly diagnosed with diabetes and has had some exposure to the signs and symptoms of hypoglycemia and hyperglycemia, but is ready for further teaching on the subject.

It is your responsibility to specify the topic of teaching.

PLANNING. After identifying patient teaching needs, you will decide how to teach about the topic. You will need to find resources for materials to use as handouts, select a time and place for teaching, and decide how to present the material based on the patient's learning preferences. In other words, you are developing a teaching plan. Box 12.2 has information on resources for handouts.

IMPLEMENTATION. When you sit down with your patient or patients and present the information in your teaching plan, you are performing the implementation portion of the nursing process. During teaching, be sure to include the following practices:

- Establish a comfortable temperature in a room without distractions.
- Ensure that the patient is in a comfortable position and is not experiencing pain or discomfort.
- Involve the patient in your teaching by asking questions, requesting feedback, and allowing the patient to ask questions. Avoid lecturing to the patient.
- Explain why the patient needs to know the information. Adults learn best when they understand the relevance of the information presented.
- Have an interpreter present if needed so that the patient can understand the teaching.
- Have the patients wear eyeglasses or hearing aids, if appropriate. Sit where the patient can see your lips as you speak. Avoid positioning yourself in front of a window or light with a glare.
- Speak clearly and distinctly, not loudly, if the patient wears hearing aids.
- Sit near the patient during teaching. Avoid standing over the patient.
- Present one piece of information at a time, allowing the patient time to absorb it before moving on.
- Arrange and present information in a simple-to-complex format.
- Explain how to perform a task, and then demonstrate as you explain it a second time.
- Give frequent positive feedback to the patient. Say things such as, "You are doing great"; "I'm so glad you remembered that, it is important"; and "Show me again how well you can do that." Avoid saying anything that discourages

Box 12.2
Resources for Patient Teaching Handouts

There are a number of different resources you can utilize when looking for specific patient teaching handouts. Some of the most prominent are the following:

- **Associations and foundations:** Look for brochures or printed information about a specific disease and self-care for that disease from organizations such as the Arthritis Foundation, American Diabetes Association, and Multiple Sclerosis Society.
- **Health departments:** City, county, and state health departments usually have patient education information available for distribution by health-care professionals. Your health-care facility may already have many of these handouts on file.
- **Patient education Web sites:** Check for information available on Web sites of universities and medical centers. Be cautious about printing and using any information that is not approved by associations or foundations. Be aware that many commercial Web sites charge you to use their patient information.

You can also create your own patient teaching handout by using information from a variety of sources. However, be careful not to copy information word for word from a Web site or existing handout. You can summarize ideas and make bulleted lists to help patients remember key ideas. Keep your handouts at about a fifth-grade reading level so that all patients can understand them. Write in short, simple sentences.

When choosing handouts, remember the following criteria:

- Handouts need to be in simple language, without the use of confusing medical terminology. A fifth-grade reading level is most appropriate for all patients.
- If medical terms must be used, they should be clearly defined.
- Keep in mind that patients may need a translation of the handout in a different language. Ask an interpreter to do this so that the information will be translated appropriately.
- Handouts should be short, between one and two pages, and in an easy-to-read type size (font). Use font size 14 or larger for patients with visual impairments.

the patient or indicates that you thought the patient was ignorant.

- Provide written materials for easy reference that are appropriate to the patient's age and reading level. The use of visual aids, even pictures, can make a difference in the retention of the information.

EVALUATING. Now you must determine if the patient has learned what you have taught. How can you tell? Have the patient restate the information you have shared. Ask questions covering the information you have presented. If you have taught the patient to perform a task, such as changing a dressing, have the patient perform the skill while you watch. You may need to give a few verbal cues as the patient performs the skill. Then have the patient repeat it again without the cues. Table 12.2 presents examples of ways to evaluate patient teaching.

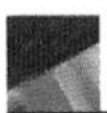

DOCUMENTATION OF TEACHING

It is very important for nurses to document the patient teaching they perform and the patient's response. This documentation is required by The Joint Commission, which is the accrediting agency for hospitals, and by third-party payers. Quality assurance departments will look for documentation reflecting topics of patient teaching and evaluation of learning. The following is an example of how to document patient teaching:

1620 Instructed on correct way to perform drsg change to L great toe. Instructed to soak foot in warm water × 20 min as ordered, pat foot dry carefully (including between the toes), apply Neosporin to suture line with sterile swab, apply sterile 4 × 4, and wrap foot with elastic bandage. Pt. returned demonstration, had mild difficulty remembering to pat dry and to dry between all toes before applying elastic bandage. To review again at 2000 dressing change. ______________ Nurse's signature and credentials

Some hospitals, home health agencies, and other health-care agencies have special patient teaching documentation forms in their electronic health records so that it is not necessary to write out the documentation in narrative format. Instead, you can fill in the columns with the topics taught; evidence of learning, either verbal or return demonstration; and any comments.

It is important to document patient teaching clearly and thoroughly. This is especially true in settings such as home health care or at a health-care provider's office where the same nurse may not see the patient again. This will allow the next nurse to know exactly what has been taught that needs to be reinforced. In additon, the Centers for Medicare and Medicaid require that home health documentation include specific descriptions of patient teaching as well as the evaluation of patient learning in order for the home health agency to be paid for any home visits that include patient teaching as a purpose for the visit.

KNOWLEDGE CONNECTION

What two nursing diagnoses apply to patient teaching? How will you position yourself during patient teaching?

Settings Connection: Medical Office

Teaching Children

When you work in a family practice or pediatric office or clinic, you may teach children of different ages about their illnesses or injuries. When teaching children, use age-appropriate information. Use a doll or teddy bear to represent the patient when explaining a procedure or treatment. Allow the child to perform the treatment on the doll or teddy bear as a return demonstration. By teaching a child what you are going to do next, you allow the child the opportunity to better understand, feel less stress, and be more compliant. Always tell the truth regarding whether or not the procedure or treatment will be uncomfortable. Take advantage of opportunities to speak at schools and day-care facilities. Emphasize a wellness or health topic, such as when and how to wash your hands.

Table 12.2
Ways to Evaluate Patient Teaching About Foot Care

Evaluation Technique	*Example*
Have the patient restate what has been taught	"Tell me what you learned about how to care for your feet because you are diabetic."
Ask questions to determine understanding	"What will you do about trimming your toenails when they grow too long?" "How will you wash and dry your feet?" "What type of shoes and house shoes will you wear?"
Ask the patient to give a return demonstration of a new task	"You change the dressing on your toe while I watch. I'll remind you of what to do if you need a hint."

Elder Care Connection

Teaching Elderly Patients

Have a caregiver or family member present during teaching, if possible. Allow plenty of time for teaching so that your elderly patient does not feel rushed. Be alert to cues that the elderly patient does not understand the teaching. He or she may put you off, saying, "I'll do it later" or "I already read it." This may occur because the patient is confused or does not understand but does not want to say so. Be very patient with elderly learners. Use plenty of repetition without getting frustrated.

Settings Connection: Home Health

Home Health Referral for Teaching

Patients who are to be discharged from the hospital but need more teaching can be referred to home health care for follow-up teaching. This requires a health-care provider's order. Be alert to the need to ask for a referral for more teaching. A home health-care follow-up often can prevent rehospitalization if the patient has not mastered information needed for self-care.

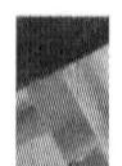

TEACHING PATIENTS ABOUT INTERNET RESOURCES

It is not uncommon to hear patients say that they, or a family member, have looked up their diagnosis on the Internet and then, when talking with them, discover that they obtained inaccurate or misleading information. In the information age, we can obtain an amazing amount of both information and misinformation. One of the newer roles of health-care professionals is to educate patients not only about their disease process, self-care, health, and wellness, but also about how to obtain accurate information using the Internet.

Use the following guidelines to help your patients find accurate information from Web sites:

- Explain that preferred sites for health-care information end in ".org," ".gov," or ".edu." Most other sites are for commercial use and often want to sell you something.
- Encourage patients to avoid reading blogs concerning disease processes or treatment. Explain that such entries are one person's experiences or opinions and are not the result of research or collective information.
- Encourage patients to use familiar sites with accurate information. For example, the Mayo Clinic and NIH.gov both are sites with understandable and credible information.
- Urge patients to avoid using sites such as Wikipedia because anyone can post information on such sites, making it subject to opinion rather than fact.
- Explain that the authors' credentials and educational background should be clearly listed.
- Tell patients to check the date of the most recent posting to be sure they are not accessing outdated medical information.
- Explain that commercial Web sites promoting a product or products with extremely positive claims are not reliable sources of factual information and should be considered doubtful unless other corroborating factual information can be found.
- Give patients alternatives to the Internet for finding quick, accurate information. Encourage them to call their pharmacist if they have questions about medications. Encourage them to read the handouts and discharge information they were given by the hospital. If they continue to have questions or concerns, encourage them to notify their physician, another health-care provider, or home health nurse.

KNOWLEDGE CONNECTION

What types of Web sites would you encourage patients to avoid when they are seeking information about their disease or self-care?

Supervision/Delegation Connection

Patient Teaching and Delegation

It is not appropriate to delegate patient teaching in any circumstances. This is in the realm of a licensed nurse only. Assistive personnel are not educated in this aspect of care; therefore, it is outside their scope of practice.

POST CONFERENCE

You completed caring for the patient who was newly diagnosed with diabetes. You had a great deal of new information to teach her. You remembered to assess her level of knowledge about diabetes and found that, because her mother also is a diabetic, she had some basic knowledge. However, you learned that her mother did not really follow diabetic diet recommendations. The patient told you that she is mostly a visual learner, so you provided her with handouts and pamphlets from the American Diabetes Association that you obtained from the diabetes educator. You were able to go over the information about diabetes, diet basics, and finger stick blood sugar tests with her during the afternoon when it was quiet. When you asked her questions about previous teaching done with her by the diabetes educator, she was able to answer them all correctly. Although she could perform a finger stick blood sugar test using a glucometer by the end of the afternoon, you recommended that she practice it again before being discharged. You also arranged for the diabetes educator to follow up with her later in the day.

Key Points

- Three common learning styles are visual, auditory, and kinesthetic.
- People can learn in every learning style—visual, auditory, and kinesthetic. However, most people prefer one style when exposed to new information and ideas. In patient teaching, address each style of learning so that the patient can absorb the information, such as providing a verbal explanation, written handouts, videos, and the demonstration of a skill.
- Many factors affect learning, including the environment, patient comfort, patient readiness, primary language of the patient, and the patient's sensory impairments.
- Even if a patient can speak and understand some English, it is best to arrange for a professional or certified interpreter with some understanding of medical terminology. Avoid using family members, especially children, as the interpreter.
- Repetition and restating are good ways to reinforce patient teaching.
- The two main purposes for patient teaching include teaching about health promotion and wellness strategies and teaching about disease processes, including treatments, medications, and self-care.
- Teachable moments occur when patients ask you questions about their illness or treatment, if you hear or observe misinformation that you correct, and when you point out cause-and-effect connections to the patient. These occur multiple times through a shift.
- You may develop a teaching plan for more formal instruction. It is developed using the nursing process and will be a part of your care plan.
- When you determine what patients need to learn, you are assessing knowledge deficits. You can evaluate how well your patient learned by asking questions, requesting a summary of what he or she learned, and asking the patient to perform a return demonstration of a skill.
- Two nursing diagnoses are used for patient teaching needs: "Deficient knowledge" and "Readiness for enhanced knowledge."
- Reliable Internet sites for health-care information generally end with ".edu," ".gov," and ".org." Blogs and commercial sites selling miracle products usually are not reliable sources of information.

Review Questions

Select the answer that is most appropriate for each of the following questions. Some questions may have more than one correct answer. Select all that apply.

1. Your patient says that he is a hands-on learner, not a book learner. You understand his primary learning style to be:
   1. auditory.
   2. visual.
   3. mixed.
   4. kinesthetic.
2. Because you know the above patient's primary learning style, your teaching will be presented:
   1. verbally only; he will learn best if you just tell him what you want him to do.
   2. by video so that he can see and hear the information as it is presented.
   3. in a variety of ways; verbally explain, give written information and videos if available, and demonstrate as you explain.
   4. as a demonstration only; he will learn best if you just show him what you want him to do.

3. As you prepare to teach your patient how to take his pulse, which of the following will be of concern to you?
   1. The television is on, visitors are talking, and someone is vacuuming in the hallway.
   2. The patient's primary language is not English.
   3. The patient is not wearing his glasses or his hearing aid.
   4. There is a large amount of clutter in the room.
   5. The patient is experiencing a significant amount of discomfort.
   6. The patient does not believe he needs any heart medications.

4. Which is an example of reinforcing previous teaching about a heart attack?
   1. Explaining for a third time to the patient about heart damage after a heart attack.
   2. Introducing information about the cause of a heart attack for the first time and leaving handouts for him to read.
   3. Asking the patient to explain to you what he wants to know about his heart attack.

5. A patient with no history of heart disease wants to keep his cholesterol at a healthy level. You will instruct him on foods high in cholesterol so that he can avoid them. Which purpose of patient teaching does this exemplify?
   1. Health promotion
   2. Wellness strategies
   3. Explaining the disease process
   4. Explaining treatment for disease

6. Which nursing intervention is LEAST appropriate for teaching a patient about a low-salt diet?
   1. Explain why the patient needs to restrict salt in her diet.
   2. Present a short lecture on the effects of excess salt in the body.
   3. Discuss information in a simple-to-complex format.
   4. Frequently praise the patient or give encouraging feedback.

ANSWERS 1. 4, 2. 4, 3. 1, 2, 3, 5, 6, 4. 1, 5. 1, 6. 2

Critical Thinking Exercises

Answers available online.

1. An elderly patient refuses to watch a demonstration on using a glucometer and performing a finger stick blood sugar test. She tells you, "My husband used one of those. I know all about it." What might be occurring?

2. A patient with heart disease needs instruction on preventing cardiac complications due to high blood pressure. Which nursing diagnosis is appropriate for this patient?

3. A patient tells you that he has looked up his disease and its treatment on the Internet. As you teach, he argues with you about basic information, saying that he did not find that on the Internet. How would you handle his patient teaching?

Additional Resources

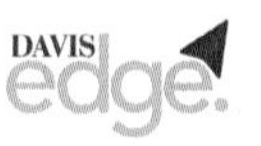

Use the scratch off code on the inside front cover of your book to access online quizzes that will help you to improve your scores on course exams and prepare for the NCLEX-PN®.

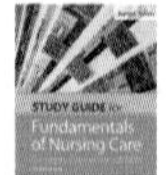

Study Guide

CHAPTER 13
Safety

KEY TERMS

Ambulate (AM-byoo-layt)
Base of support (BAYSS uv su-PORT)
Body mechanics (BAH-dee muh-KAN-iks)
Cardiopulmonary resuscitation (KAR-dee-oh-PULL-muh-nair-ee ree-SUSS-i-TAY-shun)
Center of gravity (SEN-ter uv GRA-vi-tee)
Chair or bed monitor (CHAIR OR BED MAW-ni-tor)
Code team (KOHD TEEM)
Fall assessment rating scales (FAWL ah-SESS-ment RAY-ting SCAYLZ)
Heimlich maneuver (HIGHM-lik ma-NEW-ver)
Leg monitor (LEG MAW-ni-tor)
Mass casualty event (MASS KA-zhul-tee ee-VENT)
Rescue breathing (RESS-kyoo BREE-thing)
Restraint alternatives (ris-TRAYNT awl-TUR-na-tivz)
Restraints (ris-TRAYNTS)
Safety data sheet (SAYF-tee DAY-tuh SHEET)

CHAPTER CONCEPTS

Safety
Patient-Centered Care

LEARNING OUTCOMES

1. Define various terms associated with safety.
2. Explain areas addressed by the National Patient Safety Goals.
3. Describe six factors that contribute to an unsafe patient environment.
4. Discuss strategies for preventing falls, including assessment rating scales and restraint alternatives.
5. Identify requirements for use of restraints and release of restraints.
6. Explain the acronyms RACE and PASS.
7. Describe the types of fires and extinguishers.
8. Determine actions to take when a patient is unresponsive.
9. Discuss the role of nurses in a mass casualty event.
10. Identify ways to use body mechanics to prevent injury when caring for patients.
11. Explain how lack of rest and substance use or abuse can contribute to unsafe patient care.
12. Describe ways to protect yourself from radiation hazards.
13. Discuss safe handling of chemicals and gases.
14. Identify the purpose of a safety data sheet.
15. Explain ways to protect yourself from biological hazards.
16. Discuss information found in the Connection features in this chapter.
17. Identify specific safety information.
18. Answer questions about the skills in this chapter.

SKILLS

13.1 Using a Bed/Chair or Leg Monitor
13.2 Applying Restraints
13.3 Using Body Mechanics

CRITICAL THINKING CONNECTION

Clinical Assignment

You will be caring for Mrs. Lloyd, an 82-year-old female who has been hospitalized due to a stroke. While in the hospital, she tried to get up alone and fell, resulting in a left hip fracture. Two days ago,

Continued

CRITICAL THINKING CONNECTION—cont'd

she had an open reduction and internal fixation on her hip, a surgery to repair the fractured portion of her femur and acetabulum. She is confused at times, especially at night. She nearly fell again yesterday when the bed monitor was accidentally left off of the bed and she attempted to get up. Her family is understandably very upset.

Critical Thinking Questions:

1. What patient fall assessment rating scales will you use on Mrs. Lloyd?
2. What factors contribute to an unsafe environment for the patient?
3. If a patient falls, what actions will you take as a nurse?

Safety must be foremost in your mind when you care for any patient—not only the safety of the patient, but your own safety as well. In this chapter, you will learn a variety of ways to promote safety when caring for patients. Some nurses tend to grow complacent about safety as they work year after year. Please do not allow yourself to ever become indifferent to safety awareness.

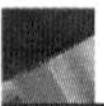

SAFE ENVIRONMENT FOR PATIENTS

Patients come to hospitals expecting to be kept safe while they are treated for and recover from illnesses. You may have heard stories about situations when that did not happen. Patients and families are devastated when additional injury or illness occurs during a hospitalization because of a lack of adequate safeguards for the patient.

At the same time, safety for nursing staff is also a major issue. Back injuries are one of the leading causes of disability among nurses. Nurses can be at risk for communicable disease and exposure to hazards such as blood and body fluids, as well as radiation. Health-care facilities develop policies to promote safety and reduce illness and injury for patients and nurses alike.

National Patient Safety Goals

A national standard for patient safety has been established by **The Joint Commission,** the organization responsible for evaluating and accrediting health-care organizations and programs in the United States. Their National Patient Safety Goals for 2017 address specific safety problems in the hospital setting, such as identifying patients correctly, improving staff communication, using medicines safely, using alarms safely, preventing infections, identifying patient safety risks, and preventing mistakes in surgery. Requirements for meeting each goal also have been established. It is up to each facility to determine ways to meet those requirements. When identifying patients in a variety of health-care settings, you need to identify the patient with two identifiers. The two identifiers can be any of the following: patient name, date of birth, medical record number, or picture. Using two identifiers will assist in eliminating potential medical errors. In this book, we will emphasize safety throughout. Specific safety issues regarding medications will be discussed in Chapters 35, 36, 37, and 38.

Factors Contributing to an Unsafe Patient Environment

When patients are hospitalized, their entire environment changes. Nothing is familiar. As nurses, we view the hospital as a comfortable place; we see it laid out in an efficient and logical pattern. However, for many patients, the hospital feels like a maze within a maze; the patient may feel confined to a tiny room miles away from anything familiar. Patients are forced to wear a hospital gown and nonslip socks, clothes that are nothing like what they are likely to wear at home. Privacy curtains that do not limit sound or smell do nothing to promote any feelings of true privacy. In addition to the strangeness of the hospital, many factors can contribute to creating an unsafe environment for patients.

Age and Ability to Understand

A hospital is threatening enough to adults, but it is an even more confusing place for very young patients and elderly patients. It is difficult for children younger than age 10 years to clearly understand what will happen and what is expected of them. If a parent can stay with the child, it helps him or her feel more secure. However, with family and work duties, that is not always possible. ***Safety: Elderly patients, especially those confused due to cognitive impairments, medications, or unfamiliar surroundings, are particularly at risk for falls. They may try to get up or walk without realizing they are attached to tubes and cords.*** Even though the nursing staff may explain these limitations, patients may not remember or clearly understand such deviations from normal.

Impaired Mobility

Patients who are unsteady on their feet or unable to bear full weight are at particular risk for injury if they attempt to **ambulate** (walk) without help. It is not uncommon for patients in the hospital to experience poor balance or general weakness after surgery or after being in bed for a prolonged period. Equipment, cords, and tubes are barriers to mobility in the hospital room, and these barriers are compounded by the patient's poor balance, weakness, or impaired mobility.

Communication

Patients who speak English as a second language may not grasp safety instructions. When you tell the patient to call for the nurse before getting up, the instruction may be unclear. Call on the telephone? Shout out? Be sure that your instructions are specific: "Press this button and tell us that you need

• WORD • BUILDING •
ambulate: ambulate – walk

to get up. Someone will come to help you." Sometimes patients do not want to bother the nurses and are hesitant to call for help. In some cultures, patients of one sex may not want a nurse of the opposite sex to assist with toileting and personal hygiene. ***Safety: Arrange for an interpreter when you give instructions if your patient does not understand English.***

Pain and Discomfort

People in pain are generally irritable and anxious. They may disregard safety precautions in an effort to be more comfortable. For example, if a patient is in pain, he or she may attempt to get back in bed after sitting up in a bedside chair to relieve the pain and fatigue even if he or she has been instructed to wait for help. Discomfort, such as a full bladder or rectum, is also a motivation for disregarding safety instructions. Patients who need to go to the bathroom may feel the need is urgent and attempt to go alone, especially if the call light is not answered promptly.

Delayed Assistance

A patient may ring the call light and then wait for assistance to the bathroom or elsewhere. But if no one answers or no one comes to assist in a timely manner, the patient may attempt to go alone. ***Safety: It is imperative that call lights be answered promptly and that assistance be quickly available to maintain a safe environment for patients.*** Although poor staffing patterns may contribute to delayed assistance for patients, nursing staff must make rapid response to requests for assistance a high priority.

Equipment

Hospital equipment is commonplace to nursing staff, who know its purpose and are familiar with its operation. However, the equipment can be upsetting to patients. When alarms go off, patients and families often become anxious, feeling that something is terribly wrong. That anxiety can create an unsafe situation for the patient. Anxiety can lead to elevated blood pressure and heart rate, which, depending on the diagnosis, can be an unsafe situation. Some patients attempt to get out of bed and go to the hallway to alert the nurses about an alarm because they are frightened by it. Even something as routine as side rails on the bed, often seen as a safety feature, can cause injury to some patients. Injuries and even deaths have resulted from entrapment of patients' heads and chests between the side rails and the bed, or between the upper and lower bed rails. Interestingly, researchers found that older, frail adults who experience confusion, pain, fecal impaction, and urinary retention are at highest risk for entrapment because they are more likely to move around in bed or try to get out of bed.

> **KNOWLEDGE CONNECTION**
> How does a delay in answering call lights contribute to an unsafe condition for your patients?

Promoting Patient Safety

It is the responsibility of all health-care staff to promote the safety of patients. Nurses have to be "on alert" at all times to detect potentially unsafe situations. It has been said that nurses make hypervigilant parents because they look at every situation and see what could happen and how injuries could occur. That is the result of protecting patients from potential harm.

Preventing Falls

One of the national goals for patient safety focuses on reducing the risk of patient harm from falls. The requirement for this goal is that each facility must have a fall reduction program, which includes ways to evaluate its effectiveness.

FALL ASSESSMENT RATING SCALES. Many facilities have developed **fall assessment rating scales—**forms that, when filled out, give a numerical rating for each patient's risk for falls. The higher the number, the greater the patient's risk (Table 13.1).

Generally, the fall assessment rating scale is completed on every patient admitted to the hospital. Facility policy will determine which patients are considered "at risk." For those patients, a system for identification and precautions is put in place. For example, a patient is admitted and is rated a 65 on the fall assessment rating scale. Facility policy states that patients rated 50 or higher are at strict risk for falls. This patient is identified by flags or stickers on the chart, the Kardex, and the patient's door to serve as reminders to all staff. Some facilities use a specially colored armband on the patients themselves. Some controversy exists over how to identify patients in a confidential way yet still alert staff to the risk of falls.

RESTRAINT ALTERNATIVES. Patients identified as "at risk" for falls may need reminders to keep them from getting up when it is unsafe for them to do so. A number of products have been developed for this purpose. They are not true **restraints,** which are vests, jackets, or bands with connected straps that are tied to the bed, chair, or wheelchair to keep the patient in one place. These **restraint alternatives** are less restrictive ways to help patients remember not to get up and try to walk, or to alert nursing staff that the patient is attempting to do so.

Monitors

One product used as a restraint alternative is the **chair monitor** or **bed monitor,** a pressure-sensitive device that generates an alarm when the patient's weight is no longer sensed, indicating that the patient is attempting to get up (Fig. 13.1a). A **leg monitor** is another type of chair monitor. It attaches to the patient's leg like a large bandage and generates an alarm when the leg is in a dependent position, indicating that the patient is attempting to stand (Fig. 13.1b). It is important to

• WORD • BUILDING •
hypervigilant: hyper – excessive + vigilant – attentive to stimuli

Table 13.1
Morse Fall Scale

Item	*Scale*	*Scoring*
1. History of falling; immediate or within 3 months	No Yes	0 25
2. Secondary diagnosis	No Yes	0 15
3. Ambulatory aid: • Bedrest/nurse assist • Crutches/cane/walker • Furniture	 0 15 30	
4. IV/saline lock	No Yes	0 20
5. Gait/transferring • Normal/bedrest/immobile • Weak • Impaired	 0 10 20	
6. Mental status • Oriented to own ability • Forgets limitations	 0 15	
Risk Level	***Morse Fall Score***	***Action***
Preventive fall precautions interventions (Level I)	0–24	Implement Level I
Modified fall risk interventions (Level II)	25–50	Implement Level II
Strict fall risk interventions (Level III)	>51	Implement Level III

Source: Reproduced with permission from Springer Publishing Company, New York, NY.

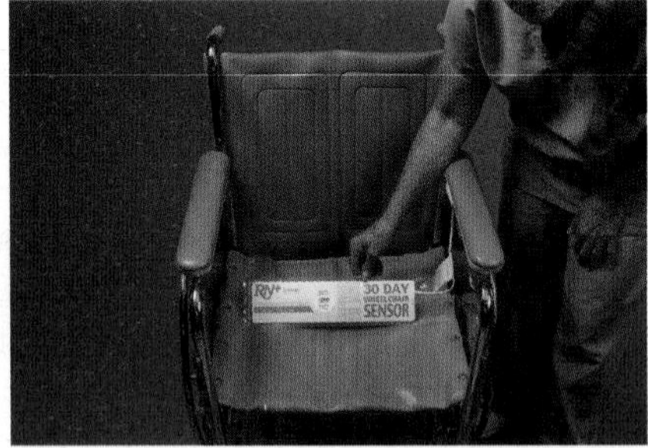

FIGURE 13.1A This chair monitor alarm will sound when no weight is detected (from Wilkinson JM, Treas LS. *Fundamentals of Nursing: Theory, Concepts & Applications*. Vol. 2. 3rd ed. Philadelphia, PA: FA Davis; 2016).

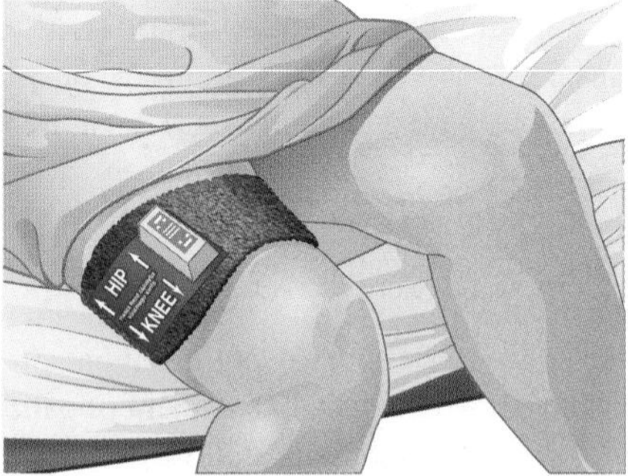

FIGURE 13.1B This leg monitor will sound an alarm when the patient is nearly vertical (from Wilkinson JM, Van Leuven K. *Fundamentals of Nursing: Theory, Concepts & Applications*. Vol. 2. Philadelphia, PA: FA Davis; 2015).

continue to check frequently on patients at risk for falls. These monitors cannot anticipate possible falls. In addition, if the pressure-sensitive pad is not moved from the bed to the chair when the patient transfers to a chair, no alarm will sound when the patient attempts to stand. Skill 13.1 (page 219) provides more information on using a bed/chair or leg monitor.

Soft Devices

Soft devices include bolsters that can be placed in the bed on either side of the patient to prevent him or her from slipping between or through the side rails. In some States, soft devices are considered restraints and do require a healthcare provider's order.

Strategies

A number of simple strategies may be used by nursing staff to help prevent falls in at-risk patients:

- Place a patient who is at risk for falls in a room near the nurse's station to make it easier for more people to see and check on him or her. Patients who are prone to falls may also benefit from sitting in a wheelchair near the nurses' station, where they can see the activity and people and where they are also easily visible.
- Stay with patients at risk for falls when they are in the bathroom or on the bedside commode. Do not leave them with the instruction to "Put on your call light when you are through," because often these patients will attempt to get up without calling for help.
- Keep the bed at the lowest level at all times except when the nursing staff is at the bedside. If there is a recurrent problem where the patient is unsafe because of repeated attempts to get out of bed, the mattress may be placed on the floor to prevent injury to the patient.
- Place the over-bed table across the wheelchair like a tray to help patients remain seated in the chair. You can also use furniture or equipment to block areas that are off limits to the patient so that he or she remains in a safe zone.
- Some patients who are at risk for falls seem to have a lot of energy and are looking for ways to stay busy. Try having them sit in a rocking chair near the nurses' station. Often the motion of rocking helps them relax as well as use pent-up energy. You can also give them simple but purposeful activities to do, such as folding washcloths or towels.
- Offer regular opportunities for the patient to go to the bathroom or to have a snack or something to drink. Sometimes patients are attempting to do one of these things when they get out of bed unsafely.
- Assess your fall-risk patients frequently for subjective complaints such as nausea, pain, or other discomfort. These patients may be trying to get more comfortable but are unable to do so safely.
- Provide back rubs and distractions, such as music or television, to help patients be more comfortable and less restless. Use a nightlight to decrease anxiety at night when surroundings are unfamiliar.

In spite of all best efforts, a fall may occasionally occur. Should you come upon a patient who has fallen, follow the steps in Box 13.1 to be sure you handle the situation appropriately.

RESTRAINTS. Other names for restraints are *protective devices* or *safety reminder devices.* Sometimes you will hear them called *Poseys* after the brand name of the first restraints on the market. Soft devices are available that fit across the patient's lap while they are sitting in a wheelchair (see Fig. 13.2). Avoid using restraints if at all possible. Try all other options first, and try them more than once. Enlist the family to help, if they are available to do so. No one wants to feel "tied down" against his or her will. Elderly and confused patients, as well as those who are very young, often cannot understand the reason for this treatment. Many long-term care facilities are moving away from using restraints and are trying alternatives to assist patients who are confused or disoriented, or who cannot understand. Never threaten patients with restraints. Instead,

Box 13.1

Actions to Take If a Patient Has Fallen

If a patient falls, it is important to know what to do. The following steps will guide you through the assessment and actions to take.

- Check the patient for obvious injuries. Look for bleeding, check level of consciousness, assess for signs of hip fracture (one leg shorter than the other and rotated outward), observe for deformities at any joint, and assess for paralysis or weakness on one side of the body.
- Call for help. It will take several staff members to move the patient off the floor. Follow facility policy for moving patients who have fallen.
- Take the patient's vital signs. The fall may be due to underlying cardiac or neurological problems such as an arrhythmia or a cerebrovascular accident.
- If the patient is not conscious, has unstable vital signs, or is not breathing or is without a pulse, call a Code Blue immediately.
- Assist the conscious patient to bed with the help of others, following facility policy.
- Notify the health-care provider. Explain what occurred and give the patient's current condition. Be prepared to take orders for x-rays and other tests.
- Document the incident according to facility policy. An incident report must be completed. Charting should include details of finding the patient, vital signs, assistance to bed, notifying the health-care provider, and orders obtained.

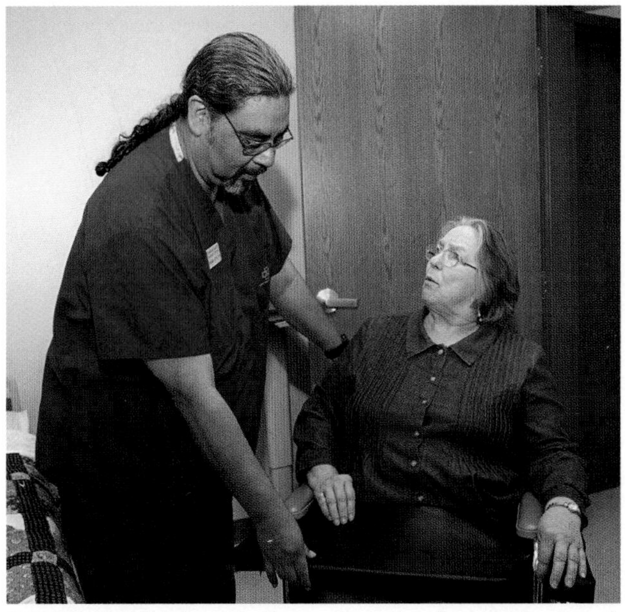

FIGURE 13.2 This lap guard keeps the patient from getting out of the wheelchair.

remind them about the purpose of the various lines, tubes, or restrictions and distract them by directing their attention to something else. For example, if a patient is pulling at his or her catheter, you could say, "I know that tube is uncomfortable, but it is necessary right now. Can I turn on the television for you?"

Students in nursing are sometimes confused about restraints. They may have seen situations on television or in movies where a patient in a mental health facility is out of control and is restrained in four-way restraints—one on each arm and one on each leg. This is a completely different situation than protecting a patient from injury or from pulling out tubes. Hospitals always use the *least restrictive environment* for patients, which means that patients are restrained only in the manner absolutely necessary to prevent harm.

In some situations, alternatives are not effective, and all other options have been exhausted. If this occurs, the first step is to speak with the patient's health-care provider. *You must have a health-care provider's order for restraints.* The order should include the type of restraint and the specific period of time it is to remain in place. Generally the order will be for no more than 24 hours.

When an order has been obtained and the restraints are in place, nursing staff are required by the Health Care Financing Administration and The Joint Commission to follow these guidelines:

- Check on the patient every 30 minutes, making sure to check the skin for redness or chafing under the restraint and the extremities for warmth and color.
- Remove the restraint every 2 hours. While the restraint is off:
  - Offer fluids to the patient.
  - Assist with toileting as needed.
  - Change the patient's position if he or she is in bed.
  - Assess the extremities for edema, capillary refill time, sensation, and function.
  - Assess skin over pressure points for integrity and erythema.
  - Assist the patient to ambulate if that is appropriate.
  - Stay with the patient the entire time the restraint is off.
- Document all actions on the appropriate flow sheet (Fig. 13.3).

There may be some variation of these guidelines from state to state due to specific laws and statutes. Facilities will have written guidelines regarding restraints, so be sure to know and follow your facility's policies.

Supervision/Delegation Connection

Delegation of Restraint Checks and Releases

When a patient has restraints applied, you can delegate the checks and releases to a certified nursing assistant (CNA) or unlicensed assistive personnel (UAP). However, you need to supervise your assistant by following up to ensure that checks are indeed being done and being documented on the flow sheet. It is very important that the patient be released from the restraints every 2 hours; otherwise, you could be accused of false imprisonment. It is your responsibility to be sure that the checks and releases occur exactly as dictated by facility policy.

Application of Restraints

It is important to use the correct restraint when you are carrying out a health-care provider's order. Several types exist: vest or jacket, waist, wrist, and mitt. Table 13.2 lists descriptions and pictures of each type of physical restraint. Chemical restraints also may be ordered and used. These are medications prescribed to prevent restlessness and anxiety in the patient who may be in an unsafe situation without the medication. They are used judiciously by health-care providers. ***Safety: No restraint, either physical or chemical, is ordered or used unless absolutely necessary to keep the patient safe. They are never used for the convenience of staff.***

It is extremely important that you know how to correctly apply restraints. You should be able to insert two fingers between the patient's body and the restraint to ensure that it is not too tight. Restraints are always tied in a quick-release knot. That way, if a patient needs immediate assistance, he or she can be quickly released from the restraint. If you struggle to master the quick-release knot, keep practicing. No other knot is acceptable when tying restraints.

Some patients have been injured or have died when restraints were applied incorrectly. Most often, instances of severe injury or death were due to choking injuries when the vest or jacket restraint was put on the patient backward. The patient then slid down in the chair or wheelchair and the tight restraint compressed the chest or throat. ***Safety: Always apply restraints according to facility policy and manufacturer's directions.***

Skill 13.2 (page 220) provides more instructions regarding the correct application of restraints.

KNOWLEDGE CONNECTION

Name three alternatives to the use of restraints. How are restraints tied? What is the reason for tying them in this manner?

Responding to a Fire

Should a fire occur in a health-care setting, it is imperative that staff know what to do and that they do it quickly and well. Fire drills are required periodically to be sure everyone practices the procedure to follow in case of an actual fire.

RESTRAINTS Q 30 MINUTE CHECKLIST							DATE: ______					
	19:00	19:30	20:00	20:30	21:00	21:30	22:00	22:30	23:00	23:30	24:00	24:30
Siderails												
Oriented/ Disoriented												
Pulse/ Circulation												
Skin Condition												
Readjust Tension												
R.O.M.												
DATE:	01:00	01:30	02:00	02:30	03:00	03:30	04:00	04:30	05:00	05:30	06:00	06:30
Siderails												
Oriented/ Disoriented												
Pulse/ Circulation												
Skin Condition												
Readjust Tension												
R.O.M.												

FIGURE 13.3 Restraint flow sheet. (Courtesy of Kingfisher Regional Hospital, Kingfisher, OK.)

Table 13.2
Types of Physical Restraints

Type of Restraint	*Description of Use*	*Picture of Restraint*
Vest	Used to protect a patient in danger of getting out of bed or out of a wheelchair or chair. Placed on the patient with the crossover in front and the straps tied to the lower portion of the back of the wheelchair. If used with the patient in bed, the straps are tied to the moveable portion of the bed frame, not to the bed rails.	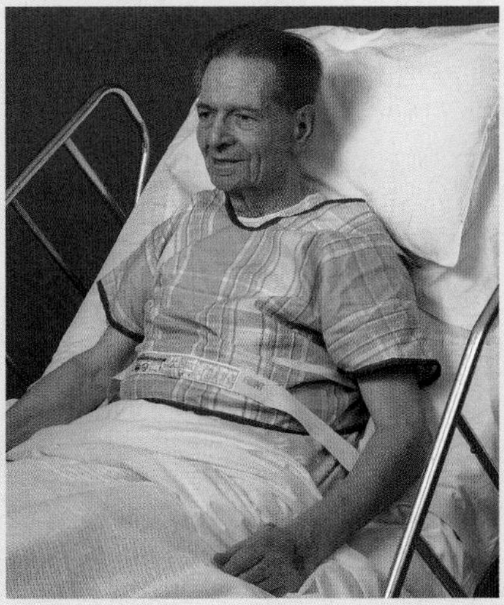

Continued

Table 13.2
Types of Physical Restraints—cont'd

Type of Restraint	*Description of Use*	*Picture of Restraint*
Waist	Used to protect a patient in danger of getting out of a bed or chair. Placed around the patient's waist, then the straps are tied to the moveable portion of the bed frame or to the lower portion of the back of the wheelchair.	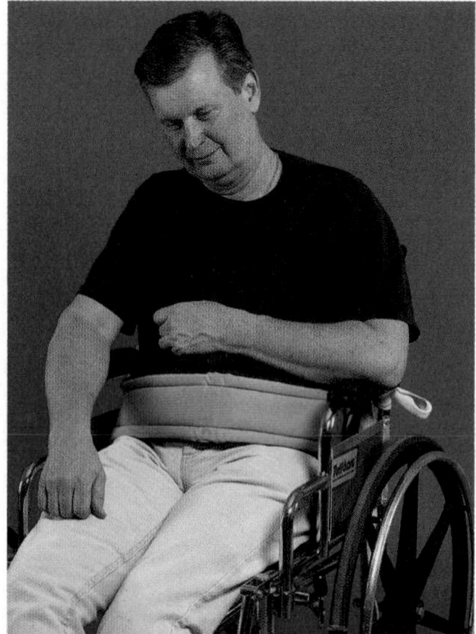
Extremity	Used to protect a patient in danger of pulling out tubes or taking off monitoring devices. Placed around the patient's wrist, then tied to the moveable portion of the bed frame and not the bed rails.	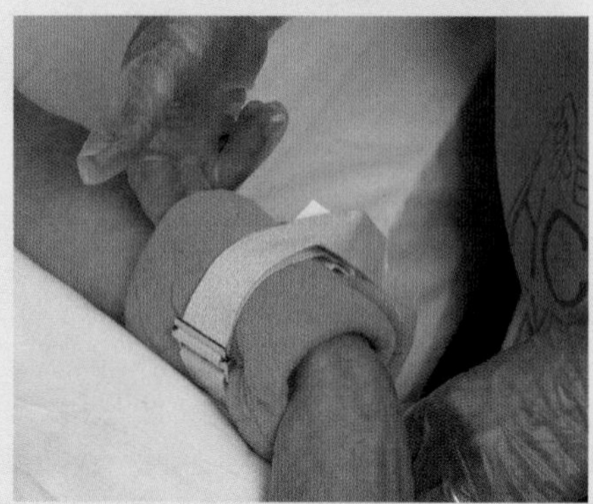
Mitt	Used to protect a patient in danger of pulling out tubes or interfering with treatments. Sometimes used to prevent scratching in patients with severe skin disorders. The patient's hand is placed within the mitt, and the mitt is secured around the wrist. The straps can also be tied to the moveable portion of the bed frame but not the bed rails.	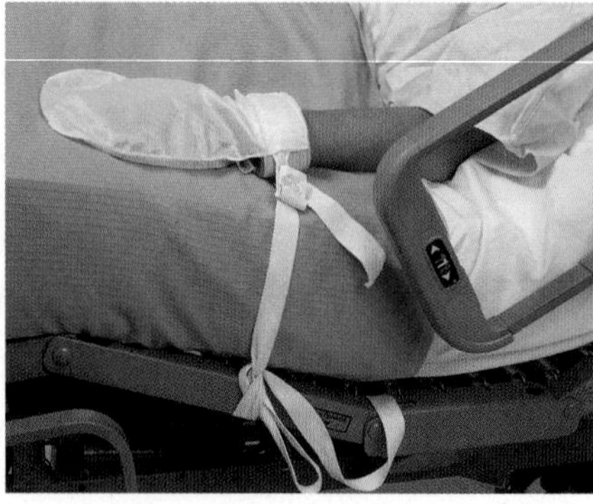

Each facility determines its own code word for a fire or fire drill. Common code words include "Code Red" and "Facility Alert, Fire Alarm Activation." The code usually is announced via the intercom or paging system. If a fire occurs, the entire facility will respond. In some cases, if the fire is not in your wing or area of the hospital, your job will be to close patient room doors and stay within your area, sealed off by fire doors that automatically close.

If the fire is in your area or you are the one to discover a fire, remember the acronym RACE and follow each letter:

- **Rescue:** Remove patients from immediate danger to a safer area of the hospital.
- **Alarm:** Sound the fire alarm according to facility policy. This may involve dialing an extension or pulling a fire alarm box. The fire department will automatically be notified.
- **Confine:** Confine the fire to one room or area. Close the doors according to hospital policy. Fire doors automatically close to help confine the fire to one wing of the hospital.
- **Extinguish:** You should only attempt to extinguish a small fire with a fire extinguisher.

The fire department will extinguish larger fires. If you need to extinguish a small fire, obtain the nearest fire extinguisher and follow the acronym PASS:

- **Pull** the pin found between the handles.
- **Aim** the nozzle of the fire extinguisher at the base of the flames.
- **Squeeze** the handles together to release the contents of the extinguisher.
- **Sweep** the nozzle back and forth at the base of the flames to extinguish the fire.

The PASS acronym is just as important to remember as RACE. It is important to know what to do before a fire occurs so that you can be ready to extinguish it in an emergency. You do not want to be trying to read the directions on the side of the extinguisher during a real fire. ***Safety: Know the fire code and procedures for each clinical facility before you begin patient care.***

TYPES OF EXTINGUISHERS. It is always important to use the correct type of fire extinguisher when attempting to fight a fire. Different types of extinguishers have different contents designed to quickly put out a specific type of fire. Fires are designated as type A, B, C, D, or K (Box 13.2), and fire extinguishers are labeled with these designations. Most fire extinguishers in health-care facilities are combination extinguishers used for the A, B, and C types of fires.

KNOWLEDGE CONNECTION

When do you use the acronym RACE? When do you need to know the acronym PASS?

Box 13.2

Types of Fires and Extinguishers

Various types of fire extinguishers are available to fight different types of fires. It is important for you to obtain the correct extinguisher for the type of fire you are fighting.

- **Type A:** Paper, wood, fabric, and trash
- **Type B:** Combustible liquids such as oil, gasoline and other petroleum-based products, and flammable gases
- **Type C:** Electrical fires such as short-circuits in wires, motor, or equipment fires
- **Type D:** Powders, flakes, or shavings of combustible metals
- **Type K:** Kitchen fires due to combustible cooking fluids such as oils and fats

Note: Most fire extinguishers are a combination of A, B, and C extinguishers that can be used to fight all three types of fires. However, each extinguisher is marked with the fires it should be used to extinguish.

Patient Teaching Connection

Teaching Safe Oxygen Use in the Home

Teach your patients in home health care or a long-term care facility about using oxygen safely. Instruct them that no open flames can be present in the same room as the oxygen source. Explain that no one can smoke, burn candles, or use an open-flame heater, all of which can cause a fire. Instruct patients to not use wool blankets or sweaters, which could generate static electricity, or electrical appliances such as shavers, which could cause a spark. Patients can use extension tubing to move around the house.

Responding to Individual Emergencies

As a student and a nurse, it is your responsibility to maintain your certification in **cardiopulmonary resuscitation** (CPR), which is a set of actions used to restart the heart or breathing of an unresponsive victim without a pulse or respirations. Recertification currently is required every 2 years. Many changes in CPR have been implemented in the past 10 years as a result of research and technology. It is very important that you be current in your training and not rely on out-of-date information. Your CPR course will include instruction and practice on the **Heimlich maneuver,** an action to relieve choking by thrusting just below a person's xiphoid process.

Some facilities may also require first aid certification, which must be kept current. Even if this certification is not required, you may wish to pursue it if you participate in community activities such as scouting, church groups, or sports teams, where injuries often occur. As nurses, we are used to having equipment and supplies at hand during an emergency

• WORD • BUILDING •

cardiopulmonary resuscitation: cardio – heart + pulmonary – lungs; re – again + suscitation – raise up

or injury. A first aid course helps you be ready to use what is available rather than what is ideal.

If, as a student, you come upon a patient who is unresponsive, it is appropriate for you to alert the emergency team. This is usually announced as a "Code Blue," but in some facilities it may be denoted as "Medical Alert, Code Blue," followed by a room number. Follow your facility policy for initiating a Code Blue. It may involve dialing a certain extension number from the room or activating an emergency call light in the room.

Once you have called the code, begin CPR or **rescue breathing** (breathing for the patient in case of respiratory arrest when the pulse still is palpable), whichever is appropriate. Continue your efforts until the **code team,** a group of specially trained personnel designated to respond to codes throughout the hospital, arrives. The code team often consists of critical care nurses, respiratory therapists, and a resident or emergency physician. The code team will take over the resuscitation efforts. When a Code Blue occurs in a critical care unit, it is not generally announced through the paging system. Instead, the critical care nurses carry out their code duties with limited assistance from other health-care staff.

While the code team is working on the patient, make notes about the time you found the patient and exactly what you did so that you can document them in the chart. Be aware of any family or friends of the patient who might be nearby during the emergency. Understandably, this is a frightening event, and family members generally know something is terribly wrong. Try to assign a UAP or CNA to stay with the family. Offer the family a private place to make phone calls, and offer them water or coffee, as well as tissues if needed. Sometimes family members are overlooked during emergencies, yet they are in great need of someone to offer kindness, empathy, and emotional support.

If you are a staff nurse on break or at lunch and a Code Blue is called for your unit, it is possible that you will be expected to return to the unit immediately to assist with other patients for the duration of the code.

KNOWLEDGE CONNECTION

Name three actions to take if you come upon an unresponsive patient. List your actions in the order in which you would perform them.

Responding to Disasters

In our current world, the term *disaster* can refer to many things: bombings, fires, blizzards, floods, tornados, hurricanes, the collapse of buildings, school shootings, bridge collapses, and anything causing mass casualties. The health-care community is always front and center when it comes to dealing with these events, whether the 9/11 terrorist attacks of 2001 or a major hurricane. In some situations, the health-care community's disaster plan was executed and all went relatively smoothly. In other situations, the planners did not anticipate all the complications that interfered with the arrival of help and supplies.

The Agency for Healthcare Research and Quality (AHRQ) defines a **mass casualty event** (MCE) as a public health or medical emergency involving thousands of victims. The office of the Assistant Secretary for Preparedness and Response, along with AHRQ and the U.S. Department of Health and Human Services, collaborated to establish guidelines for acceptable standards of care in an MCE. These guidelines help the health-care community prepare in advance for various contingencies that could occur during an MCE. The normal standards of care must shift during disasters, and these shifts have to take moral, ethical, and legal implications into account.

Not all questions are answered by these guidelines, but some of the major points addressed include using a disaster triage model, treating first those victims who are most likely to survive, how to plan for any MCE rather than specific situations, and how to adapt the use of existing facilities for various needs.

Another type of MCE is *bioterrorism,* the release of a biological or chemical agent into the air or water supply that could cause thousands of illnesses and deaths. In this situation, the health-care community must be prepared not only to deal with the MCE, but to also have to deal with a potentially contaminated water supply and a highly contagious illness. In the case of bioterrorism, the first clue that the event has occurred may be several days later when people begin presenting at various emergency departments in the area with similar symptoms, such as rapidly progressing pneumonia. In many cases, by the time serious symptoms appear, the illness is severe and difficult to treat. When a cluster of similar symptoms develops in an area, it is important that antibiotic treatment is begun at once without waiting for the usual laboratory confirmations.

Your responsibility as a student and as a nurse will be to know and follow your facility's disaster plan. Many different codes are used to indicate different types of disasters, so learn the codes used by your facility. Expect to be called in to work as an extra if a disaster occurs. It is appropriate for you to ensure the safety of your family first and then assist at your place of work. Some facilities have a plan for calling in extra help according to needs rather than having a barrage of off-duty employees arriving at once.

Real-World Connection

Participating in a Disaster During Clinical Experience

When the Murrah Federal Building in Oklahoma City was bombed in 1995, an instructor and 11 practical nursing students were at a hospital eight blocks from the site. It was a typical clinical morning until 9:01.

• WORD • BUILDING •

bioterrorism: bio – life + terrorism – unlawful violence

When the bomb exploded, the hospital swayed. Windows shattered, and glass blew into the rooms and onto patients and nursing staff. The fire alarms sounded, and the smell of smoke was everywhere. At first, the students thought something had happened just to the hospital building, but when they looked out the 11th-floor windows, a huge column of black smoke was visible where the federal building stood.

The hospital immediately went into its disaster plan. Students helped out by moving patients from damaged rooms to ones that were intact. As staff prepared for an influx of wounded, students assisted by administering routine medications, preparing supplies, and setting up additional areas for patient care if needed.

As the morning progressed, it became obvious that many had not survived the blast and that those who were more seriously injured would have to go to surgery before they came to the patient units. A young child from the day-care center was dead on arrival to the emergency room. Of course, she had no identification. A nurse described her simply by the color of her hair and the clothes she was wearing on the list of those who had perished.

The disaster plan worked exactly as it had been practiced. Everyone knew what to do and did their jobs with remarkable calm and professionalism. Each student who served that day was changed forever.

Since that time, many health-care professionals have served in response to mass casualty events such as the World Trade Center attacks, hurricanes, school shootings, bombings, tornados, and earthquakes. Be prepared, because you never know when it will happen in your world.

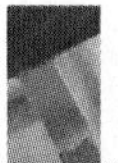

SAFE ENVIRONMENT FOR NURSING STAFF

Nursing staff in hospitals and other health-care facilities provide much of the direct patient care and therefore are exposed to safety risks, including lifting and moving patients, working with medications and chemicals, and potential exposure to contaminated blood and body fluids.

These risks can be divided into three broad categories: physical, chemical, and biological hazards. Patients may be at risk for exposure to some of these hazards as well. Nursing staff are at risk for all of them. Box 13.3 describes examples of each of these types of hazards.

> **Box 13.3**
>
> **Types of Hazards to Nursing Staff**
>
> Various types of hazards exist when you are providing nursing care. It is important to be aware of these hazards so you can protect yourself.
>
> - *Physical hazards* include injuries to back and joints; repetitive motion injuries such as carpal tunnel syndrome; exposure to lasers, which can injure the eyes if protection is not used; and exposure to radiation.
> - *Chemical hazards* include exposure to cytotoxic medications and treatments, such as those used in chemotherapy, and exposure to other chemicals, including cleaning fluids.
> - *Biological hazards* include blood and body fluids contaminated with HIV or hepatitis viruses, exposure to influenza viruses, and exposure to epidemics.

Minimizing Physical Hazards

One of the best ways to prevent physical injuries when lifting and moving anything is to use good posture and **body mechanics,** the movement of muscles of the body for balance and leverage. In addition, a number of devices are available to help move patients safely. It is important that you learn how to use these devices correctly and use them when it is appropriate so that you avoid potential injury. Chapter 16 includes more information on devices for moving patients.

The American Nurses Association developed the Handle With Care program in 2004, which advocates the availability and use of equipment to help move patients safely and reduce the number of nurse injuries. Their goal is that nurses will eventually not need to lift patients manually at all.

While working in a multidisciplinary health-care team, a nurse may encounter workplace violence. Workplace violence includes physical aggression, bullying, sexual harassment, and physical assaults. If this occurs to you as a nurse, it is important to notify the appropriate individuals. There is no need to work in an unsafe environment when caring for patients.

Body Mechanics

Body mechanics involves using the joints and leverage of the body to your advantage, working with what your body is designed to do rather than working against it. Whether you are moving patients or boxes of supplies, certain guidelines still apply. To understand how to use proper body mechanics, you have to understand the location of your **center of gravity.** This is a middle point of the body, below the umbilicus and above the pubis, around which the body's mass is distributed. You also must understand the meaning of the **base of support,** which refers to your feet and lower legs. When you are lifting or moving a heavy object, this gives your body stability and balance. The wider your base of support, the lower your center of gravity. One way to establish a solid base of support is to keep your feet shoulder-width apart.

To use good body mechanics and prevent injury to yourself, follow these guidelines:

- Plan your work carefully. Think through how to do it safely.
- Elevate your work to a comfortable level. Raise the bed so that you do not have to bend over to work, which will cause a strain on your back.
- Keep your feet shoulder-width apart, one foot slightly ahead of the other, when standing for long periods.

- Avoid twisting, which can cause strain or injury to the low back. Turn your whole body or pivot on one foot instead of twisting.
- When lifting heavy objects from a lower level, such as a low shelf or the floor, bend your knees, not your back. Squat to reach the object and keep your back straight as you flex your hip and thigh muscles to stand. In this way, you use the larger muscles of your body to support the load.
- When carrying an object, hold it close to your body with your elbows bent. If the weight is away from your body rather than close, your center of gravity shifts and your balance is affected. This increases the strain on your back muscles and makes you more likely to lose your balance and fall.
- When possible, push, pull, or slide heavy objects rather than lifting them. Push rather than pull if at all possible to prevent extra strain on your back muscles.
- Get help when you need to move or lift a patient. Figure 13.4 shows a safety decision-making chart that can help you decide when assistance is needed.

Skill 13.3 (page 221) provides more information on the proper usage of body mechanics.

Adequate Rest and Appropriate Focus

Fatigue can contribute to conditions that result in injury. If you are exhausted, you may not think as clearly as you would if you were well rested. You are at risk for making an error that could hurt both you and a patient. It is important that you get enough rest to function safely as a nurse. When you are scheduled to work, make it a priority to be rested when you arrive. One reason mandatory overtime is such a major issue for nurses is that it can contribute to unsafe practice due to lack of rest.

Other influences that contribute to unsafe practice and poor decision making include abuse of alcohol, use of prescription medications such as narcotic pain relievers, and use of illegal drugs or prescription drugs in abusive amounts. Nurses have a high rate of drug use and abuse. If you are taking narcotic medications to treat an injury or illness, speak with your instructor before you go to your clinical facility. If you believe you may have a problem with overuse of alcohol or misuse of prescription drugs, speak with an instructor or school counselor to get help. If you suspect that a coworker or staff nurse is impaired, speak confidentially with your instructor so that this person can get help. Peer assistance programs are available to nurses for help with these types of problems. By speaking up, you may help prevent a dangerous situation for patients, for yourself, or for coworkers.

Radiation Hazards

Radiation, the emission of energy in the form of rays, waves, or particles, is used to diagnose and treat some diseases.

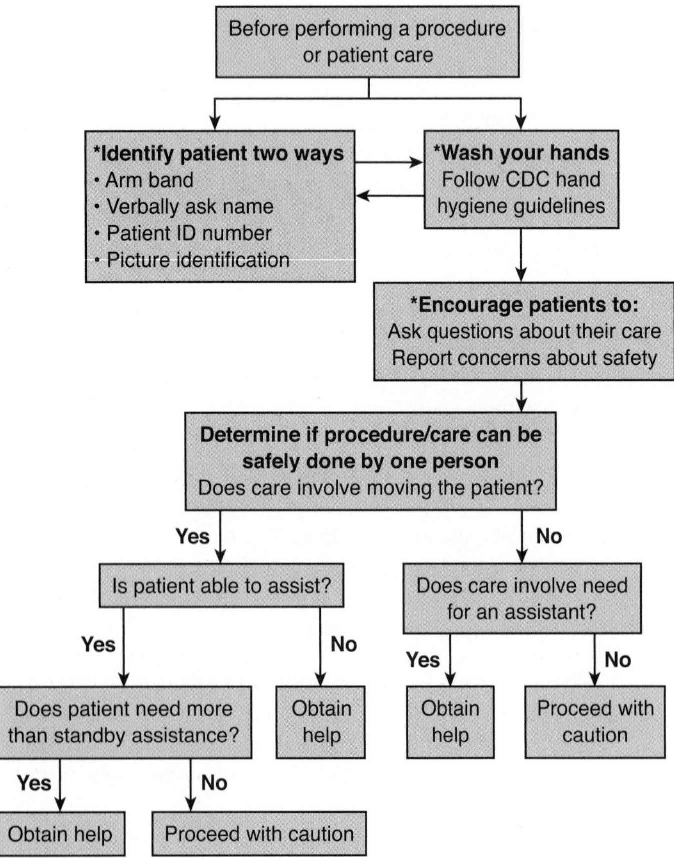

FIGURE 13.4 Safety decision-making chart.

When you care for patients treated with radiation, you may also be exposed. ***Safety: To prevent excessive radiation exposure, wear a lead apron during procedures involving x-rays and fluoroscopy. Wear a film badge if you work in a radiology area on a regular basis.*** This badge measures the amount of radiation to which you have been exposed over a period of time. If you are assigned to care for a patient with internal or implanted radiation, such as that used to treat certain cancers and thyroid conditions, limit the amount of time you spend with these patients to minimize your exposure. If you are pregnant, you should not care for these patients. Follow facility policy for alternative assignments in this situation.

Chemical Hazards

Nurses can be exposed to toxic chemicals when handling IV chemotherapy medications or other medications. Even cleaning supplies can pose hazards, especially if they spill or mix. Any time you use chemicals, you should be aware of the hazards involved. Your facility is required to have a **safety data sheet** (SDS) on file for every chemical, which contains information about potential harm caused by exposure and directions for what to do if the product gets in your eyes, on your skin, or in your mouth. These sheets are available from the manufacturers of chemicals and cleaning products. ***Safety: Know the location of the SDS sheets (usually kept in a notebook) in your facility and be aware of the hazards of the chemicals with which you work.***

Gases are ever present in the health-care environment. Oxygen is generally piped into each patient unit in the hospital. Anesthetic gases are used in the operating suites. It is important to follow safety precautions when you are around gases. No smoking or open flame is allowed in the presence of oxygen. Even static electricity can cause a spark that could ignite a fire or cause an explosion. Although oxygen is not explosive, it supports combustion. A fire burns faster and hotter in the presence of oxygen. Sheets and gowns saturated in oxygen burn very rapidly. If you work in the operating room, you will wear clothing and shoes that do not promote static electricity.

Biological Hazards

Nurses deal with the possibility of exposure to blood and body fluids containing serious, even fatal viruses. The Centers for Disease Control and Prevention (CDC), a federal agency involved in protecting patients and staff from the spread of disease, has developed guidelines to reduce this risk. These guidelines, called standard precautions and transmission-based precautions, help prevent the spread of blood-borne pathogens (see Chapter 14 for more information). ***Safety: Wash your hands before and after all patient contact and wear gloves when any risk of exposure to blood or body fluids is present.***

Needle-stick injuries have been a major route of exposure to hepatitis B and HIV for health-care workers. Safer devices such as needleless access systems, although more costly for facilities, are designed to help decrease the risk of needle-stick injuries. ***Safety: Never recap a used needle, and always use puncture-proof, labeled containers (sharps containers) for disposing of used needles and other sharps.*** Chapters 14, 34, 37, and 38 present more information about safely handling needles and sharps. Always follow CDC guidelines to help protect yourself from biological hazards.

Safety is your responsibility. Be as vigilant about your own safety as you are about the safety of your patients. Anticipate potentially unsafe situations, and take action to prevent them before they happen.

KNOWLEDGE CONNECTION

Give one example of each type of hazard encountered by nursing staff. Explain one way to minimize each hazard you have identified.

Nursing Care Plan for Patients at Risk for Falls

Safety will be a part of the care plan for many of your patients. In this example, we focus strictly on the patient's risk for falls. In many care plans, the risk for falls will be just one of several safety-related nursing diagnoses for the patient.

Assessment

It is extremely important that you recognize safety concerns for each of your patients. One of the most common is that the patient is, or could be, at risk for falling. You cannot tell if this is the case by looking at the patient. Age is not necessarily a predictor for this risk.

Use a fall assessment rating scale or other assessment tool to determine the likelihood of fall risk (see Table 13.1). Follow facility policy for scoring the scale and alerting other staff to the fall danger.

Using a fall assessment rating scale for Mrs. Lloyd, the 82-year-old female patient in the Critical Thinking Connection at the beginning of this chapter, you would identify her as a person at risk for falls because she has fallen previously, has more than one diagnosis, is weak on one side due to a stroke, and is confused at night.

Nursing Diagnoses

In assessing Mrs. Lloyd, we have determined that she is at risk for falls because of her left-sided weakness and confusion. If she does fall again, she could cause injury to her newly repaired hip fracture. The nursing diagnosis given for this patient is "Risk for falls related to left-sided weakness and confusion."

(nursing care plan continues on page 218)

• WORD • BUILDING •

fluoroscopy: fluoro – using fluorescence + scopy – examination

Nursing Care Plan for Patients at Risk for Falls—cont'd

The use of "Risk for injury" is not appropriate as a nursing diagnosis in this situation because "Risk for falls" more correctly describes her problem.

Planning

For Mrs. Lloyd, you need to find ways to prevent her from trying to get out of bed alone. Because of her confusion, left-sided weakness, and recently repaired hip fracture, you must determine interventions that will address these issues. You need some way to know when the patient is attempting to get out of bed. Some possible ways to alert staff to this situation might be:

- Apply a bed/chair monitor or leg monitor that will alarm if the patient tries to get up.
- Post reminders in the patient's room for the patient and family stating that the patient is to call for help before getting up.
- Frequently provide verbal reorientation for the patient.

You also need to enlist the nursing staff in taking extra precautions for this patient's safety. Ideas for additional precautions are:

- Post fall precautions on the door to the patient's room, in the Kardex, and in the patient's chart according to facility policy.
- Answer the patient's call light promptly so that she will not tire of waiting for help and attempt to get up alone.
- Respond to the bed/chair/leg monitor alarms immediately to prevent a fall.
- Assist the patient to ambulate to the chair or the bathroom when needed.
- Do not leave the patient alone while she is in the bathroom or on the bedside commode. Stay nearby to assist the patient back to bed.
- Keep the call light within the patient's reach at all times.
- Keep personal items within reach so that the patient does not injure herself by attempting to retrieve an item.
- Anticipate the patient's needs. Offer to assist her to the bathroom or bedside commode every 2 hours.

In Mrs. Lloyd's situation, your expected outcome is that falls will be prevented. You also want a goal of no further injury occurring to this patient during her hospitalization.

Implementation

You can now implement the interventions that you have planned.

Evaluation

To evaluate the effectiveness of your interventions, ask yourself the following questions:

- Were your interventions effective in preventing further falls?
- Did your patient avoid additional injuries during the rest of her hospitalization?

If the answer to both these questions is "yes," your interventions were successful in accomplishing your goals and outcomes. If you answered "no" to either of these questions, you must determine what went wrong and devise improved interventions for the future (see the care plan below for a summary of the care plan evaluations).

Nursing Diagnosis: Risk for falls related to left-sided weakness and confusion
Expected Outcomes: Patient will be free from injury during hospitalization.

Interventions	Evaluations
Evaluate the patient's fall risk using the Morse Fall Scale (see Table 13.1). Institute fall precautions: • Post fall precautions on the door to the patient's room, in the Kardex, and in the patient's chart according to facility policy.	Day 1: Patient was rated a 75 on the Morse Fall Scale and was identified as a high fall risk. She was placed on fall precautions immediately after admission; signs were posted on her door to indicate this.
• Apply a bed/chair monitor that will alarm if the patient tries to get up. Respond to the monitor alarm immediately to prevent a fall. • Post reminders in the patient's room for the patient and family stating that the patient is to call for help before getting up. • Provide frequent verbal reorientation for the patient. Tell her where she is and what you want her to do. • Keep needed items within her reach.	Day 3: Patient had experienced no falls or other injuries.

Nursing Care Plan for Patients at Risk for Falls—cont'd

Interventions	Evaluations
Provide assistance to the patient to prevent falls: • Answer the patient's call light promptly so that she will not tire of waiting for help and attempt to get up alone. • Assist the patient to ambulate to the chair or the bathroom when needed. Offer toileting assistance every 2 hours. • Do not leave the patient alone while she is in the bathroom or on the bedside commode. Stay nearby to assist the patient back to bed.	Day 1: Patient was on bedrest and used the bed pan. Nursing staff checked on her every 30 minutes, and she did not try to get up alone. Most of the time she would use the call light to ask for assistance, but occasionally she would call out to a staff member walking by her room. Day 2: Patient was able to get up to BR with assistance. She was still weak but was less unsteady on her feet and understood that she was not to get up alone.

Skill 13.1 Using a Bed/Chair or Leg Monitor

Assessment Steps

1. Determine the need for a monitor ***to promote patient safety.*** Follow facility policy regarding the use of monitors.
2. Assess the need for further fall prevention measures. Avoid relying too much on the monitor alone.

Planning Steps

1. Obtain the pad for the bed/chair or the patch for the patient's leg, depending on the type of monitor to be used.
2. Check to be sure the alarm is working correctly ***to prevent relying on faulty equipment.***

Implementation Steps

1. Follow the Initial Implementation Steps located on the inside back cover.
2. **For Bed/Chair Alarm:** Place the pad for the bed/chair alarm beneath the patient's buttocks. ***The pad is pressure sensitive and will alarm if the patient tries to get up or if there is no weight on it for several seconds.***
   For Leg Alarm: Place the sensor patch on the patient's thigh. ***It will alarm when the patient's leg is in a dependent position, indicating that the patient is attempting to stand.***
3. Attach control units to the monitor pads. For the bed/chair alarm, attach the control unit on the bed or the chair. For the leg alarm, attach the control unit directly to the sensor patch. ***The control units must be attached for the monitors to function.***
4. If possible, connect the control unit to the call light. Not all monitors are equipped with this function. However, when this function is in place, staff can respond more quickly because they will ***both hear the alarm and see the call light activated.***
5. Instruct the patient and family to call for assistance if the patient needs to get up. A nursing staff member will assist the patient and deactivate the alarm when needed. ***This reduces the frequency of false alarms.***
6. Disconnect the alarm before assisting the patient out of the bed or chair or before assisting the patient to stand. ***This will prevent the alarm from sounding unnecessarily.***
7. If you assist the patient from the chair to the bed (or vice versa), be sure to move the alarm sensor pad first so that the patient will be sitting or lying on the pad when he or she is in the new location. ***This helps you avoid forgetting to place the sensor pad in the new location.***
8. Reactivate the alarm by reconnecting it to the sensor ***to help prevent falls.***
9. Follow the Ending Implementation Steps located on the inside back cover.

Evaluation Steps

1. Determine the sensitivity of the alarm and adjust it to sound if the patient moves to get up. ***This will alert you as soon as the patient begins to get up.***
2. Check on the patient frequently ***to be certain that the alarm is functioning correctly and that the patient is safe.***

Sample Documentation

06/06/22 1120 Leg monitor applied to left thigh and connected to control unit. Alarm tested. Family and pt instructed to use call light for assistance before getting out of chair. ——————
—————————— Nurse's signature and credentials

Skill 13.2 Applying Restraints

Assessment Steps

1. Assess the patient's response to restraint alternatives and previous attempts to prevent harm. ***This will ensure the restraints are used as a last resort.***
2. Assess the need for restraints. Is the patient a danger to self or others? Are restraints necessary to perform a procedure or maintain tube or monitor placement?
3. Review the health-care provider's order for the type of restraint, indications for use, site of application, and duration of use of restraints. ***This will help you avoid errors when carrying out the orders.***

Planning Steps

1. Obtain the appropriate restraint, ***keeping in mind that the least restrictive restraint to prevent injury is required.***
2. Explain to the patient and family the need for restraint placement and the expected time frame for its use. ***This will encourage patient and family cooperation.***

Intervention Steps

1. Follow the Initial Implementation Steps located on the inside back cover.
2. Place the restraint on the patient. For the ***waist or belt restraint,*** place the restraint around the patient's waist without wrinkles. For the ***vest restraint,*** place the vest on in such a way that the crossover is in the front. For the ***wrist restraint,*** place the padded portion around the wrist snugly enough to prevent it from slipping off, but not tight enough to impair circulation. For the ***mitt restraint,*** place the patient's hand inside the mitt with the fingers slightly flexed. ***Correct placement prevents injury to the patient and increases the effectiveness of the restraint.***

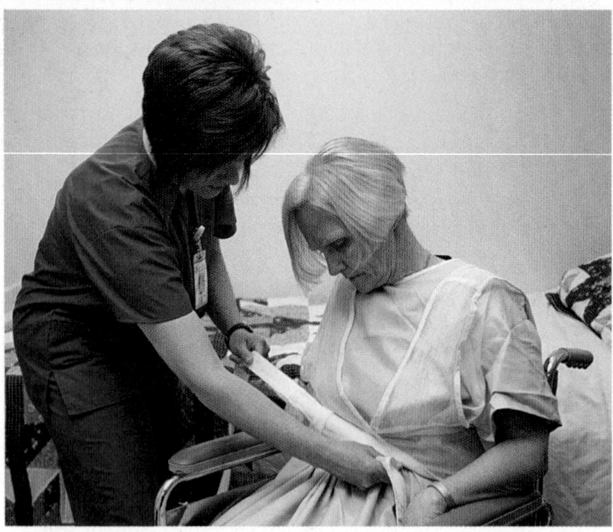

3. Ensure that the restraints are not too tight. You should be able to slide three fingers between the restraint and the patient when the restraint is applied correctly. ***This amount of space prevents injury to the patient while keeping the restraint snug.***
4. Tie the restraint ties to the moveable part of the bed frame using a quick-release knot. A quick-release knot is also called a half-bow knot. This knot will not come loose when the patient moves, but it will release completely when you pull on the loose end. ***This allows you to release the restraints quickly in case of an emergency.***

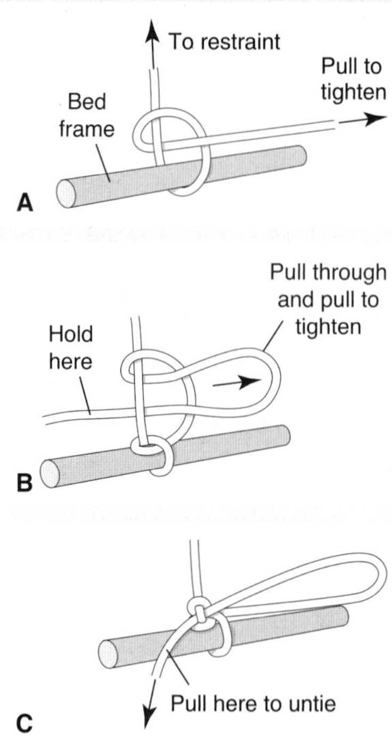

5. **Never tie restraints to side rails.** When restraints are tied to the moveable portion of the bed frame, the patient will not be injured or uncomfortable when the head of the bed is raised. ***Correct placement when tying restraints prevents injury to the patient when the bed position is changed.*** When tying restraints to a wheelchair, cross the ties in the back, then tie them to the frame of the wheelchair ***to prevent the patient from loosening the ties.***

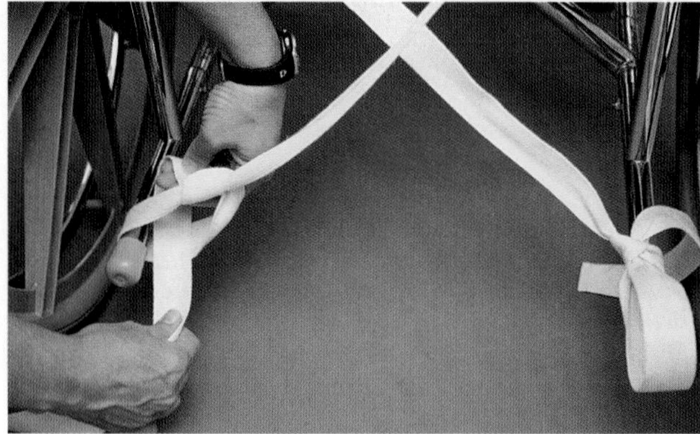

Skill 13.2 (continued)

6. Make any adjustments needed to the restraints ***to prevent discomfort or impaired body alignment.***
7. Assess the patient who is in restraints every 30 minutes ***to ensure that the patient is safe and is not being harmed by the restraint.*** Check the distal pulses if the patient is in a mitt or wrist restraint ***to ensure that circulation is not impaired.*** Assess the skin in the extremity for warmth and color, and investigate any complaints of numbness or tingling ***to ensure that nerves are not being compressed.*** Check the skin beneath the restraint for redness or chafing ***to ensure that skin integrity is not being compromised.***
8. Release the restraints every 2 hours. Assist the patient to the bathroom, offer food and fluids, and give skin care, paying special attention to the skin under the restraints. Perform passive and active range of motion to the restrained extremities. ***This allows the patient to have movement and activity while he or she is not restrained.***
9. Continue to use fall precautions for patients, even when they are restrained, ***to prevent possible injury.***
10. Follow the Ending Implementation Steps located on the inside back cover.

Evaluation Steps

1. Determine the effectiveness of the restraints. Note whether the patient is comfortable and safe with the restraints in place. Check to be sure that the restraints are not causing circulatory impairment or skin breakdown. ***This will help prevent any adverse effects due to the restraints.***
2. Determine the need for continuation of the restraints. Remove the restraints when they are no longer necessary ***to promote the least restrictive environment for your patient.***

Sample Documentation

06/06/22 1510 Right wrist restraint applied per healthcare provider's order to prevent pt from pulling out NG tube and pulling off telemetry electrodes. Remains disoriented to time and place. Right radial pulse strong at 86/min. Hand warm, capillary refill 3 seconds, color pink. Assisted to drink a glass of orange juice. Watching TV with no complaints. ——————

—————— Nurse's signature and credentials

Skill 13.3 Using Body Mechanics

Assessment Steps

1. Determine the best way to move the object. Can you push, pull, or slide, rather than lift it? ***This will help you prevent injury.***
2. If necessary, determine whether you can use a lifting device. If not, determine how much help is required. ***Obtaining assistance or using a lifting device will decrease the chance of injury while moving the patient or object.***

Planning Steps

1. Obtain the necessary lifting equipment if that is what you will use. Obtain assistance from nursing staff ***to prevent injury to yourself and others.***
2. Determine how to use your assistant(s), if needed. Keep the safety of the patient and staff as your focus.

Implementation Steps

To Obtain an Item From a High Shelf

1. Use a step stool or other safe method to comfortably reach the object. ***Trying to reach while you are on tiptoe can cause injury to your back.***
2. Tense your leg and arm muscles as you obtain the item ***to avoid using your back muscles, possibly causing injury.***

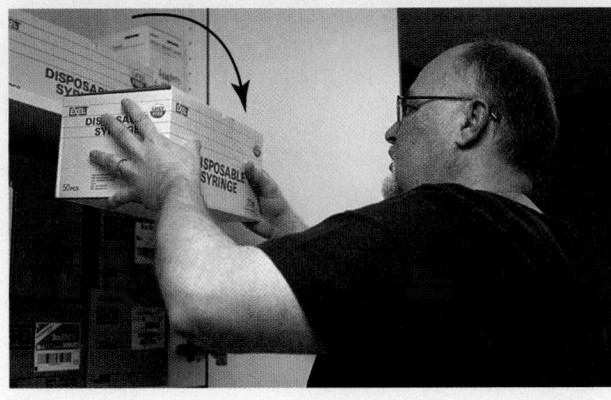

3. Lower the item to waist level for balance.
4. Step down from the stool and carry the object close to your body at waist level with your elbows flexed. ***This position is close to your center of gravity and keeps you balanced.***

To Obtain an Item From a Low Shelf or the Floor

1. Place your feet shoulder-width apart, widening your base of support ***to give you stability.***
2. Flex your hips and knees, keeping your back straight and lowering your center of gravity. Avoid bending at the waist ***because this puts strain on your back muscles.***

(skill continues on page 222)

Skill 13.3 (continued)

3. Lift the item with smooth, coordinated movements. ***Jerky movements increase your chance of accident or injury.***
4. Hold the item close to your body as you straighten your hips and knees. The larger muscles of your legs carry the load, ***which prevents injury to the smaller muscles in your back.***
5. Carry the item close to your body at waist level with your elbows flexed. ***This position is close to your center of gravity and keeps you balanced.***

To Move a Patient Up in Bed

1. Raise the bed to about your waist level ***to prevent strain on your back muscles.***
2. Stand with your feet shoulder-width apart to widen your base of support, ***which gives you stability.***

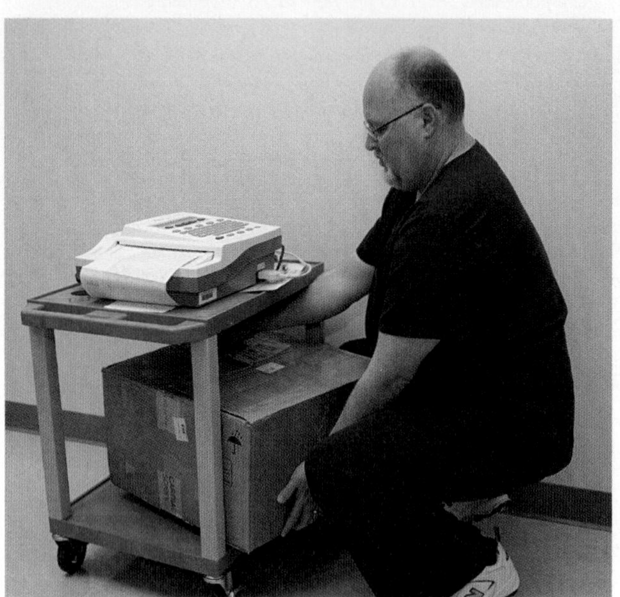

3. Turn your foot that is closest to the head of the bed so that your toes point toward the headboard. ***This helps you face the direction of movement so that you avoid twisting your back.***
4. On the count of 3, shift your weight from your lower foot to your upper foot as you move the patient up in bed. ***This prevents any twisting movements that could injure your back.***
5. Lower the bed to its lowest level ***for patient safety.***

Evaluation Steps

1. Determine the effectiveness of using good posture and good body mechanics. ***The absence of back pain and injuries validates this step.***
2. Determine if you used good decision making by getting help and/or using lift devices when appropriate.

POST CONFERENCE

When you review your care for Mrs. Lloyd, you have mixed emotions. She was not as confused as you thought she might be. She was oriented to person and sometimes to place, but not to time. She recognized her family and learned your name quickly. She remained safe during your care and did not have any more falls, so you feel good about your care. However, the sensor pad for her bed/chair alarm was not always effective. Once when you took her to the bathroom, you forgot to turn it back on when you assisted her back to bed. Her daughter-in-law noticed that the alarm was off and called it to your attention. Fortunately, Mrs. Lloyd did not attempt to get out of bed during that time. It is now easier for you to understand how her earlier fall occurred, but you have also learned the importance of checking and double-checking for safety, even on patients who are being monitored.

Key Points

- National Patient Safety Goals have been established to help decrease injury and harm to patients.
- Many factors can contribute to unsafe patient environments and must be addressed to promote patient safety.
- One of the national goals for patient safety focuses on reducing the risk of patient harm from falls. Many facilities have developed fall assessment rating scales—forms that, when filled out, give a numerical rating for each patient's risk for falls. Restraint alternatives are less restrictive ways to help patients remember not to get up and try to walk or to alert nursing staff that the patient is attempting to do so.
- Several restraint alternatives and strategies exist and can be easily implemented to keep patients safer.
- If the use of restraints is unavoidable, a health-care provider's order must be obtained first. Apply restraints correctly and check on the patient frequently. Release the restraints every 2 hours, allowing the patient to go to the bathroom. Offer food and fluids and check for any signs of skin breakdown or bruising due to the restraints.
- It is extremely important to apply restraints correctly and to tie them with a quick-release knot to prevent patient injury or even possible death.
- If a fire occurs in your area, follow the acronym RACE—**R**escue patients from danger, sound the **A**larm, **C**onfine the fire, and **E**xtinguish the fire if it is small or wait for the fire department if the fire is large.Fires are designated as type A, B, C, D, or K, and fire extinguishers are labeled with these designations. Most fire extinguishers in health-care facilities are combination extinguishers used for the A, B, and C types of fires.
- If you come upon an unresponsive patient, initiate a Code Blue or its equivalent according to your facility's policies and begin CPR or rescue breathing.
- During a mass casualty event, follow your facility's disaster plan and expect to be called in to work extra shifts.
- To use good body mechanics and prevent injury to yourself, you have to understand the location of your center of gravity and base support, which refers to your feet and lower legs.
- If you are exhausted, you may not think as clearly as you would if you were well rested. You are at risk for making an error that could hurt both you and a patient. It is important that you get enough rest to function safely as a nurse.
- Nurses and nursing staff are regularly exposed to physical, chemical, and biological hazards, so it is important to know how to minimize these hazards and protect yourself.

Review Questions

Select the answer that is most appropriate for each of the following questions. Some questions may have more than one correct answer. Select all that apply.

1. Which statement best describes the National Patient Safety Goals?
   1. They emphasize the importance of safe lifting and mandate hospitals to have equipment in place to phase out manual lifting.
   2. They address specific safety problems in the hospital setting and establish requirements for meeting each goal.
   3. They address needle-stick injuries and require hospitals to purchase needleless access devices.
   4. They identify specific communicable diseases and outline transmission-based precautions for each.

2. A newly admitted patient may be at risk for falls. While the patient is in the bathroom changing into a hospital gown, the admitting nurse would be most concerned about:
   1. ordering soft device bolsters for the bed.
   2. arranging for a bed monitor to be placed on the bed.
   3. staying near the bathroom to help the patient back to bed.
   4. determining whether to ask the doctor for an order for restraints.

3. A patient has been restrained to prevent him from pulling out his nasogastric tube. You assign a UAP to check on the patient. What directions will you give?
   1. "Check on him every 30 minutes and release him every 2 hours. Don't forget to document all your checks on the flow sheet."
   2. "Look in on the patient from the doorway every 2 hours. Make sure the tube is still in place."
   3. "Just to be extra careful, check on him every hour and ask if he needs to go to the bathroom."
   4. "Release him from the restraints every 30 minutes and document that you have done so."

4. You walk into a patient's room and find a fire involving the trash can and curtains. What will you do first?
   1. Use the call light to tell the unit clerk to activate a Code Red.
   2. Step into the hall and call for help, announcing a fire in this room.
   3. Use the telephone in the room to notify the fire department using a special code.
   4. Remove the patient from the room to a safer area of the hospital.

5. To use proper body mechanics, you need to be most concerned about:
   1. your center of gravity, your base of support, and using your leg muscles.
   2. obtaining lifting equipment, obtaining assistance, and keeping your feet apart.
   3. your center of support, base of gravity, and the position of your back.
   4. finding ways to avoid lifting and wearing a brace to protect your back.

6. During clinical, you think you see a staff nurse swallow a narcotic medicine she signed out for a patient. What will you do?
   1. Ask the staff nurse if she just swallowed that pill.
   2. Say nothing and watch the nurse to see if she acts different later.
   3. Tell a fellow student at break so you can both watch the nurse.
   4. Confidentially tell your instructor what you thought you saw.

7. While rinsing a used surgical instrument in a disinfectant called Cidex, some of the Cidex splashes on your lips and nose. Your first action is to:
   1. rinse your mouth and nose immediately with running water.
   2. consult the SDS for Cidex to know what actions to take.
   3. induce vomiting in case you accidentally swallowed any of the chemical.
   4. wash the area immediately with surgical soap and water.

ANSWERS 1. 2, 2. 3, 3. 1, 4. 4, 5. 1, 6. 4, 7. 2

Critical Thinking Exercises

Answers available online.

1. A CNA that you supervise is consistently slow in answering patients' call lights. How will you emphasize safety when discussing this with him?

2. A mass casualty event has occurred in your area. You determine that your family is safe. What actions will you now take?

3. A patient falls when trying to get out of bed alone. You are to investigate possible causes for the fall. How will you go about your investigation?

Additional Resources

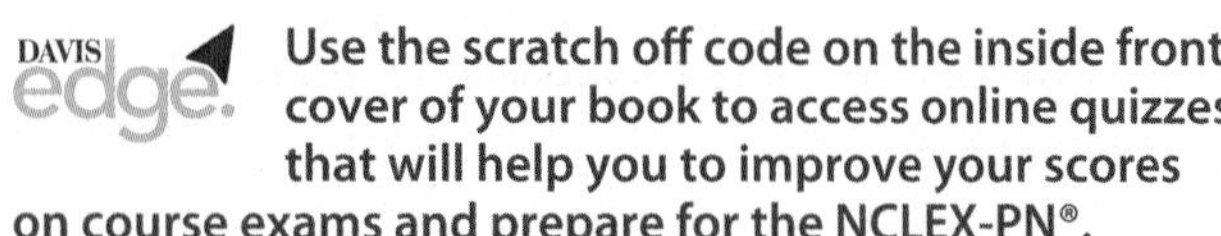

Use the scratch off code on the inside front cover of your book to access online quizzes that will help you to improve your scores on course exams and prepare for the NCLEX-PN®.

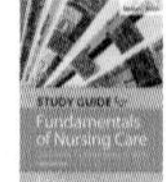

Study Guide

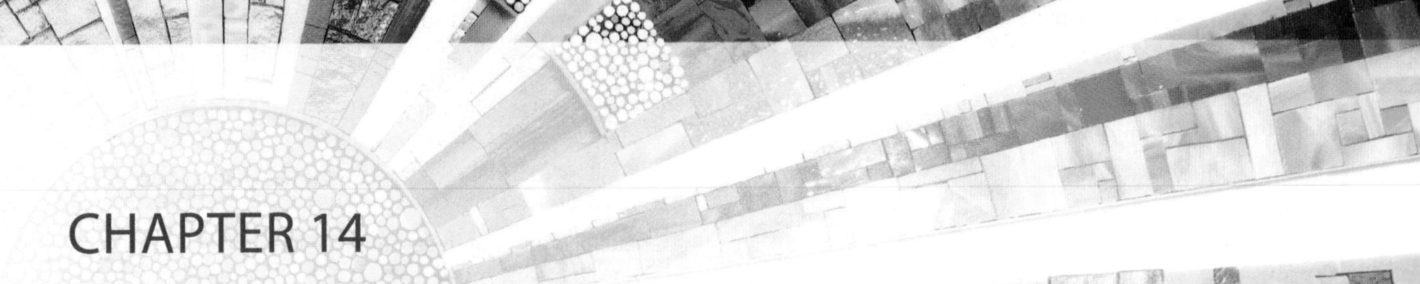

CHAPTER 14
Medical Asepsis and Infection Control

KEY TERMS

Chain of infection (CHAYN uv in-FEK-shun)
Direct contact (dih-REKT KON-takt)
Disinfectant (DISS-in-FEK-tent)
Health care–associated infection (HELLTH-KARE-a-SOH-see-ayt-ed in-FEK-shun)
Indirect contact (IN-dih-rekt KON-takt)
Localized infection (LOH-kuh-LYEZD in-FEK-shun)
Medical asepsis (MED-ih-kuhl ay-SEP-siss)
Microorganism (MY-kroh-OR-gan-izm)
Normal flora and fauna (NOR-mal FLOR-ah and FON-ah)
Pathogen (PATH-oh-jen)
Primary infection (PRY-mare-ee in-FEK-shun)
Secondary infection (SEK-un-DARE-ee in-FEK-shun)
Standard precautions (STAN-derd prih-KAW-shuns)
Systemic infection (sis-TEM-ik in-FEK-shun)
Transmission-based precautions (trans-MIH-shun BAYST prih-KAW-shuns)
Vector (VEK-tur)

CHAPTER CONCEPTS

Infection
Safety
Immunity
Patient-Centered Care

LEARNING OUTCOMES

1. Define various terms related to medical asepsis and infection control.
2. Describe five types of pathogens.
3. Identify selected common illnesses caused by microbes.
4. Illustrate the chain of infection.
5. Differentiate types of infections.
6. Compare primary, secondary, and tertiary defenses against infection.
7. Explain factors that decrease the body's defenses.
8. Differentiate between the use of standard precautions and transmission-based precautions.
9. Compare the purposes and types of transmission-based precautions.
10. Compare medical and surgical asepsis.
11. Explain nursing responsibilities for cleaning the environment and equipment.
12. Describe when and how to use hand hygiene.
13. Detail the use of standard precautions.
14. Explain ways to meet the emotional needs of patients who are isolated because of communicable disease.
15. Discuss information in the Connection features in the chapter.
16. Identify safety issues related to medical asepsis and infection control.
17. Answer questions about performing the skills in this chapter.

SKILLS

14.1 Performing Hand Hygiene
14.2 Donning Personal Protective Equipment
14.3 Removing Personal Protective Equipment

CRITICAL THINKING CONNECTION

Clinical Assignment

You are assigned to care for a 38-year-old male patient who has an infection caused by methicillin-resistant *Staphylococcus aureus* (MRSA). You know this is a highly contagious infection that is resistant to many antibiotics. It frightens you to care for this patient

Continued

CRITICAL THINKING CONNECTION—cont'd

because you are worried that you might catch the infection or take the microorganism home to your children.

Critical Thinking Questions:

1. What is MRSA?
2. What precautions would you utilize before entering the patient's room?
3. What treatment will you expect to be ordered for this patient?

When you work in a hospital as a student or as a staff nurse, you are surrounded by some virulent germs. This can be very alarming if you do not understand the causes of infection or do not know how to protect yourself and your patients from disease-causing microorganisms. In this chapter, you will learn how to protect yourself as well as how to prevent the spread of disease-causing germs to other patients or your family.

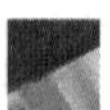

CAUSES OF INFECTION

Infections are caused by a variety of **microorganisms.** These are minuscule living bodies that cannot be seen without a microscope. Microorganisms that cause infection in humans are referred to as **pathogens.** They reproduce rapidly and can spread from one area of a person's body to another. Not all microorganisms are pathogenic, however. Many microorganisms live in and on our bodies, performing needed functions to protect us from harmful pathogens as well as helping us break down and digest food. These microorganisms are referred to as **normal flora and fauna,** which means the tiny plants and animals normally found in the human body.

Types of Pathogens

Pathogenic microorganisms are classified as bacteria, viruses, protozoa, fungi, or helminths.

Bacteria

Bacteria are one-celled microorganisms found virtually everywhere, including in the human body. It is only when they invade an area outside their normal location that problems result. For example, several bacteria live in the intestines to help the body digest food and absorb vitamins. They belong there. However, if those particular bacteria are introduced into the urethra and migrate to the bladder, they will cause a urinary tract infection.

Laboratory and Diagnostic Connection

Identifying Bacteria in the Laboratory

Bacteria are named and classified by their shape. A specimen of drainage, sputum, stool, urine, or blood is obtained and sent to the laboratory. When the specimen is examined under a microscope, the medical laboratory technologist identifies the bacterium by its shape (Fig. 14.1).

Cocci (*singular* coccus) are sphere-shaped bacteria. Sometimes they may be seen in clusters and are similar to grapes in appearance. These are known as *staphylococci.* They may also appear in chains, like a bead necklace, and are then referred to as *streptococci.* Or they may appear in pairs, like two balls side by side, which are described as *diplococci.* Bacilli (*singular* bacillus) are rod-shaped bacteria. They have a log-like appearance and may vary in length. Spirilla (*singular* spirillum) are long cells that spiral or coil, similar to a curl of long hair.

Another step in identifying which coccus, bacillus, or spirillum is under the microscope involves using a dark purple stain called a Gram stain. The slide containing the microorganism is flooded with Gram stain and then rinsed with alcohol. It is counterstained with safranin and then rinsed with water. When the slide is viewed under the microscope again, the bacteria will have taken up the stain. Those that appear either purple or blue are known as gram-positive organisms. Those that appear pink or red are identified as gram-negative organisms. The amount and type of stain the bacterium retains is dependent on the composition of its cell wall. Different medications are most effective for different types of organisms and are prescribed based on their Gram stain response.

Rickettsia are type of bacteria, but they are different from most because they can only reproduce inside the cells of the host, similar to the way viruses must reproduce. Rickettsia are often spread through the bites of insects, such as ticks and mites, which are called **vectors.** The insects are carriers of the microorganisms, and when they bite a human, the human becomes ill due to infection from the rickettsia bacteria.

Antibiotics are prescribed to treat infections caused by bacteria. There are many types of antibiotics, and each acts in a slightly different way to kill bacteria. (For more information about antibiotics and their actions, see Chapter 35.) It is important to note that antibiotics are effective against bacteria only, not against any other type of microorganisms.

Viruses

Viruses are not made up of individual cells; rather, they are very tiny parasites that live within the cells of the host and reproduce there. They can only be seen with an electron microscope because they are too small to be visualized with a standard microscope. Unlike bacteria, viruses are not endemic to the human body, and all viruses potentially cause illness.

Few antiviral medications exist at this time, and their development is targeted on the viruses that cause the most severe

• **WORD • BUILDING •**

microorganism: micro – small + organism – life form

pathogen: patho – disease + gen – producer

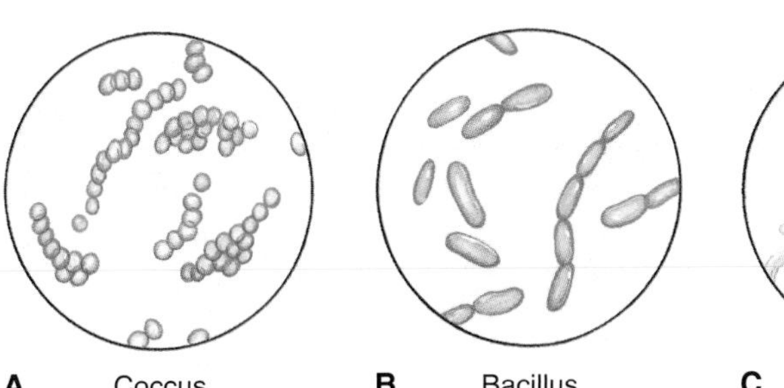

FIGURE 14.1 Bacteria identified by shapes (magnification × 2,000) (from Scanlon V, Sanders T. *Essentials of Anatomy and Physiology*. 7th ed. Philadelphia, PA: FA Davis; 2015).

illnesses. Many viral infections are mild and self-limiting, meaning they will resolve in time without medication. Some individuals, when they are ill and seek medical attention, become upset if a health-care provider does not prescribe antibiotics. However, antibiotics would not be effective against a virus. Sometimes prescribers will order antibiotics to prevent a secondary infection from occurring, but that is not necessary with every viral illness.

Protozoa

Protozoa are single-celled animals that live in water. They can be ingested by humans through water or food, and, when that occurs, protozoa cause intestinal illnesses. Some protozoa are parasites that remain in the digestive tract. They are treated with antiparasitic drugs. Other illnesses are treated with anti-infectives specific for the causative protozoan.

Fungi

Fungi may be made up of one or more cells. Not all fungi require a microscope to be seen. For example, mold on bread and mushrooms growing in the yard are both examples of fungi. Although fungi are present in the environment, they cause illness when they enter the human body through cuts or cracks in the skin. In immunosuppressed individuals, a fungal infection can become systemic, spreading throughout the entire body. Fungal infections are treated with antifungal medications available in creams, ointments, and oral and IV forms.

Helminths

Helminths are parasitic worms that can inhabit the digestive tract of humans. Some worms enter the body through the mouth, often through contaminated food. Once in the intestine, the worms may attach to the intestinal wall and absorb digested food, growing to great lengths. Other types of worms, such as pinworms, inhabit the intestines and lay eggs around the anus. The person feels intense itching in the anal area, and when he or she scratches, the eggs lodge beneath the fingernails, making it easy to spread them to others or to self-reinfect if the hands are then around the person's mouth. These worms only grow to be about ½-inch long, but they can be very numerous—to the point that they can fill up the appendix and mimic appendicitis. Helminth infestations are treated with medication, known as anthelmintics or antihelmintics, designed to kill the specific parasitic worm.

> **KNOWLEDGE CONNECTION**
> List three types of bacteria. How are viruses different from other microorganisms? Give examples of visible fungi.

Common Illnesses Caused by Microbes

Perhaps you have seen or experienced infection by some of these microorganisms. Table 14.1 provides a summary of some of the most common illnesses caused by these types of microorganisms.

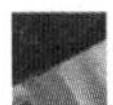

CHAIN OF INFECTION

In order for infection to spread from one person to another, a chain of events must occur. This chain of events is often referred to as the **chain of infection** (Fig. 14.2) and involves the following "links":

- An *infectious agent,* or causative organism
- A *reservoir,* or place the organism grows
- A *portal of exit,* or method by which the organism leaves the reservoir
- A *mode of transmission,* or vehicle by which the organism is transferred
- A *portal of entry,* or method by which the organism enters a new host
- A *susceptible host,* or person whose body the organism has entered

The following example will help you understand the chain of infection: A busy nurse is caring for eight patients in a hospital unit. It is a hectic day with many problems. The nurse assists the certified nursing assistant (CNA) in changing the linens in the room of Patient 1, who is hospitalized with severe diarrhea due to an infection caused by *Clostridium difficile.* The nurse wears gloves during this procedure but is unaware of a tiny hole in the finger of one glove. After the procedure, the nurse neglects to wash his hands but does use alcohol-based hand gel as he leaves the room. He then prepares oral medications for Patient 2 and

• **WORD** • **BUILDING** •
septicemia: septic – putrefying + emia – blood

Table 14.1
Common Diseases Caused by Microorganisms

Microorganism	*Disease*	*Treatment*
Bacteria		
Staphylococcus aureus	Boils, toxic shock syndrome, osteomyelitis, and MRSA, both HA and CA forms	Antibiotics, although most strains are not killed by penicillin; HA-MRSA is resistant to many antibiotics and is treated with selected IV antibiotics.
Streptococcus group A (gram-positive coccus)	Strep throat, ear infections, scarlet fever, and endocarditis; can lead to rheumatic fever, heart valve damage, transient kidney damage "Flesh-eating strep" is a rare strain causing necrotizing fasciitis that can lead to death	Antibiotics
Streptococcus group B (gram-positive coccus)	Neonatal infections, especially in premature births, causing pneumonia, meningitis, or septicemia in newborns	IV antibiotics
Clostridium perfringens (gram-positive bacillus; spore forming)	Gas gangrene in contaminated wounds—spores live in dead tissue and produce toxins that destroy more tissue, so bacteria spreads; gas forms bubbles in the dead tissue	Amputation of affected limb
Clostridium difficile (gram-positive bacillus; spore forming)	Severe diarrhea; often develops with antibiotic therapy and is called pseudomembranous enterocolitis; this is a significant nosocomial pathogen	Few antibiotics are used to treat this: vancomycin and metronidazole are two used often
Escherichia coli (gram-negative bacillus)	Normally found in the colon but can cause infection if it enters the urinary tract or other parts of the body; common cause of nosocomial infections	Antibiotics
Escherichia coli 0157:H7 (gram-negative bacillus)	Infection of colon causing bloody diarrhea and kidney failure, known as hemolytic uremic "syndrome"; can be fatal; often results from consuming undercooked ground meat	Antibiotics, dialysis for kidney failure
Mycobacterium tuberculosis (bacillus)	Tuberculosis that destroys lung tissue, leaving large cavities; drug-resistant strains are becoming more common	Antituberculosis medications
Borrelia burgdorferi (spirochete)	Lyme disease; spirochete transmitted by deer tick to human, causing flu-like symptoms, irregular heartbeat, and possible arthritis	Antibiotics
Rickettsia rickettsii (bacillus)	Rocky Mountain spotted fever spread by ticks; causes high fever, rash, and pneumonia and can lead to death	Antibiotics
Viruses		
Herpes simplex	Type 1 causes fever blisters; type 2 causes genital herpes	Antivirals such as acyclovir
Herpesvirus 3 (varicella-zoster)	Chickenpox is contracted first, and then the virus lies dormant in nerve endings; if reactivated in adults, it causes shingles that results in painful blisters along nerve pathways	Antiviral: acyclovir

Table 14.1
Common Diseases Caused by Microorganisms—cont'd

Microorganism	*Disease*	*Treatment*
Influenza	"Flu" symptoms—aching muscles, fever, respiratory congestion, cough	Antivirals such as Tamiflu and Relenza Prevention: annual flu immunization
Zika	Virus spread by Aedes mosquitoes. Once a person is infected, transmission can be spread from mother to unborn infant through sex Symptoms include fever, headache, joint pain, and muscle aches	Antipyretics, NSAIDS, and fluids
Ebola	Virus is transmitted through infected blood, body fluids, and large droplet respiratory secretions Symptoms include diarrhea, vomiting, fever, severe headache, fatigue, and muscle weakness	Provide IV fluids and electrolytes, and maintain oxygen saturation
West Nile	Virus found in birds and spread by mosquitos; causes headache and confusion in some but may be asymptomatic in others	No antiviral exists—provide supportive treatment
Fungi		
Microsporum epidermophyton	Ringworm, also known as tinea; can be found on the skin or scalp; causes itchy red, round patches Athlete's foot also caused by this fungus	Antifungals
Candida albicans	Yeast infections; called thrush when found in the mouth; often found in the vagina and may result because antibiotics kill normal bacteria, allowing an overgrowth of yeast; can cause pneumonia and heart infections	Antifungals
Protozoans		
Entamoeba histolytica	Amoebic dysentery, causes severe bloody diarrhea and can cause abscesses in body organs such as the liver, lungs, and brain	Amebicides and antibiotics
Giardia lamblia	Giardiasis, which causes diarrhea; often found in water but also may be spread through food prepared by people who have a mild case of the illness	Antibiotics
Plasmodium	Malaria; causes destruction of red blood cells and anemia; can lead to a severe form that affects the brain	Antimalarials
Helminths		
Enterobius	Pinworms; look like white threads and grow in the intestine; most common parasitic worm in the United States	Antihelmintics
Taenia	Tapeworm; may enter humans through undercooked meat containing the worm cysts; head of worm attaches to wall of intestines with suckers and grows in segments; causes bloating, constipation, or diarrhea	Antihelmintics

Source: Adapted from Scanlon V, Sanders T. *Essentials of Anatomy and Physiology.* 7th ed. Philadelphia, PA: FA Davis; 2015.

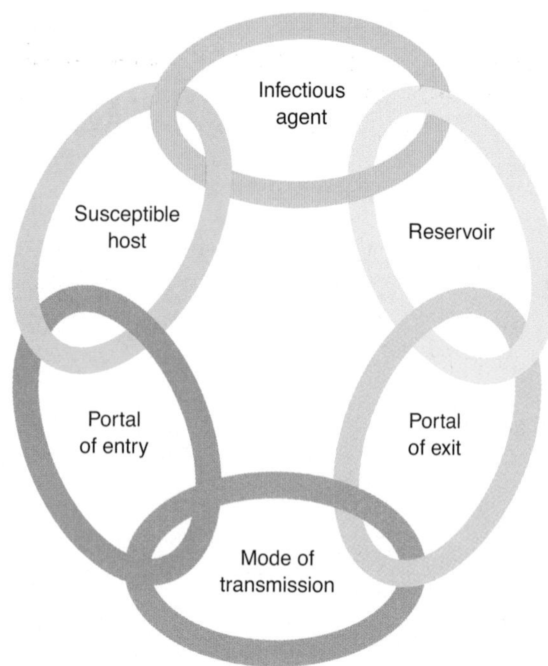

FIGURE 14.2 The links in the chain of infection, which all must be present for infection to spread (from Wilkinson JM, Treas LS. *Fundamentals of Nursing: Theory, Concepts & Applications*. Vol. 1. 3rd ed. Philadelphia, PA: FA Davis; 2016).

delivers them to the room. Patient 2 swallows the medications and later develops a *C difficile* infection as well.

In this example, the chain of infection occurred in this manner:

- **Infectious agent:** *C difficile*
- **Reservoir:** Patient 1
- **Portal of exit:** bowel movement of Patient 1
- **Mode of transmission:** nurse's hands, because this organism is not killed by alcohol-based hand gel
- **Portal of entry:** Patient 2's mouth
- **Susceptible host:** Patient 2

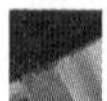 TYPES OF INFECTION

The example given above is an illustration of the chain of infection, but it is also an example of a **health care–associated infection** (HAI), which is an infection that is acquired while the patient is being cared for in any health-care setting, including home health care and long-term care. The former term for these types of infections was *nosocomial infections,* but they are now referred to as HAIs. The single most important way to break the chain of infection and to prevent HAIs is to perform hand hygiene (see Skill 14.1, page 241). Infections may be **primary infections** (initial infections caused by one pathogen only) or **secondary infections** (caused by a second, different pathogen). If a person has an infection in one area of the body (for example, in the lungs), it is described as a **localized infection.** If the infection then spreads from the lungs to other organs, it becomes a **systemic infection,** spreading through the bloodstream. When microorganisms are present and multiplying in the blood, it is referred to as *septicemia.* This condition is extremely serious, requiring aggressive treatment with IV antibiotics and support for the patient's inundated immune system. Infections may start as one type and then progress to another type. This does not mean that the causative organism changes but that the type of infection progresses to become more severe.

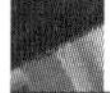 DEFENSES AGAINST INFECTION

The human body is designed to defend against invading pathogens. In fact, three "lines of defense" exist to help thwart infection. Most of us would suffer constantly with infections without this three-layer defense system, referred to as primary, secondary, and tertiary defenses.

Primary Defenses

The primary defenses include body systems, or portions of them, that block or trap invading pathogens.

- **Skin:** Intact skin protects the body from microbes that would cause disease in subcutaneous or deeper tissue. When breaks in the skin occur, such as cuts, scrapes, and burns, the resulting opening is a portal of entry for pathogens.
- **Mucous membranes:** These membranes produce sticky mucus that traps invading pathogens. In the respiratory tract, the mucus may be coughed up and expectorated or blown out of the nose, taking microorganisms with it.

  In the urinary tract, the urethra secretes mucus to trap pathogens that could enter the body through the urinary meatus. Then, the acidic urine washes the pathogens out of the body.

  In the vagina, mucus traps pathogens, preventing them from migrating into the uterus. The pH of vaginal secretions, along with the normal bacteria present in the vagina, are hostile to most microorganisms.
- **Gastrointestinal system:** The mouth provides entry into the gastrointestinal system and contains some bacteria. Saliva contains enzymes that help remove microorganisms from the teeth. Normal flora helps prevent invasion by pathogens.

  If any pathogens make it to the stomach, the strong hydrochloric acid found in digestive juices often kills them. Pathogens that enter the intestines, perhaps through food, meet with bile that breaks down and emulsifies fats, as well as killing microbes.

Secondary Defenses

The second line of defense occurs at the cellular level in reaction to toxins secreted by invading pathogens.

- **Inflammatory process:** This process is discussed in detail in Chapter 26, but a brief description is provided

• WORD • BUILDING •
tertiary: terti – third + ary – related to

here. When an injury occurs, the white blood cells release histamine and other chemicals that cause the blood vessels near the injury to dilate. This dilation results in redness and warmth in the area of injury. The blood vessels also become more permeable to allow an increased number of white blood cells, or *phagocytes,* into the injured area. These phagocytes surround the invading pathogens and consume them.
- **Elevated temperature:** The body responds to invading pathogens by creating an environment that is hostile to them. The increase of body temperature to 101°F or higher is too warm for most invading microorganisms to live and multiply. Certain microbes may take protection in spore form, but many will be killed.
- **Complement cascade:** When invading pathogens are detected in the body, complement is released. *Complement* is a group of specialized proteins that attack the pathogens by releasing chemicals that make their cell membranes rupture.

Tertiary Defenses

The third line of defense involves specialized white blood cells called *lymphocytes* that fight infection, either as B cells or T cells. These lymphocytes are found in lymph tissue, such as the spleen, thymus, lymph nodes, and tonsils. They also are circulating in the blood, searching for invading pathogens, which they identify by their surface proteins. When pathogens are found, the B and T cells signal phagocytes to destroy the invaders. The B and T cells have a major role in the antigen–antibody response.

Factors That Decrease Defenses

Have you ever noticed that you become ill more easily when you are tired and stressed? When the body is not healthy, well nourished, and well rested, the three lines of defense cannot function effectively. Box 14.1 describes factors that decrease the body's defenses against infection.

KNOWLEDGE CONNECTION

List the links in the chain of infection. What are three components of primary defenses? What are three components of secondary defenses?

PREVENTING INFECTION

When you care for patients, it is very important to be aware of the potential for spreading infection. It is your responsibility to prevent the possibility of becoming a mode of transmission in the chain of infection, spreading microorganisms from patient to patient. It is just as important that you know how to prevent infection from spreading from a patient to you.

Box 14.1

Factors That Affect the Body's Defenses Against Infection

Many factors can influence the body's ability to defend itself against infection. They include the following:
- **Age:** The immune systems of infants and young children are not yet well developed and cannot assist with defense against infection as well as the immune systems of older children and adults. In elderly individuals, the immune system gradually decreases in effectiveness, leaving them more vulnerable to invading pathogens.
- **Chemical Exposure:** Toxicity from chemicals impairs the body's defenses and ability to fight infection.
- **Chronic Illness:** The body's defenses are responding on a frequent basis to chronic illness and have no reserves to react effectively to a new infection.
- **Lack of Exercise:** Without adequate exercise, circulation slows and the flow of lymph and phagocytes decreases, interfering with their ability to destroy invading pathogens.
- **Lack of Rest:** The body needs adequate rest to repair damage and restore energy. Lack of rest increases the chance of infection occurring because the immune system cannot repair itself and function at its highest capacity.
- **Increased Stress:** When the body is frequently reacting to stressors, immune function can be impaired, which increases the risk of illness and infection (see Chapter 7).
- **Nonintact Skin:** Open wounds, such as surgical wounds, skin tears, and pressure ulcers, provide a portal of entry for microorganisms.
- **Poor Nutrition:** A diet that is lacking in fruits, vegetables, and certain dairy products negatively affects the body's defenses because it lacks vitamins and support for normal flora.

It is the responsibility of all health-care workers to be vigilant about breaking the chain of infection. ***Safety: The most effective way to break the chain of infection is to use appropriate hand hygiene.*** The Centers for Medicare and Medicaid Services have now ceased to pay for any costs related to three common HAIs. These include catheter-associated urinary tract infections due to a urinary catheter inserted during hospitalization, infections in the blood due to central line-associated bloodstream infections, and infection in the chest incision after open heart surgery. When you use appropriate precautions and good techniques, you will not contribute to HAIs.

Settings Connection: Home Health

Preventing Infection

With the rise in patients being cared for in a home health-care setting due to the aging population, it is important to maintain aseptic technique when treating patients. Patients today come home with central lines, ventilators, and IV antibiotics to continue treatment begun in the hospital. In addition, patients may return home but still require complicated wound care. You want to teach patients, families, and caregivers to maintain aseptic techniques when caring for a patient, including hand hygiene and the disposal of contaminated dressings, needles, and syringes. In the home setting, we do not always follow sterile techniques. For example, a person who does self-catheterization can clean and reuse rubber catheters in the home. It is important to make sure everything is clean, but it does not always have to be sterile in the home setting.

Precautions for Preventing the Transmission of Pathogens

The Centers for Disease Control and Prevention (CDC) is a government agency within the U.S. Department of Health and Human Services that is responsible for tracking, regulating, and educating about public health issues. In order to protect patients and health-care workers from the spread of pathogens in health-care settings, the CDC has developed precautions to be used during patient care. These precautions include both standard precautions, to be used in the care of all patients in all health-care settings, and transmission-based precautions, to be used when caring for patients with communicable diseases.

Standard precautions are a group of safety measures performed to prevent the transmission of pathogens found in the blood and body fluids. This includes performing hand hygiene, wearing appropriate protective equipment if exposure is possible, and using cough etiquette. Standard precautions are performed with all patients, whether or not an infection has been diagnosed. They protect the health-care worker from the possible transmission of illnesses spread through contact with infected blood, such as hepatitis B, hepatitis C, and HIV. They also protect patients from the possible spread of pathogens from one patient to another. Further details for following standard precautions will be discussed later in this section. Table 14.2 provides information on personal protective equipment (PPE) needed in standard precautions.

Transmission-based precautions are used to prevent the spread of known infection to patients or health-care staff. They are used when a patient has a communicable illness that can be spread through contact, through respiratory droplets, or through the air. Gowns, gloves, masks, eye protection, and possibly head covers are used to prevent transmission of pathogens. Further details for following transmission-based precautions will be provided later in this section.

Medical Asepsis

The term **medical asepsis** refers to practices performed to prevent the spread of infection. It is also sometimes described as using "clean technique." These practices, or techniques, include performing hand hygiene, maintaining a clean patient environment, using standard precautions, and using transmission-based precautions when necessary.

Medical asepsis is different than *surgical asepsis*, which refers to maintaining a sterile environment such as that found in operating rooms. *Sterile technique* means performing procedures in such a way that no pathogens will enter the patient's body when you insert tubes or give injections. You will learn about surgical asepsis and sterile technique in Chapter 22.

The following is an example of a nurse using medical asepsis: The nurse enters a patient's room to assist a patient who has used the bedside commode. The nurse washes his or her hands, puts on clean gloves, assists the patient in cleaning the genital area and then assists the patient into bed. The nurse then empties, rinses, and replaces the pan of the bedside commode. The nurse removes the gloves and washes his or her hands.

In this example, the nurse uses medical asepsis to protect himself or herself by performing hand hygiene frequently and wearing clean gloves, keeps the environment clean by emptying the bedside commode immediately, and protects the patient from possible infection by cleaning the genital area.

Clean Environment and Equipment

Maintaining a clean environment coincides with maintaining a safe environment for your patients. Clean up spills as soon as they occur for safety as well as to eliminate a breeding ground for bacteria. Wipe off dirty, dusty surfaces to decrease the possibility of microbial growth. Remove uneaten food from patient rooms to prevent possible growth of microorganisms that can cause illness.

When you clean surfaces in a health-care setting, you will use a **disinfectant** cleaning agent, which will remove most pathogens. Some viruses and spore-forming bacteria are not killed by disinfection, however. Sterilization removes all pathogens using steam under pressure, heat, gas, or chemicals. It is discussed further in Chapter 22.

After you use equipment for one patient that can be reused for another patient (for example, an IV pump), it is very important that you disinfect the equipment according to facility policy. If blood remains on a surface, even though the blood has dried, some viruses can still be present. Hepatitis B can live for up to 7 days on surfaces outside the body. In most cases, you will clean equipment after it is used and then send it to the central supply area of the hospital. It will be completely disinfected or sterilized there and made ready for use by the next patient.

• **WORD • BUILDING** •

communicable: communic – share + able – able to be
asepsis: a – without + sepsis – putrefaction

Table 14.2
Standard Precautions for the Care of All Patients in All Health-Care Settings

Component	*Use*
Hand Hygiene	Wash hands for 20 seconds using soap and water or use antibacterial hand gel unless hands are visibly soiled Avoid using hand gel if caring for a patient with illness caused by spore-forming microorganisms
Personal Protective Equipment	
Gloves	Wear when touching blood, body fluids, secretions, or items contaminated with them Wear for touching patient's mucous membranes and nonintact skin
Gown	Wear when performing procedures and patient care if there is a possibility of your exposed skin or clothing coming in contact with blood, body fluids, secretions, or excretions
Mask, eye protection, face shield	Wear during patient care procedures that could cause splashing of blood, body fluids, or secretions, such as suctioning and endotracheal intubation
Needles and Other "Sharps" (anything that could puncture a trash can liner)	Never recap a used needle, do not bend or break needles, and use safety needles whenever possible; place all used sharps in a puncture-resistant sharps container
Respiratory Hygiene/Cough Etiquette	Cover your mouth and nose with a tissue when sneezing or coughing; if tissue is unavailable, cough into your upper sleeve, not your hand, and use hand hygiene immediately after coughing or sneezing Any person entering a health-care facility with a cough, congestion, or increased respiratory secretions is to follow these recommendations

Real-World Connection

Who Is Responsible for Maintaining a Clean Patient Environment?

A nursing instructor noticed a smell in a patient room where two nursing students were caring for a debilitated patient. When she asked about it, the students replied that the patient had just used the bedside commode. The instructor told them to get some air freshener from the housekeeper's cart and use it in the room. Several hours later, the instructor returned and still noticed the smell. When she questioned the students again, they explained, "Housekeeping still has not come to empty the bedside commode." The instructor noted that this is a nursing task, not a housekeeping task. It is your responsibility to keep your patient's environment clean and free from potential pathogens.

Hand Hygiene

Nurses wash their hands repeatedly during patient care. You may not realize that there are correct and incorrect ways to perform hand hygiene. The way you are accustomed to washing your hands at home may not be the correct way to wash your hands in a health-care setting. Sometimes students even feel a bit insulted that they are expected to demonstrate a skill as basic as handwashing. However, it is extremely important to be sure that all surfaces of the hands are cleaned thoroughly to dislodge and wash away all pathogens. When you care for patients, you should avoid wearing multiple rings on your hands. Many dress codes call for only one ring, such as a wedding band, and do not allow others. When you perform hand hygiene, it is important that you clean around your ring. It is possible for microorganisms to be present in and around the sets of your rings. Skill 14.1 details the steps of hand hygiene.

WHEN TO PERFORM HAND HYGIENE. When working in a health-care setting, the possibility of spreading pathogens on your hands is great. It is one of the most common methods of transmission in the chain of infection, so it is important to wash your hands in the following situations:

- After touching blood, body fluids, secretions, excretions, or contaminated items
- Immediately after removing gloves
- Upon entering a patient's room
- Before touching the patient or tubes connected to the patient
- Between caring for two patients in the same room
- When arriving on the nursing unit
- After returning to the nursing unit from breaks or meals
- After using the restroom
- Any time your hands are visibly dirty

HAND HYGIENE GUIDELINES. In the hand hygiene guidelines from the CDC, the use of alcohol-based hand gels for cleaning

Box 14.2

Additional Information on WHO Guidelines for Hand Hygiene in Health Care

In addition to the CDC, the WHO has made recommendations regarding hand hygiene in health care. Because the WHO is a worldwide organization, its guidelines encompass situations that could be encountered in underprivileged countries as well as the United States.

- No artificial nails or nail extenders (tips) should be worn by those having direct contact with patients.
- Natural nails should be kept short, with tips less than 0.5 cm long.

In some situations, soap and clean water may not be readily available to perform a surgical scrub. The following recommendations are for using an alcohol-based hand rub instead of a surgical scrub prior to going into surgery.

- When using alcohol-based hand rub before going into surgery, wash hands first with plain soap and water to remove any visible soil. Then place 5 mL (the equivalent of three doses) into your left palm. Use the elbow of your right hand to press the dispenser.
- Dip the fingertips of your right hand in the gel for 5 seconds to decontaminate the nails.
- Then smear the hand rub up your right forearm to the elbow, using circular movements around the forearm until the rub evaporates.
- Repeat for the other arm.
- Then put 5 mL of hand rub in your left palm, again operating the dispenser with your elbow. Rub both hands together up to the wrists, covering all hand surfaces until the hands are dry.
- Total hand prep with hand gel should last 3 to 5 minutes.
- When the hands and forearms are completely dry, apply sterile gloves.

Source: World Health Organization. WHO Guidelines on Hand Hygiene in Health Care. Who.int. www.who.int/gpsc/5may/tools/9789241597906/en/index.html. Accessed June 1, 2017.

hands is recommended because they can be used when handwashing with soap and water is not optimal. Additional highlights from the guidelines include the following:

- To use alcohol-based hand gels correctly, apply the product to the palm of one hand, then rub your hands together, covering all surfaces of the hands and fingers, until the hands are dry.
- Alcohol-based hand gels should be used before and after care of each patient, just as gloves should be changed before and after each patient.
- If the hands are visibly soiled, they should be washed with soap and water.
- Hand hygiene does not eliminate the need for gloves, nor does using gloves eliminate the need for hand hygiene. Gloves reduce hand contamination by 70% to 80%, prevent cross-contamination, and protect patients and health-care personnel from infection.
- Health-care personnel should avoid wearing artificial nails and keep natural nails less than ¼-inch long if they are caring for patients at high risk for infections.

Safety: It is important to know that alcohol-based hand gels do not kill spores and are not recommended when caring for patients infected with C difficile.

The World Health Organization (WHO) has established the Guidelines for Hand Hygiene in Health Care. These guidelines are very similar to the CDC's recommendations. Box 14.2 provides additional information on the WHO guidelines.

Patient Teaching Connection

Incorporating Hand Hygiene in Patient Teaching

Avoid making the assumption that every patient knows how to correctly perform hand hygiene. When you are teaching a patient a skill, such as how to do a finger stick blood sugar test, be sure to include the correct way to wash hands in your teaching. Also, it is important to inform patients that they have every right to ask every health-care worker who enters their room to perform hand hygiene before touching the patients' wounds or tubes. If this is not automatic on the part of the health-care worker, then it is appropriate to remind the worker to clean his or her hands.

KNOWLEDGE CONNECTION

How do medical asepsis and surgical asepsis differ? What is the most effective way to break the chain of infection? When can alcohol-based hand gels be used for hand hygiene? When can they not be used?

Evidence-Based Practice

Ventilator-Associated Pneumonia in Acute Care Hospitals

Clinical Question

Do patients have a higher risk for ventilator-associated pneumonia (VAP) who receive mechanical ventilation (MV)?

Evidence

Patients who receive MV are at a higher risk for nosocomial pneumonia. VAP is a type of HAI. A patient is at risk for VAP if they are on MV for 13 to 51 per 1,000 ventilator days. A patient is also at risk for developing MRSA while on mechanical ventilation. When the patient must be frequently reintubated, is on MV for long periods, or experiences changes in heat and moisture exchange humidifiers, it increases the risk of mortality. In addition, when nursing staff use poor hand hygiene or provide poor mouth care, the risk for mortality due to VAP also increases. The risk for VAP decreases with proper hand hygiene, using gloves, and administering antibiotics as ordered. To decrease the risk for aspiration of secretions, the patient may be placed in a prone position.

Implications for Nursing Practice

The nursing implications for reducing the risk for patients developing VAP while on MV include proper hand hygiene and using protective gloves. Placing the patient in a prone position and reducing the risk for aspiration will decrease the risk for VAP.

Sources: Klompas M, et al. Strategies to prevent ventilator-associated pneumonia in acute care hospitals: 2014 update. *Infection Control and Hospital Epidemiology.* 2014;35(8):915-936. doi:10.1086/677144; Charles M, et al. Ventilator-associated pneumonia. *The Australasian Medical Journal.* 2014;7(8):334.

CDC Guidelines for Standard and Transmission-Based Precautions

Another part of medical asepsis involves following the requirements established by the CDC for preventing the transmission of communicable pathogens. The first form of protection is standard precautions that are to be used with all patients regardless of diagnosis or suspected diagnosis. The second form of protection is the use of transmission-based precautions, which requires the use of specific protective equipment when caring for patients with illnesses that are communicable through contact, respiratory droplets, or the air. It is very important to note that transmission-based precautions are always used *in addition to* standard precautions.

STANDARD PRECAUTIONS. When you perform hand hygiene, put on gloves before touching anything that is contaminated with blood or body fluids, such as when you go to empty a patient's drain; this is following standard precautions. If there is danger that the blood or body fluids in the drain could splash when it is emptied, you should also wear a face shield, mask, and gown, again following standard precautions. You should take these precautions for all patients, not just those diagnosed with hepatitis or HIV. Table 14.2 lists the components of standard precautions to be used in the care of all patients in all health-care settings. It is very important to know the correct order in which to put on the PPE and the correct order for removing it to prevent contamination of surfaces and of yourself. Skill 14.2 (page 243) describes the correct way to put on PPE, and Skill 14.3 (page 244) describes the correct way to remove PPE.

Wearing gloves is a major part of standard precautions. As a nursing student and a nurse, you will put on and remove innumerable pairs of gloves each day. For medical asepsis, including standard and transmission-based precautions, you should wear clean gloves. You use a different technique for putting on sterile gloves, which are worn for sterile procedures. How to don a sterile gown and sterile gloves, as well as how to perform sterile procedures, is covered in Chapter 22.

Gloves made of latex can cause allergic reactions in both health-care workers and patients. Most health-care facilities offer nonlatex gloves for patient care to prevent these reactions. However, it is important to be aware of latex reactions and whether you or your patients have them. The signs and symptoms of latex reactions are given in Box 14.3.

Box 14.3
Signs and Symptoms of Latex Reactions

Patients and health-care staff may react to the latex present in some gloves and other health-care supplies. Be aware of these possible reactions:

- The most common latex reaction is irritant dermatitis. The proteins in the latex irritate the skin, causing redness and itching.
- Another type of latex reaction is hypersensitivity. This allergic reaction can occur up to 48 hours after contact with latex. It causes redness and itching but is more severe than irritant dermatitis. The person also can develop hives; coughing; and itching, watery eyes.
- True latex allergy causes a serious allergic response that can lead to anaphylaxis or circulatory collapse. The person can develop swelling, hives, itching, respiratory distress, nausea, and diarrhea. If untreated, it can lead to respiratory and cardiac arrest.

Source: National Institute for Occupational Safety and Health. Latex Allergy: A Prevention Guide. NIOSH Publication 98-113. Cdc.gov. www.cdc.gov/niosh/docs/98-113. Accessed June 1, 2017.

TRANSMISSION-BASED PRECAUTIONS. Infection control is everyone's responsibility in the hospital setting. However, most hospitals have an infection control department or nurse who is responsible for following patients diagnosed with communicable diseases. The infection control nurse will set up the protective equipment supplies and post the appropriate precautions for all staff and visitors to follow. You are responsible for following the posted guidelines and ensuring that visitors and staff from other departments do so as well.

Airborne Transmission

Airborne transmission occurs when infectious particles are so small and lightweight that they can float in the air and be spread through air currents. A person entering the room could possibly inhale these particles. When you care for a patient who has a suspected or confirmed communicable disease transmitted through the air, such as tuberculosis or chickenpox, additional precautions are required. In addition to standard precautions, the nurse will wear a specific type of face mask called an N95 respirator (Fig. 14.3). These N95 respirators must be fitted to each individual to ensure that no air leaks exist. In this way, all of the air breathed by the nurse while he or she is in the room is filtered to remove airborne microorganisms.

• **WORD • BUILDING •**

dermatitis: dermat – skin + itis – inflammation

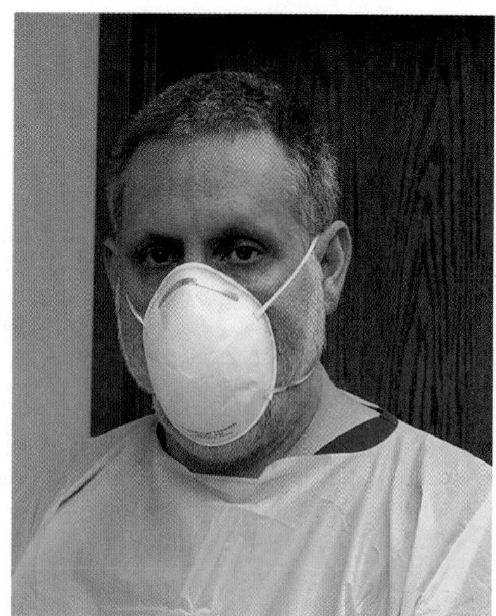

FIGURE 14.3 A nurse wearing an N95 respirator mask, which is required for the care of patients with certain respiratory illnesses.

In addition, patients with illnesses that can be transmitted via the airborne route are placed in special rooms, called *airborne infection isolation rooms,* which have a lower pressure gradient than the hallway. These rooms, formerly known as *negative pressure rooms,* are designed to prevent microorganisms from floating from the patient's room into the hallway.

Droplet Transmission

Some diseases can be transmitted from the respiratory system of one person to another through the small droplets that occur when a person coughs, sneezes, or talks. Another person could then inhale or swallow the droplets and contract the illness. It is recommended that you keep a distance of 3 feet between yourself and patients with droplet-transmitted illnesses unless you are wearing protective equipment. If two patients must share a room and one has a droplet-borne illness, the beds should be at least 3 feet apart and the curtain should be kept closed to prevent droplet spread.

When you care for a patient who has been diagnosed with a communicable disease that is spread through respiratory droplets, you would wear a mask over your mouth and nose in addition to following standard precautions. Illnesses that require this kind of protection include influenza (flu), bacterial meningitis, certain types of pneumonia, and certain streptococcal (strep) infections. In addition, you would instruct the patient to cover the mouth and nose with a tissue when coughing or sneezing. The tissue must then be discarded in a biohazard bag and not left on surfaces such as the over-bed table. The patient should perform hand hygiene after coughing or sneezing.

Direct and Indirect Contact Transmission

The most common path of microorganism transmission is by **direct contact.** This means that the microorganism spreads from one person directly to another, usually on the hands. For example, a health-care worker's hands become contaminated with a respiratory microorganism when she picks up a patient's used tissue. She then touches her face near her mouth, inhaling the microorganism, and this causes her to become ill. **Indirect contact** occurs when microorganisms leave one person (reservoir) and contaminate an object such as a blood pressure cuff (mode of transmission) that is then used on another patient (susceptible host). The second patient becomes ill because of contact with the same microorganism. Remember that you touch many surfaces in a day, including elevator buttons, door handles, and telephones, and if your hands are not clean, you can easily spread microorganisms to those surfaces that will then be touched by susceptible people.

When you care for a patient who has been diagnosed with an illness that can be transmitted by contact with infected material or surfaces touched by infected material, you will wash your hands, put on gloves, and put on a gown as you enter the room. You will wear gloves when you touch the patient's skin, even if it is intact, or when you touch items or surfaces close to the patient, such as the side rails or over-bed table. Table 14.3 summarizes the appropriate protective equipment necessary and indications for the use of transmission-based precautions.

Supervision/Delegation Connection

Supervising the Use of Medical Asepsis, Standard Precautions, and Transmission-Based Precautions

It is appropriate to delegate some care of a patient on transmission-based precautions to a CNA or unlicensed assistive personnel as long as it is within his or her scope of practice. However, it is your responsibility as the supervising nurse to ensure that all guidelines regarding medical asepsis, standard precautions, and transmission-based precautions are being followed correctly. To do that, you will need to observe the staff members carefully and evaluate them for any problems or breaches in technique. Then you will need to kindly point out any errors in technique so that your staff members will be safe from pathogens.

Psychological Aspects of Transmission-Based Precautions

An important aspect of caring for patients with illnesses requiring special precautions is to be aware of the psychological impact of being isolated from the general population. These patients often have multiple drug–resistant organisms (MDROs), such as MRSA, vancomycin-resistant enterococcus, or *C difficile,* which sound frightening to their family and friends. MRSA is not only a healthcare-associated infection, but also a community-associated infection. In this type of situation, visitors are required to put on gowns, gloves, and perhaps masks just to be allowed into the room.

Table 14.3
Transmission-Based Precautions

Type	*Required Personal Protective Equipment*	*Indications for Use*
Contact	**Put on gloves and a gown when entering the room**; wear gloves when touching patient's intact skin and the surfaces and articles in close proximity to the patient, such as side rails and medical equipment. **Plus standard precautions**	To prevent transmission of pathogens spread by direct or indirect contact; use in the presence of excessive wound drainage, fecal incontinence, and when the patient is infected with MDROs, such as MRSA, vancomycin-resistant enterococci, and *C difficile.*
Droplet	**Put on a mask when entering the room.** *Note: If the patient has H1N1 flu, an N95 respirator is required.* Instruct patient to follow respiratory hygiene/cough etiquette. **Plus standard precautions**	To prevent transmission of pathogens spread through close contact with respiratory secretions or mucous membranes; examples include influenza (flu), group A streptococcus, bacterial meningitis, rubella (German measles), and *Mycoplasma pneumonia.*
Airborne	**Put on a fit-tested N95 or higher respirator when entering the room.** Patient must be placed in an airborne infection isolation room with negative pressure. **Plus standard precautions**	To prevent transmission of pathogens small enough to be suspended in the air and spread through air currents; examples include tuberculosis, rubeola (measles), chickenpox, and severe acute respiratory syndrome.

Source: Centers for Disease Control and Prevention. Infection Control Guidelines. Cdc.gov. www.cdc.gov/HAI/settings/outpatient/basic-infection-control-prevention-plan-2011/transmission-based-precautions.html. Accessed June 1, 2017.

It is your responsibility to explain to patients and their visitors the importance of following the CDC's guidelines for transmission-based precautions. You must also enforce the precautions for everyone who enters the room to help prevent the spread of pathogens to others.

Patients diagnosed with communicable diseases and who are on transmission-based precautions tend to have less staff contact than other patients. This may be due to the fact that putting on PPE is time-consuming, so nursing staff perform all care possible while they are in the room and then leave for long periods of time. Another contributing factor is that the isolated patient cannot leave the room to walk in the hall. These patients may be lonely, feel neglected, and have fewer visitors than patients who are not in isolation. Some ways to help alleviate these feelings of seclusion include:

- Spending time talking with the patient while you are in the room. Avoid accomplishing all your tasks and then leaving immediately.
- Asking the patient if you can bring him or her anything to pass the time, such as newspapers or magazines. Many times items in the isolation room must be destroyed when the patient is discharged, so newspapers and magazines are good choices.
- Avoiding expressing distaste regarding the patient's diagnosis or having to enter an isolation room. Patients may feel rejected or unclean because of their diagnosis. Remember that the patient is a person first and that the diagnosis is secondary to his or her human needs.

KNOWLEDGE CONNECTION

When should you use standard precautions? When should you use transmission-based precautions? How can you help a patient under transmission-based precautions feel less socially isolated?

Real-World Connection

Ebola and Zika Viruses

Ebola was first discovered in humans in Africa around 1976. However, the recent outbreaks in 2014 to 2016 in West Africa were more complex in nature and spread quickly across the world. Ebola is transmitted by exposure to blood, secretions, and large respiratory droplets. People are not contagious until symptoms occur, between 2 and 21 days after being infected. The problem is that because it takes so long for the symptoms to occur, people still travel and go about their day-to-day life without even knowing they have the disease. There is no treatment for Ebola at this time. Nurses caring for Ebola patients during the recent outbreak became ill even though they followed all the precautions that were in place at the time.

Zika was first discovered in humans in Africa around 1952. Zika is transmitted by Aedes mosquitoes, and symptoms include fever, headache, and muscle aches. Infected individuals start to see symptoms between 3 and 14 days after being infected. Not all people infected with Zika will have severe symptoms. Unfortunately, transmission between a pregnant woman and her unborn child usually occurs, and these babies are often born with microcephaly.

Novel viruses will likely continue to occur. In your role as a nurse, you should be aware that when that happens the health-care community does not always have the correct answers for how to treat the virus or disease or how to protect health-care staff from related illness.

Nursing Care Plan for a Patient With a MRSA Infection (HAI)

When you plan care for patients with infections, you will need to focus not only on the type of infecting microorganism and transmission-based precautions necessary for that situation, but also on ways to support the patient's immune system to promote healing.

Assessment

You are assigned to care for Mr. Miller, a 59-year-old male who has a surgical wound infected with MRSA. He had a left total knee replacement about 1 month ago, and less than a week after discharge he developed redness, pain, and edema in his left knee. He also had *purulent,* or pus-filled, drainage oozing from the incision. He was readmitted to the hospital, where a wound culture showed the MRSA infection, and he was placed on contact precautions.

What do you assess regarding the presence of infection?

- Assess the wound for signs and symptoms of infection, such as redness, edema, or swelling, and the appearance of wound drainage. (See Chapter 26 for more information on wound assessment.) Your findings are redness of the anterior aspect of the left knee with widespread edema and a small amount of thick yellow drainage on the dressing.
- Assess vital signs, especially for elevated temperature. Your findings are blood pressure of 145/92 mm Hg, a temperature of 101.9°F, a pulse of 98, and respirations of 24.
- Do not forget to assess the sixth vital sign, pain. Remember to assess pain using a pain scale. (See Chapter 17 for more information on assessing vital signs and pain.) In this case, the patient rates his pain at a 6 on a scale of 0 to 10.
- Assess the nearby lymph nodes. Your findings are enlarged, tender lymph nodes in the groin.
- Gather information from laboratory reports. Monitor the white blood cell count because it rises above normal with a bacterial infection. Your findings are that this patient's white blood cell count was elevated but is decreasing with antibiotic therapy using vancomycin.

Nursing Diagnoses

In this situation, the nursing diagnoses should reflect any issues regarding infection—and pain—that are identified in the assessment. The nursing diagnosis for this patient are the following:

To address the MRSA infection:

- Risk for (spread of) infection related to presence of MRSA in knee wound

To address the patient's pain:

- Acute pain related to recent knee surgery and infection and edema of knee

To address the contact precautions:

- Social isolation related to contact precautions manifested by the patient's complaints of loneliness and frustration

In this chapter, we have focused specifically on nursing diagnoses that relate directly to infection and precautions. (See the Care Plan information below.)

Planning

For the nursing diagnoses of "Risk for infection related to presence of MRSA in knee wound" and "Impaired skin integrity related to open knee incision," what actions do you need to take?

- Maintain contact precautions and standard precautions to prevent the spread of MRSA to other sites and to other people.
- Wear a gown and gloves when you enter the room.
- When changing the knee dressing twice daily, inspect the wound for signs of improvement in the infection, such as decreased redness, decreasing edema, decrease in the size of the wound, and decreased drainage (see Chapter 26).
- Monitor the body's response to the IV antibiotic by tracking laboratory values, specifically white blood cell levels.
- Notify the health-care provider if signs or symptoms of worsening infection occur, including fever, increased drainage, and increased pain.

Nursing Care Plan for a Patient With a MRSA Infection (HAI)—cont'd

Interventions for the nursing diagnosis of "Acute pain related to recent knee surgery and infection and edema of knee" would include:

- Ask the patient about his pain level every 2 hours and have him rate his pain on a 0 to 10 scale (see Chapter 19).
- Administer pain medications as ordered and needed. Avoid making the patient wait for more than 5 minutes for requested pain medications.
- Teach the patient to ask for pain medication before pain becomes severe because waiting makes it more difficult to alleviate the pain.
- Determine the effectiveness of the ordered pain medication. Do the positive effects last 3 to 4 hours? If not, does the patient need something stronger? Are the side effects manageable? Notify the prescriber if changes are needed (see Chapters 36 and 37).
- Use techniques such as distraction to help relieve pain (see Chapter 19).

To address the nursing diagnosis of "Social isolation related to contact precautions manifested by the patient's complaints of loneliness and frustration," you can do the following:

- Ensure that the patient understands the purpose of contact precautions.
- Spend extra time with the patient after your nursing tasks are finished, talking with the patient about his concerns, fears, and frustrations.
- Bring in distractions for the patient as requested and allowed, such as newspapers, magazines, puzzle books, and playing cards.
- Encourage visitation by teaching the patient's family that the contact precautions should not prevent them from making visits and that it is safe to visit their loved one.
- Encourage family members and friends to use methods of distraction, such as joining the patient to watch sports events on television or playing cards or board games.

You will plan toward positive outcomes for this patient. These include:

- Resolution of the MRSA infection without spread from the knee wound to other body sites and without spread to other people.
- Management of the patient's pain to keep the rating at a 3 or below.

Implementation

You can now implement the interventions that you have planned. The Care Plan information below presents a summary of the care plan interventions.

Evaluation

To determine the effectiveness of your nursing interventions, ask yourself the following questions:

- Was the MRSA confined to the patient's knee wound?
- Was his pain managed to the degree that he was comfortable most of the time (consistently kept below a 4)?
- Were contact precautions maintained by staff and visitors?

If you can answer "yes" to these questions, you have met the outcomes goals for which you planned. If you answered "no" to any of these questions, you must determine what went wrong and devise improved interventions for the future. (See the Care Plan below for a summary of the care plan evaluations.)

Nursing Diagnosis: Risk for (spread of) infection related to presence of methicillin-resistant *Staphylococcus aureus* (MRSA) in knee wound
Expected Outcomes: Patient will identify actions to reduce risk of spread of infection by discharge from the hospital. Patient will have a healed wound within 1 month and will be free of redness and edema and be afebrile.

Interventions	Evaluations
Maintain contact precautions and standard precautions to prevent the spread of MRSA to other sites and to other people. Wear a gown and gloves when you enter the room.	Day 1: All staff maintained contact precautions. Family and other visitors were instructed about wearing a gown when entering the room and gloves if they touched the patient. Day 2: Visitors needed reminders of appropriate PPE but complied without problems. Staff continued to maintain precautions. Day 6: All visitors and staff maintained appropriate precautions. No evidence of spread of MRSA.
When changing the knee dressing twice daily, inspect the wound for signs of improvement in the infection, such as decreased redness, decreasing edema, decrease in the size of the wound, and decreased drainage.	Day 1: Moderate amount of malodorous purulent drainage on dressing, wound margins reddened, and edema of knee apparent. Wound open just above patella, measuring 3 cm by 2 cm and 2-cm deep. Day 4: Moderate amount of serosanguineous drainage noted on dressing; no odor detected. Knee less edematous and wound above patella smaller in size, 2 cm by 1.5 cm and 1.5-cm deep.

(nursing care plan continues on page 240)

Nursing Care Plan for a Patient With a MRSA Infection (HAI)—cont'd

Interventions	Evaluations
Monitor the body's response to IV antibiotic by tracking laboratory values, specifically white blood cell (WBC) levels.	Day 1: WBC count is 15,966. IV antibiotic administered every 12 hours as ordered. Day 4: WBC count is 12,854, indicating positive response to antibiotic. Day 6: WBC count is 11,220, continuing to fall in response to IV antibiotic.
Notify the health-care provider if signs or symptoms of worsening infection occur, including fever, increased drainage, and increased pain.	Day 1: Patient complains of pain, rated as a 7 on a 0–10 scale. Pain relieved to a 5 with administration of ordered narcotic analgesic. Oral temperature ranging from 100.6°F to 99.9°F. Day 4: Afebrile. Patient rates pain as a 6 before pain medication and as a 3 after medication. Day 6: Continues afebrile. Rates pain at a 4 prior to pain medication and at a 1 or 2 after medication.

Nursing Diagnosis: Acute pain related to recent knee surgery and infected wound as evidenced by rating pain a 7 on a 0–10 scale, grimacing with movement, and diaphoresis
Expected Outcomes: Patient will rate pain at a 3 or below within 72 hours. Patient will verbalize understanding of the pharmacological regimen for antibiotics and pain medication prior to discharge.

Interventions	Evaluations
Ask the patient about his pain level every 2 hours and have him rate his pain on a 0–10 scale. Administer pain medications as ordered and needed. Avoid making the patient wait for more than 5 minutes for requested pain medications.	Day 1: Patient complains of pain consistently rated as a 7 on a 0–10 scale prior to pain medication. Pain relieved to a 5 with administration of ordered narcotic analgesic. Day 4: Afebrile. Patient rates pain as a 6 before pain medication and as a 3 after medication. Day 6: Continues afebrile. Rates pain at a 4 prior to pain medication and at a 1 or 2 after medication.
Teach the patient to ask for pain medication before pain becomes severe because waiting makes it more difficult to alleviate the pain.	Day 1: Patient complains of moderate to severe pain when medicated with a narcotic analgesic. Instruct the patient regarding the need to ask for medication before the pain becomes severe. Patient verbalizes understanding. Offer pain medicine after 4 hours, and patient takes it, rating the pain at a 6. Day 4: Patient taking pain medication every 4 to 5 hours and states he is more comfortable when he does not wait too long. Day 6: Requires pain medication only every 5 to 6 hours to remain comfortable.
Determine the effectiveness of the ordered pain medication. Instruct patient regarding the effectiveness of antibiotic in helping to relieve pain as well.	Day 1: Pain medication effectiveness lasts only 3 to 4 hours but it does reduce pain during that time. Day 4: Patient complains of nausea after taking pain medication. Instructed to take it with a cracker or other food so it is not taken on an empty stomach. Day 6: Nausea relieved by taking medication with food. Pain medication continues to effectively manage his pain. Day 7: Patient verbalizes understanding of role that IV antibiotics play in resolving infection and therefore decreasing pain.

Nursing Care Plan for a Patient With a MRSA Infection (HAI)—cont'd

Interventions	Evaluations
Use techniques such as distraction to help relieve pain.	Day 1: Patient is distracted from pain only during a visit from family. As soon as they leave, he complains of increased pain and is again medicated. Day 2: Encourage patient to watch TV, read, and do crossword puzzles to help distract him from the pain. He agrees to try. Day 3: Pain is resolving some, and patient is using different things to distract himself from it.

Nursing Diagnosis: Social isolation related to contact precautions as evidenced by patient's complaints of loneliness and frustration
Expected Outcomes: Patient will participate in available social interactions during contact precautions. Patient will occupy time with allowed activities during contact precautions.

Interventions	Evaluations
Ensure that the patient understands the purpose of contact precautions. Spend extra time with the patient after your nursing tasks are finished, talking with the patient about his concerns, fears, and frustrations.	Day 1: Patient verbalizes concerns about family members being exposed to MRSA. Explain the purpose of contact precautions, and patient verbalizes understanding. Day 2: Patient expresses boredom and loneliness due to contact precautions. Brought in newspapers and magazines for the patient.
Bring in distractions for the patient as requested and allowed, such as newspapers, magazines, puzzle books, and playing cards.	Day 3: Nursing staff spends extra time as available with the patient to decrease feelings of isolation. Patient states he feels less bored and alone than earlier. Day 4: Patient plays cards with friends for most of the evening.
Encourage family members and friends to use methods of distraction such as joining the patient to watch sports events on television or play cards or board games.	Day 1: Family has visited only once and seems hesitant to go in the room. Nursing staff explains contact precautions and answered questions. Day 4: Patient playing cards with friends for most of evening. Family visits often and watches TV with patient.

Skill 14.1 Performing Hand Hygiene

Handwashing

Assessment Steps

1. Determine when to perform handwashing ***to prevent the spread of microorganisms:*** before and after donning gloves, entering and leaving patient rooms, returning to the unit after breaks and meals, coming on duty, and after using the restroom.

Planning Steps

1. Be sure that soap in a dispenser is available. *Safety: Do not use bar soap because it harbors bacteria.*
2. Obtain paper towels ***for drying your hands.***

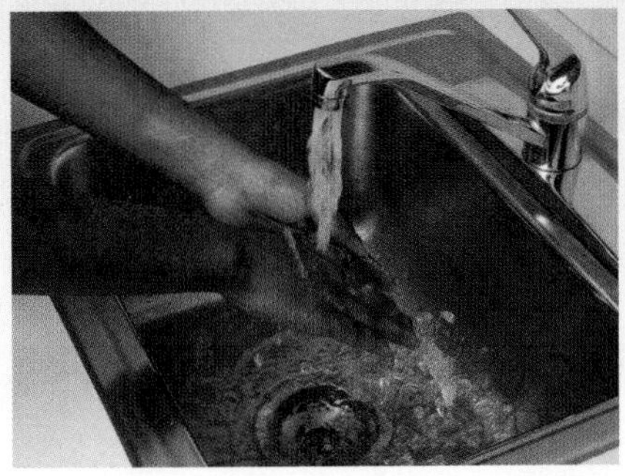

(skill continues on page 242)

Skill 14.1 (continued)

3. Push up your watch and sleeves, if necessary, ***to prevent them from getting wet.***

Implementation Steps

1. Turn on the water and adjust it to a comfortable temperature. ***Water temperature that is too hot can cause dry, cracked skin; water temperature that is too cool may not kill microorganisms.***
2. Wet your hands under running water, being careful not to touch the dirty sink with your fingertips ***to avoid contamination of your hands.***
3. Obtain a quarter-size amount (3 to 5 ml) of soap in the palm of your hand and work into a lather ***for ease of distribution over your hands and wrists.***
4. Rub the palms together using friction. Place one hand on top of the other and rub with fingers interlaced, then reverse hands and repeat. ***Friction helps dislodge soil and remove microorganisms.***

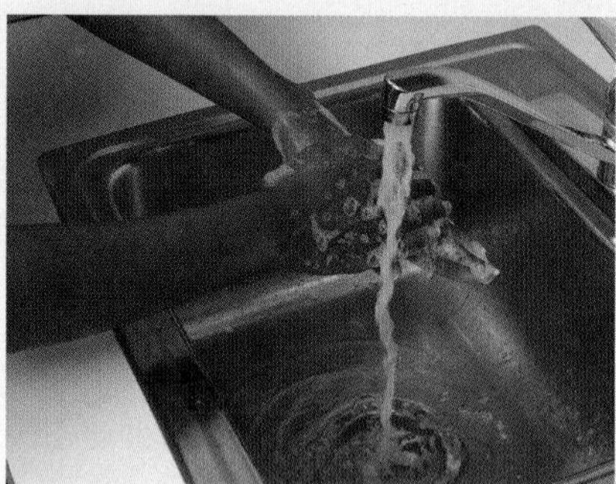

5. Rub the fingernails against the palm of the opposite hand to work the lather around and under the nails ***to loosen and remove soil from around and under the nails.***
6. Lather around each wrist ***to clean them as well as the hands.***
   Note: It is recommended that you wash for at least 20 seconds—the length of time it takes to sing "Happy Birthday" twice.
7. Rinse the hands with your fingers pointed downward, ***to allow water to run from the cleanest area downward.*** **Again, avoid touching the dirty sink with your hands** ***to prevent contamination.***
8. Obtain a clean paper towel and dry hands.
9. Obtain another clean paper towel and turn off the faucet. ***This prevents you from touching the dirty faucet handles with your clean hands.***
10. Drop the paper towels in the trash can without touching it.

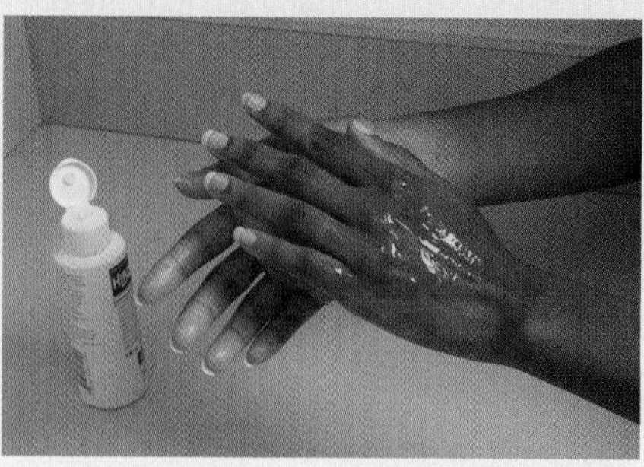

Evaluation Steps

1. Determine whether your hands touched any contaminated surfaces after you washed them. If so, repeat the handwashing procedure ***to ensure that your hands are no longer contaminated.***

Using Hand Gels

Assessment Steps

1. Determine when it is appropriate to use hand gels. The indications are the same as for handwashing except that ***you must wash your hands with soap and water if they are visibly soiled or if contamination by spore-forming microbes is likely.***

Planning Steps

1. Locate gel dispensers in patient rooms, hallways, and the nurse's station ***so that you are aware of availability when the gel is needed.***

Implementation Steps

1. Hold one hand under the dispenser and obtain the manufacturer's recommended amount of product (at least 3 ml) in the palm of your hand ***for maximum effectiveness.*** *Safety: Different manufacturers recommend different amounts of product for maximum effectiveness.*
2. Rub your hands together so that the product covers all surfaces of the hands and fingers ***to help remove microorganisms from all areas of your hands.***
3. Continue rubbing your hands together with the fingers interlaced until the hands are dry ***to remove and kill microorganisms.***
   Note: It is recommended for at least 20 seconds—the length of time it takes to sing "Happy Birthday" twice.

Evaluation Steps

1. Determine that your hands are completely dry and that the gel was spread over all surfaces of the hands and fingers ***to ensure that microorganisms from all surfaces have been killed.***

Skill 14.2 Donning Personal Protective Equipment

Assessment Steps

1. Determine the type of PPE required to maintain standard and/or transmission-based precautions. ***This will ensure that you take the proper precautions for the situation.***

Planning Steps

1. If you are allergic to latex or powder, locate latex-free or powder-free gloves ***to prevent local or systemic actions.***
2. Obtain necessary PPE for the task. Be sure you obtain the correct size of nonsterile gloves; they are generally available in small, medium, large, and extra-large. ***Correct glove size prevents open areas around the wrists where microorganisms or fluids might enter.***
3. Remain outside the patient's room or in the anteroom when donning PPE if the patient is on transmission-based precautions ***to prevent contact with fluids, air, or droplets before you have donned the appropriate PPE.***

Implementation Steps

1. Perform hand hygiene. ***Hand hygiene is necessary before donning gloves or other PPE.***

Donning Gown

1. Hold the gown by the shoulders and allow it to unfold ***to prevent contaminating the outside of the gown.***
2. Slip your arms through the gown's sleeves.

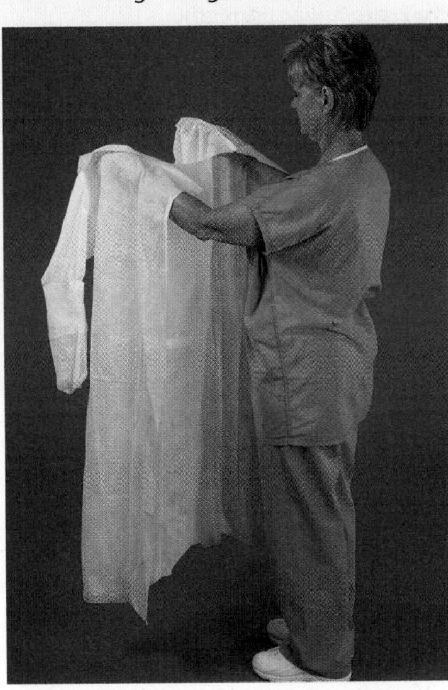

3. Pull the gown up onto your shoulders by grasping the inside of the gown at the shoulders ***to prevent touching the outside of the gown with your ungloved hands.***

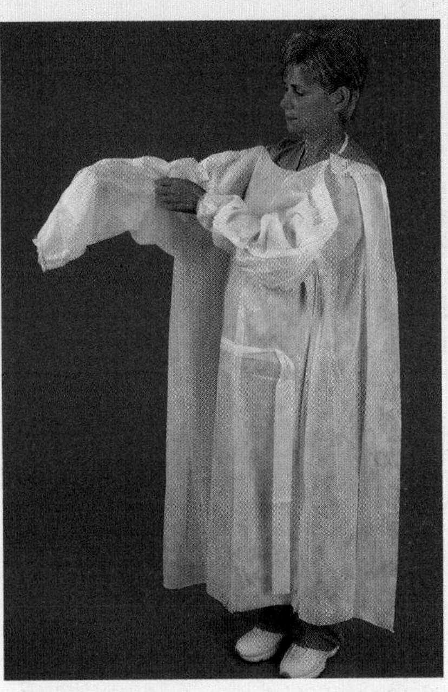

4. Fasten the gown in the back at the neck and then at the waist ***to keep your back covered.***

Donning a Mask or N95 Respirator

1. Place the mask over your mouth and nose, tie the upper ties above your ears first, and then tie the lower ties at your neck ***to protect your mouth and nose from airborne microorganisms.*** *Safety: Do not bring lower ties up on the head. This causes gaps at the side of the mask, allowing microorganisms to enter.*
2. Bend the flexible band across the bridge of the nose for a snug fit ***to prevent microorganisms from entering gaps in the mask.***
3. Pull the bottom edge of the mask down so it is below the chin ***to cover the entire mouth and nose area.***

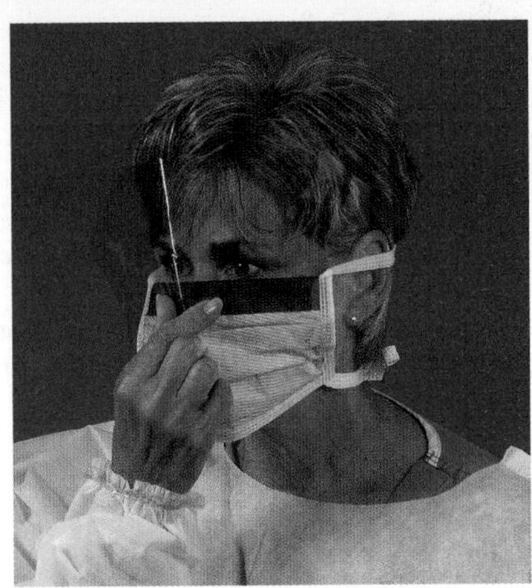

(skill continues on page 244)

Skill 14.2 (continued)

4. If using a N95 respirator, check to be sure it is fitted against your face on all sides ***to prevent microorganisms from entering any areas that gap.***

Donning Eye Protection

1. Put on goggles or face shield and adjust to fit ***to protect your eyes from splashing of blood or body fluids.***
   Note: Face shields are usually attached to the mask.

Donning Hair Cover

1. Put on the hair cover ***to protect your hair from splashing of blood or body fluids.***

Donning Shoe Cover

1. Put shoe cover on each shoe ***to protect your shoes from splashing of blood or body fluids.***

Donning Gloves

1. Pull the sleeve edges of the gloves down over the proximal half of the hand portions before donning gloves. This will help to keep the glove cuff over the gown sleeve, ***which will prevent gaps through which microorganisms may enter.***
2. Pull the first glove onto your nondominant hand, ***making it easier to put on the second glove.***
3. Pull the cuff edges of the glove up over the wrist of the isolation gown ***to prevent gaps through which microorganisms may enter.*** After adjusting the glove cuff, the gown sleeve may be pulled up slightly if necessary, but be certain to keep your wrists securely covered ***so that movement will not pull the glove and sleeve apart, exposing the wrists to contamination.***
4. Repeat for the dominant hand.

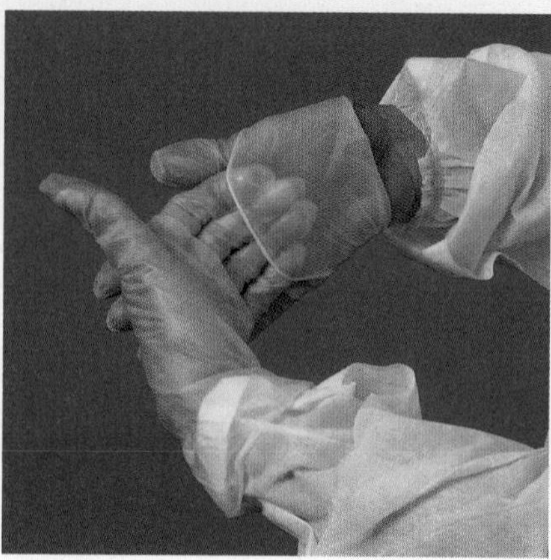

5. Change gloves if they become torn or heavily soiled and use hand hygiene before regloving ***to prevent contamination of your hands with blood or body fluids.***

Evaluation Steps

1. Evaluate your technique for donning PPE ***by determining if all steps were followed correctly.***

Skill 14.3 Removing Personal Protective Equipment

Assessment Steps

1. Determine where you will remove the PPE. Remain just inside the patient's room at the doorway ***to prevent taking contaminants into the public hallway.***

Planning Steps

1. Determine the order in which to remove PPE: gloves, goggles, gown, and then mask or respirator ***to prevent contamination during removal.***
2. Treat the outside or front side of all PPE as contaminated ***because it has been exposed to contaminants.***
3. Locate appropriate trash receptacle for disposing of all PPE ***to prevent having to carry contaminated PPE to another location.***

Implementation Steps

Removing Gloves

1. Grasp the outside of the glove on your nondominant hand with your dominant hand and pull downward to remove. ***This prevents contact of your clean hands inside the gloves with the outside of the gloves.***
2. Hold the removed glove in your dominant (and still gloved) hand. Slide the fingers of your ungloved hand under the glove on your dominant hand at the wrist. ***This protects your ungloved hand from contact with the soiled gloves.***

   Safety: Do not touch the outside of the glove with your bare fingers.
3. Peel the remaining glove off from the wrist toward the fingers. As it turns inside out, the first glove will remain within the second glove, ***allowing the soiled outsides of both gloves to be contained within themselves. You will only touch the clean inside portion of the gloves.***

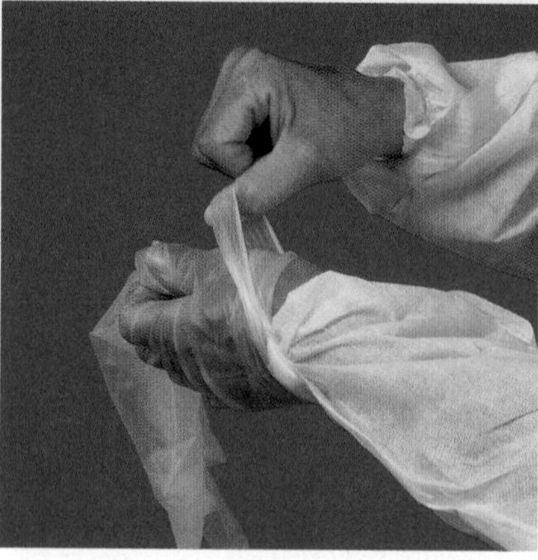

4. Drop the gloves into the appropriate waste receptacle without touching it ***to prevent contamination of your hands.***

Skill 14.3 (continued)

Removing Gown

1. Unfasten the gown ties at the neck, ***being careful not to touch any part of the front of the gown, which is contaminated.***
2. Unfasten the ties at the waist ***to allow removal of the gown.***
3. Lean forward to remove the gown. ***This helps to keep the contaminated gown from contaminating your uniform.*** Remove the gown by peeling it from one shoulder toward the hand and then the other shoulder toward that hand. The gown will turn inside out, ***keeping the soiled portions on the inside and preventing contamination.***

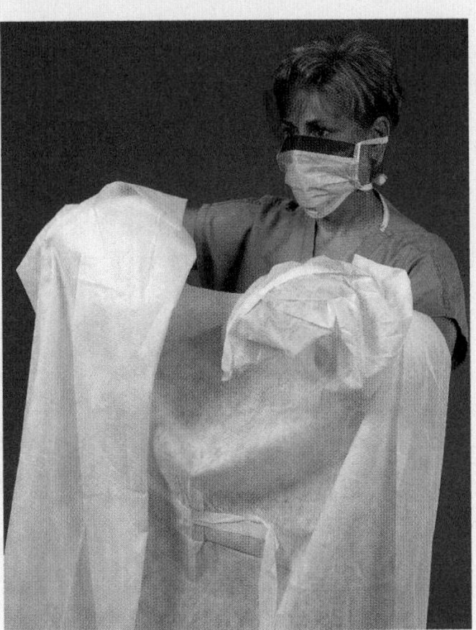

4. Hold the gown away from your body ***to prevent accidental contact with any soiled area of the gown.***
5. Roll the gown with the front exterior portion of the gown wrapped inside the rest of the gown. ***This prevents the external contaminated side of the gown from contaminating your uniform or skin.***

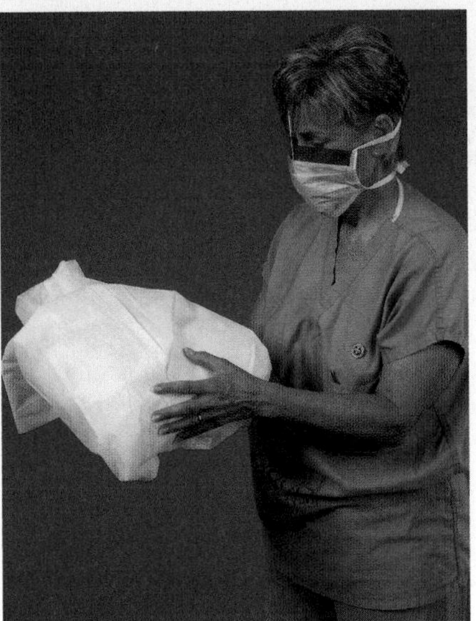

6. Drop the gown into the appropriate waste receptacle.

Removing Eye Protection

1. Touch only the earpieces of the goggles or the headband of the face shield with your bare hands. ***The remaining portions are contaminated.***
2. Remove the goggles or face shield.
3. Drop the goggles or face shield into the appropriate waste receptacle.

Removing Mask or N95 Respirator

1. Touch only the ties or elastic of the mask or N95 respirator. *Safety: Remember that the front of the mask/respirator is contaminated.*
2. Always untie the bottom ties first and then the top ties. ***This prevents the contaminated side of the mask from contaminating your neck during removal.***
3. Discard in the appropriate waste receptacle.

Remove Hair Covering

1. Slip your fingers inside the hair covering while being careful not to touch the outside of it.
2. Discard in the appropriate waste receptacle.

Remove Shoe Covering

1. Slip your fingers inside each shoe covering while being careful not to touch the outside of them.
2. Discard in the appropriate waste receptacle.
3. Perform hand hygiene immediately after removing all PPE ***to remove any microorganisms that may have been touched.***

Evaluation Steps

1. Determine that all PPE is in the appropriate waste receptacles ***to ensure that it is not a reservoir for microorganisms.***
2. Evaluate your technique for removing PPE ***by determining if all steps were followed correctly.***

POST CONFERENCE

During the conference after clinicals, you are relieved that your day has gone so well. It took you a little while to get comfortable putting on the gown and gloves before you went into your patient's room and removing them as you left his room. However, it was not long before you stopped worrying so much about the infective organism MRSA. You must have washed your hands or used hand gel at least 50 times today, but you feel certain that you have not contaminated anything. And, after being in a gown and gloves all day, plus washing your hands so much, you know you are protected and will not be taking anything infectious home with you.

Key Points

- Bacteria, viruses, protozoa, fungi, and helminths are classifications of microorganisms that cause human illnesses.
- The chain of infection illustrates how an infectious agent is transferred from a reservoir through the portal of exit via a mode of transmission to the portal of entry of a susceptible host.
- Several types of infections exist. HAIs are preventable by using appropriate hand hygiene and precautions.
- The body possesses a three-layer defense system: primary defenses involving the skin, mucous membranes, and gastrointestinal system; secondary defenses involving the inflammatory process, elevated temperature, and complement cascade; and tertiary defenses involving the B- and T-cell lymphocytes.
- Ways to prevent infection in the health-care setting include hand hygiene and use of standard and transmission-based precautions.
- Medical asepsis involves the use of the clean technique, performing hand hygiene, maintaining a clean patient environment, and using CDC precautions.
- It is extremely important to know when, why, and how to perform correct hand hygiene.
- Standard precautions are established by the CDC to prevent the transmission of pathogens in blood and body fluids. They require health-care workers to wear gloves when caring for all patients to prevent any contact with blood-borne pathogens. They also require staff to wear a gown, mask, and goggles if they risk touching or being splashed by blood or body fluids.
- Transmission-based precautions address three types of microbial spread: contact, droplet, and airborne. Transmission-based precautions are always used in addition to standard precautions.
- When caring for patients on transmission-based precautions, it is very important to address their emotional needs due to social isolation.
- MRSA is an HAI and a community-associated infection.
- Zika virus is transmitted by the Aedes mosquito. The symptoms include fever, headache, and muscle aches.
- Ebola virus is contagious and transmitted by blood, body fluids, and large respiratory droplets.

Review Questions

Select the answer that is most appropriate for each of the following questions. Some questions may have more than one correct answer. Select all that apply.

1. When you learn that your patient's infecting bacterium is identified as a gram-positive streptococcus, you know this means that:
   1. it appears in rod-shaped pairs and cannot be treated by antibiotics.
   2. it appears in sphere-shaped clusters and stains red in the laboratory.
   3. it appears as a long, coiling cell and stains blue in the laboratory.
   4. it appears in sphere-shaped chains and stains purple in the laboratory.
2. A patient complains that he feels ill and the doctor told him it was a virus but that the doctor would not give him any antibiotics. He is upset with the doctor. What is the reason for the health-care provider's action?
   1. Most viruses are immune to antibiotics.
   2. Antibiotics only kill bacteria; they do not kill viruses.
   3. Only the newest, most expensive antibiotics will kill viruses.
   4. Antibiotics are not necessary unless the viral infection is severe.

3. The most effective way to break the chain of infection is to:
   1. isolate all infected patients from remaining patients and assign only one staff member to each room.
   2. wear gowns, gloves, masks, and protective eyewear when entering every patient's room.
   3. perform effective hand hygiene according to CDC guidelines.
   4. use an N95 respirator when entering the room of any infected patient.

4. Which is true of performing hand hygiene?
   1. Use before and after a snack in the break room.
   2. Do not perform hand hygiene if you will be donning gloves.
   3. Use hand gel if your hands are visibly dirty.
   4. Use hand hygiene between providing care for two patients in the same room.
   5. There is no need to use hand hygiene if you leave a patient's room to obtain clean supplies and return immediately.
   6. Use soap and water instead of hand gel if the hands could be contaminated with spore-forming microbes.

5. A patient is placed on droplet precautions. You know his wife needs more teaching about what PPE to use when she says:
   1. "I don't need to wear a mask if I stay a foot away from him."
   2. "I will wash my hands and put on a face mask before I go into his room."
   3. "I will remove the mask just inside the door of his room."
   4. "This disease is spread through small droplets that spray out when he talks, coughs, or sneezes."

6. A nurse is caring for a 38-year-old female who was admitted with the Zika virus. The nurse understands that which of the following will be given to the patient?
   1. Antipyretics
   2. NSAIDS
   3. Fluids
   4. Morphine

7. A nurse is caring for a 78-year-old male who was admitted with the Ebola virus. The nurse understands the Ebola virus spreads by:
   1. blood.
   2. body fluids.
   3. large droplet secretions.
   4. small droplet secretions.
   5. IV fluid.

ANSWERS 1. 4, 2. 2, 3. 3, 4. 1, 4, 5, 6, 5. 1, 6. 1, 2, 3, 7. 1, 2, 3

Critical Thinking Exercises

Answers available online.

1. Create a scenario to illustrate the chain of infection. Identify each link of the chain in your scenario.

2. A patient is on droplet precautions. You are going into the room to suction her tracheostomy, which could cause splashing, and you could have contact with respiratory secretions. What PPE will you need?

Additional Resources

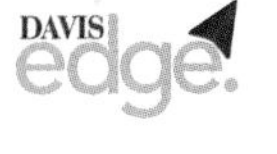

Use the scratch off code on the inside front cover of your book to access online quizzes that will help you to improve your scores on course exams and prepare for the NCLEX-PN®.

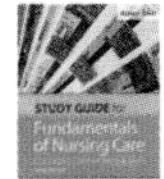

Study Guide

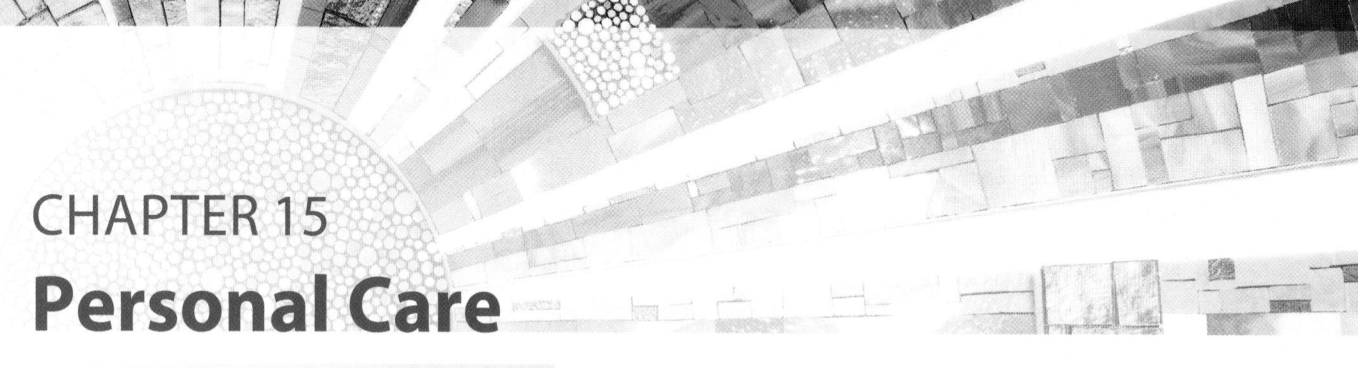

CHAPTER 15
Personal Care

KEY TERMS

Activities of daily living (ak-TIV-ih-teez uv DAY-lee LIV-ing)
Assisted care (a-SIS-ted KARE)
Bath blanket (BATH BLAN-ket)
Draw sheet (DRAW SHEET)
Excoriation (eks-koh-ree-ASH-uhn)
Hygiene (HYE-jeen)
Lesion (LEE-zhun)
Leukoplakia (LOO-koh-PLAY-kee-ah)
Lice (LYESS)
Maceration (MASS-er-RAY-shun)
Mitered corner (MYE-terd KOR-ner)
Mottling (MOT-ling)
Nits (NITS)
Ocular prosthesis (OK-yoo-lar pross-THEE-siss)
Seborrhea (seb-or-REE-ah)
Self-care (SELF-KARE)
Special mouth care (SPE-shuhl MOWTH KARE)
Tinea capitis (TIN-ee-ah kah-PEE-tiss)
Total care (TOH-tuhl KARE)
Venous return (VEE-nus rih-TERN)

CHAPTER CONCEPTS

Patient-Centered Care
Culture
Health Promotion

LEARNING OUTCOMES

1. Define various terms associated with personal care.
2. Categorize personal care tasks performed at particular times during the day.
3. Describe the benefits of bathing patients, both for the patient and for the nurse.
4. Explain factors to consider when planning patient care and bathing.
5. Describe three categories of personal care.
6. Identify types of baths and their purposes.
7. Explain guidelines and nursing responsibilities for bathing.
8. Contrast back massage with applying lotion to the back.
9. Discuss key aspects of providing oral care to unconscious and conscious patients.
10. Describe assessments to make during oral care, hair care, and nail care.
11. Explain how to remove jewelry from piercings and circumstances that could make removal necessary.
12. Discuss how to remove contact lenses, artificial eyes, and hearing aids.
13. Explain how to clean and insert an ocular prosthesis and hearing aids.
14. Identify ways to minimize noise, odors, and clutter in the patient's environment.
15. Differentiate between open, closed, and surgical beds.
16. Describe nursing responsibilities when making occupied and unoccupied beds.
17. Identify common bed positions and their purposes.
18. Discuss information found in the Connection features of the chapter.
19. Identify safety information related to personal care.
20. Answer questions about the skills in the chapter.

SKILLS

15.1 Administering a Complete Bed Bath
15.2 Administering Perineal Care
15.3 Administering a Back Massage
15.4 Administering Oral Care for an Unconscious Patient
15.5 Administering Oral Care for a Conscious Patient
15.6 Providing Denture Care
15.7 Shaving a Male Patient

SKILLS—cont'd

CRITICAL THINKING CONNECTION

Clinical Assignment

You are a male student assigned to care for an 88-year-old female patient who requires a bed bath. This is your first female patient, and you are nervous and a little embarrassed about the bath.

Critical Thinking Questions:

1. What nursing actions would you prepare for prior to giving the patient a bed bath?
2. What safety precautions would you take?
3. When setting up the supplies for the bed bath, how do you test the water in the basin?
4. As a male student, how would you approach the female patient?

So whose job is it anyway? Is it beneath a nurse to bathe patients? Is bathing a patient an ineffective use of a nurse's education? Some student nurses in the United Kingdom's Royal Academy of Nurses wanted a resolution saying that they should not be required to give baths. One student was quoted as saying, "I do not wash bottoms. There are other people to do that." The resolution was soundly defeated. In this chapter, you will learn some reasons why that happened.

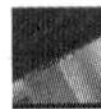

ROUTINELY SCHEDULED CARE

Most facilities have established specific times for routine care to be given. This helps to prevent missing an aspect of care. Routine care may be delegated to a certified nursing assistant (CNA) or to unlicensed assistive personnel (UAP), but it is your responsibility to be sure the care is completed. An example of generally used routine care follows:

- **Early Morning (Early a.m.) Care:** Assist with toileting. Give the patient a warm, wet washcloth to wash the hands and face. Assist with oral care if desired. Some people prefer to do oral care after they have eaten breakfast, while others prefer it before eating. Provide fresh water if allowed.
- **Morning (a.m.) Care:** This is done after breakfast. For many patients, this will include assisting with a bath. For all patients, this includes toileting, oral care, back massage, shaving, hair care, and dressing or changing the gown. Assist the patient to get out of bed if he or she is able to do so. Have the patient sit in the chair while you straighten or change the linens.
- **Afternoon (p.m.) Care:** After lunch, patients may need assistance to be comfortable to rest or to receive visitors. Assist the patient with toileting and then straighten the bed and assist the patient to a position of comfort. Provide the patient's preference of oral fluids unless contraindicated.
- **Bedtime (h.s.) Care:** Assist the patient to prepare for sleep. Assist with toileting. Offer the patient's preference of oral fluids, such as a glass of milk or juice, unless the patient is NPO or on a restricted diet or fluid allowance. Brush the teeth or remove dentures. Remove glasses and hearing aids. Give a back massage. Place needed items within reach, such as the call light, fresh water, and urinal. Straighten the room, putting away items not being used. If the patient is ambulatory, arrange furniture so that there is a clear path to the bathroom to reduce fall risk. Straighten the linens and obtain an extra blanket if needed. Dim the lights or turn them off and provide a nightlight according to the patient's preference.

KNOWLEDGE CONNECTION

What times of the day and evening are appropriate for providing a bath? Why is routine care an important part of individualized nursing care?

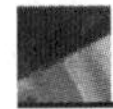

BATHING

Hygiene is a term used to describe keeping oneself clean and well groomed. When each of us prepares for the day, the activities involved—such as bathing, washing and styling hair, brushing and flossing teeth, dressing, and shaving—are referred to as **activities of daily living** (ADLs).

When people are healthy, they perform these activities themselves. When they are weak, in pain, emotionally distraught, confused, or lacking mobility, they need partial or complete assistance to accomplish ADLs.

Assisting patients with hygiene and grooming gives you the opportunity to learn a great deal about your patient as well as provide comfort. Bathing a patient offers benefits to both the patient and the nurse.

Benefits of Bathing Patients

As you provide personal care for your patients, you have the opportunity to make multiple assessments that you otherwise might miss. The following paragraphs detail the benefits of bathing to the patient and provide examples of observations to make while performing this skill.

Cleanses the Skin

As you wash, you remove dirt, bacteria, dead skin cells, sweat, and odors. Bathing is helpful not only in making the skin clean, but also in making it smell fresh and clean, as well as helping to prevent infection.

Provides an Opportunity for Skin Assessment

Bathing the skin gives you the opportunity to observe skin problems that are not obvious. Look for redness, cracking, and **maceration,** which is softened skin due to continuous exposure to moisture. This often occurs in skin crevices such as under the breasts and scrotum, in the axilla and groin areas, between the toes, and between the buttocks. Look for **excoriation,** or scrapes on the skin, that may be due to scratching or that may occur during care. Performing a bed bath also allows you to assess skin temperature to determine whether it is hot and dry, normal, or cool and clammy. In addition, you have an opportunity to notice any skin breakdown over bony prominences at its earliest stage, which could be a reddened area that does not return to normal color after pressure is removed.

Increases Circulation

During a bed bath, you will wash from distal to proximal to improve blood return from the extremities back to the heart. This is referred to as **venous return.** Assess for indications of pooling of blood, such as redness in the hands and feet; a red, warm area in the calf of the leg; or **mottling,** a purplish blotching of the skin when circulation slows greatly. While bathing the patient, you have ample opportunity to flex and extend all joints and extremities, which further stimulates the circulation and aids in preventing stiffness of joints.

Increases Sensation

If the patient is comatose or neurologically impaired, the bath provides sensory input for the brain to process, including friction from the washcloth; moisture and warmth from the water; olfactory stimulation from the clean, soapy smell; and the silky, slippery feeling of soap and suds. Even patients without neurosensory deficits tend to have decreased sensation when lying in a hospital bed. Observe for evidence of pain or discomfort during the bath, such as grimacing, pulling away from you or pushing your hand away, moaning, or verbalizing pain by saying "ouch" or "stop."

Provides Comfort and Relaxation

The feeling of cleanliness is conducive not only to comfort and relaxation, but also to rest and sleep, all of which are important to healing and restoration of health. When patients do not feel well and have to remain in a lumpy hospital bed, they soon become weary of lying there; their muscles ache and joints become stiff. Remaining in the same gown or pajamas for more than a day is unpleasant as well. They may begin to smell, wrinkle, and become uncomfortable. Assess the patient for muscle tension in the back and shoulders as you bathe the back and perform a back massage. Talk with patients about their cares and concerns. This may be when you learn that an elderly patient who lives alone is worrying about his cats or that a patient with three children is not sleeping because she is concerned about how her children are getting to and from school.

Provides Improved Self-Esteem

All of us feel better when we look and smell fresh. After bathing the patient, style his or her hair in the way the patient prefers. Assist male patients to shave or trim the beard and moustache. Assist female patients to shave the legs or axillae or apply makeup if desired. Listen as patients talk during this care. Assess the effect of illness, injury, treatment, or surgery on the person's ability to feel good about himself or herself. For example, a patient who has undergone a mastectomy may make comments about not being a real woman anymore, or a patient who has facial scarring may make comments about scaring small children. Such comments give you an opportunity to further explore the patient's feelings and self-esteem issues. Concerns about self-image are not uncommon when patients have undergone body-altering surgeries.

Contributes to the Establishment of the Nurse–Patient Relationship

Providing a bed bath is one of the most effective ways you can establish trust and rapport with your patient. There are few things that are more intimate than personal hygiene. If you demonstrate respect, preserve the patient's modesty, and show caring and compassion all while making the patient "feel so much better," you make great strides toward a stronger nurse–patient relationship. During the bath, the nurse spends an uninterrupted block of time with the patient. The patient may feel more comfortable bringing up a subject that requires extended conversation, or the patient may give hints for you to pursue further. This type of conversation does not occur easily when the nurse comes into the room to quickly change an IV or hand the patient medications to swallow. More time with the patient doing hands-on care translates into the opportunity to hear what the patient is feeling and thinking.

KNOWLEDGE CONNECTION

How does bathing a patient benefit the patient? How does it benefit the nurse?

Anatomy and Physiology Connection

Hair, Nails, and Glands

The hair and nails are considered appendages of the skin. Hair grows from the root at the base of the follicle. In the matrix of the hair root, new cells are formed and produce keratin. As they die, they are incorporated into the hair

• WORD • BUILDING •

maceration: macer – soften + ation – action
excoriation: ex – from + cori – skin + ation – action
neurosensory: neuro – related to the nervous system + sensory – related to the senses

shaft, so when you comb and brush a patient's hair, you are actually caring for dead keratinized cells. The hair functions to keep the head from losing body heat by providing insulation.

In the same way, nails grow from the nail root contained within nail follicles. The new nail cells produce a different, stronger form of keratin. When the cells die, they are incorporated into the nail. Beneath the nail is living tissue. Nails function to protect the ends of the fingers and toes and to increase the ability to pick up small objects with the fingers. When you trim a patient's nails, you are cutting off dead and keratinized cells.

The sebaceous glands secrete *sebum* (oil) onto the skin surface or into hair follicles to keep the skin and hair lubricated. Because skin is the first line of defense against invading pathogens, it is important that sebum keeps it moist and protects it from drying and cracking, which would leave an entryway for pathogens. That is why, when you bathe patients, you need to assess the skin for any open areas or cracking and why it is important to lubricate dry skin with lotion.

The sweat glands, especially the apocrine sweat glands located in the axillae and genital areas, produce sweat during stressful and emotional circumstances. The eccrine sweat glands are found over the rest of the body but are concentrated in the palms of the hands, upper lip, and forehead. They produce sweat in response to heat and exercise. When the sweat from the apocrine sweat glands remains on the skin, bacteria begin to break it down. By-products of this breakdown cause the smell we call *body odor*. When you bathe patients, you remove this sweat so that the bacteria do not have the opportunity to break it down.

Patient Preferences and Abilities

When planning personal care and bathing, you need to determine the patient's preferences regarding the time and type of bath. It is important to take into account the patient's cultural influences regarding bathing. It also is necessary to determine the patient's abilities to assist, and whether or not you will need additional nursing staff to complete the bath.

Timing

Patient care in the acute care setting tends to follow an established pattern: baths are part of morning care and therefore are done in the morning. However, not all patients want to bathe in the morning. Consider the patient who slept poorly during the night and who wants to sleep until lunchtime, the patient who normally works nights and sleeps days, or the patient who likes to bathe just before going to bed at night. It is important for you to consider the patients and their preferences regarding the time of their bath.

Students are sometimes hesitant to discuss when a patient would prefer to bathe. Some are timid and wait for the patient to ask to clean up. Others are insistent that the patient allow a bath early in the shift so that their work will flow according to the usual pattern of morning care. Some students do not really want to perform personal care, so they take any hesitancy on the part of the patient as a refusal of care.

IT'S ALL IN THE APPROACH. Most patients are ready for a fresh gown and straightened sheets in the mornings at the very least, as well as personal care such as oral hygiene and grooming. If you are hesitant as a student, your patients may decide that you do not really want to help them with bathing and dressing. If you say, "You don't want me to help you with your bath now, do you?" it is clear that you would rather not perform this task. It is important to be positive and warm in your approach to bathing and other ADLs. Avoid giving the appearance that you are really busy or are in a big hurry. Exhibit the attitude that you would desire to be shown to your own mother, father, or child. As a nursing student and as a nurse, it is your job to see that personal care needs are met. An approach to the patient who seems to delay or put off bathing is to say, "Would you like help with your bath now, or would you prefer that I come back in an hour?" This gives the patient a choice and allows for the patient to be somewhat in control of his or her own care.

Culture

In addition to considerations regarding the timing of the bath, make sure to include cultural influences. Remember that in some cultures it is not appropriate for a person to be bathed by a member of the opposite sex. Ask if it is acceptable to the patient for you to help with the bath. If it is not, arrange for someone else to do the bath. For example, if you are female and have a male patient who is from a culture that does not allow a female to bathe a male, you could ask a male nurse to give the bath to your patient. Be sure to offer to do a bath for him on one of his patients in return. It may be acceptable if a family member is present during the bath. Be respectful of cultural taboos.

In some cultures, people do not bathe daily or even every other day. Instead, weekly baths are the norm. This may be due to restricted water supplies in the country of origin or due to beliefs that more frequent exposure to water is unhealthy. Although the dominant American culture considers body odor offensive, in some countries it is completely acceptable. Again, be sure to ask permission to bathe a patient or assist with bathing.

Abilities

When determining if a patient can help with the bath, you must consider the patient's abilities. It is helpful to assess his or her ability to:

- Understand and follow directions;
- Move and turn enough to assist with the bath; and
- Tolerate the physical demands during a bath, including whether the patient is too weak, too ill, or in too much pain to participate.

KNOWLEDGE CONNECTION

How do you individualize personal care?

Settings Connection: Home Health

Personal Care Considerations in Home Health

In the home health-care setting, it is very important to respect the client's preferences regarding bathing. It is often difficult for clients to get in and out of home showers or tubs, so you may have to adapt equipment for this purpose. For example, you can use a rustproof lawn chair for the client to sit on in the shower. You can place a similar type of chair in the bathtub and use a hand-held sprayer attached to the bathtub faucet to bathe the patient. In home health care, it is often necessary to make do with what is available, even if it means pumping water from a well and then heating it on the stove in order to bathe the client.

Settings Connection: Long-Term Care

Personal Care in Long-Term Care Facilities

In long-term care, a resident's bath or shower is routinely scheduled for two or three times per week because the skin of an older person tends to be dry and fragile. However, the residents should be clean at all times. If they are incontinent, it is important to provide frequent and thorough perineal care to prevent skin breakdown and odor. They also should be assisted to wash up before and after meals.

In older adults, the sebaceous and sweat glands produce less oil and sweat. It is not necessary or desirable to bathe daily. Their skin requires frequent application of lotion to prevent dryness. They also chill easily because of decreased circulation, so keep the environment warm when you are bathing elderly patients.

Assistance

Nurses must evaluate patients' ability to participate in care as well as how much assistance they require. It is important to encourage the patient to do as much as possible but also to accurately determine what the patient is capable of doing. Sometimes this varies from one day to the next. If the patient rested poorly during the night, is in pain, is short of breath, or is excessively fatigued, he or she may be unable to do as much as on a previous day. Box 15.1 describes types of care that patients may need.

One problem encountered often in the care of hospitalized patients is that the nursing staff may think the patient can do more than really is possible. So, the staff member places a pan of water with soap in front of the patient and disappears.

Box 15.1

Types of Care

Personal care is performed in different ways: by the patient, by the staff, or by a combination of both.

- **Self-care** refers to patients who are able to perform ADLs without assistance. Most patients in hospitals or care facilities require at least some assistance.
- **Assisted care** refers to the need for some assistance with ADLs. This may mean needing another person to wash hard-to-reach areas such as the back, feet, and lower legs; assistance in helping a patient out of the tub or shower; or help obtaining necessary items for care, such as a bath basin with water.
- **Total care** means that patients are able to do very little or nothing for themselves.

When the staff person returns, he or she assumes the bath has been done and puts the supplies away. The patient may not have really had a bath.

To give thorough nursing care, you must stay close, see how the patient tolerates the activity of bathing, and help as needed. In this way, you will be sure that good nursing care is truly delivered, and your patient has truly been bathed.

Supervision/Delegation Connection

Determining Delegation of a Bed Bath

How do you decide when to delegate a bed bath? Although the bath is time consuming, you should perform it when the patient's condition is unstable, when you need more information about a patient's skin condition, when you need to evaluate the patient's capabilities to assist with personal care, or when you need to develop or strengthen the nurse–patient relationship.

Types of Baths

A bath in a hospital is different from a bath at home when a person is well. The exertion of bathing can be quite exhausting for a person who is ill. The type of bath used can be tailored to the needs of the patient (Box 15.2). When you determine which type of bath to perform, it is important to consider the patient's energy level, ability to tolerate standing or sitting for the duration of the activity, and respiratory status to tolerate steam and exertion. The health-care provider may order a specific activity level, such as complete bedrest. In that case, you must assist the patient with a complete bed bath.

A complete bed bath or towel bath requires the least effort on the part of the patient. Skill 15.1 (page 264) provides more information on administering a complete bed bath. A partial bath or assisted bath requires a minimal amount of activity by the patient. When you perform a bed bath, you will need to

Box 15.2

Types of Baths

Baths given in the health-care setting may be referred to in different ways depending on the amount of help required by the patient or the type of bath being given.

Complete Bed Bath

The patient is unable to be out of bed, so the bath is accomplished using a basin of water at the bedside. All parts of the body are washed. Generally the patient is too ill to help and the nurse performs all care.

Assisted or Help Bath

May be done in bed or with the patient sitting up in a chair. The patient participates as much as he or she is able. If the patient becomes fatigued or short of breath, or develops pain, the nursing staff finishes whatever the patient cannot reach or complete.

Partial Bath

Only selected areas of the patient are bathed. This type of bath may be done when the patient is in pain or nauseated to prevent moving him or her more than is comfortable. Generally, a partial bath includes washing the face, hands, axilla, buttocks, and perineal area, or the parts of the patient that would cause odor if not washed.

Tub Bath

In this type of bath, the patient sits in a tub of water that may or may not include whirlpool action. All of the patient's body is washed while he or she is in the tub. It is difficult for some patients to bend enough to sit down in and get out of a tub. The danger of slips and falls exists. Newer tubs are designed with doors in the side that open for entry and exit, making them less dangerous for patients.

Shower

The patient can sit on a bench or shower chair or stand under the spray of a shower. It is possible to turn the spray off while applying soap to the patient and then turn it back on to rinse. Use caution not to chill the patient. You can usually wash the patient's hair during the shower with little difficulty.

Therapeutic Baths

This is usually a tub bath given for a specific reason. It may be a whirlpool bath to remove infected or necrotic tissue from wounds. It may also involve having the patient soak in the tub with medication added to the water to soothe itching or skin disorders.

Towel or Blanket Bath

This type of bath is done with the patient in bed. It may be commercially prepared or created by the nursing staff. It includes a bath blanket, washcloth(s), and towel(s) in a large bag. The linens are saturated with a no-rinse skin cleanser. The entire bag is then heated in the microwave and taken to the bedside. The patient is covered with a regular bath blanket, which is replaced with the heated moistened bath blanket from the feet up. The patient is massaged through the warm blanket. The heated washcloths are used for the face, and the heated towels are used to cleanse the back, buttocks, and perineum.

Bag Bath

This type of bath is similar to the towel bath, but it also contains 12 to 15 washcloths that are saturated with no-rinse skin cleanser and heated in a bag in the microwave. Each washcloth is used to wash one area of the body and then discarded to prevent cross-contamination and contamination of wounds with dirty bath water. The disposable version is expensive, but the idea can be duplicated with reusable washcloths in a zip-type plastic bag.

follow certain guidelines to prevent contamination of clean areas and to keep your patient comfortable:

- Cover the patient with a **bath blanket,** a large lightweight flannel blanket, during the bath to prevent exposure. Uncover only the area of the body that you are washing, leaving the rest of the body covered. This also prevents the patient from becoming chilled during the bath.
- Fold the washcloth into a mitt around your hand (see Skill 15.1) to prevent trailing cold edges of the washcloth over the patient as you bathe him or her. This takes a bit of practice but is worth the effort to make your patient more comfortable.
- Wash from the cleanest areas to the dirtiest areas to prevent transferring bacteria from a dirty area to a clean area.
- Wash extremities from distal to proximal, which helps return blood to the heart. While patients lie in bed, blood tends to pool in the extremities. Using the distal-to-proximal motion helps move the blood in the veins back to the heart (*venous return*). This is important because when blood pools in the extremities, it increases the risk that a *thrombus,* or blood clot, may form.
- When washing extremities, start with the arm farthest away from you, then wash the nearer arm. This prevents you from reaching across an arm you have washed to reach the far arm. Your scrubs are considered dirtier than the arm you have just washed, and reaching across a clean area could possibly contaminate it. If you wash the far arm and leg first, then wash the nearer arm and leg, contamination will not be a concern.
- Change water anytime it becomes dirty, soapy, or cool. Always change the water after bathing the feet and again after bathing the buttocks and rectal area. For some patients, even tap water for a bath may be unsafe. Patients who have had surgical openings of the sternum to access the heart and lungs, known as *sternotomies,* and those with impaired immune systems may become infected

• **WORD • BUILDING** •

sternotomy: sterno – sternum + tomy – cutting

from the bacteria found in most tap water. In these cases, you may have orders to bathe the patient with sterile water or a commercially prepared towel bath (Fig. 15.1). Box 15.2 includes an explanation of a towel bath.
- Perform perineal care during the bed bath and anytime a patient has been incontinent. You can use soap and water for this care. Some commercial perineal washes are available as well. Skill 15.2 (page 266) provides more information on administering perineal care.
- Some patients are able to perform their own perineal care during the bed bath and would prefer to do so. When the bath is completed except for perineal care, it is appropriate to give the patient the washcloth and provide privacy for washing the genitals. If you say, "Now you can finish your bath," be sure the patient knows what you expect. It may be necessary to be more specific and say something like, "I will step out so you can wash your private areas."

Tub baths, showers, or therapeutic baths require the most effort because the patient must be able to sit or stand for the duration of the bath, usually 5 to 15 minutes, as well as be able to get in and out of the tub or shower. The heat of a shower or bath can cause *vasodilation,* or widening of blood vessels. This, in turn, causes a lowering of the blood pressure. As a result, it is not unusual for patients to become light-headed or dizzy, or even to faint, during a bath or shower. ***Safety: Stay with the patient during the first bath or shower after a surgery or illness in case he or she becomes dizzy or feels faint.*** You can provide privacy by working in the room while the patient is in the bathroom, but stay very near in case the patient needs help. You can delegate the responsibility of staying near and assisting the patient to a CNA or UAP, but be sure to emphasize the importance of checking on the patient often during the bath or shower and listening for the patient to call for help.

Nursing Responsibilities During Bathing

Whether or not a patient can assist with the bath, the nurse must be responsible for a variety of concerns during the bath. Your responsibilities include:

- Assessing the skin for rashes, breaks in integrity, bruising, and lesions.
- Completing the bathing process in a timely manner. Avoid leaving the patient with no gown, with a pan of water that cools off, or in the shower or tub waiting for help to get out.
- Being alert to signs of patient fatigue so that you can assist as needed. If the patient becomes short of breath or begins experiencing pain, be prepared to assume the responsibility for the bath.
- Intervening in ways to conserve the patient's energy during the tub bath or shower. Patients with respiratory illness or heart conditions may become extremely fatigued before the end of a shower or tub bath. Some ways to help conserve energy while bathing include:
  - Having the patient put on a terrycloth robe immediately after the bath or shower. This prevents the need for using energy to dry off with a towel.
  - Using a bench in the shower if the patient is unable to stand for the duration of a shower. The patient can sit during the shower and save the energy required to bend over to wash the legs and feet.
  - Using a chair or bench in the tub if the patient cannot sit all the way down in the tub and easily get back up. Use a sprayer attached to the tub faucet or showerhead to wash the patient's body.

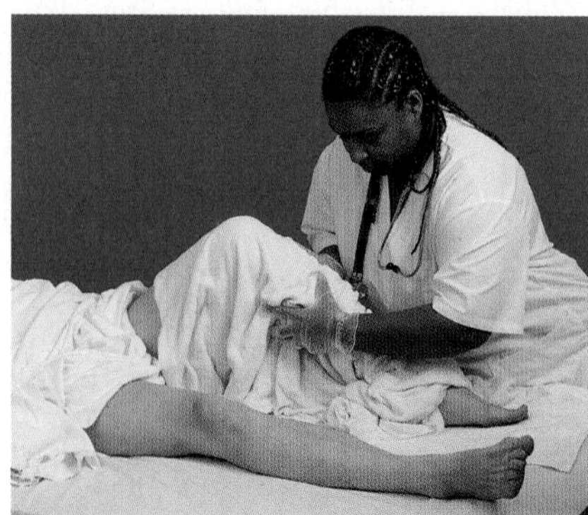

FIGURE 15.1 This nurse is administering a towel bath (from Wilkinson JM, Treas LS. *Fundamentals of Nursing: Theory, Concepts & Applications*. Vol. 2. 3rd ed. Philadelphia, PA: FA Davis; 2016).

Patient Teaching Connection

Antibacterial Versus Nonantibacterial Soaps

Debate continues over the effectiveness versus the harm regarding antibacterial soaps. Certainly, antibacterial alcohol-based hand gel is the norm in the hospital setting and has been proven to be effective through research in such settings. However, debate continues about the widespread use of antibacterial products in the home setting. A large variety of household products are now labeled as antibacterial.

Approximately 75% of antibacterial soaps contain the germ-killing ingredient triclosan. In September 2017, the FDA started to prohibit the sale of antiseptic products containing triclosan, such as antibacterial alcohol-based hand gel. However, hospitals still use 2% triclosan products with patients who are more susceptible to methicillin-resistant *Staphylococcus aureus* prior to surgery. At this time, although antibacterial soaps are still popular, there is no definite indication that they are superior to using regular soap and water.

When you teach patients to perform any skill, always include the steps of handwashing found in Chapter 14. Do not assume that everyone knows the correct way to perform handwashing, which remains the most effective way to prevent the spread of pathogens.

GROOMING

In addition to hygiene, you will assist patients with oral care, hair care, applying deodorant and lotion, dressing or putting on a clean gown, shaving, and nail care, all of which is referred to as grooming. As female patients begin to feel better, you may assist them with applying makeup as well. All of these aspects of ADLs are important to the patient's self-esteem.

Back Massage

During the bath and during evening care, perform a back massage for the patient. Not only does it help relax the patient, it also stimulates circulation. It is necessary to use lotion or oil during a back massage to prevent excessive friction on the patient's skin. Lotion rubs into the skin and is absorbed, necessitating reapplication to keep skin friction at bay.

It is important to massage the muscles, not just apply lotion to the skin (Fig. 15.2). Use the flat side of your fingers rather than your fingertips as you stroke the back to prevent uncomfortable pressure. Use the sides of the thumbs to massage the muscles. Be sensitive to tight, firm areas of muscle tension and work over those areas a bit longer than elsewhere to try to relax the muscles. Pay special attention to the area from the neck to the top of the shoulders. These trapezius muscles tighten in response to anxiety and stress. Do not neglect the lumbar and sacral areas. For many, these lower back areas fatigue quickly and receive little support while the patient lies in bed. Massage in this area also helps increase circulation and prevent pressure injuries.

Back massages may not be indicated if the patient has certain heart conditions because they can stimulate the vagus nerve and slow the heart rate. If the patient has fractures of the ribs or vertebrae, a back massage would not be appropriate because it could increase pain and put pressure on the fractured area.

Back massage is quickly becoming a lost art among nurses. They often feel that they do not have enough time to provide this care. But back massage takes very little time and is of great benefit to the patient. Skill 15.3 (page 268) provides more information on how to provide a back massage.

Oral Care

Providing oral care for patients not only freshens the mouth but also allows you to assess the mouth for problems that could be affecting the patient's nutritional and health status.

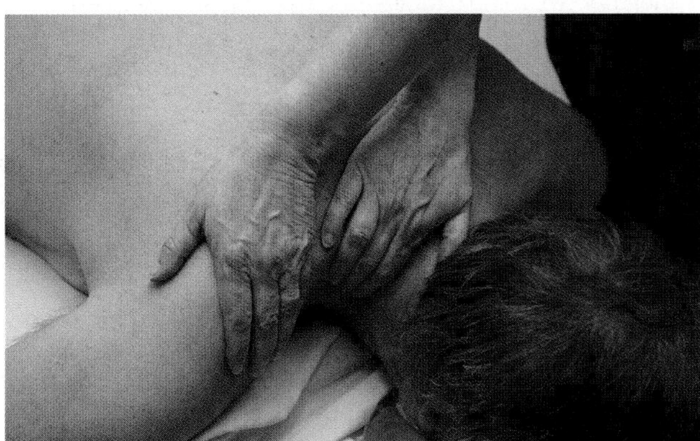

FIGURE 15.2 Correct technique for back massage.

Look for decaying, broken, or missing teeth. Observe for reddened or bleeding gums, ulcerations of the mucosa, and coating of the tongue. White patches on the tongue or oral mucosa, known as **leukoplakia,** can be precancerous lesions.

Oral Care for the Unconscious Patient

When you care for a patient who is unconscious, it still is necessary to give oral care. ***Safety: You must be careful to minimize any chance of aspiration of fluids. To do this, position the patient on either side with the bed flat. In this way, fluids can run out of the mouth instead of down the throat. Keep a suction device ready for use.*** Assess the mouth for lesions and dried mouth secretions known as *sordes*. When you clean the mouth, use the least amount of fluid possible, usually 5 mL or less, to prevent aspiration. Use a small amount of toothpaste and a brush, as well as sponge swabs to clean the mouth and teeth. Lemon-glycerin swabs are not recommended for cleaning the lips or inside of the mouth because they cause drying of the oral mucosa. If they are used over a long period of time, they may cause damage to tooth enamel. Apply water-soluble lip balm to keep the lips moist. Skill 15.4 (page 268) lists the steps of oral care for the unconscious patient.

Special mouth care is the term used for oral care for patients whose conditions result in a need for more frequent care and who need assistance for this care. Such conditions include being unable to take food or fluid by mouth (NPO), receiving oxygen by cannula or mask, having a nasogastric or feeding tube in place, and being unconscious. Special mouth care usually is performed every 2 hours, but follow your facility's policy. When the patient is unconscious, a natural reflex causes the jaw to bite down on anything inserted into the mouth. Make a padded tongue blade by wrapping several gauze squares around one end of a tongue blade and taping them in place. Then insert the padded end of the blade into the patient's mouth and turn it vertically to hold the mouth open while you perform oral care.

Oral Care for the Conscious Patient

Conscious patients may or may not be able to perform their own oral care. If the patient is unable to brush his or her own teeth, assist by putting a small amount of toothpaste on the brush and brush the teeth at a 45-degree angle to the gums. Move the brush in small circles on the inside and outside of the teeth and with back-and-forth strokes across the biting and chewing surfaces of the teeth. Assist with flossing the teeth by gently sliding a 6- to 10-inch piece of dental floss between the teeth, moving it in a backward-and-forward motion. Avoid going deeper than the gum line because this can damage the gums and cause bleeding.

If the patient is able to perform oral care, assist by setting the needed items on the patient's over-bed table. ***Safety: Remain with the patient if any danger of choking exists, such as with a patient who has swallowing difficulties.*** Skill 15.5 (page 269) lists the steps of providing oral care for a conscious patient.

Denture Care

Patients may have full dentures or partial dentures, known as a *bridge.* Partial dentures replace one or more missing teeth and often are removable for cleaning. Dental implants also replace missing teeth, but they are not removable. When cleaning full or partial dentures, be sure to handle them carefully. They are custom-made for each person, so they are expensive. They can break if they are dropped. Line the sink with a towel so that if the dentures slip while you are cleaning them, they will land on a soft surface (Fig. 15.3). Use cool water to clean the dentures because hot water can damage them. Store dentures overnight in a denture cup and water. Add a cleaning tablet if the patient desires. Avoid treating partial dentures containing metal parts with a cleaning tablet; instead, place them in water overnight. Skill 15.6 (page 270) lists the steps in performing denture care.

KNOWLEDGE CONNECTION

What are the benefits of back massage? Why is positioning important when you perform oral care for an unconscious patient?

Shaving

Both male and female patients may require assistance with shaving. Most men shave daily, and if the beard is allowed to grow for 2 or 3 days before shaving, it may become very uncomfortable. ***Safety: Patients taking anticoagulant medications, which delay blood clotting, should only be shaved with electric razors and not with blades of any kind because they could cause excessive bleeding if the patient were accidentally cut.***

When you shave a male patient with a disposable razor, always shave in the direction of hair growth to prevent causing razor burn and ingrown whiskers. When you shave a male patient with an electric razor, move the razor in circular motions over the beard for the closest shave. It is important to clean an electric razor when you are finished shaving the patient. If the razor becomes clogged with cut whiskers, it will cut poorly and be uncomfortable for the patient. To clean the razor, follow the manufacturer's instructions. Usually this involves removing the head of the razor and brushing the recesses and blades to remove debris, then replacing the head. Skill 15.7 (page 271) provides more information on shaving a male patient.

For female patients, generally the axillae and the legs are the areas shaved. Some women may need assistance to shave or pluck stray hairs on the chin or upper lip. Be aware that in many cultures women do not shave their legs or axillae, so it would not be appropriate to offer shaving assistance to them.

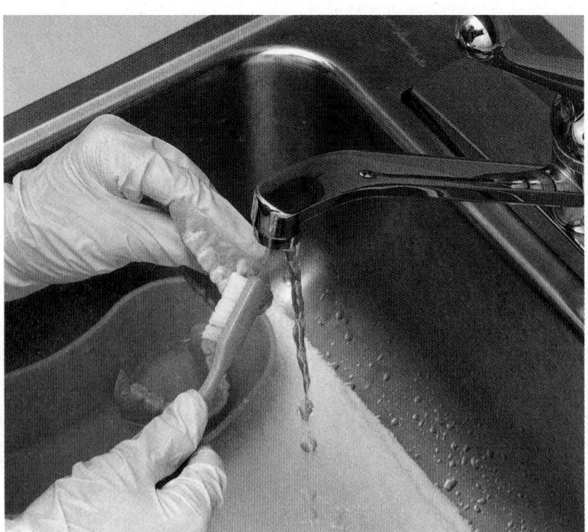

FIGURE 15.3 Correct cleaning technique for dentures. Note the towel in the sink to prevent breakage (from Wilkinson JM, Treas LS. *Fundamentals of Nursing: Theory, Concepts & Applications.* Vol. 1. 3rd ed. Philadelphia, PA: FA Davis; 2016).

Nail Care

Before performing nail care, you should assess the nails for discoloration, ridges, and redness where the skin and nail meet. Patients who are diabetic easily develop infections around nails, so look closely at both fingernails and toenails. Thick, yellowed toenails often have that appearance due to a fungal infection. Prescription medications are available to treat this, so the patient should be advised to consult a podiatrist.

Clean under the fingernails using a small wooden stick (orangewood stick) or file designed for this purpose. When you care for patients' nails, always clip them straight across and then file off any sharp corners. Clipping toenails deeply at the corners can lead to ingrown toenails. ***Safety: If the patient is diabetic, file the nails rather than clipping them to prevent accidentally clipping toe tissue. Because patients with diabetes have poor circulation, such an injury could lead to severe infection and even amputation.***

Skill 15.8 (page 272) provides more information on providing nail care.

KNOWLEDGE CONNECTION

Under what circumstance must a patient be shaved with an electric razor? How can you help prevent ingrown toenails when performing nail care? What is important to remember regarding patients with diabetes and nail care?

Hair Care

In addition to helping patients look and feel better, performing hair care gives you the chance to assess the patient's scalp for potential problems. Inspect the scalp and hair root area for the presence of **lesions,** or open areas. A round area of hair loss with a lesion may indicate ringworm or **tinea capitus,** which is a fungal infection that can affect any part of the body and can be spread from one person to another.

Dry, flaky skin on the scalp may be dandruff. The patient may need to use a special shampoo to relieve the itching and flaking that can accompany dandruff. Thick, oily scales on the scalp may be due to **seborrhea,** or an overproduction of sebum. When this occurs in infants, it is sometimes called *cradle cap*.

Inspect the hair close to the scalp for the presence of tiny parasites called **lice.** Clear bumps affixed tightly to the shaft of the hair are the **nits,** or eggs, of lice. An infestation of lice causes intense itching of the scalp as the lice burrow in to obtain nourishment. Lice are easily transmitted to others by sharing hats, combs, or brushes, or with close contact. Outbreaks of head lice are common occurrences in day-care facilities and elementary schools. Treatment with specific shampoo is required. In addition, the nits must be removed with fine combs so that they do not hatch into more lice. For this reason, the shampoo treatment is repeated approximately 1 to 2 weeks after the first treatment. Lice- and nit-treating shampoos can be toxic, so follow package instructions carefully.

African American patients who need hair care assistance require specialized hair treatment. Natural hair can mat or tangle easily and should be combed and brushed daily. It is important to apply oil to the hair and scalp, which also tends to be dry. Mineral oil or moisturizing hair cream can be used to lubricate the scalp and protect the hair. If the hair has been chemically treated with straighteners or relaxers, it can be dry and easily broken and requires special care when you comb, brush, and shampoo it. If the hair is styled in cornrows or braids, you can shampoo it in that style. Cover the hair with a stocking cap first and then shampoo through the cap.

Shampooing Hair

Patients may require assistance to keep hair clean during an illness or injury. If possible, wash the hair while the patient is in the tub or shower. Have the patient protect the eyes by holding a washcloth over them. Rinse with the patient's head tilted back to keep the shampoo from running into the eyes. If the patient cannot take a tub bath or shower, another option is using a special shampoo that does not need to be rinsed. This type of shampoo is applied to the hair, combed through, and then the hair is dried. It is not as effective as hair washing, but it does help clean the oils out of the hair.

The patient's hair also can be washed while the patient remains in bed. Skill 15.9 (page 273) provides more information on shampooing the hair with the patient in bed. To do this, a rinse-free shampoo cap and/or conditioner is available. Be sure to warm the rinse-free cap in the microwave or warm water prior to applying. Follow the manufacturer's heating instructions. Touch the cap to your wrist to ensure the temperature is not too warm before placing it on the patient's head.

Styling Hair

Style hair according to the patient's preference. Avoid using hairstyles that are not age appropriate, especially for older patients. For example, do not style a 72-year-old woman's hair in pigtails or a ponytail as you would for a young child. This is demeaning to an older woman, who deserves respect.

Caring for Piercings

Body piercing is becoming more and more popular, so you will most likely encounter patients with jewelry in piercings other than in their ears. Common piercing sites include the nose, lip, eyebrow, tongue, nipples, navel, and genitalia.

Piercings that are new must be kept clean and monitored for infections. If your patient with a piercing is unable to do this, you will need to assist. Follow instructions provided by the patient for piercing care. Soap, water, and alcohol are generally used for care of piercing sites. Assess for redness, swelling, pain, or drainage from the site, which would indicate potential infection.

Sometimes it is necessary to remove jewelry from a piercing if it could interfere with surgery; *intubation,* which involves passing a tube through the mouth to the trachea; diagnostic testing, such as magnetic resonance imaging (MRI); or catheterization. If the jewelry is made of nonmagnetic stainless steel or titanium, similar to materials used for joint replacements, it would not have to be removed for an MRI. Some piercings close quickly over a period of just a few days, so the patient may prefer that jewelry remains intact if at all possible.

Removing jewelry from piercings is not always a simple task. Kits are now available to hospitals that contain tools for removal of jewelry from piercings, along with descriptions of each of the common types of jewelry, how they are inserted, and how they should be removed. Table 15.1 provides descriptions of different types of jewelry for piercings and how to remove them.

Eye and Ear Care

Some patients wear glasses or contact lenses and may require assistance with them. Clean patients' glasses with warm water and a soft cloth. Avoid using paper towels or tissues because they can scratch the lenses. Be sure the patient knows where you have put the glasses if he or she is not wearing them. Place them within easy reach because some patients need their glasses to read or watch television.

Contact Lenses

Most patients wearing contacts will be able to remove and insert the lenses themselves. However, if it is necessary for you to remove contact lenses, follow these steps:

1. Wash your hands and put on gloves.
2. Pull down on the lower lid and place one finger across the top of the upper lid, applying gentle but firm pressure.
3. Ask the patient to blink.
4. Hard lenses will pop out between your fingers. A soft contact lens will wrinkle off the eye, and you can grasp it with your fingers. If the soft contact is not easily grasped in this manner, pull the bottom eyelid down and the top eyelid up. Then gently use your gloved finger to pull the contact down off of the *iris* (colored part of the eye) to be grasped and removed. ***Safety: Do not slide the lens down the iris with pressure as this can scratch the cornea.***

• WORD • BUILDING •

seborrhea: sebo – fat + rrhea – flow

Table 15.1
Removing Piercing Jewelry

Name of Jewelry	*Description and Removal*
Barbells	Jewelry with round knobs on each end. Some knobs are removable and some are not.
Vertical barbell	A straight shaft with round knobs on each end. At least one knob, sometimes both, will unscrew. When the knob is removed, the shaft will slip out of the piercing.
Curved barbell	A curved shaft with round knobs on each end. Only one knob will unscrew; the other is fixed. To remove, unscrew the movable knob and slide the curved shaft out of the piercing.
Circular barbell	A circular shaft with two round knobs. Both may unscrew or only one. Unscrew the removable knob and carefully slide in a circular motion to remove from the piercing.
Captive ring	A circular shaft with two ends meeting inside a single ball. To remove, use very small needle-nose type pliers. Insert them in the ring and gently separate the handles to widen the ring. As the ring ends spread open, the single ball is released. Then slide the shaft out of the piercing. *If it is difficult to slide the shaft from the piercing, apply a small amount of water-soluble lubricant to the shaft.*
Prince Albert	Essentially a curved barbell placed in a piercing of the penis. The barbell enters through a piercing in the lower portion of the head of the penis and exits through the urethra. In a reverse Prince Albert, the barbell enters the urethra and exits through a piercing in the top of the glans. Remove as you would a curved barbell.

5. Hold the lens gently and carefully while you place it in the appropriate well of the lens case, either left or right. ***Safety: Be sure you put the lenses in the correct side of the case so that the patient will not insert them into the wrong eye.***
6. Fill the wells, covering the lenses with saline or special soaking solution, according to the patient's routine.

Artificial Eyes

An artificial eye may be used in two different situations. The eye may have been *enucleated,* or complete removed, leaving only the socket. In many of these cases, a globe is implanted in the socket to restore the shape of the eye. The other situation occurs when the eye is intact but is blind, perhaps from birth or due to disease. This is referred to as a *blind globe.*

One type of artificial eye is called a *scleral cover shell.* It is like a thick contact lens that fits flush against the implanted globe or blind globe. It is made of opaque acrylic and covers the whole eye area, not just the iris. The color of the *sclera* (the white part of the eye), iris, pupil, and minute blood vessels are hand painted to match the patient's other eye. Because it is fitted over the globe, which is attached to muscles, this type of artificial eye moves in tandem with the sighted eye.

If no ocular implant is in place, the socket is flat and somewhat deep. The **ocular prosthesis** (artificial eye) is custom made to fit the socket and is hand painted with great detail to match the existing eye. This type of artificial eye does not move.

To care for these eye prostheses, follow the patient's usual care routine. If the patient is unable to remove the artificial eye for cleaning, you will need to assist. A small suction cup on a hollow handle is used to move the prosthesis to and from the orbit. While squeezing the handle of the suction cup, place it on the prosthetic eye and then release the handle. It will remain attached to the prosthesis.

To remove the prosthesis when no implanted globe is present, only an ocular prosthesis, follow these steps:

1. Wash your hands and put on gloves.
2. Dip the end of the suction cup in saline.
3. Lift the upper eyelid.
4. Squeeze the suction cup and place it on the iris of the prosthesis.
5. Stop squeezing.
6. Use the handle of the suction cup to lift the prosthesis out of the socket.

To remove the prosthesis when a natural or implanted blind globe is present, follow these steps:

1. Wash your hands and put on gloves.
2. Dip the end of the suction cup in saline.
3. Squeeze the suction cup and place it on the iris of the prosthesis.
4. Stop squeezing.
5. Raise the upper eyelid.
6. Tilt the prosthesis out from under the upper lid.
7. Lift the prosthesis out. When dealing with a natural blind globe be careful not to touch or press on the cornea, which is very sensitive.

• WORD • BUILDING •

enucleate: enucleare – to remove the kernel of

ocular prosthesis: ocular – related to the eye; pros – in addition + thesis – placed

Cleanse the prosthesis with sterile water or saline, according the patient's routine. Irrigate the eye socket with eye irrigating solution. Small amounts of mucus may gather in the socket. Assess for large amounts of thick yellow or green mucus that would indicate infection.

To replace the artificial eye, follow these steps:

1. Wash hands and put on gloves.
2. Dip the suction cup in saline.
3. Squeeze the suction cup handle and attach it to the iris of the prosthesis.
4. Stop squeezing the handle of the suction cup.
5. Ensure that the prosthesis is wet with saline or lubricating solution.
6. Lift the upper eyelid, making a gap between it and the blind globe or implant.
7. Slide the top of the prosthesis beneath the upper eyelid and release the lid.
8. Pull down on the lower lid and slide the prosthesis behind the lower lid.
9. Release the lower lid.
10. Squeeze the handle of the suction cup; it will release from the prosthesis.
11. Return the suction cup to its appropriate storage place.

Hearing Aids

A number of older patients use hearing aids and may require assistance to insert, remove, and store them. In recent years, hearing aids have become more sophisticated through the use of computer technology. Rather than magnifying all sounds, including background noises, newer types of aids can magnify voices while not increasing extra noises. Some of the newer aids must be carefully protected from moisture, including being kept in a special moisture-absorbing medium when not in use. Figure 15.4 shows different types of hearing aids.

CLEANING HEARING AIDS. If the ear mold can be separated from the hearing aid (for example, in the behind-the-ear model), turn off the aid and detach it. Clean the ear mold with warm soapy water. The in-the-canal style of hearing aid may have a screen or filter to block wax. If so, spread a clean cloth on a hard surface and gently tap the aid against the cloth to remove wax from the screen or filter. Clean other types of aids by wiping them with a damp cloth and cleaning the opening with a pipe cleaner, cotton-tipped applicator, or toothpick to remove any wax buildup.

To remove a hearing aid, follow these steps:

1. Turn off the hearing aid.
2. Turn the ear mold slightly toward the nose and lift out.
3. Store the aid in its case or moisture-control container.

To insert a hearing aid, follow these steps:

1. Check the battery by turning the hearing aid on to full volume and listening for it to whistle, which indicates that it is working.
2. If you do not hear a whistle, check the battery and replace as needed.
3. Turn off the hearing aid and lower the volume.
4. Insert the hearing aid into the ear and adjust the volume as needed.

KNOWLEDGE CONNECTION

Under what circumstances should jewelry be removed from a body piercing? How can you tell if the battery in a hearing aid is working?

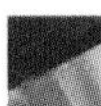

MANAGING THE ENVIRONMENT

Another aspect of patient care is making the environment comfortable and conducive to rest. This is not always easy to do given all the noise and activity found on a nursing unit.

The Patient Room

Most hospitalized patients spend the majority of their time in the patient unit or hospital room. This may be a private or semiprivate room. When a roommate is present, it is very important to provide privacy whenever you give care. This can be achieved by pulling the curtain separating the two beds and speaking in a soft voice when discussing health-care issues with the patient. If further privacy is needed, it is appropriate to move the patient to a conference room or examination room for discussion of sensitive topics.

Furniture

The hospital bed is a special type of bed designed to be placed in a variety of positions, which will be discussed later in this chapter. Both the head and the foot of the bed can be elevated. In addition, the area under the knees can be raised to prevent the patient from sliding down in the bed when the head of the bed is elevated. The mattress is covered with water-repellent material and is firmer than many home mattresses. The bed usually has rails on either side that can be raised as a safety measure to prevent falling or for the patient to grasp when turning from side to side. Often the controls for the television and the nurse call light are built into the side rails so that they are always within easy reach.

The over-bed table is designed to be placed alongside the bed or across the bed. It is wheeled for ease of movement and may have a movable top that pushes back to reveal a small storage area that is convenient for glasses, combs, and brushes. Generally it contains a mirror that the patient can use for shaving or applying makeup. A food tray is placed on this table, which is then placed across the bed so the patient can eat. It is important to remove any unpleasant sights and smells from the tabletop before placing the food tray on it. Remove anything from the over-bed table that you would not want sitting on your kitchen table during a meal, including toilet tissue, a dirty emesis basin, a urinal, trash, soiled tissues, and soiled drinking glasses or dishes from previous meals.

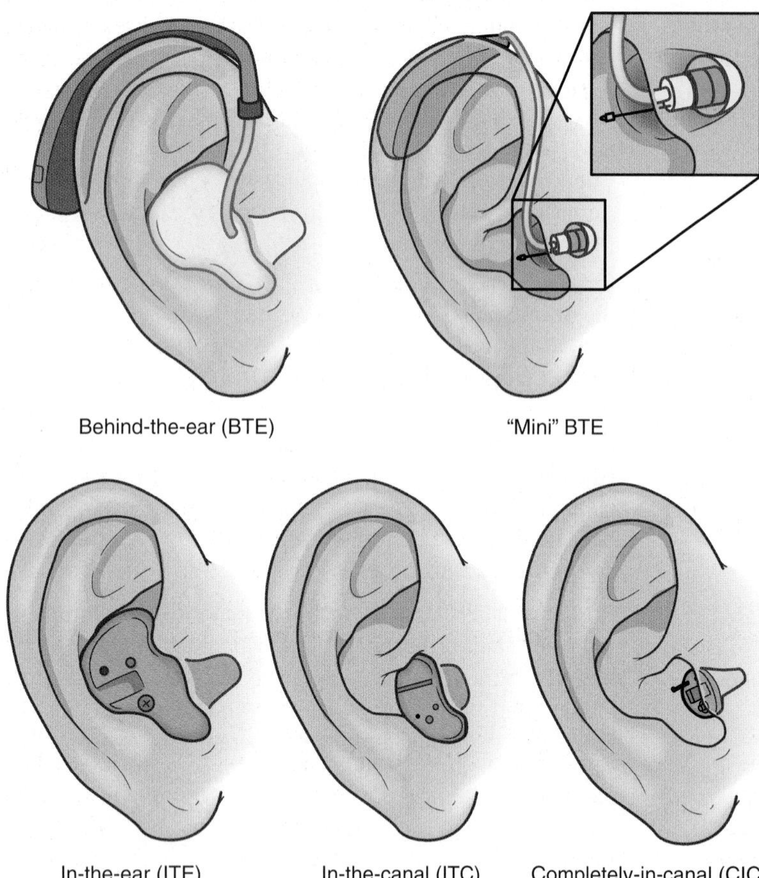

FIGURE 15.4 Five different types of hearing aids: (a) Behind-the-ear hearing aid; (b) Mini behind-the-ear hearing aid; (c) In-the-ear hearing aid; (d) In-the-canal hearing aid; (e) Completely-in-canal hearing aid. (Illustration courtesy of the National Institutes of Health, Department of Health and Human Services, https://www.nidcd.nih.gov/sites/default/files/Documents/health/hearing/nidcd-hearing-aids.pdf.)

The bedside stand usually contains three drawers and can be used for supplies, personal items, and clothing. It is difficult for the patient in bed to reach for items in the drawers, so generally infrequently needed items are stored there. When a patient leaves the room because of transfer or discharge, it is important that you empty all the drawers and ensure that personal belongings are sent with the patient. Usually a small closet is built into the area across from the bed, so clothing may be stored there as well.

Environment

The patient may have many concerns about the hospital environment that the nurse may not notice because the concerns are commonplace in the hospital. However, they are not commonplace for the patient. Some problems and ways to manage them include the following:

- **Noise:** Keep the patient's door closed or nearly closed to help block out hallway noise and activity. Avoid shouting or calling out in the hallways or from the nurse's station. If the patient wishes, keep the television or radio on for soft background noise. Answer call lights and extinguish alarms on equipment promptly.
- **Odors:** Remove and empty bed pans, urinals, bedside commodes, and emesis basins promptly. Use sprays to neutralize odors, but avoid perfumed sprays that could cause reactions in patients with respiratory disorders such as asthma. ***Safety: The health-care staff should not wear perfumes, colognes, aftershave, or scented body lotions while caring for patients. Some patients with respiratory disorders can react strongly to such scents, causing an asthma attack or difficulty breathing.***

  Sometimes food odors can be unpleasant if the patient is nauseated. Remove food trays promptly if the patient does not wish to eat. Keep the tray warm in the kitchen or other appropriate location if the patient may want it later. Empty trash promptly to prevent lingering odors in the room.
- **Clutter:** It does not take long for over-bed tables and bedside stands to become crowded with the patient's belongings and patient care supplies. In addition, patients sometimes keep food from their meal tray to eat later. The water pitcher, drinking glass, and straw should be within the patient's reach. Many hospital rooms have a plant shelf where you can put cards, vases, and potted plants. Do not remove personal items from within reach without the patient's permission. Try to arrange needed items so that they are within reach and move less frequently used items to the drawers in the bedside stand.
- **Equipment:** Hospital rooms become cluttered quickly with equipment, supplies, and visitors' belongings. It is

extremely important to keep pathways from the bed to the bathroom clear for the patient. Ensure that cords are out of the way to prevent tripping. Assist the patient in and out of bed to ensure that the IV lines and other attached tubing do not get pulled or kinked. Keep equipment against the walls if possible and out of walkways. Promptly remove equipment that is not in use.

Bedmaking

In the acute care setting, linens are changed frequently. Follow the policy at your facility for routine changes and also change the linen if the bed is soiled. When making beds, several options exist for both the unoccupied bed and the occupied bed.

UNOCCUPIED BED. The bed is considered unoccupied when the patient is out of the bed while the linens are changed. The patient may be sitting up in the chair or may have left the patient unit for therapy or diagnostic tests. Several types of unoccupied beds may be made:

- **Open bed:** This type of bed is made with the top linens fanfolded to the foot of the bed so that the patient can easily slip into the bed and pull them up.
- **Surgical bed:** This type of bed is made with the top linens fanfolded to the side of the bed (the side away from the door). When the patient returns on a stretcher, he or she can easily be moved into the bed without the top linens being in the way. The patient can quickly be covered without his or her feet getting tangled in the linens. The top sheet and blanket are spread over the patient, then tucked at the foot of the bed. Not all facilities use the surgical bed, but it is a good way to keep linens out of the way during a transfer from stretcher to bed.
- **Closed bed:** In acute care, the closed bed is only used when the patient is discharged. The room is terminally cleaned and the bed is made with fresh linens. The top linens are spread to the head of the bed to keep the bed clean. This will be converted to an open bed when staff are alerted to a patient admission.

Skill 15.10 (page 273) provides more information on making an unoccupied bed.

OCCUPIED BED. The bed is considered occupied if the linens are changed while the patient remains in the bed. This is done when the patient is unable to be out of bed. The patient is turned to one side while soiled bottom linens are loosened and fanfolded to the middle of the bed, beneath the patient. A clean fitted sheet and draw sheet are applied to the bed up to where the patient is lying. Then the patient turns to the other side, rolling over the "hump" of soiled and clean linens. The nurse goes to the opposite side of the bed and removes the soiled linens, then spreads out and tucks in the clean linens. With the patient lying on his or her back, the top soiled linens are removed and the clean ones applied. Skill 15.11 (page 275) provides more information on making an occupied bed.

NURSING RESPONSIBILITIES IN BEDMAKING. Bedmaking is often delegated to a CNA or a UAP. Whoever makes the bed, it is very important to make the bed tightly without wrinkles. Wrinkles in a poorly made bed can contribute to the development of pressure injuries as well as patient discomfort.

Making the bed in a hospital is different than making the bed at home. The number one concern is patient safety. ***Safety: Make certain the bed rails are raised on the opposite side of the bed from where you are working. Remember to raise the rails on the working side of the bed before going around the bed to the other side.*** Some facilities use mattress covers to make the plastic mattress more comfortable. Then you will most likely use a fitted sheet for the bottom sheet. Next, you will apply a **draw sheet** or turn sheet. This type of sheet is narrower than a flat sheet. Also, a flat sheet has a wide hem at the top and a narrow hem at the bottom. A draw sheet has two narrow hems on each end. Some draw sheets are wide enough to fold in half lengthwise, and some are designed to be a single layer. The draw sheet is positioned horizontally across the bed with the top edge aligned at the patient's shoulders and the bottom edge at the patient's knees.

The edge of the draw sheet is tucked between the mattress and springs on one side of the bed. When you go to the other side of the bed, grasp the draw sheet firmly in the middle with both hands. Pull the sheet tightly across the mattress and down to tuck it between the mattress and springs. Next, pull the draw sheet at the edge near the top and tuck it; follow by doing the same at the edge near the bottom. Smooth out wrinkles. A tight, smooth draw sheet is the secret to a comfortable bed.

Draw sheets are used to protect the bottom sheet from minor soiling and to help lift and turn heavier patients. A disposable or washable incontinence pad may be used to protect the bottom sheet and draw sheet from soiling. Then only the pad has to be changed instead of having to change the whole bed.

When you apply the top linens to the bed, turn the top sheet so that the seams are away from the patient and spread the sheet and blanket smoothly across the bed. Then tuck them *together* at the foot of the bed. This prevents loosening the top sheet when tucking the blanket. Go to the side of the bed and form a **mitered corner** (slanted corner) as you tuck both the sheet and blanket together. (See Skill 15.10 for details on how to form a mitered corner.) The purpose of this type of corner is to anchor the linens more firmly than if they were only tucked at the foot of the mattress.

Whether you make an occupied or unoccupied bed, it is important to cuff the top sheet over the blanket or spread to prevent rough fabric edges from irritating the skin of the patient's face and neck. Sheets and blankets are laundered in the hospital laundry or at a commercial facility and may be more stiff and scratchy than linens at home.

When making an occupied bed, the process of tucking the top linens under the foot of the mattress causes *plantar flexion* of the patient's feet (toes pointed downward). This can result in pressure injuries on the toes or contribute to *footdrop,* where the foot remains in a permanent state of plantar flexion.

Footdrop impairs the patient's ability to walk again. This is also uncomfortable for the patient and can be easily remedied by grasping the top linens above the patient's toes and pulling upward an inch or two, making room for the natural foot position.

Another consideration when making an occupied bed is that you will be placing a clean fitted sheet and draw sheet beneath soiled existing sheets. If necessary, you can place a disposable pad between the clean and soiled linens to prevent contamination.

Bed Positions

Another issue regarding the patient's environment is positioning the bed for patient comfort or for therapeutic reasons. It is important for you to be familiar with bed positions and to be able to place the bed in various positions quickly. In some situations, positioning of the bed and patient can help prevent severe shortness of breath or shock. Table 15.2 provides descriptions and uses of common bed positions.

KNOWLEDGE CONNECTION

How can you control odors in a patient's room? What bed position is used for a patient in shock? How do you keep a draw sheet tight and smooth?

Table 15.2
Common Bed Positions

Position	*Diagram*	*Use*
Flat	Head Flat Foot	Used for resting or sleeping and after certain procedures such as lumbar punctures and back surgery.
Fowler's	Fowler's position	Knees slightly elevated to prevent sliding down; used when patients want to sit up to watch TV or converse with visitors.
Semi-Fowler's	Semi-Fowler's position	Used for patients on continuous tube feedings to prevent aspiration and for comfort when patient does not wish to be completely flat.
Trendelenburg	Trendelenburg position	Used for patients who have very low blood pressure (shock) to return blood to the brain and vital organs. Keeping the head of the bed flat with the feet elevated is the preferred bed position for patients with breathing difficulty or head injury.

Table 15.2
Common Bed Positions—cont'd

Position	*Diagram*	*Use*
Reverse Trendelenburg	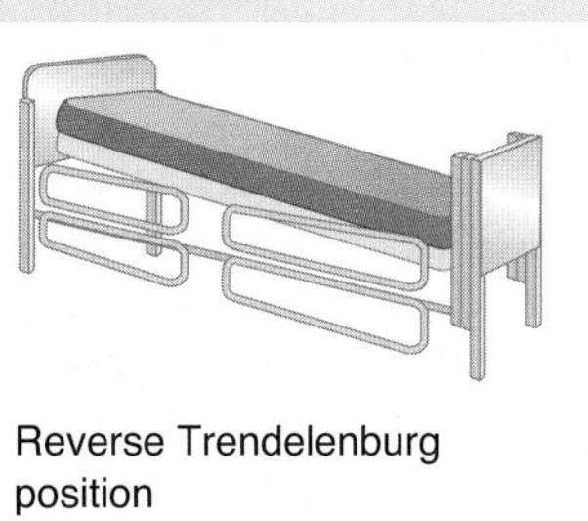 Reverse Trendelenburg position	Used to elevate the patient's head without bending at the waist for patients who have returned from procedures requiring that the legs be kept straight at the groin, such as a cardiac catheterization.

Nursing Care Plan for Personal Care for a Patient With Severe Weakness

You will often care for patients who are unable to perform their own ADLs without assistance. It is important to encourage patients to do as much as possible for themselves while still assisting before the patient becomes excessively fatigued. One day a patient may be able to do very little but another day may be able to accomplish more. You will learn to discern when to intervene and when to encourage the patient to be independent.

Assessment

You are caring for a patient who has just been admitted to a skilled nursing facility (SNF). She is 74 years old and is recovering from bacterial pneumonia. She is very weak and has come to the SNF to gain strength before she returns home. At this point she is unable to perform her ADLs without assistance and becomes short of breath with almost any exertion. She wears a hearing aid, dentures, and glasses. She is sometimes unable to control her bladder, especially when she is sleeping deeply.

Because she is new to the SNF, the staff does not know how much she can do for herself. The nurses' notes and flow sheet from the hospital indicate she was on bedrest until the day before discharge and was being given bed baths daily. She also received perineal care several times per day because of urinary incontinence.

Nursing Diagnosis

Several nursing diagnoses are related to patients who are unable to perform ADLs. In this patient's case, she needs help with bathing, grooming, and toileting. She also fatigues very easily with any activity. The nursing diagnoses for the patient would be worded as follows:

- Bathing self-care deficit related to weakness as evidenced by shortness of breath and fatigue with exertion
- Toileting self-care deficit related to weakness as evidenced by urinary incontinence when sleeping

Planning

As you plan for outcomes and care for this patient, you must focus not only on assisting her with ADLs now, but also on helping her to become more independent before she returns home. Your plan must include gradually increasing her participation in ADLs as she gains strength.

You decide that you will assist her to sit on the side of the bed during the bath. That way you can assist her back into bed if she becomes too fatigued. You will plan to evaluate her ability to help with her bath today. That way you will be able to encourage her to do more the next day.

You also plan to help her to the bathroom every 2 hours during the day to help prevent incontinence and to check the bed often while she is asleep. You will be prepared to provide perineal care should it be necessary.

Implementation

You are now ready to implement the interventions that you have planned. (The Care Plan below is a summary of the care plan interventions and evaluations.)

Evaluation

To evaluate the effectiveness of your interventions, ask yourself the following questions:

- Were your interventions effective in helping the patient perform ADLs without excessive fatigue or shortness of breath?
- Did your interventions help the patient gradually increase her ability to be independent in performing ADLs?

If you can answer both of these questions with a "yes," you have been successful in accomplishing your goals and outcomes for this patient. If you had to answer "no" to either question, you must determine what went wrong and devise improved interventions for the future.

(nursing care plan continues on page 264)

Nursing Care Plan for Personal Care for a Patient With Severe Weakness—cont'd

Nursing Diagnosis: Bathing self-care deficit related to weakness as evidenced by fatigue and shortness of breath with exertion
Expected Outcomes: Patient will gradually assume ability to bathe self prior to discharge to home.

Interventions	Evaluations
• Assist patient with partial bath while she sits on side of bed. Return to bed if she becomes too fatigued to continue. • Take cues from patient to see if she is shaky or must stop to rest often to catch her breath. If so, assist back to bed in semi-Fowler's position to complete bath.	Day 1: Patient sat on side of bed while upper body washed, rinsed, and dried. Patient asked to rest after this part of the bath and was returned to bed while you washed, rinsed, and dried her lower body. Day 3: Able to sit on side of bed for complete bath without complaints of shortness of breath or excessive fatigue.
• Ask patient to wash her face and hands on Day 1. Then ask if she feels strong enough to wash any other parts of her body. Increase her participation on Day 2 and Day 3.	Day 1: Patient able to wash face, hands, and arms. Too fatigued to do more. Day 3: Patient washed all but her back and feet. Did become somewhat short of breath washing legs.

Nursing Diagnosis: Toileting self-care deficit related to weakness as evidenced by fatigue and shortness of breath with exertion
Expected Outcomes: Patient will be able to go to the bathroom independently by discharge to home.

Interventions	Evaluations
• Assist patient to the bathroom or bedside commode every 2 to 3 hours while awake. • Perform perineal care as needed if patient is incontinent of urine. • Change incontinence pad and/or draw sheet if wet. • Provide privacy for perineal care and toileting. • Avoid saying or doing anything to embarrass patient if she is incontinent of urine.	Day 1: Patient assisted to bedside commode x4 during daytime shift. Urinated each time. Incontinent of urine 1 time while sleeping. Assisted with perineal care and draw sheet changed. Day 3: Patient asked for assistance to bathroom after meals and two other times. Able to walk to bathroom with assistance. Patient was not incontinent during day shift, but was x2 during the night.

Skill 15.1 Administering a Complete Bed Bath

Assessment Steps

1. Review the patient's chart for activity orders and position restrictions.
2. Assess the patient's ability to turn, follow directions, and remain in one position.
3. Determine the need for assistance during the bed bath.
4. Determine the patient's status: Is there pain, fatigue, or shortness of breath? Are there cultural issues to address?
5. Determine the type of bath most appropriate for this patient.

Planning Steps

1. Gather needed equipment and supplies: bath basin, towels (two or three), washcloths (two or three), soap, bath blanket, clean gown or pajamas (obtain a snap-shoulder gown if the patient has an IV line), laundry bag, and clean linens for occupied bed change.
2. Plan to give the bed bath at the time the patient prefers.
3. Plan for privacy throughout the bath by placing a "Bath in Progress" sign on the door.

Implementation Steps

1. Follow the Initial Implementation Steps located on the inside back cover.
2. Prepare the patient and the room: provide privacy, adjust the room temperature, and offer the bed pan or urinal. ***This prevents interruptions during the bath.***
3. Fill the bath basin approximately two-thirds of the way full with warm water (105°F). Test the temperature by applying water to your inner wrist to determine that it is not too warm. ***This prevents discomfort from water that is too hot or too cool.***
4. Place the basin on the over-bed table and position the table parallel to the bed.
5. Lower the side rail nearest you. Assist the patient to move closer to you.
6. Remove the blanket or bedspread. Spread the bath blanket over the top sheet. Ask the patient to hold on to the bath blanket while you remove the sheet from beneath it. ***This prevents exposure and keeps the patient warm.***
7. Untie the patient's gown and remove it. If the patient has an IV infusion that is not on a pump, slide the gown down the arm, then remove the IV bag from the stand and slide the bag through the sleeve in the same direction as the patient's hand ***to prevent the IV tubing from becoming tangled in the gown.*** If the IV infusion is on a pump, a gown with snaps or other closure on the shoulder must be used. *Safety: Do not disconnect IV tubing to change patient gowns because this can lead to infection.*

Skill 15.1 (continued)

8. Place a towel under the patient's head to protect the pillow.
9. Fold a washcloth into a mitt around your hand. To do this, dampen the cloth. Then wrap it around your hand, holding it in place with your thumb. Fold the remaining portion of the cloth over your fingers and tuck it under the edge in your palm.

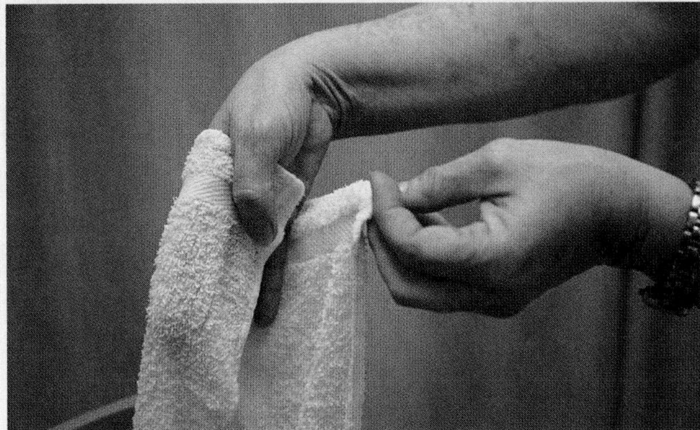

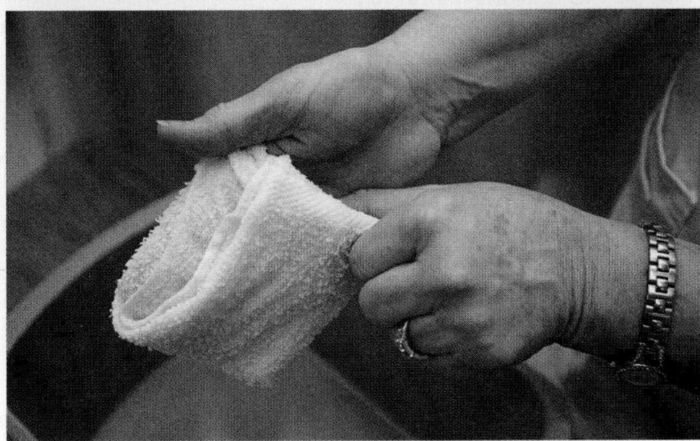

10. Wash one eye using a corner of the bath mitt. Wash from the inner *canthus* (corner of the eye) to the outer canthus ***to prevent spreading pathogens across the eye.***
11. Repeat with the opposite eye and a different corner of the washcloth.
12. Wash the face without soap. Use any special facial cleanser the patient may provide. Wash the neck and ears. Rinse the face, neck, and ears and pat dry.
13. Expose the arm farthest from you by folding the bath blanket away from the arm, but keeping the rest of the patient covered.
14. Remove the towel from beneath the patient's head and place it lengthwise beneath the far arm.
15. Wash and rinse the far hand and arm using long strokes from the hand to the axilla ***to promote venous return.*** *Safety: Support the arm joints as you lift the arm to prevent possible injury to the elbow or shoulder.* Pat the arm dry using the towel beneath it.
16. Repeat for the near arm.

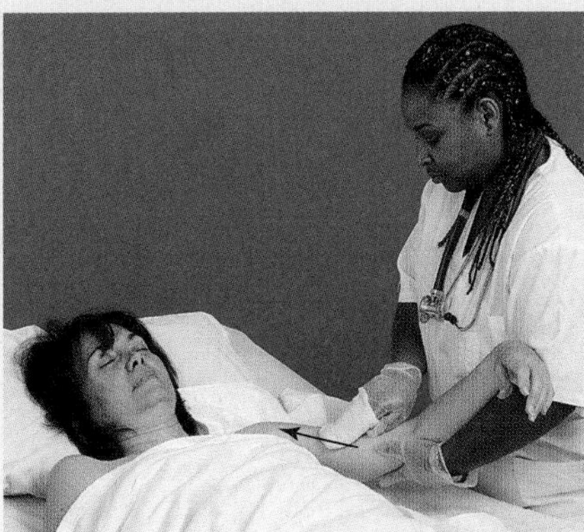

17. Apply deodorant to the axillae according to the patient's preference.

    Note: If the towel has become damp, obtain a new towel. If the water is cool or dirty, empty the basin and obtain fresh water.
18. Place the towel horizontally across the patient's chest. Fold the bath blanket back to the patient's waist. ***This protects the patient's modesty and keeps patient warm while allowing access to the chest area.***
19. Fold the towel toward the waist while you wash and rinse the chest. For female patients, lift each breast to wash and rinse beneath it. Assess for skin breakdown, which often occurs in skinfolds. Dry thoroughly beneath each breast.
20. Replace the towel over the chest and fold upward to expose the abdomen. Wash, rinse, and dry the abdomen. *Safety: If abdominal incisions are present, wash gently around dressings or tape.*

    Note: If the towel has become damp, obtain a new towel. If the water is cool or dirty, empty the basin and obtain fresh water.
21. Replace the bath blanket over the chest and fold back to expose the far leg. Place the towel lengthwise under the leg.
22. Wash and rinse the far leg, using long strokes from ankle to hip.
23. Assist the patient to bend the knee and place the foot flat on the bed. Bring the basin to the bed and place it by the patient's foot. Assist the patient to place the foot into the bath basin and allow it to soak. ***This helps soften and remove dead skin buildup on the foot and helps clean thoroughly between the toes.***

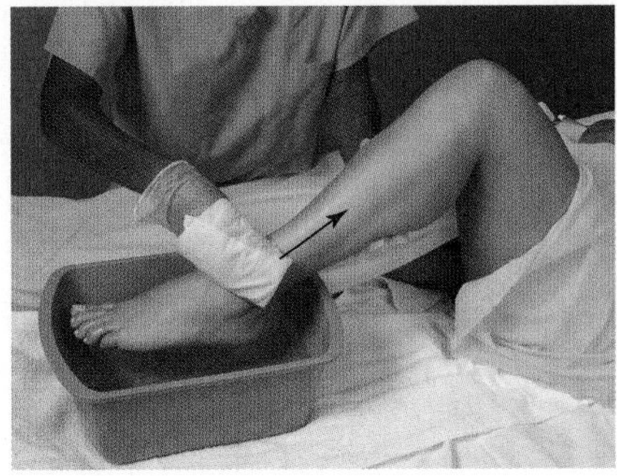

(skill continues on page 266)

Skill 15.1 (continued)

24. Wash the foot carefully. Wash between the toes and inspect for reddened areas or skin lesions.
25. Remove the basin to the over-bed table. Pat the foot and leg dry using the towel beneath the leg.
26. Repeat the procedure with the near leg.
    Note: If the towel has become damp, obtain a new towel. If the water is cool or dirty, empty the basin and obtain fresh water.
27. Assist the patient to turn onto his or her side so the back is facing you. Place a dry towel lengthwise along the back. *Safety: The far side rail should be up to prevent falling when the patient turns on his or her side.*
28. Fold the bath blanket up to expose the patient's back. Wash and rinse the back, then pat it dry with the towel. Perform a back massage (see Skill 15.3).

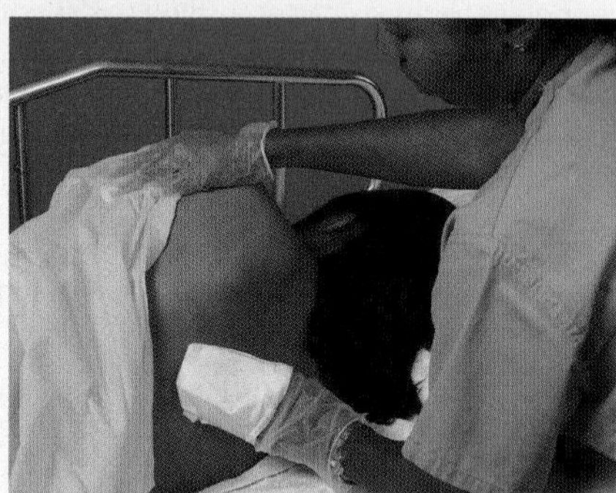

29. Wash the rectal area. Separate the buttocks and clean the area well. Assess for skin breakdown in the gluteal folds. *Safety: Wear gloves to prevent exposure to body fluids and pathogens.*
30. If the patient has been incontinent of stool, clean the area with toilet tissue first, then wash with the washcloth. *Safety: Always wash from front to back to prevent contamination with fecal matter or bacteria.*
31. Wash, rinse, and dry with towel placed along the back earlier. Cover any soiled area on the sheet with a towel or bed protector until the bath is completed and the sheets can be changed.
32. Change the water. Rinse out the basin and wipe it clean if needed. ***This prevents contamination from the basin and water when you perform perineal care.*** Obtain a clean washcloth and towel.
33. Assist the patient to turn onto his or her back and position the patient for perineal care.
34. Perform perineal care (see Skill 15.2) and remove gloves. Wash hands.
35. Reposition the bath blanket. Assist the patient into a clean gown or pajamas. If an IV infusion is present, obtain a gown with shoulder snaps or closures. If the IV infusion is not on a pump and no snap gown is available, put the IV bag through the gown sleeve first and then put the patient's arm through the sleeve.
36. Change the occupied bed (see Skill 15.11).
37. Follow the Ending Implementation Steps located on the inside back cover.

Evaluation Steps

1. Evaluate the condition of the patient's skin. Note any red or open areas or signs of pressure.
2. Evaluate the patient's condition during the bath. Did the bath tire the patient excessively? Is the patient in pain or short of breath?
3. Evaluate the patient's comfort. Is the patient clean and comfortable after the bath?

Sample Documentation

Personal care is often not documented except on a flow sheet. If abnormal findings are present, they are documented in the nurse's notes as shown below.

09/17/22 0940 Complete bed bath given. 3-cm reddened area noted on coccyx. Occlusive dressing applied. Positioned on right side. ——————

—————— Nurse's signature and credentials

Skill 15.2 Administering Perineal Care

Assessment Steps

1. Assess the need for perineal care if the procedure is not part of a complete bed bath.
2. Assess the need for clean sheets if the ones on the bed are soiled.

Planning Steps

1. Gather needed equipment and supplies: washcloths, towel, bath blanket, toilet tissue, incontinence pad, and clean sheets as needed.
2. Determine the need for assistance of another staff member to complete perineal care.

Implementation Steps

1. Follow the Initial Implementation Steps located on the inside back cover.
2. Position the patient on his or her back. Remove the blanket or bedspread and cover the top sheet with a bath blanket. Have the patient hold on to the blanket while you remove the top sheet from beneath it.

For a Female Patient

3. Turn the bath blanket so that it is in a diamond shape across the patient, with a point toward the head, one toward the feet, and the two others at the sides.

Skill 15.2 (continued)

4. Ask the patient to bend her knees and place her feet flat on the bed. Grasp one of the side points and wrap the blanket around the patient's leg and foot. Repeat with the other side. This leaves the lower point of the diamond between the patient's feet, where it can be lifted up and folded back. ***This provides warmth and privacy for the patient during perineal care.*** *Safety: Wear gloves to prevent exposure to body fluids and pathogens.*

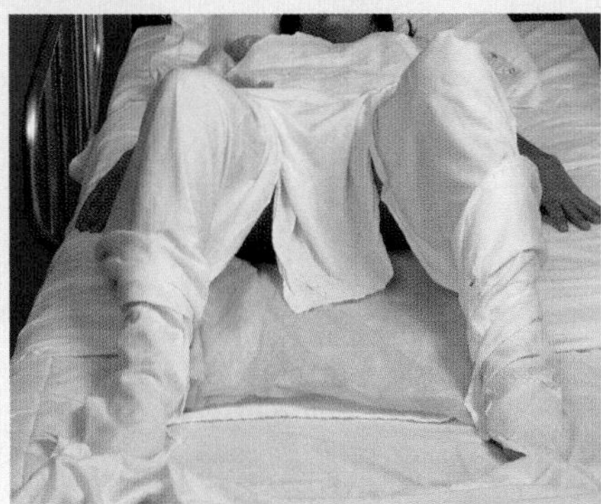

5. Use toilet paper to clean any fecal material from the perineal area, wiping from front to back. *Safety: Always wash from front to back to prevent contaminating the vaginal and urethral areas with* Escherichia coli.
6. Dampen the washcloth and apply soap or periwash. Make the washcloth into a mitt as in the procedure for a complete bed bath (see Skill 15.1).
7. Spread the patient's labia with your nondominant hand and use a different part of the washcloth to clean the far side, near side, and middle of the vulva, washing from front to back. Continue to wash the outer labia and perineum until clean.

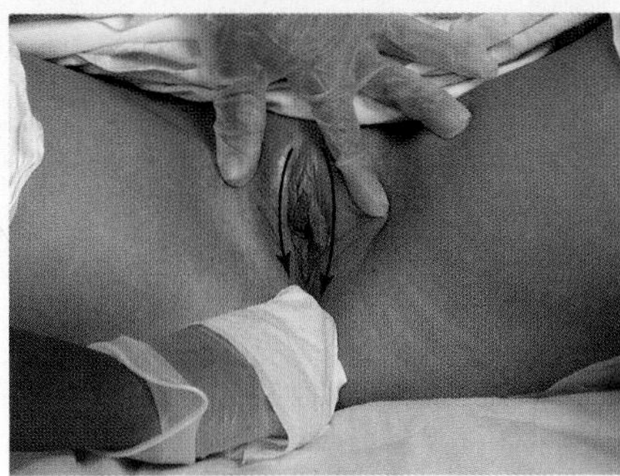

For a Male Patient

3. Place the bath blanket over the patient's chest and fold the bed linens down to expose the perineal area.
4. If the patient is uncircumcised, retract the foreskin. Wipe in a circular motion from the tip of the penis around the glans. Repeat using another area of the washcloth. Rinse and pat dry. Replace the foreskin. *Safety: It is necessary to replace the foreskin to prevent constriction of circulation and possible edema and necrosis of the glans penis.*

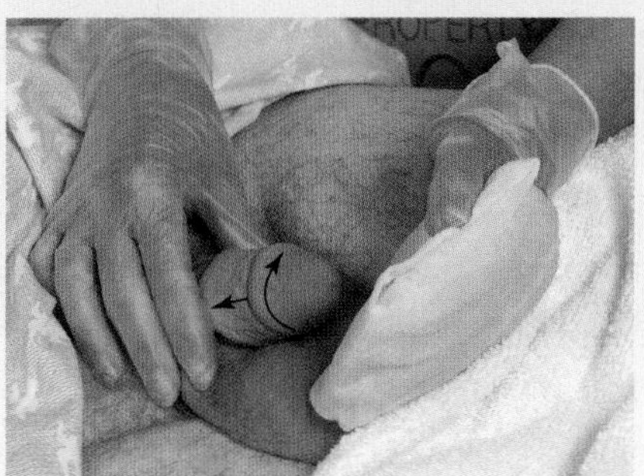

5. If the patient is circumcised, wipe in a circular motion from the tip of the penis around the glans. Repeat using another area of the washcloth. Rinse and pat dry.
6. Rinse washcloth and reapply soap or periwash.
7. Wash shaft of the penis and scrotum. Rinse and pat dry.

For Both Male and Female Patients

8. Assess skin for excoriation or maceration. ***If the patient is incontinent, the skin may break down due to exposure to urine and feces.***
9. If the patient has a catheter, use a washcloth with mild soap and water and gently wipe the catheter from the insertion site away from the body. *Safety: Hold the catheter so that no traction is placed on the tubing as you wash to prevent causing trauma to the urethra.*
10. Turn the patient to the side and clean the rectal area if you are not continuing a complete bed bath. Again, wash from front to back, rinse, and pat dry (see Skill 15.1).
11. Change the linens and bed protector as needed.
12. Follow the Ending Implementation Steps located on the inside back cover.

Evaluation Steps

1. Evaluate the patient's skin condition and frequency of incontinence.
2. Evaluate the need for skin barrier cream such as Desitin ointment.
3. Evaluate the patient's tolerance of the procedure. Did it cause shortness of breath, pain, or fatigue?

Sample Documentation

Personal care is often not documented except on a flow sheet. If abnormal findings are present, they are documented in the nurse's notes as shown below.

09/17/22 1440 Incontinent of urine and small amount of pasty brown stool. Perineal care completed. No redness, excoriation, or maceration noted. ——————
—————— Nurse's signature and credentials

Skill 15.3 Administering a Back Massage

Assessment Steps

1. Review the patient's diagnoses for contraindications to back massage, such as heart conditions, bradycardia, pulmonary emboli, and musculoskeletal disorders or fractures of the ribs and vertebrae.
2. Inspect the skin for rashes or lesions. Avoid massaging over open areas or rashes.

Planning Steps

1. Gather needed equipment and supplies: skin lotion or oil and a towel.

Implementation Steps

1. Follow the Initial Implementation Steps located on the inside back cover.
2. Position the patient on his or her side or stomach and untie gown ***to provide access to the full back.***
3. Apply lotion or oil to your hands to warm it and to avoid startling the patient by applying it directly to the back.
4. Place your hands on either side of the spine at the patient's waist with your palms and fingers flat.
5. Rub gently with continuous pressure up to the neck. With fingers flat against the patient's skin and moving in large circles, stroke from the neck to the waist.
6. Repeat Steps 3 and 4 three times, covering all of the area of the back from the spine outward. *Safety: Do not massage directly over vertebrae to prevent possible injury to the patient.*
7. Use consistent pressure that is comfortable to the patient. ***Too much pressure can cause pain or discomfort. Too little pressure can tickle the patient.***
8. Massage from the neck to the shoulder, keeping your fingers flat and sliding them down the side of the neck and along the trapezius muscle. Repeat on the other side. Note muscular tightness in this area and repeat strokes to relax the tightness.
9. Apply lotion again to reduce friction on the skin.
10. Use the sides of the thumbs, alternating between the left and right thumb, to massage around each scapula. You should feel the discrete edges of the bone without tight muscle or your thumbs bumping over muscle attachments. If this is felt, work gently but firmly over the areas to try to release them. Do not work so deep as to cause pain or discomfort to the patient.
11. Massage with the sides of the thumbs from near the spine outward, alternating between your left and right thumb to cover from the low back to the shoulder. Repeat on the other side.

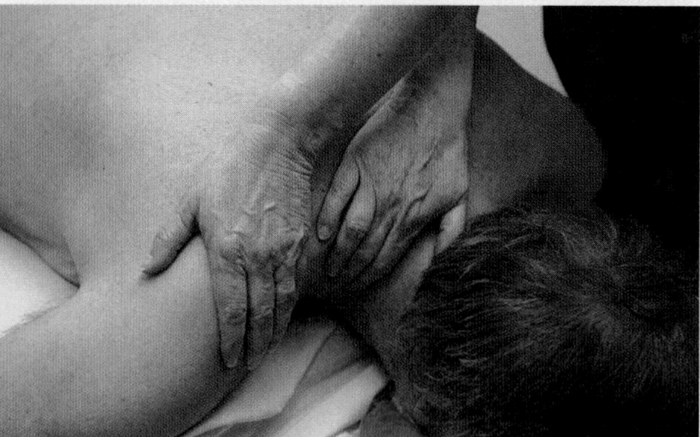

12. Massage over the low back in small circles using the flat part of your fingers.
13. Massage with long strokes from the low back to the neck with your hands flat. Then make large circles outward on either side of the spine, moving back down to the low back. Repeat three times.
14. Wipe off any excess lotion or oil.
15. Follow the Ending Implementation Steps located on the inside back cover.

Evaluation Steps

1. Evaluate your patient's level of relaxation and comfort. Offer to lower the lights and provide quiet for rest after massage.
2. Evaluate the need to work on a particular area further if the patient complains of continued tightness.

Sample Documentation

Personal care is often not documented except on a flow sheet. If abnormal findings are present, they are documented in the nurse's notes as shown below.

09/17/22 2140 2140 Back massage given. Pink area noted on left scapula, which disappeared after massage. States she is "relaxed and ready to sleep." ——————
—————— Nurse's signature and credentials

Skill 15.4 Administering Oral Care for an Unconscious Patient

Assessment Steps

1. Assess the condition of the mouth to see if there are any bridges, dentures, broken teeth, or lesions.
2. Assess gag reflex by placing a tongue blade on the back of the tongue. If gag reflex is present, it is safe to proceed. If gag reflex is not present, do not put liquids in the patient's mouth. Use only sponge swabs to clean the lips, mouth, and tongue.

Planning Steps

1. Determine the type of oral care devices to use.
2. Gather needed equipment and supplies: sponge swabs, towel, suction equipment, padded tongue blade, bed protector, emesis basin, water or dilute mouthwash, and an irrigation syringe.

Skill 15.4 (continued)

3. Determine the need for personal protective equipment. Obtain gloves and mask with face shield and gown if there is risk of splashing of body fluids.

Implementation Steps

1. Follow the Initial Implementation Steps located on the inside back cover.
2. Put the bed in the flat position unless contraindicated.
3. Turn the patient on his or her side with a bed protector and towel under the head and the emesis basin at the cheek. *Safety: Attach the oral suction device to the suction tubing. Turn on the wall suction to "regular" or "continuous," not "intermittent," and test it to be sure it is in working order.*
4. Moisten the sponge swab with a small amount of water and squeeze out excess ***to prevent aspiration of water.***

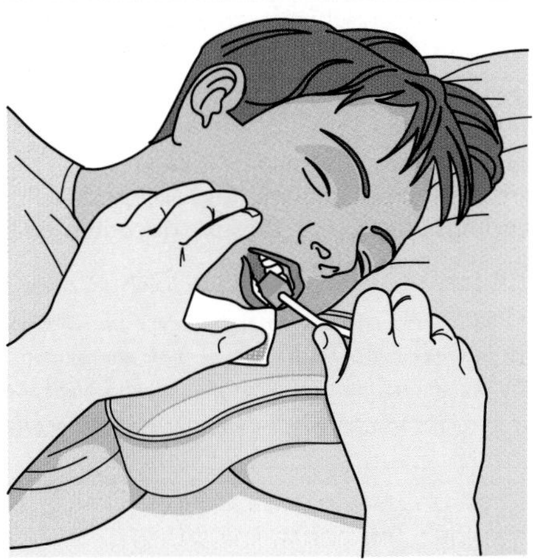

5. Insert the padded tongue blade and turn it vertically between the teeth to hold the mouth open. ***It is a natural reflex to bite down when something is placed in the mouth.***
6. Use the sponge swabs or a soft toothbrush with a small amount of toothpaste to brush all surfaces of the teeth and tongue. Brush the teeth at a 45-degree angle to the gumline. Use the swabs to clean between the cheeks and gums where mucus may collect. Use separate swabs for different parts of the mouth ***to prevent cross-contamination.***
7. Irrigate the mouth with approximately 10 mL of water or dilute mouthwash using the irrigation syringe. Allow the fluid to drain into the emesis basin or suction it out if necessary.
8. Apply water-soluble lip balm to the lips. *Safety: Do not apply petroleum-based products to lips. If the patient is on oxygen, it can cause burns. If the patient aspirates it, it can cause pneumonia.*
9. Remove the basin and dry the patient's face. Empty and rinse the basin and toothbrush if used. Return to appropriate storage location. Dispose of sponge swabs in biohazard trash.
10. Follow the Ending Implementation Steps located on the inside back cover.

Evaluation Steps

1. Evaluate the cleanliness of the patient's teeth and mouth. Examine the condition of the mouth after care for evidence of trauma or bleeding.
2. Evaluate the need to provide oral care more frequently because of mouth breathing and drying of mucous membranes.

Sample Documentation

Personal care is often not documented except on a flow sheet. If abnormal findings are present, they are documented in the nurse's notes as shown below.

09/17/22 0815 Oral care given. Gag reflex intact. 1-cm red area with 1-mm yellow center noted on left cheek. Health-care provider notified. ——————— Nurse's signature and credentials

Skill 15.5 Administering Oral Care for a Conscious Patient

Assessment Steps

1. Assess the mouth for lesions, broken teeth, gum disease, sordes, and color of mucous membranes.
2. Ask the patient about his or her usual oral care. Does the patient use mouthwash, floss, or whitening products?

Planning Steps

1. Gather needed equipment and supplies: toothbrush, toothpaste, dental floss, emesis basin, towel, drinking glass, water, and mouthwash if desired.
2. Determine the need for personal protective equipment. Obtain gloves and mask with face shield and gown if there is risk of splashing of body fluids.

Implementation Steps

1. Follow the Initial Implementation Steps located on the inside back cover.
2. Assist the patient to sit upright in a chair or the bed.
3. Place emesis basin, water in glass, toothbrush, and toothpaste on the over-bed table.
4. Place a towel across the patient's chest.
5. Moisten the toothbrush in the water and apply a pea-sized amount of toothpaste on the toothbrush.
6. Hold the emesis basin under the patient's chin, or have the patient do this if he or she is able.
7. If the patient is able to brush his or her teeth, hand the patient the toothbrush and stay near in case he or she needs assistance or becomes choked.

(skill continues on page 270)

Skill 15.5 (continued)

8. If the patient is unable to brush his or her own teeth, begin brushing by holding the bristles at a 45-degree angle to the teeth. Brush in small circles over all the inner and outer tooth surfaces. *Safety: Allow the patient to spit out mouth contents as often as needed to prevent choking. Have suction apparatus available if aspiration is a concern.*

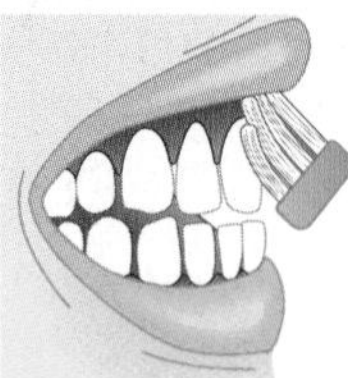

9. Brush the biting and chewing surfaces of the teeth in a back-and-forth motion.

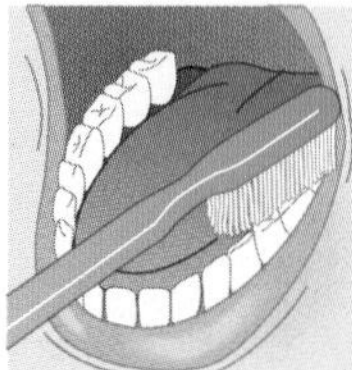

10. Ask the patient to stick out the tongue and gently brush it to remove debris. ***This makes it less likely to stimulate the gag reflex when you brush the tongue. Food and bacteria on the tongue are the usual cause of bad breath.***
11. Hand the patient the glass of water for rinsing the mouth.
12. Assist the patient to floss between the teeth. Use 6 to 10 inches of dental floss. Wrap the ends around the middle fingers of each hand or use a floss holder.
13. Slide the floss between the teeth and move back up. Avoid going too forcefully and injuring the gums. Bend the floss around each tooth to floss all sides.
14. Offer diluted mouthwash if desired.
15. Assist the patient to wipe the mouth with the towel. Remove, empty, and clean the toothbrush and emesis basin. Return them to the appropriate storage area.
16. Moisturize the lips.
17. Follow the Ending Implementation Steps located on the inside back cover.

Evaluation Steps

1. Evaluate how the patient tolerated the procedure. Did the patient complain of pain, fatigue, or shortness of breath?
2. Evaluate the appearance of the teeth and gums. Are they clean, and is the mouth fresh?
3. Evaluate for any trauma or bleeding due to brushing teeth or possible gum disease.

Sample Documentation

Personal care is often not documented except on a flow sheet. If abnormal findings are present, they are documented in the nurse's notes as shown below.

09/17/22 0815 Assisted with oral care. Able to rinse own mouth but not brush teeth. Gums pink and mucous membranes moist and pink. C/O fatigue at end of procedure.
——————— Nurse's signature and credentials

Skill 15.6 Providing Denture Care

Assessment Steps

1. Determine the type of dentures the patient wears. Are they full plates or partials? Upper and lower plates?
2. Inspect the inside of the mouth for lesions or evidence of poorly fitting dentures.
3. Inspect dentures for cracks or loose or broken teeth.

Planning Steps

1. Gather needed equipment and supplies: denture cup, toothbrush, toothpaste or denture cream, towel, mouthwash if desired, and gauze 4×4s.
2. Determine the need for personal protective equipment. Obtain gloves. Also obtain a mask with face shield and gown if there is risk of splashing of body fluids.

Implementation Steps

1. Follow the Initial Implementation Steps located on the inside back cover.
2. Line the sink with a towel ***to prevent damage if dentures accidentally slip.***
3. Don gloves. *Safety: You will be exposed to body fluids that could contain pathogens.*
4. Remove the upper dentures by using a gauze 4×4 to grasp them. ***The gauze keeps the dentures from slipping in your gloved hands.***
5. Rock the dentures gently from side to side to loosen and then pull them down and out. If necessary, place one gloved finger above the upper plate against the gum and press downward to break the suction so you can remove the dentures.

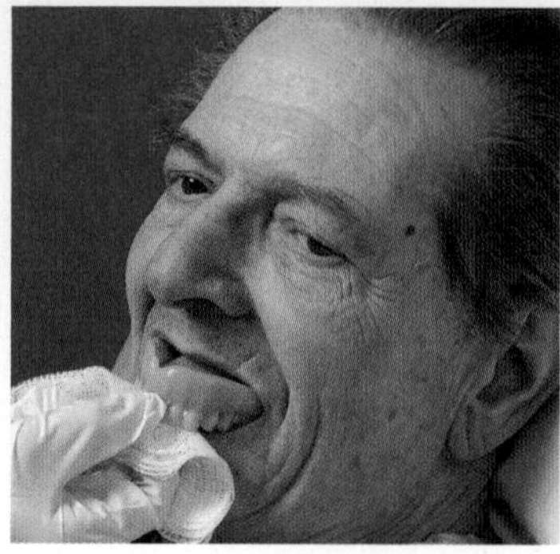

Skill 15.6 (continued)

6. Remove the lower plate by grasping it with a gauze 4×4 and lifting up and out.
7. Place the dentures in a denture cup and take to the sink.
8. Rinse with cool water. ***Hot water can damage or warp dentures.***
9. Squeeze a small amount of toothpaste or denture cream onto the toothbrush.
10. Brush the tooth surfaces and all other surfaces of the upper dentures. Repeat for the lower dentures. ***Food can become trapped between the gums and the dentures, so all surfaces must be thoroughly cleaned.***
11. Rinse the dentures again with cool water. Do not dry them because ***dentures are easier to insert if they are moist.***
12. Have the patient rinse his or her mouth with water or dilute mouthwash ***to remove any food trapped between the gums and the cheeks.***
13. Apply denture adhesive to the inner surfaces of the plates if the patient wishes.
14. Replace the upper denture by sliding it into the mouth and pushing up with the thumb on the palate of the denture to obtain a good seal.
15. Replace the lower denture by tilting it slightly, sliding it into the mouth, and pressing it gently downward into place.

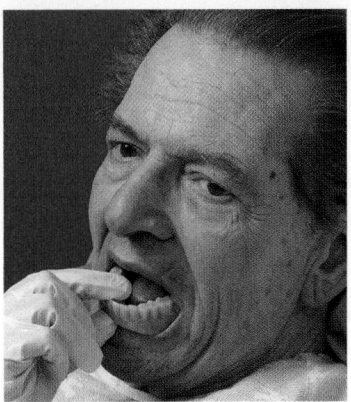

16. Place the towel in the dirty laundry and return the denture cup, toothbrush, and toothpaste to the bedside stand.
17. Follow the Ending Implementation Steps located on the inside back cover.

To Store Dentures for the Night

Follow the steps above to remove and clean the dentures. Place them in the denture cup and cover them with cool water. If the patient wishes, place a denture tablet in the water first, allow it to dissolve, and then add the dentures. Assist the patient to rinse his or her mouth with water or diluted mouthwash.

Evaluation Steps

1. Evaluate the condition of the patient's mouth without the dentures. Are there any lesions or reddened areas?
2. Evaluate the dentures themselves. Are they in good repair? Does the patient need to consult a dentist?

Sample Documentation

Personal care is often not documented except on a flow sheet. If abnormal findings are present, they are documented in the nurse's notes as shown below.

09/17/22 1020 Dentures removed, cleaned, and placed in denture cup for the night. Dark pink crusted area noted at the left corner of the mouth. Denies pain or discomfort.
—————————— Nurse's signature and credentials

Skill 15.7 Shaving a Male Patient

Assessment Steps

1. Assess the beard area for lesions, eczema, or ingrown whiskers.
2. Determine the type of razor to use. Check the chart to see if the patient is on anticoagulants. If that is the case, you must use an electric razor.

Planning Steps

1. Gather needed equipment and supplies: disposable razor, shaving cream, towel, washcloth, basin of water, and aftershave if desired *or* the patient's electric razor with cleaning tools, preshave lotion, and aftershave if desired.
2. Determine the need for personal protective equipment. Obtain gloves. Also obtain a mask with face shield and gown if there is risk of splashing of body fluids.

Implementation Steps

1. Follow the Initial Implementation Steps located on the inside back cover.

For Using a Disposable Razor

2. Fill the basin with warm water. Moisten the washcloth and place it on the beard for 1 to 3 minutes. ***This helps soften the beard and lift the whiskers.***
3. Apply a liberal amount of shaving cream to your hand. Spread the cream over the patient's beard and moustache area for 1 to 3 minutes.
4. Rinse and dry your hands.
5. Don gloves. *Safety: You will be exposed to body fluids that could contain pathogens.*

(skill continues on page 272)

Skill 15.7 (continued)

6. Remove the cover from the disposable razor. Begin shaving on the cheeks. Shave in the direction of hair growth ***to prevent irritation and ingrown hairs.***

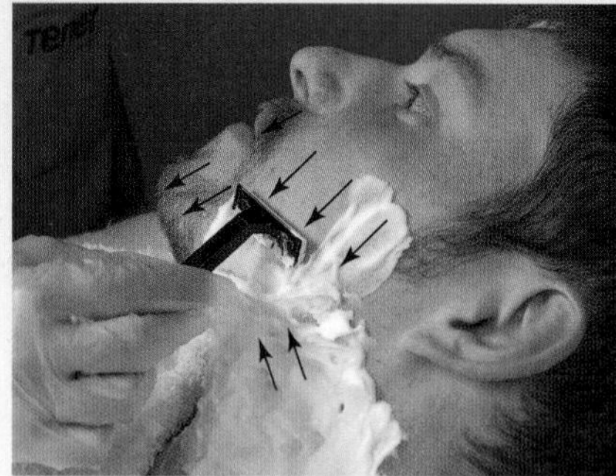

7. Shave the neck in an upward direction ***to prevent causing ingrown hairs or irritation to the skin.***
8. Shave the moustache area if patient desires. Have the patient pull his upper lip over his teeth ***to increase access to the area between the nose and lip.***
9. Shave chin from lower lip downward. Use caution shaving the contour of the chin because it is easy to nick.
10. Rinse the razor frequently while shaving. ***Avoids clogging the blade.***
11. Wipe the patient's face with a wet washcloth. Pat dry with towel. Check for any missed areas and touch up if needed.
12. Apply aftershave lotion if desired.
13. Follow the Ending Implementation Steps located on the inside back cover.

For Using an Electric Razor

2. Apply preshave lotion ***to lift the whiskers.***
3. Turn on the razor and shave the cheeks using a circular motion. You may need to go over an area more than one time.
4. Shave the moustache area in a downward motion.
5. Shave the neck in a circular upward motion ***to prevent causing ingrown hairs or irritation to the skin.***
6. Apply aftershave lotion if desired.
7. Clean the razor by removing the head and brushing out debris with the small brush supplied with the razor. Replace the head and return the razor to the appropriate storage area.
8. Follow the Ending Implementation Steps located on the inside back cover.

Evaluation Steps

1. Evaluate the closeness of the shave. Is there razor burn or nicks?

Documentation

Personal care is often not documented except on a flow sheet. If abnormal findings are present, they are documented in the nurse's notes.

Skill 15.8 Providing Nail Care

Assessment Steps

1. Assess the condition of the nails: the length, redness around nails, splitting or cracking of nails, and thickness or discoloration.
2. Review the chart for a diagnosis of diabetes or peripheral vascular disease. *Safety: For these diagnoses, file nails only. Do not clip or cut because of the risk of damaging tissue that might not heal.*

Planning Steps

1. Gather needed equipment and supplies: a basin with warm water, an orangewood stick, lotion, nail clippers, and an emery board.
2. Plan to do nail care for both hands and feet unless it is contraindicated.
3. Determine the need for personal protective equipment. Obtain gloves if needed. Also obtain a mask with face shield and gown if there is risk of splashing of body fluids.

Intervention Steps

1. Follow the Initial Implementation Steps located on the inside back cover.

For Fingernails

2. Assist the patient to sit up in bed or a chair.
3. Place the patient's hands in the basin of warm water one at a time for 5 to 20 minutes to soak and soften the nails and cuticles. Perform nail care on the first hand after it has soaked, while the other hand is still soaking.
4. Have the patient lay his or her hands on the towel spread on the over-bed table.
5. Using the pointed end of the orangewood stick, clean beneath the nails. Use the flatter end to push back the cuticles.
6. Clip the nails (unless contraindicated) straight across. ***Nails that are rounded are more likely to ingrow.***
7. Use the emery board to file the corners ***so that they are not sharp to prevent scratching.***
8. Apply lotion to the patient's hands and forearms and massage into the skin.

For Toenails

2. Assist the patient to bend the knees and soak the feet in the basin one at a time for 5 to 20 minutes. Perform nail care on the first foot after it has soaked, while the other foot is still soaking. Change the water after cleaning each foot.
3. Place a towel on the bed and have the patient put his or her foot on the towel.
4. Clip the toenails (unless contraindicated) straight across. File straight across with an emery board to prevent scratching.

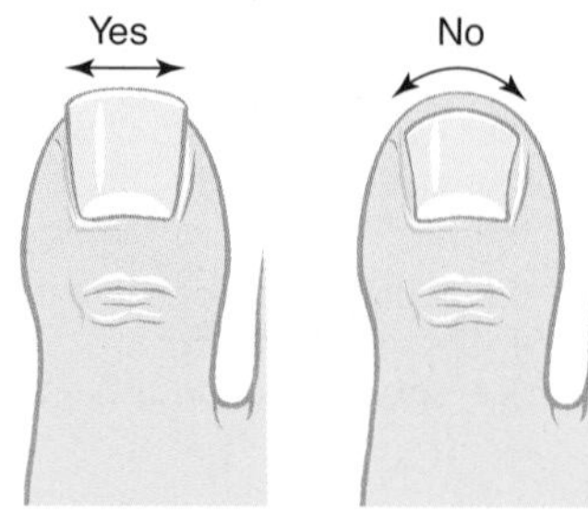

Skill 15.8 (continued)

5. Dry the feet well, paying special attention to the areas between the toes ***to prevent maceration of the skin.***
6. Apply lotion to the feet but not between the toes.
7. Clean and return equipment to its appropriate storage location.
8. Follow the Initial Implementation Steps located on the inside back cover.

Evaluation Steps

1. Evaluate the appearance of the fingernails and toenails. Are there any ingrown nails or infected or inflamed areas? Report as appropriate.
2. Evaluate the effectiveness of the nail care. Does the patient need to be seen by a podiatrist?

Sample Documentation

Personal care is often not documented except on a flow sheet. If abnormal findings are present, they are documented in the nurse's notes as shown below.

09/17/22 1530 Nail care given for hands and feet. Left foot has 2-mm reddened area between 2nd and 3rd toes. Health-care provider notified. ——————— Nurse's signature and credentials

Skill 15.9 Shampooing Hair Using a Rinse-Free Shampoo Cap With the Patient in Bed

Assessment Steps

1. Check hair for mats, tangles, and any scalp lesions.
2. Review the chart for any contraindications to shampooing the hair using a rinse-free shampoo cap in bed.

Planning Steps

1. Gather needed equipment and supplies: rinse-free shampoo cap; rinse-free conditioner (optional); a brush, comb, or hair pick; and gloves.
2. Determine the need for personal protective equipment. Obtain gloves if needed.
3. Warm the shampoo cap using a microwave according to the packaged instructions. ***You must be careful not to overheat.***

Implementation Steps

1. Follow the Initial Implementation Steps located on the inside back cover.
2. Assist the patient to the high Fowler's position unless contraindicated.
3. Comb through hair to remove tangles.
4. Apply the rinse-free shampoo cap on the patient's hair. Begin to work the shampoo through the hair.
5. Remove the rinse-free shampoo cap and dry the patient's hair with a bath towel.
6. Comb gently through the hair. Remove tangles by working from the ends of the hair toward the scalp ***to prevent pulling.***
7. Use a hair dryer if desired by the patient, or allow to air dry. Style according to the patient's wishes.

Evaluation Steps

1. Evaluate the condition of the scalp and hair. It should be soft and clean without flakes or oil.
2. Evaluate how the patient tolerated the activity. Did it cause fatigue, pain, or shortness of breath?

Sample Documentation

Personal care is often not documented except on a flow sheet. If abnormal findings are present, they are documented in the nurse's notes as shown below.

09/17/22 2045 Hair shampooed and dried. Bedrest maintained. Tolerated activity but became short of breath as hair was being dried. ——————— Nurse's signature and credentials

Skill 15.10 Making an Unoccupied Bed

Assessment Steps

1. Assess the patient's ability to be out of bed during the linen change. Review the chart for activity level.
2. Determine linens needed for the bed change.

Planning Steps

1. Plan to change linens when the patient will be out of bed, either sitting up in a chair or off of the unit for therapy or a procedure.
2. Gather needed equipment and supplies: mattress pad (if needed), fitted sheet, draw sheet, bed protector (if in use), flat sheet, blanket or spread (if needed), pillowcase, and laundry bag or hamper.
3. Determine the need for personal protective equipment. Obtain gloves if needed.

Implementation Steps

1. Follow the Initial Implementation Steps located on the inside back cover.

(skill continues on page 274)

Skill 15.10 (continued)

2. Remove the spread or blanket. Don protective gloves and other protective gear if sheets or bedspread are soiled. If it is not soiled, fold it carefully and place it over the back of a chair to be put back on the bed. If it is soiled, place it in the laundry hamper or bag.
3. Fold soiled top linens to the center of the bed. Check for any personal belongings that might have been left in the bed, such as glasses, a gown, or a book.
4. Loosen the fitted bottom sheet and fold it to the middle of the bed. Remove the pillow from the pillowcase and place the pillow in a chair.
5. Place all soiled linen in a laundry bag or hamper. *Safety: Do not allow the soiled linens to touch your scrubs to prevent contamination. NEVER put soiled linen on the floor because this spreads microorganisms.*
6. If the mattress is damp or soiled due to incontinence, spray with a disinfectant spray and wipe with a clean washcloth ***to prevent contaminating the clean linens.***
7. Unfold the fitted bottom sheet to cover the half of the mattress closest to you and slide the corners over the mattress corners.
8. Unfold the draw sheet and center it so that it will cover an area from the patient's shoulders to his or her knees. ***This keeps the patient centered on the draw sheet for turning and moving.***
9. Tuck the draw sheet between the mattress and springs.

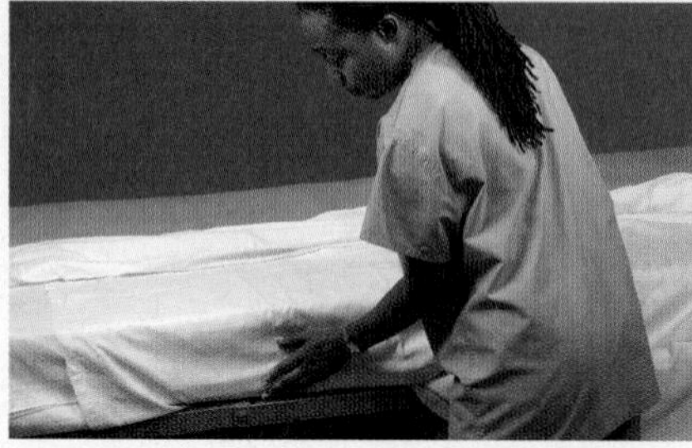

10. Go to the other side of the bed and spread the bottom sheet over the remainder of the bed. Slide the corners over the corners of the mattress.
11. Spread the draw sheet across the bed. Grasp the draw sheet in the middle and pull tightly across and down. Tuck it between the mattress and the springs. Grasp the draw sheet near the upper edge, pull, and tuck. Repeat near the lower edge of the draw sheet.
12. Unfold the top sheet to cover the half of the mattress closest to you. ***This keeps you from walking around the bed several times during the procedure, conserving your energy.*** Ensure that the seams (rough edge of hem) are up, or away from the patient, ***to prevent scratching of the patient by the rough edges.***
13. Unfold the blanket or spread to cover the half of the mattress closest to you. Position so that the blanket is approximately 4 inches below the top edge of the flat sheet ***to make a cuff over the rough edges of the blanket.***
14. Tuck blanket and sheet together under the foot of the bed, between the mattress and the springs. ***This prevents you from loosening the sheet when you tuck the blanket separately.***

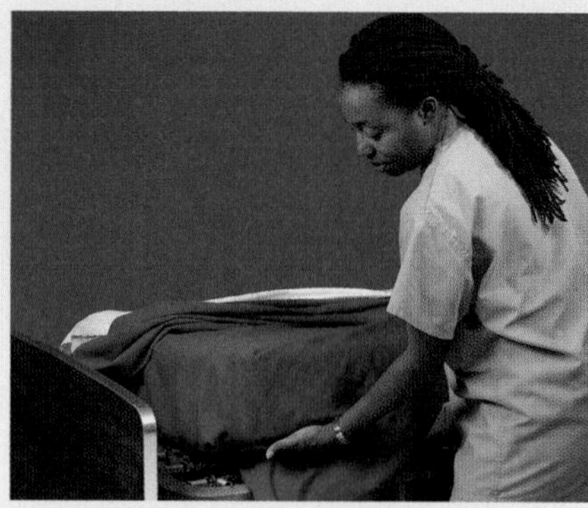

15. Make a mitered corner by grasping the sheet and blanket together at a 45-degree angle to the foot of the bed. Lay the angled portion on the bed and tuck the lower edge of the blanket and sheet under the mattress. Then let the angled portion of the blanket and sheet hang freely. You should have a tight, slanted corner at 45 degrees from the end of the mattress. ***This keeps the sheet and blanket from pulling out as the patient moves and turns.***

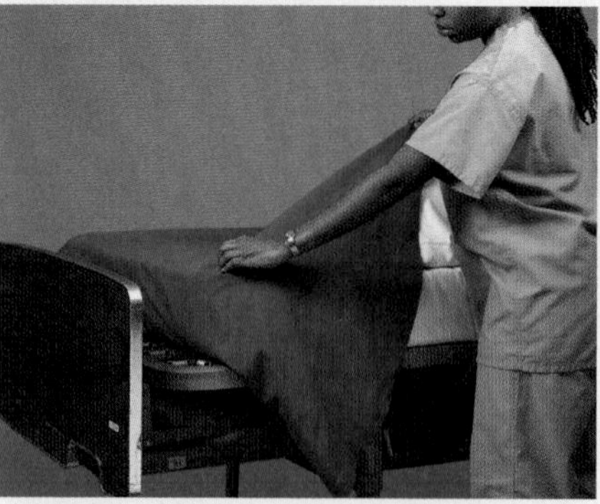

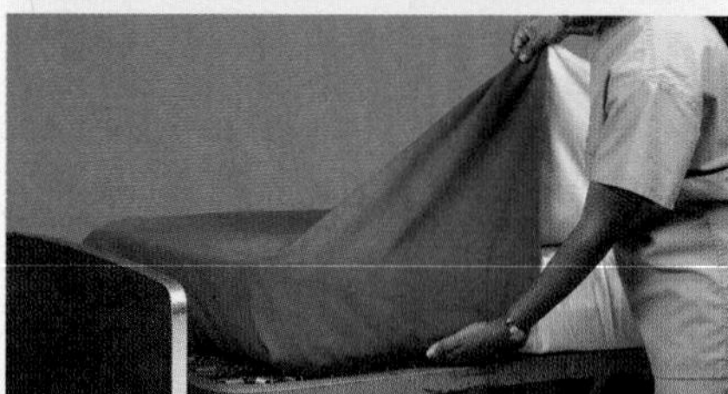

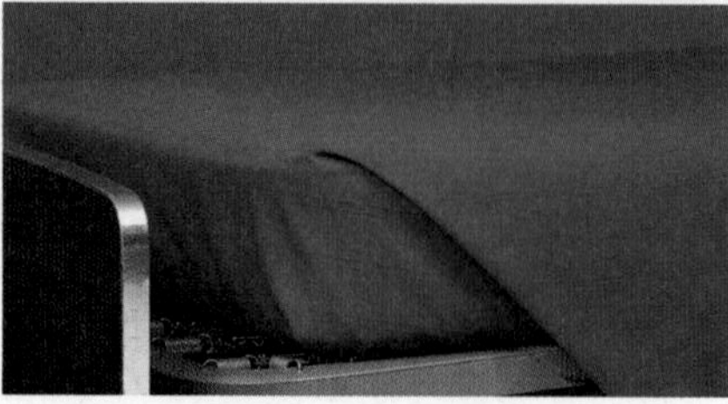

16. Repeat Steps 13–15 on the other side of the bed.
17. Cuff the top sheet over the blanket at the head of the bed. All seams and rough edges should be away from the patient.
18. Replace the pillowcase by holding the pillow lengthwise and pinching the bottom corners together. Slide the pillow into the case while it is lying on the bed. Release the corners when they are aligned with the pillowcase corners. ***This prevents you from holding the pillow next to***

Skill 15.10 (continued)

your scrubs or under your chin, which could cause contamination.

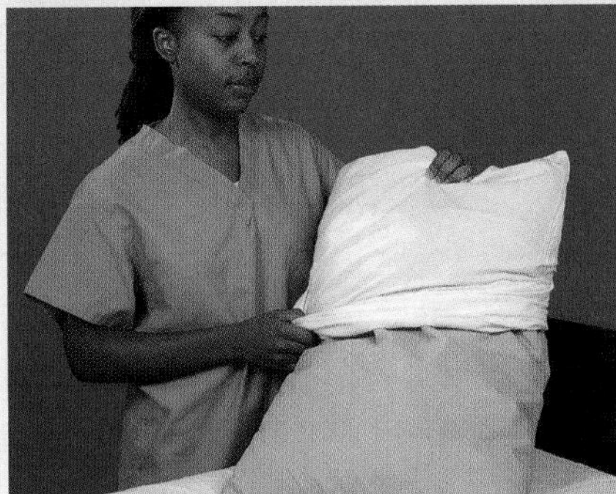

19. Place the pillow so that the opening of the pillowcase is away from the door.

For an Open Bed

Follow Steps 1–19 above and then fanfold the top linens to the foot of the bed ***to make it easier for the patient to get into the bed.***

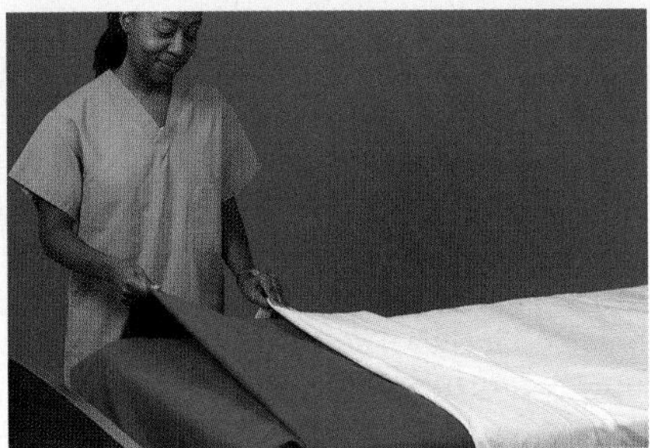

20. Assist the patient into bed and ensure comfort.
21. Follow the Ending Implementation Steps located on the inside back cover.

For a Surgical Bed

Follow Steps 1–13 above and then fanfold the top linens to the side of the bed away from the door. ***This allows a patient returning on a stretcher to be easily moved into the bed.*** Once the patient is in the bed, you will tuck in the top sheet and blanket together at the foot of the bed and make mitered corners at each side.

14. Assist the patient into bed and ensure comfort.
15. Follow the Ending Implementation Steps located on the inside back cover.

Evaluation Steps

1. Evaluate the bed for smooth, tight linens and corners.

Documentation

This type of information is generally documented only on a flow sheet.

Skill 15.11 Making an Occupied Bed

Assessment Steps

1. Review the patient's chart for activity level. Those on bedrest will need an occupied bed change.
2. Assess the patient's ability to remain on his or her side while you change the bed.

Planning Steps

1. Determine if another staff member is needed to help during the bed change. It is not uncommon for this procedure to take two staff members.
2. Gather needed equipment and supplies: fitted sheet, draw sheet, bed protector (if in use), flat sheet, blanket or spread, pillowcase, and laundry bag or hamper.
3. Determine the need for personal protective equipment. Obtain gloves if needed.

Implementation Steps

1. Follow the Initial Implementation Steps located on the inside back cover.
2. Remove the spread or blanket. Don protective gloves and other protective gear if sheets or bedspread are soiled. If it is not soiled, fold it and place it over the back of a chair to be put back on the bed. If it is soiled, place it in the laundry hamper or bag.
3. Leave the top sheet in place unless it is soiled. If it is soiled, replace it with a bath blanket and place it in the laundry hamper or bag.
4. Assist the patient to move to the far side of the bed and to turn away from you. *Safety: Be sure that the far side rail is up to prevent the patient from falling.*
5. Ensure that no tubes or wires are tangled in the linens.
6. Lower the side rail closest to you and loosen the bottom linens. Tightly fold the linens toward the patient and tuck them next to him or her.
7. Unfold the clean fitted sheet and slip the corners over the mattress corners. Unfold the draw sheet and tuck it under the mattress, positioning it from the patient's shoulders to his or her knees. ***This keeps the patient centered on the draw sheet for turning and moving.***

(skill continues on page 276)

Skill 15.11 (continued)

8. Fanfold the fitted sheet and draw sheet toward the patient. Tuck them beneath the tightly folded soiled linens. *Safety: If there is a danger that the soiled linens are wet or could contaminate the clean ones, place a towel or waterproof pad between the clean and dirty linens.*

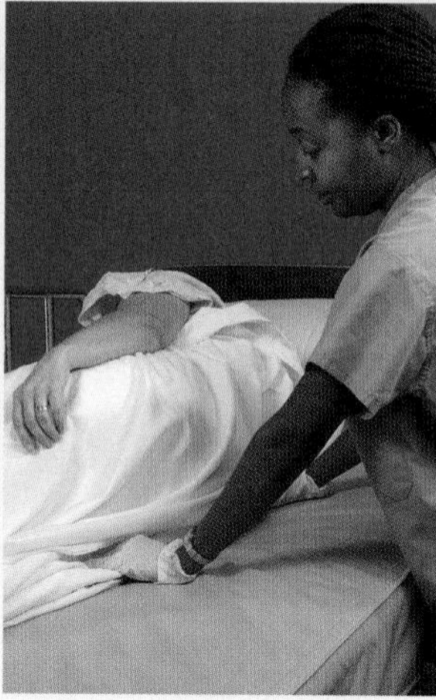

9. Put up the side rail and assist the patient to turn to the other side of the bed. Warn the patient that he or she will be rolling over the "hump" of both clean and used linens. Place the pillow beneath his or her head for comfort.
10. Go to the other side of the bed and lower the side rail. Pull the soiled linen off of the bed and put it in the laundry bag or hamper. *Safety: Do not allow the soiled linens to touch your scrubs to prevent contamination. NEVER put soiled linen on the floor because this spreads microorganisms.*

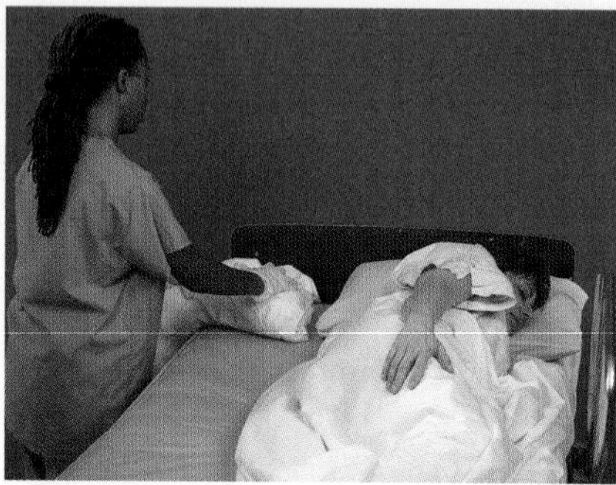

11. Spread the fitted sheet and draw sheet across the bed. Slip the corners over the mattress corners. Smooth the draw sheet by grasping the middle and pulling tightly across and down. Tuck it between the mattress and springs. Repeat with the top and bottom edges of the draw sheet. ***This helps make a tight bed with fewer wrinkles, which is more comfortable for the patient.***

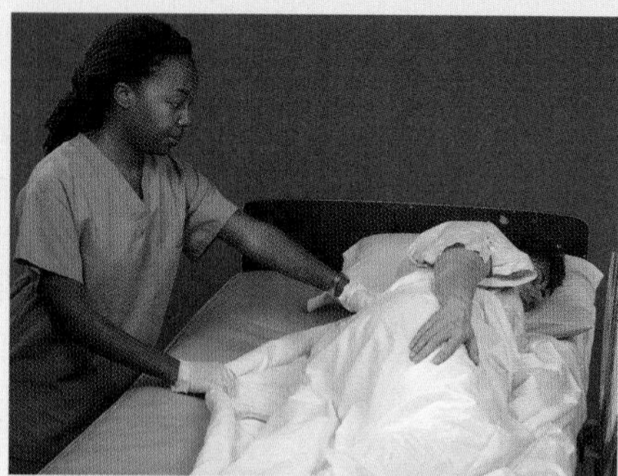

12. Assist the patient to turn onto his or her back in the center of the bed.
13. Unfold the clean top sheet so that it is centered on the bed. Be sure the seams are away from the patient.
14. Remove the bath blanket by pulling it from beneath the clean top sheet. Put it in the laundry bag or hamper and avoid touching it to your scrubs.
15. Replace the blanket or spread so that it is centered on the bed and the top edge is approximately 4 inches lower than the top edge of the sheet.
16. Tuck the sheet and blanket together at the foot of the bed. Make a mitered corner (see Skill 15.10).
17. Go to the other side of the bed and tuck the sheet and blanket together at the foot of the bed. Make a mitered corner.
18. Grasp the top linens over the patient's feet and pull up approximately 3 inches. ***This prevents plantar flexion of the foot leading to footdrop.***
19. Cuff the top sheet over the edge of the blanket ***to prevent any rough edges from being against the patient's skin.***
20. Change the pillowcase (see Skill 15.10) and replace the pillow.
21. Ensure that the patient is comfortable.
22. Follow the Ending Implementation Steps located on the inside back cover.

Evaluation Steps

1. Evaluate the patient's level of comfort in the bed. Is it free of wrinkles?
2. Evaluate the patient's tolerance of the procedure. Are there any complaints of pain, fatigue, or shortness of breath?

Documentation

Personal care is often not documented except on a flow sheet. If abnormal findings are present, they are documented in the nurse's notes.

POST CONFERENCE

As you attend post conference after clinicals, you think about all the things you learned about your patient during her bath today. She really opened up to you about some of her health problems and concerns. In fact, she was thrilled to have you take care of her today and was not upset at all that you were a male nursing student. Also, during the bath, you noticed a fine raised rash on her back that you showed to your instructor. It turned out to be a reaction to an antibiotic that could have gotten much worse if you had not noticed it. When you evaluate your nursing actions, you feel good about caring for this patient and meeting her needs, even the most basic needs of bathing and grooming. You do not at all feel that you wasted your valuable time by bathing this patient.

Key Points

- Providing personal care for patients gives you the unique chance to make multiple observations about their skin, hair, and mouth as well as an unparalleled opportunity to establish the nurse–patient relationship.
- When you plan personal care, it is extremely important to learn about the patients' preferences regarding timing of care, their cultural influences, and their capabilities to assist with care.
- There are many ways to bathe patients, from a complete bed bath for a helpless patient to a shower with minimal assistance. Different types of baths require various amounts of participation on the part of the patient. It is the nurse's responsibility to know the appropriate way to bathe a patient based on each person's individual needs.
- Back massage has many benefits for the patient, including promoting relaxation, relieving muscle tension, and stimulating circulation. Back massage is far more than rubbing lotion on a patient's back. Nurses should make every effort to provide this care for their patients.
- When you provide oral care for unconscious patients, it is very important to prevent aspiration. Keep the patient positioned on the side during oral care and be prepared to use suction to remove fluids if necessary.
- Assess the hair and scalp for contagious conditions such as tinea capitus (ringworm) and lice. Give special care for the hair of African American patients, both in combing and in shampooing.
- Expect to care for patients with body piercings. Be prepared to remove jewelry from piercings only if necessary because of infection or possible interference with surgery, intubation, catheterization, or diagnostic testing.
- Nurses may need to remove, clean, and insert contact lenses, ocular prostheses, and hearing aids, and they need to know the steps involved in each procedure.
- Minimizing negative aspects of the patient's environment, such as odor, noise, and clutter, as well as providing clean, fresh bed linens, is a valuable part of patient care.
- Most facilities have established specific times for routine care to be given. This helps to prevent missing an aspect of care.
- Personal care is performed in different ways: by the patient, by the staff, or by a combination of both. The three types of care are self-care, assisted care, and total care.
- When giving care for a patient who is unconscious or conscious, you must be careful to minimize any chance of aspiration of fluids. Assess the mouth for lesions and dried mouth secretions.

Review Questions

Select the answer that is most appropriate for each of the following questions. Some questions may have more than one correct answer. Select all that apply.

1. The circulatory effect of venous return is accomplished by bathing:
   1. the back along the trapezius muscles.
   2. the extremities in a distal-to-proximal direction.
   3. the arm farthest away from you first, then the nearer arm.
   4. the extremities in a proximal-to-distal direction.
2. The staff nurse says that your patient refused her bath yesterday and really needs one today. The patient says she is too exhausted to have a bed bath and just wants to sleep. Your best response would be:
   1. "That's fine. Sleep is more important than a bath, anyway."
   2. "I will do your bath first, then you will sleep better."
   3. "I have other patients to care for, so we need to do your bath now."
   4. "You rest now, and I will come back in about an hour to do your bath."

3. You are giving evening care to your patient. What care will you provide?
   1. Assist with toileting
   2. Give a warm, wet washcloth for washing hands and face
   3. Change the gown
   4. Offer a back massage
   5. Straighten the linens and get an extra blanket
   6. Brush or comb hair
   7. Remove glasses, dentures, and hearing aids
   8. Ensure that needed items for the night are within reach

4. In which situations would it be inappropriate for the nurse to delegate the patient's personal care to a CNA or UAP?
   1. A patient whose vital signs are unstable
   2. A patient who requires total care
   3. A patient whose capabilities to assist with personal care are unknown
   4. A patient who is from a different culture
   5. A patient who has a worsening skin condition

5. You know a patient with diabetes needs more teaching about nail care when he says:
   1. "My daughter can cut my toenails so they are rounded without any sharp edges."
   2. "I won't clip my toenails anymore. I will just file them."
   3. "Any reddened area on my feet can be a problem, so I will tell the doctor if I see any."
   4. "I don't want to risk even a small cut on my toes or feet."

6. The nurse is taking care of a 78-year-old male patient who is bedridden. Which type of bath would be appropriate for the patient?
   1. Partial bath
   2. Complete bed bath
   3. Tub bath
   4. Bag bath

7. A patient receiving a nasogastric tube feeding will have which common bed position?
   1. Flat
   2. Fowler's
   3. Semi-Fowler's
   4. Trendelenburg

8. The bed-bath supplies the nurse would plan for when caring for a patient are:
   1. Washcloths
   2. Towels
   3. Nail file
   4. Bath blanket
   5. Bath basin

9. When cleaning a hearing aid, you should do which of the following?
   1. Turn off the hearing aid
   2. Turn the earlobe slightly away from the nose and lift up
   3. Store the aid in its case
   4. Store the aid in an open area within the patient's reach

ANSWERS 1. 2, 2. 4, 3. 1, 4, 5, 7, 8, 4. 1, 3, 5, 5. 1, 6. 2, 7. 3, 8. 1, 2, 4, 5, 9. 1, 3

Critical Thinking Exercise

Answers available online.

1. A CNA that you supervise tells you that a female patient from India refuses to take a bath. The CNA whispers to you that the patient has strong body odor and needs to shave her armpits. How will you handle this situation?

Additional Resources

Use the scratch off code on the inside front cover of your book to access online quizzes that will help you to improve your scores on course exams and prepare for the NCLEX-PN®.

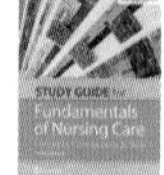

Study Guide

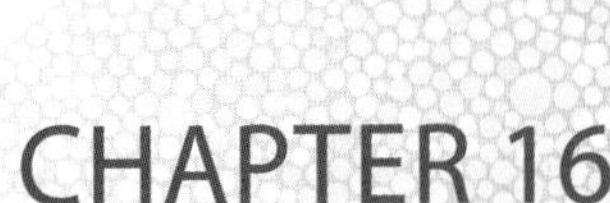

CHAPTER 16
Moving and Positioning Patients

KEY TERMS

Contracture (kon-TRAK-chur)
Dorsiflexion (DOR-sih-FLEK-shun)
Footdrop (FOOT-drop)
Fowler's position (FOW-luhrz po-ZIH-shun)
Lateral position (LAT-er-ruhl po-ZIH-shun)
Logroll (LOG-rohl)
Orthopneic position (or-THOP-nee-ik po-ZIH-shun)
Orthostatic hypotension (OR-tho-STAT-ik HYE-poh-TEN-shun)
Plantar flexion (PLAN-tar FLEK-shun)
Position of function (po-ZIH-shun uv FUNGK-shun)
Prone position (PROHN po-ZIH-shun)
Semi-Fowler's position (SEM-ee-FOW-luhrz po-ZIH-shun)
Shearing (SHEER-ing)
Sims' position (SIMZ po-ZIH-shun)
Supine position (soo-PYEN po-ZIH-shun)
Syncope (SING-ko-pee)
Transfer (TRANS-fer)
Trochanter roll (troh-KAN-ter rohl)

CHAPTER CONCEPTS

Patient-Centered Care
Safety

LEARNING OUTCOMES

1. Define various terms associated with moving and positioning patients.
2. Describe the effects of immobility on seven body systems.
3. Enumerate nursing measures to prevent complications of immobility in these body systems.
4. Describe the psychological effects of immobility and nursing measures to prevent psychological complications.
5. Discuss the importance of positioning patients correctly and performing frequent position changes.
6. Identify commonly used patient positions.
7. Explain the purposes and focus of the Handle With Care campaign established by the American Nurses Association.
8. Describe devices available to increase safety and ease of transferring patients.
9. Enumerate guidelines for performing a manual patient transfer.
10. Contrast types of specialty beds and their purposes.
11. Summarize the importance of assisting a patient to dangle prior to transfer or ambulation.
12. Discuss assisting patents with ambulation and potential complications.
13. Identify proper body mechanics for protecting yourself and the patient.
14. Discuss information found in the Connection features in the chapter.
15. Identify safety information related to moving and positioning patients.
16. Answer questions about performing the skills in the chapter.

SKILLS

16.1 Performing Passive Range-of-Motion Exercises
16.2 Positioning Patients
16.3 Moving a Patient Up in Bed
16.4 Turning a Patient in Bed
16.5 Transferring a Patient From Bed to a Stretcher, Chair, or Wheelchair
16.6 Transferring a Patient With a Mechanical Lift
16.7 Assisting a Patient to Dangle
16.8 Assisting With Ambulation

CRITICAL THINKING CONNECTION

Clinical Assignment

You will be caring for a 56-year-old male patient who is paralyzed in both legs as the result of a spinal cord injury from a motor vehicle accident. He is currently in the rehab unit. He is unable to turn himself in bed and spends part of each day in a motorized wheelchair. The nurse tells you in report that skin breakdown is a major concern and that he has an Envella bed to help prevent it. The nurse also tells you that the patient has had difficulty adjusting psychologically to his limited mobility.

Critical Thinking Questions:

1. How often will you turn the patient?
2. What is a major concern you will have when getting the patient up to the wheelchair?
3. If the patient develops pressure injuries, where are the most common areas the patient may develop pressure injuries?

The human body is intended to move in order for a person to remain healthy, and every organ in the body depends on movement for optimal function. Physiological and psychological changes can result as consequences of immobility. This chapter will help you determine what to do for patients with mobility problems and how to help prevent further complications from immobility.

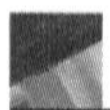

EFFECTS OF IMMOBILITY

Immobility occurs as a result of lack of activity and movement, which may occur when a person is ill and less active than usual. When movement is restricted, body systems immediately react—and they continue to react as long as immobility persists. When a patient is placed on prolonged bedrest, for reasons such as coma, multiple trauma, long intensive care stays, severe weakness, and overwhelming infection, even more complications can result. However, it is important to recognize that complications resulting from bedrest and immobility, although numerous, are preventable.

It has been recognized for many years that immobility and prolonged bedrest have adverse effects. As early as 1947, an article about the dangers of immobility was published in the *British Medical Journal.* In 1967, the *American Journal of Nursing* published the often-cited article, "The Hazards of Immobility," detailing the effects of immobility on each body system. Prior to these publications, it was common for medical authorities to prescribe strict bedrest for many days or even weeks. Now we know that the longer a patient remains inactive, the more his or her chances of developing complications increase. Such complications include the following:

- Blood clots
- Pneumonia
- Bone demineralization
- Kidney stones
- Constipation
- Pressure injuries
- Urinary retention
- Depression

You, as a nurse, have an important responsibility for ensuring that the complications resulting from immobility are minimized and for maintaining patient mobility when possible.

Physiological Effects

It is essential that individuals remain active to maintain optimal functioning of all body systems. As a nurse, you will be responsible for anticipating and minimizing the effects of inactivity and immobility on your patients. Table 16.1 summarizes the effects of immobility on various body systems.

Effects of Immobility on the Musculoskeletal System

When a patient is unable to move about, he or she can suffer from *muscle atrophy,* which means that muscle decreases in size, tone, and strength as a result of disuse. Along with the muscle tissue, connective tissue such as ligaments and tendons undergoes structural and functional changes after 4 to 6 days of immobility. These changes lead to decreased joint flexibility, decreased range of motion, and **contractures,** or shortening and tightening of the muscles due to disuse. This is why your muscles feel weak when you have been ill and have remained in bed for several days.

Osteoporosis is a condition that occurs due to loss of bone minerals; it leads to an increased risk of skeletal fractures. Immobility increases the risk of osteoporosis because a lack of activity and weight-bearing results in a loss of calcium from the bones. This bone demineralization can begin as early as 2 to 3 days from the onset of immobility. The calcium leaves the bones and enters the bloodstream, placing the patient at increased risk for kidney stones because the excess calcium in the blood must then be filtered out by the kidneys.

NURSING MEASURES TO PREVENT MUSCULOSKELETAL COMPLICATIONS. The most basic nursing measure to prevent musculoskeletal complications is to maintain proper body alignment, which means to keep the head, trunk, and hips positioned in a straight line. The legs should be positioned so that the toes always point in the same direction as the anterior or ventral side of the body. This is accomplished by preventing the legs from rotating in the hip sockets either medially

• WORD • BUILDING •

bone demineralization: bone – bone; de – loss + mineral – mineral salts + ization: action

contracture: con – together + tract – draw + ure – process or action

osteoporosis: osteo – bone + por – passage + osis – condition

Table 16.1
Effects and Complications of Immobility

Body System	*Effects of Immobility*	*Potential Complications*
Musculoskeletal system	Decreased muscle strength and muscle mass; shortening and tightening of connective tissue; calcium leaves the bones, resulting in weakness and brittleness	• Muscle atrophy • Footdrop • Contractures • Osteoporosis
Cardiovascular system	Decreased cardiac output; pooling of blood in the extremities; increased cardiac workload	• Orthostatic hypotension • Blood clots in extremities • Blood clots traveling to lungs, heart, and brain
Respiratory system	Decreased respiratory muscle strength and decreased lung expansion; impaired oxygen and carbon dioxide exchange; pooling of respiratory secretions	• Atelectasis • Hypoxemia • Hypostatic pneumonia
Gastrointestinal system	Decreased peristalsis; decreased appetite; increased intestinal gas	• Constipation • Flatulence • Distention
Urinary system	Pooling of urine in the renal pelvis; incomplete emptying of the bladder; increased calcium in the blood to be filtered by the kidneys	• Urinary tract infection • Renal calculi
Integumentary system	Decreased oxygen and nutrients to tissues; skin and capillaries compressed between the bed and bony prominences	• Pressure injuries
Neurological system	Decreased oxygenated blood circulating to nerves trapped between the bed and bone; decrease in normal cues and activities; decreased balance when initially out of bed	• Compression neuropathy • Impaired level of consciousness • Confusion
Psychological effects	Decrease in normal social interaction; decrease in independent activity	• Depression • Anxiety • Impaired sleep

or laterally. The arms should be maintained in correct alignment with the shoulders and trunk and not allowed to fall forward in a "slump-shouldered" position, which causes the thorax to curve in an unnatural manner. Correct body alignment should be maintained while the patient is in the **supine position,** in all variations of side-lying positions, and even while sitting. When lying in the supine position, the patient's ankles should be flexed approximately 90 degrees so that the toes point toward the ceiling. This is referred to as **dorsiflexion** of the foot. If the toes are allowed to fall toward the foot of the bed, the proper dorsiflexion of the ankle is lost and permanent plantar flexion of the foot develops, a condition known as **footdrop.** This condition will be discussed further in this chapter.

One common nursing measure that is used to combat the physiological effects of immobility is the use of *range-of-motion (ROM) exercises,* which are a series of activities designed to move each joint through all of its natural actions. To decrease the incidence of muscle atrophy and contractures, it is necessary to maintain muscle mass and healthy bones. Use these actions to help prevent muscle contractures and osteoporosis:

- Perform ROM exercises every 8 hours to maintain muscle strength and flexibility as well as joint flexibility. These may be active or passive exercises (Box 16.1).
- Ensure that you support the weight of the extremity at the joints during passive ROM exercises (see Skill 16.1, page 295).
- Correctly apply any supportive or therapeutic devices for maintaining proper body alignment, such as a trochanter roll or footdrop splint, and follow the orders for their use exactly. A **trochanter roll** is a rolled towel or cylindrical device placed snugly against the lateral aspect of the patient's thigh to prevent the leg from rotating outward. Some facilities use *footdrop boots,* a splintlike padded

Box 16.1

Active Versus Passive Range-of-Motion Exercises

ROM exercises are used in a variety of situations. They may be active or passive depending on who is moving the extremity.

- Active ROM exercises are performed by the patient without physical nursing assistance. The nurse may remind or encourage the patient to perform the exercises, but the patient is able to move all extremities independently.
- Passive ROM exercises are done with the nurse performing the exercising of the patient's joints while providing proper support to the patient's extremity. Passive exercises are indicated when a patient is too weak to move his or her own extremities or when one or more extremities are paralyzed.

device that supports the foot in proper plantar flexion and suspends the heel over a small pocket of air, thereby reducing the risk of pressure injuries and *footdrop*.
- Assist patients out of bed and with ambulation as soon as orders permit to limit the demineralization of bones.

Effects of Immobility on the Cardiovascular System

Bedrest results in a 50% reduction of blood flow to the legs and contributes to *venous stasis,* or pooling of blood in the veins of the lower legs. When a patient is lying down rather than sitting or standing, the heart actually has to work harder to pump blood throughout the body. This is because the muscles in the legs normally contract as you walk, sit, and stand, helping return venous blood from the lower extremities to the heart. When those skeletal muscles are not in use, the heart must work harder to pump blood throughout the body, increasing its workload. This is also a contributing factor to the pooling of blood in the legs, which can lead to blood clots.

When a patient is confined to bed, he or she may develop a blood clot, which may then dislodge and travel through the vein. One type of blood clot is called deep vein thrombosis (DVT), which is a clot that develops in the deep veins of the legs. These types of clots can impair circulation in the limb. Other clots may develop in the more superficial veins of the legs but are less of a threat to limb circulation.

Any stationary clot or clot fragment may dislodge and enter the circulation. It is then referred to as an *embolus,* or a traveling blood clot. The clot breaks away from the vein wall in the leg and travels through the bloodstream. As the embolus travels through the venous system back to the heart and lungs and into the arterial blood flow, there is a risk that it will become lodged in a small arterial capillary that supplies blood to vital organs, such as the lungs, heart, and brain. Once the embolus becomes lodged so that it blocks blood flow to a portion of a vital organ, oxygen and nutrients are prevented from reaching the tissue, resulting in the death of the affected cells. When it occurs in the lungs, it is referred to as a *pulmonary embolus* (PE); in the heart it is known as a *myocardial infarction* (MI), or *heart attack;* and when it occurs in the brain it is termed a *cerebrovascular accident* (CVA), commonly known as a *stroke.* An embolism to any of these three vital organs may result in death. An embolism has been identified as the most preventable cause of death during hospitalization.

Orthostatic hypotension, also known as *postural hypotension,* is a decrease in blood pressure that occurs when a patient changes from a reclining or flat position to an upright position, such as sitting or standing, and is common after a patient has been restricted to bedrest. As a result of slow or insufficient vasoconstriction once the patient becomes vertical, blood pools in the lower extremities and abdominal organs, which results in a drop in the blood pressure and inadequate circulation to the brain. This can cause the patient to become dizzy, pale, clammy, or nauseated because the blood pressure drops more than normal and the heart rate increases more than normal in an effort to pump blood to the head. If the blood pressure falls too far, the patient may experience **syncope,** or *fainting.* If the patient exhibits any of these signs upon standing, assist him or her to a sitting or reclining position.

The patient is most likely to experience orthostatic hypotension the first few times he or she gets up after a surgery or any other procedure requiring bedrest for several hours. This is why it is extremely important for you, the nurse, to be with any patient the first time he or she gets out of bed. If dizziness or syncope occurs, you will be there to prevent injury to the patient.

NURSING MEASURES TO PREVENT CARDIOVASCULAR COMPLICATIONS. To prevent the formation of venous thrombosis, it is important to keep the blood from pooling in the legs, where clots most commonly form. To do so, follow these guidelines:

- Encourage movement of the extremities. If the patient is unable to do so, you will perform passive ROM exercises (see Skill 16.1).
- Apply ordered devices to prevent pooling of blood in the legs. These include *antiembolism stockings,* which are close-fitting elastic stockings that usually cover the whole leg, and *sequential compression devices* (SCDs). SCDs are air-filled sleeves that are wrapped around the patient's lower legs and connected to a pump that inflates and deflates each area of the sleeve in a sequence designed to move blood in the legs toward the heart. (See Chapter 33 for more information about antiembolism stockings and SCDs.)

To help decrease the workload of the heart and prevent orthostatic hypotension, it is important to gradually move the patient from a lying position to a sitting or standing position. Use these actions to prevent orthostatic hypotension:

- Encourage movement of the extremities, especially dorsiflexion and plantar flexion of the feet, which will cause

• WORD • BUILDING •
embolus: embolos – stopper

muscle contraction that will help push the blood in the veins back to the heart. If the patient is unable to move his or her extremities, perform passive ROM exercises to promote muscular pressure on the veins to assist the flow of blood back to the heart.

- Change the patient's position frequently to improve blood return to the heart from the rest of the body.
- If possible, change the patient's position from horizontal to vertical. Elevate the head of the bed as much as possible or allow the patient to sit in a chair if permissible.
- Remain with the patient the first few times he or she gets out of bed. Follow procedures for assisting the patient to dangle (see Skill 16.7, page 305) before allowing the patient to stand.

KNOWLEDGE CONNECTION

Describe an adverse effect on the musculoskeletal system of the patient with limited mobility. Identify two nursing measures to assist in maintaining joint flexibility and muscle strength of the patient with limited mobility. What is orthostatic hypotension?

Effects of Immobility on the Respiratory System

When the patient is unable to move about and take deep breaths, the result is a decrease in lung expansion and respiratory muscle weakness. As an individual rests in bed, he or she tends to take shallow breaths that limit the expansion of the lungs. Pneumonia and *pulmonary emboli,* or blood clots in the lungs, are adverse respiratory conditions that can occur in immobilized patients. They are preventable, so it is extremely important for you to use appropriate nursing measures as discussed in this chapter.

Hypostatic pneumonia is a type of lung infection that occurs when a patient is immobile. Secretions pool in the lungs, and the warm, dark, moist environment is ideal for bacterial growth, resulting in an infection. Health care–associated infections (HAIs), once called *nosocomial infections,* are preventable in today's health-care settings. (See Chapter 14 for more information on HAIs.) Because such illnesses are preventable, some insurers are refusing to pay costs related to certain HAIs. It is extremely important that you know what to do to prevent such illnesses and utilize your nursing knowledge to be proactive.

Atelectasis, the collapse of lung tissue affecting part or all of a lung, can occur due to the inability of the lung to fully expand. It also may occur when a patient does not take full, deep breaths to keep the alveoli open. When the alveoli collapse, oxygen and carbon dioxide exchange is impaired, resulting in lowered oxygen in the blood, or *hypoxemia.*

NURSING MEASURES TO PREVENT RESPIRATORY COMPLICATIONS. To prevent atelectasis and pneumonia, it is necessary to increase lung expansion, strengthen respiratory muscles, improve oxygen and carbon dioxide exchange, and improve the effectiveness of coughs. Use these actions to prevent respiratory secretions from pooling in the lungs:

- Turn the patient from side to side at least every 2 hours to permit lung expansion.
- Elevate the head of the bed 45 degrees or more to promote lung expansion (see Table 16.3 later in this chapter).
- Encourage cough and deep breathing exercises every hour while the patient is awake (Box 16.2).
- Encourage the patient to use an incentive spirometer, taking 10 to 20 deep breaths every hour to expand the lungs in an attempt to reach a preset level of inspiratory volume (see Chapter 28). An incentive spirometer is a device used to encourage patients to take deep breaths because it provides visual feedback. The spirometer consists of one to three chambers, each containing a small ball or platform. As the patient inhales, expanding the lungs, the ball or platform in the chamber rises. The greater the volume of air that is inhaled, the higher the number of balls or platforms that rise, and the farther they rise (Fig. 16.1).

Box 16.2

Turning, Deep Breathing, and Coughing

Assisting a patient to turn, deep breathe, and cough is a frequent nursing intervention. This important action helps prevent respiratory and circulatory complications of immobility.

- **Turning:** Turn the patient from side to side at least every 2 hours and make him or her comfortable. This stimulates circulation to help prevent blood clots and prevents stasis of fluids in the lungs.
- **Deep breathing:** Instruct the patient to take a long, slow, deep breath; hold it for 3 seconds; and then exhale slowly. This should be repeated at least five times. This serves to expand the lungs and increase gas exchange.
- **Coughing:** Instruct the patient to inhale using long, slow, deep breaths. Hold for 3 seconds and then cough forcefully on the third or fourth expiration. Repeat at least five times. This also helps to prevent stasis of fluid in the lungs.

Effects of Immobility on the Gastrointestinal System

When patients are not able to be physically active, they may have a decreased appetite. However, because they are healing from illness or injury, good nutritional intake is extremely important (see Chapter 23). The major effect of immobility on the gastrointestinal system is the lack of *peristalsis,* or natural movement of the intestines. Again, without activity, the smooth muscle of the intestines is less active. This generally results in constipation, flatulence, and distention, and it may also cause indigestion and lack of appetite.

• WORD • BUILDING •

atelectasis: atel – incomplete + ectasis – expansion

hypoxemia: hypo – deficient + ox – oxygen + em – blood + ia – condition

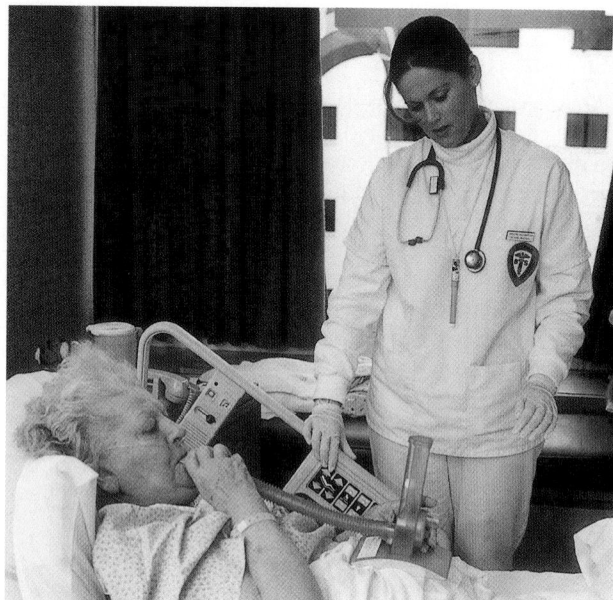

FIGURE 16.1 A patient using an incentive spirometer to expand her lungs and prevent respiratory complications of immobilization (from Williams LS, Hopper PD. *Understanding Medical Surgical Nursing*. 5th ed. Philadelphia, PA: FA Davis; 2015).

When peristalsis slows, food moves more slowly through the gastrointestinal tract, allowing the colon to absorb too much water. When too much water is absorbed from the food, the result is dry, hard feces.

NURSING MEASURES TO PREVENT GASTROINTESTINAL COMPLICATIONS. To help prevent constipation, intestinal gas, and lack of appetite, it is important that you encourage appropriate food and fluid intake. Muscle contraction and exercise help to stimulate peristalsis, making it important to ensure as much movement and physical activity as allowed, even when the patient is ordered to be on bedrest. Use these measures to help prevent gastrointestinal discomfort for your patients:

- As soon as the health-care provider's orders allow, assist the patient to get up in a chair or ambulate at least three to four times daily. Encourage the use of a bedside commode or getting up to the bathroom rather than using a bedpan.
- While the patient is on bedrest, ensure that the patient repositions at least every 2 hours and encourage active ROM exercises or provide passive ROM to all joints at least once every 8 hours.
- Place the patient in a sitting position to defecate on the bedpan or bedside commode, allowing gravity to assist in the elimination process. (See Chapter 30 for more information about digestive elimination.)
- Inquire about the patient's food likes and dislikes.
- Help the patient select well-balanced, nutritious meals from the menu.
- Encourage the patient to choose foods with fiber to help prevent constipation. Include fresh fruits and vegetables, raw if possible, to add fiber.
- Encourage fluid intake of 8 ounces or more every 2 hours to help prevent constipation unless the patient is on a fluid restriction. Be sure to offer and bring fluids that the patient likes to drink.
- Instruct the patient to avoid drinking fluids through a straw if intestinal gas is a problem. Each time the patient swallows a sip of fluid, he or she also swallows a straw full of air.
- Assess and document the activity level of bowel sounds and the frequency and characteristics of bowel movements. (See Chapter 30 for more information on assessing the digestive system.)
- If a patient has not had a bowel movement in 3 days, administer a laxative or enema according to the health-care provider's orders. If there is no order, you need to obtain one. The exception to this situation is when the patient's normal elimination routine at home is less frequent than every 3 days.
- Provide a laxative or stool softener, as needed, according to the health-care provider's orders.

KNOWLEDGE CONNECTION

How can the HAIs hypostatic pneumonia and pulmonary emboli be prevented? Name one complication of the gastrointestinal system of a patient with limited mobility.

Effects of Immobility on the Urinary System

The patient who is lying in bed is at risk for a urinary tract infection because urine can pool in the renal pelvis of the kidney. Normally when a person is upright, urine moves from the renal pelvis into the ureters and then to the bladder. Bedrest interferes with this normal movement of urine. In addition, the patient is at risk for developing kidney stones, or renal calculi, because excess calcium in the blood is filtered out by the kidneys.

When a patient must void on a bedpan or use a urinal while remaining in bed, he or she is less likely to completely empty the bladder, resulting in urinary retention. This retained urine provides an excellent medium for bacteria to proliferate, possibly causing a bladder infection that can spread to the remaining urinary tract.

NURSING MEASURES TO PREVENT URINARY COMPLICATIONS. To avoid urinary stasis and prevent urinary tract infection and renal calculi, use these measures:

- Provide adequate fluid intake to prevent concentrated urine. Again, offer beverages of the patient's choice and encourage intake of 8 ounces or more every 2 hours unless he or she is on a fluid restriction.
- Assist the patient to urinate in a sitting position to encourage full emptying of the urinary bladder. Male patients may be able to urinate best if they are allowed to stand at the bedside. Be sure to obtain a health-care provider's order allowing this activity if the patient is on bedrest.

- Assess the patient's output. He or she should void at least every 8 hours. If the patient who is properly hydrated is unable to void, he or she may need to be catheterized to drain the bladder.

Anatomy and Physiology Connection

When a patient is immobile, many systems are affected (see Table 16.1). Often the changes in one system will affect other systems in a negative way. An example of this occurs when the skeletal system is affected, and this impacts the urinary system as well.

As a result of immobility, the skeletal system no longer needs to support the body for activity and weight-bearing, which is what keeps bones strong. Because of negative feedback, the brain allows calcium, a mineral needed for bone strength, to leave the bones in larger amounts than usual. The calcium then enters the bloodstream, causing the blood to have higher amounts of calcium than normal. This is called *hypercalcemia.*

The excess calcium circulating in the blood goes to the kidneys where normally it is filtered out into the urine. If too much calcium is present for the kidneys to effectively remove it, the calcium collects, forming one or more kidney stones. One stone is called a *renal calculus.* More than one stone is referred to as *renal calculi.*

The lack of calcium in the bone (demineralization) leaves the bones porous and brittle. This condition is known as *osteoporosis* and can occur due to a lack of weight-bearing exercise as well as to immobility. People with osteoporosis can have bone fractures without any injury or trauma causing them. Their bones may break more easily from a stumble or fall than in those without osteoporosis. The vertebrae of the spine may collapse, causing compression fractures, which are extremely painful.

Effects of Immobility on the Integumentary System

When a patient is immobile and consistent pressure is applied to the same area of the body, the blood flow to that area is reduced or is stopped entirely. When this occurs, the skin and underlying tissue die. This is referred to as a *pressure injury,* also called *skin breakdown* or a *decubitus ulcer.* The area may be red at first, but the skin will continue to deteriorate if the circulation to the area does not improve. Shearing of the skin will further destroy the integument. **Shearing** occurs when the skin layer is pulled across muscle and bone in one direction while the skin slides over another surface, such as a bed sheet, in the opposite direction. This shearing and friction on the skin can cause abrasions and open areas.

Patients on prolonged bedrest are especially at risk for developing pressure injuries. (See Chapter 26 for more information on pressure injuries.) Special support surfaces and specialty beds have been developed to help alleviate this risk, such as air-fluidized beds, low-air-loss beds, and combination beds.

It can be difficult to turn patients with multiple trauma and other musculoskeletal conditions. As a result, some beds have been developed that turn from side to side so that the patient has less chance of developing respiratory and cardiovascular complications while on bedrest. Table 16.2 provides information about different types of support surfaces and specialty beds.

NURSING MEASURES TO PREVENT INTEGUMENTARY COMPLICATIONS. To prevent skin breakdown and to maintain skin integrity, use these guidelines:

- Provide adequate nutrition because tissue cannot repair itself without proper nutrients (see Chapter 23).
- Reposition patients in bed at least every 2 hours and those in a wheelchair every hour if they are unable to turn or shift their own weight.
- Inspect bony prominences for redness at least every 2 hours. If you find areas of redness, massage around them but not on the areas themselves. (See Chapter 26 for more information about pressure injuries and their treatment.)
- Use mild soaps for cleansing the skin, followed by gentle but thorough drying to help maintain skin integrity.
- Provide an appropriate surface for the patient, such as a mattress overlay, specialized mattress, or specialty bed.

KNOWLEDGE CONNECTION

How does immobility contribute to the formation of kidney stones? List two ways you can help prevent urinary complications of immobility. What is shearing? What can result from it?

Effects of Immobility on the Neurological System

When a patient is immobile, several neurological complications may result. The patient may become less mentally alert, and their vision may be less clear. Balance and coordination will decrease as immobility persists. In addition, if the patient is not turned and positioned appropriately, nerves may be compressed between the bones and the firm surface of the bed, resulting in impaired nerve function called *compression neuropathy.* The most common site for compression neuropathy in the lower extremities of the immobile patient is the peroneal nerve at the fibular head. Compression of this nerve can result in footdrop, which causes the foot to point in the downward position of **plantar flexion.** This condition can be permanent and will prevent the patient from being able to walk normally when he or she is able to ambulate. Footdrop also may be caused by injury, paralysis, and a weakness of the muscles and nerves of the foot.

• **WORD • BUILDING •**

decubitus: decumbere – lie down

NURSING MEASURES TO PREVENT NEUROLOGICAL COMPLICATIONS. To prevent adverse effects of immobility on the neurological system, it is important to take measures to maintain alertness, visual acuity, and balance. Use these measures to promote normal neurological function:

- Determine the patient's level of consciousness by asking specific questions related to person, place, and time. (See Chapter 21 for more information on assessment of level of consciousness.)
- Use a foot splint or high-topped tennis shoes to keep the patient's feet in a natural position; this promotes the ability to bear weight and walk normally.
- Perform neurological checks to determine changes in the patient's neurological status. (See Chapter 21 for details on how to assess the patient's neurological condition.)
- Provide clues to the correct date and time in the room. Keep a calendar and clock within the patient's line of vision. Open the curtains to allow the patient to observe the weather and the season.
- If the patient is confused about time, place, or person, gently reorient him or her by supplying the correct information.

Table 16.2
Support Surfaces and Specialty Beds

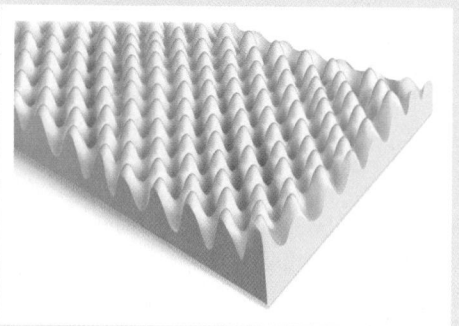

Surface/Bed	*Description*	*Figure*
Support Surfaces		
Mattress overlays	Applied to the top of the mattress; may be filled with air or gel, or made of foam	Eggcrate mattress
Specialized mattresses	Mattresses containing special foam, such as "memory foam" or chambers containing air that can be controlled with a dial	Synergy® Air Elite mattress 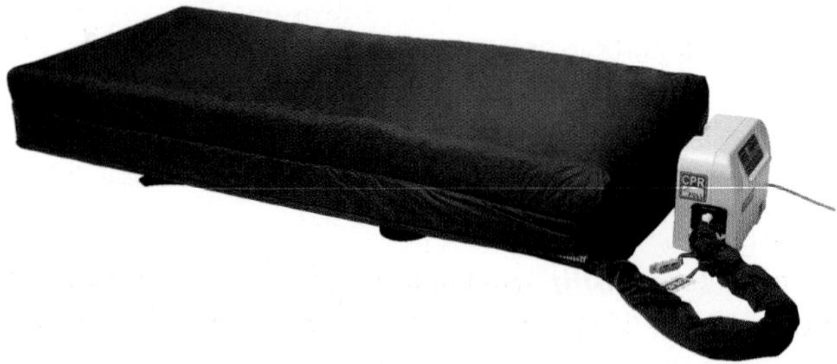
Specialty Beds		
Air-fluidized bed	An encased mattress filled with small round beads coated in silicone to prevent clumping; air is pumped through the bed, which causes the beads to mimic liquid; patient rests on a thin sheet within the air-fluidized compartment	Envella air-fluidized therapy system 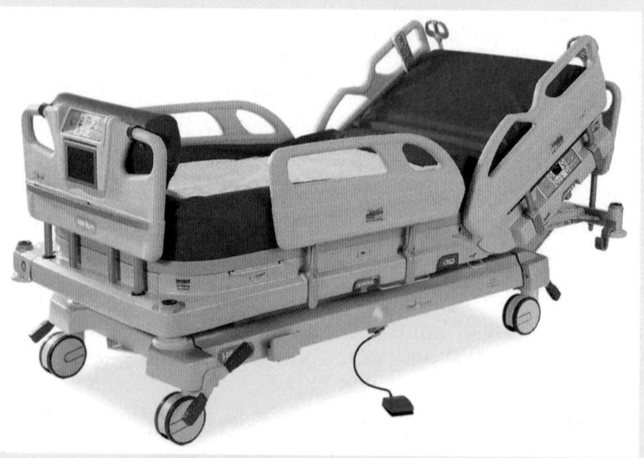

Table 16.2
Support Surfaces and Specialty Beds—cont'd

Surface/Bed	*Description*	*Figure*
Combination low-air-loss and lateral rotation bed	A combination bed is a low-air-loss type of bed with lateral rotation to prevent pressure on any one area; each pocket is filled with air that can be inflated or deflated; can be utilized with a ventilator-assisted patient	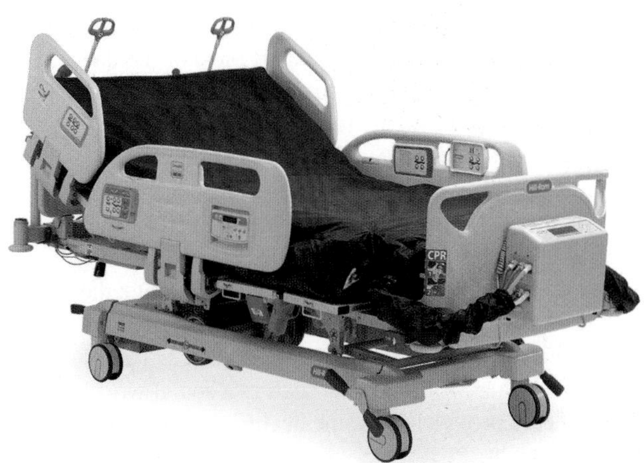
Continuous lateral-rotation bed	Special type of bed frame that allows the entire bed to turn from side to side; mattress is low air loss; bed can be programmed to turn by degrees at set intervals	TotalCare® SpO2RT 2 bed 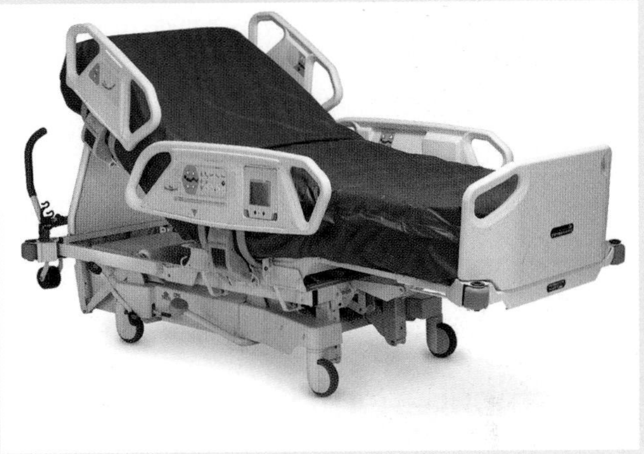

For example, if the patient thinks it is Tuesday, you might say, "Today is Thursday. You have been here for 2 days now," to help the patient reorient to time.

Psychological Effects of Immobility

Psychological effects of immobility will differ with each individual. Depression, anxiety, hostility, and fear are common adverse effects of immobility. Restricted mobility affects the patient's self-image, independence, and ability to meet his or her own needs. If a person has always taken care of himself or herself and now must rely on others for simple activities such as washing his or her face, the patient may be frustrated or embarrassed. In addition, he or she may be concerned about finances, work, and family issues. The patient may feel isolated because of limited social interactions. He or she may feel rejected or forgotten because others do not come to visit as often as desired.

Sensory deprivation may also occur when a patient must lie in bed all day and all night, especially if the patient is alone in the room. With decreased sensory stimulation, the patient may experience auditory or visual hallucinations.

It is possible that patients will have difficulty sleeping when they are unable to get out of bed and be active. They may be restless and irritable, and they may take out their frustrations on you. Should this occur, do not take any outburst by the patient as a personal attack. Try to put yourself in the patient's place and empathize with his or her feelings. Then use your nursing skills to help the patient find ways to occupy time and to sleep better. (See Chapter 19 for more information about promoting rest and sleep.)

Nursing Measures to Prevent Psychological Complications

To help prevent depression, anxiety, and fear and to promote feelings of self-worth, use these nursing measures:

- Minimize sensory deprivation by ensuring that the patient has distractions to keep himself or herself occupied.

These include television, radio, books, magazines, newspapers, and puzzles.

- When you are with the patient, try to involve his or her senses with pleasant smells, tastes, sounds, and sights.
- Help improve the patient's sleep pattern by encouraging him or her to remain awake and alert most of the day. Keep window curtains or blinds open in the daytime to allow natural light into the room.
- Encourage and allow the patient to do as much as possible for himself or herself during patient care, such as helping with their bath, performing active ROM exercises when able, and making decisions about their care.
- Allow the patient to express concerns. Encourage the patient to talk about the things that are worrying him or her. Be kind and listen without giving advice. Take steps to involve other professionals, such as a social worker, pastoral care provider, or home health caregiver, if appropriate.
- Encourage visits with family and friends. Try to schedule care around visitors if the patient has few guests. Allow visitors to participate in care if they wish to do so and the patient wishes them to be involved.

KNOWLEDGE CONNECTION

How can you promote mental alertness in an immobilized patient? What are some common psychosocial effects of immobility?

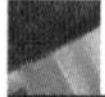

POSITIONING PATIENTS

When patients are unable to move independently, you will need to provide assistance in position changes to prevent complications that are associated with immobility. Traditionally, the gold standard for frequency of position change of immobile patients has been every 2 hours, although some patients may need to be repositioned more frequently.

Assisting Patients With Position Changes

It is important to maintain good body mechanics when positioning patients to prevent injury to the patient and staff. (See Chapter 13 for more information on body mechanics.) ***Safety: For safe patient handling, always lock the wheels of the equipment. Elevate the bed to a comfortable working height for you. After patient care, place the bed in the lowest setting with the wheels locked to prevent possible injury when the patient gets out of bed.***

As a general rule, patients who need assistance with positioning will need position changes at least every 2 hours when on bedrest. If the patient is confined to a wheelchair and cannot shift position independently, you will need to adjust his or her position in the wheelchair every hour. Patients who are at risk for skin breakdown may need even more frequent position changes. This includes patients who are thin, dehydrated, malnourished, or immobile. In most situations, you will position all extremities so that they will maintain their function and flexibility.

The term **position of function** means placing the extremities in alignment to maintain the potential for their use and movement. Positioning for function will help prevent undue pressure on nerves and help prevent discomfort, pain, and nerve damage. Many simple positioning devices are available to help maintain good alignment and prevent excessive pressure on joints and nerves. Positioning devices include pillows, hand rolls, arm boards, and foot splints. When you are placing a patient's extremity in the position of function, avoid direct pressure over bony prominences, compromised tissue, or pressure injuries. You may need to use additional padding on positioning devices to prevent pressure.

Patient Teaching Connection

Explaining to Promote Cooperation

When you care for a patient who has mobility problems, always make a point to explain what you will be doing for the patient. Many patients who require positioning assistance may be sedated from surgery, or they may have decreased levels of understanding because of a CVA, head injury, or dementia. When you give instructions as to how the patient can help with the position change, be sure those instructions are at an appropriate level of understanding for the patient. (See Chapter 12 for more information on patient teaching.) The patient will be more cooperative and less likely to resist during repositioning when he or she understands what is to be done. It is important to remember that, no matter how well a patient is positioned, it is necessary to reposition at least every 2 hours and possibly more frequently if the patient is unable to move himself or herself.

Selecting Appropriate Positions and Positioning Devices

In many situations, you will decide which position to use for procedures and to promote comfort for your patients. Specific positions are used for specific purposes. Table 16.3 identifies the common patient positions, describes each, and lists the purposes for which they are used.

When you position patients, it is very important that you support the limbs and areas of the body not in contact with the bed. You will accomplish this by using pillows and other positioning devices. The placement of these devices is discussed in Skill 16.2 (page 298). Table 16.4 describes commonly used positioning devices, their purposes, and their placement. Box 16.3 describes how to make these positioning devices out of common items.

Table 16.3
Common Positions and Their Purposes

Position	*Description*	*Purposes*
Supine	Lying on the back with arms at sides	For physical examination, resting in bed, undergoing anesthesia
Dorsal recumbent	Lying on the back with arms at sides, legs apart, knees bent, and feet flat on the bed	For physical examination of abdomen and genitalia, perineal care, examination during labor
Trendelenburg	Lying on back with arms at sides, bed positioned so that foot is higher than the head	During some abdominal surgeries to shift abdominal contents upward
Reverse Trendelenburg	Lying on back with arms at sides, bed positioned so that head is higher than foot but with no flexion at waist	After certain angiography procedures, allows head of bed to be elevated without causing pressure on the femoral artery During certain abdominal surgeries to shift abdominal contents downward
Lateral	Lying on the left or right side, supported behind back and between knees and ankles with pillows, in good body alignment	For patient comfort and to promote lung and cardiac function To relieve pressure on bony prominences of the coccyx and sacrum
Left Sims'	Lying on left side in semiprone position with right leg flexed and drawn up toward the chest; left arm is positioned along the patient's back	For rectal examinations and for administering enemas
Right Sims'	Lying on right side in semiprone position with left leg flexed; right arm is positioned along the patient's back	To relieve pressure on bony prominences of coccyx and sacrum
Fowler's	Semi-sitting position with various degrees of head elevation with knees slightly elevated	Purposes vary based on elevation
Low Fowler's	Head of bed elevated 30 degrees	To prevent aspiration during tube feeding
Semi-Fowler's	Head of bed elevated 45 degrees	To comfortably watch television or converse with visitors After abdominal surgeries to relieve tension on incision To assist patients who have difficulty breathing
High Fowler's	Head of bed elevated 90 degrees	To eat and drink without risk of choking To assist patients who have difficulty breathing
Orthopneic	Sitting upright with head of bed elevated 90 degrees or on the side of the bed with feet flat on the floor; patient leaning slightly forward with arms raised and elbows flexed, supported on an over-bed table	To assist patients in severe respiratory distress by allowing chest to expand to maximum capacity for moving air in and out of the lungs
Prone	Lying on stomach with head turned to the side	To improve oxygenation in patients with acute respiratory distress To relieve pressure on the back, coccyx, and hips
Lithotomy	Lying on back with knees flexed above the hips and legs supported in stirrups	For vaginal examinations, delivery of neonate, pelvic and gynecological surgery and procedures

Box 16.3

Making Positioning Devices From Common Objects

You can make positioning and supportive devices out of common objects that may be available in a home health care client's home. These work as well as more expensive commercial alternatives.

- **Arm board:** You can cover a piece of balsa wood with foam or a washcloth for padding and make an arm board. To increase comfort, add a wrist roll fashioned like a hand roll from a washcloth folded in half. Place under the patient's wrist to support the wrist and increase comfort. Use this to keep the arm straight if an IV is inserted near a joint.
- **Blanket roll:** To make a blanket roll, roll a small blanket into a firm roll. Use this to keep the patient lying on his or her side.
- **Hand roll:** You can make a hand roll by folding a washcloth in half, then rolling it into a log shape. Tape the ends in place to prevent unrolling of the hand roll. Use this in the palm of the hand to prevent contractures of the fingers.
- **Foot splint:** It is possible to improvise and fashion a foot splint to prevent footdrop by placing a blanket roll at the patient's feet. You can make a blanket roll by rolling a small blanket into a firm roll approximately the width of the patient's feet.
- **Trochanter roll:** You can make a trochanter roll by tightly rolling a sheet or blanket securely and placing it against the lateral side of the thigh to prevent outward rotation of the hip and leg.

Table 16.4

Positioning Devices

Positioning Device	*Purpose*	*Placement*
Pillow	Used to keep the head in proper alignment with the spine and reduce excessive pressure on nerves caused by stretching of the neck	Under the head and shoulders when in a supine position
	Used to relieve pressure on the lumbar spine and increase comfort	Under the knees in a supine position
	Used to maintain proper alignment of the hips and legs and to pad bony prominences	Between the knees and ankles in a lateral position
	Used to reduce rotation of the spine and maintain proper spinal alignment	At the back in a lateral position
Arm board	Used to prevent flexion of a joint, such as when an IV catheter is near the joint	Wrist or elbow
Blanket roll	Used to support the back or soles of the feet	Place blanket roll firmly at the patient's back or at the soles of the feet
Hand roll	Used to maintain a position of function of the hand and fingers of a patient with decreased movement of the hand and fingers	In the palm of the hand
Foot splint	Used to maintain a position of function of the feet in relation to the legs of a patient with decreased movement and strength of the lower extremities	Against the soles of the feet
Stirrups	Positioning for vaginal surgery, pelvic examination, or delivery of infant	Place feet in the stirrups to position the lower legs and feet in a lithotomy or dorsal recumbent position
Trochanter roll	Used to prevent external rotation of the legs	At the lateral side of the hip and thigh

KNOWLEDGE CONNECTION

How can you help prevent footdrop? What is the gold standard for frequency of position change of the immobile patient while he or she is on bedrest? Frequent repositioning of the immobile patient can prevent which complications? What is the first thing the nurse should do after approaching the patient prior to repositioning?

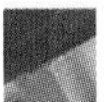

MOVING AND LIFTING PATIENTS

An enormous task required of the nursing staff is the safe handling and movement of patients. Nursing has one of the highest rates of musculoskeletal injuries related to the work environment compared to other occupations, resulting in a number of nurses leaving the profession. In addition, many of the nurses who remain in the profession have left bedside nursing because of the physical demands of direct patient care. Researchers suspect that many musculoskeletal injuries that occur to nursing staff are unreported. It is very important that you learn how to protect yourself from injury by using proper body mechanics (discussed in Chapter 13) and how to safely lift and move patients.

Safe patient handling is of great concern not only to nurses but also to their employers and their professional organizations. In the workplace today, there is a new emphasis on ways to replace manual lifting with equipment designed to assist nursing staff with lifting and moving patients.

The American Nurses Association (ANA) has instituted the Handle With Care campaign in response to the significant number of musculoskeletal disorders reported by nurses. The purpose of the campaign is to build an industry-wide program in health care to prevent musculoskeletal injuries. Since these changes have been put in place, there has been a marked decrease in reported lifting-related injuries in the health-care workplace. The ANA has published "Safe Patient Handling and Mobility," which includes interdisciplinary standards for lifting and moving patients across the continuum of care. At this time, a bill has been introduced in the U.S. House of Representatives to require safe patient handling programs in all health-care facilities and to eliminate manual lifting. Many health-care facilities have now instituted "no lifting" programs to relieve nursing staff of the need to lift patients, instead using lifting equipment such as sit-to-stand lifts, hydraulic lifts, and battery-operated lifts. It is your responsibility as a nursing student and later as a nurse to learn how to correctly use such equipment. Although it might at times seem faster to move patients manually, the saved time is not worth the risk of a debilitating injury caused by lifting more weight than your body can tolerate.

Devices for Lifting and Moving Patients

Various types of equipment are available to assist in the movement of patients, such as transfer belts, nylon friction-reducing devices, and slide boards, as well as partial- or full-weight-bearing assistive devices, including sling-type, battery-operated patient lifts. Overhead ceiling lift devices are becoming the equipment of choice in new hospital construction and remodeling projects.

Moving Patients in Bed

When patients are unable to move or turn themselves in bed, the nursing staff must do this for them. An overhead *trapeze bar,* a triangular device suspended above the patient on an overbed frame, allows the patient to lift some or all of his or her weight off of the bed, which is helpful when moving the patient up in bed or turning the patient (see Skill 16.3, page 299).

TURNING A PATIENT. Draw sheets are helpful to move and turn the patient in bed. A draw sheet can be untucked and used for turning the patient. Before turning a patient on his or her side, it is recommended to move the patient toward the side of the bed opposite of the direction in which you will turn the patient. For example, if you wanted to turn a patient onto his or her left side, you would first move the patient toward the right side of the bed. Then, when the patient is turned, he or she will be positioned in the center of the bed, rather than at the edge (see Skill 16.4, page 300).

LOGROLLING A PATIENT. When a patient has undergone spinal surgery or has a spinal injury, it is necessary to turn his or her body as one unit. This procedure is known as a **logroll** because the patient is turned in the same way a log would be rolled. Three nursing personnel are required to correctly logroll a patient. One stands at the patient's head, one stands at the patient's waist, and one stands at the patient's thighs. The staff member standing at the head controls the turn. He or she gives directions and counts to three before the move occurs. ***Safety: It is very important that all three staff members turn the patient at the same time. Failure to do so can cause damage to the patient's spine, which could potentially result in paralysis.*** When the count is given, all three staff members move the patient to the side of the bed that is opposite the direction in which he or she will be turned. Then the two staff members not standing at the head of the bed move to the opposite side of the bed to turn the patient toward them. Again, the person at the head directs the turn. He or she supports the patient's head and neck during the turn. On the count of three, the patient is turned as one unit, using a draw sheet to keep his or her neck, shoulders, and hips in alignment during and after the turn (see Skill 16.4).

Transferring Patients

You will often assist patients out of bed to sit in a chair or to move from the bed to a stretcher or wheelchair for transport to another area of the hospital. It is very important that you know the correct way to **transfer,** or move patients from one place to another, in a way that is safe both for you and for the patient.

Before attempting to transfer a patient, you need to know how much assistance the patient will require. If the patient can stand but is unsteady on his or her feet, you will provide only minimal assistance. However, if the patient cannot stand on both feet, perhaps because one side is paralyzed, you will need to provide a great deal of assistance to prevent the patient from falling to his or her weak side. If the patient is unable to bear weight, you will transfer the patient using a lift. To accomplish this, you will need the assistance of one or more people. If you are transferring a patient from the bed to a chair or wheelchair, always place the chair or wheelchair on the patient's strong side. For example, if the patient has left-sided weakness, place the chair or wheelchair on the patient's right side. When you assist this patient from the wheelchair to the bed, place the wheelchair so that the patient is transferring toward his or her strong side. In other words, the bed should be on this patient's right side.

TRANSFER BELTS. Once you know the amount of assistance the patient will need, you will then determine which assistive devices might be useful for the transfer. If the patient can fully or partially bear weight, you will need to use a transfer belt, also called a gait belt. This device is constructed of strong webbed fabric that is placed around the patient's waist during transfers or ambulation. It provides a place for you to grasp the patient without holding onto clothing that could tear or come loose if the patient loses his or her balance.

SLIDE SHEETS. Slide sheets are nylon friction-reducing devices made of thin webbed nylon sheets slightly smaller than the surface of the hospital bed (see Skill 16.4). A slide sheet is placed beneath the patient, allowing the patient to move easily from the bed to a stretcher or up in the bed (Fig. 16.2). Always use caution, because these nylon devices are intended to require minimal staff exertion. Skill 16.5 (see page 302) provides the steps needed to use a slide sheet to move a patient from the bed to a stretcher.

SLIDE BOARDS. Slide boards, also called transfer boards, are another method used to transfer a patient from the bed to a stretcher or a stretcher to the bed. A slide board is a hard, thin, flat plastic board that can be used with a draw sheet or plastic trash bag to help reduce friction (Fig. 16.3). The patient is turned using the draw sheet, and then the board is

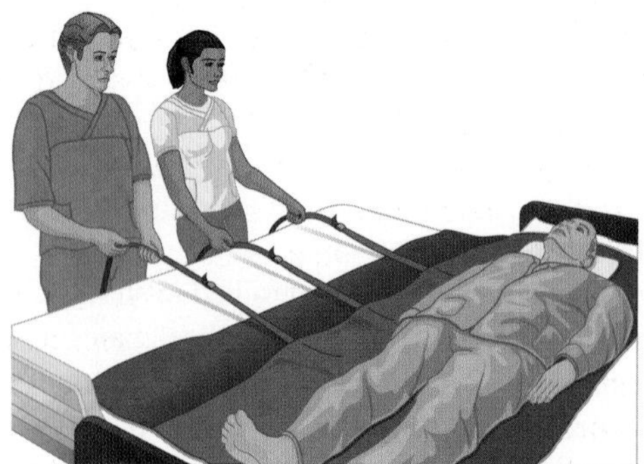

FIGURE 16.2 Once the slide sheet is positioned under the patient, two nurses stand on the far side of the stretcher and pull the patient from the bed to the stretcher (from Wilkinson JM, Treas LS. *Fundamentals of Nursing: Theory, Concepts & Applications*. Vol. 2. 3rd ed. Philadelphia, PA: FA Davis; 2016).

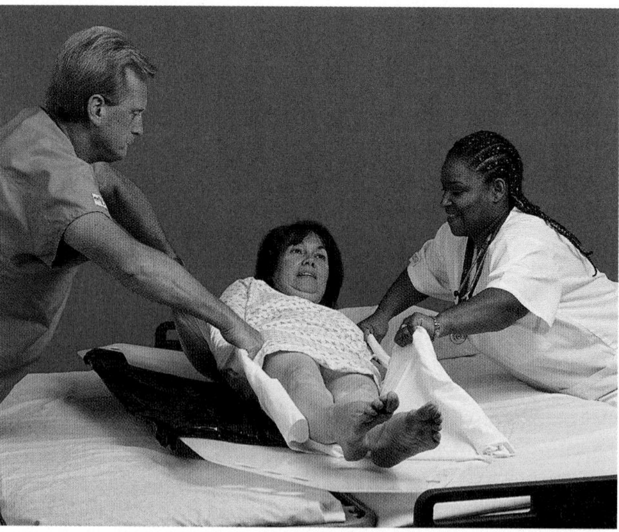

FIGURE 16.3 This patient is being moved with a slide board and draw sheet, which decreases the workload on the nurses as well as preventing friction on the patient's skin (from Wilkinson JM, Treas LS. *Fundamentals of Nursing: Theory, Concepts & Applications*. Vol. 2. 3rd ed. Philadelphia, PA: FA Davis; 2016).

placed on the bed next to the patient, spanning the space between the bed and the stretcher. The patient is turned onto the slide board, and the health-care providers use the sheet to simultaneously slide the patient across the board from the bed to the stretcher.

SIT-TO-STAND LIFTS. Partial-weight-bearing assistive devices, also known as sit-to-stand lifts, are useful when transferring a patient who is in need of assistance, such as those who are weak, elderly, or recovering from surgery. These devices may be used to transfer the patient from the bed to the chair, the bedside commode, or the bathroom. The patient is assisted to a standing position on the locked device (Fig. 16.4). Some devices have seats, while others have slings to support the patient during the transfer. The device is unlocked for transport. The patient is then wheeled to the chair, bedside commode, or bathroom. The device is locked, and the transfer is made.

LIFTS. Sling-type, battery-operated patient lifts are used for the non-weight-bearing patient. The patient is rolled to the side, and a sling constructed of a thin webbed material is positioned beneath him or her according to the manufacturer's recommendations. Several different types of slings are available, and proper training is critical for safe use of all transfer assistive devices. The sling is attached to the battery-operated lift device, which raises the patient into a sitting position above the level of the bed. The lift is stabilized with a wide base of support and moved to the desired location. During this time the patient is sitting in the sling, and then he or she is gradually lowered to a chair or wheelchair. When the patient has been transferred from the bed to a chair and will require assistance for transfer back to the bed, the sling is left in place beneath the patient. When the patient is later transferred

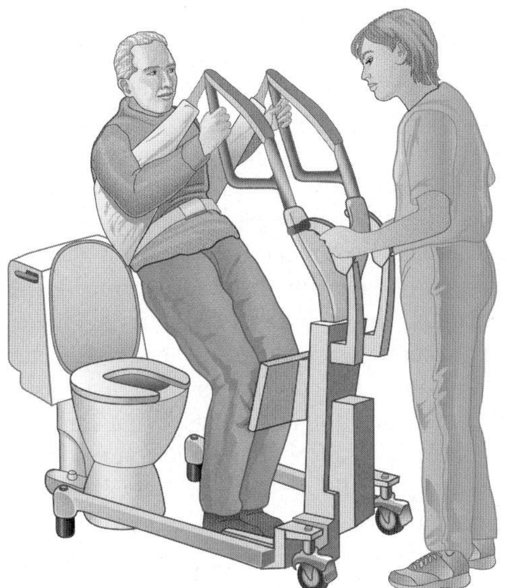

FIGURE 16.4 A sit-to-stand lift is used to move the patient from a sitting to a standing position (from Wilkinson JM, Treas LS. *Fundamentals of Nursing: Theory, Concepts & Applications*. Vol. 2. 3rd ed. Philadelphia, PA: FA Davis; 2016).

back to the bed, the sling is then removed. Sling-type, battery-operated patient lifts are the device of choice if a patient has fallen to the floor and requires assistance to be returned to the bed or a chair. Using this device after a patient has fallen reduces the chance of staff or patient injury.

Battery-operated lift devices are preferred because the nursing staff does not have to lever the patient's weight. Older models of lifts are not battery operated but operate using hydraulics. While these require some effort to lever weight on the part of the nursing staff, they are far preferable to lifting a patient without assistance (Fig. 16.5). These lifts operate in the same way as discussed previously, except that once the patient is centered in the sling and it is attached to the lift, you must pump a lever to lift the patient into a sitting position above the bed surface. Once the patient is transferred to the desired location, a valve is turned that releases air, gently lowering the patient into the chair or wheelchair (see Skill 16.6, page 304).

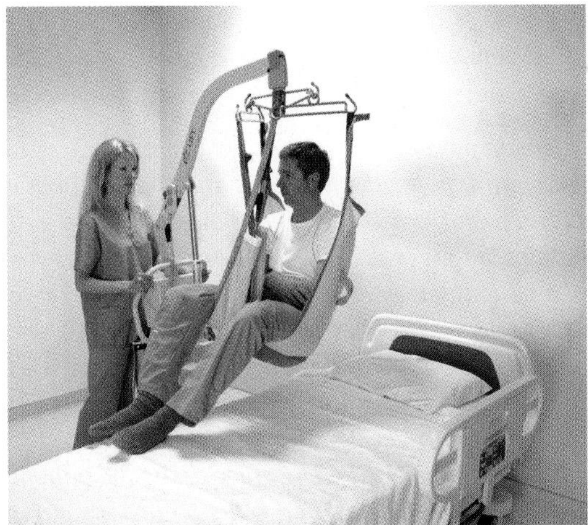

FIGURE 16.5 A mechanical lift is used to transfer patients who cannot easily be transferred by the nursing staff (from Wilkinson JM, Treas LS. *Fundamentals of Nursing: Theory, Concepts & Applications*. Vol. 1. 3rd ed. Philadelphia, PA: FA Davis; 2016).

Overhead ceiling lift devices are becoming more popular in the safe patient handling campaign. These devices require tracks in the ceiling for patient lifts. These lifts are being incorporated into new hospital construction or remodeling projects. A sling is placed under the patient and attached to the lifting device prior to transfer. Overhead ceiling lifts require even less staff exertion than battery-operated models, which require health-care providers to push the device supporting the patient during the transfer.

Real-World Connection

Safety Tips for Stretchers

An elderly patient was in the radiology department after completion of a CT scan. He needed to be moved from the CT scan table to a stretcher. The stretcher was placed against the CT scan table and locked. A second nurse who was unaware that the stretcher had been locked pressed the foot lock and inadvertently unlocked the bed. The patient fell between the CT table and the stretcher during the transfer when the stretcher moved unexpectedly. ***Safety: Always verify that the stretcher or bed wheels do not roll by physically attempting to move the stretcher or bed.***

Manual Transfers

Although the use of assistive devices is recommended in the ANA's safe patient handling initiative, such devices may not always be available. ***Safety: If you must transfer a patient without an assistive device (called a manual transfer), you must use proper body mechanics.*** Proper body mechanics includes using a wide base of support and standing close to the object being moved, keeping your back straight, and avoiding twisting your torso. Use your thigh muscles instead of the muscles in your back (again, see Chapter 13 for a review of proper body mechanics). Remember to explain to the patient what you will do and instruct him or her about what to do during the transfer (see Skill 16.5).

When you perform a manual transfer to move a patient from a bed to a stretcher, a draw sheet or bath blanket is helpful. First, assess the situation to determine the number of staff members required to safely transfer the patient. Consider the patient's weight, level of consciousness, and physical ability. For patients who can assist with the transfer, use a draw sheet. Roll the patient and place the draw sheet under the patient, extending from the shoulders to the thighs. If the patient is unable to assist with the transfer, you can use a bath blanket under the patient from the head to the feet and then grasp the bath blanket to move the patient to the stretcher.

KNOWLEDGE CONNECTION

What is the primary purpose for using patient lift devices? What is the first thing a nurse does when preparing to use a patient lift device?

Supervision/Delegation Connection

Safety in Numbers

When you are manually moving or transferring patients, it is imperative to carefully assess each situation. Be sure that you have the proper number of staff available to assist with the move. Although you can delegate transferring patients to unlicensed assistive personnel (UAPs) and certified nursing assistants, it is important that you are aware of the patient's abilities. If the patient is unsteady, heavy, or weak or paralyzed on one side, then at least two members of the nursing staff should assist with the transfer. It may be necessary to delegate additional nursing staff to assist with safe patient movement or transfer to prevent patient or staff injury.

Assisting With Ambulation

Patients needing assistance with ambulation should move from the supine position to the standing position in stages to avoid possible dizziness, orthostatic hypotension, and syncopal episodes. To safely move a patient from the supine to the standing position, raise the head of the bed and then assist the patient to sit on the side of the bed to ensure that the patient is able to tolerate the change in position. The patient's feet should be firmly on the floor or a footstool. This process is referred to as *dangling* (see Skill 16.7, page 305). If the patient becomes dizzy while dangling, assist him or her back to the **Fowler's** or **semi-Fowler's position** on the bed. If the dizziness continues, lower the head of the bed to the low Fowler's position if doing so is not contraindicated for this patient. Once the dizziness has passed, return the patient to the Fowler's position. Check the patient's pulse and blood pressure prior to attempting to assist the patient to dangle again. Next, allow the patient to dangle for 1 to 3 minutes and then check their pulse and blood pressure. If the patient does not experience dizziness and the pulse and blood pressure do not change significantly, allow the patient to proceed to a standing position with staff support available. However, if the pulse rate increases more than 20 bpm, the blood pressure drops more than 20 mm Hg, or the patient experiences dizziness, assist the patient back to a sitting position, lift the legs onto the bed, and lower the head of the bed slightly. Remain with the patient. In 1 to 3 minutes, recheck the pulse and blood pressure. Notify the health-care provider of the patient's vital signs and response to dangling.

After the patient is able to dangle without adverse reactions, you will assist him or her to a standing position. ***Safety: Be certain that the patient is wearing nonskid footwear.*** Place your feet in front of the patient's feet and your knees against the patient's knees to provide stability when he or she is moving from a sitting to a standing position. A transfer belt may be helpful as it provides a place to grasp hold of the patient. If the patient experiences dizziness, assist him or her back to a sitting position. When the patient is able to stand without dizziness, proceed with ambulation. Stand at the patient's side for support. If a transfer belt is used, hold the belt tightly near the patient's body. If a transfer belt is not used, provide support by securely placing one arm around the patient at the waist and grasping the patient's forearm that is nearest you with your other hand. Begin by slowly ambulating the patient short distances, such as to the bedside commode, bathroom, or door of the patient's room, as the patient tolerates. Take into consideration that the patient will need enough stamina to ambulate back to the bed (see Skill 16.8, page 306).

If the patient begins to fall, pull him or her toward your body and allow the patient to slide down your leg to the floor. As you lower the patient, bend your knees. Keep your back straight as you lower the patient to the floor. ***Safety: Do not attempt to hold a patient upright if he or she loses consciousness or is falling. This will only injure you and possibly injure the patient.***

Lifting and Moving Obese Patients

Some patients are *obese,* which means that they are more than 30% overweight. When you lift and move these patients, you must take care to protect yourself and the patient from injury. Be sure to use equipment approved for the weight of the patient. Enlist the help of coworkers to move large patients and to prevent injuries. It may be necessary to obtain specialized equipment designed to lift and move patients who weigh in excess of 300 pounds (136 kg).

Protecting Yourself and Your Patients

Your knowledge of transfer techniques and body mechanics and the use of transfer devices are keys to protecting yourself and your patients from injury. In addition, one mark of a good nurse is the ability to anticipate possible problems and take steps to prevent those problems, such as in the following scenario:

> *A female patient puts on her call light and asks to use the bathroom for the first time after having abdominal surgery. Nurse A is busy and sends a UAP to assist the patient but gives the UAP no particular instructions. The patient becomes dizzy and nearly faints on the way to the bathroom. Nurse B thinks through the patient's situation and realizes that the patient's blood pressure is running a bit low and that she has not been out of bed for over 24 hours. Nurse B, although busy, goes in with the UAP. They first assist the patient to dangle and then assist her to the bathroom, carefully monitoring her responses.*

Which nurse would you rather have caring for your loved one? Which nurse would you rather be?

Skill 16.1 Performing Passive Range-of-Motion Exercises

Assessment Steps

1. Check the chart for any contraindications to full range-of-motion (ROM) exercises.
2. Assess the patient for complaints of pain, nausea, and the need for toileting before beginning exercises. If the patient complains of pain or nausea, medicate and wait 30 minutes before performing ROM exercises. Assist with toileting as needed before starting the exercises.

Planning Steps

1. Obtain a bath blanket or use the top sheet and blanket to cover the patient during exercises. Keep all parts of the patient covered except the limb you are exercising ***to preserve dignity and keep the patient warm.***
2. Ensure that equipment is away from the bed to allow enough space for abduction of the limbs ***to prevent injury during exercise.***
3. Plan to repeat each exercise 5 to 10 times. Plan to move each joint to the maximum extent of its motion. *Safety: If you meet resistance during exercise, stop at that point. Do not force a joint or exercise a joint beyond the point of pain.*

Implementation Steps

1. Follow the Initial Implementation Steps located on the inside back cover.
2. Exercise the neck:
   - Place your hands on either side of the patient's head, gently move the chin to the chest, and then return it to a neutral position ***to flex the neck muscles.***
   - Lift the patient's head so that the chin is pointed toward the ceiling and return it to a neutral position ***to extend the neck muscles.***
   - Turn the patient's head to the left side, return it to a neutral position, then turn it to the right side, and return it to a neutral position ***to rotate the neck.***

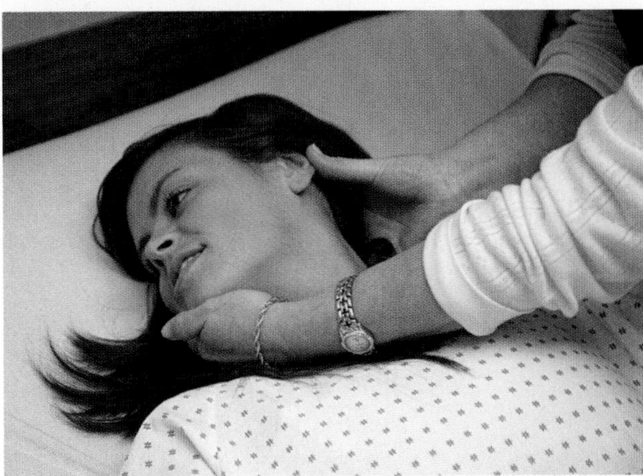

   - Tilt the patient's head to the right side, moving the ear toward the shoulder. Repeat for the left side. *Safety: Move the neck gently and carefully because bone spurs can be dislodged and cause neurological damage if neck motion is forced.*
3. Exercise the shoulder:
   - Place your hands so that one is above and the other is below the patient's elbow. Keeping the patient's arm straight, lift it up until the inner elbow is even with the patient's ear and return it to the patient's side. ***This will extend the shoulder.***

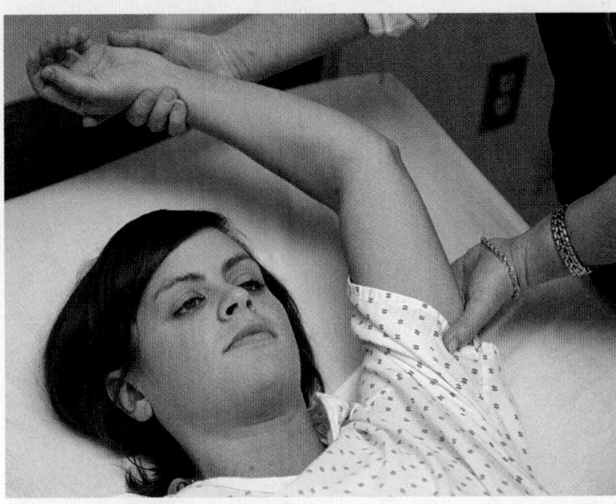

   - Move the patient's arm away from his or her body to a 90-degree angle ***to abduct the shoulder.***

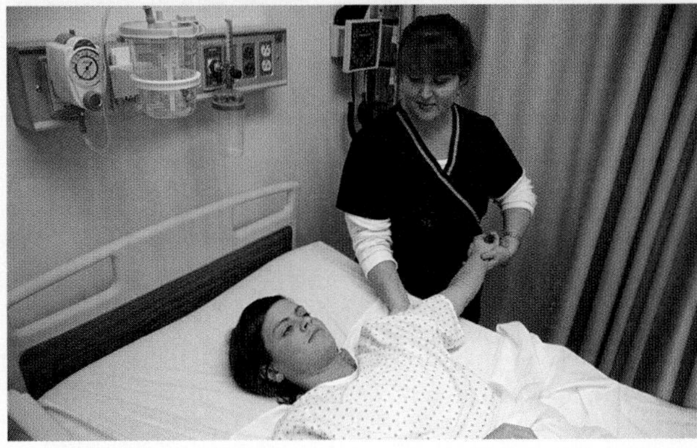

   - Return the patient's arm to the side of his or her body ***to adduct the shoulder.***
   - With the elbow slightly bent, move the patient's hand to his or her opposite shoulder ***to internally rotate the shoulder.***
   - Return the patient's arm to the side of his or her body with elbow flexed ***to externally rotate the shoulder.***
4. Exercise the elbow:
   - With your hands still in place, bend the patient's elbow, moving the patient's hand toward his or her shoulder to flex the elbow.
   - Return the patient's hand to the side of his or her body to extend the elbow.
   - Turn the patient's lower arm so that the palm is upward ***to supinate the arm.***

(skill continues on page 296)

Skill 16.1 (continued)

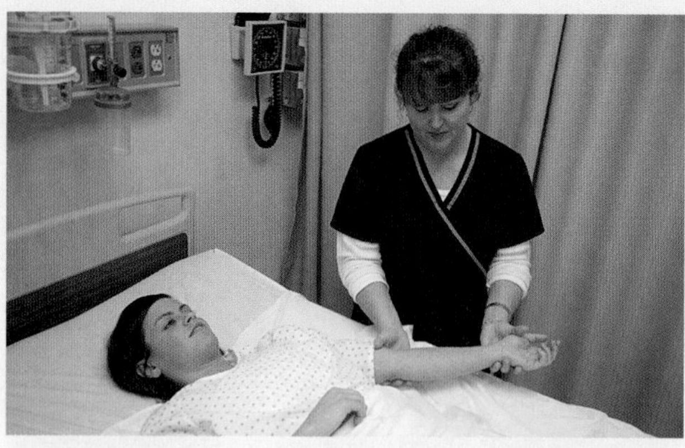

- Turn the patient's forearm so that the palm is downward ***to pronate the arm.***

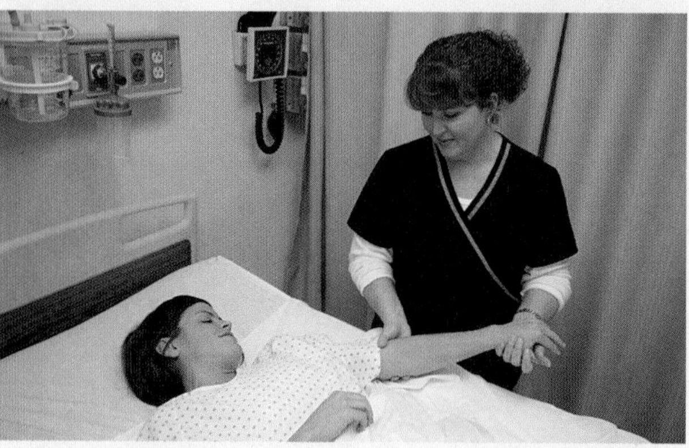

5. Exercise the wrist:
   - Place one of your hands above and the other below the patient's wrist. Bend the patient's wrist so that the palm is at a 90-degree angle to the forearm to flex the wrist. Return the wrist to the neutral position.
   - Then gently bend the wrist so that the palm is facing upward to hyperextend the wrist. Return to the neutral position.

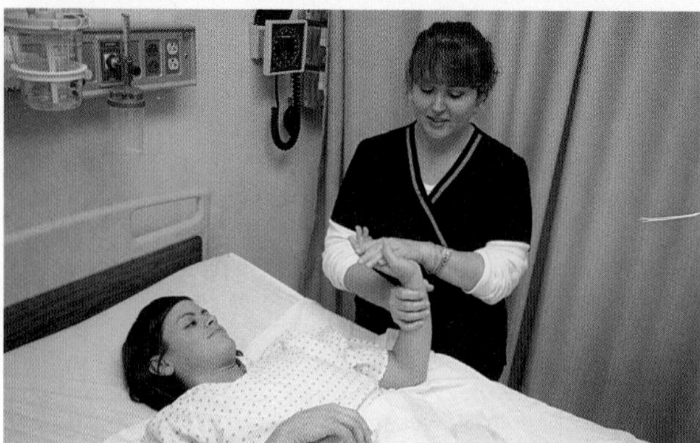

- Tilt the wrist to the thumb side ***to perform radial deviation*** and return it to the neutral position.
- Tilt the wrist to the little finger side ***to perform ulnar deviation*** and return it to the neutral position.

6. Exercise the fingers and thumb:
   - Grasp the patient's fingers and separate each from the adjacent ones ***to abduct the fingers.***
   - Bring each finger close to the adjacent ones ***to adduct the fingers.***
   - Place your hand over the patient's hand and close it into a fist ***to flex the fingers.***
   - Straighten the patient's fingers to extend the fingers.
   - Touch each fingertip to the thumb tip ***to perform opposition of the thumb.***
   - Move each finger and the thumb in a circular motion ***to circumduct the fingers and thumb.***
7. Exercise the hip and knee:
   - Place one hand under the patient's calf just below the knee and the other under the heel of the patient's foot. Slowly bend the hip and knee, keeping the lower leg parallel to the bed, ***to flex the hip and knee.*** Return to the resting position.

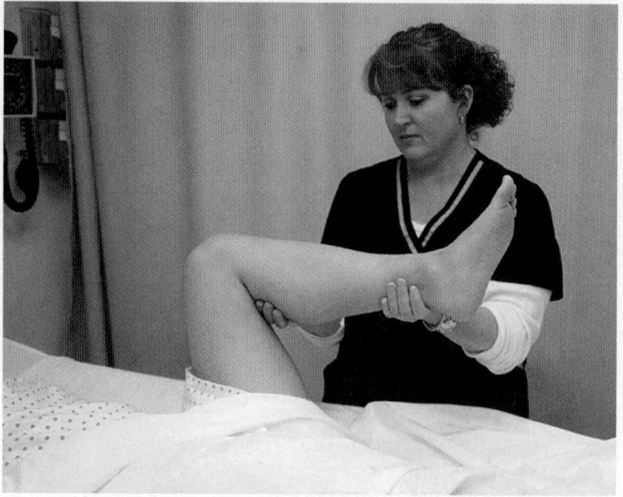

- Keeping the patient's upper leg, knee, and lower leg straight, place one hand beneath the knee joint and the other hand under the lower leg and move the leg from the midline of the body outward to the side as far as is comfortable to abduct the hip. *Safety: If the upper leg and lower leg are not kept straight, slight rotation will occur at the knee joint and may injure the anterior cruciate ligament (ACL).*
- Move the leg back to the midline and cross it over the other leg ***to adduct the hip.*** *Safety: Do not bring the leg beyond the midline of the body if the patient has had a total hip replacement because this could cause dislocation of the artificial hip.*

Skill 16.1 (continued)

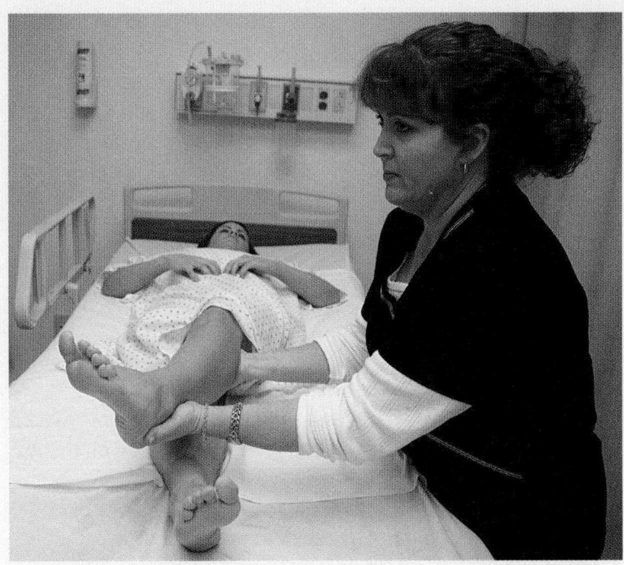

- Maintain your hand positions and roll the leg inward until the great toe touches the bed ***to internally rotate the hip.*** *Safety: If the upper leg and lower leg are not rolled as a single unit, you may injure the ACL.*
- Maintain your hand positions and roll the leg outward until the little toe touches the bed ***to externally rotate the hip.*** *Safety: If the upper leg and lower leg are not rolled as a single unit, you may injure the ACL.*

8. Exercise the ankle and foot:
   - Place one of your hands above the patient's ankle and one on the sole of the patient's foot. Gently push the foot back so that the toes are pointing toward the patient's head ***to dorsiflex the foot.***
   - Gently pull the patient's foot forward so the toes are pointing toward the foot of the bed ***to plantar flex the foot.***
   - Turn the sole of the foot inward toward the midline ***to invert the foot.***

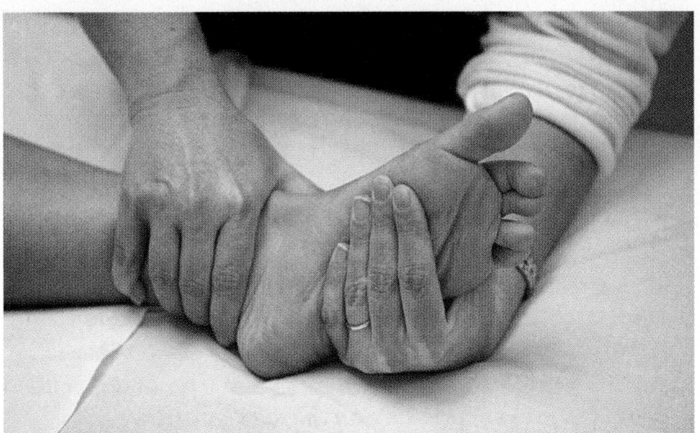

   - Turn the sole of the foot outward toward the outside of the body ***to evert the foot.***

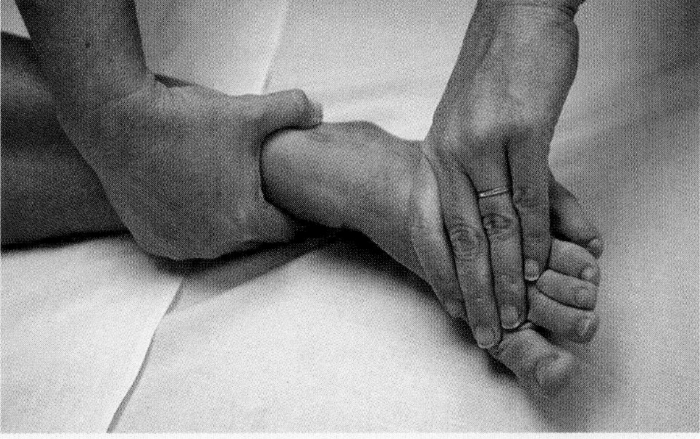

   - Gently move the foot in a circular motion ***to circumduct the ankle.***
   - Separate the toes from the adjacent ones ***to abduct the toes.***
   - Bring the toes together with the adjacent ones ***to adduct the toes.***
   - Place your hand over the patient's toes and bend them downward to flex the toes and straighten them ***to extend the toes.***
9. Follow the Ending Implementation Steps located on the inside back cover.
10. Document and report any abnormal ROM to the charge nurse or health-care provider.

Evaluation Steps

1. Determine whether any joints were resistant to full ROM movement. If so, note which joint(s) and at what degree was resistance found.
2. Evaluate how well the patient tolerated the exercise. Did he or she complain of pain or discomfort? If so, during the exercise of which joint(s)? Did the patient grimace or show any other sign of discomfort?

Sample Documentation

04/09/22 1630 Passive ROM performed to all joints. Grimaced when left shoulder extended and internally rotated. Resistance met when left shoulder extended to approx 140°. No resistance noted when left shoulder internally rotated. ——————————

—————————— Nurse's signature and credentials

Skill 16.2 Positioning Patients

Assessment Steps

1. Determine the position the patient has most recently been in and then determine the position to use next or the position most appropriate for the patient's needs.
2. Determine if any positions are contraindicated for this patient.
3. Determine the number of people needed to change the patient's position. If the patient is heavy or unable to help, obtain assistance and use an assistive device.

Planning Steps

1. Obtain slide sheets or other type of assistive device, if needed.
2. Enlist the assistance of one or more nursing personnel as needed.

Implementation Steps

1. Follow the Initial Implementation Steps located on the inside back cover.

For the Supine Position

2. Assist the patient to turn onto his or her back ***into a position for sleeping or resting.***

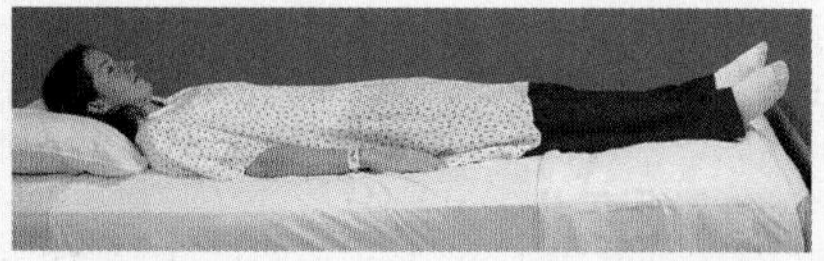

3. Place pillows beneath the patient's head, arms, and knees ***for comfort and to support the joints.*** *Safety: Slightly elevate only the forearms, not the upper arms. Elevation of the upper arms will pull the shoulders out of correct body alignment.*
4. Elevate the head of the bed slightly if it is more comfortable for the patient.
5. Follow the Ending Implementation Steps located on the inside back cover.

For the Fowler's Position

2. Assist the patient to the supine position.
3. Elevate the head of the bed:
   - 45 to 60 degrees for the Fowler's position ***for watching television or talking with visitors.***
   - 30 to 45 degrees for the low Fowler's or semi-Fowler's position ***for reading or resting.***
   - 60 to 90 degrees for the high Fowler's position ***for eating meals or to facilitate easier respirations.***

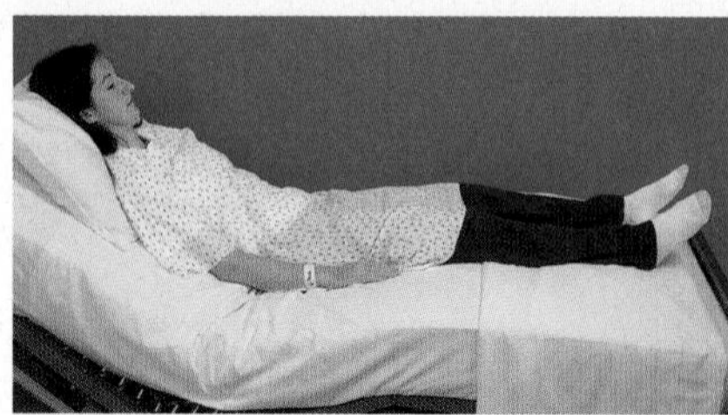

4. Place pillows behind the patient's head and under his or her knees ***for comfort and to support the joints.*** *Safety: Elevate the knees only slightly because pressure against the back of the knees may restrict circulation to the lower legs and increase risk of thrombus formation.*
5. Follow the Ending Implementation Steps located on the inside back cover.

For the Lateral Position

2. Assist the patient to turn onto his or her right or left side ***to relieve pressure on the back and on the sacral and coccygeal areas.*** *Safety: When turning patients, it is helpful to flex the patient's knees first. If the patient cannot assist with this, flex his or her knees yourself. Once you begin to turn the patient, the flexed knees will extend beyond the patient's body and help to pull the weight of the legs during the turn. This action decreases the amount of effort required to turn the patient.*
3. Flex the knee of the upper leg and rest it on a pillow placed between the patient's legs ***to prevent pressure areas from developing on the knees and ankles.***
4. Place a pillow under the patient's head and pull the lower shoulder just ***slightly*** forward ***to prevent pressure on the joint and nerves.***
5. Fold a pillow lengthwise and place it at the patient's back. Tuck the edges of the pillow beneath the patient's back. ***This keeps the patient on his or her side. If the patient leans backward, the pillow will stay tucked behind him or her.***

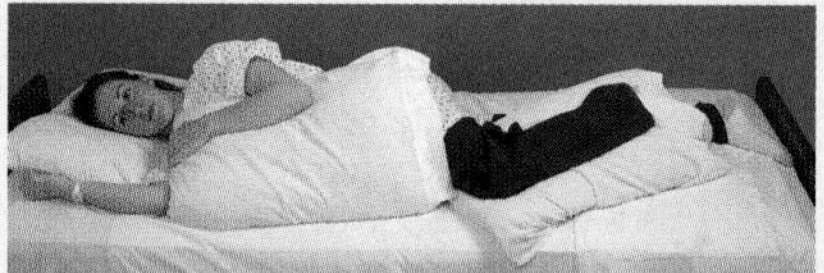

6. For the ***lateral oblique position,*** follow the steps above except place the top leg behind the body ***to prevent pressure on the trochanter.***

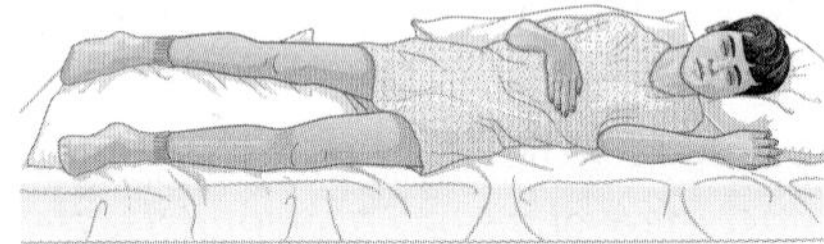

7. Follow the Ending Implementation Steps located on the inside back cover.

For the Left Sims' Position

2. Assist the patient onto his or her left side and then move the patient so that he or she is lying partially on his or her stomach. Turn the patient's head to the right ***for comfort.***
3. Flex the right arm at a 90-degree angle at the elbow and support it with a pillow ***for comfort and to support the joint.***
4. Flex the right leg and place the thigh on a pillow, keeping the left leg resting on the bed with the knee slightly flexed. ***This allows access to the rectal area and the sigmoid colon for rectal examinations and administration of enemas.***
5. Pull the left shoulder slightly back so that it is not under the patient ***to prevent pressure on the joint and nerves.*** The left arm will rest along the patient's back ***for comfort.***

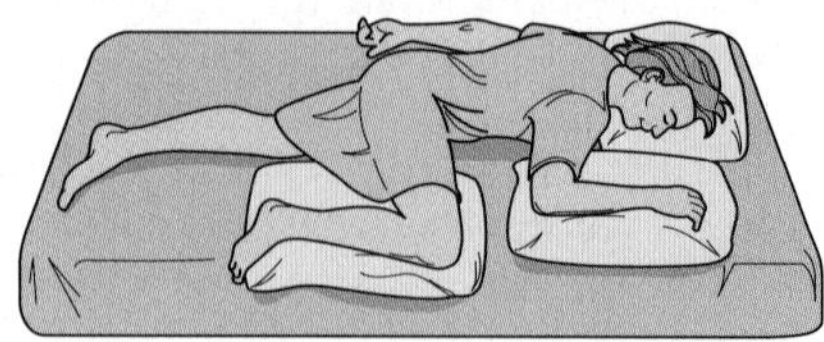

Skill 16.2 (continued)

6. Follow the Ending Implementation Steps located on the inside back cover.

For the Prone Position

2. Assist the patient to the lateral position and then onto the abdomen, with his or her head turned to the side ***for comfort.***
3. Move the arms to a 90-degree angle at the elbow and support them on pillows ***for comfort and to support the joints.***
4. Place a small pillow or folded towel beneath the patient's abdomen ***to relieve pressure in the low back.***

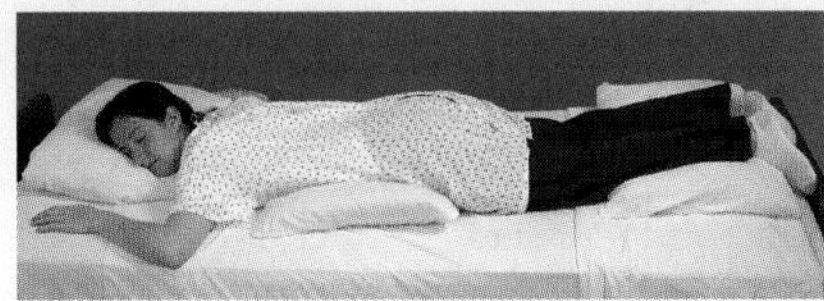

5. Follow the Ending Implementation Steps located on the inside back cover.

Evaluation Steps

1. Determine if the patient is in good body alignment after being positioned. Make any changes needed to support the body and joints in good alignment.
2. Evaluate the patient's level of comfort. If the patient is not comfortable, make adjustments to promote comfort, such as moving pillows or joints.
3. Evaluate how well the patient tolerated the position change and note any complaints of pain or discomfort. Take steps to relieve pain if it persists after the position change.

Sample Documentation

04/11/22 1830 Assisted to rt lateral position and supported with pillows. C/O discomfort in left arm and shoulder, relieved by pillow placement. ———————
——————— Nurse's signature and credentials

Skill 16.3 Moving a Patient Up in Bed

Assessment Steps

1. Determine which assistive device would be most appropriate to decrease the chance of injury to your patient, your coworkers, and yourself.
2. Determine how much the patient can assist you.

Planning Steps

1. Obtain the appropriate assistive device, such as a slide sheet.
2. Enlist assistance from a coworker if needed.

Implementation Steps

1. Follow the Initial Implementation Steps located on the inside back cover.
2. Lower the head of the bed to as flat as the patient can tolerate. ***It is easier to move the patient on a horizontal plane than to move him or her uphill.***
3. Remove the pillow from under the patient's head and position it vertically next to the headboard ***to protect the patient's head when moving him or her up in bed.***

Moving the Patient with a Draw Sheet Only

4. Stand on one side of the bed with a coworker on the opposite side. Both you and your coworker should follow these steps:
   - Roll the draw sheet up until it is close to the patient's body to more easily lift and move the patient.
   - Grasp the draw sheet near the patient's shoulders and hips to help you move the patient's center of gravity.
   - Instruct the patient to flex his or her neck, bend the knees, and place his or her feet flat on the bed. Ask the patient to grasp the trapeze bar over the bed if one is available. Tell the patient to push against the bed with his or her feet on the count of 3. ***In this way, the patient can assist with moving his or her body, reducing strain on you and your coworker.***
   - Stand with your front foot pointed toward the head of the bed and your back foot pointed toward the side of the bed ***to use the correct body mechanics and reduce the possibility of injury.***
   - On the count of three, shift your weight from your back foot to your front foot while lifting the patient with the draw sheet and moving him or her up in bed. ***This uses the muscles in your legs, not your back, to move the patient.***
5. Follow the Ending Implementation Steps located on the inside back cover.

Moving the Patient with a Slide Sheet

4. Turn the patient to one side and place a slide sheet or large plastic bag beneath the draw sheet, positioned so that it reaches from the patient's shoulders to below the hips. ***This helps you move the patient's center of gravity.***
5. Turn the patient to the opposite side and smooth the slide sheet evenly beneath the draw sheet.
6. Stand on one side of the bed with a coworker on the opposite side. Both you and your coworker should follow these steps:
   - Roll the draw sheet up until it is close to the patient's body to more easily lift and move the patient.
   - Grasp the draw sheet near the patient's shoulders and hips.
   - Instruct the patient to flex his or her neck, bend the knees, and place his or her feet flat on the bed. Tell the patient to push against the bed with his or her feet on the count of three. In this way, the patient can assist with moving his or her body, reducing strain on you and your coworker.
   - Stand with your front foot pointed toward the head of the bed and your back foot pointed toward the side of the bed to use the correct body mechanics and reduce the possibility of injury.
   - On the count of three, shift your weight from your back foot to your front foot while lifting the patient with the draw sheet and moving him or her up in bed. This uses the muscles in your legs, not your back, to move the patient.
7. Turn the patient from side to side to remove the slide sheet. Remember to flex the patient's knees prior to turning him or her.

(skill continues on page 300)

Skill 16.3 (continued)

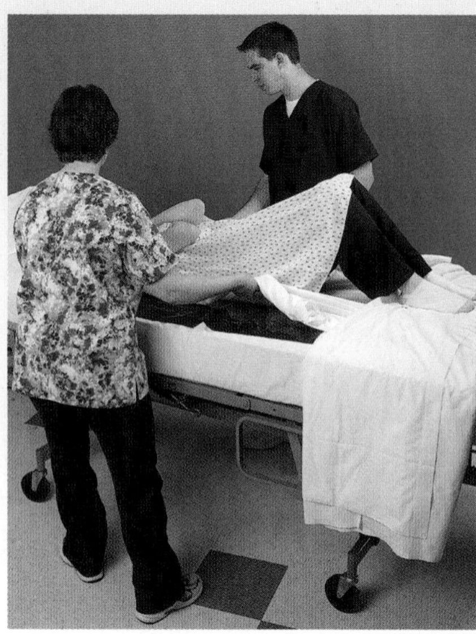

8. Follow the Ending Implementation Steps located on the inside back cover.

Evaluation Steps

1. Determine if the patient is positioned in good body alignment after moving him or her up in the bed.

Documentation

Moving a patient up in bed is often not documented except on a flow sheet. If abnormal findings are present, they are documented in the nurse's notes.

Skill 16.4 Turning a Patient in Bed

Assessment Steps

1. Determine the amount of assistance needed. *Safety: When logrolling a patient, you will need three staff members—one at the patient's head and yourself plus another coworker at the patient's body.*
2. Determine onto which side you will turn the patient, based on previous positions.

Planning Steps

1. Obtain a slide sheet, large plastic bag, or plastic film to use as a friction-reducing device.
2. Enlist the assistance of another person if needed.

Implementation Steps

1. Follow the Initial Implementation Steps located on the inside back cover.
2. Place the patient in the supine position with the head of the bed lowered to ***allow you to work with gravity when turning the patient.***

Turning with a Draw Sheet

3. Turn the patient to one side and place a slide sheet or large plastic bag beneath the draw sheet, positioned so it reaches from the patient's shoulders to below the hips. ***This helps you move the patient's center of gravity.***
4. Turn the patient to the opposite side and smooth the slide sheet evenly beneath the draw sheet.
5. Move the patient to the right side of the bed if you are turning him or her onto his or her left side. ***This gives room for the patient to be turned and remain in the center of the bed, not up against the side rail.*** Reverse this step if you are turning the patient to his or her right side. *Safety: Remove the plastic bag or plastic film from beneath the patient at this point to prevent it from holding moisture against the patient's skin.*
6. Flex the patient's knees to help pull the body weight into the turn. Or you may move the patient's right leg over his or her left leg if you are turning the patient to the left ***to help keep the patient's weight in the center.*** Reverse this if you are turning the patient to his or her right side.
7. Move his or her right arm across the chest to keep the weight of the patient in the center. Again, reverse if turning in the opposite direction.
8. Position his or her left shoulder so that it is abducted and externally rotated ***to prevent it from becoming trapped under the patient during the turn.***
9. Stand with your feet shoulder-width apart ***to provide a wide base of support.*** Place one foot more forward than the other so you can shift your weight as you move the patient.
10. Grasp the draw sheet with one hand near the patient's shoulders and just below his or her hips ***to allow you to move the patient's center of gravity.*** Use the draw sheet to turn the patient.

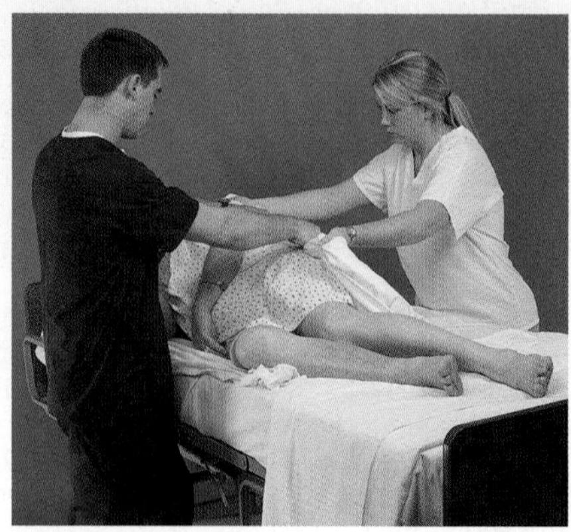

Skill 16.4 (continued)

11. On the count of three, bend your knees and hips and shift your weight from the back foot to the front foot. Your coworker on the opposite side of the bed will shift his or her weight from the front foot to the back foot as the patient comes toward him or her. ***This allows both you and your coworker to use good body mechanics while smoothly moving the patient.***
12. Reposition the patient's left shoulder slightly forward ***to prevent pressure on the joint and nerves.*** Reverse this if the patient is being positioned on the right side.
13. Position with pillows as described for positioning the patient in the lateral position in Skill 16.2.
14. Follow the Ending Implementation Steps located on the inside back cover.

Logroll the Patient

3. A slide sheet should already be in place beneath the patient ***to facilitate turning the body as a single unit.***
4. Have one coworker stand near the patient's head ***to be responsible for keeping the head and shoulders in alignment with the rest of the body.***
5. Stand even with the patient's waist and have your remaining coworker stand at the patient's thighs ***to ensure that the patient's body remains aligned during the turn.*** Lower the side rail closest to you.
6. Instruct the patient to cross his or her arms across the chest ***to keep them protected during the turn.***
7. All three coworkers should grasp the slide sheet closely to the patient's body. On the count of three, move the patient toward you and your coworker as one unit. *Safety: Do not allow different parts of the spine to move at different times because this can cause damage to a spine that has been injured or surgically repaired. This allows the patient to be in the center of the bed once turned.*
8. Raise the side rail. You and your coworker now move to the opposite side of the bed. Lower the side rail nearest you. Place a pillow between the patient's legs and, if allowed, replace the pillow under his or her head without moving the head out of alignment with the spine.
9. You and your coworker face the patient, standing with your feet shoulder-width apart, one foot slightly ahead of the other. While placing your weight on your forward foot, bend at the hips, flex your knees, and grasp the draw sheet on the opposite side of the patient.
10. The coworker who is controlling the patient's head and shoulders counts to three. On the count of three, each staff member moves the patient using the draw sheet in one fluid motion ***to prevent twisting or torque on the patient's spine.*** The patient's head and hips should be kept in a straight line at all times ***to prevent damage to the spinal cord.***

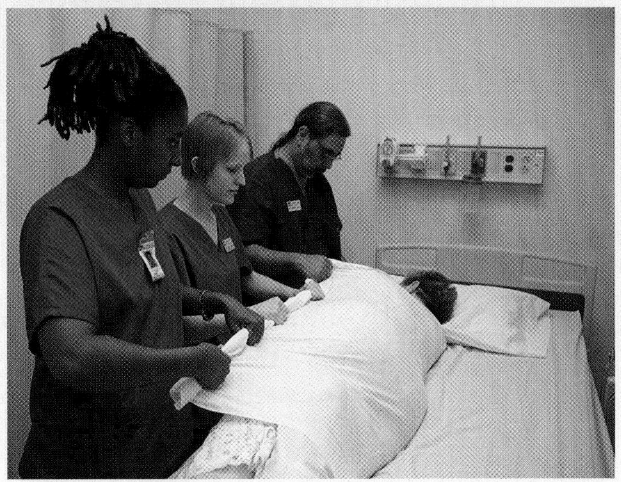

11. Prop the patient on his or her side using a pillow or rolled blanket. Keep the head and hips in a straight line. It usually is necessary to place a pillow between the patient's knees and ankles to prevent the top leg from pulling forward, causing the hip to be out of alignment.
12. Follow the Ending Implementation Steps located on the inside back cover.

Evaluation Steps

1. Determine if the patient remained in a straight line during the turn.
2. Evaluate the effectiveness of the three staff members working together.
3. Evaluate the position and comfort of the patient.

Sample Documentation

05/12/22 1915 Logrolled to left side without c/o discomfort or pain. Body alignment maintained. ———— ———————— Nurse's signature and credentials

(skill continues on page 302)

Skill 16.4 (continued)

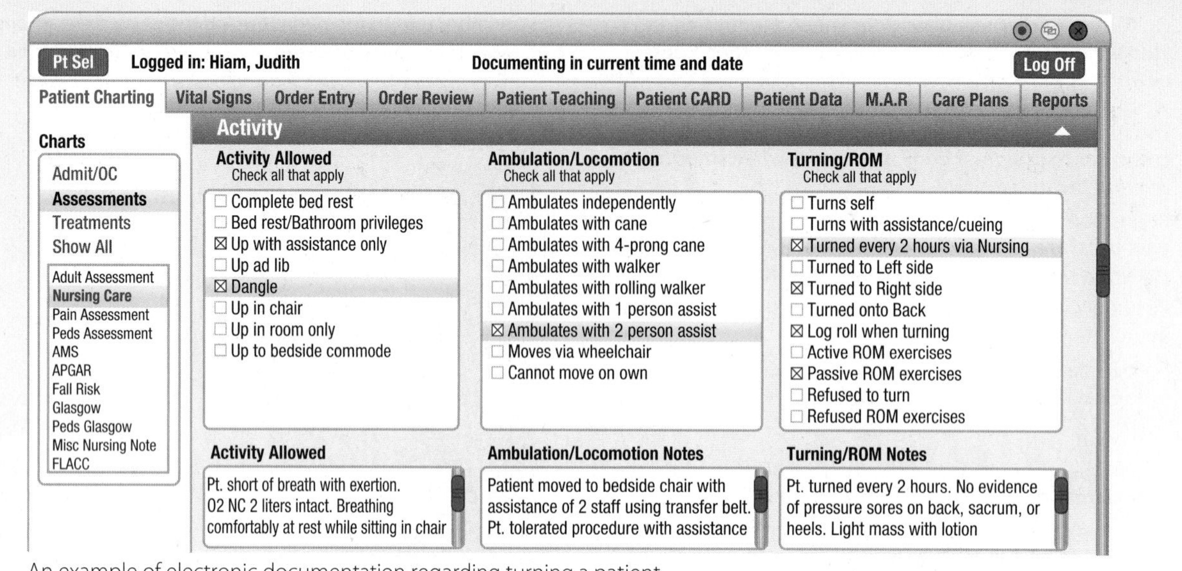

An example of electronic documentation regarding turning a patient.

Skill 16.5 Transferring a Patient from a Bed to a Stretcher, Chair, or Wheelchair

Assessment Steps

1. Assess the patient's ability to help with the transfer.
2. Determine the need for an assistive device, such as a slide sheet.
3. Determine the need for coworker assistance.
4. Assess the patient for complaints of pain, discomfort, or nausea. Administer ordered medications as appropriate.
5. Assess the patient for weakness on one side of the body.

Planning Steps

1. Obtain needed equipment: a transfer belt and a friction-reducing device (i.e., a slide sheet or slide board), as well as a gown or robe and nonskid slippers if you are transferring the patient to a chair or wheelchair.
2. Enlist the assistance of coworkers as needed.
3. Determine the number and types of tubes and equipment attached to the patient. Plan to protect them during the transfer ***to prevent tangling or pulling loose of tubes or equipment.***
4. If the patient has a weak side, position the chair or wheelchair on the patient's strong side. ***This allows the patient to bear weight on his or her strong side during the transfer, reducing the chance for loss of balance and falls.***
5. Prepare the equipment as needed for transfer via stretcher or wheelchair. For example, unplug the IV pump or obtain a rolling IV pole, obtain an E-cylinder of oxygen if the patient is on continuous oxygen, and disconnect suction.

Implementation Steps

1. Follow the Initial Implementation Steps located on the inside back cover.

Transferring to a Stretcher

2. Lock the wheels on the bed and lower the head of the bed.
3. Turn the patient from side to side to place the slide board, slide sheet, or large plastic bag beneath the draw sheet.
4. Move the patient close to the side of the bed where the stretcher will be placed, keeping a sheet or blanket over the patient ***to preserve modesty and provide warmth.***
5. Lower the side rail and position the stretcher firmly against the bed. Raise or lower the bed so that it is the same height as the stretcher. *Safety: Lock the wheels on the stretcher to prevent possible injury to the patient and the nursing staff.*
6. *Safety: If the patient has a Foley catheter, avoid raising the catheter drainage bag above the level of the patient's bladder, which can result in backflow of urine into the bladder, increasing the risk of urinary tract infection.*
7. Stand on the far side of the stretcher with a coworker. Lean against the stretcher as an added measure to ensure that the stretcher does not move away from the bed during transfer.
8. Pull the patient onto the stretcher using the slide sheet or slide board.
   - If using a slide sheet, lay the straps of the sheet across the stretcher. Both you and your coworker will grasp the straps of the slide sheet and, on the count of three, pull steadily. ***This will move the patient across to the stretcher with minimal effort since friction is reduced.*** You can leave the slide sheet in place until the patient returns to the bed and then remove the slide sheet by turning the patient from side to side.

Skill 16.5 (continued)

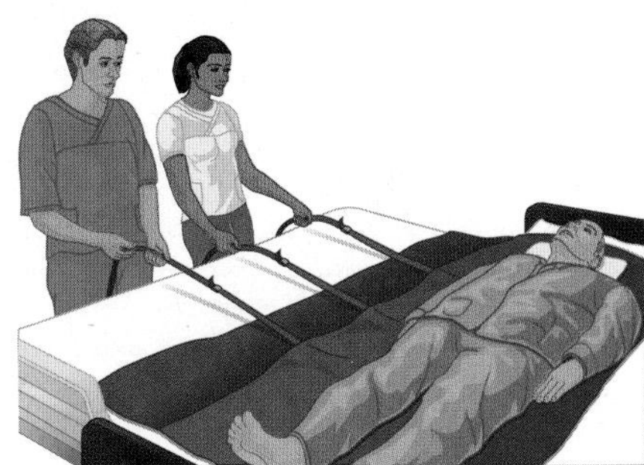

- If using a slide board, have the patient flex his or her neck to keep the head up. Pull on the draw sheet, moving the patient across the slide board and onto the stretcher. Remove the slide board. *Safety: To secure the patient on the stretcher, reach across the patient and grasp the draw or slide sheet. Pull it snugly across the patient's trunk and pelvis, similar to a cocoon. Secure the stretcher's lap belt across the patient's pelvis and raise both stretcher rails, ensuring that the patient is covered.*

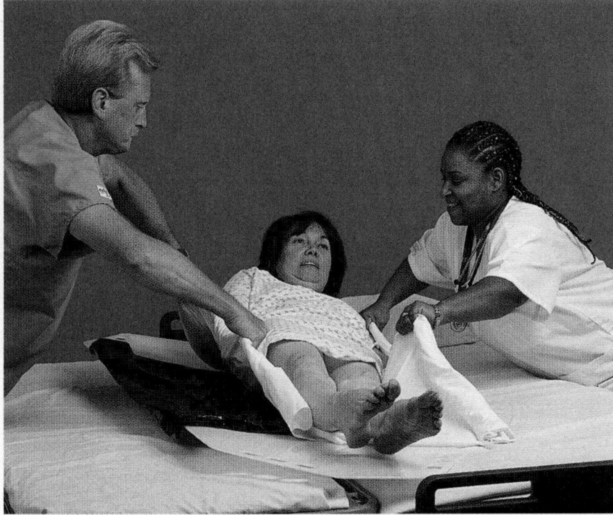

9. Follow the Ending Implementation Steps located on the inside back cover.

Transferring to a Chair or Wheelchair

2. Assist the patient into a robe or a second gown with the opening to the front ***to cover the patient's exposed back and protect modesty.*** Apply nonskid slippers to the patient's feet to reduce risk of falling.
3. Apply a transfer belt to the patient ***to provide a way to hold onto the patient during the transfer.***
4. Raise the head of the bed to a sitting position ***to prevent the patient from having to move himself or herself to the sitting position.*** Place one hand on either side of the patient and grasp the transfer belt. *Safety: Lock the wheels on the bed and lower it to the lowest position to prevent injury to the patient.*
5. Explain exactly how you are going to get the patient up, instructing him or her how to assist in the process. ***This helps to reduce anxiety and increase cooperation during the transfer.***
6. Stand facing the bed with one foot forward of the other. Maintain a wide base of support. Flex your knees and hips. ***This gives you a wide base of support and maintains good body mechanics for the transfer.***
7. On the count of three, move the patient to a sitting position on the side of the bed with his or her feet resting on the floor. Ensure that the patient is not dizzy or nauseated and is ready to proceed. Assist the patient to put on nonskid footwear and a robe.
8. Stand facing the patient with your feet against his or her feet and your knees against his or her knees ***to keep the patient's feet from slipping or the knees from buckling.***

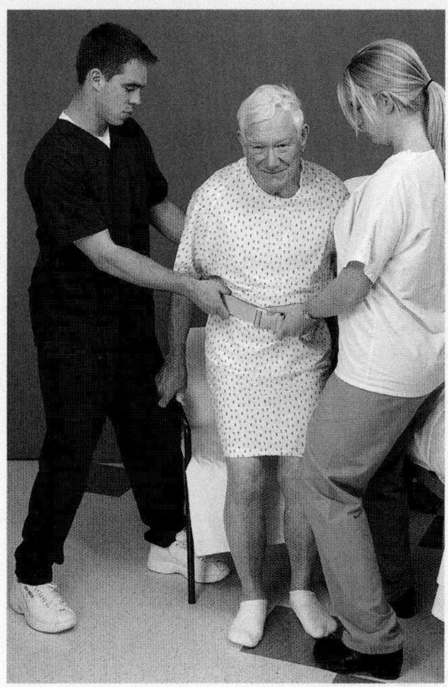

9. Flex your hips and knees as you grasp the transfer belt on either side of the patient's waist. ***This gives you the ability to hold the patient near his or her center of gravity.***
   Note: If two people are assisting, each one grasps the transfer belt at the patient's waist and places one foot and knee against the patient's foot and knee.
10. Instruct the patient to hold onto your shoulders, not your neck, ***to prevent injury to your neck or upper back.*** Straighten your knees and hips and bring the patient to a standing position.
11. Wait briefly for the patient to adjust to a standing position. Turn the patient to align with the wheelchair or chair. *Safety: Ensure that your feet and the wheelchair footrests are out of the way to prevent the patient from tripping.*
12. Have the patient step back until he or she feels the chair or wheelchair against the back of the knees and then grasp the chair arms and gently lower him or her into the chair. Keep your back straight, flexing your hips and knees as the patient sits in the chair ***to use your leg muscles, not your back muscles, and prevent possible injury.*** Ensure that the patient's hips are positioned against the back of the chair ***so that proper body alignment is maintained.***

(skill continues on page 304)

Skill 16.5 (continued)

13. Place the patient's feet on the footrests and cover the patient's lap with a sheet or blanket ***to protect modesty and provide warmth.***
14. Follow the Ending Implementation Steps located on the inside back cover.

Evaluation Steps

1. Determine if the transfer occurred safely and smoothly. If not, what problems occurred and how could they be prevented?
2. Determine how well the patient tolerated the activity. Did he or she become frightened, anxious, or dizzy?

Sample Documentation

11/04/22 2040 Transferred to chair with assist of one. Pivoted on R leg and maintained balance well. Resting comfortably in chair, call light within reach. ——— Nurse's signature and credentials

Skill 16.6 Transferring a Patient With a Mechanical Lift

Assessment Steps

1. Determine where the patient is to be moved.
2. Determine the need to move furniture and equipment to have a clear pathway for the lift.
3. Assess the patient for concerns regarding use of the lift and movement out of bed.

Planning Steps

1. Obtain the lift and sling.
2. Enlist the assistance of at least one coworker. *Safety: Always have at least two members of the nursing staff operating the lift and moving the patient.*

Implementation Steps

1. Follow the Initial Implementation Steps located on the inside back cover.
2. Roll the patient side to side and place the sling beneath the patient so that it starts at the shoulders and ends at the knees. *Safety: Position the sling carefully so that the patient is completely supported when he or she is being lifted and moved.*
3. Fasten the sling around the patient's legs according to the manufacturer's instructions.
4. Position the lift at the side of the bed with the wheels in the widest position ***to increase the base of support.***
5. Attach the sling to the lift. ***Note: The shorter chains attach to the top openings of the sling and the longer chains to the lower grommets. This pulls the patient up to a sitting position when the lift is activated.***
6. Activate the lift to slowly raise the patient. This may involve pushing a button or pumping a lever.

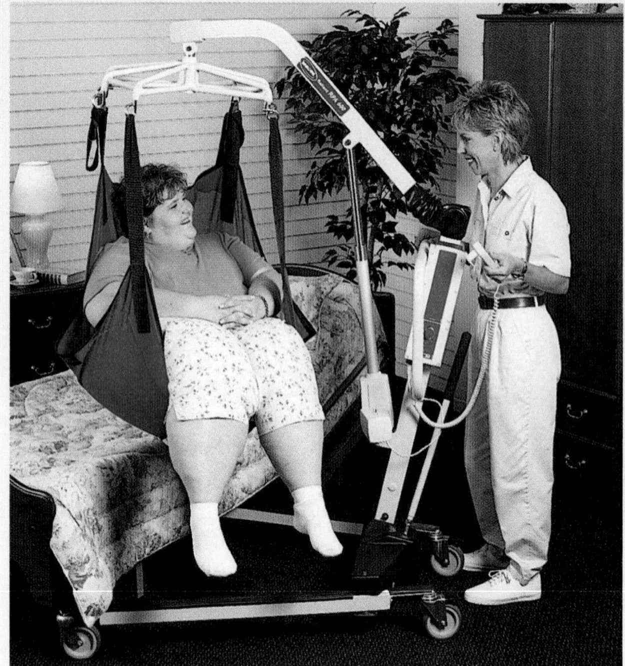

7. Slowly pull the lift away from the bed once the patient is above the level of the bed. *Safety: Two members of the nursing staff are required; one person holds onto the patient in the sling and guides him or her, and the other person pushes the lift.* The person guiding the patient in the sling explains to the patient each movement that is about to occur to prevent increasing fear and anxiety. He or she also makes frequent eye contact with the patient, observing for signs of fear, and offers reassurance.

Skill 16.6 (continued)

8. Push the lift to the desired location and align it so that the patient is over the chair.
9. Release the valve that slowly lowers the lift while your coworker guides the patient into the chair. Ensure that the patient's hips are positioned against the back of the chair ***to ensure proper body alignment.***
10. Detach the sling from the lift and store the lift in the designated area ***to prevent blocking high-traffic areas.***
11. Leave the sling in place beneath the patient until he or she is returned to the bed. Then turn the patient side to side and remove the sling.
12. Follow the Ending Implementation Steps located on the inside back cover.

Evaluation Steps

1. Determine the effectiveness of the transfer. Was the patient safely positioned in the sling? Were you able to move the patient with a minimum of swaying? Was the patient aligned well with the chair or bed before he or she was lowered into it?

Sample Documentation

10/14/22 1135 Transferred via lift from bed to wheelchair. C/O anxiety as lift was raised. Reassured by UAP and guided throughout transfer. Resting comfortably in wheelchair. Call light within reach. —————— Nurse's signature and credentials

Skill 16.7 Assisting a Patient to Dangle

Assessment Steps

1. Check the health-care provider's order for the patient's activity level.
2. Assess the patient for complaints of pain rated a 5 or above on a 10-point scale prior to dangling. If this is the case, medicate the patient according to the health-care provider's orders and wait until the pain decreases to assist the patient to dangle.
3. Assess the patient's pulse and blood pressure while he or she is in the supine position.

Planning Steps

1. Enlist the assistance of a coworker if help is needed.

Implementation Steps

1. Follow the Initial Implementation Steps located on the inside back cover.
2. Elevate the head of the bed until the patient is in a sitting position. ***This prevents the patient from having to move from a lying to sitting position prior to dangling.*** Apply a transfer belt ***to give you something to hold onto as you assist the patient to dangle.***
3. Place one hand on either side of the patient and grasp the transfer belt.
4. On the count of three, move the patient to a sitting position on the side of the bed. Ensure that the patient is not dizzy or nauseated and is ready to proceed.
5. Lower the bed so that the patient's feet rest on the floor. ***Allowing the feet to rest on the floor prevents pooling of blood in suspended lower extremities, which will occur if the feet are not supported.***

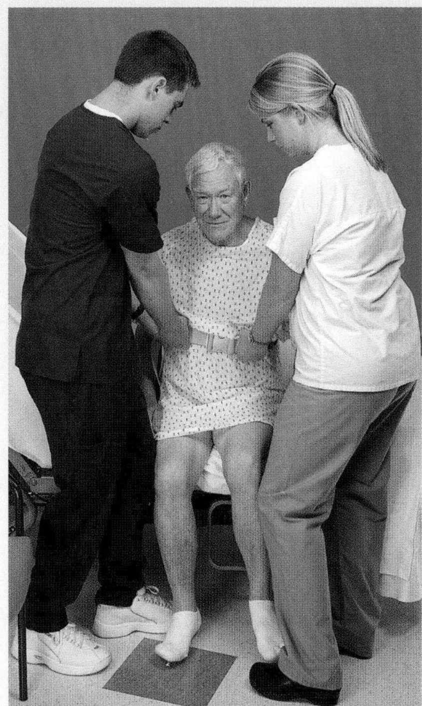

6. Assess the patient's pulse and blood pressure for an increase or decrease of more than 20 bpm or 30 mm Hg. Assess the patient for complaints of dizziness, nausea, or pain. *Safety: If the patient's vital signs are outside these parameters or if he or she complains of these symptoms, immediately assist the patient to Fowler's or low Fowler's position to prevent possible syncope and injury. If the dizziness continues, lower the head of the bed until the dizziness passes. Then return the patient to the Fowler's position and repeat steps 4 to 6.*

(skill continues on page 306)

Skill 16.7 (continued)

7. Remain with the patient while he or she dangles for 1 to 3 minutes and assist the patient to put on his or her robe and nonskid footwear. If the patient tolerates this process, it is safe to proceed with transferring the patient to a chair or wheelchair (see Skill 16.5) or to assist the patient with initial ambulation if there is a health-care provider's order to do so (see Skill 16.8).
8. When the dangling process is complete, return the patient to bed and assist him or her to a supine position.
9. Assess pulse and blood pressure again, comparing them to your findings when the patient was supine and sitting.
10. Follow the Ending Implementation Steps located on the inside back cover.

Evaluation Steps

1. Evaluate the patient's response to dangling. Did the pulse and blood pressure remain stable with position change? Did the patient complain of pain, dizziness, or nausea?

Sample Documentation

11/04/22 0935 Assisted to dangle on side of bed. P - 66, BP - 112/76 in supine position. P - 74, BP - 120/80 when dangling. Denies c/o nausea, pain, or dizziness. Remained on side of bed for 6 min, then assisted to supine position in bed. P - 76 and BP - 122/78 after return to bed. ——————
—————————— Nurse's signature and credentials

Skill 16.8 Assisting With Ambulation

Assessment Steps

1. Check the health-care provider's orders for activity level.
2. Assess the patient for complaints of pain, discomfort, nausea, or dizziness. Take appropriate action if complaints exist, and delay ambulation if needed.
3. Determine the need for coworker assistance during ambulation.

Planning Steps

1. Obtain a transfer belt according to facility policy.
2. Obtain the patient's robe and nonskid footwear.
3. Prepare the equipment as needed for ambulation. For example, unplug the IV pump or obtain a rolling IV pole, obtain an E-cylinder of oxygen if the patient is on continuous oxygen, and disconnect suction.

Implementation Steps

1. Follow the Initial Implementation Steps located on the inside back cover.
2. Assist the patient to dangle (see Skill 16.7). ***If the patient is able to tolerate dangling, you can then proceed with ambulation. If not, follow the procedure in Skill 16.7.***
3. Assist the patient to put on his or her robe and nonskid footwear ***to prevent possible slips and falls.***
4. Fasten a transfer belt around the patient's waist. *Safety: The belt should be snug without being too tight. You should be able to insert three fingers between the belt and the patient to prevent injury to the patient.*
5. Assist the patient to a standing position. Stand slightly behind and next to the patient, holding the transfer belt on the patient's far side and near side. *Safety: This gives you control of the patient if he or she should start to fall.*

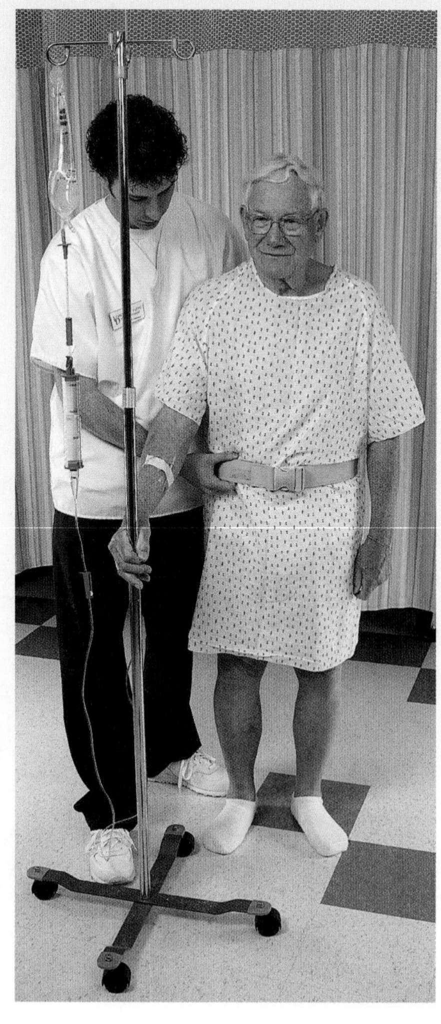

Skill 16.8 (continued)

6. Walk with the patient, ensuring that tubes and equipment are out of the way of the patient's feet and legs to prevent tripping. A second person may be needed to assist with the IV or a catheter drainage bag.
7. Observe the patient during ambulation for shortness of breath, fatigue, complaints of dizziness, or increasing pain. ***These symptoms indicate intolerance of ambulation.***
8. Return the patient to the bed or chair after he or she has ambulated the prescribed distance or if the patient becomes symptomatic.

Breaking a Fall

9. If the patient begins to fall or faint, pull him or her toward you. Lower yourself and the patient to the floor. *Safety: Do not attempt to keep the patient upright. Do not bend your back; rather, bend your forward leg and allow the patient to slide down the inner aspect of your leg to the floor. Avoid letting the patient's weight slide down the front of your lower leg because this can hyperextend your knee joint and cause injury.*
10. Call for assistance. *Safety: Do not attempt to get the patient back up by yourself.*

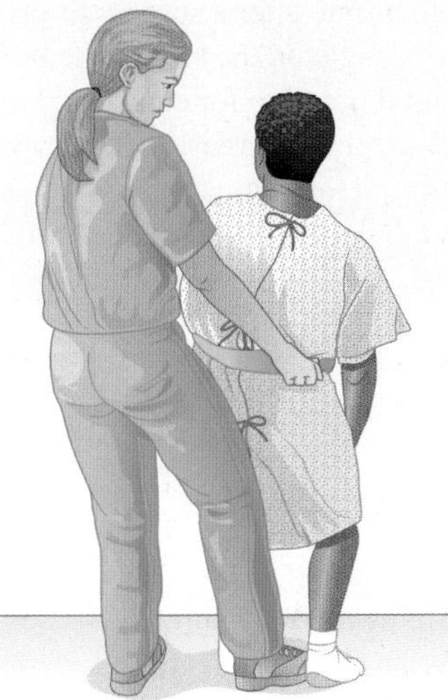

11. Obtain a set of vital signs ***to determine if the patient has a lowered blood pressure or pulse rate.***
12. Assist the patient back to bed using a lift or other equipment ***to prevent injury to yourself and the patient.***
13. Follow the Ending Implementation Steps located on the inside back cover.

Evaluation Steps

1. Determine the effectiveness of your preparation. Did you use a transfer belt with the correct fit? Did you grasp it in the correct manner?
2. Evaluate ambulation. Did the patient tolerate it without problems? Were you focused on the patient at all times? Did equipment or tubes get in the way during ambulation?
3. Evaluate your response to a fall. Did you protect the patient from actually falling? Did you lower him or her gently to the floor? Did you protect yourself from injury in the process, using good body mechanics?

Sample Documentation

11/12/22 1720 Assisted to ambulate in hallway, gait belt in use. Amb approx 14 feet. C/O of dizziness and began to sag. Lowered gently to floor by nurse without hitting floor or walls. BP - 88/60, P - 116, R - 28. ——————
—————— *Nurse's signature and credentials*

11/12/22 1735 Assisted from floor via lift and returned to bed. BP - 100/68, P - 100, R - 24 when returned to bed. Health-care provider notified. ——————
—————— *Nurse's signature and credentials*

POST CONFERENCE

Your clinical experience in the rehab unit has been educational. You share with your clinical group in post conference that you now know how to use a battery-operated lift and that you understand the use of an Envella bed to help prevent pressure injuries in patients at risk for skin breakdown. You describe how the bed works to blow air through the microbeads within it to reproduce a fluid-like surface for the patient. You share that your patient was very depressed about his paralysis and would barely interact with you. While you found this frustrating, you also understood his reactions. By the end of the second day, he was a little more responsive, but you agreed with the staff nurse that he would need counseling to deal with the changes in his life.

Key Points

- Immobility negatively affects every body system, causing complications such as blood clots, kidney stones, bone demineralization, pressure injuries, pneumonia, urinary tract infections, constipation, confusion, and depression.
- Nurses must anticipate such complications and be proactive by implementing measures to prevent them. These nursing interventions include performing passive ROM exercises, turning the patient frequently, encouraging the patient to cough and deep breathe often, applying antiembolism stockings and sequential compression devices as ordered, assisting the patient to dangle and ambulate, using therapeutic devices correctly, encouraging food and fluid intake, preventing urinary retention, and utilizing specialty beds and mattresses.
- Positioning patients correctly requires knowledge not only of the position but also of the appropriate supportive devices and their correct locations. Positioning patients to maintain function is extremely important to their recovery.
- When you position patients, it is very important that you support the limbs and areas of the body not in contact with the bed. The common positions to promote comfort for your patients are supine, dorsal recumbent, Trendelenburg, reverse Trendelenburg, and lateral.
- Nurses must use good body mechanics when moving and positioning patients to prevent injury to themselves and to the patients. They must know about available assistive devices for lifting and moving patients, including how to use them to decrease the risk of musculoskeletal injury.
- The ANA has instituted the Handle With Care campaign in response to the significant number of musculoskeletal disorders reported by nurses. The purpose of the campaign is to build an industry-wide program in health care to prevent musculoskeletal injuries.
- Assistive devices for lifting and moving patients include slide sheets, transfer or gait belts, slide boards, sit-to-stand lifts, battery-operated lifts, and overhead ceiling lifts.
- When performing manual transfers, the nurse must be ever vigilant to keep the patient and himself or herself from injury. Always set up the transfer so that the patient is moving toward his or her strong side.
- When a patient is immobile and consistent pressure is applied to the same area of the body, some beds have been developed that turn side to side so that the patient has less chance of developing respiratory and cardiovascular complications while on bedrest.
- Before a patient stands to transfer to a chair or to ambulate for the first time after a surgery or procedure, assist him or her to dangle on the side of the bed and check the pulse and blood pressure for changes.
- Always take the time to assist patients who are getting out of bed for the first time or if complications during transfer or ambulation are possible. Anticipate potential problems and be proactive in preventing them.

Review Questions

Select the answer that is most appropriate for each of the following questions. Some questions may have more than one correct answer. Select all that apply.

1. Which of the following would not be considered a consequence of immobility affecting the musculoskeletal system?
   1. Decreased muscle strength
   2. Muscle atrophy
   3. Skin breakdown
   4. Contractures
   5. Pressure injuries
   6. Increased bone weakness

2. Number the following steps for assisting a patient to dangle in the correct sequence.
   1. The patient becomes dizzy while dangling.
   2. Take the patient's vital signs and document.
   3. Raise the head of the bed.
   4. Explain to the patient what you are going to do.
   5. Assist the patient to a resting position on the bed.
   6. Assist the patient to a dangling position.

3. For the safest patient transfer, which devices are the best to use?
   1. Transfer belt
   2. Wheelchair
   3. Webbed nylon sheets
   4. Stretcher
   5. Overhead ceiling lift

4. The purpose of the Handle With Care campaign, which is supported by the ANA, is to:
   1. require all hospitals to install ceiling lifts for every patient.
   2. increase awareness of musculoskeletal injuries to nurses and establish a fund for their care.
   3. compile research about the types and frequency of injuries that occur to nurses during their working life.
   4. prevent injuries to nurses by increasing the use of assistive devices for moving and lifting patients.

5. A male patient in the supine position is:
   1. lying flat on his back with legs extended and arms to the side.
   2. resting in bed with the head of the bed elevated 45 degrees.
   3. lying on his side with legs flexed.
   4. resting in bed with the head of the bed elevated 90 degrees.

6. The ideal method for transferring a patient includes which of the following steps?
   1. Assessing the situation and the environment
   2. Ensuring that one of the transfer team members is a strong male
   3. Properly using transfer or lift devices
   4. Using the appropriate number of staff members
   5. Explaining the procedure to the patient

7. The purpose of dangling is to:
   1. check for changes in vital signs with position changes.
   2. determine the patient's response to being suspended in a lift sling.
   3. prevent possible syncope and injury.
   4. place the patient in position so that he or she will be in the center of the bed after being turned.
   5. determine the patient's ability to bear weight on both legs during a transfer.
   6. determine if it is safe for the patient to ambulate or transfer.

8. A nurse is caring for an obese 87-year-old patient with respiratory distress. The nurse understands the best position to place the patient in and selects the proper bed by which of the following positions?
   1. Semi-Fowler's position
   2. Prone position
   3. Sims' position
   4. Compella position
   5. Envella position
   6. High Fowler's position

9. The nurse understands that the best supportive devices for pressure injuries are which of the following?
   1. Trochanter roll
   2. Foot splint
   3. Pillow
   4. Arm board
   5. Hand roll

ANSWERS 1. 3, 5, 2. 4: 1; 3: 2; 6: 3; 1: 4; 5: 5, 2: 6, 3. 1, 3, 5, 4. 4, 5. 1, 6. 1, 3, 4, 5, 7. 1, 3, 6, 8. 4, 6, 9. 1, 2, 3, 4, 5

Critical Thinking Exercise

Answers available online.

1. While you are walking, the patient suddenly gasps and loses consciousness. What should you do?

Additional Resources

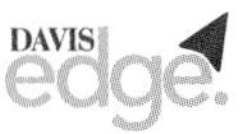

Use the scratch off code on the inside front cover of your book to access online quizzes that will help you to improve your scores on course exams and prepare for the NCLEX-PN®.

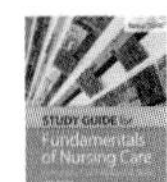

Study Guide

CHAPTER 17
Vital Signs

KEY TERMS

Afebrile (ay-FEB-ryel)
Auscultatory gap (aws-KUL-ta-TOR-ee GAP)
Biot respirations (bee-OH RES-pih-RAY-shunz)
Bradycardia (BRAY-dih-KARD-ee-ah)
Bradypnea (BRAD-ip-NEE-ah)
Cheyne-Stokes respirations (CHAYN-STOHKS RES-pih-RAY-shunz)
Diastole (dye-ASS-tuh-lee)
Diastolic pressure (dye-uh-STOL-ik PREH-shur)
Dyspnea (disp-NEE-ah)
Eupnea (yoop-NEE-ah)
Febrile (FEE-bril)
Hypertension (HYE-per-TEN-shun)
Hypertension, primary (HYE-per-TEN-shun, PRY-mare-ee)
Hypertension, secondary (HYE-per-TEN-shun, SEK-un-DARE-ee)
Hypotension (HYE-poh-TEN-shun)
Hypothermia (HYE-poh-THUR-mee-ah)
Orthopnea (or-THOP-nee-ah)
Pulse deficit (PULS DEF-ih-sit)
Pulse pressure (PULS PREH-shur)
Sphygmomanometer (SFIG-moh-ma-NOM-uh-ter)
Stridor (STRYE-dor)
Systolic pressure (siss-TOL-ik PREH-shur)
Tachycardia (TAK-ih-KAR-dee-ah)
Tachypnea (TAK-ip-NEE-ah)

CHAPTER CONCEPTS

Patient-Centered Care
Safety
Health Promotion
Assessment

LEARNING OUTCOMES

1. Define various terms associated with assessment of the six vital signs.
2. Describe the six vital signs, their significance, and their normal ranges.
3. Identify times when vital signs should be assessed.
4. Describe internal and external factors affecting body temperature.
5. Identify the advantages and disadvantages of temperature assessment routes.
6. Identify nursing care for patients with fever.
7. Describe the various peripheral pulse sites and factors affecting pulse rate.
8. Distinguish the scale for measuring peripheral pulse volume.
9. Distinguish the difference between inspiration and expiration.
10. Identify factors affecting respiratory rate and abnormal respiratory patterns.
11. Outline the four circulatory qualities and how they determine blood pressure.
12. Identify factors affecting blood pressure
13. Contrast the effects of hypertension and hypotension on the body.
14. Describe how to assess and document pain.
15. Identify nursing interventions regarding vital signs appropriate in specific scenarios.
16. Discuss information found in the Connection features in this chapter.
17. Identify safety information related to vital signs.
18. Answer questions about the skills in this chapter.

SKILLS

17.1 Assessing Body Temperature by Various Routes
17.2 Assessing the Radial and Apical Pulses
17.3 Assessing Peripheral Pulses
17.4 Using Doppler Ultrasound to Assess Nonpalpable Pulses
17.5 Assessing Respirations
17.6 Assessment of Blood Pressure
17.7 Assessment for Orthostatic Hypotension
17.8 Assessing Oxygen Saturation

CRITICAL THINKING CONNECTION

Clinical Assignment

While caring for your patient in clinical, you take his vital signs with an automatic vital sign machine at 8 a.m. and get T – 98°F, P – 64, BP – 126/74, and SpO_2 – 98% on room air. Manually, you assess the respiratory rate at 19 breaths per minute. When asked about pain, your patient says he is having abdominal incision pain at a 2 on a scale of 0 to 10. Your patient has a good morning and is sitting up in the chair reading when you take his vital signs with the same machine at noon. The readings are T – 96.6°F, P – 51, BP – 94/46, and SpO_2 – 70% on room air. When you repeat vital signs with the machine, you get similar readings. The respiratory rate is 17, and pain assessment response is a 3.

Critical Thinking Questions:

1. Why would you notify the health-care provider regarding his abnormal vital signs?
2. How you would determine the vital sign readings could be inaccurate?
3. Why would it be beneficial to take the vital signs manually rather than relying on the machine?
4. What should be your next course of action?

The human body responds physiologically to all stimuli, both internal and external. External stimuli include air, sunshine, environmental temperature, sound, electricity, and any number of stimuli found outside the body itself. Internal stimuli include hormones, enzymes, electrical conduction of impulses along nerve pathways, gases, and pH. To provide appropriate nursing care to a patient, the nurse must know how the patient's body is physiologically responding. One of the basic ways to determine this is to assess the patient's vital signs. In this chapter, you will learn not only how to assess vital signs, but also how to relate them to vital physiological functions of the body. You will learn the implications of abnormal readings and the appropriate nursing care to provide.

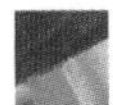

THE SIX VITAL SIGNS

Vital signs, the fundamental measurement of life signs, include five objective measurements and a sixth subjective measurement. The five objective measurements include the following:

1. Temperature (T)
2. Pulse (P)
3. Respirations (R)
4. Blood pressure (BP)
5. Oxygen saturation (SpO_2)

The sixth vital sign is the subjective measurement:

6. Pain

The five objective vital signs tell how certain systems are functioning, provide data regarding the patient's overall condition, and provide a baseline against which you can measure even subtle changes. Although subjective, the assessment of pain is important because this feeling of distress can have effects on pulse, respirations, and blood pressure (BP), and it serves as a warning that tissues are actually being injured or about to be injured. In fact, pain is one of the primary reasons individuals seek medical care, and it gives us insight as to what may be wrong with the patient's health.

You will *assess,* or measure, vital signs often because it is a quick and efficient way to monitor a patient's physiological condition, identify new problems, and determine if an intervention should be performed or if prior interventions were effective. It is important to remember that vital signs are only of value when they are accurate. The inaccurate measurement of vital signs can result in a range of serious problems, from failure to detect deterioration in the patient's condition all the way to death.

It is important to understand that vital signs must be evaluated in conjunction with the patient's overall condition. Even though vital signs are one of the most important and frequent assessments that you will make, they do not always reflect changes occurring in the patient's condition. For example, a patient with a serious respiratory illness such as pneumonia may still have a respiratory rate within the normal range. Therefore, further assessments such as breath sounds and chest x-ray are required to detect deviations in function. Remember to always look at the whole patient, not just his or her vital signs.

Supervision/Delegation Connection

There Are Times When You Should Not Delegate Vital Signs

Vital sign assessment is commonly delegated, but because the skill of measuring vital signs is simple to perform and is performed many times a day, day after day, it is possible to take the process and the delegation of vital sign assessment for granted and to become totally dependent on unlicensed assistive personnel (UAP) for their measurement. Although it is appropriate in most cases to delegate this task to a certified nursing assistant or UAP, keep in mind that vital sign assessment is ultimately your responsibility. You are responsible for analyzing the vital sign findings and for determining when further action is necessary whether or not you take the vital signs yourself. These are the *vital signs of life* that indicate when your patients' conditions begin to change.

There are times when you should assess a patient's vital signs or reassess them after someone else has already taken them, including the following:

- After administration of IV medications that may affect the vital signs
- When vital signs are markedly different from the patient's normal range

• **WORD** • **BUILDING** •

respiration: respir – breathe + ation – action

- With a change in level of consciousness
- When the patient is in an unstable postoperative condition
- If there is uncontrolled bleeding
- When the patient has pale, cold, and clammy skin
- Any time you suspect hemorrhage, shock, stroke, pulmonary embolism, heart attack, or any other serious condition
- Any time you suspect the validity of the vital signs reported to you or the vital signs do not seem to match the patient's condition
- Any time your "gut tells you to"

Occasionally there are times when you cannot identify a patient's problem but something just does not seem right with his or her condition. Never ignore those feelings. It has been proven that we can subconsciously detect subtle changes in a patient's condition without being able to consciously identify the change. It is always better to repeat vital sign assessment and find nothing out of the ordinary than to miss a problem because you did not reassess. Learn to trust your intuitive instincts that tell you the vital signs should be reassessed. Your patient's condition may be dependent on it.

There are designated times to assess vital signs. Most hospitals have a routine schedule of once every 8 hours unless the health-care provider orders it more frequently or the nurse determines that there is sufficient reason to measure them at shorter intervals. It is standard to measure vital signs when a patient is admitted to the facility, and they are considered part of the initial shift head-to-toe assessment. Box 17.1 lists other times to assess vital signs.

Further guidelines for assessment of vital signs include the following:

- Use the appropriate equipment for each patient, such as a child BP cuff for a toddler or a large adult cuff for an obese patient.
- Be familiar with normal ranges for different ages.
- Always compare vital signs with previous vital sign ranges for that specific patient.
- Know the patient's medical history, medications, and therapies because sometimes they can have predictable effects on vital signs.
- Understand and interpret the vital sign findings.
- Record and communicate significant vital sign changes to the health-care provider as well as to the nurse on the next shift.
- Minimize environmental effects on vital signs, such as waiting 15 to 30 minutes after the patient has a cold drink to assess oral temperature.

KNOWLEDGE CONNECTION

List at least five times or situations when you should assess vital signs rather than delegate them. List at least five guidelines regarding the assessment of vital signs.

Box 17.1 When to Assess Vital Signs

Every facility will have designated or set times to assess vital signs, such as a specific time on each shift. However, there are many additional situations and circumstances in which it is important that you assess a patient's vital signs. It is your responsibility to identify when it may be necessary to perform this common but important assessment. Additional times to assess vital signs include, but are not limited to, the following:

- On admission to the hospital
- At each visit to a clinic or emergency room
- At each home health or hospice visit
- Every 8 hours or according to hospital policy
- According to health-care provider's orders if they are more frequent than hospital policy
- Any time a patient complains of feeling unusual or different
- When you suspect a change in condition
- Before, during, and after administering medications or treatments that affect any of the physiological controls of temperature, pulse, respiration, or oxygen saturation
- Before, during, and after blood product transfusion
- Before, during, and after a surgical procedure or invasive diagnostic procedure
- At least every 4 hours whenever one or more vital signs are abnormal
- A second time, or more, when a vital sign assessment finding is significantly different from the last assessment
- Every 5 to 15 minutes when the patient's condition is unstable, such as after delivery, surgery, or trauma

Note: Vital signs are routinely assessed only once a week or once a month in long-term care facilities, such as nursing homes, depending on facility policy.

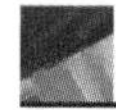

BODY TEMPERATURE

Body temperature is the difference between the amount of heat the body produces and the amount of heat that is gained or lost to the external environment. The core temperature, the temperature of the deeper structures and tissues, is normally slightly warmer than that of the more superficial body tissues. The core temperature is the most important measurement to maintain as it determines the conditions in which the brain, heart, and other internal organs must survive.

Measurement of the true core temperature is accomplished with a sterile thermometer probe inserted into the pulmonary artery, heart, or urinary bladder. However, in most circumstances it is adequate to measure the body temperature using a clinical thermometer and less-invasive methods, which are presented in this chapter. The body's surface, or skin, temperature is typically assessed by laying your hand on the patient to determine if their skin is warm, hot, cool, or cold, as well as whether it is dry or moist.

• WORD • BUILDING •

thermometer: thermo – heat + meter – measure

Scales of Temperature Measurement

Health-care providers measure body temperature using either the Fahrenheit scale or the centigrade scale, also known as the Celsius scale. Figure 17.1 shows a comparison of the two scales, and Box 17.2 presents a conversion formula.

Thermogenesis

The production of heat is known as *thermogenesis.* One of the ways the human body produces heat is through the processes occurring after the ingestion of food: digestion, absorption, breakdown, and synthesis of proteins. Because the intake of food results in the increase of these metabolic functions, the production of heat increases. In other words, body heat is a by-product of metabolism. More heat is produced as metabolism speeds up, and less is produced when metabolism slows down. The *basal metabolic rate* is the amount of heat produced by the body when at total rest. Because an increase in metabolism results in more heat production, any physical activity that increases the metabolism will also increase heat production. Muscle contraction normally produces about 25% of body heat in the resting state. Shivering, an involuntary skeletal muscle response, can raise heat production to four to five times normal. Depending on the level of exertion, exercise can increase the metabolic rate up to 50 times normal, thus explaining why you feel so "hot" when performing moderate to heavy exercise.

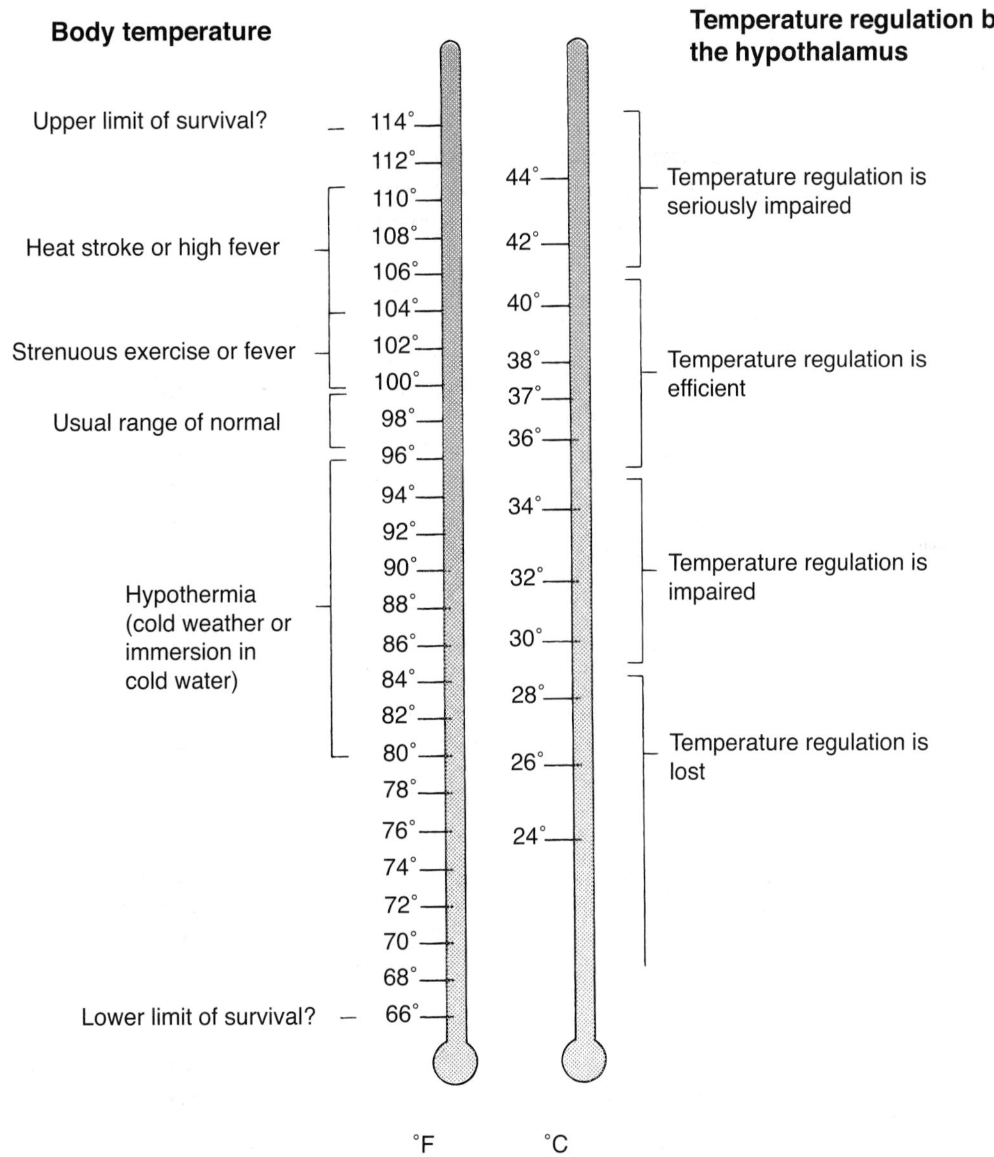

FIGURE 17.1 Ranges of normal and abnormal body temperatures in degrees Fahrenheit and degrees Celsius (from Scanlon V, Sanders T. *Essentials of Anatomy and Physiology.* 7th ed. Philadelphia, PA: FA Davis; 2015).

• WORD • BUILDING •

thermogenesis: thermo – heat + genesis – generation

Box 17.2

Fahrenheit-to-Celsius Conversion Formula

To convert Fahrenheit to Celsius, subtract 32 from the Fahrenheit reading and multiply by 5/9.

$$C = (F - 32) \times 5/9$$

Example: $(104°F - 32) \times 5/9 = 40°C$

To convert Celsius to Fahrenheit, multiply the Celsius reading by 9/5 and add 32.

$$F = (C \times 9/5) + 32$$

Example: $(40°C \times 9/5) + 32 = 104°F$

Numerous other factors influence heat production, including the hormones thyroxine, produced by the thyroid gland; epinephrine and norepinephrine, secreted by the adrenal medulla; and adenosine triphosphate, which is an energy source produced in all cells during cellular respiration. The liver is always metabolically active and produces 15% to 20% of body heat in the resting state.

Settings Connection: Long-Term Care

Older Adults and Body Temperature

Older adults also may have a difficult time maintaining normal body temperature because of the limited amount of subcutaneous fat cells available to insulate their internal organs. In these individuals, any type of circulatory impairment will inhibit the vasoconstriction and vasodilation aspects of controlling body temperature.

Thermoregulation

Thermoregulation, or the regulation of body temperature, is primarily controlled by the part of the brain known as the *hypothalamus.* When the hypothalamus functions correctly, it maintains a comfortable core temperature known as the *set-point.* When this set-point is exceeded, signals are sent, causing the body to sweat and the blood vessels to dilate. This vasodilation brings more blood to the skin's surface for increased heat loss through radiation, resulting in reduction of temperature. The sweat helps to reduce temperature through evaporation. When sweat production is high enough to be seen on the skin, it is termed *diaphoresis.*

The hypothalamus also has capabilities to increase heat production by causing muscles to shiver and to conserve body heat by constricting vessels in the body's outer surface layers and extremities. This vasoconstriction helps to redirect the majority of blood flow to the vital organs, primarily the brain and heart, to maintain adequate core temperature.

Factors Affecting Body Temperature

Many internal and external factors affect body temperature. Some of the common factors are environment, time of day, gender, physical activity and exercise, medications, food or liquid intake, stress, and illness.

Environment

The climate and temperature of the environment affect the body temperature accordingly. If the environment is hot, the body temperature will tend to be higher; when the environmental temperature is cold, the body temperature will tend to be lower.

Time of Day

The body has a "time clock" or rhythm of its own, known as the *circadian rhythm.* The body's physiological functions vary somewhat over the 24-hour day. Most individuals' body temperature will drop 0.5°F to 1°F lower between midnight and dawn and raise 1°F to 2°F in the late afternoon and evening, thus explaining why children always seem to get "sicker" after the typical health-care provider's office closes in the afternoon.

Gender

Only slight differences are found in the ranges of normal vital signs for men versus women. However, women tend to have a slight rise in body temperature during ovulation. This is due to the rising level of progesterone, a hormone that prepares the uterus for pregnancy.

Physical Activity and Exercise

During activity and exercise, muscles require fuel in the form of glucose to metabolize or burn for energy. As mentioned earlier in the chapter, the more metabolism increases, the more heat the body produces. Thus, exercise raises the body temperature and inactivity lowers it.

Medications

Various medications affect the body temperature. Stimulants such as ephedrine increase the body's metabolism and thus raise body temperature. Other medications such as acetaminophen lower an elevated temperature.

Food Intake

Because calories are burned, providing fuel for metabolism, the amount, type, or lack of food ingested can directly affect the body temperature. Hot and cold fluids can have mild effects on the oral temperature reading for 15 to 30 minutes after ingestion.

Stress

Individuals who are anxious or stressed may tend to have a slightly higher body temperature due to stimulation of the sympathetic nervous system. This results in production of excessive amounts of hormones such as epinephrine, which will raise the body's metabolic rate, including the temperature.

• WORD • BUILDING •

vasodilation: vaso – blood vessel + dilation – spreading out

diaphoresis: diaphoresis – perspiration

Illness

Various diseases and injuries can directly affect the hypothalamus, resulting in changes in body temperature. Common conditions affecting body temperature include inflammatory processes and infections caused by bacteria or viruses, fluid loss, central nervous system tumors, head injuries, and heat stroke.

> **KNOWLEDGE CONNECTION**
>
> Explain what is meant by set-point. Identify at least five factors that can affect body temperature. Describe how the body regulates its temperature.

Types of Thermometers

Various types of clinical thermometers may be used to assess the body temperature, including the plastic nonmercury thermometer, disposable chemical-strip thermometer, electronic thermometer, tympanic thermometer, and temporal artery thermometer (Fig. 17.2). Plastic nonmercury thermometers have a digital readout, with oral, axillary, and rectal settings, requiring you to preset the correct route before taking the temperature. Some disposable chemical-strip thermometers are designed for topical application to the skin, and others are designed for oral or axillary use. Electronic thermometers may be used to assess oral, axillary, or rectal temperatures. The tympanic thermometer is used only for measurement of the temperature of the tympanic membrane in the ear. Temporal artery thermometers are used to scan the temporal artery of the head for blood temperature. ***Safety: There is much controversy related to the accuracy of chemical-strip, tympanic, and temporal thermometers, in other words, those thermometers that measure body temperature externally. It is pertinent that you follow the manufacturer's instructions carefully and always double-check the temperature if you suspect that the reading is not accurate.***

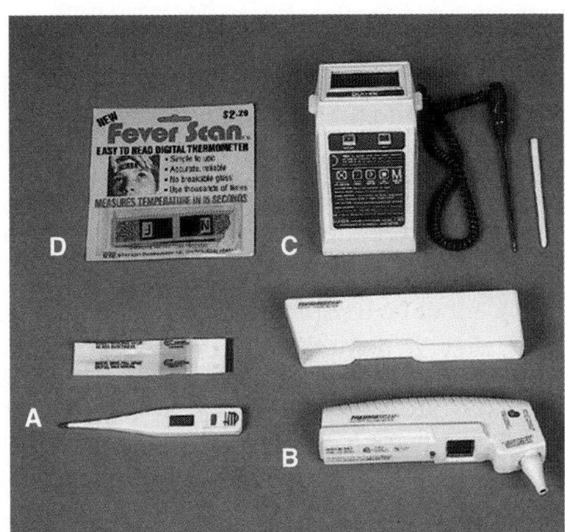

FIGURE 17.2 Types of thermometers. (a) Nonmercury thermometer; (b) Tympanic thermometer; (c) Electronic thermometer; (d) Digital-tape or other paper-strip thermometer (from Wilkinson JM, Treas LS. *Fundamentals of Nursing: Theory, Concepts & Applications*. Vol. 1. 3rd ed. Philadelphia, PA: FA Davis; 2016).

Disposable thermometer sheath covers should be used each time a plastic nonmercury, electronic, or tympanic thermometer is used in order to prevent cross-contamination.

Routes of Temperature Assessment

Body temperature is most accurate when measured at sites where there is a rich blood supply. The common routes used to measure temperature are the oral, axillary, tympanic, skin, temporal artery, and rectal routes. The oral route is considered to be the best, noninvasive method to obtain an accurate reading. The thermometer is placed deep into the sublingual pocket under the tongue, usually 1.5 to 2 inches. The *axillary route* consists of placing the thermometer under the arm, in the armpit. The tympanic route requires the use of a special thermometer that is designed to fit into the ear canal and measures the temperature of the tympanic membrane. A scanning thermometer may also be used to measure the temperature of the blood by scanning the temporal artery.

For continuous, noninvasive monitoring of body temperature, a temperature probe or chemical-strip thermometer may be applied to the skin. In intensive care units, it is sometimes important to continuously monitor the patient's core temperature by inserting a sterile catheter probe into the pulmonary artery. Each route has advantages and disadvantages that are listed in Table 17.1. Skill 17.1 (see page 331) covers how to assess body temperature by various routes.

Oral

To accurately measure an oral temperature, you must make certain the patient has not eaten, drunk, or smoked within the last 15 to 30 minutes. After applying a disposable thermometer cover sheath, the thermometer should be placed deep into the sublingual pocket under the tongue. Make sure the patient is able to hold the thermometer in place with his or her tongue. If not, select another route for temperature assessment.

If a plastic nonmercury thermometer or an electronic thermometer is used, it should be left in place until it signals the assessment is complete (usually an auditory sound); generally this takes less than a minute. Single-use oral paper thermometers vary in length of time required, so read the instructions carefully before using them.

Axillary

The axillary route is used for patients who cannot hold the oral thermometer in place or for patients for whom the oral route might pose a safety risk, such as a patient who is having seizures. Place either a plastic nonmercury thermometer or an electronic thermometer under the arm in the axilla. Make sure

• **WORD • BUILDING** •
temporal: tempor – temples (of the head) + al – related to

Table 17.1
Advantages and Disadvantages of the Various Temperature Assessment Routes

Route	*Advantages*	*Disadvantages*
Oral	More accurate Convenient and easily accessible Simple	Risk of body fluid exposure Affected by smoking, drinking hot or cold liquids, and oxygen administration Not for infants, small children, or confused or unconscious patients
Skin	Does not require position change Convenient, safe, easily accessible, and comfortable for patient Provides continual assessment to reflect changes quickly Good for use with newborns Unaffected by eating, drinking, or smoking	Affected by perspiration Reflects surface rather than core temperature Affected by severe environmental temperatures
Tympanic membrane	Convenient, easily accessible, and comfortable for the patient Good for use with newborns Quick (less than 5 seconds) Good for patients with difficulty breathing or on supplemental oxygen Often can be performed without disturbing a sleeping patient Unaffected by eating, drinking, or smoking	Inaccurate if probe is not pointed directly at the tympanic membrane The walls of the ear canal are cooler than the tympanic membrane Correct placement is difficult in children's ear canals Affected by environmental factors such as radiant heaters or incubators Cannot be used for patients with ear infections or after ear surgery Higher cost of equipment
Temporal artery	Quick (less than 5 seconds) Easy, noninvasive, and comfortable for the patient Good for use with small children Does not require positioning Unaffected by eating, drinking, or smoking	Affected by perspiration Inaccurate if hair is thick on the forehead or if adequate contact with skin is not maintained during assessment Higher cost of equipment
Axillary	Safe and noninvasive Can be used with unconscious patient	Temperature will be at least 1°F less than core temperature Changes in temperature are slower to be reflected
Rectal	Most accurate Provides core temperature Reflects temperature changes quickly	Source of embarrassment for patient Requires positioning of patient Risk of body fluid exposure Risk of rectum perforation, especially in newborns Cannot be used for patients with diarrhea, severe hemorrhoids, or rectal surgery
Internal catheter probe	Most accurate Provides core temperature Continual monitoring	Most invasive Requires sterile technique Risk of vessel perforation and infection

the thermometer bulb or tip is encased within the axilla and does not protrude behind the arm. Leave it in place until it signals the temperature has been read, usually less than 1 minute.

Tympanic

The tympanic thermometer is an infrared device used with a disposable cover over the tip of the speculum. Gently pull the pinna up and back on an adult and down and back on a small child younger than 3 years. The speculum should be inserted gently into the ear canal, pointing the tip toward the mandible on the opposite side of the face and making a seal between the ear and the speculum. After pushing the indicated button on the device, it takes only 1 to 2 seconds to read the temperature. To improve accuracy, some manufacturers recommend repeating this assessment two to three times and then recording the highest reading because the lower readings indicate the infrared beam was not aimed directly at the eardrum but at the sides of the ear canal.

Skin

If using a disposable topical chemical-strip thermometer, peel off the backing and apply the sticky side of the thermometer directly to clean, dry skin. If using a special thermometer with a skin probe, tape the probe to the skin and observe the continual temperature readout. ***Safety: If the skin probe is part of a radiant heating device, such as those used on newborns, make certain to set the temperature alarms so that the infant is not at risk for being overheated to dangerous levels.***

Rectal

You may use a nonmercury thermometer that is designated specifically for just one patient for rectal use. Insert the thermometer into a disposable plastic thermometer cover sheath and lubricate the tip of the thermometer with a water-soluble lubricant. While wearing gloves, insert the thermometer into the rectum approximately 1 to 1 1/2 inches for an adult, 1/2 to 1 inch for a child, and 1/2 inch for an infant. Leave the thermometer in place until it signals that assessment is completed, which will take less than 1 minute. ***Safety: Because of the risk of intestinal perforation, this route is not recommended as the route of choice.***

Temporal Artery

A special thermometer is used to scan the temporal artery temperature. While pressing the scan button with your thumb, place the probe on a dry forehead and move slowly across the width of the forehead and temple. Then lift the probe off the skin and touch it to the neck just behind the earlobe. It is important to follow the manufacturer's instructions for use to increase accuracy.

Normal Body Temperatures by Selected Routes

The normal range for core temperatures varies from 97°F to 99.6°F (36.1°C to 37.5°C), with the average being 98.6°F (37°C). The oral, tympanic, and temporal artery routes are the most common routes used to measure the temperature and should provide close to the same readings, within about 0.5 degrees (Table 17.2). The rectal route provides the closest to the core temperature and is approximately 1°F higher than the oral temperature. The axillary route temperature is approximately 1°F lower than the oral temperature.

Elevated Temperature

Various terms are used to indicate an elevated body temperature, including *fever, pyrexia,* and *hyperthermia.* The term **febrile** is used to indicate the state of having a fever, and **afebrile** is used to indicate the state of being without fever. *Hyperthermia* is more commonly used to describe serious elevations above 105°F (40.5°C).

Fever is the body's natural way of protecting itself from bacteria, viruses, other microorganisms, and foreign bodies that invade the body and threaten its state of health. After these invaders enter an area of the body in which they do not belong, the body stimulates specialized white blood cells whose purpose is to ingest the invaders. These specialized blood cells, known as *phagocytes,* secrete pyrogens, which stimulate secretion of prostaglandin hormones. The prostaglandin hormones trigger the hypothalamus to raise the set-point for body temperature in an effort to prevent replication of the offending microorganisms, in other words, to raise the temperature high enough to inhibit microorganism reproduction. To assist in raising the temperature, the body tries to conserve body heat through surface vasoconstriction. This can cause the patient to feel chilled or cold. Muscles may begin to involuntarily contract, known as *shivering,* as the body attempts to increase its metabolic rate to reach the new temperature set-point. As the new set-point is attained, the fever also stimulates production of interferon, which is the body's natural defense mechanism against invading viruses.

Because fever is the body's natural defense against infection, it is accepted practice to allow the fever to accomplish its purpose unless it becomes too high. Most health-care providers will not attempt to reduce fever until it elevates above 102°F (38.9°C). ***Safety: Temperature elevations above 105°F (40.5°C) can result in damage to body cells.*** Fever may occur and be constant, or it may come and go in differing patterns.

Table 17.2
Normal Temperature Equivalents by Site

	Oral	*Tympanic*	*Rectal*	*Axillary*
Fahrenheit	98.6°	98.6°	99.6°	97.6°
Celsius	37°	37°	37.5°	36.4°

Signs and Symptoms of Fever

Every patient with a fever will not present in the same manner. Some of the common signs and symptoms that may indicate fever include the following:

- Flushed face
- Dry hot skin
- Dry mucous membranes
- Elevated pulse rate and rapid respirations
- Glassy or droopy eyes
- Increased irritability or restlessness
- Photophobia, which means the eyes have increased sensitivity to light
- Thirst
- Headache
- Myalgia (muscle aches)
- Lethargy or drowsiness
- Diaphoresis
- Anorexia
- Nausea
- Confusion, especially in children and the elderly
- Seizures, especially in infants and children

Nursing Care for Patients With Fever

When caring for a patient with fever, you will want to perform the following:

- Assess all vital signs at least every 2 hours *or more often depending on the degree of abnormality.*
- Provide allowed fluids frequently and measure intake and output as soon as fever is detected. It is important to remember that your patient will have an additional need for adequate fluid intake (up to 3 liters per day) to allow for proper cell function and to prevent dehydration. If you detect signs that the patient is dehydrating or is not taking adequate oral fluids, it is your responsibility to notify the health-care provider for possible IV fluid orders.
- Take extra care to offer foods the patient likes and to offer five to six smaller feedings rather than the routine three meals per day. This will provide your patient with the nutritional needs necessary to accommodate his or her increased metabolic rate.
- Provide mouth and skin care to prevent dryness. Apply petroleum jelly to lips and lotion to skin. A cool washcloth may be applied to the eyes, forehead, or neck. A tepid sponge bath may be given to ease the patient's discomfort as long as you are careful to avoid chilling the patient and causing shivering, which will actually raise the temperature (see Chapter 18, Skill 18.4).
- Encourage limited activity and rest to reduce the amount of heat produced through physical activity.
- Encourage the patient to use minimal covers unless shivering occurs. Then a single blanket may be used in an attempt to prevent shivering. Avoid use of multiple blankets, which can help to raise body temperature.
- Apply cloth-covered ice packs to the forehead or neck, axillae, and groin for high fevers, making sure to avoid causing shivering.
- If the patient is perspiring, keep gown and linens clean and dry to avoid chilling.
- Administer *antipyretic,* or fever-reducing, medications as ordered. Common antipyretics used include salicylates, acetaminophen, and ibuprofen.
- In patients with higher fevers, it may become necessary to provide supplemental oxygen to meet the body's increased metabolic needs.
- In severe cases, a fan or water-circulating cooling blanket may be used.

KNOWLEDGE CONNECTION

Describe how and why the body raises its temperature during illness. List at least four signs and symptoms of fever. Explain at least three nursing actions you should take when a patient exhibits fever.

Patient Teaching Connection

Children With Viruses: No Aspirin!

It is important to educate your patients regarding the proper medications to use for fever reduction in children. Acetaminophen or ibuprofen may be used for fever in children. ***Safety: Avoid all salicylate use, including aspirin, in children less than 15 years of age because of the increased risk of Reye's syndrome.*** Reye's syndrome is an acute and potentially fatal childhood disease, affecting the central nervous system and liver, that has been associated with administration of aspirin to children with viruses.

Hypothermia

Hypothermia, or a core temperature below 95°F (35°C), slows body metabolism. Although hypothermia may be induced deliberately to reduce the body's need for oxygen during neurological or cardiac surgeries, prolonged or severe periods of hypothermia can result in death. Mild hypothermia is treated with warm clothes or blankets and ingestion of warm drinks such as broth or soup. ***Safety: Because up to 40% of body heat can be lost through the head, coverings such as a hat or scarf can dramatically help reduce heat loss.*** More severe hypothermia generally is treated with additional measures such as heating blankets, hot water bottles, warmed IV fluids, or warm baths. Patients with severe hypothermia should be brought up to normal temperature slowly because of the risk of irregular heart rhythm and shock.

PULSE

The heart's four chambers rhythmically contract and relax. With each contraction of the ventricles, oxygenated blood is forced out of the left ventricle through the aorta to be delivered to the body's arteries. The amount of blood discharged from the left ventricle with each contraction is known as the *stroke volume.* This pumping action of the heart results in a fluid wave of blood that travels through the arteries as they rhythmically expand and contract. This arterial fluid wave can be palpated as a gentle pulsing, tapping, or throbbing sensation at various points over the body; this is called the *pulse.* The pulse corresponds to the contractions or beats of the heart and is counted by the number of beats per minute (bpm). The volume of blood pumped from the heart in 1 minute is known as the *cardiac output.* The average adult heart pumps approximately 5 liters per minute.

The central or primary pulse site, the *apical pulse,* is located over the apex of the heart where the contraction is the strongest (Fig. 17.3). The apex of the heart, the cone-shaped end of the left ventricle, actually touches the anterior chest wall at or near the fifth intercostal space. This spot is known as the point of maximum impulse (PMI) and is located 3 to 4 inches to the left of the sternum, generally in the fifth intercostal space, at the midclavicular line. In a child, it may be found in the fourth or fifth intercostal space. You should be able to feel the PMI with your fingertips. The PMI is the site over which you will place your stethoscope to auscultate, or listen to, the apical pulse.

Although less convenient to assess, the apical pulse is the most accurate pulse because both heart sounds can generally be heard and it provides information about the valves and contraction of the atria and ventricles that cannot be detected when assessing peripheral pulses. The apical pulse can be auscultated even when peripheral pulses cannot be detected. It is assessed for a full minute to listen for irregularities. When auscultating the heart sounds, you normally hear two sounds called the S_1 and S_2, or "lubb-dupp." Together, these two sounds represent one complete heartbeat. If both the S_1 and S_2 or lubb-dupp sounds are heard clearly and distinctly, the volume or strength of the apical pulse is described as *distinct* or *strong.* If both heart sounds cannot be heard distinctly, it is described as *distant* or *muffled.*

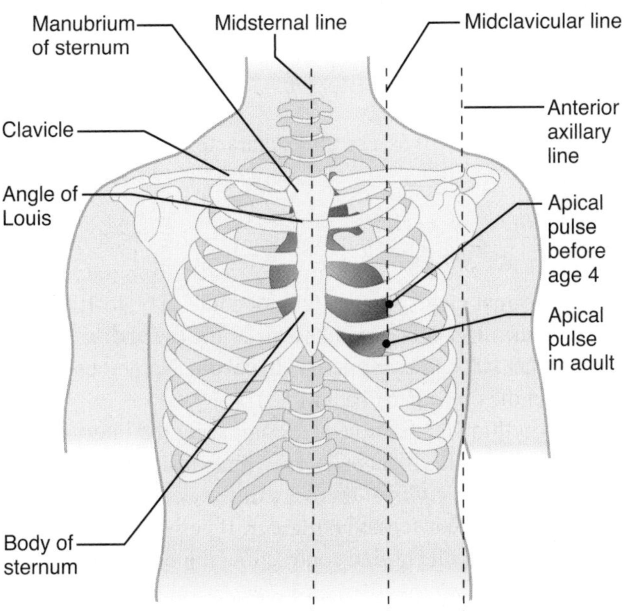

FIGURE 17.3 Location of apical pulse in adults and children (from Wilkinson JM, Treas LS. *Fundamentals of Nursing: Theory, Concepts & Applications.* Vol. 1. 3rd ed. Philadelphia, PA: FA Davis; 2016).

The apical pulse should be the same rate as the peripheral pulses, but if the heart does not pump effectively, blood flow may not be strong enough to consistently deliver a fluid wave to the more distant pulse sites from the heart. Often this occurs when the pulse is irregular, resulting in an apical pulse rate that is faster than the radial pulse. When the radial pulse is slower than the apical pulse, this is known as a **pulse deficit.** For example, the heart rate may be 83 bpm but the radial pulse is only 77 bpm. This would be a pulse deficit of 6 bpm and should be recorded and reported. The number of the pulse deficit, 6 bpm in the previous example, represents the number of heartbeats in which the force of the heart's contraction fails to produce a pulse wave strong enough to be felt at, or *perfuse* to, the radial pulse site. Beats that do not perfuse are ineffective in circulating the blood. Skill 17.2 (see page 333) presents more information on assessing the radial and apical pulses.

Anatomy and Physiology Connection

What Makes the Heart Beat?

Contraction of the heart is a function of the cardiovascular system, but the rate of contraction is regulated by the medulla oblongata, which is located in the brainstem of the central nervous system. In a normal healthy heart, contraction of the heart, or the heartbeat, initiates in the sinoatrial node in the top of the right atrium in the form of an electrical impulse. The impulse is conducted through the atrium on the electrical conduction pathway, causing the atria to depolarize and contract. The impulse continues on the electrical conduction pathway through the atrioventricular (AV) node in the right ventricle. From there, the impulse is transmitted through the bundle of His and the Purkinje fibers throughout both ventricles. Once the impulse has been transmitted through both ventricles, the ventricles depolarize and contract. As the ventricular contraction begins, the AV valves, also known as the *tricuspid* and *bicuspid valves,* slam shut, causing the first heart sound: the longer, lower-pitched sound known as the S_1 or "lubb." As soon as the ventricles begin relaxation, the semilunar valves, also known as the *pulmonary* and *aortic*

• **WORD • BUILDING** •

auscultate: auscultare – to listen attentively

valves, close, causing a shorter and sharper sound: the S_2 or "dupp." Thus, the pattern of normal heart sounds is a rhythmic "lubb-dupp...lubb-dupp...lubb-dupp."

Peripheral Pulse Sites

There are various other pulse sites where the pulse may be palpated by applying gentle fingertip pressure over the artery against the underlying bone. These sites are known as the *peripheral pulses* (Fig. 17.4). The peripheral pulse sites include the following:

- **Temporal:** can be used when radial pulse is not accessible
- **Carotid:** used in cardiac arrest and cardiopulmonary resuscitation (CPR)
- **Brachial:** used to measure BP; can be used to assess pulse rate in small children
- **Radial:** routinely used for pulse rate assessment
- **Femoral:** used to determine circulation to the leg, cardiac arrest
- **Popliteal:** used to determine circulation to the lower leg

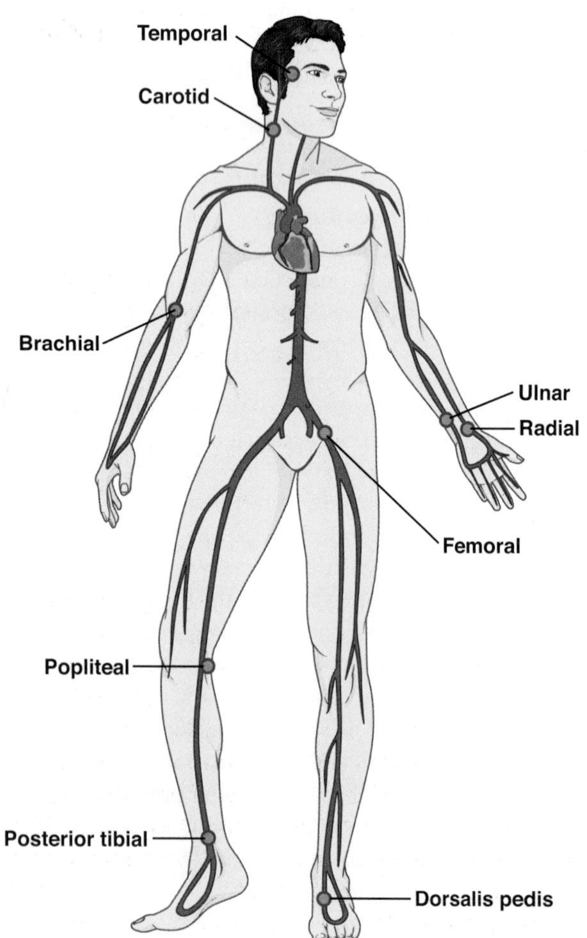

FIGURE 17.4 Peripheral pulse sites (from Wilkinson JM, Treas LS. *Fundamentals of Nursing: Theory, Concepts & Applications*. Vol. 1. 3rd ed. Philadelphia, PA: FA Davis; 2016).

- **Posterior tibialis:** used to determine circulation to the foot
- **Dorsalis pedis:** used to determine circulation to the foot

The temporal pulse can be felt over the temporal bones on the sides of the head. The carotid pulse is located on the sides of the neck between the trachea and the sternocleidomastoid muscle. The brachial pulse is found in the medial elbow crease of each arm, known as the antecubital space. The radial pulse runs parallel to the radius bone on the thumb side of the wrist. The femoral pulse can be palpated along the groin crease at the top of the thigh. The most difficult pulse to locate is the popliteal, found behind the knee. When palpating the popliteal pulse, first have the patient slightly flex the knee. To feel the dorsalis pedis pulse, place your fingertips at the space between the great toe and the second toe. Move the fingers proximally until they rest over the metatarsals of the foot. The posterior tibialis pulse is located by laying your fingertips on the medial aspect of the ankle, directly behind the medial malleolus bone.

Any of the peripheral pulses can be used to assess the heart rate, but the easily accessible radial pulse is the most commonly used site; if it is weak or cannot be felt, then the apical pulse is auscultated. Use the apical pulse for assessing pulse rate in children under the age of 3 years, when the radial pulse is weak or has irregular rhythm, and prior to administering heart rate–altering medications such as digoxin. The peripheral pulses are generally assessed for strength or volume, comparing the right and left sides for equal strength. During CPR, the carotid artery is easily palpated to determine the presence of a pulse. ***Safety: Never palpate both carotid pulses at the same time because this can drop the pulse and BP.*** Skill 17.3 (see page 334) presents more information on assessing peripheral pulses to detect circulation.

Pulse Assessment

As a nurse, you will assess three characteristics of the pulse:

1. Rate
2. Rhythm
3. Volume (strength)

The normal range of pulse rate for adults is 60 to 100 bpm. A pulse less than 60 bpm is known as **bradycardia;** a pulse greater than 100 bpm is termed **tachycardia.** Numerous factors can affect the pulse rate (Table 17.3).

The rhythm is determined by comparing the intervals between the beats. If all the beats are evenly spaced, the rhythm is described as *regular*. If there are differences in the interval lengths, the pulse is termed *irregular*. If peripheral pulses are palpated with each cardiac contraction, the blood fluid wave

• WORD • BUILDING •

femoral: femor – femur + al – related to

proximal: proxim – nearest + al – related to

Table 17.3
Factors Affecting Pulse Rate

Factor	*Effect*
Age	Newborns: 120–160 bpm 1–2 years: 90–120 bpm 3–18 years: 80–100 bpm Adults: 60–100 bpm
Emotions, hormones, and stress	Stimulate sympathetic nervous system, increasing pulse rate
Medications	Can either increase or slow pulse rate Drugs such as digitalis or propranolol slow the rate, while epinephrine and theophylline increase the rate
Caffeine and nicotine	Increase the rate
Exercise	Increases the rate during activity Long-term training and conditioning, as in athletes, will slow the rate Well-conditioned athletes may have a pulse rate less than 60 bpm
Meditation, rest, and sleep	Lower the pulse rate
Circadian rhythm	Pulse rates are slowest from predawn hours to dawn and faster as the day progresses toward evening
Blood volume decreased, as in hemorrhage and dehydration	Hemorrhage and dehydration will increase the pulse rate in an effort to more quickly transport the oxygen carried by red blood cells to the body tissues
Blood volume increased, as in fluid overload	Fluid overload will cause pulses to be full and bounding; sometimes faster
Body temperature	As body temperature increases, each degree Fahrenheit results in increasing the heart approximately 10 bpm As the body cools, each degree results in slowing the pulse by 10 bpm
Hypoxia	Increases the pulse rate
Cardiovascular disease	Different diseases can raise, lower, or make the pulse irregular
Increased intracranial pressure	Typically lowers the pulse rate and may cause it to be irregular

is reaching the pulse points, or is *perfusing*. Volume or strength of a radial pulse is somewhat subjective in its description. A scale of 0 to 3 is generally used to assess pulse volume (Table 17.4). If the palpated pulse is easily detected, it is generally described as strong or 2+. This would be considered a normal finding. A pulse that is faint and difficult to feel is categorized as weak or 1+. If the pulse is so weak that slight fingertip pressure on the pulse site results in the pulse disappearing, the pulse is classified as *thready* or *feeble*. A thready pulse disappears, or *obliterates*, because an inadequate volume of blood is being ejected from the heart with each contraction. In other words, the pumping action of the heart is too weak to deliver an adequate blood fluid wave to the peripheral pulse sites. The result of this problem is decreased delivery of oxygen and nutrients to the tissues, thus preventing optimal functioning of tissues, organs, and systems. A pulse that is very strong and does not disappear, even with moderate pressure, would be classified as a full, *bounding*, or 3+ pulse.

If a pulse is not detectable by palpation, it is termed *absent* or rated as a 0. If this occurs, your next step is to palpate for the next *proximal* pulse in that extremity. If you cannot feel the next proximal pulse either, proceed up the limb to the next proximal pulse until you detect the peripheral pulse that is farthest away from the heart. For example, if you cannot palpate the dorsalis pedis pulse, palpate for the posterior tibialis pulse, and if unable to feel it, palpate for the popliteal pulse, and finally the femoral pulse. While

Table 17.4
Scale for Measuring Peripheral Pulse Volume

Description of Pulse	*Scale and Terms*
Pulse feels very strong and full and is easily counted; does not obliterate even with moderate pressure.	3+ or bounding
Pulse is easily detected, feels strong, and is easily counted; can be obliterated with moderate pressure. This is considered the normal finding.	2+ or strong
Pulse feels weak and can be obliterated with slight pressure.	1+ or weak
If the pulse is so faint and weak that it is difficult to feel it long enough to count the rate, an additional descriptor may be used.	*Thready*
Pulse is not detectable.	0 or absent

assessing for these pulses, there are further assessments you should perform on the extremity *distal* to the pulse site, including skin color, skin temperature, sensation, and capillary refill time.

- Is the color a healthy pink, or is it pale or cyanotic, indicating impaired circulation?
- Is the temperature of the skin warm, as it should be? Or is it cool or cold, again indicating impaired circulation?
- Does the patient have adequate sensation in the distal aspect of the extremity? Can he or she differentiate between dull and sharp sensations as you apply the stimuli to the distal portion of the extremity? You may use something soft, such as a gentle brush of your fingertip or a tissue across the patient's skin. You can use something like a pencil eraser or the side of the barrel of your ink pen. Use something that is relatively sharper, such as a pin or the pointed tip of a pencil or ink pen, to provide a sharp stimulus.
- What is the *capillary refill time?* This is assessed by gently squeezing a nailbed of the extremity to empty the capillaries of blood. The nailbed will turn pale until you remove the pressure, after which it should return to a pink color as the capillaries refill with blood. Normally this will occur within 3 seconds in an adult and within 5 seconds in an elderly patient. If it takes longer to refill, this is an indication that there is circulatory impairment. In a patient whose nails are thickened and yellowed or one who is wearing nail polish, you may press the tip of the finger or toe to assess capillary refill.

After assessing the extremity for proximal pulses and other signs of adequate circulation, obtain a *Doppler ultrasound machine*, a device that uses sound waves to determine if blood flow is present. Listen for the most distal peripheral pulse that you were unable to palpate to confirm that there is adequate arterial blood flow to the site. Skill 17.4 (see page 335) describes the use of Doppler ultrasound to assess nonpalpable pulses.

KNOWLEDGE CONNECTION

List eight peripheral pulse sites. Name three characteristics of the pulse you should assess. What would be your concern if you found the femoral pulse to be weak or absent? Explain how to assess capillary refill.

RESPIRATION

Respiration is the interchange of oxygen (O_2) and carbon dioxide (CO_2) between the atmosphere and the body; it involves both external respiration and internal respiration. *External respiration* is the exchange of these gases between the lungs' alveoli and the blood found in the capillaries that surround the alveoli. *Internal respiration* is the process of exchanging gases between the circulating blood and the tissue cells that make up the body. The movement of air into and out of the lungs is known as *ventilation*. The mechanics of respiration involve the act of breathing in, termed as *inhalation* or *inspiration*, and breathing out, described as *exhalation* or *expiration*. Although the act of breathing is a function of the respiratory system, it is regulated by the central nervous system, specifically by the medulla oblongata and the pons, two structures of the brainstem, and by chemoreceptors in the carotid and aortic bodies. The *carotid body* is a section of the carotid artery wall, and the *aortic body* is a section of the aortic arch wall, both of which contain chemical receptor sites that detect decreases in the blood level of O_2, known as hypoxemia. When hypoxemia is detected, electrical impulses are generated and sent via nerves to the medulla, which will then increase the respiratory rate or depth as needed to correct the hypoxemia.

• WORD • BUILDING •

ventilation: ventilat – airing + ion – action
inspiration: in – inside + spir – breathe + ation – action

Inspiration

To effect inspiration, the medulla sends an impulse via the phrenic nerves to the diaphragm muscle and along the intercostal nerves to the intercostal muscles, telling the muscles to contract. The contraction of the diaphragm causes it to flatten and move downward, while the contraction of the intercostal muscles results in pulling the ribs upward and outward, enlarging the chest cavity.

Expiration

Once the medulla stops sending the motor impulses to inhale, the intercostal and diaphragm muscles begin to relax, once again shrinking the thoracic or chest cavity to the smaller, pre-inhalation state and compressing the lungs. The elastic connective tissue of the alveoli recoils somewhat like a rubber band, forcing the air that is mostly CO_2 out of the alveoli so that it can be exhaled and returned to the atmosphere.

Assessing Respiration

The only equipment required to assess respiration is a watch with a second hand. Assess respiration for the following:

- Rate per minute
- Depth
- Rhythm
- Pattern
- Respiratory effort

Because individuals can voluntarily control their breathing for short intervals of time, it is best to assess the respirations without the patient's awareness. This may be accomplished by positioning the patient's arm across his or her chest or abdomen. Feel for the radial pulse and hold the pulse site while you assess first the respirations and then the radial pulse. It will appear that you are simply taking the patient's pulse, and this will help to distract the patient from concentrating on his or her breathing. While pressing two fingers against the pulse site, count the respiratory rate for 30 seconds, multiply it by 2 for a 1-minute rate, and then continue to palpate the radial pulse site to assess the pulse rate. If the patient is very ill or respirations deviate in any manner from the norm, assess for a full minute.

Rate

Each respiration consists of one inspiration and one expiration. Observe the rise and fall of the chest or abdomen to count the rate. The normal rate for adults is between 12 and 20 bpm. When the rate, depth, rhythm, pattern, and respiratory effort fall within normal parameters, the term **eupnea** is used to describe the respirations. **Bradypnea** describes a respiratory rate below 12 respirations per minute; when the rate exceeds 20 respirations per minute, the term is **tachypnea.**

When the breathing rate slows, it results in a decreased intake of O_2 that can result in a deficiency of O_2 in the tissues and cells. When respirations cease or are absent, this is known as *apnea*. You have only a brief window of 3 to 5 minutes in which to restore respirations before brain damage and death occur.

Because the heart and lungs work together to provide circulation of nutrients and oxygen, the factors that affect the heart rate generally affect the respiratory rate as well. For example, as fever raises the pulse rate, it will also increase the respiratory rate. Breathing speeds up in an attempt to meet the body's increased metabolic needs and to remove excess heat. For every 1°F rise in body temperature, the respiratory rate increases approximately four breaths per minute. Table 17.5 presents further factors that affect the respiratory rate.

Depth

The depth of respiration is observed by the amount of chest expansion with each breath and is related to the volume of air that is inhaled. The average amount of air inhaled in one breath is between 300 and 500 mL and is known as the *tidal volume,* which can be assessed with special equipment. Without special equipment, you can only observe the rise and fall of the chest to provide a subjective measurement of the depth, usually described as shallow, normal, or deep.

Table 17.5
Factors Affecting Respiratory Rate

Factor	*Effect*	
Age	Normal rates:	
	Newborns:	30–60
	Infants:	20–40
	Children:	20–30
	Adolescents:	14–25
	Adults:	12–20
Smoking	Increase	
Environmental temperature	Heat: Increase Cold: Decrease	
Exercise and exertion	Increase	
Rest, sleep, and meditation	Decrease	
Pain, anxiety, stress, and fear	Increase	
Medications, such as narcotics and sedatives	Decrease	
Drug overdose, such as aspirin	Increase	
Respiratory diseases, such as asthma and emphysema	Increase	
Metabolic acidosis, such as caused by diabetes	Increase	
Metabolic alkalosis, such as caused by severe vomiting	Decrease	
Increased intracranial pressure	Decrease	

Rhythm and Pattern

The rhythm of normal respirations is one that is regular, or has evenly spaced intervals between the respirations. When the intervals are not consistent, you assess them as irregular. When the rhythm is irregular, further assess the respirations to determine if the respirations fall into certain patterns, as described in Table 17.6.

Respiratory Effort

Respiratory effort refers to the amount of work required to breathe. Normally, the act of breathing is effortless and is performed unconsciously. An individual who is having labored or difficult breathing is said to be having **dyspnea.** The severely dyspneic patient will usually appear frightened, anxious, or worried. The first thing you may notice when you look at the patient is a "wide-eyed" or startled appearance. This may be indicative that the impaired gas exchange has progressed to the point of hypoxemia or hypoxia. *Hypoxemia* is the term used to denote a decreased oxygen level in the blood. If hypoxemia is not relieved, *hypoxia,* or decreased delivery of oxygen to the tissues and cells, occurs.

Often the patient does not appear to have dyspnea until he or she begins to exert energy, which increases the body's metabolic demand for oxygen. Exertional dyspnea only occurs during activities such as speaking, eating, repositioning, or ambulating. Another sign of difficult breathing is use of the accessory respiratory muscles: the neck and abdominal muscles. It is important to assess which activities result in exertional dyspnea, document findings in the patient's record, and report such findings to the RN supervisor.

Some patients find it too difficult to breathe unless positioned in an upright position, such as sitting or standing. This condition is known as **orthopnea.** More information about nursing care of the patient with orthopnea can be found in Chapter 28.

Related Characteristics

Other respiratory assessments go hand in hand with those previously detailed, including the audible sounds during ventilation and the breath sounds that are auscultated with a stethoscope:

- **Stertorous** breathing refers to noisy, snoring, labored respirations that are audible without a stethoscope.
- **Adventitious sounds** are abnormal sounds that may be heard when auscultating the lungs with a stethoscope and include wheezes, rales or crackles, rhonchi, and stridor.
- **Wheezes** are musical, whistling sounds that may be audible without a stethoscope or heard only during auscultation.
- **Crackles or rales,** are adventitious sounds that may be auscultated with a stethoscope and are the result of air moving over secretions in the lungs. Crackles are short, choppy, popping, snapping, or raspy sounds that may resemble the sound made by rubbing strands of hair between your thumb and index finger. Crackles may be classified as fine or coarse depending on their characteristics.
- **Coarse or rhonchi** are continuous, low-pitched, rattling or bubbling, snoring or sonorous wheezing sounds that can be auscultated when there is partial obstruction of the larger airways due to secretions or tumor.
- **Stridor** is an audible, high-pitched crowing sound that results from partial obstruction of the airways.

You will learn more about auscultating breath sounds in Chapter 21. Skill 17.5 (see page 336) provides additional information on assessing respirations.

Table 17.6
Abnormal Respiratory Patterns

Pattern	*Explanation*	*Graph of Pattern*	*Associated With*
Cheyne-Stokes respirations	Respirations begin shallow, gradually increase in depth and frequency to a peak, and then begin to decrease in depth and frequency until slow and shallow; this is followed by a period of apnea lasting from 10 to 60 seconds. Pattern is repetitious.	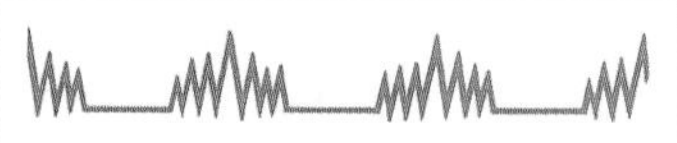	Children: may be a normal pattern Adults: usually ominous—coma, heart failure, head injury, drug overdose, or impending death
Kussmaul's respirations	Respirations are increased in rate and depth, with long, strong, blowing or grunting exhalations.	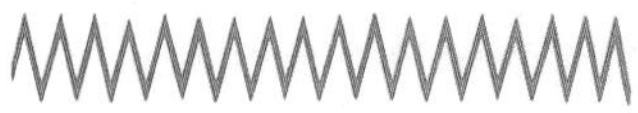	Diabetic ketoacidosis and renal failure
Biot's respirations	Respirations are grouped as several shallow breaths followed by variable-length periods of apnea.	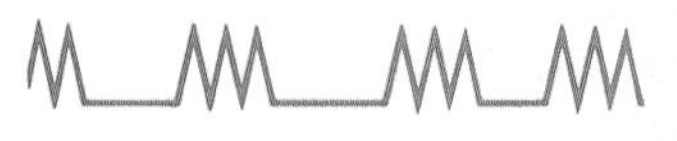	Meningitis and central nervous system disorders

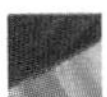

BLOOD PRESSURE

BP is the measurement of the pressure or tension of the blood pushing against the walls of the arteries in the vascular system. The amount of pressure is determined by a combination of the following four circulatory qualities:

1. Strength of the heart contraction, or pumping action of the heart
2. Blood viscosity, or thickness
3. Blood volume
4. Peripheral vascular resistance, or elastic recoil ability of the blood vessel walls

The stronger the contraction of the heart, the greater the volume of blood pumped out of the heart into the arteries. The amount of blood ejected from the heart in one contraction is known as the *stroke volume.* The volume of blood pumped from the heart in a full minute is termed the *cardiac output.* The greater the cardiac output, the higher the BP will be. Conversely, the lower the cardiac output, the lower the pressure will be.

When the heart contraction is weaker or the blood volume is decreased, such as in cases of dehydration or hemorrhage, the BP will decrease. Some conditions that decrease the heart's contraction strength include congestive heart failure and myocardial infarction (commonly known as a heart attack), which ultimately damage the heart muscle, rendering the contraction of the muscle weaker.

Pregnancy, on the other hand, increases the blood volume, and when there is a higher fluid volume within the vascular system, BP will naturally rise. During exercise, the heart beats faster in an effort to help meet the increased demand for oxygen and as a result raises BP. When the arterial walls are nonelastic or constricted, the BP will increase. An example of this is *arteriosclerosis,* otherwise known as hardening of the arteries, which is a gradual process that happens to everyone as they progress through the life span.

Laboratory and Diagnostic Connection

Hematocrit Impacts Blood Pressure

When there is a higher proportion of red blood cells (RBCs) to blood plasma, the viscosity of the blood is increased, which causes the BP to rise. A diagnostic test known as the *hematocrit* is a measurement of this concentration of RBCs in the plasma. Loss of fluids, such as occurs in dehydration, results in a higher hematocrit, while overhydration decreases the hematocrit percentage. Normal ranges are as follows:

- Newborns: 46%–68%
- Children 3 months–6 years: 35%–49%
- Children 7–15 years: 32%–42%
- Adult females older than 18 years: 36%–48%
- Adult males older than 18 years: 42%–52%

Factors Affecting Blood Pressure

The patient with a family history of hypertension (elevated BP) or other circulatory system problems is more likely to develop hypertension than the patient who does not have a family history of circulatory problems. Diseases such as diabetes and kidney disease also can affect BP. Other factors that affect a person's BP include the following:

- **Age:** The average systolic pressure in newborns is around 40 mm Hg. BP gradually increases throughout the life span.
- **Race:** Hypertension tends to have a higher incidence in African Americans, especially males.
- **Exertion or exercise:** Both cause the heart rate and cardiac output to go up, which then raises the BP.
- **Rest:** When a person is at rest, the parasympathetic system is stimulated and lowers the BP.
- **Circadian rhythm:** BP naturally lowers during sleep, increases with waking until peak is reached in the afternoon, and begins to lower during the evening.
- **Anxiety, stress, and emotions:** These factors stimulate the sympathetic nervous system, raising BP.
- **Medications**: These agents can directly or indirectly lower or raise BP; includes herbs and prescription, over-the-counter, and illicit drugs.
- **Nicotine and caffeine:** Nicotine can raise BP long term, while caffeine only raises BP for a short interval.
- **Obesity:** BP is higher in some overweight and obese individuals.
- **Level of hydration:** Dehydration, which leads to volume loss, tends to lower BP; overhydration, which leads to volume increase, tends to raise BP.
- **Hemorrhage:** Loss of volume lowers BP.
- **Increased intracranial pressure:** This condition raises BP.

Components of a Blood Pressure Reading

The measurement of BP involves assessment of two values:

1. **Systolic pressure,** which is the measurement of the force exerted by the blood against the walls of arteries during contraction of the heart ventricles. This time during which the ventricles are contracted is known as *systole* and is the time when the pressure is the highest.
2. **Diastolic pressure,** which is the measurement of the pressure exerted by the blood on the artery walls while the heart ventricles are not contracting. This is the lower of the two pressures. The time during which the ventricles are at rest is known as **diastole.**

There is a simple word association you can use to help you remember which pressure term relates to the resting state of the heart ventricles. When the ventricles are not contracting, the heart is resting or having down time. *Diastolic* pressure equates with *down* time.

BP is measured in millimeters of mercury (mm Hg) and is written as a fraction. If the systolic pressure is 120 mm Hg and the diastolic pressure is 72 mm Hg, the BP is written as 120/72 mm Hg, or just 120/72. The systolic pressure will always be the highest reading and is documented as the top number of the fraction, with the diastolic pressure written as the bottom number.

Pulse pressure is the measurement of the difference between the systolic and diastolic pressures (subtract the smaller number, the diastolic, from the larger number, the systolic) and normally is between 30 and 50 points. A pulse pressure less than 30 or greater than 50 is considered abnormal. An example of a normal pulse pressure of 40 is seen in a BP of 112/72 mm Hg.

The normal range for adult BP is between 100/60 and 120/80 mm Hg. When the systolic pressure rises above 120, it is considered to be *elevated* (Table 17.7).

Hypertension is the term used to describe a systolic reading consistently above 130 or a diastolic reading consistently over 80. To make the medical diagnosis of hypertension, the elevation must be documented on at least two or more separate occasions.

Blood Pressure Equipment

BP is assessed using a stethoscope and a BP cuff, otherwise known as a **sphygmomanometer** (pronounced *sfig'-moe-man-om'-et-er*), which comes with an aneroid or electronic pressure manometer, or gauge.

Sphygmomanometer

The aneroid sphygmomanometer consists of an inflatable rubber bladder that holds air, a cloth cuff that covers the bladder and is long enough to wrap around the extremity, rubber tubing from the bladder to the gauge to indicate the pressure, and rubber tubing from the air bladder to a bulb that is used to pump up the air bladder. A screw valve that is attached proximally to the squeezable bulb allows you to fill and empty the air from the bladder as you observe the pressure manometer. The aneroid gauge must be calibrated every 6 months to remain accurate, so make certain the needle is on zero before using a cuff.

An electronic sphygmomanometer has a transducer that uses sound waves to determine the pressure and a digital gauge to provide the readout, and it automatically inflates and deflates. There is neither a squeezable bulb nor a need for a stethoscope when using an electronic cuff.

The sphygmomanometer may be mounted on the wall above the patient's bed or on an automatic vital sign machine. It also is available as a smaller, portable cuff unit. Box 17.3 provides additional information regarding automatic vital sign machines, and Figure 17.5 shows the different BP cuff types.

The cuffs also come in different sizes, and the correct size must be used to accurately assess the BP. If the cuff is too large the reading will be erroneously low, and if it is too small the reading will be erroneously high. The width of the BP cuff should cover approximately two-thirds of the upper arm. Figure 17.6 shows a BP cuff containing an inflatable bladder.

Table 17.7

Categories of Blood Pressure Levels in Adults*

Category	*Systolic (top number)*		*Diastolic (bottom number)*
Normal	Less than 120	*and*	Less than 80
Elevated	120–129	*or*	Less than 80
High BP			
Stage 1	130–139	*or*	80–89
Stage 2	140 or higher	*or*	90 or higher

*Measured in millimeters of mercury (mm Hg)

Source: American Heart Association. High Blood Pressure. Heart.org. *http://www.heart.org/HEARTORG/Conditions/HighBloodPressure/GettheFactsAboutHighBloodPressure/The-Facts-About-High-Blood-Pressure_UCM_002050_Article.jsp#.Wo2rgZPwbow.* Accessed November 10, 2018.

Box 17.3

Automatic Vital Sign Machines

Automatic vital sign machines have the capability to assess multiple data simultaneously, including:

- BP
- Temperature
- Pulse rate
- SpO_2

Some machines are capable of displaying trends in vital signs. You can preset intervals at which the machine is to measure the vitals, as well as set automatic high and low alarms to warn of abnormal findings. You can print the vital signs for posting in the patient record. These machines are convenient for frequent vital sign assessment schedules, such as postoperative and blood product transfusion schedules. ***Safety: Manually assess vital signs as needed to validate machine accuracy.***

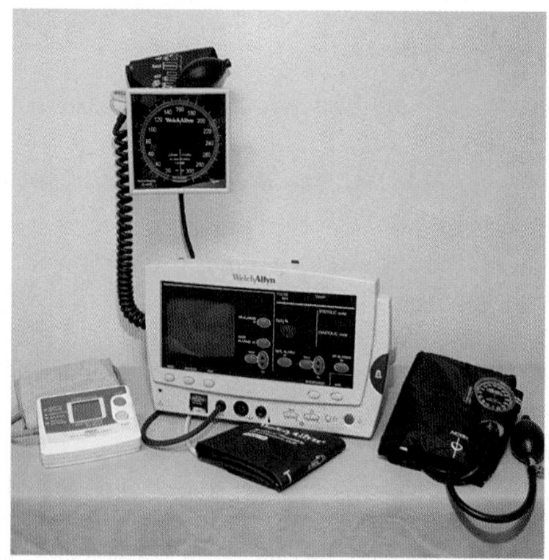

FIGURE 17.5 *Front row, left to right:* A digital sphygmomanometer, an automated vital signs monitor, and an aneroid manometer and cuff. *Back center:* A wall-mounted aneroid manometer and cuff.

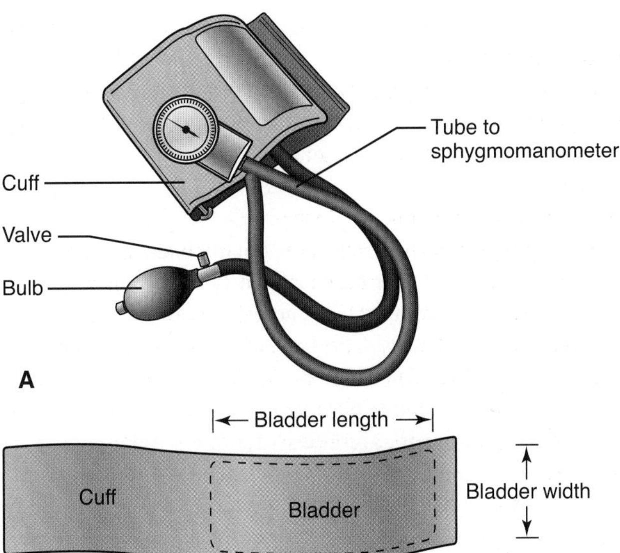

FIGURE 17.6 BP cuff showing placement of the inflatable bladder within the cuff (from Wilkinson JM, Treas LS. *Fundamentals of Nursing: Theory, Concepts & Applications*. Vol. 1. 3rd ed. Philadelphia, PA: FA Davis; 2016).

Stethoscope

A stethoscope has a sound-transmitting chest piece consisting of a bell and a diaphragm, which attaches to rubber tubing that leads to two hollow metal tubes (binaurals) with earpieces attached to the ends. The earpieces are placed in the ears corresponding to the angle of the ear canals and should point *toward* the face when the stethoscope is in place. The chest piece is placed against the patient's skin. The bell is used to auscultate the lower-pitched sounds, such as the heart sounds, and other low-frequency sounds (Fig. 17.7), while the larger flat side, known as the diaphragm, is used to auscultate higher-pitched sounds, such as the lung sounds, bowel sounds, and usually BP. Sometimes heart sounds may be better heard using the diaphragm. Note that some stethoscopes do not have a bell, thus requiring that the diaphragm be used, with lighter pressure for lower-pitched sounds and more pressure for higher-pitched sounds.

Assessment Sites

BP is normally assessed with the cuff around the upper arm and the stethoscope over the brachial artery at the *antecubital* site, on the inner aspect of the elbow. It also can be performed by wrapping the cuff around the lower arm and placing the stethoscope over the radial pulse. However, certain conditions prevent you from using these sites, including the following:

- Amputation of the arm
- Mastectomy on the selected side
- Presence of a shunt for renal dialysis on the selected side
- Casts, braces, or dressings on the selected side
- Recent vascular surgery or trauma on the selected side
- In some cases, the presence of an IV infusion on the selected side

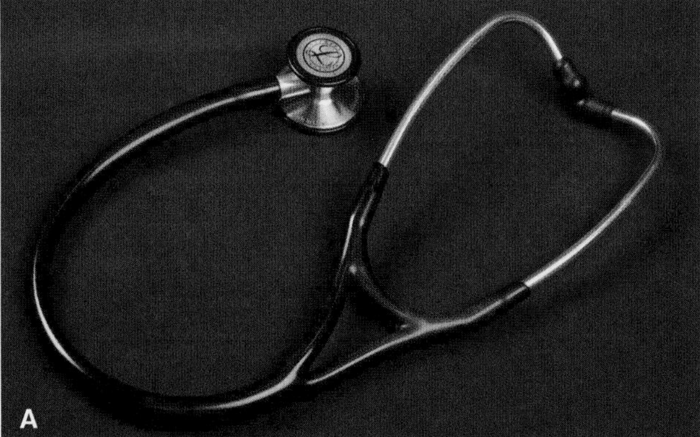

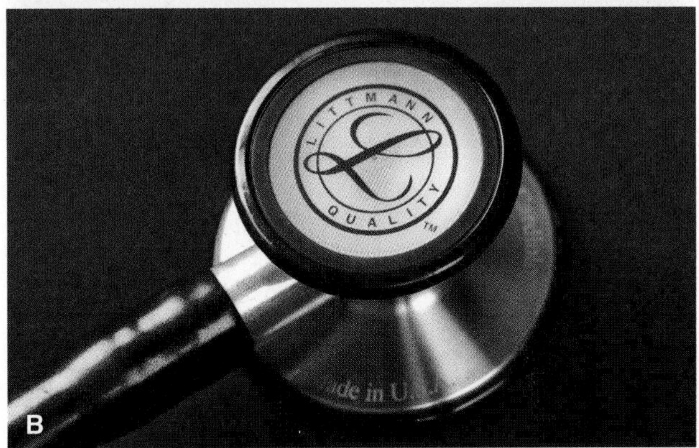

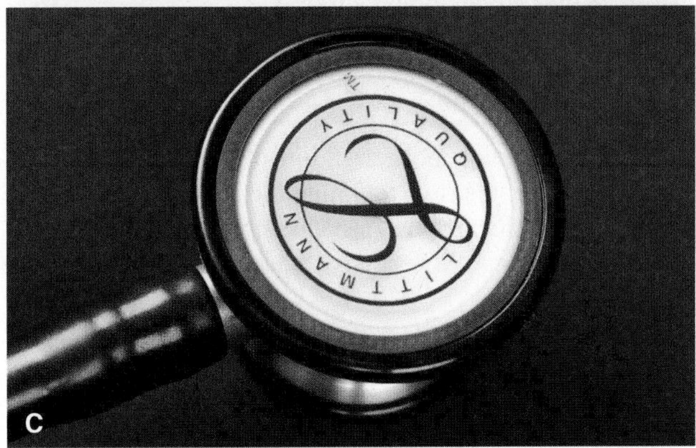

FIGURE 17.7 Stethoscope. (b) The concave side, known as the bell, is used for auscultating lower pitched heart sounds. (c) The flat side, known as the diaphragm, is used for auscultating higher pitched heart sounds, BP, lung sounds, and bowel sounds (from Wilkinson JM, Treas LS. *Fundamentals of Nursing: Theory, Concepts & Applications*. Vol. 1. 3rd ed. Philadelphia, PA: FA Davis; 2016).

When conditions prevent you from assessing BP on either arm, it can be measured on the leg by wrapping the correct-size cuff around the midthigh (Fig. 17.8), with the cuff bladder on the posterior aspect of the thigh and the tubing exiting the cuff distally (toward the knee), and placing the stethoscope over the popliteal artery behind the knee. The systolic pressure may register 20 to 30 mm Hg higher in the leg than in the arm, but the diastolic pressure should be about the same.

Korotkoff's Sounds

Upon inflation of the cuff and accompanying compression of the artery, the flow of blood is not audible with a stethoscope.

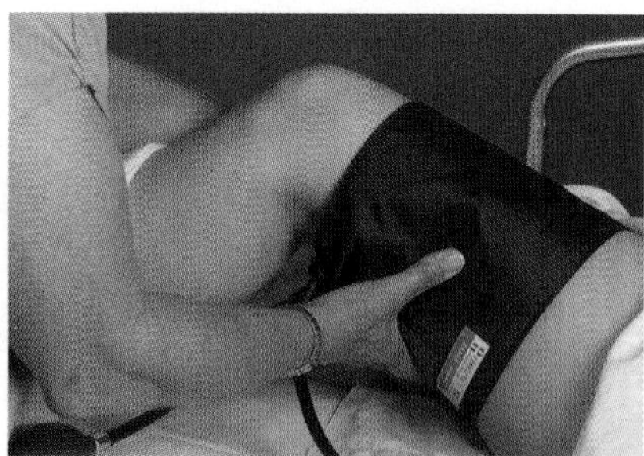

FIGURE 17.8 Position the cuff bladder on the posterior aspect of the thigh with the bottom edge 1 to 2 inches (2.5–5 cm) above the popliteal fossa, centering the arrow on the cuff directly over the popliteal artery. Wrap the cuff snugly around the thigh (from Wilkinson JM, Treas LS. *Fundamentals of Nursing: Theory, Concepts & Applications*. Vol. 1. 3rd ed. Philadelphia, PA: FA Davis; 2016).

As you begin to deflate the cuff and allow the return of blood flow, you will hear the tapping sounds representing this blood flow. These are known as *Korotkoff's sounds,* named after the Russian physician who first described the sounds heard over an artery during cuff deflation. There are five Korotkoff's sounds:

- **First sound:** a clear, rhythmic tapping sound gradually increasing in intensity
- **Second sound:** a soft, swishing or murmuring sound representing turbulent blood flow
- **Third sound:** a sharper, crisper rhythmic sound
- **Fourth sound:** a softening or muffling of rhythmic sound
- **Fifth sound:** silence

You may or may not hear all five of the sounds that represent different stages of returning blood flow, but the first sound heard is documented as the systolic pressure, and the point at which you last hear any sound is documented as the diastolic pressure.

Measurement of Blood Pressure

After selecting the site for assessment and determining the correct size cuff, bare the arm, and wrap the cuff around the extremity about 1 to 2 inches above the auscultation site for your stethoscope. While palpating the arterial pulse distal to the cuff, close the screw valve and squeeze the bulb to rapidly pump the inflatable cuff up to 80 mm Hg for an adult. Now continue to slowly pump the pressure up about 10 mm Hg at a time until you can no longer feel the pulse, noting the point at which you lose the pulse. Then deflate the cuff and wait 2 minutes. Place your stethoscope over the arterial pulse and keep the chest piece of the stethoscope flat against the bare skin. Pump the cuff up to approximately 20 to 30 mm Hg above where you last felt the pulse. For example, if you last felt the pulse at 116 mm Hg, pump the cuff up to 136 to 146 mm Hg. It is uncomfortable for the patient and may cause erroneous readings to pump the pressure up to 180 or 200 mm Hg when pressure is not that high. Slowly unscrew the valve to release air from the cuff bladder at 2 to 3 mm Hg per second, while listening for Korotkoff's sounds. Record the number at which you hear the first Korotkoff sound and the number at which you hear the last sound. Write it as a fraction, such as 118/76. If you hear the sounds all the way to zero on the manometer, record the number at which the sound decreased in amplitude as well as the zero, such as 126/74/0. Further description of BP assessment is found in Skill 17.6 (see page 337).

Auscultatory Gap

When assessing the BP in some patients with hypertension, you may hear a 30 mm Hg "gap" in the Korotkoff sounds. For example, you may hear the first Korotkoff sound beginning at 162 mm Hg and then hear nothing but silence as the needle drops to 138 mm Hg, at which the Korotkoff sounds return and continue until you lose them for good at 74 mm Hg. This silence and the return of sounds is known as an **auscultatory gap.** If you do not adequately inflate the cuff while palpating, this gap can be missed and an erroneously low BP reading recorded. An error of this nature might result in failure to identify an elevated BP that requires treatment. Use caution to palpate carefully and then inflate to 30 mm Hg above that point. If an auscultatory gap is detected, record the number at which it began and ended, for example, a BP of 162/74 with an auscultatory gap of 162 to 138.

Hypertension

Normally, the arterial walls are elastic, with stretch and recoil abilities to accommodate the changing volume of blood in the cardiovascular system. However, as arteriosclerosis progresses through the years, the gradual loss of elasticity in the arterial walls results in less stretch and recoil. The heart has to work harder to pump the blood through the cardiovascular system as the rigidity of the artery walls increases. The rise in BP that results is known as **primary hypertension** or *essential hypertension.* When there is a renal or endocrine disease process that results in elevation of BP, it is termed **secondary hypertension.**

Hypertension is a widespread health problem in the United States, and because there are frequently few or no symptoms, it often goes untreated. Thus, it is important that you educate your patients and encourage them to have annual BP screenings. Also teach your patients the risk factors that contribute to the occurrence of hypertension (Box 17.4).

Treatment of Hypertension

Treatment of hypertension usually involves a number of lifestyle changes, such as reducing dietary intake of salt and fat, weight loss, smoking cessation, reduction or cessation of excessive alcohol intake, stress reduction, and increasing physical activity and exercise, as well as the use of medications when lifestyle changes are not adequate. Left untreated, hypertension can result in permanent damage to the following:

- Brain, in the form of a stroke
- Heart, in the form of congestive heart failure or myocardial infarction (heart attack)
- Kidneys, resulting in kidney failure
- Retinas of the eyes, resulting in loss of vision

Box 17.4

Risk Factors for Hypertension

It is important to identify an individual's risk factors for development of hypertension. Common risk factors include the following:

- Positive family history of hypertension
- Smoking
- Chronically high stress level
- Moderate to heavy alcohol consumption
- Obesity
- Elevated cholesterol levels in the blood

Hypotension

When BP suddenly falls 20 mm Hg to 30 mm Hg below the patient's normal BP or falls below the low normal of 100/60 mm Hg, it is considered **hypotension.** However, it is important to note that some perfectly healthy individuals normally run BPs in the lower ranges, such as a person with a small body build or an athlete in good physical condition. This is one reason why it is necessary for you to always be familiar with your patient's normal range of vital signs. What would be abnormal for one patient, and require treatment, might be normal for another patient, with no need for treatment.

Normally, the peripheral arteries have enough elasticity and recoil to constrict and provide for a slight increase in BP to counteract the forces of gravity when a person rises from a lying position to a sitting or standing position. In older adults, much of this elasticity has been lost, thus slowing or reducing the constriction of the arteries, allowing the blood to pool in the lower extremities upon standing. As a result, BP drops, sometimes enough to result in dizziness and syncope (fainting). When position changes result in a systolic pressure greater or equal to 15 mm Hg or the diastolic pressure falls 10 mm Hg, this is known as *orthostatic hypotension,* also known as *postural hypotension.* Patients who are dehydrated, have anemia, or have been limited to bedrest for extended periods of time; those who are receiving medications such as narcotic analgesics, sedatives, and anesthesia medications; and elderly patients are especially prone to orthostatic hypotension. Skill 17.7 (see page 338) provides information on the assessment of orthostatic hypotension.

Safety: It is advisable to teach these patients to slowly sit up from a reclining position and then to sit on the edge of the bed for several minutes to allow their BP to balance before standing up. After he or she has stood up, you should encourage the patient to stand for several seconds before walking away from the bed to make sure that he or she is not going to faint.

If a patient becomes faint due to hypotension, the initial treatment is to lay the person in a *modified Trendelenburg* position. This is a supine position in which the feet are elevated above the level of the heart. This increases the blood flow to the brain. A *full Trendelenburg position,* where the head is lower than heart level, is no longer recommended.

An extremely serious condition results when hypotension is due to hemorrhage or shock. Immediate medical intervention is necessary to provide adequate blood supply and oxygen to the life-sustaining organs.

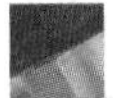

OXYGEN SATURATION

When oxygen enters the blood, it binds with hemoglobin in the RBCs to be transported to and made accessible to the cells of the body. Normally, 96% to 100% of the hemoglobin in arterial blood is bound with oxygen molecules. This saturation level is measured with an electronic pulse oximeter by attaching the plastic clip sensor to the fingertip, the earlobe, the bridge of the nose, or—when circulation is adequate—the toe. Special sensor probes can be applied to the forehead, the palm, or the sole of the foot of an infant. The LED emits light and then calculates the measurement of the reflected light waves to monitor the pulse saturation, known as the SpO_2. A digital readout displays the results. The pulse oximeter can be applied and read intermittently, or it can be applied for continual monitoring.

The selected assessment site should have adequate blood flow, and it should be clean and dry because moisture interferes with accuracy. Artificial nails do not allow accurate assessment because the LED cannot read through them, so remove dark fingernail polish to allow for accurate readings. Patient movement also interferes with accuracy. Finger probe assessment findings are produced in less than 30 seconds, and earlobe sensors deliver results in less than 15 seconds. If the results are below 90%, the RN supervisor should be notified. For further instructions regarding assessment of oxygen saturation, see Skill 17.8 (page 339).

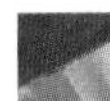

PAIN ASSESSMENT

Acute pain is pain that has a sudden onset, may have severe symptoms, and runs a shorter course than *chronic pain,* which is of longer duration or is ongoing with little change or progression. Pain has been considered one of the vital signs for only a few years, but acute pain can have such dramatic effects on the pulse, respirations, and BP that it is important to assess pain along with the rest of the vital signs. Chronic pain does not affect the other vital signs in the same manner that acute pain can. The characteristics of pain that should be assessed include the following:

- Site or location
- Characteristics, such as sharp, dull, constant, intermittent, stabbing, cramping, or burning
- Severity based on a specified pain scale

Site or Location

It is important to inquire where the pain is located. It is easy to assume that a patient who has undergone a surgical procedure performed on the left leg is having pain in the left leg, when the fact may be that the patient has a headache, a backache from lying in the bed, or abdominal pain related to intestinal gas. Always ask the location of the pain.

It also is important to know that patients may use terminology differently than you do. For example, a patient may deny pain when asked if he or she "has any pain." Further inquiry may find that the patient is having "discomfort," "cramping," or "tenderness." Some patients feel that "pain" is something that is intolerable, therefore thinking their discomfort does not really qualify as pain. Be thorough when assessing pain and use more than one term. You might ask, "Are you having pain or discomfort anywhere?"

Characteristics

When the patient indicates he or she is having pain, ask for an additional description of the type of pain. Is the pain sharp or dull? Is it cramping or stabbing? The patient's description sometimes helps you to differentiate between conditions or possible sources of the pain. For example, a complaint of "heaviness" in the chest or the patient stating that "it feels like an elephant is standing on my chest" describes a different and potentially more serious type of pain than might be expected if the patient were to say that "it is only tender when I cough or sneeze."

Pain Scale

Use a pain scale, such as a scale of 0 to 10, with 0 being "no pain" and 10 being the "worst pain you can imagine," when assessing the patient's pain. Because pain is a subjective matter for the patient, use of the numerical scale allows for introduction of a certain amount of objectivity. After pain medication has been given, it is important to reassess the patient's pain using the same pain scale used before treatment of the pain so that you can objectively determine whether or not the medication was effective. This is part of the evaluation phase of the nursing process. For young children or patients with impaired cognition, you probably will use the Wong-Baker FACES Pain Rating Scale, which consists of a picture of a series of faces that show varying degrees of comfort, from smiling, to frowning, to crying (Fig. 17.9). The child can point to the picture that matches his or her pain level (Fig. 17.10).

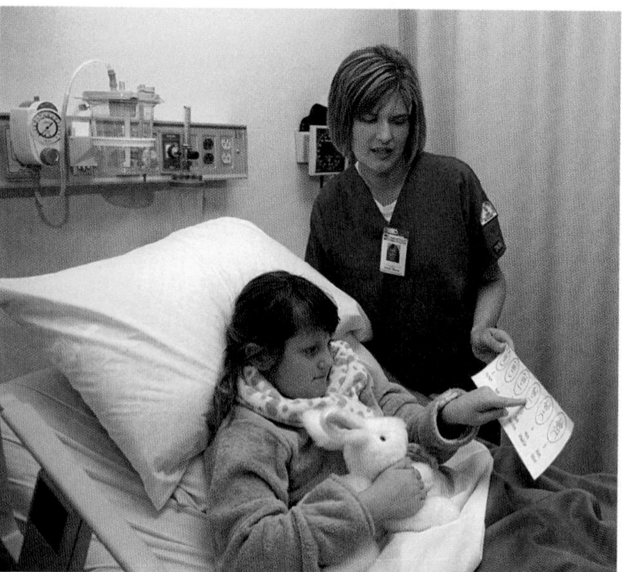

FIGURE 17.10 A nurse using the FACES pain rating scale for pain assessment in a child.

The FLACC scale is a behavioral pain assessment tool for pediatric patients ranging from 2 months to 7 years old. This tool measures 5 different categories for assessing pain: face, legs, activity, cry, and consolability, with scores ranging from 0 to 10. This tool is used in conjunction with patient assessment of the infant or child. This tool is also used with pediatric patients with cognitive development delays.

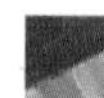

DOCUMENTING VITAL SIGNS

Vital signs are generally documented on a flow sheet designed solely for this purpose. Refer to Figure 17.11 for a sample electronic flow sheet. Most facilities also require that vital signs be documented in the nurse's notes.

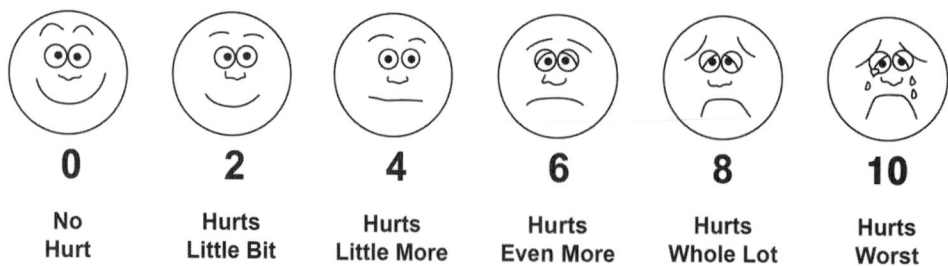

FIGURE 17.9 Wong-Baker FACES Pain Rating Scale (from Wong-Baker FACES Foundation. Wong-Baker FACES® Pain Rating Scale. Available at: http://www.WongBakerFACES.org. Accessed October 18, 2017).

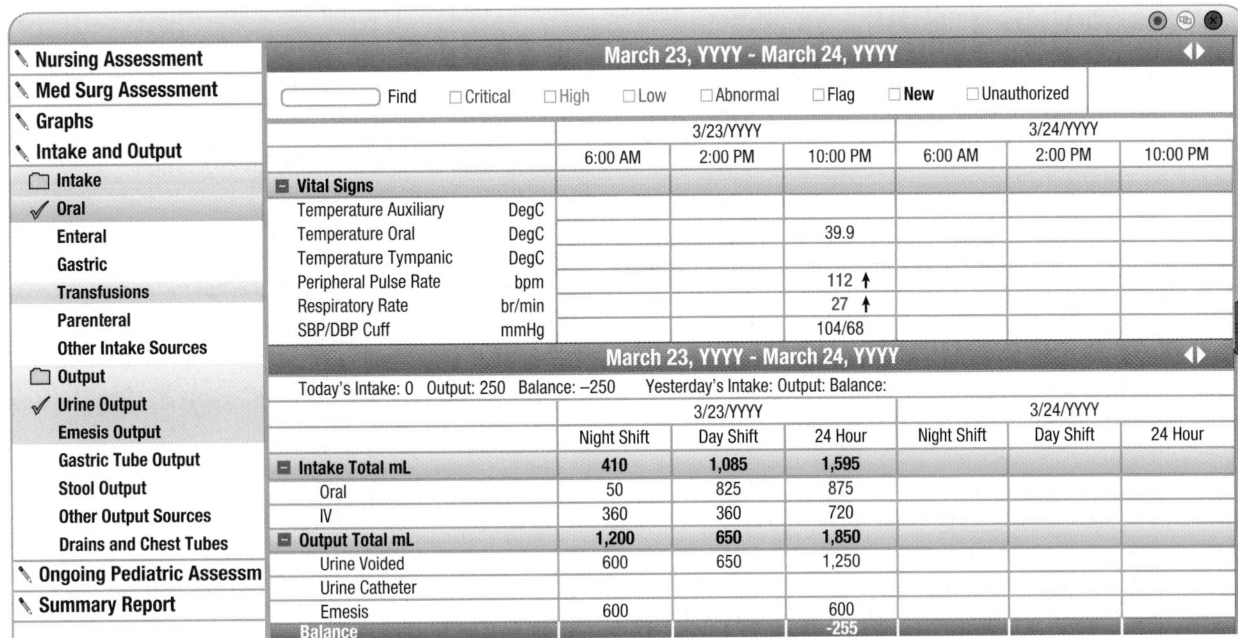

Nursing Assessment
Med Surg Assessment
Graphs
Intake and Output
Intake
Oral
Enteral
Gastric
Transfusions
Parenteral
Other Intake Sources
Output
Urine Output
Emesis Output
Gastric Tube Output
Stool Output
Other Output Sources
Drains and Chest Tubes
Ongoing Pediatric Assessm
Summary Report

March 23, YYYY - March 24, YYYY

Find ☐Critical ☐High ☐Low ☐Abnormal ☐Flag ☐**New** ☐Unauthorized

		3/23/YYYY			3/24/YYYY		
		6:00 AM	2:00 PM	10:00 PM	6:00 AM	2:00 PM	10:00 PM
Vital Signs							
Temperature Auxiliary	DegC						
Temperature Oral	DegC			39.9			
Temperature Tympanic	DegC						
Peripheral Pulse Rate	bpm			112 ↑			
Respiratory Rate	br/min			27 ↑			
SBP/DBP Cuff	mmHg			104/68			

March 23, YYYY - March 24, YYYY

Today's Intake: 0 Output: 250 Balance: –250 Yesterday's Intake: Output: Balance:

	3/23/YYYY			3/24/YYYY		
	Night Shift	Day Shift	24 Hour	Night Shift	Day Shift	24 Hour
Intake Total mL	**410**	**1,085**	**1,595**			
Oral	50	825	875			
IV	360	360	720			
Output Total mL	**1,200**	**650**	**1,850**			
Urine Voided	600	650	1,250			
Urine Catheter						
Emesis	600		600			
Balance			-255			

FIGURE 17.11 A sample electronic flow sheet.

Skill 17.1 Assessing Body Temperature by Various Routes

Assessment Steps

1. Determine which route will be the most appropriate to use with this patient.
2. Review the patient's chart to determine his or her range of temperature.
3. Determine which type of thermometer would be best for use with this patient.

Planning Steps

1. Obtain supplies: thermometer and thermometer sheath or disposable probe cover and tissue, lubricant, and gloves if assessing temperature via the rectal route.
2. If using an electronic or tympanic thermometer or automatic vital sign machine, check the low battery light.

Implementation Steps

1. Follow the Initial Implementation Steps located on the inside back cover.
2. If assessing temperature by the ***oral route,*** determine whether the patient has had anything hot or cold to drink or has smoked within the last 15 minutes. If so, wait another 20 to 30 minutes before assessing temperature. ***This helps to ensure accuracy.***
3. Position the patient appropriately. For the ***oral, axillary, temporal,*** **or** ***tympanic route,*** position the patient in a sitting or supine position. For the ***rectal route,*** position the patient in the Sims' or lateral position. Be certain to provide privacy if you are assessing temperature by the rectal route.
4. If you are using a nonmercury thermometer, apply the appropriate thermometer sheath or probe cover. ***This prevents cross-contamination.***
5. ***Oral route:*** Place the thermometer under the tongue, deep into the sublingual pocket, and leave in place until it signals assessment is complete. Make sure the patient closes his or her lips. ***This helps to prevent falsely low temperatures.***

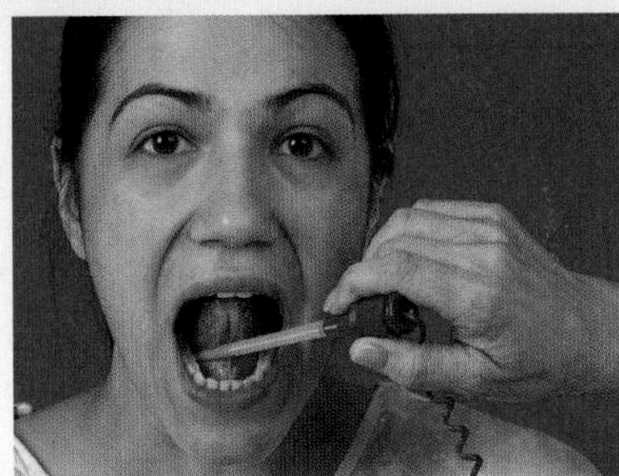

Axillary route: Place the thermometer in the axilla, making certain the tip of the thermometer is covered by the arm posteriorly. Leave the thermometer in place until it signals assessment is complete.

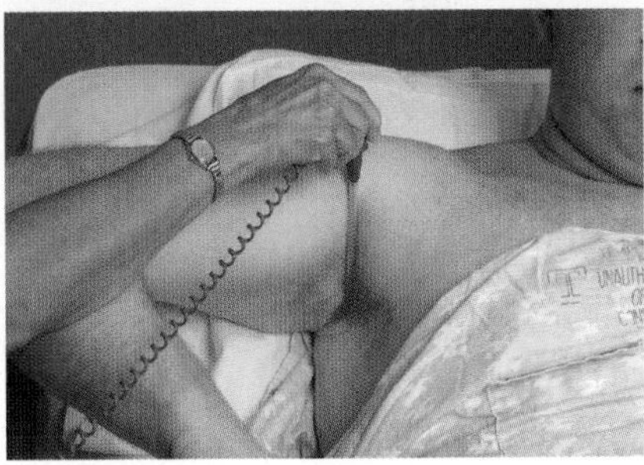

(skill continues on page 332)

Skill 17.1 (continued)

Temporal route: Make sure the skin is dry, place the probe lightly against the forehead skin, scan the thermometer across the forehead and left or right temple area, and then lift the probe and briefly touch it to the area just behind the ear lobe. Then release the button from the thermometer.
Tympanic route: Apply the probe cover. While pulling the pinna upward and back in an adult or downward and back in a small child, gently insert the probe into the ear canal, pointing the probe toward the mandible on the opposite side of the face. Depress the button on the handheld unit and observe the temperature readout.

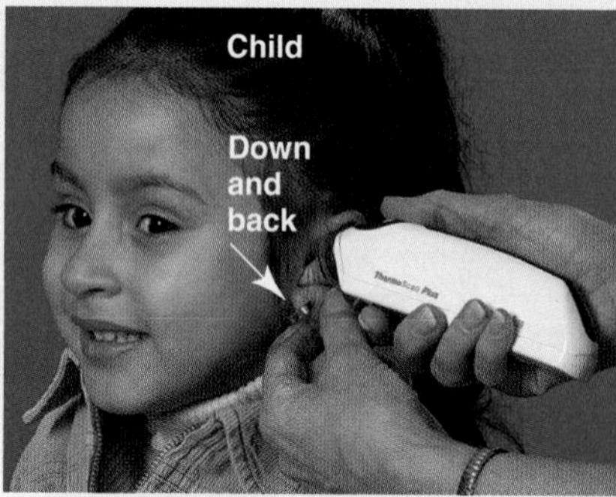

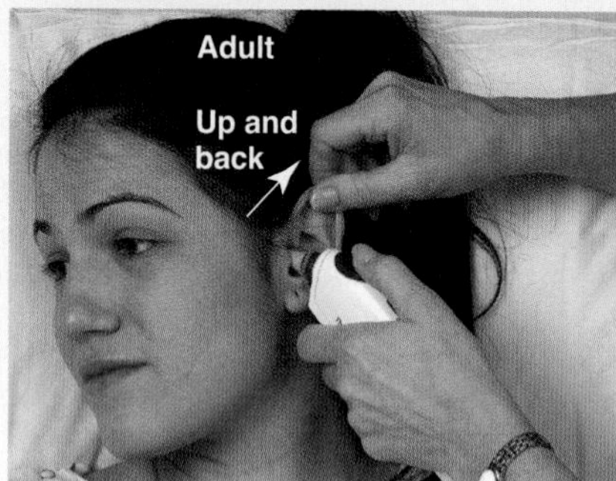

Rectal route: *Safety: Apply gloves.* Lubricate the tip of the thermometer sheath or probe cover with water-soluble lubricant. **This makes insertion easier.** *Safety: Carefully insert the thermometer 1 to 1 1/2 inch into the rectum of an adult, taking care not to perforate the rectum.* Hold the thermometer in place until it signals assessment is complete.

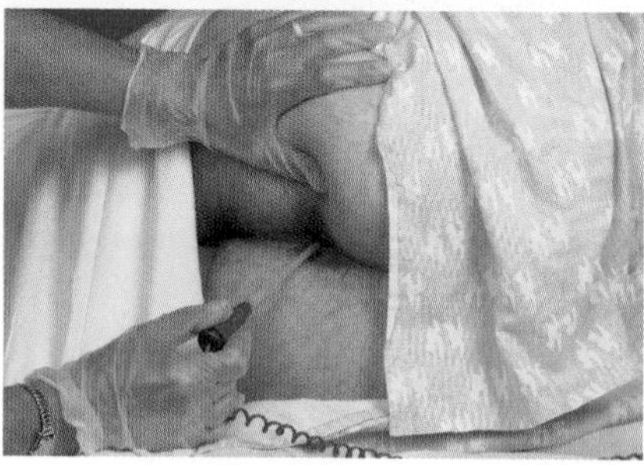

6. Remove the thermometer, and then remove the sheath and dispose of it. If using an electronic or tympanic thermometer, eject the probe cover into the trash and return the thermometer to the charger. Read the temperature.
   Rectal route: Wipe the anus with tissue to remove excess lubricant. Remove gloves.
7. Write down the temperature and route.
8. Follow the Ending Implementation Steps located on the inside back cover.
9. Document temperature and route on a graphic sheet and in the nurse's notes in the following manner:
   Oral route: 98.6°F
   Tympanic route: ^{T}98.6°F
   Axillary route: ^{ax}97.6°F
   Rectal route: ^{R}99.6°F

Evaluation Steps

1. Compare the temperature reading with previous readings.
2. Compare the temperature route with the equivalent oral route.
3. Evaluate if the temperature correlated with any signs and symptoms displayed.
4. If the temperature is abnormal, decide what nursing action may now be necessary.
5. Report abnormal findings according to facility policy.

Sample Documentation

09/18/22 0800 T - ^{ax}98.6°F. ______________
______________ *Nurse's signature and credentials*

Skill 17.2 Assessing the Radial and Apical Pulses

Assessment Steps

1. Review the patient's chart to determine previous pulse rate and site obtained.
2. Review the medication administration record for any medications that may affect pulse rate or assessment site. ***Some cardiac medications require assessment of an apical pulse.***
3. Determine which pulse site is to be assessed.

Planning Steps

1. Be certain a watch or clock with a second hand is available. Obtain a stethoscope if assessing the apical pulse. ***Being prepared saves time and effort.***
2. Plan to wait 5 minutes if the patient has recently ambulated. ***This allows the rate to return to its resting rate.***

Implementation Steps

1. Follow the Initial Implementation Steps located on the inside back cover.

Radial Pulse

2. Rest the patient's forearm comfortably across the abdomen if he or she is supine, or on the arm of the chair if he or she is sitting in a chair, with the palm facing down. ***The pulse is easier to detect if the patient's arm muscles are relaxed. The palm-down position allows you to place your hand on top of the wrist and easily curve your fingers around the radius to access the radial pulse.***
3. Gently grasp the wrist, placing the first and second fingertips over the radial artery. Apply slight pressure until a recurring pulse is felt.

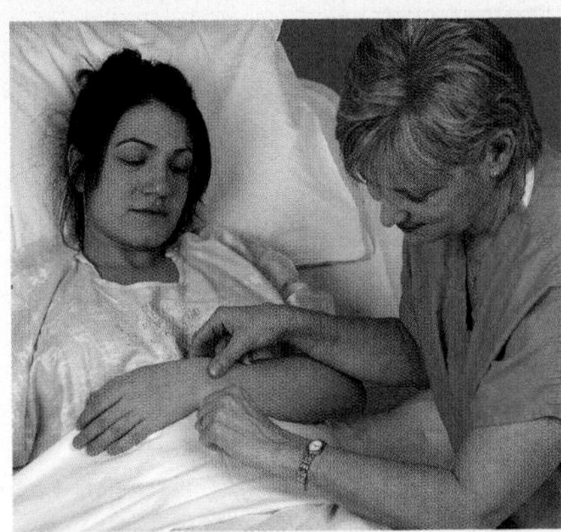

4. While observing the second hand of your watch, count the pulse for 60 seconds, noting any irregularity and volume or strength of pulse. *Safety: An experienced nurse can count the rate for 15 seconds and multiply times four, or count the rate for 30 seconds and multiply times two. However, as a student, you should always assess the pulse for a full minute until you have more experience. This will help to prevent errors because of subtle irregularities that may not be detectable by an inexperienced student. Even experienced nurses should count the pulse for a full minute if there are any irregularities.*
5. Follow the Ending Implementation Steps located on the inside back cover.

Apical Pulse

2. Elevate the head of the bed or have the patient sit upright and lean forward slightly, unless contraindicated, ***to better position the heart against the anterior chest wall for easier auscultation.***
3. Being careful to preserve the patient's modesty, loosen the patient's gown to allow access to the left side of the chest. Palpate the fifth intercostal space on the left side of the sternum. Do this by palpating the angle of Louis (felt as a prominence between the top of the sternum and the body of the sternum, two to three fingerbreadths below the suprasternal notch). Move a fingertip to the left of the sternal prominence, into the second intercostal space. Placing a finger in each space, count down to the fifth intercostal space. Walk your fingers laterally to the midclavicular line. Palpate for the PMI. ***The apical pulse of most adults will be located in the fifth space but may vary and be located in either the fourth or sixth space.***
4. Place the bell of the stethoscope directly on the skin, over the PMI. ***This is the point where the heart contraction is felt, making it easier to hear the apical pulse clearly.*** If you do not hear the apical pulse clearly using the bell, you may want to use the flat diaphragm to see if this helps.
5. Listen to determine that both S_1 and S_2 are detected and note the strength or volume of both sounds by determining whether the S_1 or S_2 sound is muffled, distant, or distinct. Also note any third or fourth extra sounds. Listen to the rhythm, noting any irregularities and whether they are "regular irregularities," such as a skip every fifth beat.
6. Count the rate for a full minute. This is always the length of time used when auscultating the apical pulse. It helps to better detect any arrhythmias.
7. While continuing to auscultate the apical pulse, palpate the radial pulse with your free hand. Feel and listen concurrently for another minute to determine that the radial and apical pulses are the same, without a pulse deficit. If there is a difference in the two pulse rates, solicit help from a second nurse. One nurse then counts the apical pulse while the second nurse counts the radial pulse concurrently for 1 minute, using the same watch second hand. Document both rates and the amount of the difference (pulse deficit).
8. Rearrange the patient's gown and position for comfort.
9. Record pulse rate, rhythm, and strength or volume for use in later documentation.
10. Follow the Ending Implementation Steps located on the inside back cover.
11. Document pulse rate and characteristics on a graphic sheet and in the nurse's notes.

Evaluation Steps

1. Evaluate whether the findings are consistent with the patient's condition and any expected therapeutic effects of prescribed medications.
2. Determine if further action needs to be taken.
3. Report abnormal findings according to facility policy.

Sample Documentation

05/17/22 2215 Apical pulse - 84, regular and distinct. No pulse deficit. ————
———— *Nurse's signature and credentials*

06/11/22 1430 Apical pulse - 76, regular and distinct. Radial pulse - 69, irregular and weak. Pulse deficit of 7 beats per minute. ————
———— *Nurse's signature and credentials*

Skill 17.3 Assessing Peripheral Pulses

Assessment Steps

1. Review the patient's chart for previous findings and any record of a disease process that may affect the strength and equality of peripheral pulses.

Planning Steps

1. Plan to use Doppler ultrasound if any pulse is not palpable.

Implementation Steps

1. Follow the Initial Implementation Steps located on the inside back cover.
2. As you palpate each pulse, be sure to palpate both left and right pulses and compare the strengths.
   - ***Temporal pulse:*** Using two fingertips, palpate over the temple area, lateral and superior to the eye. Some facilities do not require that the temporal pulse be assessed as part of the peripheral pulses.

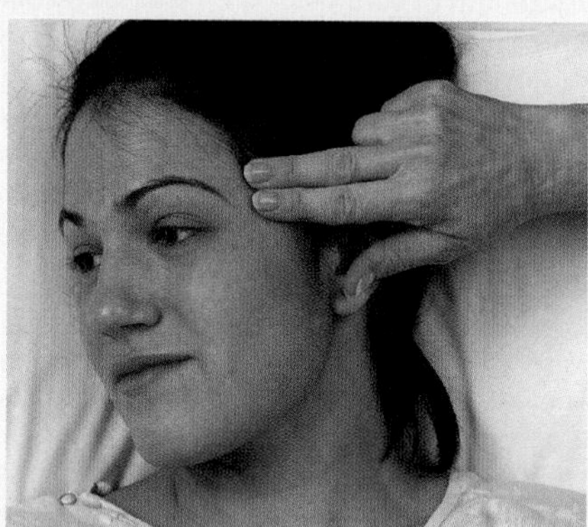

- ***Carotid pulse:*** Using two fingertips, gently palpate to the side of the trachea, in the depression between the trachea and sternocleidomastoid muscle on the side of the neck. *Safety: NEVER palpate both carotids simultaneously or press hard enough to impair blood flow to the brain, because this has been known to result in a stroke.*

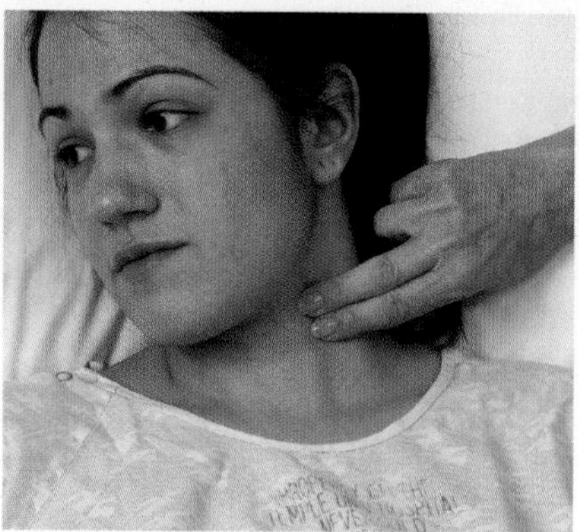

- ***Brachial pulse:*** Using two fingertips, palpate the brachial artery in the antecubital area.

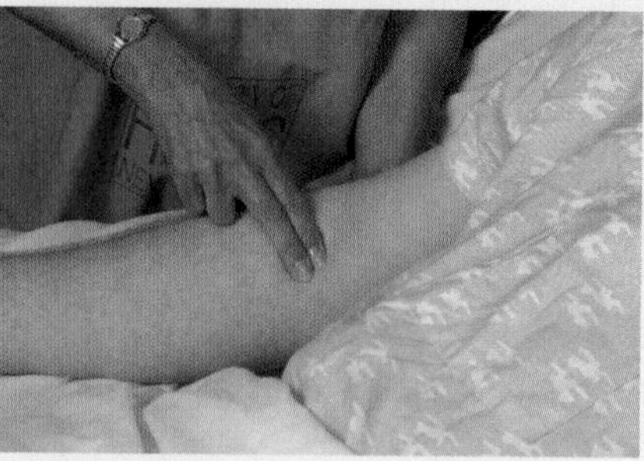

- ***Radial pulse:*** Using two fingertips, palpate the radial pulses in both wrists.

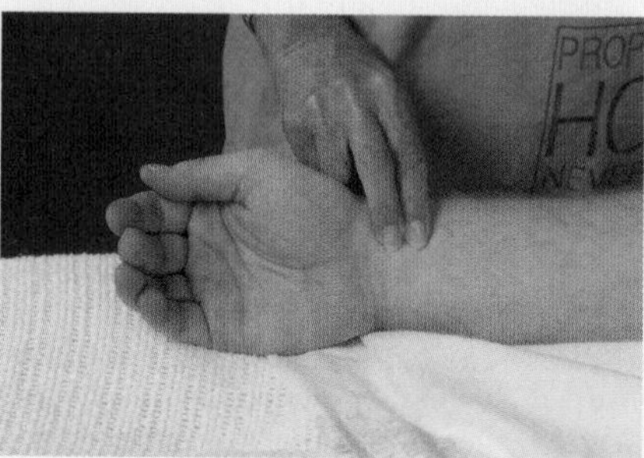

Note: If assessing peripheral pulses only to determine adequate circulation to the extremities, it may not be necessary to count the rate. There may not be a need to palpate the more proximal brachial pulses if the more distal radial pulses both are strong.

- ***Femoral pulse:*** Using two or three fingertips, palpate firmly in the midline of the groin crease. ***This pulse is deeper than most pulses.***

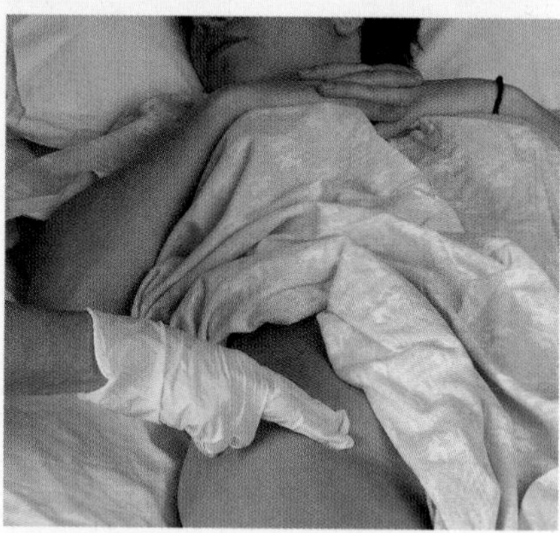

- ***Popliteal pulse:*** Using two or three fingertips, palpate behind the knee in the middle of the popliteal fossa.

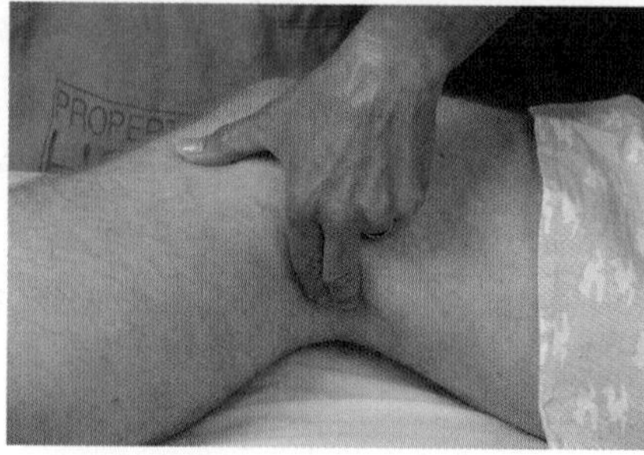

Skill 17.3 (continued)

- ***Posterior tibialis pulse:*** Place two or three fingertips on the medial aspect of the ankle, just below the malleolus.

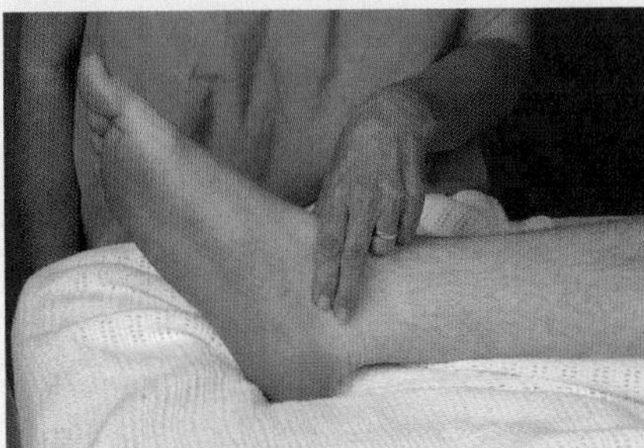

- ***Dorsalis pedis pulse:*** Place two or three fingertips gently on the dorsal aspect of the foot, on a line extending from between the great toe and the second toe. Follow the groove between the extensor tendons proximally until the pulsation is felt over the dorsal surface of the foot.

Note: If assessing peripheral pulses only to check circulation to the extremities, there may be no need to palpate the more proximal femoral and popliteal pulses if the more distal dorsalis pedis or posterior tibialis pulse is strong.

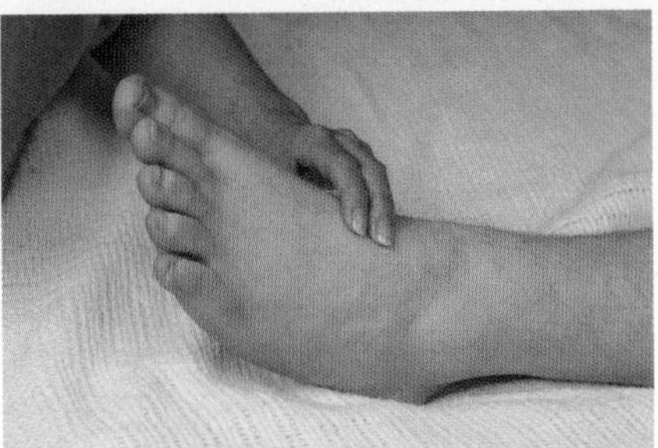

3. Record pulse rhythm and equality of strength for use in later documentation. ***This improves accuracy in documentation.***
4. Follow the Ending Implementation Steps located on the inside back cover.
5. Document pulse characteristics on the flow sheet or in the nurse's notes as soon as possible.

Evaluation Steps

1. Evaluate if distal peripheral pulse findings were within the patient's range of normal and are consistent with the patient's condition.
2. Report abnormal findings that are inconsistent with the patient's condition.

Sample Documentation

05/03/22 1730 Radial and pedal peripheral pulses strong and equal bilaterally. ———————— Nurse's signature and credentials

Skill 17.4 Using Doppler Ultrasound to Assess Nonpalpable Pulses

Assessment Steps

1. Assess the need for use of Doppler ultrasound. ***If pulses are palpable, the use of Doppler is not required. If pulses are not palpable, Doppler is used to determine adequate circulation to an extremity.***

Planning Steps

1. Obtain a Doppler ultrasound machine and transmission gel. Check the low battery light on the Doppler. ***Being prepared saves time and effort.***

Implementation Steps

1. Follow the Initial Implementation Steps located on the inside back cover.
2. Apply a small dab of transmission gel over the pulse site to be assessed or to the transducer probe on the Doppler. ***This improves the clarity of sound.***
3. Turn on the Doppler.
4. Using only light pressure, hold the transducer probe against the skin over the pulse site. Move the transducer probe only enough to locate the strongest pulse sound.

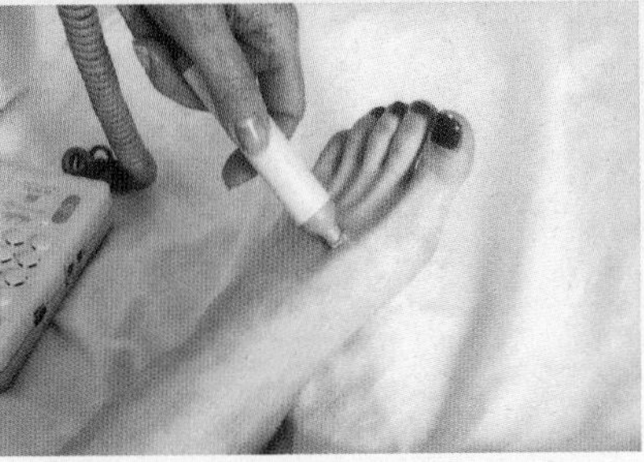

5. After assessing the pulse, clean the gel from the patient's skin and from the transducer probe with a dry cloth or tissue. Then clean the transducer probe surface with a damp cloth only. ***Harsh chemicals will damage the transducer.***
6. Follow the Ending Implementation Steps located on the inside back cover.
7. Document the pulse and the need to use Doppler ultrasound in the nurse's notes.

(skill continues on page 336)

Skill 17.4 (continued)

Evaluation Steps

1. Evaluate if the pulse findings were within the patient's range of normal and consistent with the patient's condition.
2. Report that a pulse was obtainable only with Doppler ultrasound.

Sample Documentation

01/14/22_1845_Unable to palpate left pedal pulse. Doppler used to obtain rate of 80. Left foot pink & warm, with 3-second capillary refill. ———————— Nurse's signature and credentials

Skill 17.5 Assessing Respirations

Assessment Steps

1. Review the patient's chart for the previous range of respirations and disease conditions that might influence respiratory efforts.

Planning Steps

1. Plan to wait 5 minutes after physical activity by the patient before beginning assessment.

Implementation Steps

1. Follow the Initial Implementation Steps located on the inside back cover.
2. Position the patient in the supine or sitting position. Grasp his or her wrist as you would if you were assessing the radial pulse. Position the arm across the patient's abdomen or chest. ***This distracts the patient from your assessment of his or her respirations.***

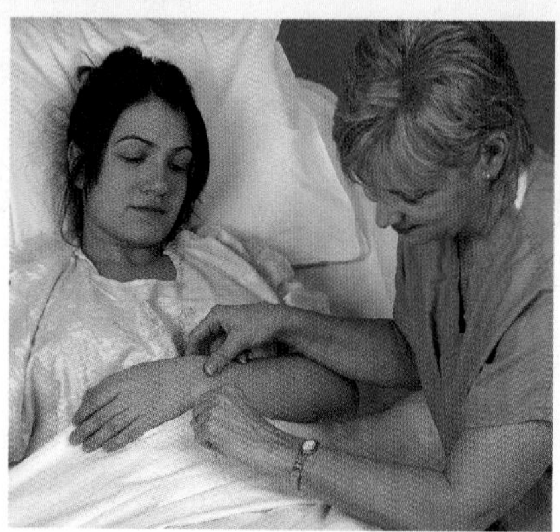

3. While observing the passage of 1 minute on your watch, observe the rise and fall of the patient's chest, counting an inhalation and expiration as one complete breath. Count the rate of respiration for 1 full minute, noting rhythm, depth, and effort. *Safety: An experienced nurse can count the rate for 15 seconds and multiply times four, or count the rate for 30 seconds and multiply times two. As a student, you should always assess the respirations for a full minute until you have more experience. This will help to prevent errors because of subtle irregularities that may not be detectable by an inexperienced student.*
4. Write down the rate, rhythm, depth, and effort for use in later documentation.
5. Follow the Ending Implementation Steps located on the inside back cover.
6. Document respiratory rate on a graphic sheet and the rate, rhythm, depth, and effort in the nurse's notes.

Evaluation Steps

1. Evaluate if respiration findings were within the patient's range of normal and consistent with the patient's condition.
2. Report abnormal findings according to facility policy.

Sample Documentation

12/03/22 0315 R - 16 regular, shallow, effortless. Skin pink. SpO_2 - 97% on room air. ———————— Nurse's signature and credentials

Skill 17.6 Assessment of Blood Pressure

Assessment Steps

1. Determine when and how frequently to take the patient's BP.
2. *Safety: Assess if there is a contraindication to taking the BP on either arm.* If the patient has undergone a mastectomy or removal of the lymph nodes, or has a hemodialysis shunt or an IV infusion on either side, that side should not be used for BP assessment. If both arms are contraindicated, assess the BP in the thigh using a thigh cuff.
3. Assess which size BP cuff is needed. ***It should cover two-thirds of the arm circumference (distance around the arm) to obtain an accurate BP.***
4. Review the range of BP readings recorded in the patient's chart. ***This shows the BP trend, which helps to indicate how high to inflate the cuff.***

Planning Steps

1. Gather supplies: sphygmomanometer with a cuff and stethoscope. *Safety: Clean the stethoscope earpieces and chest piece with alcohol. If the facility does not use individual patient BP cuffs that are left in each patient's room, clean the multiuse cuff with the facility's approved disinfectant to prevent cross-contamination. Being prepared saves time and effort.*
2. Unless it is an emergency, plan to allow the patient at least 5 minutes of inactivity and at least a 30-minute interval between smoking or consumption of caffeine and BP assessment. ***This allows the BP to stabilize after the hemodynamic changes caused by physical movement and stimulants such as caffeine or nicotine.***

Implementation Steps

1. Follow the Initial Implementation Steps located on the inside back cover.
2. Support the patient's arm at the level of his or her heart with the palm facing upward. ***The BP may erroneously increase by as much as 20 mm Hg if the arm is not supported.***
3. Roll or push up the sleeve of the patient's gown to expose the bare upper arm ***for more accurate placement of the cuff.***
4. Snugly wrap the cuff around the upper arm, centering the inflatable bladder over the brachial artery. If using the forearm, center the arrow over the radial artery. Position the bottom edge of the cuff approximately 1 inch above the antecubital space in an adult and less than 1 inch in a child. Make certain the gauge is attached to the cuff or positioned at the same height as the cuff. ***The center of the cuff bladder must be positioned over the brachial artery to obtain an accurate reading. Placing it 1 inch above the antecubital space leaves room for placement of the stethoscope diaphragm. The gauge position can affect the accuracy of the reading.***
5. Close the screw valve by turning it clockwise ***to direct the air into the cuff bladder.*** If this is the ***first*** assessment of BP on this patient, use Step 6, the palpation step, to determine how high to inflate the cuff. If recent measurements of BP were recorded in the chart or you have assessed it yourself previously, the palpation step is not required and you may skip to Step 7 (unless the BP is variable).
6. Palpate the brachial pulse with two fingertips while rapidly compressing the bulb to inflate the cuff to 80 mm Hg. Then slowly continue inflating the cuff 10 mm Hg at a time until the pulse is no longer palpable. Make a mental note of the number at which the pulse was lost so that you will know how high to inflate the cuff when you assess the BP, which will be 20 to 30 mm Hg higher than the point where you could no longer palpate the pulse. Then screw the valve counterclockwise and quickly deflate the cuff. ***This helps to indicate how high to pump the cuff.***
7. Wait 2 minutes before reinflating the cuff, allowing arm veins to refill.
8. Place the stethoscope earpieces into your ears with the angle of the earpieces pointing toward your face. This positions the earpieces correctly within the ear canals so that ***sounds can be heard more clearly.*** Place the chest piece over the brachial artery. If you are using the bell, apply gentle pressure to hold the stethoscope in place. If you are using the flat diaphragm, press more firmly until a seal is made with the skin. ***This makes it easier to hear Korotkoff's sounds.***

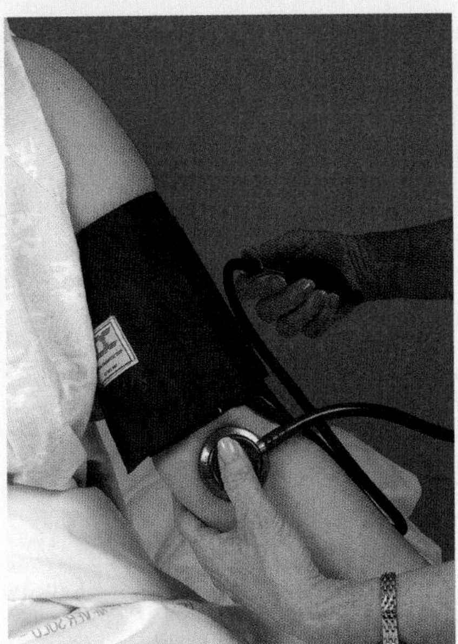

9. Screw the valve clockwise to close it; ***this allows air to enter the cuff bladder.*** Compress the bulb until the cuff is inflated to the desired number.
10. Slowly turn the screw valve counterclockwise, letting the cuff deflate 2 to 3 mm Hg per second while you listen for the first Korotkoff sound. ***If you deflate the cuff too rapidly, you may miss the first sound, causing the BP to appear to be lower than it really is.***
11. Make note of the number at which the first sound is heard and continue to listen as the cuff slowly deflates. Note the number at which the last sound is heard. Make certain that there are no further sounds for 10 to 15 mm Hg.
12. Deflate the cuff rapidly and completely. ***This allows restoration of circulation to the arm.***
13. Remove the cuff and straighten the patient's gown.
14. Record in your pocket notes the BP and any auscultatory gap detected. Transcribe it to the chart as soon as possible.
15. Follow the Ending Implementation Steps located on the inside back cover.
16. Document BP on a graphic sheet in the nurse's notes and in the patient's care plan. ***By graphing the BP, trends as well as any abnormal values may be identified.***

(skill continues on page 338)

Skill 17.6 (continued)

Evaluation Steps

1. Evaluate if BP is within the patient's expected range. Is the BP elevated? Is it dangerously low?
2. Report abnormal BP findings according to facility policy.

Sample Documentation

08/03/22 1600 BP – 114/66 in left arm, supine. ——— ——— Nurse's signature and credentials

Skill 17.7 Assessment for Orthostatic Hypotension

Assessment Steps

1. Review the range of BP readings recorded in the patient's chart so that you know how high to inflate the cuff. ***This helps to indicate how high to pump the cuff and whether the patient requires assessment for orthostatic hypotension.***
2. *Safety: Assess if there is a contraindication to taking the BP on either arm.* If the patient has undergone a mastectomy or removal of the lymph nodes, or has a hemodialysis shunt or IV infusion on either side, that side should not be used for BP assessment. If both arms are contraindicated, assess the BP in the thigh using a thigh cuff.
3. Assess which size BP cuff is needed. Make certain the inflatable bladder width covers two-thirds of the upper arm. ***A cuff that is too small will produce a falsely elevated reading, and one that is too large will result in a falsely low pressure.***

Planning Steps

1. Gather supplies: sphygmomanometer with a cuff and stethoscope. *Safety: Clean the stethoscope earpieces and chest piece with alcohol. If the facility does not use individual patient BP cuffs that are left in the patient's room, clean the multi-use cuff with the facility's approved disinfectant to prevent cross-contamination. Being prepared saves time and effort.*
2. Unless it is an emergency, plan to allow at least 5 minutes of inactivity once the patient is placed in the supine position and at least 30 minutes following smoking or consumption of caffeine before assessing BP. ***This allows stabilization of BP after the hemodynamic changes that occur with movement and stimulants such as caffeine and nicotine.***

Implementation Steps

1. Follow the Initial Implementation Steps located on the inside back cover.
2. Place the patient in the supine position and wait 5 minutes before taking BP. ***This allows the pressure to stabilize after activity.***
3. Support the patient's arm at the level of his or her heart with the palm facing upward. ***Positioning the arm above or below the heart level may cause an inaccurate BP measurement.*** Avoid allowing the patient to hold up his or her own arm; ***tensing of the arm muscles will raise the systolic pressure.***
4. Roll or push up the sleeve of the patient's gown to expose the bare upper arm. ***This provides better visualization of the antecubital area for placement of the stethoscope. Also, the BP reading is more accurate when performed directly on bare skin as opposed to taking it over layers of fabric.***
5. Snugly apply the cuff to the upper arm as for assessment of BP. ***A cuff applied too loosely will result in a false elevation in the BP measurement.***
6. Close the screw valve by turning it clockwise. ***This prevents air from escaping from the cuff as the bulb is pumped.***
7. Palpate to locate the patient's brachial pulse. ***Placement of the stethoscope diaphragm directly over the brachial pulse produces a louder, clearer BP.***
8. Rapidly inflate the BP cuff approximately 20 to 30 mm Hg above the point at which you can no longer palpate the brachial pulse. ***The artery is now occluded, preventing blood from flowing into the distal arm.***
9. Slowly unscrew the valve, allowing the cuff to deflate. Note the reading at which you once again are able to feel the brachial pulse. ***This is known as the palpated systolic pressure, which should be slightly lower than the auscultated systolic pressure.*** Then rapidly deflate the cuff completely. This allows the blood trapped in the veins to be released and restores arterial circulation to the distal arm.
10. Place the stethoscope earpieces in your ears directed toward your face. ***Sound is better transmitted when the earpieces follow the direction of the ear canals.***
11. Place the chest piece over the brachial artery. Make certain the stethoscope hangs free from your ears and does not touch the bed or linens. ***Allowing the stethoscope to rub against the bed or linens causes noise that can prevent the hearing of Korotkoff's sounds.***
12. Screw the valve clockwise once again ***so that the cuff will hold air.***
13. Compress the bulb until the cuff is inflated to approximately 20 to 30 mm Hg above the palpated systolic pressure. ***This helps to ensure detection of the initial Korotkoff sound.***
14. Slowly turn the screw valve counterclockwise, letting the cuff deflate 2 to 3 mm Hg per second while listening for Korotkoff's sounds.
15. Make note of the number at which the first Korotkoff sound is heard and continue to listen as the cuff slowly deflates. Note the number at which the last Korotkoff sound is heard. Continue to listen for more sounds, allowing the gauge to drop another 10 to 15 mm Hg. ***This helps to ensure accuracy.***
16. Deflate the cuff rapidly and completely. ***This allows circulation to resume to the arm.***
17. Leave the cuff in place on the arm.
18. Record the BP and the patient's position, to be documented in the chart after completion of assessment.
19. Lower the bed and have the patient sit up on the side of bed with his or her feet flat on the floor for 1 minute.
20. Retake the BP while the patient sits upright. ***Normally the pressure should increase just slightly as the cardiovascular system works a little harder to pump blood to the head, which now is higher than the heart.***

Skill 17.7 (continued)

21. Write down the BP and the patient's position, to be documented in the chart after completion of assessment.
22. Assist the patient to stand at the side of the bed and wait for 1 minute. *Safety: Observe the patient for dizziness and assist him or her to bed should it occur.*
23. Retake the BP while the patient is standing.
24. Have the patient sit down on the side of the bed and remove the cuff.
25. Write down the standing BP, to be documented in the chart after completion of assessment.
26. Clean the cuff and wash your hands. ***This helps to reduce cross-contamination. BP cuffs have been shown to carry significant levels of microorganisms.***
27. Follow the Ending Implementation Steps located on the inside back cover.
28. Document the BP on a graphic sheet in the nurse's notes and in the patient's care plan ***to inform other nurses and staff members.***

Evaluation Steps

1. Evaluate if the BP showed a normal pattern of increase:
   - Sitting BP slightly higher than supine BP
   - Standing BP slightly higher than sitting BP
2. Or if the BP dropped 20 mm Hg, showing an abnormal pattern of decrease:
   - From supine BP to sitting BP
   - From sitting BP to standing BP
3. *Safety: If orthostatic hypotension is indicated, instruct the patient to call for assistance before attempting to get out of bed.*
4. Report abnormal findings according to facility policy.

Sample Documentation

03/27/22 1230 Assessed for orthostatic hypotension. Supine BP - 122/76. Sitting BP - 110/68. Standing BP - 98/58. C/O dizziness upon standing. Assisted back to bed. Dizziness abated within 1 min. Instructed to call for assistance before getting out of bed to avoid falls. Verbalized she would be sure to call for help. Bed rails raised times two. Call light within reach. Bed in lowest position. ——————— Nurse's signature and credentials

03/27/22 1250 Dr. Smith phoned with results of BP assessment. New order received to assess BP supine, sitting, & standing every 4 hours. ———————
——————— Nurse's signature and credentials

Skill 17.8 Assessing Oxygen Saturation

Assessment Steps

1. Review the patient's chart for the previous range of SpO_2 and disease conditions that might influence respiratory gas exchange. Assess the patient's hemoglobin level. ***A low hemoglobin level reduces the oxygen-carrying capacity of the blood.***
2. Assess whether the patient has a health-care provider's order for supplemental O_2.
3. Determine which site will be used for the next assessment: fingertip, earlobe, nose, toe, or forehead.

Planning Steps

1. Obtain a pulse oximeter with appropriate sensor to be used for the selected site. Check the low battery light. ***Being prepared saves time and effort.***
2. Plan to assess the SpO_2 with O_2 on (if applicable) or on room air if no supplemental oxygen is being delivered.

Implementation Steps

1. Follow the Initial Implementation Steps located on the inside back cover.
2. If using an extremity, assess the patient's finger or toe for adequate capillary refill to ensure adequate circulation to the site to be assessed. ***A digit without adequate circulation would not provide an accurate oxygen saturation level.***
3. Prepare the site. The site should be clean and dry. Remove the patient's nail polish if you are using a finger or toe for assessment. ***Polish interferes with accurate measurement.***
4. Apply the appropriate sensor to the site that was selected for assessment.

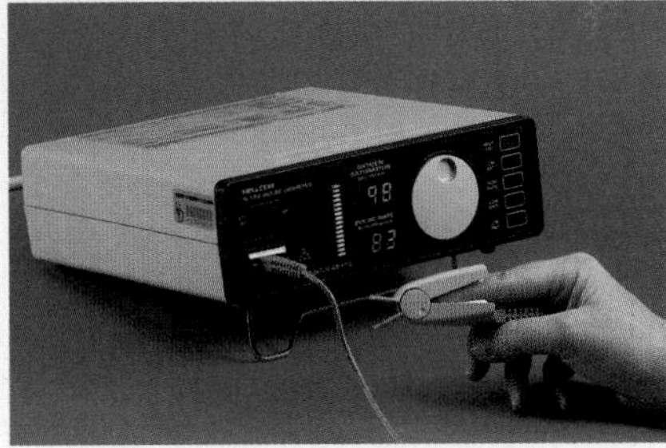

5. Turn on the oximeter and check that preset alarms for high and low SpO_2 are set.
6. Read the digital readout and record for later documentation.
7. Remove the sensor if this is a one-time assessment. If assessment is to be continual, leave the sensor in place. *Safety: Inspect and change the location of the sensor every 2 hours to prevent tissue necrosis from prolonged pressure.*
8. Follow the Ending Implementation Steps located on the inside back cover.
9. Document SpO_2 on a graphic sheet or flow sheet and in the nurse's notes.

(skill continues on page 340)

Skill 17.8 (continued)

Evaluation Steps

1. Evaluate if SpO_2 findings were within the patient's range of normal and consistent with the patient's condition.
2. Report abnormal findings according to facility policy.

Sample Documentation

12/9/22 0845 SpO_2 - 94% on room air. ——— *Nurse's signature and credentials*

12/11/22 0900 SpO_2 - 97% with O_2 @ 2 L/min via NC ——— *Nurse's signature and credentials*

POST CONFERENCE

You provided care for your patient who, according to the automatic vital sign machine, had abnormal vital signs at noon. When evaluating your nursing care, you review the actions you took:

- You reviewed the 8 a.m. vital signs: BP – 126/74 mm Hg, T – 98°F, P – 64, R – 19, SpO_2 – 98% on room air, pain at a 2.
- You compared the 8 a.m. vital signs to those obtained at noon using the automatic vital sign machine, which were BP – 94/46 mm Hg, T – 96.6°F, P – 51, and SpO_2 – 70% on room air, indicating dramatic differences from those obtained at 8 a.m.
- You further assessed the patient and found him to be awake, alert, oriented, and smiling; skin pink, warm, and dry; oral mucosa and nail beds pink; respirations normal depth, regular, and effortless at 13 breaths per minute; and radial pulse regular at strong 69 bpm.
- Because the results from the automatic vital sign machine did not match the rest of your assessment, you performed manual reassessment of vital signs with an aneroid BP cuff, plastic nonmercury thermometer, and portable pulse oximeter, with the following results: BP – 122/78 mm Hg, T – 98.4°F, AP – 69, SpO_2 – 96%.
- Because the newest assessment of vital signs more closely matched the patient's other assessment findings as well as previous vital sign baseline, you determined that the automatic vital sign machine was inaccurate and removed it from use until repairs and calibration could be completed.

This event reinforced in your mind the importance of looking at all of the assessment data and performing manual assessments rather than always depending on automatic vital sign machines or looking at just one piece of data.

Key Points

- There are six vital signs: temperature, pulse, respirations, BP, oxygen saturation, and pain assessment.
- Assess all vital signs every 2 hours or more often depending on the degree of abnormality. Do not encourage the use of covers because they can raise the body temperature. If a patient has a high fever, you can apply a cold washcloth or ice pack wrapped in a washcloth to the forehead or neck and groin.
- The normal range for core temperatures varies from 97°F to 99.6°F (36.1°C to 37.5°C), with the average being 98.6°F (37°C).
- It is important to continuously monitor the patient's temperature. When monitoring temperature, remember to select the best method by ease of use, comfort, and accuracy.
- The peripheral pulse sites include temporal, carotid, brachial, radial, femoral, popliteal, posterior tibialis, and dorsalis pedis (pedal).
- The normal range for the adult pulse is 60 to 100 bpm.
- A scale of 0 to 3 is generally used to assess pulse volume. Depending upon how strong or weak the pulse is will determine if the patient has too much or too little blood or normal.
- Inspiration is when you breathe in, and expiration is when you breathe out. Each respiration consists of one inspiration and one expiration.
- The normal range for adult respirations is 12 to 20 breaths per minute. Age, smoking, exercise, medications, and environmental temperature are all factors that affect the respiratory rate.
- The four circulatory qualities are the strength of the heart contraction, blood viscosity, blood volume, and peripheral vascular resistance. BP is determined by stroke volume and preload.
- The normal ranges for BP in adults are a systolic pressure between 100 and 120 mm Hg and a diastolic pressure between 60 and 80 mm Hg.

- For some individuals, there are BP factors that an individual has no control over. These include heredity, gender, age, and race. Some individuals can control BP by diet, rest, exercise, and hydration.
- Hypertension involves three areas: elevated, primary hypertension, and secondary hypertension. Hypertension begins at a systolic pressure above 130 and diastolic pressure above 80. Hypotension begins at a systolic pressure below 100 and diastolic pressure below 60.
- Pain is normally assessed using a pain scale of 0 to 10 (or other facility-approved scale) for adults and a scale using a series of facial expressions for children.

Review Questions

Select the answer that is most appropriate for each of the following questions. Some questions may have more than one correct answer. Select all that apply.

1. In which of the following situations would it be inappropriate to delegate the vital sign assessment?
   1. Routine vital signs on a patient with pneumonia
   2. A patient whose level of consciousness has gone from alert to responding only to pain stimuli
   3. A teenager admitted with influenza A whose temperature 2 hours ago was 100.6°F orally
   4. A confused and lethargic patient brought to the emergency room after being involved in an automobile accident
   5. An adult patient who becomes diaphoretic and pale and complains of sudden onset of severe left chest pain while ambulating in the hallway

2. Which of the following objective vital signs, all taken on adults, have one or more components that fall outside of typical normal ranges?
   1. BP – 118/66 mm Hg, T – 99.2°F, P – 74 regular and strong, R – 17, O_2 sats – 99%
   2. BP – 98/62 mm Hg, T – 98.2°F, P – 98 regular and strong, R – 20, O_2 sats – 97%
   3. BP – 142/92 mm Hg, T – 98.4°F, P – 62 regular and bounding, R – 14, O_2 sats – 96%
   4. BP – 120/74 mm Hg, T – 100.6°F, P – 86 regular and strong, R – 24, O_2 sats – 98%

3. Uncontrolled hypertension can result in permanent damage of which organs?
   1. Heart and eyes
   2. Pancreas and spleen
   3. Large intestine and skeletal structures
   4. Brain and kidneys
   5. Urinary bladder

4. You must assess the temperature of an 89-year-old female who is confused, hostile, and combative. Which route would be most appropriate to use?
   1. Rectal
   2. Oral
   3. Temporal
   4. Axillary

5. Upon assessing the vital signs of a 56-year-old male, you find that he has an apical pulse of 71 bpm and a radial pulse of 62 bpm. Which of the following numbers would be correct to document as the pulse deficit?
   1. 0
   2. 3
   3. 7
   4. 9
   5. 133

6. A 68-year-old African American female is admitted for hypertension. She is at risk for hypertension based on which of the following?
   1. Smoking
   2. Obesity
   3. Lower cholesterol level in the blood
   4. Moderate to heavy alcohol consumption
   5. Low stress level

7. The nurse would refrain from taking a BP on which of the following areas?
   1. Amputation of the arm
   2. Mastectomy on the affected side
   3. IV infusion on the selected sites
   4. Presence of a shunt

8. The disadvantages of the oral and skin temperatures assessment routes for an adult patient include which of the following?
   1. Risk of body fluid exposure
   2. Affected by severe environmental temperatures
   3. Not affected by smoking
   4. Not for confused or unconscious patients

ANSWERS 1. 2, 4, 5. 2. 3, 4. 3. 1, 4. 4. 3. 5. 4. 6. 1, 2, 4. 7. 1, 2, 3, 4. 8. 1, 2, 4

Critical Thinking Exercise

Answers available online.

1. Enumerate possible vital signs and other findings that might indicate a patient has impaired circulation.

Additional Resources

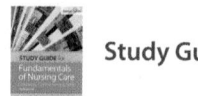

DAVIS edge Use the scratch off code on the inside front cover of your book to access online quizzes that will help you to improve your scores on course exams and prepare for the NCLEX-PN®.

Study Guide

CHAPTER 18

Applying Heat and Cold Therapies

Patricia Perryman

KEY TERMS

Aquathermia pad (ah-kwa-THUR-mee-ah PAD)
Cellulitis (sell-yoo-LYE-tiss)
Contraindication (KON-truh-in-di-KAY-shun)
Deep venous thrombosis (DEEP VEE-nus throm-BOH-siss)
Edema (uh-DEE-muh)
Hemostasis (HEE-moh-STAY-siss)
Indication (IN-di-KAY-shun)
Interstitial space (IN-ter-STISH-uhl SPAYSE)
Metabolism (muh-TAB-uh-lizm)
Pallor (PAL-or)
Permeable (PER-mee-ah-buhl)
Phagocytosis (FAG-oh-sye-TOH-siss)
Phlebitis (fle-BYE-tiss)
Rebound phenomenon (REE-bownd fe-NOM-e-non)
Tepid (TEP-id)
Vasoconstriction (VAY-zoh-kon-STRIK-shun)
Vasodilation (VAY-zoh-dye-LAY-shun)
Vessel lumen (VESS-uhl LOO-min)

CHAPTER CONCEPTS

Patient-Centered Care
Comfort

LEARNING OUTCOMES

1. Define various terms associated with applying heat and cold.
2. Contrast the physiological effects of local heat and cold applications.
3. Identify at least four uses for heat therapy.
4. Explain how application of heat can support healing.
5. Detail the nursing assessments to make prior to, during, and after application of heat therapy.
6. Describe a minimum of three interventions for cold therapy.
7. Compare the methods of heat and cold application.
8. Summarize the nursing assessments pertinent to cold applications.
9. Teach a patient how to make a simple cold pack using only a washcloth and a zip-type plastic bag.
10. Perform patient teaching regarding application of heat and cold.
11. Identify appropriate nursing interventions when applying heat and cold to a patient with specified health conditions.
12. Discuss information found in the Connection features in this chapter.
13. Identify specific safety information.
14. Answer questions about the skills in this chapter.

SKILLS

18.1 Application of Dry or Moist Heat
18.2 Application of Aquathermia Pad (K-Pad)
18.3 Administering a Sitz Bath
18.4 Application of Cold Packs

CRITICAL THINKING CONNECTION

Clinical Assignment

You will be caring for a 72-year-old female who has developed sepsis due to a bladder infection. She has an overwhelming infection in her bloodstream. Her temperature has been spiking to 103.8°F (39.8°C). The health-care provider has ordered a cooling blanket to be applied when the patient's temperature exceeds 104°F (40.0°C).

Continued

CRITICAL THINKING CONNECTION—cont'd

Critical Thinking Questions:

1. Describe how to correctly apply a cooling blanket.
2. How would you monitor the patient's temperature while she is on the blanket?
3. Identify parameters to use when maintaining the blanket.
4. How do you tell if the patient is becoming too cold?
5. How would you intervene if the cold therapy is causing injury to the patient's skin?

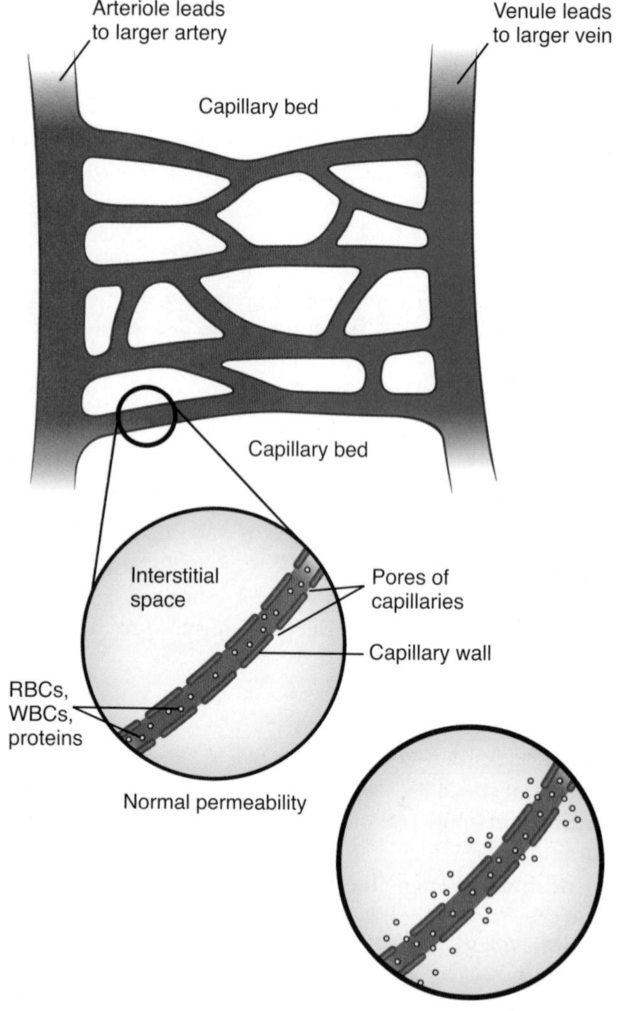

FIGURE 18.1 Vasodilation and increased permeability.

The terms *heat* and *cold* probably seem basic and nonthreatening to you. The concepts behind the terms are simple, but the effects that heat and cold can have on the body tissues and their functions are dramatic.

When we refer to environmental heat and cold, meaning the effects of weather, excessive exposure can result in severe trauma or death. In smaller, controlled doses, heat and cold are used as therapeutic applications to specific parts of the body for both local and systemic effects. The local effects of heat and cold applications impact the body's cutaneous layers where the heat or cold is applied, including the underlying subcutaneous tissue, muscles, and vascular structures, as well as their functions. Systemic effects of heat and cold involve more than a specific area and can affect all body systems. An example of this would be raising body temperature with the application of warm packs or a warm bath.

In this chapter, you will develop a better understanding of the uses and benefits of these therapies and the complications that can result if safety measures are not carried out. You will also learn how to correctly apply various heat and cold therapies and to make appropriate assessments pertinent to each.

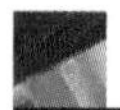

HEAT THERAPY

The local application of heat to an area of the body results in **vasodilation** of the blood vessels underlying the area (Fig. 18.1). This means there is an increase in the size of the cavity or space inside the blood vessel, known as the **vessel lumen,** allowing for an increased flow of oxygenated and nutrient-rich blood to the site. The pores in the capillary walls also become more **permeable,** which means they open wider. This allows increased passage of plasma, oxygen-carrying red blood cells, nutrients, and white blood cells from the capillaries into the spaces between cells, known as the **interstitial spaces,** and to the cells themselves.

Indications for Heat Therapy

Most circumstances require a health-care provider's order for application of heat therapy. Some facilities provide standing procedures regarding heat application. Some facilities allow nurses to apply a warm compress in specific situations, such as inflammation of a vein due to IV therapy, a condition known as **phlebitis.** It is your responsibility to be familiar with your employer's policies and procedures regarding heat application. Unless there is a standing order or protocol for the procedure, be certain to obtain an order from the health-care provider.

There are numerous **indications** for heat therapy, or situations in which it should be used, including:

- Relaxation of muscle spasms,
- Pain relief,
- Support of the healing process,
- Reduction of edema once it has stabilized (stopped increasing), and
- Elevation of body temperature.

• WORD • BUILDING •

subcutaneous: sub – under + cutaneous – skin
vasodilation: vaso – blood vessel + dilation – expansion
phlebitis: phleb – vein + itis – inflammation

Relaxation of Muscle Spasms and Pain Relief

Heat therapy relaxes muscles that are in spasm, such as tight or tense muscles that might result from driving an automobile for a long distance or standing for extended periods of time at work. For example, the use of a hot tub or whirlpool bath often relieves the tired and sore muscles of a snow skier on a once-a-year vacation.

Support of the Healing Process

When heat is applied to an inflamed site, the resulting increased blood flow delivers adjunct *phagocytes,* which are defensive white blood cells, to the wound site. These defensive white blood cells perform **phagocytosis,** meaning they surround, engulf, and digest the offending microorganisms and debris in the cells and exudate, which helps to prevent infection. The increased blood flow delivers the extra oxygen and nutrients that are needed to support the increased **metabolism,** or the chemical and physical processes required to build and maintain body tissues. Without the increased metabolism, the tissue does not heal properly in a timely manner.

Reduction of Edema

Sometimes an acute injury results in a large amount of edema, such as you might see with a sprained ankle. **Edema** is the term for swelling that occurs when excessive fluid leaves the vascular system and remains in the interstitial spaces. This presence of extra fluid in a space where it does not normally reside increases the pressure on nerve endings, resulting in pain and discomfort. Applying heat at this stage of inflammation will simply increase the amount of swelling and therefore is contraindicated. After 48 to 72 hours, once the edema stabilizes, heat may then be applied to dilate the capillaries and veins so that they can carry away the excess fluid, thus reducing the edema.

Elevation of Body Temperature

Application of heat is helpful in raising the body temperature for comfort as well as for patients with *hypothermia*, a condition that occurs when an individual's core temperature drops below 95°F (35°C). Warm packs and warming blankets may be used to help the patient feel warmer and raise lowered body temperatures. In extreme cases of hypothermia, the health-care provider may even order an intravenous infusion of warm normal saline to help raise the body temperature.

Contraindications for Heat Therapy

Although heat is appropriate therapy for the above-listed indications, there are certain **contraindications** for heat therapy, or situations in which heat should not be used. If heat is used in a situation in which it is contraindicated, it may result in harm or damage. For example, if heat is used on new injuries, it will result in more edema than would normally occur with the injury. Thus, heat is contraindicated and should never be used on new trauma or damage to tissue. Further contraindications for heat therapy are listed in Box 18.1.

Box 18.1

Contraindications to Heat Applications

Heat applications should be used judiciously because there are specific situations and conditions in which it is unwise or actually detrimental to apply heat. This list is not all-inclusive.

- **Suspected appendicitis:** Use of heat therapy to the right lower abdomen during acute appendicitis could cause enough increased blood flow to the area to result in a ruptured appendix.
- **Bleeding wound or injury:** Applying heat to a bleeding wound or injury would dilate the vessels, increasing the bleeding.
- **Newly injured joints:** Heat increases edema, making joint mobility more difficult.
- **Large areas of the body in certain cardiac patients:** Extensive heat application can result in massive vasodilation to the superficial skin and subcutaneous layers, depriving the major organs, such as the brain, heart, lungs, and kidneys, of adequate blood supply, which can cause serious damage.

KNOWLEDGE CONNECTION

Explain the physiological effects of local heat application. Describe how application of heat can support the healing process.

Methods of Heat Application

Heat can be delivered as dry or moist heat (see Skill 18.1, page 351). Because water is a better conductor than air, moist heat penetrates quicker and deeper into the tissues than dry heat does. There are numerous methods of delivering heat therapy, including the following:

- Commercial heat packs
- Heating pads
- Aquathermia pads
- Warming blankets

All the above application methods can be used dry or with a moist towel, except the warming blanket, which is dry. Additional methods of applying moist heat include the following:

- Hot compresses
- Soaks
- Sitz baths
- Whirlpool baths

Safety: Never use microwaves to heat compresses because of the dangers of burns.

Local heat application is generally used just long enough for maximum vessel dilation to occur, which is 20 to 30 minutes, and heat is reapplied every 2 to 3 hours as ordered.

Safety: Leaving heat packs in place longer than 45 minutes can cause constriction of vessels instead of dilation, which is known as rebound phenomenon.

• **WORD • BUILDING •**

phagocytosis: phago – eat + cyt – cell + osis – condition

In other words, the treatment results in a worsening of the original condition rather than improving it.

KNOWLEDGE CONNECTION

Identify the duration of heat application and the time between applications to maximize the healing effects. Describe rebound phenomenon.

Commercial Heat Packs

Many companies manufacture easy-to-use heat packs, which are activated by squeezing, striking, or twisting the plastic package. ***Safety: Again, be certain to place some type of cloth barrier between the patient's skin and the heat pack.***

Heating Pads

Electrical heating pads are rarely used in hospitals and long-term care facilities because of the risk of burns. Most facilities require the patient to sign a release of responsibility form before allowing him or her to use a heating pad brought from home. If you do use a heating pad, make sure to use only the low and medium temperature settings to prevent burns. ***Safety: Never place heating pads under the patient because the heat cannot dissipate and may result in a severe burn. Do not apply a heating pad to an infant or a sleeping or confused patient.***

Aquathermia Pads

An **aquathermia pad** (K-pad) is a device with a small, electrically heated water storage tank and two tubes connected to a network of tubing within a disposable pad. The warmed, distilled water is pumped from the storage tank and circulates back and forth between the water tank and the pad (Fig. 18.2). These pads can be used continuously because they can maintain a specific temperature, which reduces the chance of accidental burns.

The temperature of the water is controlled by the temperature dial on the tank and can be set between 98°F (37°C) and 105°F (40.5°C). The most common temperature setting used is 105°F (40.5°C). ***Safety: A key must be used to set the temperature dial to prevent inadvertent changing of the temperature. Monitoring skin for hot spots should be done frequently.***

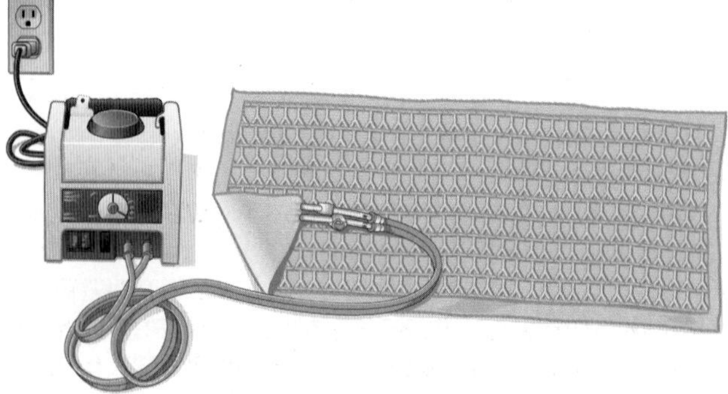

FIGURE 18.2 Aquathermia pads circulate water in the interior of the pad to create a constant temperature (from Wilkinson JM, Treas LS. *Fundamentals of Nursing: Theory, Concepts & Applications.* Vol. 1. 3rd ed. Philadelphia, PA: FA Davis; 2016).

Some K-pads are designed to be used dry; others are made moist by wetting the absorbent outside layer of the pad. The most common uses for a K-pad are treatment of blood clots in the lower leg, a condition known as **deep venous thrombosis,** and inflammation and infection of the skin and underlying tissue, a condition known as **cellulitis.** Make certain that the health-care provider's order includes the temperature setting, whether the pad should be moist or dry, how long the application is to remain in place, and time between heat treatments.

Skill 18.2 (page 352) presents more information on applying an Aquathermia pad.

Warming and Cooling Blankets

There are numerous types of heating blankets, including forced-air warming blankets and water-circulating blankets. Some of these blankets have a temperature setting to gradually raise or lower body temperature as needed.

The most common uses for warming blankets are to warm the body either during surgery or postoperatively and to raise the body temperature of an individual exposed to environmental conditions, such as snow, cold temperatures, or submersion in cold lake water. When the blanket is used as a cooling blanket, the temperature is set to a cooler temperature to reduce high body temperatures due to disease or heat stroke. Depending on their design, warming and cooling blankets may be placed underneath or over the patient, while others are designed to be placed both under and over the patient at the same time. ***Safety: The patient's vital signs and core temperature are constantly monitored while these blankets are in use. Follow the manufacturer's instructions for use and maintenance of these blankets.***

Real-World Connection

How Much Good Can the Application of Heat Really Accomplish?

In the 1980s, in the midst of a freak blizzard in Oklahoma, an ambulance radioed a small rural hospital that they were bringing in a 32-year-old female patient who, the night before, had been beaten unconscious and thrown out of a car into a deep snow drift, where she had lain in single-digit temperatures for approximately 10 to 12 hours wearing only jeans, a shirt, oxford tie shoes, socks, underwear, and a medium-weight parka. Her clothes were snow-laden and frozen solid. Her pulses were not palpable, and respirations were barely discernible. Her apical pulse was faint and irregular. There was no audible or palpable blood pressure, and her temperature registered "below 86°F (30°C)" on the rectal core temperature probe. Her skin was gray and mottled.

Although it was believed that there was little hope for her survival, the nurses and health-care provider teamed up to do everything they could. After removing the patient's frozen clothing, the health-care provider ordered warmed blankets, as this was before warming blankets were widely available, and warmed and humidified oxygen. He also ordered warm wash cloths placed on the top of her head, under both axillae, on each inguinal area, and on both feet. The nurses monitored the patient's level of consciousness, vital signs, and electrocardiogram (EKG) monitor strips continually. The patient remained unresponsive even as her body temperature slowly rose over the next 4 hours to 91°F (32.7°C) and then to 92°F (33.3°C). Within 6 hours, her core temperature finally reached 95°F (35°C), and she was speaking coherently. She suffered some minor frostbite on her fingers, earlobes, and toes, but otherwise she recovered fully within 72 hours. Once the patient was awake and alert, the nurses learned a fact that probably played an important role in her survival: She was a full-blooded Eskimo who had lived all her life in Alaska. She was just in Oklahoma visiting friends when she suffered the life-threatening event.

Hot Compresses

Dip gauze or a cloth in a hot solution (type and temperature ordered by the health-care provider), wring it out, and apply to an inflamed area. Use sterile gloves, supplies, and technique if the skin is not intact. Otherwise, the simple clean technique is adequate. (See Chapter 22 for information regarding sterile technique.)

Warm Soaks

For warm soaks, submerge the patient's body part in a pan of warm water or use a whirlpool with water between 105°F and 115°F (40°C to 46°C). Warm soaks are useful for increasing the circulation to the extremities to aid healing, as is needed with infection of the foot.

Sitz Baths

The sitz bath is a source of comfort, increases blood flow to support healing, and cleanses to aid in prevention of infection. They are commonly used for patients recovering from vaginal childbirth or hemorrhoid surgery. A special plastic basin is filled with warm water and set on the toilet. The bucket or bag is filled with warm water between 105°F and 110°F (40°C to 43°C) and hung 18 to 24 inches (45.7 to 60.9 cm) above the patient's hips. The water drains via tubing that extends to the basin and snaps in place in the bottom of the basin (Fig. 18.3).

After the patient sits down on the basin in the toilet, the tubing is unclamped, which allows warm water to flow into the basin, causing a gentle swirling of warm water to bathe the patient's perineum. This is usually continued for 10 to 15 minutes. The nurse must stay in close proximity of the

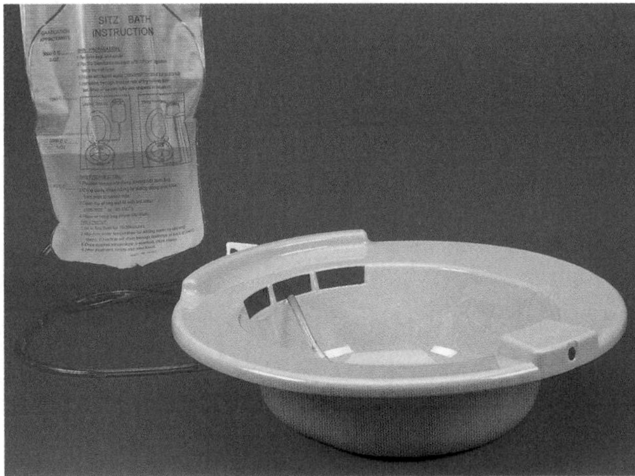

FIGURE 18.3 A sitz bath soaks the patient's perineal area (from Wilkinson JM, Treas LS. *Fundamentals of Nursing: Theory, Concepts & Applications*. Vol. 1. 3rd ed. Philadelphia, PA: FA Davis; 2016).

patient during the first exposure of the sitz bath. The sitz bath causes vasodilation in the perineal area and causes blood to pool in the pelvic region. ***Safety: When the patient stands after completion of the sitz bath, close monitoring is required to make certain the patient does not suffer a drop in blood pressure upon standing.***

This is known as *orthostatic hypotension* and results in decreasing blood flow to the brain, which causes the patient to become faint or fall. The nurse should take a set of orthostatic vital signs to assess for this potential. Skill 18.3 (page 353) provides more information on administering a sitz bath.

Whirlpool Baths

Generally, whirlpool baths are administered by physical therapists, but some facilities such as long-term care facilities delegate use of the whirlpool to nursing. A *whirlpool* is a large stainless steel or porcelain tub with powered jets that circulate the water around the patient. The tub must be filled with water above the level of the power jets before the pump is turned on or water will be sprayed everywhere. The baths are very relaxing and can be used for routine bathing, wound care, debridement, relaxation, or loosening of tight muscles and stiff joints prior to physical therapy treatments. ***Safety: Children and elderly, confused, or sedated patients must NEVER be left alone in a whirlpool tub because the depth of water makes drowning a real risk. Significant vasodilation may occur, and patients must be assessed for orthostatic hypotension.***

A tub or whirlpool is typically used as a source of cleansing for a patient, although they can become the source of serious and even life-threatening infections, known as *health care–associated infections (HAIs)*, which you learned about in Chapter 14. If the tub is not disinfected properly before and after each use, it can become a source for serious contamination. This is a vital step because of the increasing numbers of serious HAIs, such as methicillin-resistant *Staphylococcus aureus*, *Clostridium difficile,* and vancomycin-resistant *enterococcus.* In long-term care facilities, such as nursing homes, whirlpool tubs are commonly used for routine bathing of many residents. Hospitalized patients and the elderly residents in long-term facilities already have decreased immunity and are more susceptible to infection than the average individual. Nurses must work to prevent the transmission of infection to other patients and residents as part of daily nursing care.

KNOWLEDGE CONNECTION

What are the risks of different methods of heat application? Which type of heat penetrates the deepest, dry or moist? Identify the risks associated with the use of whirlpool baths.

Nursing Care During Heat Therapy

Safety: The safety of the patient must be a primary concern during heat therapy. Assess the patient's age, cognitive level of function, orientation, sedation, sensory impairment, and impairment of circulation for risks prior to heat therapy. Certain diseases such as diabetes and peripheral vascular disease impair circulation to the extremities. Patients with these conditions may be more susceptible to burns. Before application of any type of heat therapy, you must assess the patient's skin for temperature, color, sensation, edema, and integrity. Remember that sterile technique must be used for broken skin when applying hot compresses.

Elder Care Connection

The Skin of Seniors Is Fragile

Two populations require extra caution when applying heat therapy: elderly individuals and children. Elderly patients often have reduced tactile sensation due to the loss of touch receptors. Their skin is thinner and drier, making it more susceptible to damage the tissues. ***Safety: The temperature of the heat application should be lowered to a setting between 95°F and 100°F to reduce risk of tissue injury. The skin condition should be assessed more frequently, every 5 to 10 minutes.***

Safety: If using electrical equipment, assess the condition of the equipment and the electrical cord for defects. Do not use cords that are frayed or have a scratched insulation layer, which allows wires to show. Make sure the plug is securely attached to the cord. Make certain that electrical cords are placed where they will not cause someone to trip over them. Advise patients to use heating pads only while they are awake and for no longer than 30 minutes at a time.

Carefully check the temperature of the heating device before applying it to the patient. The temperature setting should be in accordance with the health-care provider's order, usually around 105°F (40.5°C). Instruct the patient to notify the nurse quickly if the heat application becomes too warm. After initiation of the heat therapy, reassess the area and surrounding skin within 5 minutes, noting if the skin is bright red or blistering. Check the site every 10 to 15 minutes until treatment is completed. Skin should be pink or light red, but never bright or dark red. Place the patient's call light within reach before leaving the room. When a K-pad is ordered continuously, assess the site at least hourly.

Safety: Before placing a patient in a whirlpool tub, disinfect the tub thoroughly to prevent cross-contamination from the previous patient. Use a lift to transfer patients in and out of the tub, which will help to prevent falls. Check the temperature of the water and make sure it is not too hot before lowering the patient into the tub. Again, never leave elderly patients, children, patients with diminished mental capacity, or sedated patients alone in a whirlpool tub. Take care to heat the environment to a comfortable temperature to prevent chilling of your patient. Use a bath blanket or towels to appropriately drape your patient during transfer; this provides for modesty as well as warmth preservation.

If using a warming or cooling blanket, be certain to place the blanket either over or under the patient as instructions indicate. Observe the patient temperature monitoring device closely to avoid raising or lowering the temperature too quickly. Monitor the patient's vital signs, level of consciousness, and condition of skin at least every 30 minutes. An EKG monitor is generally applied to observe heart rhythm during systemic heating or cooling.

Always reassess the skin after removal of the heat source to evaluate the patient's response. Ask the patient if the therapy helped. Was the treatment effective? Did it do what you intended? Did it help to reduce discomfort? If it was a whirlpool for wound care, did it débride the wound of all slough and debris? Evaluation of the effectiveness of treatment is always necessary to provide data for use in determining whether the plan of care needs modification.

Patient Teaching Connection

Heating Pad Use Carries Risk

In the home setting, it is more common to use heating pads as the primary source of heat therapy. The patient and family should be taught how to safely apply and monitor the heating pad. Points to include in teaching are:

- ***Safety: Inspect the cord and pad for fraying or bare wires.***
- Assess the site for color and warmth to touch.
- ***Safety: Set a timer for no longer than 20 to 30 minutes.***
- Use a low or medium setting. ***Safety: Avoid the highest setting.***
- Check the skin under and around the heating pad every 10 minutes for excessive redness or signs of blistering.

- ***Safety: Never allow the patient to lie on top of the heating pad or sleep while using it.***
- Avoid use of petroleum products on the skin during heat application.
- Avoid use of a heating pad on a new injury or trauma and on bleeding wounds.
- Avoid use on areas that continue to swell.

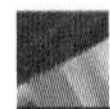

COLD THERAPY

Local application of cold to a site causes **vasoconstriction,** or narrowing, of the veins and capillaries. The pores in the capillary walls become less permeable to the passage of fluid from the vessels to the interstitial space. These processes result in decreased blood flow to the area. When used systemically, cold lowers the body temperature, which slows metabolism. Cooling the body below normal temperature has been used in cardiovascular surgery and neurosurgery to decrease the tissue oxygen demand. This helps preserve heart and brain cells that otherwise might die from lack of oxygen, known as *ischemia,* at normal body temperature and metabolic rate.

Indications for Cold Therapy

A health-care provider's order is required for application of most cold therapies, although it is generally accepted that cold packs may be applied to new localized injuries seen in the emergency room. You should check your facility's policy before using cold therapy without an order. Cold packs are used for prevention of edema, control or stoppage of bleeding, pain relief, numbing of sensation, reduction of muscle spasm, and reduction of fever. Table 18.1 compares and contrasts the effects of cold application versus those of heat application.

Prevention of Edema

Application of cold therapy is generally the treatment of choice for injuries that tend to swell, such as a sprained ankle or bone fractures, or the overuse of a joint, such as in tennis elbow. It is commonly used after joint surgeries and neck and throat surgeries. The vasoconstriction reduces the amount of fluid that leaves the capillaries and leaks into the interstitial space, which results in less edema. Cold therapy is recommended for the first 48 to 72 hours after an injury that can result in swelling.

Hemostasis

The vasoconstriction caused by application of cold also helps to stop active bleeding, or produce **hemostasis.** Cold therapy is useful after trauma, dental surgery, and tonsillectomies, as well as to stop nosebleeds.

Pain Relief

Cold applications are helpful when applied to painful sites such as hemorrhoidectomy or skeletal surgery incisions, perineal lacerations and episiotomies due to childbirth, the forehead and occipital areas for headaches, and the face for sinus congestion pain. Much of the pain relief effects result from the prevention of edema, which causes increased pressure on nerve endings. Many health-care providers have found ice packs effective in helping to relieve migraine headaches, facial pain from temporomandibular joint problems, and chronic back and neck muscular spasms when medications do not.

Numbing Sensation

Application of cold therapy is useful for numbing a particular area, such as to relieve itching of insect bites or allergic rashes. It is also used to relieve the stinging or burning sensation of minor burns such as sunburn.

Reduction of Muscle Spasm

It used to be thought that only heat applications would relieve muscle spasms, but now we know that cold applications also help to interrupt the cycle of muscle tension and spasms. Cold therapy is the treatment of choice if the spasm is acute.

Fever Reduction

When an individual has a fever, the body's metabolism increases, and, as a result, more calories and oxygen are required to maintain the increased metabolism. Once the fever becomes so high that the body cannot provide adequate supplemental calories and oxygen, the brain may suffer permanent damage if the fever is not reduced quickly.

One of the most effective and noninvasive methods of reducing high fever in both children and adults is the application of cold therapy. Ice packs may be placed on the forehead, in the axillae, and on the inguinal areas. The packs cool the blood as it courses through the major vessels to the extremities and through the abundant vascular supply to the face and head. A tepid tub or sponge bath, with water temperature from 65°F to 90°F (18°C to 32.2°C), may also be used, but chilling should be avoided. When the patient is chilled too rapidly, he or she will begin to shiver, which can raise rather than lower body temperature.

For extremely high fevers that do not come down with either of the above methods, the health-care provider may order cold water irrigation, known as *lavage,* of large body cavities such as the stomach or colon. Intravenous infusion of cold normal saline may also be given in an effort to reduce the fever.

KNOWLEDGE CONNECTION

What are five uses of cold therapy? How does local application of cold help with hemostasis? What does systemic cooling of the body do to the basal metabolic rate?

• WORD • BUILDING •

vasoconstriction: vaso – vessel + constriction – squeezing
ischemia: isch – hold back + emia – blood

Table 18.1
Effects of Local Heat and Cold Applications

Heat	*Cold*
Vasodilation	Vasoconstriction
Increases blood flow to site	Decreases blood flow to site, decreasing bleeding
Increases inflammatory response Delivers increased number of red and white blood cells, oxygen, and nutrients to aid healing	Decreases inflammatory response Slows bacterial growth
Increases capillary permeability	Decreases capillary permeability
Increases cellular metabolism	Decreases cellular metabolism
Will *increase* edema if used during the first 48 hours following trauma Will *decrease* edema if used after edema has stabilized	Helps prevent edema
Relaxes muscles	Relaxes muscles
Decreases pain	Decreases pain Numbs sensation

Methods of Cold Application

Cold applications include refillable ice bags or collars, refreezable commercial cold packs, chemical cold packs, cold compresses, and tepid baths (Fig. 18.4). Cold, like heat, can be applied dry or moist. Moisture increases the depth and rate of cold penetration. Skill 18.4 (page 353) provides more information on the application of cold packs.

Refillable Ice Bags, Collars, and Gloves

Refillable ice bags may be made of rubber or waterproof paper, with clamp or foldable closures. Bags should be filled one-half to two-thirds full with ice and some water. Do not overfill the bag or you will find it difficult to mold the bag to the appropriate body part. Then expel the remaining air from the bag and hook the closure.

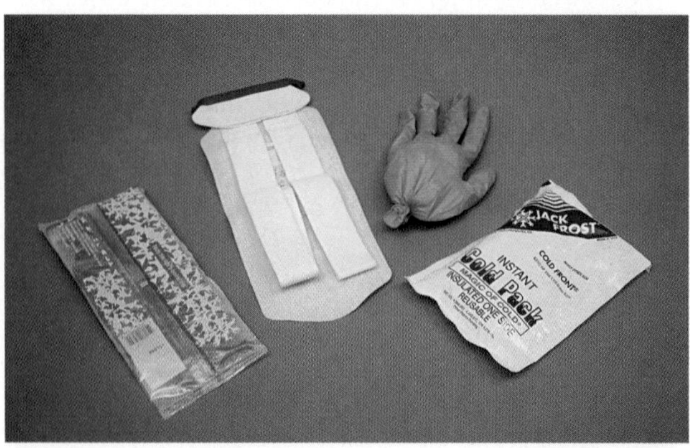

FIGURE 18.4 Cold applications. From left to right: (a) Refreezable gel pack; (b) Disposable refillable ice pack; (c) Small glove-filled ice pack; (d) Instant chemical cold pack.

Some facilities use disposable rubber gloves and fill them with ice. They are secured by tying the glove opening in a knot, as you do a balloon. These smaller ice packs are good for use on the perineum, fingers, and nose, and on small children. Use some type of barrier between the ice bag and the skin to prevent tissue damage.

Refreezable Commercial Cold Packs

These commercial packs are generally filled with a gel-like substance that hardens while remaining malleable when chilled in the freezer. They warm with use, necessitating refreezing after 20 to 30 minutes. The advantage is their ease of use.

Chemical Cold Packs

Chemical cold packs may be smaller than refillable ice bags and must be activated. Instructions for activation are printed on the container and usually require squeezing or twisting the bag until the chemicals mix and become cold. They are only good for one application and then must be discarded.

Cold Compresses

Cold compresses can be made by wetting a folded washcloth, placing it in a zip-type plastic bag, and placing it in the freezer for a short period. Or you may use a bowl of ice water and simply dip the washcloth into the water, wring it out, and apply the washcloth to the site. If the skin is not intact, the compress should be made using sterile water and sterile dressings such as gauze 4×4s.

Tepid Baths

Tepid (cool but not cold) baths are used mostly for reduction of body temperature when use of medication is undesirable or ineffective. Either a tub bath or pan of water for sponging the patient can be used. Reassess temperature every 15 minutes to determine the effectiveness of the intervention. Stop the tepid bath when the body temperature is slightly above normal because the temperature will continue to decrease slightly after completion of the bath. ***Safety: Avoid chilling the patient to the point of shivering, which raises body temperature.*** Tepid baths may be repeated if the body temperature does not adequately come down after 15 minutes.

Nursing Care During Cold Therapy

Assessment of the skin is done prior to application of the cold therapy, noting the integrity, sensation, temperature, and color of the skin. ***Safety: Always use a thin cloth barrier between the ice pack and the patient's skin to prevent frostbite and damage to the tissues.*** Leave cold packs in place no longer than 20 to 30 minutes. When cold therapy is left in place too long, the vasoconstriction continues, depriving tissues of oxygen and nutrients to the point of injury and necrosis. The patient may complain of pain or a burning sensation. If the pack is left in place until skin temperature drops to 60°F, rebound phenomenon may be seen: Vasodilation occurs in an attempt to prevent the tissue damage. ***Safety: Assess the skin for pallor or mottling every 10 to 15 minutes during therapy.*** **Pallor** appears pale or white; mottling occurs in irregular blotches, usually a mixture of pallor and blue or purplish-blue. When using cold therapy for local effect only, the patient may require a blanket to cover the rest of the body, or the room temperature may need to be raised a few degrees to prevent chilling discomfort. Limit time in a tepid bath to 20 to 30 minutes to prevent overcooling to the point of shivering.

Evaluate the effects of the cold therapy. Did it achieve the intended results? Has the bleeding stopped? Did it relieve the pain or reduce the fever? Always assess the patient's response to cold therapy for untoward effects because individuals sometimes react differently than expected. When using cold to reduce fever, be certain to assess the body temperature after 10 minutes of tepid bathing or ice packs.

KNOWLEDGE CONNECTION

Describe the assessments you should make prior to application of cold. How do they differ from assessments during the treatment? What assessments do you make to determine the effectiveness of the cold therapy? How frequently should you reassess body temperature during a tepid sponge bath for fever reduction?

Skill 18.1 Application of Dry or Moist Heat

Assessment Steps

1. Review the health-care provider's order and nurse's note on the last heat application. ***This will help to determine the type of heat delivery device to use and how the patient tolerated the previous treatment.***
2. *Safety: Assess the patient's age and cognitive level of function, orientation, sedation, sensory impairment, and impairment of circulation to determine if there are any contraindications.*
3. *Safety: Assess the site where heat is to be applied, noting the appearance, color, presence of edema, temperature of site and surrounding skin, and integrity of skin, as well as any patient discomfort. This provides a baseline against which you can measure the effects of the application.*

Planning Steps

1. Obtain the correct type of heat delivery device, such as commercial gel, or chemical pack, and a barrier or protective covering such as a towel. ***Planning saves time and effort.***

Implementation Steps

1. Follow the Initial Implementation Steps located on the inside back cover.
2. **If using a commercial gel pack:** *Safety: Follow instructions on the gel pack for heating.*
If using a disposable commercial chemical pack: *Safety: Activate the chemical pack according to pack instructions.*
3. *Safety: Check the temperature against your wrist and allow the patient to test it against his or her wrist to make certain it is not too hot.*
4. *Safety: Apply the heat delivery device to the appropriate site using a dry protective cloth covering or barrier device to prevent burns.* If moist heat is ordered, apply a warm moist towel to the skin. Lay the heat delivery device on the moist towel, making certain it does not directly touch skin, and ***cover the device with a dry towel to help maintain the heat.***
5. After 5 minutes, reassess the site for bright redness of skin to make certain it is not too hot. *Safety: Continue to reassess the skin every 10 to 15 minutes, asking the patient about discomfort. If the skin becomes dark red or bright red or the patient complains that it is too hot, remove the heat pack immediately.* Otherwise, leave the heat pack in place for the ordered length of time.
6. Follow the Ending Implementation Steps located on the inside back cover.
7. Document the condition and each assessment of the skin along with the heat application in the nurse's notes.

Evaluation Steps

1. Remove the heat pack after the appropriate length of treatment. Assess the site for objective data such as color, temperature, and edema.

(skill continues on page 352)

Skill 18.1 (continued)

2. Assess the subjective data related to effectiveness of the heat application by asking the patient about any change in discomfort/comfort level at the site.

Sample Documentation

12/03/22 1430 Complained of sacral discomfort rated a 7 on a scale of 0 to 10. Described it as muscle "tightness." Dry heat applied using disposable chemical pack wrapped in towel to sacral area for 30 minutes as ordered. Skin intact, pink, without edema, warm to touch. States heat seemed to relieve much of the muscle tightness & discomfort down to a 2.
__________ Nurse's signature and credentials

Skill 18.2 Application of Aquathermia Pad (K-Pad)

Assessment Steps

1. Review the health-care provider's order and previous nurse's note. ***This provides needed data, such as temperature setting and the patient's response to the last treatment.***
2. *Safety: Assess the patient's age and cognitive level of function, orientation, sedation, sensory impairment, and impairment of circulation to determine if there are any contraindications.*
3. Assess the patient's discomfort level and assess the site for color, temperature, edema, and integrity of skin. ***This provides a baseline against which to measure effectiveness of treatment.***
4. Examine the K-pad and cord for defects. ***This helps to reduce accidents.***
5. *Safety: Review the manufacturer's instructions for use of the K-pad.*

Planning Steps

1. *Safety: Make certain there is an electrical outlet that can be reached in such a manner that the cord will lay where it will not cause falls.*
2. Obtain the disposable pad that attaches to the K-pad unit and distilled water to fill the tank. ***Preparation saves time and effort.***

Implementation Steps

1. Follow the Initial Implementation Steps located on the inside back cover.
2. Fill the tank to the indicated level with distilled water. Do not overfill.
3. Attach the disposable pad by connecting the two tubes on the pad to those extending from the K-pad unit. ***This allows water to flow from the K-pad unit into the pad.***
4. *Safety: Using the designated key, set the temperature dial to the ordered setting, usually 98°F to 105°F (37° to 40.5°C). This helps to prevent burns.*
5. Allow 10 to 15 minutes for the unit to heat the distilled water that is circulating through the maze of tubes inside the pad. If the health-care provider has ordered "moist" heat, carefully pour several ounces of water on the absorbent side of the pad until the surface is completely moistened. Otherwise, leave the pad dry. ***Moist heat penetrates deeper and quicker than dry heat.***
6. Place the pad on the appropriate body part. If it is ordered on an extremity, secure with ties or wrap it with a towel to help hold it in place. *Safety: Do not use pins. Pins will make holes in the tubes inside the pad.*
7. *Safety: Assess the site every 10 to 15 minutes, noting any changes in the color and temperature of the skin. Ask the patient about any discomfort to make certain the pad is not too hot.*
8. Follow the Ending Implementation Steps located on the inside back cover.
9. Document the condition and each assessment of the skin along with the heat application. Include the temperature at which the K-pad is set.

Evaluation Steps

1. After completion of treatment, evaluate for effectiveness. Did it achieve the desired results? Did it help the problem for which it was applied? Reassess for objective data, including color, temperature, edema, and integrity of skin. Assess subjective data: Did the heat make a difference in how the site felt?

Sample Documentation

04/13/22 0830 Dry K-pad to left lower leg for 30 minutes, temp – 105°F. Skin intact, mildly pink, warm to touch, midcalf measures 17.5 cm compared to right @17 cm. States the calf still aches, a 3 on a scale of 0 to 10. Pedal pulses strong and equal bilaterally. Capillary refill 5 seconds in left and 3 seconds in right foot. __________
__________ Nurse's signature and credentials

Skill 18.3 Administering a Sitz Bath

Assessment Steps

1. *Safety: Determine if this is the patient's first sitz bath or a subsequent sitz bath. If patient has had a previous treatment, review the nurse's note regarding the prior bath to determine how the patient responded. You will need to know if the patient became faint afterward.*

Planning Steps

1. **If using a regular tub:** Prepare the tub by disinfecting it ***to prevent cross-contamination.***

   If using a disposable portable sitz bath: Gather needed equipment and supplies: sitz bath tub, clean gown, two towels, a washcloth, and any other personal items the patient may need. ***Preparation saves time and effort.***
2. Heat the bathroom ***to prevent chilling.***
3. *Safety: Review the manufacturer's instructions for use.*

Implementation Steps

1. Follow the Initial Implementation Steps located on the inside back cover.
2. **If using a regular tub:** Fill the tub approximately 4 to 5 inches deep with warm water between 105°F and 110°F (40.5°C and 43°C). ***The water must be deep enough to adequately cover the perineum.*** *Safety: Water hotter than 110°F (43°C) can burn the patient.*

   If using a disposable sitz bath: *Safety: Fill the water container with warm water between 105°F and 110°F and prime the tubing to remove air from the line.*

   Clamp the tubing. Hang the container on a hook or IV pole to a height approximately 18 to 24 inches above the toilet seat. Insert tubing from the water container through the designated opening in the sitz basin and snap it into grooves in the bottom of the basin. Place the basin on the toilet rim. *Safety: Fill the basin with warm water between 105°F and 110°F.*
3. **For regular tub:** *Safety: Assist patient to get into the tub. This reduces risk of falls.*
   For disposable sitz bath: Assist patient to sit on the toilet and basin with the perineum immersed in the water. Unclamp the tubing and allow water to drain from the water container into the basin. As the basin fills, the excess water will drain through the overflow opening and into the toilet.
4. Make certain the patient does not become chilled. A bath blanket or towel may be draped around his or her shoulders ***for added warmth.***
5. *Safety: Inform the patient to avoid standing unassisted after completion of the sitz bath. Make certain the patient can reach the call light. If this is the first time he or she has used the sitz bath, remain close enough to the bathroom door so that you can be summoned if the patient begins to feel faint.*
6. After completion of the sitz bath, assist the patient to stand and dry off as needed.
   For regular tub: *Safety: Disinfect the tub to reduce risk of cross-contamination.*
   For disposable sitz bath: Clean the basin, dry it, and return it to its storage area. Rinse the water container with cool water. Unclamp the tube and hang it in the shower to drain. ***This leaves the basin ready for the next use.***
7. Follow the Ending Implementation Steps located on the inside back cover.
8. Document the sitz bath in the nurse's notes or on the flow sheet.

Evaluation Steps

1. Assess the perineal area for edema, color, and drainage, and ask the patient about discomfort level.

Sample Documentation

06/24/22 2100 Assisted with portable sitz bath. Water 107°F. Treatment lasted 10 minutes. Dried and assisted back to bed. Perineum still slightly edematous with no bruising. Episiotomy with good approximation and light red edges. States the sitz bath "sure did feel good." No complaints of weakness or pain. ————
———— Nurse's signature and credentials

Skill 18.4 Application of Cold Packs

Assessment Steps

1. Review the health-care provider's order and previous nurse's note on the last cold application. ***This will help to determine the type of cold delivery device to use and how the patient tolerated the previous treatment.***
2. *Safety: Assess the patient's age and cognitive level of function, orientation, sedation, sensory impairment, and impairment of circulation to determine if there are any contraindications.*
3. Assess the site where cold is to be applied, noting the appearance, color, presence of edema, temperature of site and surrounding skin, integrity of skin, and any patient discomfort. ***This provides a baseline against which to measure the effects of the application.***

Planning Steps

1. Obtain the correct type of cold delivery device, such as a reusable ice bag, collar, glove, or a commercial gel or chemical pack, and a barrier or protective covering such as a towel. ***Being prepared saves time and effort.***

Implementation Steps

1. Follow the Initial Implementation Steps located on the inside back cover.
2. **If using ice bag, glove, or collar:** Fill one-half to two-thirds full of ice. Remove excess air and close the device. ***This allows the ice bag to conform to the application site.***

(skill continues on page 354)

Skill 18.4 (continued)

If using commercial gel pack: Remove the gel pack from the freezer.
If using disposable commercial chemical pack: Activate the chemical pack according to pack instructions, usually by striking, twisting, or squeezing the container.

3. Apply cold delivery device to the appropriate site using a ***dry*** protective cloth covering or barrier device ***to prevent tissue damage.*** If ***moist*** cold is ordered, apply a moist towel to the skin. Lay the cold pack on top of the moist towel, making certain it does not directly touch skin, and cover it with a dry towel. ***Moist cold penetrates faster and deeper than dry cold.***
4. *Safety: After 5 minutes, reassess the site for pallor or mottling of skin to make certain it is not too cold. Continue to reassess skin every 10 to 15 minutes, asking the patient about discomfort.* If skin becomes pale or mottled or the patient complains the cold pack is too cold, remove the pack immediately to prevent frostbite. Otherwise, leave the cold pack in place for the ordered length of time.
5. Follow the Ending Implementation Steps located on the inside back cover.
6. Document the skin assessment and cold application.

Evaluation Steps

1. Remove the cold pack after the appropriate length of treatment. Assess the site for objective data such as color, temperature, sensation, and edema.
2. Assess the subjective data related to effectiveness of the cold application by asking the patient about any change in discomfort/comfort level at the site. Did the cold pack help the pain?

Sample Documentation

03/03/22 1230 Complained of right ankle discomfort rated a 6 on a scale of 0 to 10. Described pain as throbbing. Applied dry cold pack using disposable chemical pack wrapped in towel to right ankle for 20 minutes as ordered. Ankle skin intact, pink with bruising, 1+ pitting edema, toes warm to touch with brisk capillary refill, pedal pulses equally strong. States the cold pack reduced pain to a 3.
——————— Nurse's signature and credentials

POST CONFERENCE

You cared for your patient with sepsis and a highly elevated temperature. When you evaluate how you did on this assignment, you find that you did pretty well and are pleased with your performance. You had remembered to read the accompanying instructions to the cooling blanket and applied the blanket accordingly. You also located and read the facility policy for this skill and found there were no discrepancies between the manufacturer's instructions and the facility policy. You reviewed the specific parameters of the health-care provider's order as well. By remembering to assess the patient's skin before, during, and after the treatment, you were able to determine that no injury occurred. You knew to remain with the patient so that you could assess her vital signs at the frequency dictated by facility policy and monitor the patient for signs of excessive cold, level of consciousness, and condition of her skin at 10 minutes and then every 30 minutes thereafter until the fever was adequately reduced. You were relieved that the patient responded appropriately and did not exhibit any problems. To document the care, you recorded the patient's vital signs on the graphic sheet in the chart and charted your assessment findings in the nurse's notes according to facility policy.

Key Points

- Local application of heat results in vasodilation and increased permeability of capillaries.
- Indications for heat therapy include relaxation of muscle spasms, pain relief, reduction of inflammation, support of the healing process, reduction of edema once it has stabilized, and elevation of body temperature.
- Application of heat increases metabolism.
- ***Safety: Contraindications for the use of heat therapy include suspected appendicitis, bleeding wound, new injury or trauma, and application of heat over large areas of the body in certain cardiac patients.***
- Local cold applications result in vasoconstriction and decreased permeability of capillaries.
- Indications for use of cold therapy include prevention of edema, hemostasis, pain relief, numbing of sensation, muscle relaxation, and reduction of fever.
- Risks for injury from cold therapy include tissue damage, frostbite, and hypothermia.
- ***Safety: Nursing assessments pertinent prior to heat and cold applications include patient's age and cognitive level of function, orientation, sedation, sensory impairment, and impairment of circulation; the appearance, color, presence of edema, and temperature of skin; and whether or not the patient experienced any discomfort.***
- ***Safety: Nursing assessments pertinent during and after heat and cold applications include appearance, color, presence of edema, and temperature of skin, as well as whether or not the patient experienced any change in comfort or discomfort level.***

Review Questions

Select the answer that is most appropriate for each of the following questions. Some questions may have more than one correct answer. Select all that apply.

1. A patient has an erythematous area at the site where you just discontinued an IV infusion. There is no edema, but the patient complains of the site being very tender. Which of the following would be the treatment of choice?
   1. Telling the patient the tenderness will subside without treatment
   2. Administering a sitz bath
   3. Applying an ice pack
   4. Applying a warm pack

2. Which of the following treatments would possibly help relieve a patient's discomfort from a muscle spasm in her lumbar area?
   1. Immersion in a whirlpool
   2. Administration of a tepid sponge bath
   3. Application of a warm pack
   4. Application of a cold pack

3. A child has a minor cut on her scalp that continues to ooze blood after the wound is cleansed. Which type of heat or cold application would be appropriate in this situation?
   1. Examination glove filled with ice
   2. Sterile warm compress
   3. Tepid sponge bath
   4. Warm K-pad
   5. Cooling blanket

4. During a heat application, which of the following assessment findings would indicate the heat pack should be removed immediately?
   1. Skin is pale pink.
   2. Skin is dark red.
   3. Temperature of the site is slightly warmer than surrounding skin.
   4. Patient denies discomfort.
   5. Skin is starting to look "bubbly."
   6. Skin is hot to the touch.

5. During a cold application, which of the following assessment findings would indicate the cold pack should be removed immediately?
   1. Skin is pink.
   2. Skin is white.
   3. Skin is mottled.
   4. Patient complains of a "burning" sensation.
   5. Skin is very cool to the touch.
   6. Patient states the itching from the rash site is decreasing.

6. The nurse understands that local heat application can cause which of the following?
   1. Vasodilation
   2. Increased cellular metabolism
   3. Vasoconstriction
   4. Relaxed muscles
   5. Decreased pain
   6. Decreased blood flow to the site

7. The nurse is preparing a sitz bath for a postpartum mother. The nurse understands the water must be hung to what level?
   1. 18 to 24 inches
   2. 15 to 20 inches
   3. 17 to 25 inches
   4. 10 to 22 inches

8. The nurse understands that which of the following methods are moist heat?
   1. Hot compresses
   2. Soaks
   3. Sitz baths
   4. Whirlpool baths

ANSWERS 1. 4 , 2. 1, 3, 4, 3. 1, 4. 2, 4, 6, 5. 2, 3, 4, 6. 1, 2, 4, 5, 7. 1, 8. 1, 2, 3, 4

Critical Thinking Exercises

Answers available online.

1. Melonie Jones, a 68-year-old female, is diabetic and suffers from the complications of neuropathy and impaired peripheral vascular circulation. As a result, she has poor circulation to and decreased sensation in her feet. She has fractured her left ankle so badly that she will require a cast once the edema has gone down. The health-care provider has ordered ice packs to the left ankle for 30 minutes every hour. What precautions must you take and what assessments are pertinent for you to make before, during, and after each cold application? Explain your answer.
2. A 19-year-old male sprained his right ankle while playing basketball yesterday. He tells you that his ankle has swollen to nearly double its size since he went to bed last night. He wants to apply a heat pack to help the edema resolve so that he can play in the game tomorrow. What do you tell him?

Additional Resources

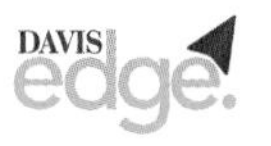

Use the scratch off code on the inside front cover of your book to access online quizzes that will help you to improve your scores on course exams and prepare for the NCLEX-PN®.

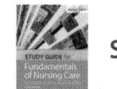

Study Guide

CHAPTER 19

Pain Management, Rest, and Restorative Sleep

KEY TERMS

Acute pain (a-KYOOT PAYN)
Adjuvant (AD-joo-vant)
Analgesic (AN-al-JEE-zik)
Chronic pain (KRON-ik PAYN)
Circadian rhythm (ser-KAY-dee-an RITHM)
Controlled substance (kon-TROHLD SUB-stans)
Cutaneous pain (kyoo-TAY-nee-us PAYN)
Deep somatic pain (DEEP soh-MAT-ik PAYN)
Effleurage (EF-luh-RAHJ)
Endorphin (en-DOR-fin)
Holistic (hoh-LIS-tik)
Intractable pain (in-TRAK-tah-buhl PAYN)
Neuropathic pain (noo-ro-PATH-ik PAYN)
Nociceptor (NOH-see-SEP-tor)
Patient-controlled analgesia (PCA) (PAY-shent-kon-TROHLD AN-al-JEE-zee-ah)
Phantom limb pain (FAN-tom LIM PAYN)
Prostaglandins (PROS-tah-GLAN-dins)
Radiating pain (RAY-dee-ay-ting PAYN)
Referred pain (rih-FERD PAYN)
Restorative sleep (rih-STOR-uh-tiv SLEEP)
Substance P (SUB-stans P)
Visceral pain (VIH-ser-uhl PAYN)

CHAPTER CONCEPTS

Comfort
Sleep and Rest
Patient-Centered Care

LEARNING OUTCOMES

1. Define various terms associated with pain management, rest, and restorative sleep.
2. Explain the gate control theory.
3. Describe the role that endorphins play in pain perception and relief.
4. Compare the different types of nociceptive and neuropathic pain.
5. Outline the factors that affect pain and pain perception.
6. Paraphrase how to thoroughly assess pain.
7. Correlate acknowledgment and acceptance of pain to treatment of pain.
8. Identify at least three nonpharmacological methods of pain relief.
9. Characterize restorative sleep.
10. Enumerate sleep requirements for different age groups.
11. Name six specific factors that affect sleep.
12. Describe interventions you might use to promote sleep.
13. Discuss information found in the Connection features in this chapter.
14. Identify specific safety information.
15. Answer questions about the skills in this chapter.

SKILLS

19.1 Application of TENS Unit

CRITICAL THINKING CONNECTION

Clinical Assignment

You are assigned to care for a patient who had a left above-the-knee amputation 3 days ago. He has been restless and has not slept well. Today he is very tired and irritable, especially with his wife, who earlier in the day voiced frustration with her husband's moodiness and went home in tears. He has difficulty rating his pain when you try to evaluate it and finally tells you, "I must be nuts because what really hurts is my left foot—only it isn't there!"

Continued

CRITICAL THINKING CONNECTION—cont'd

Critical Thinking Questions:

1. What interventions will you use to relieve his pain?
2. What type of pain does he exhibit?
3. How would you explain the need for restorative sleep?
4. Explain the measures you would use to assist him to rest and sleep.

The management of pain and discomfort is imperative for one to truly rest and experience restorative sleep, that which helps the body to regain strength and return to a healthful state. In this chapter, you will learn different methods to decrease and relieve your patient's pain and provide comfort, as well as ways to help the patient to experience beneficial rest and sleep.

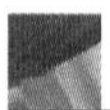

PAIN

Pain serves as a warning sign indicating that actual damage has occurred or that the potential exists for damage of tissue. Pain can be a sensory and/or an emotional experience, is complex with many components, and means different things to different people. The human response to pain varies not only from culture to culture, but also from individual to individual. As you learned in Chapter 17, pain is so important that it is known as the fifth vital sign.

Nature and Physiology of Pain and Its Transmission

Pain can have negative effects on and can even destroy numerous aspects of a patient's life. Pain can make it difficult to:

- Perform activities of daily living,
- Rest and experience restorative sleep,
- Eat,
- Perform normal body movements and exercise,
- Maintain family relationships,
- Work or maintain a job,
- Have a social life or maintain friendships,
- Maintain cognitive abilities, and
- Focus on spiritual beliefs.

Thus, it is important to develop an understanding of pain and how you can assist your patients with pain relief and development of coping skills for dealing with unrelieved pain. Your beliefs regarding pain will affect how you respond to patients and, as a result, impact your patients' lives. We encourage you to open your mind and begin to view pain **holistically,** which includes viewing the physical, mental, social, and spiritual aspects of a person as parts of the integrated whole being. This will prepare you to best meet your patients' pain relief needs.

One of the core things to remember about a patient's pain is that pain is always *what the patient says it is.* If the patient says the pain level is an 8 on a scale of 0 to 10, with 10 being the worst pain one can imagine, then the pain is an 8. It does not make a difference if the patient *does not appear* to be in pain or if you think the source of the pain should not cause *that much* pain. *It is what it is* to the patient, and that is what you will want to treat.

Gate Control Theory

In the 1960s, researchers proposed a theory that helps to explain the transmission and perception of pain and how even nonpharmaceutical interventions can relieve the pain. The theory purports that the transmission of pain impulses to the central nervous system is controlled by a "gate" that opens and closes in response to sensory input. The gate must be open for the pain impulse to be transmitted to the brain and interpreted as pain. When the gate is closed, the nerve impulse for pain is blocked from transmission.

It is thought that the thalamus can open and close the gate in relationship to stress and anxiety: An increase in stress can cause the gate to open, while decreased stress and anxiety can close the gate. Stimulation of the broad nerve fibers is thought to close the gate, while stimulation of the narrow nerve fibers is thought to open the gate. The broader nerve fibers are stimulated by things such as exercise, heat, cold, massage, and transcutaneous electrical nerve stimulation (TENS). The smaller, narrow nerve fibers are directly stimulated by injury and damage to the tissues. Thus, when tissue damage or injury stimulates the narrow nerve fibers, it makes sense when a person naturally begins to rub the painful site in an effort to relieve some of the pain. An example is when you bang your elbow against the corner of a cabinet, the first reaction is usually to grab the elbow and rub it vigorously. This helps to relieve the pain.

Thoughts and emotions are also believed to have an effect on opening and closing the gate by stimulating endorphin production. **Endorphins** are natural body chemicals produced by the brain in response to pleasant thoughts or feelings, exercise, laughter, sex, and massage. They act similarly to morphine and produce feelings of euphoria, well-being, and pleasure. They bind to the opiate receptor sites, which help to close the gates and block the transmission of pain to the central nervous system. Long-distance runners sometimes experience what they describe as "hitting the mark" or a "runner's high" that allows them to continue running more miles without experiencing any discomfort or pain. Think of a time when you and a friend or relative have gotten tickled about something, began laughing, and just could not stop laughing for several minutes. Afterward, you probably felt very good and quite relaxed, with a positive sense of well-being. You might have even said something like, "Boy, did I need that!" This feeling is thought to be a direct result of endorphins.

• WORD • BUILDING •

holistic: hol – entire + istic – related to a belief system

> **KNOWLEDGE CONNECTION**
> Name some of the effects pain can have on one's daily life. What is meant by the *gate control theory?* Describe the role of endorphins and their effects on pain perception and pain relief.

Classifications of Pain

There are many different classifications of pain. Pain that comes on suddenly and has a short duration (less than 6 months) is known as **acute pain.** Pain that lasts longer than 6 months is termed **chronic pain.** *Intermittent pain* is pain that comes and goes at intervals. **Intractable pain** refers to pain that cannot be relieved, is incurable, or is resistant to treatment. **Referred pain** is pain felt in an area other than where the pain was produced. An example of referred pain is the pain that is felt in the left arm, jaw, and shoulder that often occurs from the lack of oxygen to the heart muscle during a myocardial infarction (heart attack). Figure 19.1 shows specific sites of referred pain. **Radiating pain** is pain that begins at a specific site and shoots out from or extends to a larger area beyond the site of origin.

Nociceptive Pain Versus Neuropathic Pain

Pain is derived in one of two ways:

1. From the stimulation of nerve pain receptors, called **nociceptors**
2. From damage to the nerves themselves

Nociceptors are randomly dispersed throughout the skin, subcutaneous tissue, and muscular tissue. These nerve pain receptors can be stimulated by temperature changes, tissue damage, and certain chemicals. Two of these chemicals that can stimulate the nerve pain receptors are substance P and prostaglandins, which are released during injury and damage to tissue. **Substance P** plays a role in eliciting localized tissue reactions similar to inflammation. **Prostaglandins** are hormones that act in the immediate area to initiate inflammation by sensitizing local pain receptors. The resulting pain is known as *nociceptive pain* and is generally localized within a specific area, from which the receptors send impulses to the central nervous system via afferent nerve pathways. Nociceptive pain also may result from surgery or injury. Nonsteroidal anti-inflammatory drugs help to block the production of prostaglandins, thus reducing the pain. Common examples of nonsteroidal anti-inflammatory drugs include ibuprofen and aspirin. Neuropathic pain occurs due to destruction of peripheral nerves or the central nervous system itself. This destruction may be the result of an injury or a chronic disease, such as diabetes mellitus or AIDS, or from chronic vitamin B_{12} deficiency. This pain may extend beyond the local region to encompass a broadening area of discomfort that follows along the pathway of the damaged nerves.

NOCICEPTIVE PAIN. Nociceptive pain can be broken down into three different types:

1. **Cutaneous pain** is pain that is more superficial or pertaining to the skin's surface and underlying subcutaneous tissue. An example is a paper cut or a mild burn.
2. **Visceral pain,** sometimes known as *soft tissue pain*, is the pain experienced from stimulation of deep internal pain receptors. Examples include pain that results from traumatic injury or surgery, or with metastatic invasion of the soft tissues such as the skin, muscles, and organs. It is generally described as an ache or a cramping-type pain, and it can be intermittent or continuous.
3. **Deep somatic pain,** also known as *osteogenic pain*, is bone, ligament, tendon, and blood vessel pain. The pain may be diffuse and of longer duration than cutaneous pain. Bone cancer, fractures, and arthritic-type diseases are common sources of this type of pain. Your patient may describe it as pain with movement.

NEUROPATHIC PAIN. **Neuropathic pain** is the burning, stabbing, or sometimes deep ache that your patient describes when there is nerve compression caused by pressure from tumors, lymphedema, or compression fractures of the spine. Nerve destruction can cause sharp, jagged, knifelike pain, burning, prickly pins and needles, and even numbness. An example of this numbness is diabetic neuropathy. During the late stages of diabetes, a patient may develop total numbness of the feet that is extremely uncomfortable and dangerous for the patient.

One type of neuropathic pain is **phantom limb pain,** which feels as though the pain is coming from an extremity that has been *amputated,* meaning that it has been surgically or traumatically removed. A common example of phantom pain is the complaint of foot pain after the lower leg and foot have been surgically amputated.

> **KNOWLEDGE CONNECTION**
> Differentiate between nociceptive pain and neuropathic pain. Describe three types of nociceptive pain.

Factors Affecting Pain

There are various factors that affect pain and its expression. They include the following:

- Ethnic and cultural beliefs
- Developmental stage
- Individual values
- Previous pain experiences

• **WORD • BUILDING •**

nociceptor: noci – pain + ceptor - receptor
prostaglandin: prosta – prostate + gland – gland + in – suffix for organic compounds
cutaneous: cuta – skin + neous – relating to
visceral: viscera – abdominal organs + al – relating to

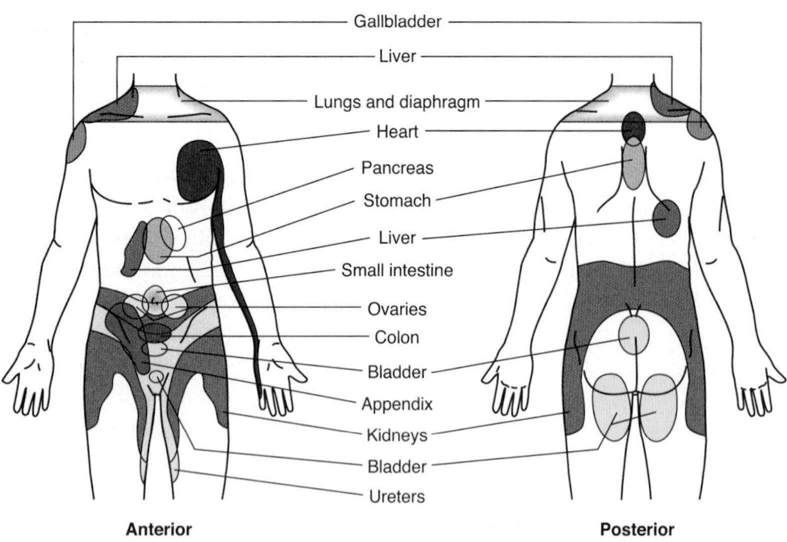

FIGURE 19.1 Sites of referred pain (from Williams LS, Hopper PD. *Understanding Medical-Surgical Nursing*. 5th ed. Philadelphia, PA: FA Davis; 2015).

- Personal support system
- Emotions
- Fatigue

Ethnic and Cultural Beliefs

One's culture and ethnicity can dictate how the pain experience is outwardly expressed. Individuals from some cultures often feel that pain should be suffered in silence, while other cultures may embrace the verbalization of pain, such as moaning, as a means of comfort. Individuals from other cultures may not traditionally verbalize pain but instead express pain with facial expressions and gestures. Age can also influence how an individual deals with pain; for example, in some cultures, older individuals may tolerate discomfort in order to fulfill work duties, while those of younger generations may find it acceptable to complain of discomfort and to use medication for relief.

While it is important to consider the patient's cultural beliefs, you should never assume that a patient will react in the same manner as another patient of that particular cultural or ethnic group.

Developmental Stage

Infants and children experience the same levels of physiological pain but are less able than adults to express or articulate what they are feeling. Infants usually respond with loud or shrill crying, changes in facial expression, waving their arms wildly, kicking their legs, and increases in pulse and respiratory rates. Older children may respond much like infants or may only whimper when experiencing pain. Their pain response may be affected by previous pain experiences. As children get older and have a better grasp of language, they are better able to verbalize pain or discomfort. Part of a child's expression of pain may directly relate to a lack of understanding of what is happening to him or her, anxiety, and fear.

Pain perception does not change with advancing age, nor is it natural for elderly individuals to have more pain simply because they are aging. When older adults suffer from multiple chronic and acute diseases, these individuals sometimes believe that they are expected to hurt more as they become more elderly. As a consequence, they may suffer in silence.

Individual Values and Previous Pain Experiences

Some individuals value stoicism. Some want to be independent and not rely on others to assist with their pain relief. Some individuals are simply very private regarding their personal feelings. Others may believe that being stoic about pain is illogical and unnecessary, or they may feel free to express their discomfort to anyone and everyone.

A patient may respond to pain based on his or her previous pain experiences. Regardless of a patient's values or previous pain experiences, it is your responsibility to educate the patient and ensure understanding regarding methods and availability of pain relief for that patient. To better understand your patient's pain, it is helpful to identify your own personal values regarding pain and to consider your previous pain experiences. How did you respond when you were in pain? What are your values regarding pain?

Personal Support System

Individuals who do not have a personal support system of family or friends may cope with pain differently than those who can depend on the support and assistance of a spouse, loved ones, or close friends. This is especially true for children, who generally do better if a parent remains with them at all times. Even though the patient has a personal support system, if those support individuals are absent or are far away, the patient may experience more discomfort along with a sense of loneliness. Or the patient may simply find the pain experience to be more stressful without someone close by.

Emotions

All emotions affect the level and tolerance of pain and discomfort. Unpleasant emotions, such as anxiety, stress, loneliness, and fear, generally increase the patient's perception of pain or decrease his or her tolerance of pain. Conversely, positive emotions, such as joy, happiness, and love, are more apt to decrease the perception of pain or render the patient more tolerant of the pain.

Fatigue

Patients who are not resting well or are fatigued will usually have an increased perception of pain as well as a lower capacity to cope with the pain. When patients experience continual pain, they relate that the pain worsens in the evening and night unless they rest or nap during the day.

Responses to Pain

The body responds to pain physiologically, psychologically, and behaviorally. Initially pain stimulates the sympathetic nervous system, which initiates the fight-or-flight response. A patient's pulse, respiratory rate, and blood pressure may rise. The pupils dilate, as do the cerebral blood vessels, delivering more blood to the brain to increase awareness. If the pain continues for days or weeks, the body begins to adapt to the pain, allowing the parasympathetic nervous system to reverse many of the sympathetic system responses, returning vital signs, pupils, and cerebral blood vessels back to normal. Thus, there are signs and symptoms that may be noted in acute pain that are not seen in chronic pain. Table 19.1 presents signs and symptoms of acute and chronic pain.

KNOWLEDGE CONNECTION

Describe five factors and how they affect pain perception and pain relief. Compare the signs and symptoms of acute pain to those of chronic pain.

Management and Treatment of Pain

Before pain can be effectively treated, you must acquire as much information about the pain as possible, known as a pain assessment. It is important to know a number of things about the complaint of pain, including:

- **Level or extent of the pain:** Consistently use the same pain scale, such as a scale of 0 to 10, with 0 being none and 10 being the worst pain the patient can imagine.
- **Site of pain:** Be specific. For example, do not state that the pain is just in the abdomen, but in which quadrant; not just in the back, but whether it is right, left, or midline, and whether it is in the cervical, thoracic, lumbar, or sacral area of the back; and not just in the leg, but whether it is right or left; whether it is in the foot, ankle, calf, thigh, or groin; and whether it is anterior, lateral, or posterior.
- **Characteristics of the pain:** Is it sharp, dull, intermittent, constant, burning, cramping, stinging, aching, or pressure like? Does it feel like a vice grip, knifelike, pulling, tension or tightness, or spasmodic?
- **Whether the pain is acute or chronic:** When did it begin?
- **What elicits the pain:** Does eating, deep breathing, palpation, coughing, sneezing, repositioning, movement, or activity bring about the pain?
- **Patient's desires in relation to the pain:** This includes whether the patient wants medication or prefers nonpharmacological methods of pain relief.

The use of a pain scale for assessment of pain was covered in Chapter 17.

Acknowledgment and Acceptance

The first step in assisting your patient to obtain maximum pain relief is letting the patient know that you believe that he or she is in pain. Remember that the patient is the *expert* about whether or not he or she is suffering, not the health-care provider. You should be the expert in relieving the pain, not interpreting whether or not the patient is really hurting. Listen to how the patient describes the discomfort and verbally acknowledge that you understand that he or she is hurting. After obtaining a complete description of the patient's pain, be quick to respond with relief measures. Explain to the patient your intent; let the patient know what you are going to do to effect pain relief for him or her. If it is too soon for medication, be certain to offer other methods of relief and distraction. Never tell the patient that it is too soon for more medication and leave his or her needs unmet. There is always something that you can do to help reduce discomfort.

Nonpharmaceutical Methods

There are numerous ways to decrease pain or the perception of pain. The Agency for Healthcare Research and Quality has printed guidelines encouraging health-care providers to incorporate nonpharmaceutical methods of pain relief in situations that are appropriate, such as lower levels of discomfort in which the patient desires to avoid use of medication. When the pain is beyond mild levels, these nonpharmaceutical methods should serve as an adjuvant along with pharmacological therapies. **Adjuvant** means to assist or aid another treatment, therefore increasing the effectiveness.

HOT AND COLD PACKS. Both heat and cold therapy are especially good sources of relief for musculoskeletal pain and discomfort. When pain is due to an acute trauma or injury, cold therapy will help prevent swelling and thereby reduce discomfort. Cold therapy also is effective in disrupting the transmission of pain impulses in both acute and chronic pain. Heat is rarely used on new injuries due to the fact that it will dilate the vasculature in the area and increase swelling, which results in more pain. Heat is more commonly used for chronic pain and muscle spasms. More information regarding the use and effects of hot and cold packs is included in Chapter 18.

MASSAGE AND EFFLEURAGE. Cutaneous relief measures such as massage and effleurage are simple to provide but can be extremely effective in some painful conditions. **Effleurage** is the repetitive gentle, gliding stroking of your fingertips over the surface of the skin. This technique is particularly effective during back massage to relax muscles or used on the

Table 19.1
Signs and Symptoms of Pain

	Physiological Signs	*Behavioral Signs*	*Psychological Signs*
Acute	Recent onset Diminishes with healing **Fight/flight response:** Heart rate increases Respirations increase Systolic blood pressure increases Pupils dilate **As it worsens:** Diaphoresis Blood pressure drops Syncope Pupils constrict	Wincing or facial grimacing Moaning or crying Restlessness, such as nervous finger tapping or foot bouncing Rigid body posture Slow movement Holding or guarding the area Worsens during anxiety/fear Rocking or pacing	Reduced attention span Focused only on pain Anger Fear or anxiety Irritability
Chronic	Onset longer than 6 months ago Few or none Pupils may constrict Vital signs may not change	Lassitude Impaired mobility/activity Sleep disturbance Withdrawal from family and friends	Low self-esteem Depression Fatigue Anger Irritability

head to reduce tension headaches. You can use both hands to stroke two side-by-side circles over the abdomen of a woman in labor to decrease her discomfort from contractions. Firmer massage of muscles is often helpful to reduce limb, neck, and back pain. This method of relief is thought to stimulate the closing of the gate and production of endorphins that you read about earlier in this chapter.

TRANSCUTANEOUS ELECTRICAL NERVE STIMULATION. A TENS unit is a battery-powered device that you apply to the skin over the painful area (Fig. 19.2). It is about the size of a small pager, with lead wires and electrode pads. The device delivers electrical stimulation to the large-diameter nerve fibers, which is thought to work similarly to massage by closing the gate and stimulating the production of endorphins. The frequency and strength of impulse delivery are controlled by gradually increasing the dials on the TENS unit to a level at which the impulses are described as "gentle tapping" by the patient. The impulses should not be strong enough to feel like an irritant or produce discomfort. Skill 19.1 (page 369) provides instructions regarding application of a TENS unit.

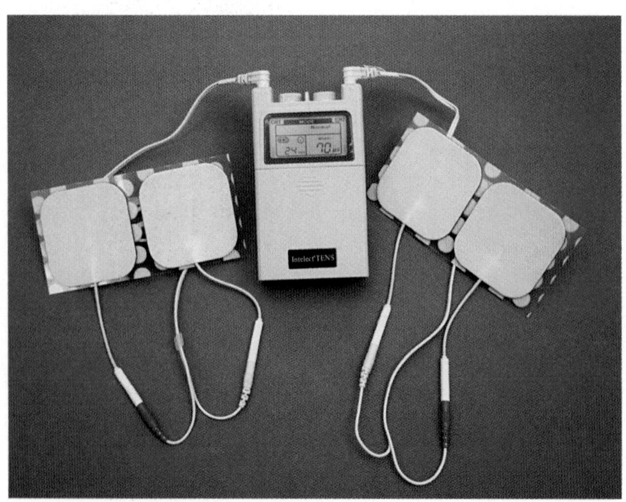

FIGURE 19.2 A TENS unit.

ACUPRESSURE AND ACUPUNCTURE. Acupressure involves applying fingertip pressure, and acupuncture is the insertion of ultrafine needles into specific body areas; both are thought to stimulate endorphin production. Further explanation is found in Chapter 11.

RELAXATION. Helping a patient relax can be done in a number of ways, two of which we will explain here: progressive relaxation and guided imagery. *Progressive relaxation* is a systematic process of using the mind to actually relax the patient's muscles from the top of the head to the toes. Focusing the patient's conscious mind on the tightening and relaxing of muscles interferes with perception of pain impulses, and the physiological reaction of muscle relaxation can directly relieve some types of pain. The patient lays in bed in the most comfortable position he or she can find with the eyes closed. You verbally direct the patient to focus on specific muscles, first tensing and then relaxing them, beginning at the head and progressing to the toes (Box 19.1). There are also many commercial tapes and compact disks that can be purchased and utilized for progressive relaxation.

Guided imagery is another method of using the mind to help control the body and guide the patient toward a more relaxed

Box 19.1

Progressive Relaxation

Instruct the patient to find a comfortable position, dim the lights, close the door, and reduce as much noise and distraction as possible. Using a quiet voice, verbally guide the patient in the following steps, beginning with the top of the head:

- Take a deep breath, breathing in slowly through your nose. Feel your chest and stomach rise until they can't rise any further. Exhale slowly through your mouth. Feel your chest and stomach relax. (Repeat the deep breath two or three times.)
- Focus on the top of your head. Feel the tightness of the skin and muscles. Contract those muscles. Feel how tight they are.
- Now, relax the top of your head. Feel all the tightness and tension drain away. Feel them leaving your body as you exhale. Let the top of your head just go limp. Feel it totally relaxed and limp. Feel any discomfort leave your body as you breathe out. Doesn't it feel good to relax?

Continue to use this same phrasing on the successive parts of the body as you progress to the toes. Include the following body parts:

Forehead	Tongue	Shoulders	Hips	Calves
Eyes	Chin	Chest and back	Pelvis	Ankles
Cheeks	Neck	Stomach	Thighs	Feet and toes

Most patients are either asleep or very relaxed by the time you reach the toes. This is particularly effective for anxious or stressed patients, those who cannot seem to fall asleep, and those who are in pain. It takes a few minutes of your time, but your patients will benefit from it, thus making it very rewarding for you.

state. This process can help the patient feel more in control of emotions and thought processes and provide relief of discomfort and induction of rest or sleep. Guided imagery can be done verbally or by use of tapes or compact disks. Using verbal suggestions, you direct the patient's thoughts to a place that is pictured as comfortable, calming, relaxing, and perfect. By asking the patient to use several of his or her senses, the body seems to respond as though what is imagined is real. A picturesque location, such as a beach, garden, mountaintop, or forest, is described in great detail as the patient lies quietly with the eyes closed. The patient is asked to visualize the specified place and to feel all the comforts of this place as you describe them in a soft, quiet, melodious voice (Box 19.2).

DISTRACTION. Some patients will respond to distraction; others will not. If distraction works, it helps to take the patient's mind off the pain and focus on something else. This simply decreases the conscious awareness of the pain. It should not be used as the sole method of pain relief, but it is a good aid to analgesics (pain medications). Distraction is at work when a patient is talking and laughing with visitors but asks for pain medication only a few minutes after the visitors leave. It can be accomplished through use of different senses as well as the cognitive mind, including the following:

- **Visual distraction:** watching television or reading a good book

Box 19.2

Guided Imagery

The following is an example of a scenario to use for guided imagery:

Close your eyes and take a deep, deep breath. As you exhale, feel all your stresses and discomforts leave your body. Picture in your mind a beautiful white sandy beach, close to the ocean, with lots of palm trees. You are lying comfortably in a hammock made of the softest silk fabric that you have ever felt. Feel its silkiness, its soothing caress on your skin. Feel how it supports your body. Let your body relax against the silk. Let it support you in complete and utter comfort. See the soft, puffy, white clouds as they drift lazily overhead. Watch their shapes as they change from one shape to another. Feel the warmth of the sun on your face, on your arms. It is just the perfect temperature, with the cool tropical breeze that blows gently across your skin. It's such a peaceful place. Breathe in the fresh tropical air and smell the ocean. Hear the waves as they lap onto shore and then trickle back to the sea. Listen as the birds echo their sweet calls, each a little different, soothing in their own ways. Hear the palm leaves rustle in the breeze. Smell the tropical flowers and see their vibrant colors. What a perfect place to be, a place where you can rest.

- **Auditory distraction:** listening to music or someone reading aloud; an infant will often respond to soft whispering or singing close to his or her ear while being held or rocked
- **Tactile distraction:** receiving a back rub, having the hair brushed, rocking, receiving hugs, holding a pet, playing with a toy, or taking a warm bath; an infant may respond to being patted or effleurage on the cheek or back of the neck, around the ear, or on the back
- **Intellectual distraction:** conversing with another individual; working; doing a Sudoku, crossword, or other type of puzzle; or playing card games

KNOWLEDGE CONNECTION

Who is the expert on the pain level the patient is experiencing? What characteristics should you assess during pain assessment? Discuss at least four methods of nonpharmacological pain relief.

Pharmaceutical Methods

There are various classifications of medications that are effective against pain, including nonsteroidal anti-inflammatory drugs (NSAIDs), nonopioids, opioid narcotics, and adjuvant drugs. These medications can be used alone or in conjunction with nonpharmaceutical methods of pain relief.

• WORD • BUILDING •

analgesic: an – not + algesic – feeling pain

NONOPIOID ANALGESICS. Nonopioids are nonnarcotic pain relievers used for mild to moderate pain. Acetaminophen is one of the most common; it is available over the counter and is used alone as well as in combination with other drugs such as codeine or hydrocodone for more severe pain. Besides having analgesic effects, acetaminophen has *antipyretic* (fever-reducing) effects. The maximum dosage allowed in adults is 4 grams (4,000 milligrams) every 24 hours. Even though it is an over-the-counter drug, acetaminophen can cause *hepatotoxicity* (damage to the liver) and death.

Real-World Connection

Over-the-Counter Pain Relief Carries Risks

A 19-year-old female was brought into the emergency room unresponsive and died a short time later from liver failure, secondary to acetaminophen overdose. She had been having recurring headaches for several weeks and had been taking acetaminophen around the clock in an effort to obtain relief. She thought that since it was a common, over-the-counter drug, one that you could "even give to infants," it was harmless. She failed to follow the dose limits printed on the label, and it ended tragically in the loss of her life.

NONSTEROIDAL ANTI-INFLAMMATORY DRUGS. NSAIDs are a medication class that helps to reduce inflammation and pain by preventing the release of inflammatory mediators, such as histamine, serotonin, prostaglandins, and leukotrienes, at the site of injury or inflammation. NSAIDs are useful in relieving cutaneous pain, visceral pain, and deep somatic pain. The most common over-the-counter drugs in this class are ibuprofen, naproxen, and aspirin, all of which have anti-inflammatory, analgesic, and antipyretic effects. Aspirin also has antiplatelet effects, which means that it decreases platelet clumping, which is the first step in clotting. Aspirin is commonly used for its *antiplatelet* effects to reduce risk of clotting in patients who might be prone to heart attacks or strokes, such as a patient with an elevated cholesterol level or hypertension. The dosage of aspirin is reduced from that used for analgesic, antipyretic, and anti-inflammatory purposes, which is 600 to 650 milligrams several times a day, to a mere 81 to 300 milligrams once a day. Because these drugs can cause severe gastric irritation and bleeding, they should be administered with food.

OPIATE/OPIOID ANALGESICS (NARCOTICS). When nonopioid medications are ineffective in relieving moderate to severe pain, opiates or opioids may be needed. They usually are effective in relieving visceral pain and deep somatic pain. These analgesics work by binding with opiate receptors and stimulating the brain's production of enkephalin and beta-endorphin, compounds that decrease pain perception. They come from opium and its derivatives, known as opiates; they also come in synthetic forms, known as opioids. They are **controlled substances** and therefore require a prescription to obtain them. All controlled, or *scheduled,* drugs have greater capacity for addiction and abuse and are regulated by federal law. Meperidine, codeine, hydromorphone, morphine, and fentanyl are some of the more common drugs used in this class. Please note that meperidine use should be avoided in patients older than 65 years of age and in those patients with renal function impairment because of production of normeperidine, a metabolite that can cause adverse side effects by irritating the cerebrum. Cerebral irritation can range from minor mood alterations to seizures in patients who do not have adequate kidney function to remove the products of drug breakdown.

Opiates and opioids can be administered by the oral, rectal, and transcutaneous routes; they also are used extensively via the intramuscular and IV routes for intense pain. Along with pain relief, they may cause side effects of nausea, vomiting, constipation, itching, sedation, and even respiratory depression and pupil constriction in higher dosages. Patients with chronic or acute pain are often prescribed opiates or opioids. Although opiates and opioids are shown to be effective for chronic and acute pain, they are prescribed too often and can lead to addiction and overdose. If a patient becomes only minimally responsive, administer the antagonist naloxone (Narcan) to counteract the opiate/opioid effects. You want to check the patient's vital signs, including respiratory rate, before giving an opiate or opioid. Use caution when giving opiates or opioids to patients who are prescribed sedative medication. This will cause the respiratory rate to decrease, leading to respiratory depression and failure.

These drugs may be administered, within preset boundaries, by the patient, who controls the frequency and administration of his or her pain medication, a process known as **patient-controlled analgesia** (PCA). It uses a computerized IV infusion device consisting of a pump, a large syringe containing the analgesic, IV tubing, and a push button that the patient presses for delivery of analgesic (Fig. 19.3). The health-care provider orders the maximum dosage and the intervals at which the drug may be administered, and the nurse or pharmacist calibrates the PCA pump accordingly. Initially, the nurse administers a larger dose known as the loading dose, or *bolus,* which provides an optimum blood level to get the pain under control. Then the patient pushes the hand-controlled button whenever he or she feels additional pain relief is needed. The preset dose limits and intervals (lockout times) prevent the patient from overdosing. The PCA offers the patient a sense of control over his or her own medication and provides more consistent pain relief with less medication. Figure 19.4 shows a sample of electronic documentation regarding the use of PCA. Box 19.3 lists additional advantages of PCA.

ADJUVANT ANALGESICS. Adjuvant analgesics are classes of medication that produce pain relief either through a mechanism different than traditional analgesics or by

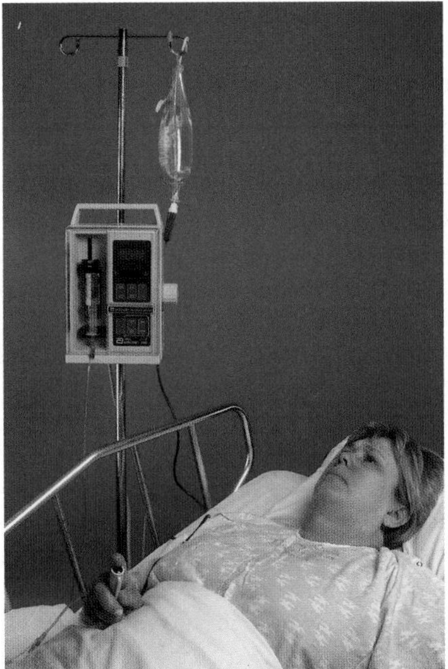

FIGURE 19.3 A woman pushes the button on her PCA pump to deliver pain medication (from Wilkinson JM, Treas LS. *Fundamentals of Nursing: Theory, Concepts & Applications*. Vol. 2. 3rd ed. Philadelphia, PA: FA Davis; 2016).

Box 19.3

Advantages of Patient-Controlled Analgesia

There are numerous advantages of using patient-controlled analgesia, and it is helpful to explain these benefits to the patient and the patient's family. Proper explanation will generally improve compliance as well as understanding, which both are necessary to achieve the optimal benefits of this type of pain control. The following are some of these advantages:

- Provides patient with control over pain relief
- Reduces waiting for nurse response
- Avoids repeated injections
- Provides rapid relief via IV route
- Reduces anxiety and fear that pain will get out of control
- Allows for more frequent and evenly controlled pain relief
- Allows for smaller dosing, ultimately resulting in use of less medication
- Enables patient to achieve more comfortable ambulation over a continuum of time, therefore reducing complications of immobility

potentiating or increasing the effects of opiates, opioids, and nonopioid drugs. Two examples are anticonvulsants and antidepressants. A blood level of anticonvulsants and antidepressants must be reached and maintained before pain relief will be noticed; this generally takes 2 to 3 weeks. Anticonvulsants, such as gabapentin and carbamazepine, and antidepressants, such as amitriptyline, are used to treat nerve pain, which is a complication found in diabetics. Skeletal muscle relaxants, benzodiazepines, and caffeine are helpful in relieving pain due to muscle spasms. Antispasmodics or anticholinergics are used to treat pain from intestinal colic.

KNOWLEDGE CONNECTION

Compare the different ways NSAIDs, nonopioids, and narcotic opiates/opioids work to effect pain relief. List three categories of adjuvant medications that are sometimes used in pain relief. Explain what *controlled* or *scheduled drug* means. What are the benefits of using PCA?

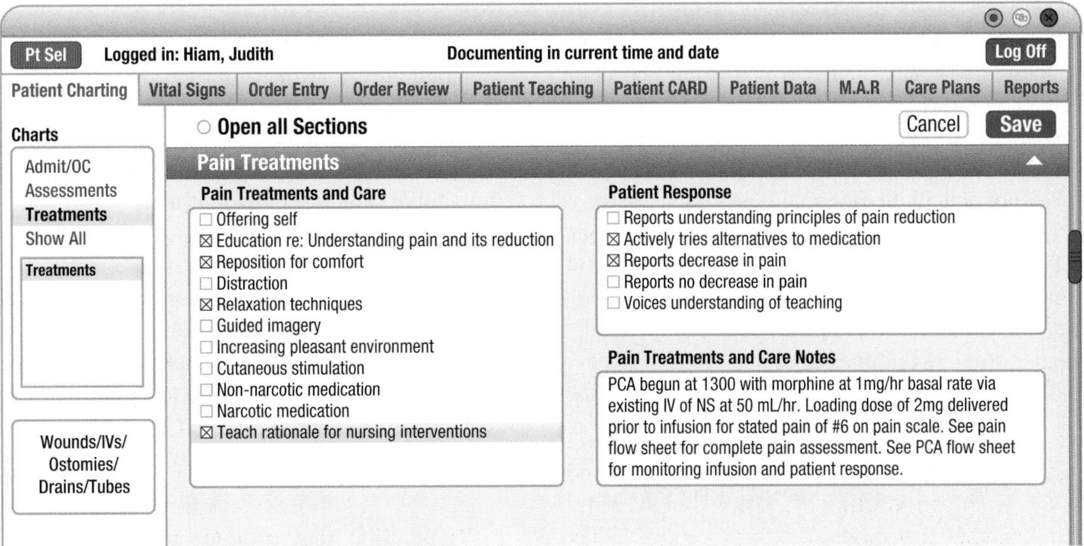

Pt Sel Logged in: Hiam, Judith Documenting in current time and date Log Off

Patient Charting | Vital Signs | Order Entry | Order Review | Patient Teaching | Patient CARD | Patient Data | M.A.R | Care Plans | Reports

Charts

Admit/OC
Assessments
Treatments
Show All

Treatments

Wounds/IVs/Ostomies/Drains/Tubes

○ Open all Sections Cancel Save

Pain Treatments

Pain Treatments and Care
☐ Offering self
☒ Education re: Understanding pain and its reduction
☒ Reposition for comfort
☐ Distraction
☒ Relaxation techniques
☐ Guided imagery
☐ Increasing pleasant environment
☐ Cutaneous stimulation
☐ Non-narcotic medication
☐ Narcotic medication
☒ Teach rationale for nursing interventions

Patient Response
☐ Reports understanding principles of pain reduction
☒ Actively tries alternatives to medication
☒ Reports decrease in pain
☐ Reports no decrease in pain
☐ Voices understanding of teaching

Pain Treatments and Care Notes
PCA begun at 1300 with morphine at 1mg/hr basal rate via existing IV of NS at 50 mL/hr. Loading dose of 2mg delivered prior to infusion for stated pain of #6 on pain scale. See pain flow sheet for complete pain assessment. See PCA flow sheet for monitoring infusion and patient response.

FIGURE 19.4 Electronic documentation of PCA.

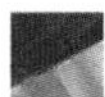

REST AND RESTORATIVE SLEEP

Rest and restorative sleep not only are necessary for pain relief and comfort, but are also imperative for good physiological, psychological, and emotional health. **Restorative sleep** is that which allows an individual to awaken feeling rested, refreshed, rejuvenated, and energized, ready to meet new challenges. *Resting* may or may not involve sleep. It is any time that an individual feels relaxed and free from anxiety, such as when visiting with a loved one he or she has not seen in a long time, laughing during a funny movie, reading a good book, or napping. When napping, a person is disturbed by external noises and awakens easily, but during restorative sleep the individual experiences a partial loss of consciousness and is more difficult to arouse. During restorative sleep, external noises may be incorporated into dreams that will not cause the individual to awaken.

What Happens During Restorative Sleep?

It is impossible to maintain good health without adequate restorative sleep, because this is when the brain works to repair the small injuries to the body, mind, and emotions that occur as part of the natural wear and tear of daily living, including such things as cellular repair and synthesis of protein. Of course, during illness and trauma there is much more damage that must heal before the body can be restored to optimum health. Without adequate rest and restorative sleep:

- Healing is slow and incomplete;
- Immunity decreases;
- Pain tolerance decreases;
- Fragile emotions and impatience affect relationships;
- Cognitive functions are impaired, making concentration difficult, resulting in poor decision making;
- Work performance suffers; and
- Accidents increase dramatically.

The brain also uses sleep time to *sort out* all the data that were received by the senses while awake, determining which information is important to keep and which is unimportant and can be purged. The trivial things such as hearing a car horn honk or smelling the aroma of dinner as you cooked probably are forgotten. If the brain identifies new information as useful, then it not only will process and store the new data, but also will associate it with previously acquired and stored knowledge. This allows the individual to learn more and better apply the new data in different ways. This explains a mind and body mechanism that you probably have experienced: worrying about a problem but finding yourself unable to decide what to do about it. So, rather than continue to fight with yourself over the matter, you decide to go to bed and worry about it tomorrow. The next morning when you awaken, the solution to the problem just comes to you. This occurs because the central nervous system was sorting and processing all the data perceived yesterday while you slept.

Sleep Cycle

The body has a 24-hour cyclical pattern known as the **circadian rhythm,** during which body metabolism and functions increase and decrease in rhythmic patterns. For example, body temperature usually is lowest in the predawn hours and highest in the late evening hours, which is why children tend to spike fevers more in the evening and early nighttime hours, after the health-care provider's office has closed.

Sleep is cyclical and alternates with longer periods of wakefulness. Two sleep cycles have been identified: *non–rapid eye movement (NREM) sleep* and *rapid eye movement (REM) sleep*. NREM sleep involves four stages and is considered the deepest and most restful sleep cycle (Table 19.2). It makes up approximately 60% of an infant's sleep time and 80% of an adult's. These sleep cycles are repeated several times a night depending on the length of time spent in sleep. Antianxiety and sleep-promoting medications can interfere with REM sleep, preventing the individual from feeling "rested" even after having slept several hours.

> **KNOWLEDGE CONNECTION**
>
> Compare rest with restorative sleep. What are the central nervous system functions that occur during sleep? Differentiate between REM sleep and NREM sleep.

Amount of Sleep Required

The body requires different amounts of sleep depending on the person's age, health, and fatigue level. The average number of hours of sleep required in healthy individuals is:

- **Newborns:** 16 to 18 hours per day
- **Infants up to 2 years:** 12 to 14 hours per day, including naps
- **Children 3 to 6 years:** 12 hours per day, including naps
- **Children 7 to 12:** 10 hours per night
- **Adolescents:** 8.5 to 9.5 hours per night
- **Young adults:** 7.5 to 8 hours per night
- **Older adults:** gradually decreases to 5.5 or 6 hours per night, may begin to nap

Societal pressures to earn more money and participate in extracurricular activities tend to lead us to think we must work longer hours and be doing something all the time, which interferes with the sleep and rest requirements of children and adults alike. Studies show that most Americans do not get enough sleep and complain that they feel sleepy during the day. These studies also show that automobile accidents and on-the-job injuries increase dramatically in sleep-deprived people. Statistics indicate that nursing errors increase during the last 4 hours of 12-hour shifts. Because of this, it is important that you evaluate your sleep and work habits. How much sleep is optimum for you? Do you get adequate sleep so that you do not feel sleepy the next day?

• WORD • BUILDING •

circadian rhythm: circa – about + dian – day; rhuthmos – to flow

Table 19.2
Stages of REM and NREM Sleep

NREM Sleep	
Stage I	Relaxation begins during Stage I, as metabolism and vital signs begin to slow. The lightest sleep occurs, lasting only a few minutes. The individual is easily aroused and, if awakened, feels as if he or she has been daydreaming.
Stage II	Relaxation deepens as metabolism continues to slow. The individual begins to experience sound sleep, but arousal is still relatively easy. Stage II lasts 10 to 20 minutes.
Stage III	Stage III lasts 15 to 30 minutes. Deep sleep begins as muscles are now completely relaxed. The parasympathetic nervous system slows vital signs further and the body becomes immobile. Arousal is more difficult.
Stage IV	It becomes very difficult to arouse the person during this deepest sleep, which lasts 15 to 30 minutes. If the individual is sleep deprived, more time will be spent here. The body rests and is restored during this deep sleep. Even though the eyes are still, dreaming may occur during this stage.
REM Sleep	
REM sleep occurs at the end of each NREM cycle. The first cycle occurs about 90 minutes after sleep begins. Rapid eye movement begins and vital signs fluctuate. The brain is very active and is engaged in vivid dreaming that may be remembered after awakening occurs. The duration increases with each cycle, averaging 20 minutes. REM sleep is not as restful as NREM sleep.	

KNOWLEDGE CONNECTION

How much sleep does a newborn require? A school-age child? A young adult?

Patient Teaching Connection

We Need to Educate Parents About Sleep

It is important that you educate parents regarding sleep requirements of infants and children in an effort to promote better health and increase the learning abilities of school-age children. Teach parents to establish a time for going to bed and to be consistent in its enforcement. This sometimes requires limiting a child's participation in extracurricular activities to only one or two per week. Explain that certain bedtime rituals are helpful in gaining cooperation from the child; these rituals may include the following:

- Giving a warm bath at a set time
- Brushing the child's hair or applying lotion to the child's skin
- Giving each family member good-night kisses
- Allowing the child to select a stuffed animal or doll to sleep with
- Reading a bedtime story or Bible verses to the child
- Saying a bedtime prayer

The use of such rituals helps establish more regular sleep habits for children. Teach parents that the use of nightlights may be helpful to allay fears of the dark.

Factors Affecting Rest and Restorative Sleep

There are many factors that affect the body's ability to rest and obtain the restorative sleep that it needs. The factors may be physiological, emotional, or environmental. Chronic sleep deprivation can result in fatigue, irritability, slow response time, blurred vision, headaches, forgetfulness, and confusion.

Lifestyle

Components of a lifestyle that many view as normal may have detrimental effects on rest and sleep. Caffeine, nicotine, alcohol, and sleep-inducing medications all can impair the body's ability to get adequate sleep. Caffeine and nicotine interfere with the initiation of sleep, whereas alcohol causes awakening during the night. Individuals who work the night shift often have difficulty getting enough sleep during the day. Exercise is conducive to sleep when it is performed early in the day but inhibits sleep in most people if performed within 1 to 2 hours of bedtime. Individuals who work in high-stress jobs often complain of continual problems sleeping.

Stress and Anxiety

All humans experience stress and anxiety and often take those stresses and worries to bed with them at night. Stress can prevent one from falling asleep and cause one to awaken during the night.

Environmental

Environmental temperatures that are too warm or cold, hospital noises and bright lights, waking the patient for nursing care, and other hospital routines interfere with a patient's ability to sleep. An uncomfortable hospital bed also can play havoc with a patient's comfort and sleep. Patients in intensive care units commonly complain of interruption of sleep due to noise produced by hospital staff; other patients; and equipment, such as bright lights, beeping sounds, alarms, telephones, and pagers.

Illness and Health Problems

Individuals who have health problems, illnesses, or injuries may suffer symptoms that interfere with their sleep, including the following:

- Pain or discomfort
- Shortness of breath or dyspnea
- Itching
- Reflux of gastric contents into throat
- Sinus drainage, congestion, or coughing
- Fever or diaphoresis
- Frequent elimination

Sleep Disorders

Various sleep disorders also interfere with the body's ability to obtain adequate restorative sleep (Table 19.3). The effects of these disorders range from annoying to life threatening. A constant singular positive airway pressure (CPAP) breathing machine is used for people who suffer from chronic sleep apnea. The CPAP and bilevel positive airway pressure (BiPAP) machines utilize pressurized air to open up the airway and keep the throat from closing during sleep. When someone stops breathing during his sleep, he will awaken from his sleep gasping for air. A person suffering from chronic sleep apnea will not remember the episode and may suffer with chronic fatigue due to restless sleep. The CPAP can be set for a single pressure, whereas the BiPAP can be set to the timing of how the patient breathes. If the patient's breath falls below the desired number during sleep, the BiPAP will force pressurized air into his lungs to help open up his airway. The CPAP or BiPAP device is placed around the bridge of the nose and mouth and secured to the back of the head with Velcro straps. Always follow the manufacturer's directions when applying a CPAP or BiPAP device.

Interventions to Promote Restorative Sleep

Promotion of sleep is an important nursing function that is sometimes overlooked. Most interventions are easy and simple to perform and produce increased comfort, cleanliness, and relaxation. They can also assist normal body functions and make the environment more conducive to sleep.

Prepare the Environment

Prepare the patient's room by modifying the room temperature to the patient's preference. Some individuals prefer a slightly cooler temperature for sleeping; others may have difficulty staying warm at night and want the temperature set a bit warmer. Provide blankets and pillows as desired by the patient. Clear the pathway from the door to the bed and from the bed to the bathroom. Turn on a nightlight or provide dim lighting that is enough to ensure safety and orientation in an unfamiliar environment but not enough to disturb sleep. Close the room door to reduce noise.

Comfort

To provide comfort at bedtime, begin by washing the patient's face and hands, detangling and brushing the hair, brushing the teeth, and moistening the lips with petroleum

Table 19.3
Sleep Disorders

Disorder	*Description*
Bruxism	Grinding of teeth during sleep
Insomnia	Chronic inability to fall asleep or stay asleep
Narcolepsy	Condition causing uncontrollable, recurrent daytime episodes of sleepiness; can hinder driving and operating dangerous equipment
Night terrors	Nightmares in children that cause awakening and fear
Restless legs syndrome	An intolerable crawling sensation in the legs that results in an irresistible urge to move the legs
Sleep apnea	Inability to maintain breathing while sleeping; the patient usually snores, accompanied by periods of apnea lasting from 10 seconds to 2 minutes; can be life-threatening
Somnambulism	Sleepwalking; has the potential for serious consequences
Sundowning	Confusion and disorientation in elderly patients that occurs in the evening hours; the patient is at higher risk for injury

jelly, if needed. Offer a snack if hungry and offer fresh water or cold or warm milk if preferred. Assist the patient with toileting as needed. Assess to determine if the patient has any pain or discomforts that require medication. Straighten and remove wrinkles in gown and bed linens, reposition the patient, and provide support with pillows.

Relaxation

One of the easiest ways to help a patient relax is by administering a back massage. Another intervention that helps to relax the patient is providing range-of-motion exercises, which stretch the muscles and stimulate the circulation. Playing soft, relaxing music is a good source of relaxation for some patients, while other individuals prefer meditation to initiate the relaxation process. Ask about the patient's concerns. Sometimes a patient needs validation of his or her feelings or needs to vent frustration or worries. Learn to be an active listener. Often 5 minutes spent listening and expressing empathy is all it takes to help a patient begin to relax.

Pain Relief

Pain must be relieved in order for a patient to sleep soundly and deeply. If analgesics are required, they should be administered. There is a common myth perpetuated by some nurses: "The patient could not be hurting too badly. He complained of pain but was asleep when I got there with his pain medication. So I didn't give it to him." It is totally possible for some patients to sleep even though they are in pain. Sleep is sometimes exactly what the body needs to heal. Remember that much repair and healing takes place during sleep. The residual effects of general anesthesia can affect the level of consciousness of a patient for 24 to 48 hours. If a patient is drowsy or falls asleep after requesting pain medication, do not ignore his or her request for pain relief. Treat the pain.

Sleep Medications

Some patients just cannot sleep when hospitalized, no matter what interventions you try. Most health-care providers will order sleep medication that may be used on an as-needed basis. They are effective for short-term use, but they interfere with sleep with chronic use. It is always better for the patient if you can promote sleep without medications that can interfere with REM sleep. ***Safety: Monitor the patient for sleep walking, fatigue, and dizziness while taking sleep medications.***

Supervision/Delegation Connection

The Delegation of Tasks Does Not Relieve You of Your Responsibilities

Delegation of most of the nonpharmaceutical interventions to certified nursing assistants and unlicensed assistive personnel is common and acceptable. However, it is important that you perform assessments as needed to determine the patient's usual sleep habits and to identify what problems may be preventing the patient from sleeping. It is also your responsibility to work with the patient and other staff members to determine which nonpharmaceutical interventions would be most appropriate.

Skill 19.1 Application of TENS Unit

Assessment Steps

1. Review the health-care provider's order for site of application, settings for the TENS unit, and length of treatment. ***This reduces the risk of administering incorrect treatment.***
2. Assess the patient's knowledge level regarding a TENS unit. ***This determines patient learning needs.***

Planning Steps

1. Gather needed equipment and supplies: TENS unit, battery, lead wires, electrodes, conduction gel if the electrodes are not precoated, and tape if the electrodes are not self-adhesive. ***Preparation saves time and effort.***
2. Assess the patient's level of pain or discomfort using a scale of 0 to 10. ***Using the same pain scale each time allows for more consistent pain measurement.***

Implementation Steps

1. Follow the Initial Implementation Steps located on the inside back cover.
2. Insert the battery and lead wires into the TENS unit, making certain the unit is turned off ***to prevent premature delivery of electrical impulses.***
3. *Safety: Apply conductive gel to electrodes that are not precoated to ensure conduction and prevent shocks due to noncontinuous conduction.*
4. Secure the electrodes to their designated sites. If necessary, use tape to hold the electrodes in place.
5. Turn on the TENS unit. Instruct the patient to inform you as soon as he or she can feel the tingling sensation.
6. Gradually increase the amplitude according to the patient's response. Inform the patient that he or she should tell you when it feels like a gentle tapping.

The electrical impulses should be well within the patient's comfort range. Caution the patient to avoid trying to "tolerate it at higher, more uncomfortable amplitudes." ***Discomfort prevents complete relaxation and tightens muscles, which increases pain.***

7. Assess the patient's comfort level every 15 minutes during the first hour of use. If the health-care provider's order states to leave the TENS unit on longer than 1 hour, continue to assess the patient's comfort level every 1 to 2 hours. ***This helps to assess the effectiveness of the treatment.***

(skill continues on page 370)

Skill 19.1 (continued)

8. At the designated time, turn the unit off before removing the electrodes. ***Removing the electrodes while the unit is still on can result in shocks from current, which are uncomfortable.***
9. Remove the adhesive electrodes and wipe the patient's skin to remove gel.
10. Follow the Ending Implementation Steps located on the inside back cover.

Evaluation Steps

1. Assess how the patient tolerated the treatment, along with the level of discomfort according to a scale of 0 to 10.

Sample Documentation

04/22/22 1530 States right & left. lumbar area is tight and hurting, a 6 on a scale of 0 to 10. TENS unit applied to left and right lumbar area, pulse mode, and amplitude. ——— Nurse's signature and credentials

04/22/22 1630 TENS unit removed. States lumbar pain is now 2 on 0 to 10 scale. ——— Nurse's signature and credentials

POST CONFERENCE

Other students are aware that your patient was angry and that his wife left in tears. They ask if the patient was difficult for you. You explain that your patient was experiencing phantom pain that he would not describe because he thought it was impossible to feel pain in his amputated foot. Your evaluation of your clinical day is very positive. It felt good to relieve his fears by explaining phantom pain to him. Several interventions helped him relax, especially the back massage. After medicating him with an ordered opiate for pain, he slept soundly for 3 hours and woke up refreshed. He was much more pleasant and wanted to call his wife to apologize.

Key Points

- The gate control theory purports the transmission of pain impulses to the central nervous system by a "gate" that opens and closes in response to sensory input.
- Pain is always what the patient says it is. The patient is the expert on his or her pain.
- Pain is a warning sign that something is wrong or that tissue damage has occurred or is about to occur. The body responds to pain physiologically, psychologically, and behaviorally.
- Pain is classified as either nociceptive or neuropathic.
- Nociceptors are randomly dispersed throughout the skin, subcutaneous tissue, and muscular tissue. These nerve pain receptors can be stimulated by temperature changes, tissue damage, and certain chemicals.
- Neuropathic pain is the burning, stabbing, or sometimes deep ache that your patient describes when there is a nerve compression caused by pressure from tumors, lymphedema, or compression fractures of the spine.
- Factors that affect pain are ethnic and cultural beliefs, developmental stage, individual values, previous pain experiences, personal support system, emotions, and fatigue.
- Management and treatment of pain may include acknowledgment and acceptance, hot and cold packs, massage, TENS unit, acupressure and acupuncture, relaxation, distraction, nonopioid analgesics, NSAIDs, opiate/opioid analgesics, and adjuvant analgesics.
- Pain can affect numerous aspects of a patient's life, including activities of daily living, sleep, nutrition, activity level, family relationships, job performance, social life, cognitive abilities, and spiritual beliefs.
- Rest and restorative sleep are necessary for pain relief, comfort, and physiological, psychological, and emotional health.
- Factors that affect rest and restorative sleep include lifestyle, stress level, environmental factors, illness, and sleep disorders.
- Sleep cycles include both REM and NREM sleep.
- Interventions that promote sleep include preparing the environment, providing comfort, relaxation, active listening to patient concerns, and medications as needed.

Review Questions

Select the answer(s) that is most appropriate for each of the following questions. Some questions may have more than one correct answer. Select all that apply.

1. Pain can indicate which of the following?
   1. Damage has occurred to tissue.
   2. Edema is increasing and placing pressure on nerve endings.
   3. The wound is healing normally.
   4. Circulation to the site is adequate.
   5. There is a potential for damage to the tissues.

2. Which of the following individuals is the expert regarding the amount of pain Brad Monett is experiencing?
   1. The nurse
   2. The health-care provider
   3. Brad
   4. The pain clinic representative

3. Christy Leigh is complaining of a burning, searing pain along the lateral aspect of her left foot. When you assess Christy's foot, you see no wounds or abnormalities. She tells you that she has not injured the foot but has been having this pain intermittently for approximately 1 month. Upon reviewing her chart, you read that Christy has severe diabetes. Which type pain do you think Christy is having?
   1. Neuropathic pain
   2. Cutaneous pain
   3. Visceral pain
   4. Nociceptive pain

4. Alex Ganner has pancreatic cancer in the advanced stages and has been at home. He has been attempting to get relief of severe abdominal pain with prescription opioids for 6 days, but the pain is not responding. He finally agrees to be admitted for treatment of pain. Which type of pain is Mr. Ganner experiencing?
   1. Cutaneous pain
   2. Neuropathic pain
   3. Chronic pain
   4. Intractable pain
   5. Referred pain

5. Marissa Jones suffers from a sleep disorder that awakens her during the night, and she is experiencing chronic fatigue. Which sleep disorder is Marissa suffering?
   1. Insomnia
   2. Somnambulism
   3. Sleep apnea
   4. Narcolepsy

6. Which of the following are NSAIDs?
   1. Hydrocodone
   2. Codeine
   3. Ibuprofen
   4. Naproxen
   5. Meperdine
   6. Aspirin

7. Joseph Walker is suffering from chronic back pain and is requesting pain medication. Upon reviewing his medical administration record, you notice it is too early to have pain medication. What nonpharmacologic methods can you use to relieve his pain?
   1. Massage
   2. Hot and cold packs
   3. Transcutaneous electrical nerve stimulation
   4. Acupressure
   5. Relaxation

Fill-in-the-Blank Questions

8. Captain Julius James, a veteran of the Vietnam War, lost his right foot in combat. He is hospitalized with pneumonia, and you are assigned to admit and care for him during your shift. While interviewing Captain James, he tells you that he has right foot pain a lot in the evenings. You would document this as ________________ pain in the admission assessment.

9. You are administering medications to Ruth Smith, who has severe arthritis in most of the joints of her hands and lower extremities that causes her significant joint and muscle pain. Her medication administration record shows that she is to receive 800 milligrams of ibuprofen three times per day for this pain. You know that ibuprofen is not a narcotic and is classified as a(n) ____________ because of its anti-inflammatory effects.

ANSWERS 1. 1, 2, 5. 2. 3. 3. 1. 4. 4, 5. 5. 3. 6. 3, 4, 6. 7. 1, 2, 3, 4, 5. 8. Phantom. 9. NSAID

Critical Thinking Exercise

Answers available online.

1. It is 1:00 a.m., and one of the elderly patients on your unit is unable to sleep tonight. He tells you that he is worried about his cat at home. He knows his neighbor is feeding the cat each day, but he is concerned that the cat is lonesome without him. You know that the patient needs restorative sleep to help him recover from a urinary tract infection. What interventions might you try to help him get some rest?

Additional Resources

DAVIS edge. Use the scratch off code on the inside front cover of your book to access online quizzes that will help you to improve your scores on course exams and prepare for the NCLEX-PN®.

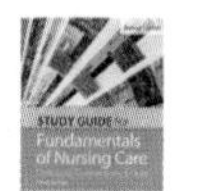
Study Guide

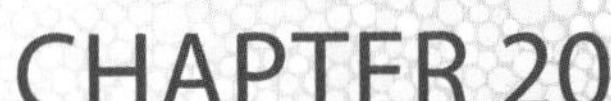

CHAPTER 20
Admission, Transfer, and Discharge

KEY TERMS

Admission process (ad-MI-shun PRAH-sess)
Discharge instruction form (DISS-charj in-STRUK-shun FORM)
Discharge planning (DISS-charj PLAN-ing)
Discharge process (DISS-charj PRAH-sess)
Leaving AMA
Medication reconciliation (med-i-KAY-shun REE-kon-si-lee-AY-shun)
Separation anxiety (SEP-uh-RAY-shun ang-ZYE-uh-tee)
Terminal cleaning (TER-mi-nuhl KLEE-ning)
Transfer summary form (TRANS-fer SUM-uh-ree FORM)

CHAPTER CONCEPTS

Patient-Centered Care
Culture

LEARNING OUTCOMES

1. Define various terms associated with admission, transfer, and discharge.
2. Identify four common patient reactions to admission.
3. Describe therapeutic nursing interventions that will demonstrate respect and compassion for common reactions to admission.
4. Explain the importance of making the patient feel welcome during the admission process.
5. Relate specific ways you can enhance communication in a culturally diverse patient population.
6. Discuss components of the admitting procedure.
7. Discuss the importance of completing an admission orientation checklist and personal belongings inventory.
8. Outline nursing responsibilities and appropriate interventions during the patient discharge processes.
9. Describe the discharge process, including the discharge summary.
10. Discuss the significance of medication reconciliation as part of the discharge process.
11. Compare the transfer of a patient to another facility to a transfer within the same facility.
12. Identify appropriate documentation for admission, transfer, and discharge scenarios.
13. Discuss information found in the Connection features in this chapter.
14. Identify specific safety information.

CRITICAL THINKING CONNECTION

Clinical Assignment

You will be caring for a 67-year-old male who fell on the ice and shattered his right femur. He had surgery to repair it, using plates, screws, and wire. He cannot bear any weight on his right leg for a minimum of 8 weeks. He is married, but his wife is in poor physical health and is unable to care for him. As soon as you arrive on the floor, you learn that he is to be discharged today because his insurance will no longer pay for hospitalization. No decisions have yet been made about where he will go upon discharge.

Continued

CRITICAL THINKING CONNECTION—cont'd

Critical Thinking Questions:

1. When does discharge teaching for the patient begin?
2. How would you coordinate care for the patient since his wife is unable to care for him?
3. Describe how you would advocate for the patient.

Many individuals have never been admitted to a hospital as a patient nor even had a loved one hospitalized. Maybe you have not been through this traumatic experience or have not thought about hospitalization being traumatic. Maybe it does not seem like it is a big deal to become hospitalized. However, those who either have been a patient or have attended a close friend or relative while he or she was hospitalized know differently.

In this chapter, you will learn some possible patient reactions and how you can respond to them to decrease the trauma for your patients and their loved ones. You will also learn the guidelines and processes of admitting, transferring, and discharging patients. At the end of this chapter, you will be better prepared to meet your patients' needs during these periods of transition.

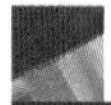

ADMISSION

As the nurse, you have the opportunity, ability, and responsibility to make admission less stressful for your patients. It is during the **admission process** that you will make your first impression on the patient, one that either can help improve your patient's stay or make it a negative experience. This is the time to begin establishing rapport and a trusting relationship with the patient.

A patient can be admitted from the physician's office as a direct admit to the hospital. When a patient is being admitted from the physician's office, the doctor will contact the hospital and speak with the hospitalist (a general hospital doctor). If the physician has hospital privileges, then he or she will write doctor's orders for the hospital nurses so they can go ahead and start the admission process. A direct admission can vary from hospital to hospital, so it is important to contact the hospital for more information. If the nurse is receiving or giving information regarding a transfer, it is important to document the name of the nurse information was taken from or given to. The nurse will inform the patient of the transfer and calm any fears they have.

It is so important for you to begin the process of admission with the most positive approach possible. ***Walk into the room with a smile on your face.*** Make it a requirement for yourself! Make a conscious effort to avoid letting unpleasantries, such as being short-handed or behind schedule, show in your speech, facial expression, or body language. It is amazing how easily expressions can sometimes be read or interpreted. Avoid sighing or taking an obvious deep breath as if fatigued, frowning or pinching your lips together, grinding your teeth, and rolling your eyes—all things one may do without thinking about it when one is stressed or busy. The patient will remember this as his or her first impression of you, making it difficult, if not impossible, to develop the rapport that you desire and need in order to be therapeutic with your patient. Speak kindly and respectfully to the new patient. Remember that he or she is likely to be nervous and concerned about having to be admitted to the hospital. One of your responsibilities is to begin to relieve this nervousness and begin the process of developing a trusting rapport that will enhance the patient's recovery and comfort level. Introduce yourself and include your credentials so that the patient will know whether you are a registered nurse, licensed practical/vocational nurse (LPN/LVN), student nurse, or someone from another department such as the business office or laboratory. Shake the patient's hand (Fig. 20.1). This provides a form of physical contact that is not threatening or demeaning and exhibits a welcoming approach.

Make brief eye contact and speak at a rate that does not sound hurried. Address the patient by his or her surname, such as Mr. or Mrs. Stephens. Avoid the use of first names unless the patient specifically asks you to address him or her by first name. Avoid using terms of endearment such as "honey" and "sweetie." It is unprofessional to use these endearments for adults even though you may not mean them in a negative way. Use of these terms may be considered condescending or patronizing, especially for those patients who are from an older generation than you.

Reactions to Admission

When admitting a patient, make certain that he or she is made to feel welcome. It is very difficult to establish rapport and a trusting relationship with a patient who feels that he or she is viewed by staff as a burden and not welcome. The patient does not need to know how busy you are or how badly your day might have gone. He or she is focused on his or her own health situation during admission. Box 20.1 presents some of the possible reactions your patients may experience during admission and hospitalization.

Fear

Fear of the *unknown* is something most individuals have experienced at different points in their lives. With hospitalization, there are so many variables that most individuals have little or no knowledge of what is going to happen to them. This fear of the unknown probably is one of the most common responses your patients will exhibit. Fear of the unknown comes under *safety and security* in Maslow's hierarchy of human needs and can result in insecurity if the unknowns are not revealed in a timely manner. Some of the

• **WORD • BUILDING •**

hospitalist: hospital – related to a guest + ist – member of a profession

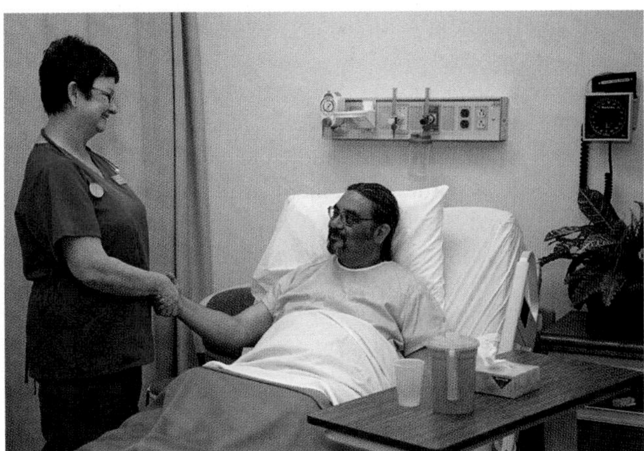

FIGURE 20.1 Making a good first impression helps the process of establishing rapport and trust with the patient.

questions plaguing a patient during admission may include the following:

- What is wrong with me? What is my unknown diagnosis? What does it mean?
- What tests, procedures, treatments, or surgeries will I undergo?
- Will there be discomfort or pain?
- Who are all these people who keep coming into my room, one after another?
- How long will I have to be here?

It is helpful if you tell the patient what you are about to do, explain what he or she can expect, and ask if there are any questions you might answer. Reducing the number of unknowns for your patient will lower his or her fear and stress levels and gain better compliance.

If the patient is a child, allow the parent to hold the child for as much of the admission process as you can. Physically get down to the child's level rather than towering above the child. In other words, if the child is sitting on mother's lap, squat down or pull up a chair, but put yourself at eye level with the child so that you are not intimidating simply because you are "taller" than the child. Remember to smile and talk softly and slowly. It is often helpful to allow the child to hold and become familiar with supplies or equipment that will be used in his or her care. For example, allow the child to take a teddy bear's tympanic temperature or listen to mommy's heart with your stethoscope (Fig. 20.2). Never tell the child that a procedure will not hurt unless it is the truth. It is important to be honest and admit that it "will hurt a little bit." You can then follow up with the child by describing what can be done to decrease the discomfort. If you tell the child that something will not hurt and it does, you instill distrust rather than trust and damage your credibility with the child.

Anxiety

Anxiety is another *safety and security* concern in Maslow's hierarchy. The physician, nurse practitioners, physician assistants, and nurses may view the patient's diagnosis as a common occurrence that is easily treated, with the expectation the patient will recover quickly and return to normal routines. However, the patient most likely will not have the knowledge that his or her caregivers possess, and the diagnosis probably will not feel common or simple. Fear of the diagnosis can result in high levels of anxiety, especially if it is something as serious or frightening as cancer. It is important to remember that the layperson usually does not know what you mean when you tell him that you are going to "auscultate" his lungs. This may sound invasive or scary to the patient because he may not be familiar with medical terminology. The most common way to reduce this anxiety is to always explain what you are about to do *before* you do it, even the simple things such as "listen to your lungs." Avoid the use of medical terminology and use layperson's terms whenever possible. And when you do use medical jargon with adults, explain what those words mean in terms they will understand. Never assume that adults know medical terminology unless you know that it is a fact.

Anxiety can also develop due to separation from familiar surroundings and significant others; this is known as **separation anxiety.** Most individuals prefer to recover from illness or injury at home, where they are most comfortable and where care can be provided by family or loved ones rather than strangers.

A patient may worry about responsibilities as well, such as who will care for his or her children or other dependent loved ones, such as an elderly parent or pets, or who will run

> **Box 20.1**
> **Common Patient Reactions to Admission**
>
> Becoming a patient in a hospital or outpatient clinic is always stressful. Even when it may bring relief, comfort, or even a cure, it is still not the most relaxing situation in which to find oneself. So many things are unfamiliar—the environment, the diagnosis or illness, the diagnostic testing and treatment it requires, the staff with whom the patient does not have an established relationship, the facility routines that will be imposed upon the patient, and the extent of the ensuing financial cost it will bring. The list of unknowns for the patient is endless, and each unknown has the potential to invoke unexpected or unusual reactions from the patient. Some of the more common reactions include the following:
>
> - Fear of the unknown, which could be caused by a new diagnosis, tests or procedures, pain or discomfort, or even health-care providers who are strangers
> - Anxiety, which could be caused by problems with child care during hospitalization, effects of hospitalization on job, the cost and expenses of hospitalization, and separation from familiar surrounds and significant others
> - Loss of control over things such as attire, modesty, privacy, daily schedule of activities, and diet
> - Loss of identity, because the patient may feel he or she is just one of many patients, a patient number, or a diagnosis

• WORD • BUILDING •
diagnosis: dia – through + gnosis – knowledge

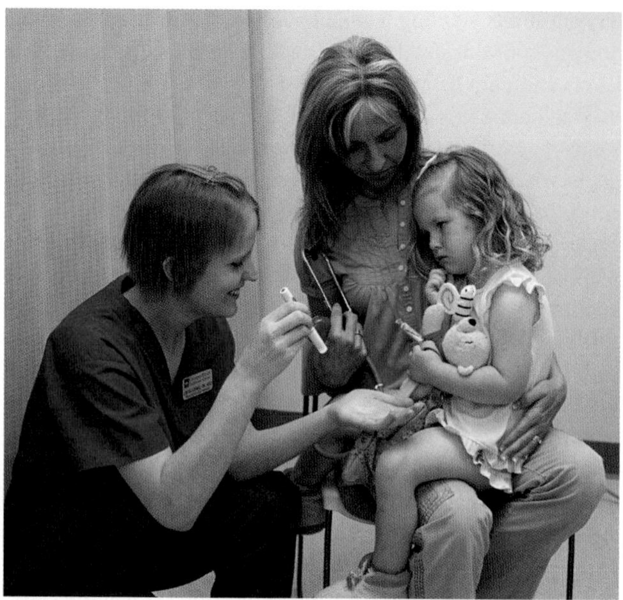

FIGURE 20.2 Attempt to familiarize the child with the stethoscope, penlight, or other equipment to reduce the child's anxiety.

his or her business or farm while he or she is hospitalized. Individuals may not have strong support systems or family members who live nearby. The patient may not have anyone whom the patient feels he or she can depend on to help with these responsibilities.

A common cause of anxiety is financial concern. The patient may worry about the cost of hospitalization if there is no insurance coverage, the added expense of missing work, or the expense of hiring someone to care for his or her dependents. It is often a problem for those without insurance to purchase their prescriptions. Thus, you will need to make a list of all medications that the patient is taking and inquire if there are other medications that have been prescribed that he or she is not taking because of preference or expense. It is important to identify these problems and involve appropriate hospital resources as soon as possible. Social workers can generally assist the patient with some of these types of problems.

Real-World Connection

Separation Anxiety Is Real

Separation anxiety is particularly common in children and older adults. Young children are dependent on and accustomed to having their needs met by their parents or guardians, with whom they usually have a trusting relationship. The younger the child, the more dependent the child will be on the parent or guardian. The older adult may have been married to his or her spouse for 40 or 50 years, sometimes rarely or never having been separated from the spouse overnight. If the older adult is dependent on a spouse, child, or other designated caregiver, separation from the caregiver can cause severe anxiety and loneliness.

To help decrease anxieties, encourage the patient to ask questions and look for signs of understanding as you answer those questions. Provide a brief but factual explanation of the patient's diagnosis. Avoid the use of medical terminology unless it is clear the patient understands it; otherwise, use layperson's terms. Reassure the patient whenever possible without giving false reassurance. Encourage a child's parent or guardian to stay with the child if at all possible to reduce separation anxiety. Ask the parent to bring a couple of toys or a favorite blanket from home to help familiarize the room for the child. The patient who is elderly may also be comforted by allowing a family member to stay.

If policy allows, provide a recliner or cot to allow the family member to obtain rest while staying with the patient. Offer a pillow and blanket, towel and washcloth, coffee or tea, and the option of ordering a meal to be delivered to the room if that is possible. Do whatever you can to accommodate the loved one staying with your patient; not only will this make him or her more comfortable, but it will help your patient to experience less anxiety and heal faster. A good nurse takes care of the family as well as the individual patient.

Loss of Control

Another response common to hospitalization is loss of control, and it, too, comes under Maslow's *safety and security* needs. There is generally a steady stream of individuals at the patient's bedside. Visitors can come from the laboratory, radiology department, and business offices; they can be interns and residents; and they can be nurse assistants, primary care nurses, or a registered nurse case manager. And this is only a partial list of hospital staff who can visit the patient at the bedside. They all ask numerous questions, many of them repeated by several individuals, leading patients to complain of repetition. Surveys indicate that one of the most common patient complaints is a "lack of communication" among health-care providers. Effective communication by health-care providers can prevent some of this question duplication. Pay attention to what has already been documented by others.

Many of the questions are of a private nature, some being very personal to the point of discomfort for the patient, and the patient may feel the answers to some of the questions are not the business of health-care providers. If your patient feels this way, explain why some of the more personal questions are asked and how they may be applicable to his or her care. Also, make certain the door to the patient's room is closed when interviewing the new patient. Avoid asking questions out in the hall, at the nurse's station, or at any site where other individuals could overhear.

Other aspects of hospitalization that may make a patient feel a loss of control include the following:

- Sharing a room with another patient
- Sleeping in a different bed
- Using a different toilet
- Eating whatever food is provided regardless of how it was prepared

- Being forced to accommodate the facility's "schedule" for meals, waking and sleeping, health-care provider's rounds, diagnostic tests, etc.
- Being awakened during the night for the provision of nursing care
- Being disturbed by the "normal" hospital noises

ATTIRE AND MODESTY. Other areas where loss of control may be felt include attire, modesty, and privacy. For example, when a patient is admitted for certain tests, surgeries, or procedures, the nurse may request that the patient wear a hospital gown rather than the patient's personal pajamas. It may seem a small issue to you, but to the patient it may represent a loss of control. Whenever possible, allow the patient to wear his or her own pajamas or gown if the patient has a preference.

Take care to protect the patient's modesty while assisting the patient to dress or undress as well as during examinations, tests, and treatments. Failure to do so can result in substantial patient embarrassment. It is important to remember that your patient may view exposure of his or her own body differently than would a health-care provider. It is not an everyday occurrence for patients to view and handle other people's bodies as it is for you. Demonstrate sensitivity and respect by preserving your patient's modesty at all times. If it is necessary for the patient to wear a typical hospital gown, be vigilant in keeping the gown edges together and overlapping in the back, tying the strings to keep the gown closed as much as possible. Use drapes to prevent unnecessary exposure during delivery of nursing care. Always knock before entering the patient's room. If the curtain is pulled, ask for permission to enter. While providing personal care, protect the patient's modesty by closing the door and pulling the privacy curtain around the bed. Avoid exposing more of the patient's body than is necessary; use a sheet or bath blanket for coverage, if needed. Allow the patient to do as much changing of his or her own clothes as possible. Encourage independence unless there are restrictions in activity. Let the patient wear his or her own pajamas if possible and allow underwear to remain in place unless contraindicated. If the patient must wear a hospital gown, use a second gown put on backward to serve as a robe for added modesty.

There is no excuse for walking down a hallway and seeing patients exposed simply because doors have not been closed, gowns have not been tied, robes have not been used, or a sheet or blanket has not been placed over the patient's lap while sitting in a wheelchair or room chair. This is too common an occurrence in most facilities. As a nurse, go to all lengths to preserve your patients' privacy and modesty.

An older adult may be mortified when the gender of the nurse differs from his or her gender. In certain cultures, it is even prohibited for a female to provide nursing care for a male and vice versa. It is pertinent to make efforts to accommodate patients who feel strongly about this issue, especially for personal body functions such as bathing and toileting. When you must provide care to a patient of different gender than yourself, be vigilant to demonstrate respect and provide for privacy as much as possible while delivering nursing care. This will help to establish rapport in a situation that may be uncomfortable for the patient of a different gender.

Patient Rooms

Although private rooms are now more commonly available to patients, in some hospital settings there is still the possibility that the patient will have to share a room with a stranger. Generally, the two patients not only share a room, but they also share bathroom facilities and are able to overhear each other's conversations with health-care providers and families. These situations can cause undue stress and feelings of loss of control for the patient.

If caring for a patient who is sharing a room, pull the curtain between the beds, stand near the head of the bed while conversing with the patient, and strive to keep the volume of your voice low when discussing sensitive issues. At times, it may be prudent to take the patient to a private examination room before divulging devastating or sensitive test results. It may be possible to arrange for the roommate to be taken for a walk or a ride in a wheelchair to allow more privacy for personal interaction with the patient.

DECISION MAKING. Allow the patient to make decisions when possible, even seemingly small ones such as the following:

- "Do you prefer ice water or tap water in your pitcher?"
- "Do you prefer your drinks with or without a straw?"
- "Would you like to leave your socks on?"

Provide choices and let the patient feel that he or she maintains some control over the situation as much as possible.

Loss of Identity

Some patients feel a loss of identity when they are hospitalized. It is easy to see how it develops. They now have a room number, a patient number, and a call light that they must use to obtain assistance. They are now one of many patients and are often forced to wait for what they might consider to be routine services, such as the following:

- The performance of a test or procedure
- The delivery of pain medication
- The delivery of their lunch tray
- Their call light being answered
- Visits from their health-care provider
- Assistance with bathing
- Linen changes

Explain to the patient why you are placing an identification band on his or her wrist. Make it a priority to learn the new patient's name quickly and call him or her by Mr., Miss, Ms., or Mrs. along with their last name. As stated before, avoid calling patients by first name unless requested to do so. This is especially important to show respect to patients who are older than you and grew up as part of a different generation. Never refer to patients by a room number or a disease or condition. Calling the patient by his or her name helps maintain identity and eases the patient's feeling of being "just another number."

> **KNOWLEDGE CONNECTION**
> What age groups of patients are most prone to suffer separation anxiety? How can you help to relieve this anxiety?

Cultural Considerations

Patients will come from many different cultures and may have values, attitudes, beliefs, traditions, and customs that deviate from yours. They may not view the place of religion in daily life in the same way that you do or see the medical world as you see it. These cultural differences can magnify the problems of fear, anxiety, loss of control, and loss of identity. Fear and anxiety can increase if the patient feels that he or she will not be treated in a culturally acceptable manner. When someone of a different culture provides the patient's care, the patient may be concerned that cultural rituals surrounding religion, hygiene, manner of dress, nutrition, and even food preparation may not be possible. This can increase the feelings of loss of control and loss of identity. Cultural differences can also cause additional problems by hindering verbal and nonverbal communication with the patient (Box 20.2). It is extremely important not only that you are aware of these differences, but also that you display sensitivity and respect for patients' beliefs whether or not you agree with them. Acceptance is necessary to establish a trust-based rapport with your patients.

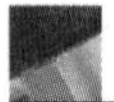

ADMITTING PROCEDURE

The patient's chart is initiated during the admitting process and includes various admission forms specific to each facility's policies and procedures. Admitting office staff obtains demographic data, such as the patient's:

- Full name
- Social Security number
- Age
- Date of birth
- Residential address
- Telephone number
- Next of kin name and contact information
- Religious preference
- Place of employment
- Insurance and billing data
- Physician's name
- Reason for admission
- Whether or not the patient has an advanced directive

Authority to Treat

Each facility has a form that must be completed and signed, granting permission for treatment. If the patient is a minor, the authorization for treatment must be signed by a parent or legal guardian. As you learned in Chapter 3, it is legal for an individual younger than age 18 years to sign authorization for treatment if he or she is an emancipated minor. The age at which an individual is no longer considered a minor differs from state to state. In most states, the patient may provide authority to treat at age 18 years.

Identification Bands

Either the nurse or the admission office personnel applies an identification wristband containing patient name, room number, hospital identification number, age, birth date, and physician's name. The identification wristband stays on the patient throughout the entire hospitalization. ***Safety: This identification band is one of the methods used to identify the patient prior to any procedure or administration of medications. If the***

Box 20.2

Culturally Savvy Communication

Communication between nurses and those with whom we share some of the same ethnic and cultural backgrounds, and maybe even similar religious beliefs, is not always easy or as clear as we think it is. It is of particular importance when there are cultural differences between two individuals, especially if there is a language barrier that exacerbate the problem. Work hard to become a culturally savvy communicator; it will bring unforeseen rapport, respect, trust, and rewards.

- Always address your patient by Mr., Mrs., Miss, or Ms. and his or her last name. Never use a first name to address a patient unless the patient requests it.
- Avoid the use of slang.
- Use simple, common, proper English.
- If there is a language barrier, provide an interpreter. Only use the patient's relatives to interpret if requested by the patient or there is no one else available.
- Do not attempt to use ethnic dialects unless you are fluent in the language.
- Use eye contact judiciously. Some cultures consider it disrespectful or a challenge to authority to look someone in the eye.
- Position yourself so that the patient can see your face and read your lips if necessary.
- Pay attention to the patient's facial expressions and other nonverbal communication. This may help you determine when the patient does not understand your communication.
- Exhibit respect for the patient's beliefs regarding health care, family, traditions, and religion.
- Clarify information when you do not understand what the patient has said.

patient is allergic to any medications, herbs, or foods, an allergy identification band is also applied. Different color bands are also used to indicate food and drug allergies, latex allergy, fall risk, and limb alert. The colors used may vary from state to state, although an allergy band may be bright red or yellow so that it is more easily noticed.

Nursing Responsibilities During Patient Admission

Once the patient is brought to his or her room, you have numerous tasks to perform as part of the admission process. If the patient's condition warrants direct admission from the physician's office or the emergency room without going to the admitting office, send a family member to the admitting office to complete the paperwork.

Introduction

When greeting the patient and family, remember to smile genuinely and introduce yourself, including your credentials. If the identification band has already been applied, check the band for confirmation of identity. If a band has not yet been applied, do so at this time. If there is a roommate, introduce the patients to each other. It is important to be courteous and respectful in your interactions with the new patient. The impression you make may be the lasting impression that goes home with the patient.

Orient the patient and family to the room, showing them how to obtain assistance and operate various room furnishings; also show them the availability and location of amenities (Box 20.3).

Admission Kit

Most hospitals have a basic admission kit that consists of a water pitcher or carafe, drinking glass, wash basin, emesis basin, soap dish, and box of tissues (Fig. 20.3). Make certain the admission kit is present at the bedside table; if it is missing, retrieve one from the supply room. Also provide a bedpan and urinal as appropriate. If the health-care provider's orders indicate the patient may have oral fluids, fill the pitcher with water and ice according to the patient's preference.

Provide the patient assistance as needed with undressing and donning either a hospital gown or his or her personal pajamas, ensuring privacy by closing the room door and pulling the privacy curtain. If the patient is able to perform this task without your assistance, allow her or him to do so. This reduces some of the initial embarrassment the patient may feel.

Personal Belongings Inventory

Complete an inventory of clothing and personal items, such as eyeglasses, dentures, and hearing aids, that have been brought to the hospital. These items may be kept at the bedside. Instruct the patient to send all valuables, such as money, credit cards, or jewelry, home with family members. If there is no family member available or the patient desires to keep valuables at the hospital, review with the patient the hospital's policy for storing valuables. Inventory the valuables and

Box 20.3

Admission Orientation Checklist

Each patient should be oriented upon admission to reduce anxiety and promote patient compliance. By providing the patient with a proper orientation, you allow the patient to maintain a better sense of control over the hospital experience, which is conducive to healing and a sense of well-being. Orientation of the patient to his or her room and hospital routines should include the following information:

- Location of the nurse's station in relation to the patient's room
- How to use the call light, intercom system, and emergency call light. *This is a good time to inform the patient of the health-care provider's orders regarding whether or not the patient is allowed to get out of bed.*
- Location of the bathroom
- How to use the telephone
- How to operate the bed. ***Safety: Explain that the bed should be kept in its lowest position.***
- How to adjust the lighting
- How to operate the television and radio
- Location of personal care items; closet and drawer space for patient's belongings
- Times meals are served and any dietary restrictions ordered by the health-care provider
- Location of the cafeteria and snack machines
- Hours that you will be his or her nurse and how often your visits are to be expected
- Any policies that apply to the patient or family, such as visitation times, cell phone usage, or tobacco use policy
- When the health-care provider normally makes visits

Safety: Make certain the patient is wearing an identification band and any necessary allergy alert band. Explain to the patient that each individual who provides care for the patient should check the name on the ID band as well as use a second identifier prior to delivery of all care. This will help to reduce the patient's irritation at repeatedly being asked to state his or her name. Plus, should a staff member fail to read the ID band as required, it provides the patient with the additional control of "offering the ID band for verification" to ensure that the staff member does indeed have the correct patient before beginning a treatment or administering medication.

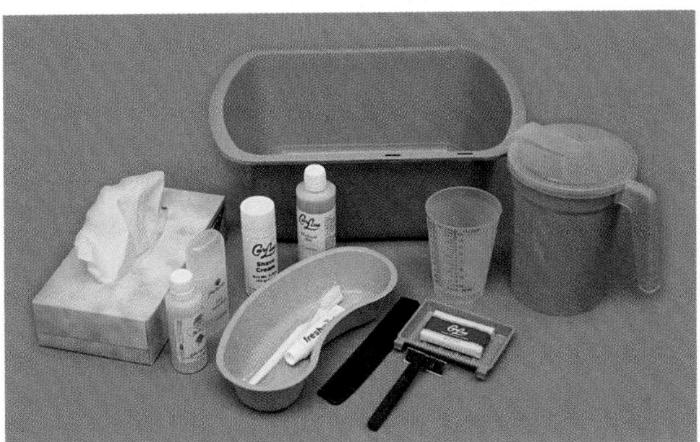

FIGURE 20.3 Typical items that might be found in a hospital admission kit.

list them using only general descriptions. You cannot, with certainty, tell by simply observing a piece of jewelry whether it is real gold, silver, platinum, diamond, or zirconium. Whatever you list on the inventory is what the hospital is responsible for returning to the patient. It does not matter what subjective information the patient may tell you; you must document only objective data, that which you can see with your own eyes and state factually. For example, rather than writing "24-carat yellow gold ring with 1-carat diamond," write "gold-colored ring with clear stone." Then document whether the patient kept their valuables at the bedside or placed them in a valuables envelope in the hospital safe. In order to provide extra protection against patient claims for "lost valuables," some facility policies require a second nurse's signature as witness of the valuables placed in the envelope. A copy of the inventoried items kept at the bedside should be given to the patient, and another copy should be placed in the patient's chart.

Data Collection

An initial assessment database includes both objective and subjective data and is completed by interviewing the patient and performing physical assessment of all body systems. Objective data are those that you can perceive or measure, such as something you can hear, see, touch, or smell. Subjective data are those that only the patient can perceive and tell you about, such as pain, family history, or the patient's feelings. Inquire why the patient is seeking health-care services. It is often enlightening to hear the patient's perspective, which may provide clues as to needed patient teaching. During the interview, it is important to obtain a thorough patient medical and surgical history, as well as a social history, including the following:

- Diseases, injuries, and surgeries experienced by the patient
- Family medical history
- Food, drug, seasonal, latex, or environmental allergies
- Current prescription and over-the-counter medications, herbs, nutritional supplements, and illicit/recreational drugs
- Pertinent health habits practiced by the patient, such as a special diet, use of sleep aids, smoking and tobacco use, alcohol use, dependence on laxatives for regular bowel movements, or use of assistive devices
- List of the patient's complaints, such as discomfort, nausea, weakness, congestion, shortness of breath, fatigue, or itching
- Living arrangements, such as whether there are stairs in their house and whether they live alone, with a spouse, in an assisted living facility, and/or with children
- Employment and type of work performed

The initial physical assessment should include:

- Vital signs, including blood pressure, temperature, pulse, respirations, and oxygen saturation level, as well as pain level, location, and characteristics
- Level of consciousness
- Orientation to person, place, time, and situation
- Auscultation of heart, breath, and bowel sounds
- Assessment of bowel and bladder status and habits
- Examination of pupils, mucous membranes, and skin
- Peripheral pulses, capillary refill, color, temperature, range of motion, and strength of all extremities
- Actual weight and height, which should be assessed because most individuals are inaccurate when they are asked their weight and height

This assessment provides a baseline against which changes in patient condition, both improvement and deterioration, can be measured. (For further information regarding physical assessment, see Chapter 21.)

Supervision/Delegation Connection

Admission Assessments

The Joint Commission, an accrediting agency for health-care facilities, requires each patient to be assessed by a registered nurse (RN) upon admission, although portions of the assessment may be delegated to the LPN/LVN. A few assessments may be delegated to the certified nursing assistant, such as the assessment of vital signs, weight, and height.

Inquire about and answer any questions or concerns the patient or family may have. If you do not know the answer to a particular question, be honest and say you do not know. Then find out the answer and report back to the patient as soon as possible. Work to convey confidence as well as competence in order to help establish the trust and rapport that is so important.

Analyze Data

You will then compile and analyze the collected data to identify the actual problems the patient has, as well as any potential problems the patient is at risk for developing. These identified problems are used in the development of their plan of care.

Although it may sound strange, **discharge planning** should be initiated during the admission process. You should collect data regarding the patient's living arrangements, physical limitations, and ability to perform activities of daily living, such as bathing, dressing, toileting, and meal preparation. This provides you with a better picture of the patient's current needs as well as needs that must be addressed in planning for discharge.

The patient's chart is compiled and health-care provider's orders are noted and carried out according to protocol. You should explain any diagnostic tests and treatments that are ordered, assist the patient in collection of specimens such as urine or sputum, and arrange for transportation to the laboratory or radiology department. After explaining a test or procedure to the patient, observe for objective and subjective signs of understanding or confusion. This is part of the nursing process known as evaluation.

KNOWLEDGE CONNECTION
Describe the objective and subjective components of an initial assessment database.

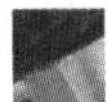

DISCHARGE

The primary goal when a patient is hospitalized is to keep the patient's stay in the hospital as short as possible without endangering the patient's health. Discharge planning that has been ongoing since admission helps to make the discharge process go smoothly. The typical **discharge process** involves the following:

- Obtaining a physician's order
- Notifying the business office of impending discharge
- Reconciling the patient's medications
- Providing discharge instructions, prescriptions, and appropriate patient teaching
- Assisting the patient to gather his or her personal belongings and valuables
- Documenting the patient's condition, including vital signs
- Assisting the patient to the car
- Documenting the time of discharge and method of transportation
- Notifying housekeeping so that the room can be cleaned

Some facilities require the discharging nurse to schedule the patient's follow-up appointment with the physician, nurse practitioner, or physician's assistant as a patient courtesy. The social worker may schedule the patient with helpful support groups.

Discharge Planning

Discharge planning should begin during or shortly after admission to the hospital and continue until the patient is discharged from the hospital. You and the patient work together and systematically plan how to best meet the patient's needs after hospitalization. Discharge planning may involve the following:

- Teaching about the patient's illness and how it may impact the patient's life
- Teaching dietary alterations to meet the patient's needs
- Teaching safe and effective use of medications
- Teaching how to perform treatments, such as the assessment of finger stick blood sugar levels, colostomy irrigation, or dressing changes
- Teaching methods of adaptation for daily living
- Recommending various support groups, such as the Mastectomy Support Group or Alcoholics Anonymous
- Providing the patient with a list of available community resources, such as Meals on Wheels or Women, Infants, and Children Services
- Making referrals to appropriate agencies such as home health care or hospice
- Assisting the family to find a long-term care or assisted living facility that will meet their needs

KNOWLEDGE CONNECTION
When should you begin discharge planning for each patient?

Physician's Discharge Order

When the physician feels the patient is well enough to be discharged, a discharge order is written. If a patient becomes unhappy with his or her care, decides against treatment, or for any other reason simply decides to leave the hospital before the physician authorizes a discharge, this is known as "leaving against medical advice" or **leaving AMA.**

If the patient decides to leave AMA, your responsibility is to attempt to reason with him or her and to explain why it is not in his or her best interest to leave without authorization of the physician. If that fails to convince the patient to stay, you will ask the patient to sign a Leaving AMA form, which releases the hospital and physician from responsibility for the patient's health status after he or she leaves. If the patient refuses to sign the leaving AMA form, document in the nurse's notes that the form was offered but the patient refused to sign it. Most facilities require you to notify the attending physician regarding the situation.

Reconcile Medications

One of the most important discharge responsibilities of the nurse is **medication reconciliation.** The medication list must be reconciled with the prescription and over-the-counter medications the patient was taking at home and with their health-care providers' orders while the individual was a patient in the facility. Patients often have more than one health-care provider providing care and writing medication orders. This can result in health-care providers writing orders for similar drugs or for drugs that are contraindicated, meaning they are not supposed to be administered together. It is not uncommon for the patient who has a primary health-care provider as well as one or more specialists to have the same or similar medications prescribed by more than one health-care provider. With the use of generic drug names and multiple trade names, the patient most likely would not know that they were the same drug. ***Safety: It is the nurse's responsibility to use caution when comparing the names of medications the patient is taking prior to admission as well as comparing them***

• WORD • BUILDING •
medication reconciliation: medic – healing + ation – action; re – back + conciliation – bring together

to any new orders or dosage changes ordered at discharge. The nurse compares the medications that the patient was taking at home to the medications the patient is to take after discharge to ensure the following:

- There are no duplications in ordered medications.
- Dosages are correct and any differences or changes in dosage were intended.
- All previous home medications have been either continued or discontinued, not overlooked.
- Prescriptions have been provided for new medications.
- A written list of medications is provided to the patient.

This safety measure was adopted in an effort to decrease medication omissions and duplications and potential drug interactions.

Discharge Instructions

When the physician writes a discharge order for a patient, the nurse completes a **discharge instruction form,** which includes:

- When to return to the physician's office for follow-up
- A list of medications and how to take them and what side effects to watch for
- Required modifications or restrictions of diet or activity level
- Signs and symptoms of worsening condition that warrant physician notification
- Care or treatment that the patient is to continue at home

Figure 20.4 presents an example of a discharge instruction form.

After reviewing the discharge instructions verbally, ask the patient for questions and verify understanding of information. Once the patient acknowledges understanding, have the patient sign the discharge instruction form. Give one copy to the patient and place one copy in the patient chart. In the nurse's notes, you should document that instructions were reviewed verbally and given in writing, noting the patient's response to the instructions.

Patient Teaching Connection

Discharge Teaching

You are in the process of preparing a patient for discharge from the hospital in 2 days. The patient has been started on a new medication, nitroglycerin, for heart-related chest pain, known as angina. It is your responsibility to teach the patient what he needs to know so that he can safely and correctly take the new medication. You must teach him to protect the nitroglycerin from light and moisture to maintain its *efficacy*—its ability to achieve its desired effect. Explain that the drug is not to be taken after the expiration date on the bottle. Teach the patient to always take the medication with him when he leaves home. Explain that the drug is taken *sublingually,* which means that it is placed underneath the tongue to dissolve and should never be swallowed. Tell him to place one tablet under his tongue as soon as he begins to have chest pain. If chest pain is not relieved, tell him that he is to repeat the tablet every 5 minutes for a maximum of three tablets. If the chest pain has not resolved after three tablets, he is to contact the physician or go immediately to the emergency room. Discuss the safety of having another individual drive the patient to the physician's office or emergency room to prevent risk should the patient lose consciousness while driving himself. Explain to the patient that the nitroglycerin may cause a headache as a side effect.

This information generally needs to be given verbally and written down for later reference. Ask for clarification that the patient understands.

Notification of Business Office

As soon as you are aware of an impending discharge, you should notify the business office so that records can be assessed for completeness. If the patient has health insurance, a form authorizing the release of information to the insurance company will be checked for the patient's signature. If the patient does not have health insurance, it is important to make payment arrangements with the patient. Notifying the business office as soon as possible allows time to complete the necessary paperwork before the patient is ready to leave.

Gathering of Belongings and Valuables

In preparation for discharge, assist the patient to gather personal belongings together. Make certain any assistive devices such as eyeglasses, hearing aids, and dentures are safely placed with the personal belongings. Check to see if the patient has valuables locked in the hospital safe. Remember to have the patient sign the form for the receipt of the valuables and then sign the form yourself. If necessary, obtain a cart on which to place the patient's belongings, as well as any gifts and flowers, to take them to the car.

Final Nursing Responsibilities

Discontinue any equipment and tubes that are to be removed prior to discharge and assess the patient's vital signs if they have not been assessed within the last hour. Document the patient's condition and vital signs in the nurse's notes, along with the time the patient actually leaves and the method of transportation. Most facility insurance carriers require that patients be taken to the car in a wheelchair to reduce the risk of falls or injury.

Make sure to notify housekeeping so that the room can be given **terminal cleaning.** This includes disinfecting the bed, furniture, bathroom, sink, and floor. The bed must be made with fresh linens and the room prepared for admission of the next patient.

• **WORD** • **BUILDING** •

efficacy: efficacy – ability to accomplish

TAKE THIS SHEET WITH YOU WHEN YOU RETURN TO YOUR DOCTOR

DISCHARGE INSTRUCTIONS

Name ______________ Age ________ Doctor ______________ Pharmacy ______________

Discharge Date/Time ______________ Diagnosis ______________

MEDICATIONS ALLERGIES ______________

SPECIAL INSTRUCTIONS:

____

____

____

____

Nurse's Signature ______________

Patient/Guardian Signature ______________

DIET ______________

WOUND CARE

Keep clean and dry
May shower
Watch for signs of Infection
(redness, pain, swelling, temperature, drainage)

ACTIVITY INSTRUCTIONS:
(driving, sex, lifting, walking, exercise, etc.)

____

____

____

RETURN TO CLINIC: ______________

Call for Appointment:
Dr. S. Arthurs 375–3752
Dr. T. Stough 263–7263
Dr. J. Gerber 263–7263
Dr. R. Matson 375–3433
Dr. B. Krablin 375–7935

Meds sent with patient Yes _____ No _____

Discharged by: w/c _____ amb. _____ carrier _____

DISCHARGE ASSESSMENT

Discharged to: _____ home _____ N.H.

BEHAVIOR
___ alert
___ anxious
___ confused
___ oriented
___ lethargic

CIRCULATORY
___ no difficulty
___ edema
___ numbness
___ dizziness
___ palpitations
___ angina
___ anemia
___ bruising

URINARY
___ no difficulty
___ incontinence
___ hematuria
___ UTI
___ urostomy

ELIMINATION
___ no difficulty
___ constipation
___ diarrhea
___ incontinence
___ ostomy
___ bleeding
___ laxative

MOBILITY
___ self
___ with help
___ cane/walker
___ bedfast

VISION
___ no difficulty
___ glasses
___ blurring

HEARING
___ no difficulty
___ limited

SPEECH
___ no difficulty
___ aphasic

NEUROLOGICAL
___ no difficulty
___ incoordination
___ parathesis
___ weakness

MUSCULOSKELETAL
___ no difficulty
___ pain/stiffness
___ contractures
___ arthritis
___ prosthesis

RESPIRATORY
___ no difficulty
___ dyspnea
___ cough
___ sputum
___ asthma
___ breath sounds
___ R
___ L

P ___ R ___
T ___ BP ___

GASTROINTESTINAL
___ no difficulty
___ dysphagia
___ nausea
___ vomiting
___ pain
___ bleeding

SKIN
___ warm
___ cold
___ dry
___ clammy
___ diaphoretic
___ pale
___ color pink
___ flushed
___ cyanosis
___ turgor

COMMENTS:

____

____

____
(RN's Signature)

FIGURE 20.4 An example of a discharge instruction form. (Courtesy of Kingfisher Regional Hospital, Kingfisher, OK.)

> **KNOWLEDGE CONNECTION**
> Summarize the steps of the discharge process. What subjects should be included in discharge teaching? List the information that should be included in the nurse's discharge note.

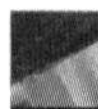

PATIENT TRANSFER

An improvement or deterioration in the patient's condition may necessitate transferring the patient from one unit to another within the same facility or from the hospital to another facility, such as a long-term care facility or specialty hospital. A transfer from the hospital to another facility includes completion of discharge as well as transfer papers.

Transfer Within the Facility

The simplest transfer is the transfer of a patient from one unit to another unit within the same facility. To complete this type of transfer you will need to:

- Obtain the physician's order for transfer.
- Explain the reason for the transfer to the patient and family.
- ***Safety: Reconcile the patient's list of medications, both prescription and over the counter, with any home medications and new health-care provider's orders to ensure that nothing has been duplicated or omitted.*** The list is then reviewed with the nurse receiving the patient at transfer. (This is another safety requirement of The Joint Commission's 2013 National Patient Safety Goals.)
- Gather the patient's personal belongings, medications, nursing supplies, and complete chart.
- Complete a **transfer summary form,** which is used to document the patient's condition and the reason for transfer, and a comprehensive list of the patient's medications.
- Phone a full report of the patient's condition and plan of care to the receiving nurse on the new unit.
- Document the time of transfer in the nurse's notes.
- Transfer the patient with all his or her belongings and chart to the new unit.

Discharge planning may involve multiple disciplines. Although generally the nurse or a specified discharge planner coordinates this process, it typically involves some of the following health-care team members to effectively develop a plan that meets all the patient's needs after discharge:

- Physical therapist
- Occupational therapist
- Speech therapist
- Dietitian
- Social worker
- Home health nurse
- Ostomy nurse

Transfer to Another Facility

The process of transferring a patient to another facility is more complex. After obtaining the physician's transfer order, notify the business office of impending transfer. Assist the patient in arranging for transportation, such as calling for an ambulance or notifying a family member if the patient can go via private automobile. Some facilities require both a transfer summary form and a discharge summary to be sent to the receiving facility. You are responsible for knowing the facility's policies and procedures. If you are uncertain what the policy is, refer to the facility policy and procedure book.

A transfer summary form is prepared that contains information about the patient's condition and vital signs at time of discharge; discharge instructions that include a list of the patient's discharge medications, diet, activity restrictions, patient teaching that has been done, and follow-up appointments; time of transfer; and method of transportation. This form usually is completed by the transferring nurse, and a copy is sent with the patient to the receiving facility. Some facilities may also require the social worker to complete a transfer information record. Another document commonly sent with the patient transferring to another facility is a document called a *discharge summary.* The physician completes this document, which summarizes the patient's condition, diseases, pertinent diagnostic results, medications and treatments, as well as where the patient is to go after discharge and follow-up treatment plans.

Any valuables in the hospital safe should be sent with the patient and notation made in the hospital chart and the transfer record. Make certain the patient has signed consent to release medical information to third parties to comply with the Health Insurance Portability and Accountability Act. All patient records that are sent with the patient should be sealed in a large manila envelope to protect confidentiality. Some facilities prefer to send the data via fax machine. It is important to phone the receiving facility and inform them of the impending transmission. This helps ensure that the proper personnel receive the medical records.

> **KNOWLEDGE CONNECTION**
> List the different health-care providers who may contribute to the discharge planning of a patient. Describe the information that should be included in a transfer summary.

POST CONFERENCE

At your post conference, you have many thoughts to share. Several students are frustrated to learn that your patient was discharged not based on the physician's determination but based on the insurance company's rules. As you evaluate your clinical performance, you question if you did all you could for this gentleman. Did you:

- Explain what was happening to the patient?
- Gather all his belongings, including his valuables from the safe?
- Listen to his discharge instructions when presented by the staff nurse?
- Ensure that he had all his discharge instructions, list of all current medications, and prescriptions with him when he left?
- Relay any questions or concerns about discharge to the appropriate staff person?
- Act in a calm, reassuring manner even if you were rushed?
- Encourage him about the rehabilitation program he is about to begin?

If you strongly feel the patient is not ready for discharge, it is your responsibility as patient advocate to discuss your concerns and possible options with the physician. Sometimes there does not seem to be a resolution to the problem. If this is the case, it is difficult to see your patient discharged before he seems ready to go, but you will have done all you can do to help the patient transition from the hospital to his next destination.

Key Points

- The first impression you make on your patient is made during admission and can either help improve your patient's stay or make it a negative experience.
- Four common reactions to admission are fear, anxiety, loss of control, and loss of identity.
- Some therapeutic nursing interventions that can improve the admission process for your patient include using effective communication, introducing yourself and other direct health-care providers, orienting the patient to the hospital room and typical hospital routines, and providing as much information as possible regarding the patient's stay in the facility.
- A few specific ways to enhance communications when there are cultural or language differences between two individuals involve avoiding the use of slang, paying attention to the patient's facial expressions and other nonverbal communication, and using eye contact judiciously.
- The admission process includes obtaining authority to treat; applying identification bands; assisting the patient to change into a hospital gown or pajamas; orienting the patient and family to the environment; taking an inventory of clothing, personal items, and valuables; providing a basic admission kit and carafe of water if allowed; completing the initial assessment database; and compiling the patient chart.
- Separation anxiety is common in children and older adults.
- Discharge planning begins at or shortly after admission.
- The discharge process includes obtaining a physician's order, notifying the business office, reconciling the patient's medications, assisting the patient to gather personal belongings and valuables, discharge teaching, documenting the patient's condition along with time of discharge and method of transportation, notifying housekeeping, and creating a discharge summary.
- The medication reconciliation during discharge is a safety measure that was adopted in an effort to decrease medication omissions and duplications and potential drug interactions.
- Transferring within the facility is the simplest transfer of a patient from one unit to another unit within the same facility.
- Transferring to another facility is more complex than transfers within a facility. It includes obtaining a physician's transfer order, notifying the business office, calling the other facility, giving a report to the obtaining RN, and assisting in arranging for transportation.

Review Questions

Select the answer that is most appropriate for each of the following questions. Some questions may have more than one correct answer. Select all that apply.

1. The first impression you make on the patient:
   1. will not affect the outcome of the hospitalization.
   2. can be a negative one.
   3. is not important.
   4. can lead to improving the patient's stay.
   5. can be the first step in establishing rapport with the patient.
   6. is partially determined by your facial expression.
   7. is partially determined by the time you take to explain things to the patient during the admission process.

2. Which of the following data should be included in a discharge summary?
   1. List of discharge medications
   2. Activity restrictions
   3. Patient's condition
   4. Follow-up appointment
   5. Diet
   6. Discharge teaching that has been done

3. Children and older adults are more prone to:
   1. feeling a loss of identity.
   2. experiencing separation anxiety.
   3. feeling a loss of control.
   4. adapting more readily to admission to a health-care facility.

4. You can help prevent loss of identity for your patients by:
   1. calling them "honey," "sweetie," or other endearments.
   2. addressing them by title and surname.
   3. referring to them as a room number to protect privacy.
   4. referring to them by their diagnosis.
   5. addressing all patients with their first name to provide a sense of familiarity.

5. Which of the following should be included on an admission orientation checklist?
   1. How to use the call light
   2. Times meals will be served
   3. Location of the nurses' supply room
   4. How to raise the height of the bed
   5. How busy it is on the unit and that you may not be available as much as you would like to be
   6. Location of the bathroom
   7. Two methods staff will use to check the patient's identity before each procedure or medication administration

6. Which of the following will enhance communication with a patient from a different culture?
   1. Make jokes about the patient's beliefs and traditions to put the patient at ease
   2. Clarify information when you do not understand what the patient has said
   3. Use simple, common, and proper English
   4. Avoid the use of slang
   5. Make eye contact at all times while conversing with the patient
   6. Demonstrate respect for and acceptance of the patient's cultural and religious differences
   7. Attempt to emulate the dialect and accent of the different culture

7. The nurse is treating a patient with pneumonia on the medical-surgical floor. The nurse understands separation anxiety is common in which age group?
   1. Adolescents
   2. Children
   3. Older adults
   4. Young adults

8. At what point before discharge should discharge planning begin?
   1. Upon admission
   2. Right before discharge
   3. Right before social services visits the patient
   4. In the emergency room

9. When admitting a patient to the medical-surgical floor, the nurse knows what information should be found on a patient identification band?
   1. Medical record number
   2. Name
   3. Date of birth
   4. Address
   5. Room number
   6. Phone number
   7. Allergies

10. Mrs. Jones is admitted to the hospital for pneumonia. While taking care of Mrs. Jones, you know some common patient reactions to admission are which of the following?
    1. Fear of the unknown
    2. Anxiety
    3. Loss of control
    4. Loss of identity

ANSWERS 1. 2, 4, 5, 6, 7, 2. 1, 2, 3, 4, 5, 6, 3. 2, 4. 2, 5. 1, 2, 6, 7, 6. 2, 3, 4, 6, 7. 2, 3, 8. 1, 9. 1, 2, 3, 5, 7, 10. 1, 2, 3, 4

Critical Thinking Exercise

Answers available online.

1. You are completing a valuables inventory for a new patient. The patient tells you that the ring is platinum with a 1.5-carat diamond and six emeralds that are a total of 1.2 carats. How can you objectively describe the ring on the inventory? Why would it be a problem to describe it as it is written in this question?

Additional Resources

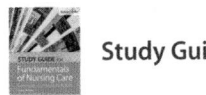

Use the scratch off code on the inside front cover of your book to access online quizzes that will help you to improve your scores on course exams and prepare for the NCLEX-PN®.

Study Guide

CHAPTER 21

Physical Assessment

Patricia Williams

KEY TERMS

Accommodation response (uh-KOM-uh-DAY-shun ree-SPONS)
Adventitious breath sounds (AD-ven-TI-shus BRETH SOWNDZ)
Atelectasis (AT-eh-LEK-tah-siss)
Auscultation (AWS-kul-TAY-shun)
Cheilitis/chelosis (kye-LYE-tiss/kee-LOH-siss)
Consensual reflex (kon-SEN-shoo-uhl REE-fleks)
Crackles (KRAK-elz)
Dysphagia (dis-FAYJ-ee-ah)
Dysphasia (dis-FAYZ-ee-ah)
Eructation (e-ruk-TAY-shun)
Excursion (eks-KER-shun)
Guarding (GAR-ding)
Halitosis (ha-lih-TOH-siss)
Jaundice (JAWN-diss)
Lethargy (LETH-uhr-jee)
Ophthalmoscope (ahf-THAL-muh-skohp)
Otoscope (OH-toh-skohp)
Palpation (pal-PAY-shun)
Paresthesia (PAR-es-THEE-zee-ah)
Percussion (per-KUSH-uhn)
Peristalsis (pair-iss-TALL-siss)
PERRLA
Ptosis (TOH-siss)
Retractions (ree-TRAK-shunz)
Rhonchi (RONG-kee)
Signs (SIGHNZ)
Solar lentigines (SOH-luhr len-TIJ-i-neez)
Sordes (SOR-dez)
Stridor (STRY-dohr)
Symptoms (SIMP-tuhmz)
Turgor (TER-gor)
Wheezes (WEE-zuhz)

CHAPTER CONCEPTS

Patient-Centered Care

LEARNING OUTCOMES

1. Define various terms associated with physical assessment.
2. Describe five purposes of physical assessment.
3. Differentiate between a comprehensive health assessment, a focused assessment, and an initial head-to-toe shift assessment.
4. Discuss the important of and the various ways to foster rapport and communication when interacting with patients.
5. Summarize the six techniques used for physical assessment, including their correct performance.
6. Describe adaptations in assessment techniques that are necessary due to the age, size, or condition of the patient.
7. Explain the significance of abnormal assessment findings.
8. Identify assessment techniques and assessment findings relative to specific health conditions.
9. Relate each component of assessment to its associated body system(s).
10. Distinguish the different components to be examined during an initial head-to-toe shift assessment.
11. Differentiate between normal and abnormal assessment findings of each body system.
12. Explain how to document an initial head-to-toe shift assessment.
13. Discuss information found in the Connection features in this chapter.
14. Identify specific safety information.
15. Answer questions about the skills in this chapter.

SKILLS

21.1 Measuring a Patient's Height
21.2 Measuring a Patient's Weight
21.3 Measuring an Infant's Weight and Length
21.4 Performing a Shift Assessment
21.5 Performing a Basic Neurological Examination
21.6 Auscultating Breath Sounds
21.7 Auscultating Heart Sounds
21.8 Assessing Visual Acuity Using a Snellen Standard Eye Chart, Snellen E Chart, or Preliterate Chart

CRITICAL THINKING CONNECTION

Clinical Assignment

You are assigned to care for a 62-year-old male patient with congestive heart failure and emphysema. The staff nurse came in to do a shift assessment. She checked the oxygen flowmeter and the IV pump and site, listened to his heart, listened to the anterior lung fields, and checked his ankles for edema. She tells the patient, "Everything looks good," and leaves the room. As you care for him, you notice that he becomes short of breath when he is turning or moving in the bed. When you listen to his posterior lung sounds, you hear crackles throughout. You also notice edema over his low back area when he is turned. When you check his vital signs, his blood pressure has elevated some in the past 4 hours and is now 158/88.

Critical Thinking Questions:

1. Instead of stating "Everything looks good," how would you inform the patient of his current condition?
2. As the nurse, what interventions would you do after you noticed posterior crackle lung sounds?
3. When calling the health-care provider to give her or him an update, explain in detail a situation, background, assessment, and recommendation (SBAR) report.

As a nurse, your goal for all nursing care will be to provide care that is coherent, or logically connected to the patient's actual condition. What does this really mean? If nursing care is to be of any benefit to your patient, the care must be relevant to that specific patient and his or her needs and problems. It is important to remember that not all patients, even those with the same diagnosis, will have the same needs. That is the beauty of the human body: Even though we are technically similar to each other, we each have highly individualized differences. For example, you could line up 20 healthy individuals who all have "normal breath sounds," yet all 20 individuals' breath sounds will sound slightly different when you listen with your stethoscope. Regardless of this fact, it will be necessary for you to identify the presence of any abnormal breath sounds in all 20 of these patients.

How can you meet the individual needs of a patient if you are unaware of how that patient is different from another? The full value of each and every task, procedure, and skill you perform as a nurse is dependent on whether or not you can accurately assess the patient's condition prior to, during, and after completion of the task, procedure, or skill. In this chapter, you will learn how to perform physical assessment in a thorough manner, to critically evaluate the assessment findings, and to determine the significance of abnormal findings.

WHAT IS PHYSICAL ASSESSMENT?

As you learned in Chapter 4, assessment is the first step of the nursing process and is ongoing throughout the nurse-patient relationship. It is the process you use to collect physical data that are relevant to the patient's health. To collect physical data about the patient's current condition, you will perform a physical examination of the patient, using four of your senses: sight, smell, hearing, and touch.

Purpose of Physical Assessment

Assessments are performed for several purposes:

- To establish the patient's current condition, a baseline against which future changes may be measured
- To identify problems the patient may have or have the potential to develop
- To evaluate the effectiveness of nursing interventions
- To monitor for changes in body function
- To detect specific body systems that need further assessment or testing

Three Levels of Physical Assessment

A *comprehensive health assessment* involves an in-depth assessment of the whole person, including the physical, mental, emotional, cultural, and spiritual aspects of the patient's health. The data, or information about the patient, are collected through physical examination and interview that may take as long as 2 hours to complete. This assessment is generally performed when a patient is admitted. The depth of assessment and the specific data to collect vary from facility to facility. The comprehensive assessment is generally performed by the admitting registered nurse (RN) in a hospital setting. The responsibility for admission assessment for long-term care facilities may vary.

A *focused assessment* is less encompassing and involves an examination and an interview regarding a specific body system, such as examining solely the integumentary system or the respiratory system. It provides a cluster of data about just the one body system being assessed, which usually is the system involved in the illness or injury. Focused assessments are performed when time constraints allow you to check only the system or systems related to the patient's disease process or when performing reassessment of a system in which abnormal findings were obtained earlier.

An *initial head-to-toe shift assessment* provides you with a quick overall assessment of the patient's condition to establish a baseline against which you can compare later assessments. This baseline is necessary for you to be able to identify changes in the patient's condition, such as whether it is improved or has deteriorated. An initial head-to-toe shift assessment consists of performing a focused assessment of the following systems in a sequence beginning at the head and moving down to the toes:

- Neurological
- Cardiovascular
- Respiratory
- Integumentary
- Gastrointestinal
- Genitourinary

- Muscular
- Skeletal

An initial head-to-toe shift assessment also includes a specific assessment of the patient's:

- Vital signs, including pain and oxygen saturation (SpO_2)
- Appearance
- Speech
- Safety risk factors
- Tubes and equipment
- Comfort or complaints
- Needs

Although the immune system is not assessed in depth, it should be mentioned because the vital signs, along with the focused assessments of the eight systems included in an initial shift assessment, will provide you with a meager amount of information that also relates to the patient's immune system.

> **KNOWLEDGE CONNECTION**
> Explain the differences between a comprehensive health assessment, a focused assessment, and an initial head-to-toe shift assessment. List the eight systems and seven specific items to assess during an initial head-to-toe shift assessment.

When Is Physical Assessment Performed?

Assessment is an ongoing process that the nurse performs every time he or she encounters a patient, even when passing the patient walking down the hall. The nurse should always be looking and observing for changes in any aspect of the patient's condition. This continual assessment may not be recorded unless the nurse encounters what he or she determines to be a change from previous assessments. For the most part, though, the physical assessments we are talking about in this chapter are performed at typical times, including the following:

- On admission (comprehensive, in depth)
- At the beginning of each shift (shorter, more focused)
- When the patient's condition changes
- When evaluating the effectiveness of nursing care
- Any time things do not *feel right*

When assessment findings are outside the normal range for the specific patient, they are considered to be abnormal. Abnormal findings should be reassessed within at least a 4-hour window and sooner depending on the severity of the finding. Some abnormal assessment findings are minor or even may be expected, while others are totally unexpected or represent potentially serious conditions. For example, if a patient admitted with an upper respiratory illness is noted to have developed an occasional dry cough, you might request that he or she let you know if it gets worse. Then you would reassess the cough within 4 hours to determine if it has worsened, improved, or remains the same. ***Safety: But if you assess a fever of 103°F (39.4°C), you must not only take immediate action to treat the fever, but also reassess the temperature within an hour to see if further intervention is required.***

> **KNOWLEDGE CONNECTION**
> Which of the three types of assessment are done on admission? At the beginning of each shift? How often should you reassess abnormal findings?

Six Assessment Techniques

You will begin your assessment with a method that produces *subjective* data: interviewing or asking questions of the patient. You will continue to collect the subjective data from the patient or family member throughout the assessment, even as you begin to collect objective data.

> **KNOWLEDGE CONNECTION**
> **S**ubjective data (symptoms) is what the patient **S**ays, and **O**bjective data (signs) is what the nurse **O**bserves.

Five additional techniques are used to collect *objective* data in the performance of physical assessment. They include inspection or observation, palpation, percussion, auscultation, and olfaction. They are performed in this order, *except when you are conducting an abdominal assessment; when conducting an abdominal assessment, auscultation comes before palpation and percussion so that bowel sounds are not altered.*

Although you may use additional tools to assist you in assessment, the most important tools you will need are your eyes, ears, hands, nose, and critical thinking ability. When use of the four senses produces evidence of illness or injury, the findings are objective and measurable and are classified as **signs.** When evidence of illness or injury is verbalized by the patient, the findings are subjective, not directly measurable, and classified as **symptoms.** In other words, signs of disease are those that can be detected by the nurse, while symptoms of disease are apparent only to the patient, so they must be verbally communicated by the patient to the nurse.

Interviewing

An inordinate amount of data is obtainable solely by interviewing or asking questions of the patient. You will ask questions to determine the patient's:

- Personal identity and demographics
- Details regarding current condition, including complaints, problems, concerns, and the specific reason the patient is seeking medical care at this time

• WORD • BUILDING •

percussion: percuss – striking + ion – action
palpation: palpa – stroking + tion – action

- Medical history
- Social history
- Food and drug allergies
- Height and normal weight
- Expectations for hospitalization

As you learned in Chapter 6, rapport and trust are influential during the interviewing process. It is difficult to convince a patient who does not trust you to impart personal feelings or information. Box 21.1 lists ways to foster rapport and communication. Unless the patient is uncomfortable with it, make frequent eye contact with the patient while conversing. In addition to paying attention to what the patient says, remember to observe nonverbal behavior. If you see nonverbal evidence that does not correlate with what the patient says, assess further to clarify. For instance, a patient may deny pain but winces when you palpate the epigastric area. Inquire if the area is tender or hurts: "Does it feel uncomfortable when I press here?" Some patients interpret pain as something different and more severe than discomfort or tenderness. Ask if the patient has experienced "indigestion," "nausea," "reflux," or "heartburn," or use any other terminology that could elicit further information that might relate to the observed nonverbal behavior.

THERAPEUTIC COMMUNICATION. Remember to utilize the therapeutic communication techniques you learned in Chapter 6, as they will help you in establishing and maintaining rapport and interpersonal relationships. Avoid communication blocks that might discourage interaction and feedback. ***Safety: If there is a language barrier, make all efforts to obtain the assistance of an interpreter to avoid miscommunication and omission of important data.***

Box 21.1

Ways to Foster Rapport and Communication

When meeting and talking with a patient, it is important to establish a trusting, professional relationship. The following techniques can be used to foster rapport and communication with your patient:

- Smile
- Greet the patient using his or her surname
- Provide for privacy
- Introduce yourself and explain your intent
- Exhibit an open and relaxed posture
- Be professional
- Demonstrate active listening
- Be attentive to the patient's responses and needs
- Be aware of cultural influences and restrictions
- Be sincere
- Be nonjudgmental
- Use touch purposefully and judiciously

Inspection

Inspection is the visual observation of anything about the body that you can see with the naked eye or with the assistance of other equipment, such as a penlight, an otoscope, or an ophthalmoscope (Fig. 21.1). A penlight is used for assessment of pupil constriction of the eyes and examination of the oral and nasal mucous membranes. An **otoscope** is a lighted instrument used to inspect the lining of the nose, tympanic membranes, and ear canals. An **ophthalmoscope** is a lighted instrument used to assess or examine the internal structures of the eyes. Without using any other equipment, you can use your powers of observation to inspect the patient's:

- General appearance
- Affect
- General body shape and size
- Posture
- Pupil size
- Color and condition of skin, sclera, and mucous membranes
- Respiratory efforts
- Skin for beads of perspiration
- Muscle movements and coordination
- Size and shape of abdomen
- Extremities for edema
- Equipment and tubes

Settings Connection: Medical Office

Preparing an Otoscope and Ophthalmoscope in a Medical Office

When you work in a health-care provider's office or clinic, you may be responsible for preparing the otoscope and ophthalmoscope for use. First, assess the patient's age and size to determine what equipment to use. The health-care provider will use an ophthalmoscope to examine the inside of the eye and an otoscope to examine the inside of the ear and to look up inside the nose. Both of these scopes have lights in them to help visualize the internal structures of the eye and ear. These light bulbs may have to be replaced if they burn out, and that may be your responsibility. Always check the scopes to be sure the lightbulbs are working before they are used on a patient. The health-care provider will need disposable speculum covers to go over the speculums to examine the ear and nose. Be sure there is an adequate supply of these in the examination rooms. Wipe off the scopes after use with an alcohol wipe or according to the manufacturer's directions to prevent cross-contamination.

• WORD • BUILDING •

otoscope: oto – ear + scope – examine
ophthalmoscope: ophthalmo – eye + scope – examine

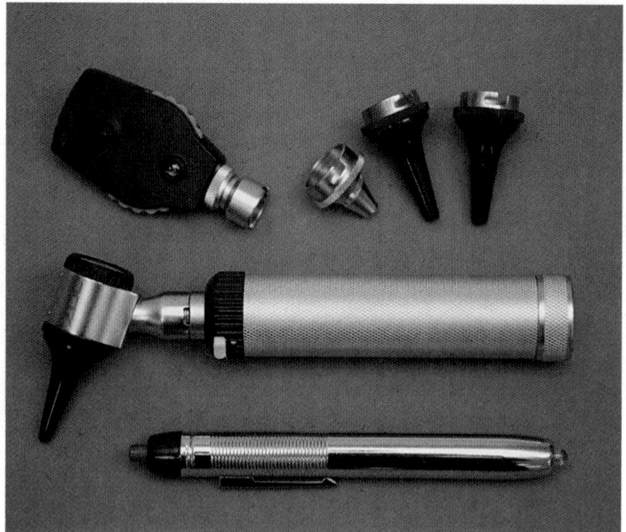

FIGURE 21.1 Front row: Penlight. Second row: Otoscope for assessing the tympanic membrane of the ear. Third row, left to right: Ophthalmic head to convert otoscope to ophthalmoscope for assessing the internal eye and retina; nasal speculum for assessing the nasal passageway; two sizes of otic speculum for assessing the ear.

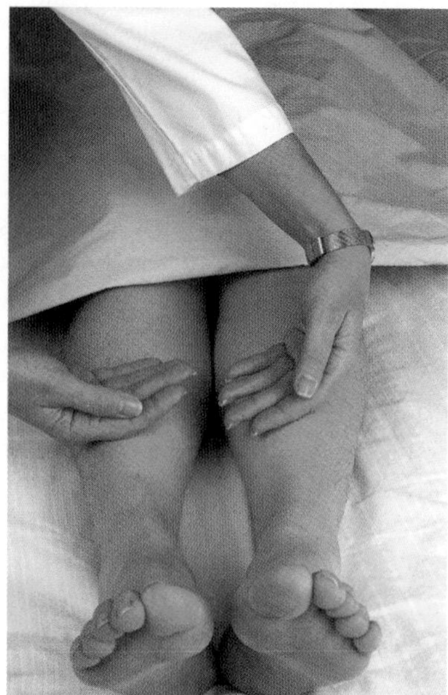

FIGURE 21.2 Use the dorsal aspect of the hand, which is more sensitive, to detect subtle differences in skin temperature (from Dillon PM. *Nursing Health Assessment: The Foundation of Clinical Practice.* 3rd ed. Philadelphia, PA: FA Davis; 2016).

WEIGHT AND HEIGHT. Although you may obtain a patient's verbal estimation of body weight and height/length, there are times that you will need to verify the data by weighing and measuring the patient. The weight may be assessed using bed scales or stand-alone scales, on which the height can also be measured. Some facilities require that all patients be weighed and have their height measured during admission. Other times when assessment of weight and height/length may be ordered include the following:

- For a newborn infant
- For assessment of nutritional or growth status
- For assessment of dehydration or fluid excess
- To determine the effectiveness of diuretic medications
- For calculation of certain medication dosages

Information on measuring a patient's height/length and weight can be found in Skill 21.1 (page 415) and Skill 21.2 (page 415). Skill 21.3 (page 416) presents the procedure for obtaining the length and weight of an infant.

Palpation

Palpation is the application of your hands to the external surfaces of the body to detect abnormalities of the skin or tissues lying below the skin, that is, to examine by touch or feel. By application of the fingertips, you can detect the following:

- Skin turgor
- Growths on or below the skin
- Edema
- Size and location of body parts
- Distention of the bladder or abdomen
- Firmness versus softness of tissue, such as muscle rigidity
- Location and strength of pulses
- Temperature, texture, and moisture of the skin
- Pain/discomfort

The dorsal or back surface of the hand provides for more sensitive assessment of temperature changes in the lower extremities (Fig. 21.2).

Palpation is classified according to the depth of tissue compression:

- Light palpation only depresses the tissue between 1 and 2 cm.
- Moderate compression depresses the tissue between 2 and 3 cm.
- Deep palpation depresses the tissue between 4 and 5 cm. This type of palpation is only done by the RN.

Using the palmar surface of the hands, you can palpate for masses below the skin surface and accumulation of fluid in the peritoneal cavity called *ascites;* you can also determine if palpation elicits pain anywhere on the body. When palpating the abdomen after auscultation, observe the patient's face for grimacing and feel for tensing of the abdominal muscles, both of which may indicate discomfort. When an area of discomfort is detected in the abdomen, you may want to assess further for what is known as rebound tenderness. This is done by applying moderately deep pressure, holding it for a couple of seconds, and then quickly releasing the pressure from the abdomen. Reflexive tensing of abdominal muscles or verbalization of *increased pain* with the *release* of pressure is termed *rebound tenderness,* which is common in appendicitis.

Real-World Connection

Cultural Beliefs in Assessment

It is important to consider cultural beliefs regarding the use of physical touch and modesty. Some cultures maintain differing views regarding exposure of and touching of the body, and your sensitivity to these views is critical. For example, members of some cultures may only remove his or her underwear in emergency situations. Members of other cultures may prefer health-care providers of the same gender or exhibit extreme modesty. Other patients may not like to be touched until permission has been obtained; some cultural norms make patients distrustful and cautious with nurses and health-care providers until they know them better. Others may frown on public displays of affection and touching.

Percussion

Percussion is the technique used least for assessment. **Percussion** involves striking body parts with the tips of the fingers to (Fig. 21.3):

- Elicit sounds that can help locate and determine the size of structures beneath the surface
- Identify whether the structure is solid or hollow
- Detect areas containing air or fluid

Auscultation

Auscultation is listening to the sounds produced by the body. Some sounds may be heard with the naked ear, such as belching, also known as **eructation;** passing of *flatus* or rectal gas; loud wheezing or gurgling; and loud bowel sounds. Most typically, auscultation is thought of as using a stethoscope to assess the quieter sounds made by the heart, lungs, intestinal tract, and arteries of the neck. The bell side of the stethoscope (the cupped smaller piece) is used to assess low-pitched sounds such as abnormal heart valve sounds, known as *murmurs,* and the rushing of blood through a vessel such as the carotid artery, known as a *bruit.*

The bell should be held lightly against the skin. Avoid pressing firmly or you will not be able to detect the sounds. The larger flat piece, or diaphragm side of the stethoscope, is used to assess high-pitched sounds, such as the normal heart sounds (S_1 and S_2), breath sounds, and bowel sounds. The diaphragm should be pressed firmly against the skin. To help you remember which side of the chest piece to use for different sounds, remember that the *little side (bell) is for lower* sounds and the *larger side (flat) for higher* sounds. Box 21.2 presents further stethoscope usage hints.

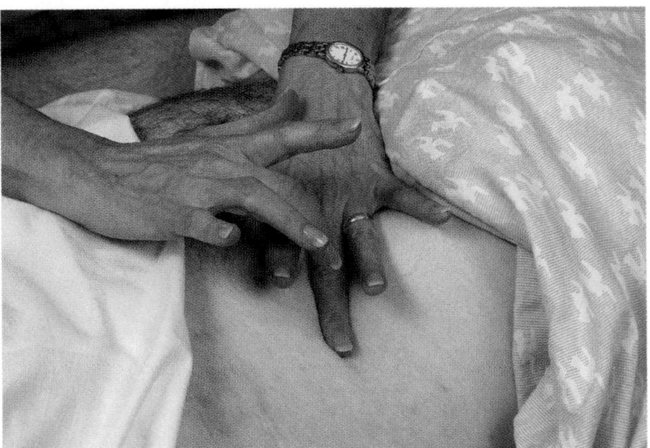

FIGURE 21.3 To perform percussion of the abdomen or chest, strike the stationary middle finger with the tip of the curved middle finger of the opposite hand, allowing the moving hand to flex freely at the wrist. This allows the finger to strike in a hammerlike manner that produces the best sound (from Wilkinson JM, Treas LS. *Fundamentals of Nursing: Theory, Concepts & Applications.* Vol. 1. 2nd ed. Philadelphia, PA: FA Davis; 2016).

Olfaction

Olfaction, or the sense of smell, is used to detect odors characteristic of different health problems. For example, the smell of a patient's breath often can be revealing. A patient with bad breath, known as **halitosis,** may have poor oral hygiene, a sinus infection, or gastric upset. Individuals with high stress levels often have sour-smelling breath. A patient with kidney failure and uremia may have the smell of ammonia or urine on the breath. A smoker usually has a characteristic smoker's breath, just as one who has consumed alcohol may have a strong alcohol odor on breath. A patient with liver disease may have breath that has either a musty or a sweet odor. When the breath smells like acetone or has a fruity smell, it may be an indicator of diabetes that is out of control.

Infectious drainage generally has a foul odor. The stools of a patient with cystic fibrosis usually are extremely foul smelling. Stools containing old blood have a very characteristic odor to them. *Cerumen,* or earwax, even has its own

Box 21.2

Tips for Stethoscope Use

When using a stethoscope, it is important to use it correctly or the results you get from your assessment may not be accurate. Keep the following tips in mind:

- Point the earpieces forward toward your face
- Clean the chest piece with alcohol between patients
- Clean the earpieces between staff usage
- The chest piece must be rotated to the bell or the diaphragm side to hear
- Apply light pressure to the bell
- Apply firm pressure to the diaphragm
- Apply the chest piece directly to skin, not clothing
- To improve sound transmission:
  - Use a stethoscope with dual tubing rather than single tubing
  - If the tubing is 28 inches or longer, remove the chest piece and trim the tubing to a length between 22 and 27 inches
  - Avoid tubing contact with clothing/rails

characteristic odors with some diseases. Cerumen that smells mousy may be indicative of a *Proteus* infection, while cerumen that has a putrid smell is due to a *Pseudomonas* infection. Cancer often has its own characteristic odor, sometimes detectable in an advanced stage that has yet to be diagnosed. Researchers are doing studies regarding the use of dogs and their acute sense of smell for detection of cancer in patients.

The sense of smell is stronger in some individuals than others. Some individuals have such an acute sense of smell that they can detect the odor of normal menstrual flow, even in women with scrupulous hygiene. Some health-care providers are even able to differentiate the odor of strep throat from other throat infections. However, not all individuals have a sensitive sense of smell. For instance, someone with severe nasal allergies may have a more difficult time detecting odors than someone who does not have these allergies.

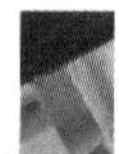

ASSESSMENT COMPONENTS RELATED TO EACH BODY SYSTEM

There are numerous components to be assessed to evaluate each body system. Table 21.1 presents a breakdown of assessments by body system.

Table 21.1
Assessment Components Related to Body Systems

System	*Components Assessed*
Neurological	Vital signs and level of consciousness Orientation Facial symmetry Pupillary size and reaction Ability to follow simple commands Speech Hand grip Feet flexion
Cardiovascular	Blood pressure and pulse Skin color, moisture, and temperature Color of mucous membranes Jugular vein distention Heart sounds Peripheral pulses Capillary refill of extremities Edema Color and temperature of extremities Clubbing of fingertips Activity tolerance Results of laboratory tests, such as blood counts, cardiac enzymes, and bleeding and clotting studies Results of radiological tests, such as chest x-ray Results of other tests, such as electrocardiogram
Respiratory	Respiratory rate and characteristics Respiratory effort Respiratory pattern Symmetry of excursion SpO_2 Breath sounds Use of accessory respiratory muscles Shape of chest Retractions Cough and sputum Skin color Color of nailbeds Tolerance for activity Laboratory test results, such as arterial blood gases Radiological test results, such as chest x-ray

Table 21.1
Assessment Components Related to Body Systems—cont'd

System	*Components Assessed*
Integumentary	Skin color, texture, moisture, and temperature Turgor Skin integrity, including pressure points and lesions Surgical incisions
Gastrointestinal	Anorexia Nausea or vomiting Shape or distention of abdomen Consistency of abdomen Bowel sounds Bowel elimination Incontinence Flatus
Genitourinary	Last voiding Distention of bladder Frequency, burning, or urgency Color and clarity of urine Incontinence
Musculoskeletal	Range of motion in joints Presence of contractures Strength of hand grip Strength of foot flexion Ability to sit up or turn to side

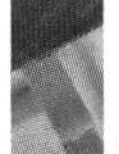

PERFORMING AN INITIAL HEAD-TO-TOE SHIFT ASSESSMENT

Gather the necessary equipment to perform the assessment, including a stethoscope, sphygmomanometer, thermometer, pulse oximeter, and penlight. Upon entering the patient's room, ask any visitors to step out into the hallway or waiting room. Remember to assess the patient's identity with two identifiers. Close the door, provide privacy, and explain what you are about to do. Give the patient time to empty the bowel or bladder if needed. If you require urine or stool specimens, now is a good time to collect them. Be careful to protect the patient's modesty by keeping the patient covered with a sheet, except for the body part that is being assessed. Make certain the room temperature is comfortable for the patient. Maintain a professional demeanor at all times. Speak in a relaxed tone of voice and exhibit a relaxed facial expression. These preparatory steps serve to gain the patient's cooperation and decrease his or her anxiety. Skill 21.4 (page 417) provides the steps of a shift assessment.

General Appearance

Note the patient's general appearance upon entering the room. In what position do you find the patient? Does the patient appear to be comfortable? Are there any signs of respiratory distress? Is there an indication of fear in the patient's face, such as wide eyes? What is the patient's skin color? Does the patient respond to the stimulus of your voice? Is the patient fidgeting? Is he or she unkempt? Visiting with guests? What indicators of mood or emotional tone are noted? Is the patient smiling or frowning? Research has related increased stress levels to a decrease in an individual's immunity. Is the patient making eye contact as is appropriate to his or her culture? Is the patient *mouth-breathing,* or breathing through the mouth, rather than through the nose?

Vital Signs

Begin each head-to-toe shift assessment by assessing the patient's six vital signs: temperature, pulse, respirations, blood pressure, SpO_2, and pain level. Because the vital signs serve as important indicators of numerous processes occurring throughout the body, their assessment serves to establish a basic foundation of the patient's condition, possibly alerting you to problems or areas of concern that you may want to assess in more depth. The vital signs, except the SpO_2 and pain, along with the general appearance of the patient, can also serve as possible indicators of infection and may relate to the functioning of the immune system.

Temperature

An elevated temperature can direct your attention to infection or injury to the hypothalamus, the portion of the central nervous system that helps regulate body temperature. If the immune system is working correctly, it raises the body temperature whenever there are signs of microorganism invasion of the body. Hypothermia might indicate exposure to an environment that was too cold or a disorder of the body's temperature-regulating mechanisms. In a newborn, hypothermia may identify that the infant is not yet able to regulate body temperature. It also can be a sign of sepsis or severe hypothyroidism, or it can be a result of trauma.

Pulse

Pulse assessment may reveal hypovolemia, due to either dehydration or blood loss. An elevated pulse rate can possibly indicate pain, anxiety, fear, stress, physical exertion, low blood pressure, infection, effects of medication, and many other conditions.

Respirations

Assessment of respirations provides detail about the patient's respiratory system as well as the acid-base balance of the blood. The rate and depth of respirations may provide insight into the patient's pain intensity and level, anxiety or fear, or recent exertion.

Blood Pressure

Blood pressure provides data associated with the cardiovascular system. As we age, atherosclerosis (hardening of the arteries) increases, contributing to the widening of the pulse pressure, or the difference between the systolic and diastolic readings. Blood pressure also relates information regarding the kidneys, which excrete renin, a major component in the control of blood pressure. Blood pressure also provides us with data relating to the level of hydration or fluid volume within the cardiovascular system. A pulse pressure of 20 mm Hg or less may be indicative of severe dehydration. In a patient who has fluid overload, blood pressure will be increased.

SpO_2

The patient's SpO_2 level provides further insight as to the state of oxygenation.

Pain

Pain assessment includes the site of pain, characteristics of the pain, and strength of the pain, which can affect assessment of the other vital signs. Include any body language the patient may exhibit supporting the idea that he or she is in pain, such as facial grimacing; rubbing, holding, or guarding any particular part of the body, such as the abdomen or head; or any additional verbal sounds such as moaning. Pain also can direct you to problems in any of the body systems. The intensity and characteristics of pain can relate the severity of illness or injury and also detail the effectiveness of pain medication.

Neurological Examination

The vital signs also play a major role in a neurological assessment because they relate to the function of the central nervous system, as all of them are controlled by the brain except the SpO_2. The medulla and the pons control the respiratory rate portion of oxygenation. The hypothalamus controls the body temperature and the autonomic nervous system, which controls the blood pressure and pulse. The medulla oblongata extends some control over the blood pressure and pulse.

Additional aspects of a basic neurological assessment will be performed throughout the head-to-toe process. However, when the components of the neurological assessment are performed together as a single assessment, this is commonly known as a *neuro exam.* Box 21.3 lists all the components of a basic neurological examination. Skill 21.5 (page 418) details the steps of performing a basic neurological examination.

Head and Neck

As you begin the actual physical assessment, begin assessing at the head and work in a sequential order toward the toes. Begin by assessing the skin color, which provides data about the circulatory and respiratory systems. Pallor indicates poor circulation or anemia, while cyanosis indicates hypoxia.

Level of Consciousness

One of the first steps is to identify the patient's level of consciousness (LOC), a function of the neurological system. The LOC is used to assess if the patient is alert. Note if the patient is awake or asleep. Is the patient alert or lethargic? **Lethargy** means drowsiness or mental sluggishness.

How do you determine if a patient is truly alert or if he or she is simply awake? A patient who is wide awake and responds to questions spontaneously is classified as alert. If the patient does not respond to verbal stimulus, the next level of stronger stimulus to use is tactile, or touch. If the patient still does not respond to the tactile stimulus, then you will use the third and strongest level of stimulus, which is pain. Slight pressure (absolutely NO rubbing, as this can cause blistering and injury to the skin) on the sternum or pressure on a nailbed will produce discomfort. Careful use of one of the painful stimuli will determine if the patient is responsive or not. A patient who is heavily sedated may not respond, but otherwise, if the patient does not respond to a painful stimulus, the patient is considered to be *comatose,* or in a state of unconsciousness from which he or she cannot be aroused. The Glasgow Coma Scale, a scale used to assess LOC, is shown in Table 21.2.

If the patient is responsive to stimuli, you will then assess the patient's orientation level. There are four spheres of orientation to assess: person, place, time, and situation. To gather these data, ask the patient questions that will demonstrate the patient's knowledge regarding all four spheres. The

• **WORD • BUILDING •**

atherosclerosis: athero – fatty plaque + scler – hard + osis – condition

Box 21.3

Components of a Basic Neurological Examination

The following are components of a *basic* neurological examination only. A more advanced neurological evaluation can include various other assessments.

- Vital signs
- Level of consciousness
- Orientation to four spheres
- Pupil size, round, equality, and reaction to light
- Facial symmetry
- Speech clarity and appropriateness
- Response to simple commands
- Movement and strength of four extremities

easiest and most basic questions include questions similar to the following:

- **Person:** "What is your name?" or "Who is the president of the United States?"
- **Place:** "Can you tell me where you are?"
- **Time:** "What is today's date?" or "What day is it?"
- **Situation:** "What problem brought you to the hospital?" or "Do you know why you are here?"

With practice and experience, you will learn to garner the same information from the conversation you have with the patient without having to ask the same questions each time you want to assess orientation. For example, the patient says, "The night nurse told me that Dr. Smith was going to discharge me either Tuesday or Wednesday." If this is accurate information, it is clear that the patient is oriented to person, place, time, and situation.

Documentation of LOC might appear as "awake, alert, oriented to person and time, disoriented to place and situation." Using acceptable abbreviations to chart the same information would look something like this: "AAO to person and time, disoriented to place and situation." Documentation for a patient who is awake, alert, and oriented to all four spheres would look like this: "AAOX4."

Eyes

Next, assess the eyes. The sclera should be smooth, white, and glistening. In dark-skinned patients, the sclera may have a normal, slightly darker cast around the outside edges. Abnormalities might include redness or a bloodshot appearance, which can be a sign of inflammation, lack of sleep, or allergies. Yellowish-orange color of the sclera is normally an indication of elevated bilirubin, known as **jaundice.** Gently pull down

Table 21.2

Glasgow Coma Scale

Function Assessed	*Patient's Response*	*Score*
Eye response	Opens spontaneously	4
	Opens to verbal command	3
	Opens to pain stimulus	2
	No response	1
Motor response	Reacts to verbal command	6
	Reacts to localized pain	5
	Flexes and withdraws from pain	4
	*Positions to decorticate posturing	3
	**Positions to decerebrate posturing	2
	No response	1
Verbal Response	Oriented, converses	5
	Disoriented, converses	4
	Uses inappropriate words	3
	Makes incomprehensible sounds	2
	No response	1

*Arms flexed to chest, hands clenched into fists and rotated internally, feet extended: Indicates problem is at or above the brainstem. Also known as *flexor posturing.*

**Arms extended, hands clenched into fists, wrists flexed, and forearms severely pronated (internally rotated): Indicates the problem is at the level of the midbrain or pons and is the more ominous of the two postures. Also known as *extension posturing.*

The total points possible ranges from 3 to 15. The highest possible score is 15, indicating the patient has full level of consciousness; is awake, alert, and oriented; and follows simple commands. The lower the score, the higher the degree of neurological impairment.

Source: Teasdale G, Jennett B. Assessment of Coma and Impaired Consciousness: A Practical Scale. *Lancet.* 1974;304:81-84, with permission.

the lower eyelids to observe the conjunctival sacs, which normally are pink and moist. Tissue redness, or *erythema,* may indicate inflammation and possibly infection. If the conjunctiva is receiving less oxygen than it requires, the naturally pink conjunctival sac may appear to be *cyanotic,* or blue. The cornea and lens should be clear and smooth. Older adults may have an opaque white ring around the outer edge of the cornea, known as *arcus senilis* (Fig. 21.4). Abnormalities include cloudiness, which is a sign of infection or vitamin A deficiency, and opaqueness of the lens, which usually is a cataract. Young adults may have cataracts, but they occur more frequently in older adults.

PUPILS. Normally pupils are black, round, between 3 and 7 mm in diameter, and equal in size and reaction (Fig. 21.5). If the pupils are different sizes, it is called *anisocoria.* Unless it is a congenital abnormality that the patient was born with, anisocoria is indicative of neurological impairment. Observe the eyelids for drooping, or **ptosis,** of one side. This is most commonly associated with paralysis from a stroke.

After assessing the pupils for size and shape, you will use a penlight to assess the equality of direct response to light, consensual response to light, and accommodation. To assess direct pupil response to light, dim the room lights, which allows the pupils to dilate slightly so that they are easier to detect. Then briefly shine the penlight in one eye and observe the response of the pupil in that eye. Remove the light, allowing the pupil to dilate back to normal size. Then shine the light into the same eye a second time while observing the pupil in the opposite eye. It should constrict at the same rate and to the same size as the first pupil. Because the optic nerve divides, or *bifurcates,* at the distal end, stimulation of the nerve by shining a light in either eye should cause both pupils to rapidly constrict simultaneously and equally, known as the **consensual reflex** or *consensual response.* Repeat the process for the opposite eye.

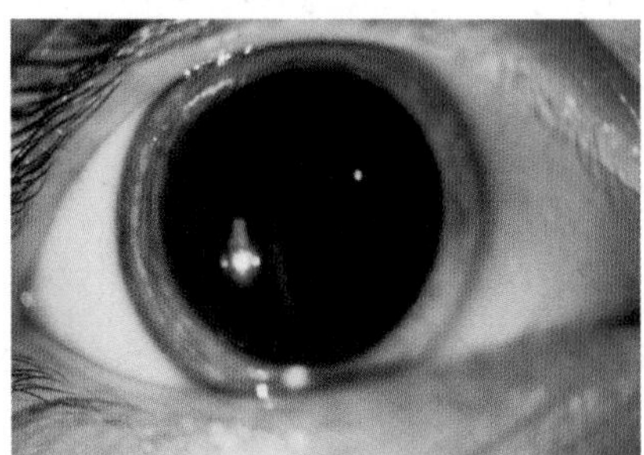

FIGURE 21.4A Normal lens (from Dillon PM. *Nursing Health Assessment: The Foundation of Clinical Practice.* 3rd ed. Philadelphia, PA: FA Davis; 2016).

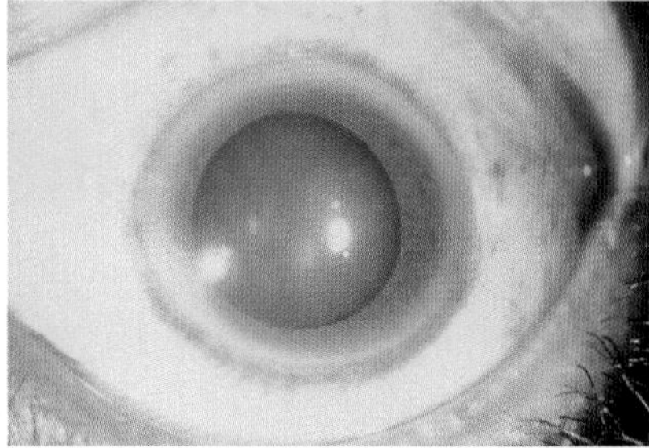

FIGURE 21.4B Arcus senilis (from Dillon PM. *Nursing Health Assessment: The Foundation of Clinical Practice.* 3rd ed. Philadelphia, PA: FA Davis; 2016).

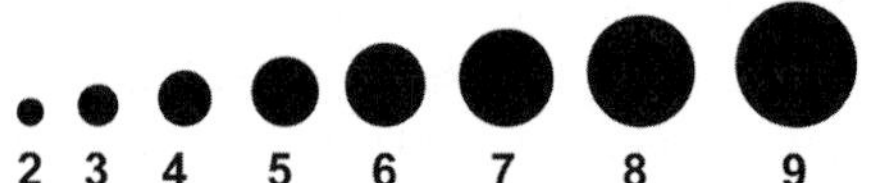

FIGURE 21.5 Pupil size in millimeters (from Myers E, Hopkins T. *LPN Notes.* 4th ed. Philadelphia, PA: FA Davis; 2016).

Next, you will assess for the **accommodation response,** which measures the eye muscles' ability to focus on an image up close and in the distance. Hold your finger in front of the patient's face and ask the patient to focus on your finger as it moves. Slowly increase the distance between the patient's face and your finger to approximately 1.5 to 2 feet. The pupils should both dilate to allow in more light to see better at a distance. Then slowly move your finger closer to the patient's face until your finger nearly touches the patient's nose. The pupils should both constrict because they will not require entrance of as much light to see something up close. A difference in the rate of constriction or size of the pupils, failure to constrict simultaneously, or failure to accommodate can be indications of neurological impairment. Document that the pupils are bilaterally brisk and equally reactive to light and accommodation as "pupils equal and round and reactive to light and accommodation," or **PERRLA.**

Oral Mucous Membranes

Use a penlight to examine the oral mucous membranes for color, integrity, moisture, and odor. Normally the mouth, tongue, and gums should be intact, pink, and moist. A dry mouth is an indication of inadequate hydration, but it also may be a side effect of certain medications. Erythema is an indicator of inflammation, and pallor is a sign of poor circulation or anemia. If the mucosa is erythematous and tender with white patches, it may be due to *Candida albicans,* a fungus commonly known as yeast. Cyanosis indicates either hypoxia or severe vasoconstriction.

Observe for ulcerations, lesions, coating of the tongue, bleeding of gums, and poor oral hygiene. Halitosis may be due to poor oral hygiene, stomach problems, or a sinus or oral infection. Small, painful ulcerations may be due to a virus, stress, or trauma. Painless ulcerations can be a sign of syphilis. White lesions and erythema of the tonsils are due to infection. Severe ulcerations or growths on the oral mucosa may be cancerous. An ulceration that has perforated the hard palate or roof of the

• WORD • BUILDING •

anisocoria: aniso – unequal + coria – pupils
ptosis: ptosis – dropping
bifurcate: bi – two + furcate – fork

mouth may be indicative of cocaine use (Fig. 21.6). Reddish-purple or hemorrhagic-appearing gums may be a sign of leukemia. Receding gums can be a sign of periodontal problems. A black, hairy appearance on the tongue indicates a fungal infection (Fig. 21.7), while a red, beefy-looking tongue is a sign of pernicious anemia (Fig. 21.8). A smooth, painful tongue is termed *glossitis* and can be due to inflammation or a side effect of medication. ***Safety: Assess that the patient is able to swallow. Difficulty swallowing is known as dysphagia and puts the patient at risk for aspiration.***

Lips

Observe for **cheilitis** (also known as ***chelosis***), or inflammation of the lips, as well as excessive dryness and cracking, all of which may be due to wind chapping, braces, dentures, dehydration, or seasonal allergies. A patient who repeatedly licks his or her lips or a patient who excessively applies lip balm may show the same signs of dryness or cracking. Sun exposure without sunscreen lip protection also can cause excessively dry and peeling lips. Fissures or cracking at the corners of the mouth are known as *cheilosis* and usually are related to vitamin B deficiencies.

If the lips are grossly swollen, especially if the edema occurred rapidly, the patient may have angioedema (Fig. 21.9), which is associated with serious allergic reactions such as anaphylaxis, a life-threatening allergic response. Allergic angioedema of the lips is usually seen along with other facial swelling and hives. It requires immediate medical treatment.

Lip color is also informative. Cherry-red lips may be a sign of carbon monoxide poisoning and acidosis. Pale lips are associated with anemia, but when the pallor is *circumoral,* meaning that it encircles the mouth area, it may indicate scarlet fever.

The objective data gathered in assessment of the lips provide you with information regarding the patient's nutritional status and hydration level.

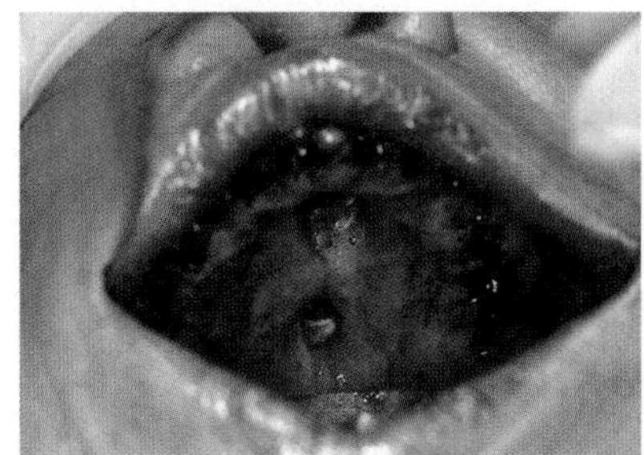

FIGURE 21.6 Perforation of hard palate as a result of cocaine use.

Teeth

Does the patient have dentures? Is the patient without teeth, or *edentulous?* Inspect for excessive dental cavities, or *caries.* Are the teeth and mouth clean? Dried mucus or food caked on the lips and teeth is termed ***sordes*** and can easily be treated with good oral hygiene. ***Safety: Research has related poor oral hygiene to health-care facility–acquired pneumonia as well as an increased risk of developing heart disease.*** Inquire if the patient has any difficulties chewing or eating. An elderly individual with dentures may not wear the dentures anymore because of poor fit. He or she may complain that the dentures rub sores when worn. Problems of this type may indicate special dietary needs.

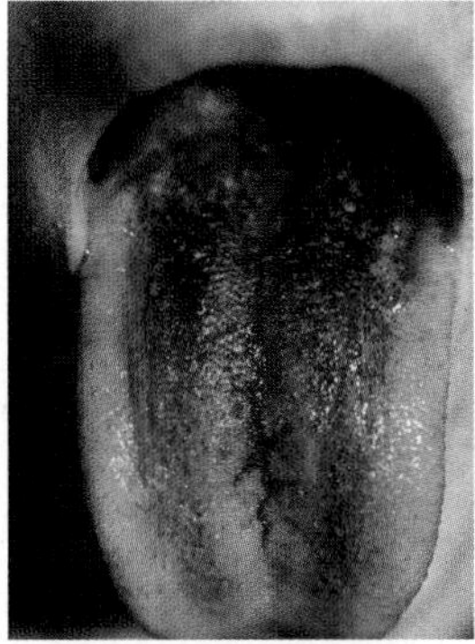

FIGURE 21.7 Black, hairy tongue caused by fungal infection.

Speech

Is the patient's speech appropriate, clear, and easy to understand? Or is it rambling, incoherent, inappropriate, or slurred? Some patients who have had strokes or other types of brain damage may be able to understand spoken and written words. The patient may even know what he or she wants to say but cannot say the actual words. This is known as *aphasia* and usually is frustrating to the patient.

An individual who has difficulty coordinating and organizing the words correctly in a sentence may be suffering from an impairment known as **dysphasia.** Patients with dementia

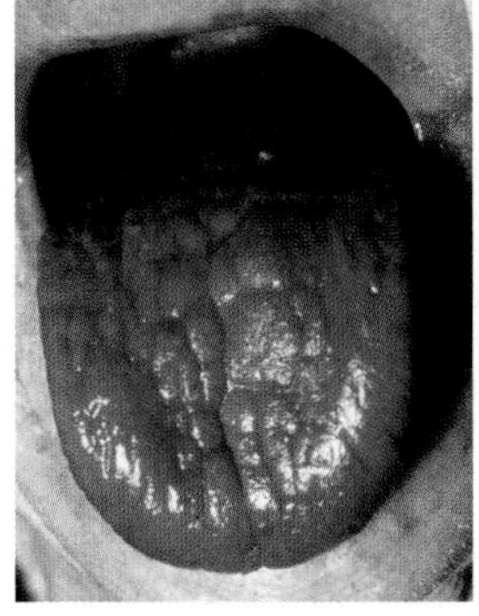

FIGURE 21.8 Red, beefy tongue due to pernicious anemia.

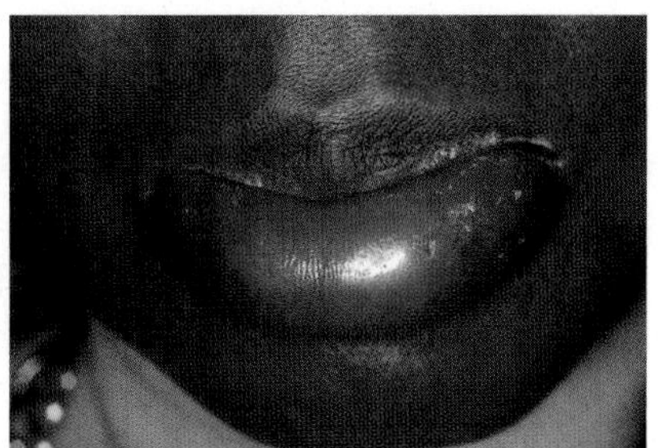

FIGURE 21.9 Angioedema caused by an allergic response.

may have difficulty finding the right words to express themselves (expressive aphasia) or may have difficulty in understanding what is being communicated to them (receptive aphasia) and therefore become confused and frustrated. ***Safety: Impairment of speech often is related to impairment of the central nervous system, including dysphagia (difficulty in swallowing), which can lead to aspiration.***

Neck

Are the jugular veins *distended,* or full enough that you can see them? If they are distended, this is indicative of fluid overload of the cardiovascular system, as in congestive heart failure (CHF). When you detect distended jugular veins, it necessitates further assessment, including auscultating breath sounds, weighing the patient, and reviewing the fluid intake and urine output for balance. Make note if the patient has a tracheostomy, as tracheostomies require special assessments and nursing care.

Dressings and Equipment on the Head and Neck

The patient may have dressings, incisions, supplemental oxygen, nasogastric tubes, tracheostomy tubes, or artificial airways in place on the head or neck. Assess their status and make certain all equipment is operating correctly.

> **KNOWLEDGE CONNECTION**
> What findings can be noted by just observing as you enter the patient's room? Which vital signs provide information about each of the eight body systems mentioned? Which portion of the head and neck assessment pertains to the neurological system? The level of hydration? Circulation? What does PERRLA stand for? Explain how to assess the consensual reflex and what it means. How is accommodation assessed?

Chest and Abdomen

Chest

As you move down to the chest area, observe the chest during respiration, noting the characteristics and pattern of respirations. Do they appear effortless? Or does the patient appear to have shortness of breath or difficulty breathing, known as *dyspnea?* Does difficulty breathing in the supine position, known as *orthopnea,* force the patient to sit upright to ease the breathing? Even if you do not observe these problems, inquire if the patient has had any shortness of breath. Also ask the patient if he or she has a cough. If so, is it frequent or occasional? Is it a dry cough, known as a *nonproductive cough,* or does it produce sputum, known as a *productive cough?* If it is a productive cough, what amount of sputum is produced? What is the viscosity (thickness) of the sputum? Is it yellow, green, white, or clear, or is it blood-tinged? Is the sputum frothy or pink-tinged? Both of these are indicative of pulmonary edema as a result of worsening CHF. Blood-tinged sputum may be due to tuberculosis, and rust-colored sputum is common with pneumonia. Does the patient produce sputum each and every time he or she coughs? Or is it only a few times a day? Does the cough occur mostly at night? This is known as a *nocturnal* cough and may be a sign of pulmonary edema and CHF. Does the patient have to sleep sitting up due to orthopnea? This is often seen in patients with chronic obstructive pulmonary disease.

Also observe the respiratory rhythm and pattern. Is the breathing within normal parameters? If so, the term for this is *eupnea.* Or do you observe a pattern of respirations such as Biot's, Cheyne-Stokes, or Kussmaul's respirations? Table 21.3 lists different patterns of respirations and their meanings. Observe for equal chest expansion, or **excursion,** of both sides as the patient inhales. A more exact way to determine if the excursion of both sides of the chest is equal is to place both of your hands vertically on the patient's back with both thumbs on the spine at the level of the 9th or 10th ribs. Have the patient take a deep breath while observing the increasing distance that develops between your thumbs, noting whether or not both hands raise the same distance. Lack of or decreased excursion on one side of the chest can be caused by severe pneumonia or lung (alveoli) collapse, known as ***atelectasis.*** If one side does not expand, it might be documented as "excursion absent on the [designated either left or right] side." If the right side does expand but not as well as the left side, you might document it as "decreased excursion of right side" or "right side excursion less than left side."

Note whether the patient uses the normal respiratory muscles (the diaphragm, chest, and abdominal muscles) or the accessory respiratory muscles (the sternocleidomastoid, scalene, trapezius, intercostal, and rhomboid muscles). Patients with chronic respiratory diseases such as emphysema often require use of these accessory respiratory muscles to breathe and develop a barrel-shaped chest. The shoulders should be the same height. Notice the shape of the anterior, lateral, and posterior aspects of the thorax. When viewing the thorax from the lateral view, there should be a slight convex curve of the midthoracic area and mild concave curve noted at the lumbar area. If the lumbar concavity is increased, it is known as *lordosis.* When the convexity of the midthorax is increased, it is called *kyphosis.* The older adult may develop severe kyphosis and a stooped posture, which must be taken into consideration when auscultating breath sounds and heart sounds. When viewing the spine from the posterior, the vertebrae should be midline and straight. Curvature to either the left or right is called *scoliosis.*

Make note whether the patient's chest wall appears depressed, or sunken in, between the ribs or under the xiphoid process when the patient inhales. These abnormal movements are called **retractions** and indicate acute respiratory problems that need attention.

LANDMARKS FOR AUSCULTATION. To accurately place the stethoscope for auscultation of breath and heart sounds, it is necessary to be familiar with the landmark terms and to know their locations (Fig. 21.10). Anteriorly, there are three vertical

Table 21.3
Respiratory Patterns

Pattern	*Characteristics*	*When Seen?*	*Illustration*
Eupnea	Normal rate and pattern: regular, equal-depth respirations	Normal conditions	
Tachypnea	Increased respiratory rate	Fever, stress, fear, anxiety, pain, exercise, hypoxia	
Bradypnea	Abnormally slow respiratory rate	Opioid medications, sedatives, brain damage, metabolic alkalosis	
Kussmaul's	Abnormally deep and rapid respirations, rhythm regular, blows off excess CO_2	Compensatory breathing mechanism seen during periods of metabolic acidosis	
Cheyne-Stokes	Cyclic breathing: Depth of respirations begins as very shallow, then each respiration gradually increases in depth until reaching a peak, at which time the depth begins to decrease with each breath until the depth is barely discernible; then there is a period of apnea, from 10 to 60 seconds in length, after which the cycle begins again	Increased intracranial pressure, brain damage, impending death	
Biot's	A sequence of several breaths of equal depth that alternate with periods of apnea	Brain damage	
Apnea	Temporary or periodic absence of breathing	Cheyne-Stokes respirations, sleep apnea, sudden infant death syndrome	

lines of reference: the midsternal line and the left and right midclavicular lines. Laterally, there are also three vertical lines of reference: the anterior axillary line, midaxillary line, and posterior axillary line. Posteriorly, the three vertical lines include the midspinal line and the left and right scapular lines.

AUSCULTATION OF BREATH SOUNDS. To help you hear the breath sounds, assist the patient to sit on the side of the bed or in the high Fowler's position. If the patient cannot sit up, try to place the patient in at least a semi-Fowler's position, if tolerated. Otherwise, place the patient in the supine or lateral position for lung auscultation.

Warm the diaphragm or flat surface of the stethoscope with your hands. Place the diaphragm directly against the skin and listen from the top or apex of each lung to the base,

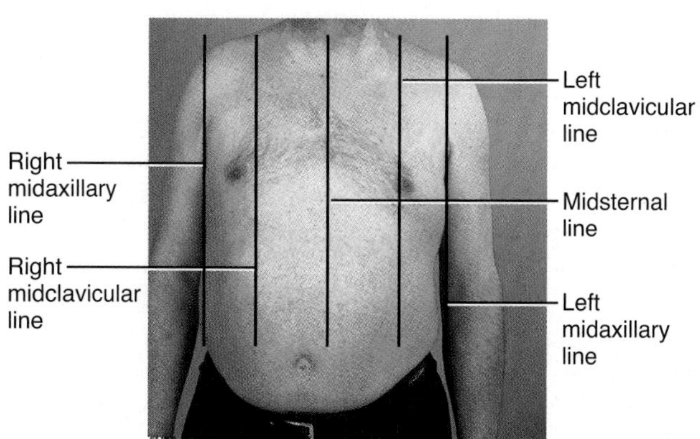

FIGURE 21.10A Vertical lines drawn to indicate anterior chest landmarks (from Wilkinson JM, Treas LS. *Fundamentals of Nursing: Theory, Concepts & Applications*. Vol. 1. 3rd ed. Philadelphia, PA: FA Davis; 2016).

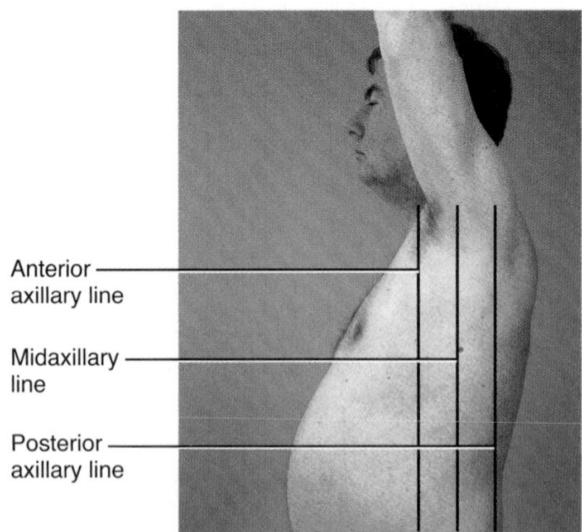

FIGURE 21.10B Vertical lines indicating lateral chest landmarks (from Wilkinson JM, Treas LS. *Fundamentals of Nursing: Theory, Concepts & Applications.* Vol. 1. 3rd ed. Philadelphia, PA: FA Davis; 2016).

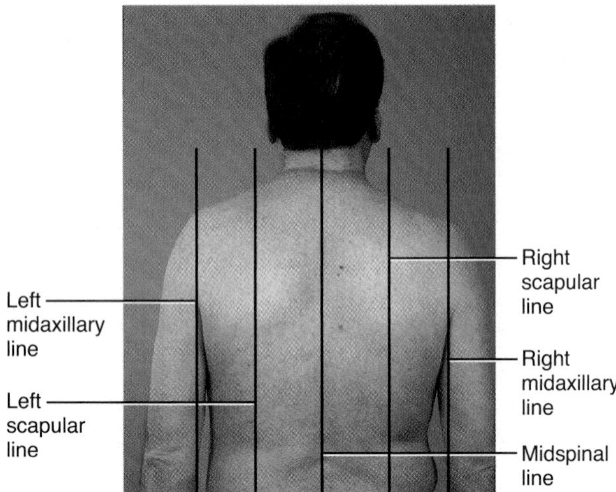

FIGURE 21.10C Vertical lines indicating posterior chest landmarks (from Wilkinson JM, Treas LS. *Fundamentals of Nursing: Theory, Concepts & Applications.* Vol. 1. 3rd ed. Philadelphia, PA: FA Davis; 2016).

alternating sides. Avoid listening through the gown or clothing; you will be able to hear more clearly and better detect abnormalities when the diaphragm is placed directly on the skin. Auscultate the breath sounds anteriorly, laterally, and posteriorly using the flat diaphragm side of your stethoscope. To perform this assessment correctly, you must know where the five lobes of the lungs are located.

Anatomy and Physiology Connection

The Lungs

Anteriorly, the superior, cone-shaped portion of each lung is known as the *apex* and extends approximately 1 inch above the medial aspect of the clavicle. The bottom, or base, of each lung is located at the sixth intercostal space in the midclavicular line. The bases extend down to the eighth intercostal space on the lateral aspect of the chest (Figs. 21.11 and 21.12). On the posterior aspect of the thorax, the apexes of the lungs begin at the first intercostal space, just below the first thoracic vertebrae. The bases of the lungs are located at approximately the 10th intercostal space, just below the 10th thoracic vertebrae, but extend down to the 12th intercostal space upon deep inspiration. There are two lobes in the left lung and three lobes in the right lung, but only the upper and lower lobes can be auscultated posteriorly. The right middle lobe is positioned where it can *only* be accessed from the anterior and lateral aspects. The acronyms used to designate the five lobes are as follows: *LUL* is used for the left upper lobe, *LLL* for the left lower lobe, *RUL* for the right upper lobe, *RML* for the right middle lobe, and *RLL* for the right lower lobe.

When you auscultate breath sounds, listen for a complete respiration, both the inspiratory and expiratory phases, at each site. You should hear the air moving into the lungs and out of the lungs, and there should be equality of breath sounds comparing the left to the right. As you move the stethoscope over different areas of the chest, listen to the pitch and duration of the sounds and the length of the inspiratory phase compared to the expiratory phase. Sounds heard over different portions of the chest will vary in these three characteristics.

The sounds heard over the bronchi, located under the manubrium, will have a shorter inspiratory phase and longer expiratory phase and will sound louder and slightly harsher than other breath sounds. These are the bronchial breath sounds.

Over the middle chest and sternum, you will hear the bronchovesicular sounds, which have equal inspiration and expiration phases. They are quieter than the bronchial sounds and are less harsh sounding.

The vesicular sounds can be heard over the periphery of the lungs. They have a longer inspiratory phase than expiratory phase and are softer rustling sounds.

Abnormal and Adventitious Breath Sounds. If there are fewer breath sounds on one side, this is known as decreased breath sounds. When secretions and exudate from pneumonia solidify in lung tissues, this is known as consolidation, and may result in absence of breath sounds in that lobe. If there are no breath sounds, you will note them as absent. **Adventitious breath sounds** are abnormal breath sounds. They include crackles, rhonchi, wheezes, pleural friction rub, and stridor.

Crackles, also formerly called rales, are discontinuous, usually heard during inspiration, and may be either fine or coarse. These adventitious breath sounds may be caused by the movement of air over secretions in the lung or the sudden

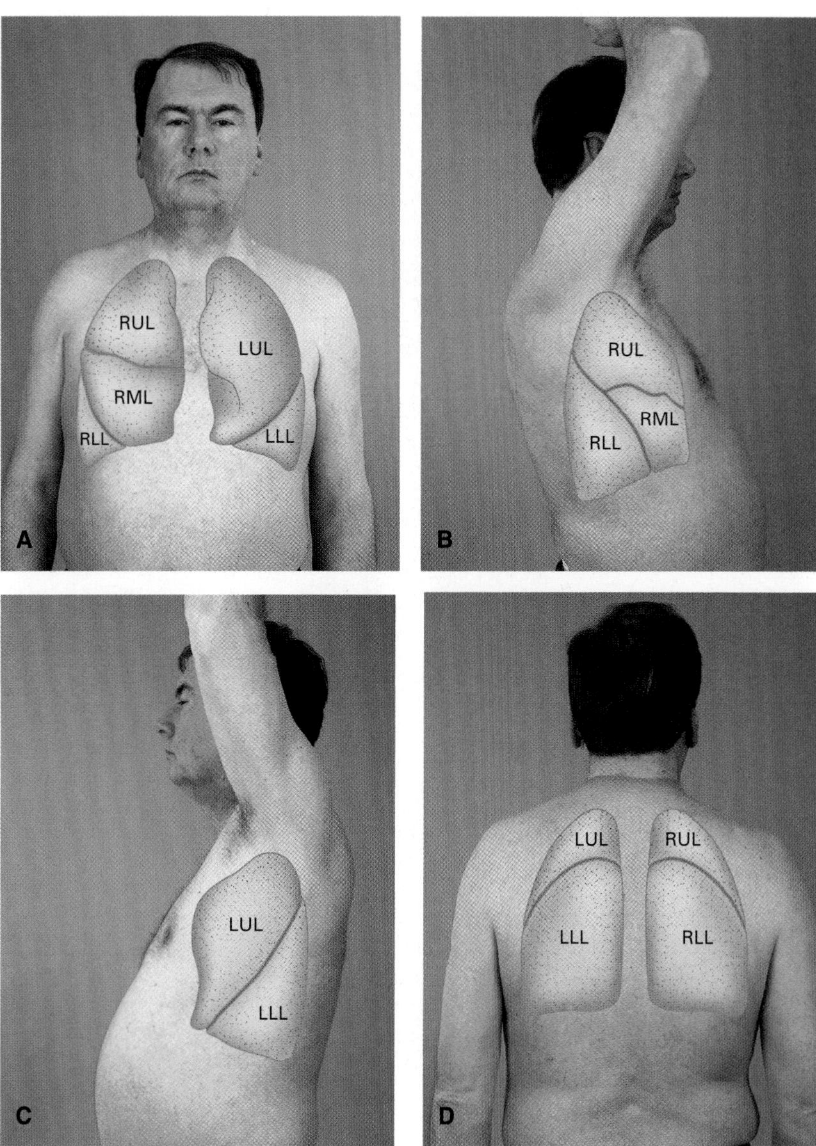

FIGURE 21.11 (a) Anterior view of both lungs' lobes; (b) Lateral view of right lung lobes; (c) Lateral view of left lung lobes; (d) Posterior view of both lungs' lobes (from Dillon PM. *Nursing Health Assessment: The Foundation of Clinical Practice.* 3rd ed. Philadelphia, PA: FA Davis; 2016).

opening of alveoli that have been closed. Crackles cannot be cleared by coughing. To learn to distinguish the sound of fine crackles, try rubbing several hairs together between your fingers just in front of your ear.

Rhonchi include sounds described as snoring, rattling, gurgling, squeaking, and low-pitched wheezes and are caused by either secretions or partial occlusion of the airways. They are deeper and more rumbling sounds than crackles and usually are heard during expiration. Rhonchi are intermittent and may clear by having the patient cough. They can be caused by secretions in the airway, tumors, and partial airway obstruction.

Wheezes are continuous melodious, musical, or whistling sounds. They are due to constriction of the airways and can be inspiratory or expiratory.

A *pleural friction rub* is a grating, creaking sound that is due to inflamed, edematous pleural surfaces rubbing together during breathing. These sounds are often heard during the first couple of days of lung inflammation.

Stridor usually can be heard with or without use of a stethoscope and is a sign of a life-threatening upper airway obstruction caused by a foreign body, tumor, swelling, or bronchial spasms. ***Safety: Stridor is a shrill, high-pitched, harsh, crowing sound and requires immediate intervention. Note that this sound is heard on inspiration.*** Small children who are prone to croup may present in the emergency room with stridor.

Placement of Stethoscope. Figure 21.13 illustrates the sequencing and positioning of stethoscope placement for auscultation of breath sounds. Anteriorly, listen to the apex of the left lung and then listen to the corresponding site on the right. The air movement should sound the same. Make note if one side exhibits decreased or increased sounds compared to the other side or exhibits adventitious sounds. Place the

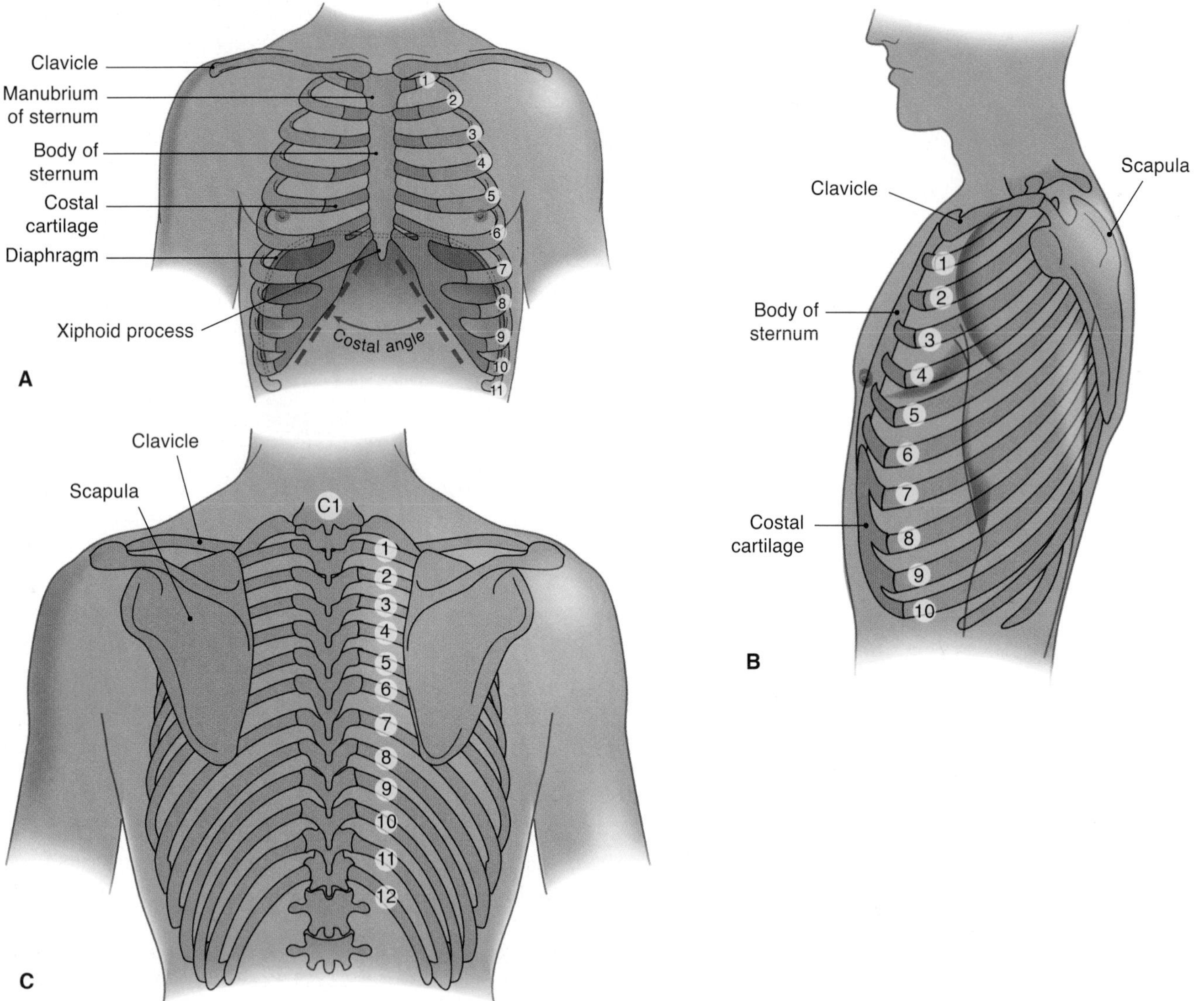

FIGURE 21.12 (a) Anterior view of chest with landmarks and ribs numbered; (b) Left lateral view of chest with landmarks and ribs numbered; (c) Posterior view of chest with landmarks and ribs numbered (from Dillon PM. *Nursing Health Assessment: The Foundation of Clinical Practice.* 3rd ed. Philadelphia, PA: FA Davis; 2016).

stethoscope on the next lower intercostal space to listen, and then cross over to the corresponding space on the opposite side. You will be able to auscultate all five lobes on the anterior chest. Posteriorly, listen from the apexes of the lungs downward toward the bases, alternating from side to side. Remember that listening laterally is important, too.

The breath sounds provide objective data regarding the function of the respiratory system. To document that breath sounds are equal and clear to auscultation, meaning that no adventitious sounds or abnormalities are identified, chart something like "breath sounds clear to auscultation in all 5 lobes." Skill 21.6 (page 418) provides further details regarding auscultation of breath sounds.

KNOWLEDGE CONNECTION

What are the landmarks of the anterior, lateral, and posterior thorax? How many lobes are there in the lungs? Where can you access the sounds of each of these lobes: anteriorly, laterally, or posteriorly? What are the types of adventitious breath sounds? What does each mean? What intercostal space level indicates the bases of the lungs anteriorly? Posteriorly? How many sites of placement for the stethoscope are there for anterior assessment? Posterior assessment? What is the most life-threatening adventitious breath sound?

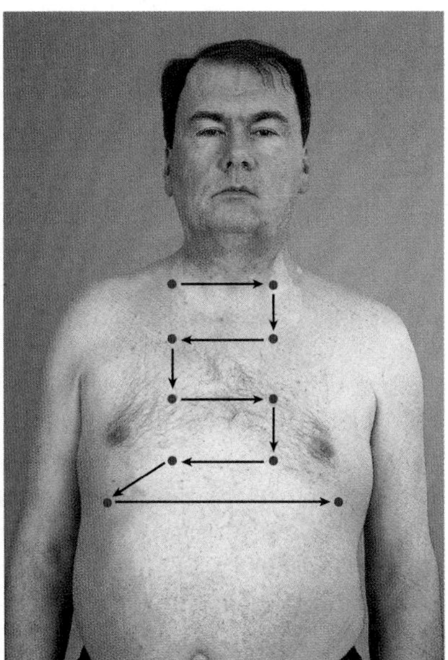

FIGURE 21.13A Sequence of anterior auscultation sites (from Dillon PM. *Nursing Health Assessment: The Foundation of Clinical Practice.* 3rd ed. Philadelphia, PA: FA Davis; 2016).

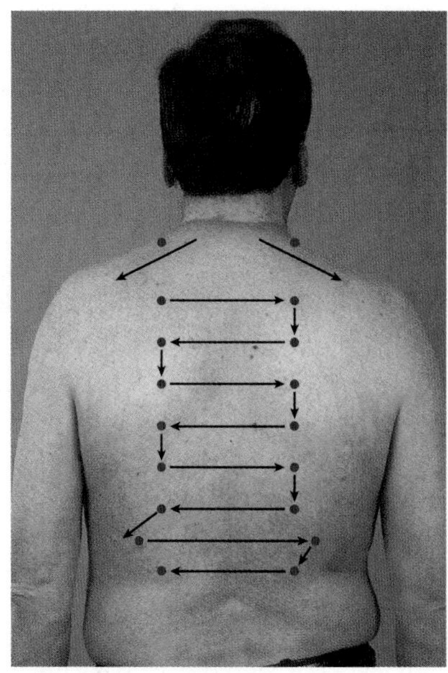

FIGURE 21.13C Sequence of posterior auscultation sites (from Dillon PM. *Nursing Health Assessment: The Foundation of Clinical Practice.* 3rd ed. Philadelphia, PA: FA Davis; 2016).

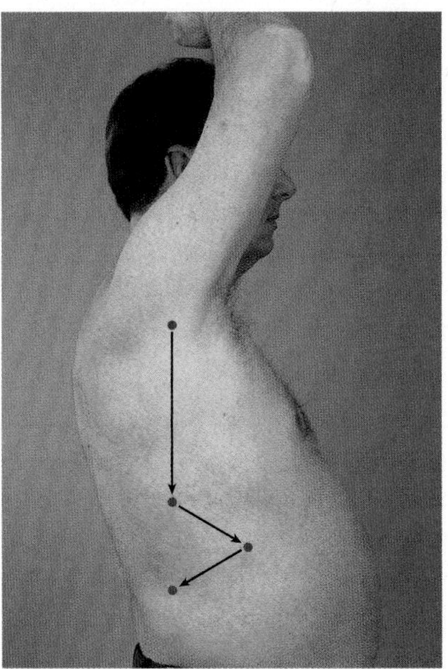

FIGURE 21.13B Sequence of lateral auscultation sites for both sides (from Dillon PM. *Nursing Health Assessment: The Foundation of Clinical Practice.* 3rd ed. Philadelphia, PA: FA Davis; 2016).

AUSCULTATION OF HEART SOUNDS. The preferred position to auscultate heart sounds is sitting, but they also can be heard using the left lateral or supine position. As you prepare to listen to the heart sounds, inspect the upper chest for an implanted pacemaker or central-line port. When implanted under the skin, either of these two devices will be visible as a firm, raised area in the shape of the implanted device. A port is a round device about 2 cm in diameter and provides intermittent or continual IV access. A pacemaker and an implanted defibrillator is an approximately 3-cm by 4-cm rectangular-shaped box. It provides an automatic electrical impulse stimulus to initiate cardiac contraction when the patient's electrical conduction system is impaired.

Inspect and palpate the chest wall at the fifth intercostal space in the left midclavicular line for a pulsation. For most patients, this is the spot just inferior to the left nipple. It is easier to observe in thinner individuals. This location is known as the point of maximum impulse (PMI) because it is located over the apex of the left ventricle, which pumps the blood out of the heart to the rest of the body. This is the site where you can best hear the mitral valve and where you will auscultate the apical pulse (AP) for rate, rhythm, and strength (Fig. 21.14). Three other sites are used to auscultate the heart sounds and hear the aortic, pulmonic, and tricuspid valves clearly:

- The aortic valve is best heard at the second intercostal space just to the right of the sternum and is known as the *right base heart sound.*
- The pulmonic valve can be auscultated at the second intercostal space just to the left of the sternum and is known as the *left base heart sound.*
- The tricuspid valve is best heard at the edge of the sternum, at the level of the fourth intercostal space just to the left of the sternum, and is known as the *left lateral sternal border (LLSB) heart sound.*

The first heart sound, known as the S_1 or *systolic sound,* is the louder, prolonged dull sound, usually of a lower frequency. Its source is ventricular contraction and the closure of the mitral and tricuspid valves. The S_1 is the "lubb" of the rhythmic "lubb-dupp" sound of the heartbeat.

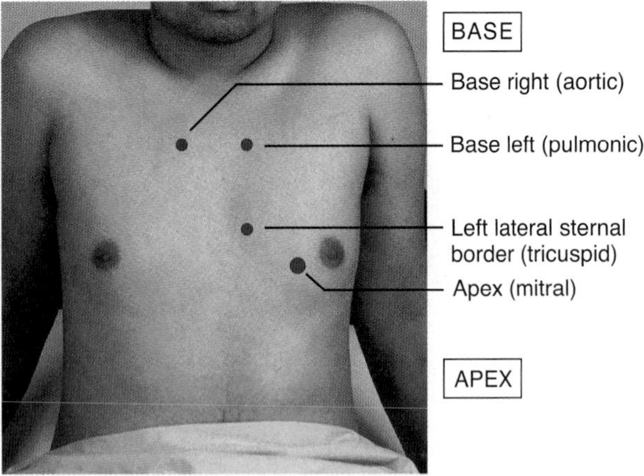

FIGURE 21.14 Cardiac auscultation sites (from Dillon PM. *Nursing Health Assessment: The Foundation of Clinical Practice.* 3rd ed. Philadelphia, PA: FA Davis; 2016).

After the S_1, there is a short pause before the second heart sound, the S_2. Also termed the *diastolic sound,* the S_2 is shorter and higher pitched than the S_1, and it results from the closure of the aortic and pulmonary valves. The S_2 serves as the "dupp" of the "lubb-dupp" heart sound. Figure 21.15 illustrates where these sounds appear on an electrocardiogram.

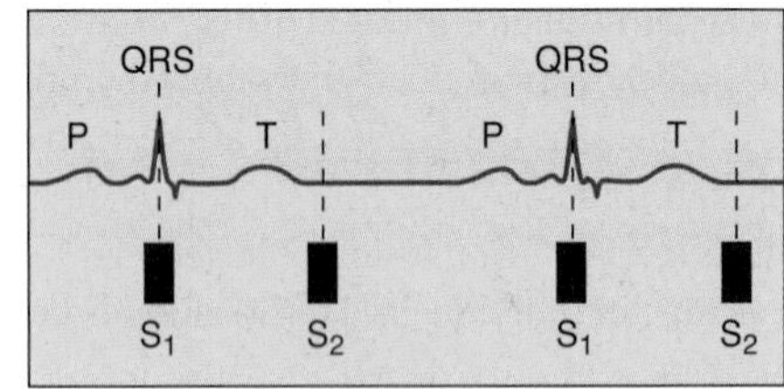

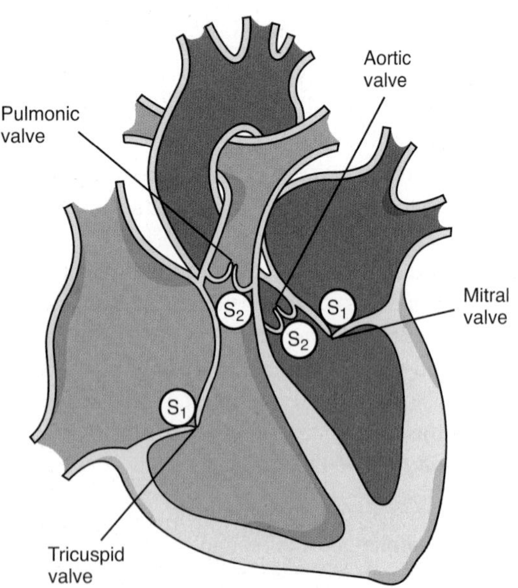

FIGURE 21.15 Occurrence of heart sounds shown on electrocardiogram. S_1 is heard at the beginning of systole; S_2 is heard at the beginning of diastole (from Williams LS, Hopper PD. *Understanding Medical-Surgical Nursing.* 5th ed. Philadelphia, PA: FA Davis; 2015).

Apical Pulse

The AP is assessed for rate, rhythm, and strength. To assess the AP, place the diaphragm of the stethoscope directly on the skin over the PMI and listen for both the S_1 and S_2, or "lubb-dupp." Remember, in identifying the S_1 and S_2, the S_1 will be the louder of the two sounds. The combination of the two sounds will equal one complete heartbeat. Some nurses find it helpful to close their eyes while auscultating heart sounds. This decreases sensory input and makes it easier to focus on the heart sounds.

Take the pulse for a full minute to provide a wider window of opportunity to detect abnormalities. ***Safety: Taking the AP pulse rate for 1 full minute is the standard of practice, as it is the most accurate and concise evaluation of an irregular pulse rate. The AP rate is required immediately prior to the administration of multiple medications related to irregular heart rhythms.*** Note the rate and also compare the length of the intervals between the heartbeats. If they are all regularly or evenly spaced, the rhythm is said to be regular. If there is any variance in the length of time between beats, the rhythm is noted as irregular. The third assessment of the heart sounds is the strength of the beats. If both the S_1 and S_2 are clearly and distinctly heard, the strength may be documented as strong or distinct.

If you have a hard time hearing the AP, have the patient lean forward and slightly to the left side, bringing the heart closer to the chest wall for better sound. If the sounds are still hard to hear or you can only hear one of the two sounds, document that the AP strength is muffled or distant. A weak AP may be a sign that the heart is not pumping adequately, as in CHF.

As you listen to the AP, also feel the radial pulse (RP) to determine if they are the same rate. If the RP is slower than the AP, it is documented as a *pulse deficit.* This is a common finding in patients with atrial fibrillation. If a pulse deficit is detected, seek another nurse to count the RP at the same time you are counting the AP to determine how many beats' difference there is between the two pulses. Once you are more experienced, you may become skilled enough to count both the AP rate and the number of skips at the RP site without the assistance of a second nurse, but it generally works best to utilize a second nurse to assist you. If there is a pulse deficit, be certain to also document it; for example, "AP – 71, RP – 67, pulse deficit of 4."

If you hear extra heart sounds, they may be due to a murmur. A *murmur* may present as a swishing, rumbling, or blowing sound, or it may be soft, loud, or booming. Some murmurs are normal, especially in children and young adults. Other murmurs are indicators of valvular problems or a congenital heart defect. Murmurs may be heard during systole or diastole and are classified on a scale from 1 to 6. Murmurs are often difficult to auscultate, especially for the inexperienced nurse. As you progress in your clinicals and learn more about medical-surgical diseases, you will begin to increase your skills at murmur detection. As you begin clinicals, simply listen carefully and, if you think you are hearing extra heart sounds, solicit assistance from your instructor to clarify the sounds you hear. Skill 21.7 (page 419) presents further details regarding the auscultation of heart sounds.

> **KNOWLEDGE CONNECTION**
> What is the PMI? Where do you assess the base heart sounds? The AP? What are the names of the two heart sounds? How long do you listen to assess the AP rate? What is a pulse deficit?

Abdomen

As you progress down from the chest, you will next assess the abdomen. You will begin with inspection, move to auscultation of bowel sounds, and finally end with palpation and percussion if desired. This particular sequence of assessing the abdomen should always be followed. It is important that you auscultate the bowel sounds before you palpate the abdomen. If you deviate from the sequence and palpate the abdomen before auscultating the bowel sounds, you can stimulate bowel sounds that were not originally present, creating inaccuracy in your assessment findings.

First, inspect the shape and size of the abdomen, noting whether it is flat, rounded, or distended. Be certain to also gather subjective data by asking the patient if there is any problem with pain, indigestion, gas, nausea, vomiting, or *anorexia* (a lack of appetite). Anorexia, with its lack of nutritional intake, may contribute to decreased immunity. As people age, metabolism slows, activity decreases, and calorie requirements naturally decrease. Therefore, the appetite of older adults decreases over time. Be cautious and do not confuse a naturally lighter appetite of an older adult with anorexia. Also, a small child obviously will not require the amount of caloric intake needed by a teenager or adult. ***Safety: When inspecting and palpating the abdomen and pulsations are observed, do not continue to palpate the abdomen due to possibility of an aortic aneurysm.***

BOWEL SOUNDS. After visualization of the abdomen, auscultate the bowel sounds with the stethoscope, using the diaphragm. Mentally divide the abdomen in four equal quadrants, using the umbilicus as the midpoint (Fig. 21.16).

Begin listening in the right lower quadrant, then the right upper quadrant, then the left upper quadrant, and lastly the left lower quadrant. This pattern will track the ascending colon up to the transverse colon, and then to the descending colon and sigmoid. Place the stethoscope firmly against the skin and listen for clicks or gurgles. These are the sounds of **peristalsis,** the wavelike muscular contractions of the intestines that move intestinal contents through the alimentary canal, where absorption of nutrients and water takes place, toward the rectum for elimination.

There should be between 5 and 30 clicks, or gurgles, per minute in each of the four quadrants, and they should be somewhat high pitched, which is known as *active* bowel sounds. Fewer than 5 clicks or gurgles per minute in any quadrant is termed *hypoactive* bowel sounds, the result of slowed peristalsis, which can be caused by opioids, anesthesia, bedrest or decreased physical activity, infection in the peritoneal cavity, and bowel obstruction. The slower the peristalsis, the longer food remains in the intestines; this allows the large intestine to absorb more of the water from the food, making the remaining waste drier and harder. Therefore, a patient with hypoactive bowel sounds is more prone to constipation. More than 30 clicks or gurgles per minute is termed *hyperactive* bowel sounds and is the result of excessive peristalsis. Hyperactive bowel sounds may result from intestinal infection, irritable bowel disease, early bowel obstruction, and laxatives. This state of hyperactivity can cause cramping and rapid passage of food through the alimentary canal so that the colon does not have time to absorb the water from the digested food, leaving it in a liquid form to be expelled via the rectum, known as diarrhea. Some inflammatory diseases cause such excessive hyperactivity of the bowel that there is poor food absorption as a result of the severe diarrhea. If *gurgling* bowel sounds are loud enough to hear without a stethoscope, it is termed *borborygmus.*

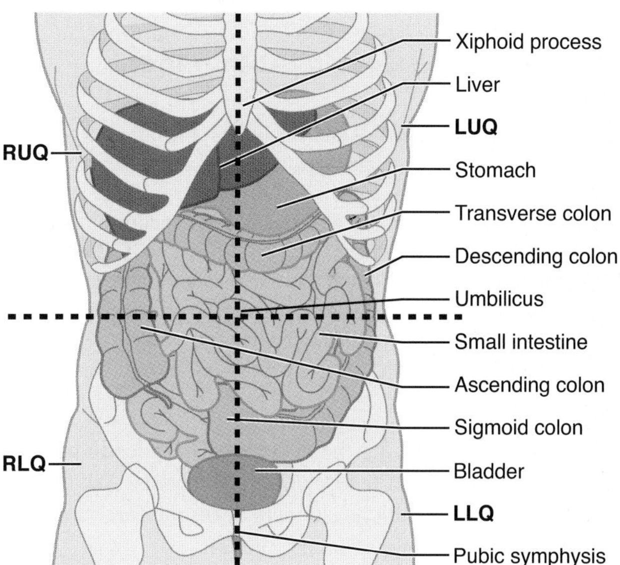

FIGURE 21.16 The four abdominal quadrants (from Wilkinson JM, Treas LS. *Fundamentals of Nursing: Theory, Concepts & Applications.* Vol. 1. 3rd ed. Philadelphia, PA: FA Davis; 2016).

A complete absence of bowel sounds may be due to late bowel obstruction, infection of the peritoneal cavity, or a paralytic ileus postoperatively. Therefore, it is important to be absolutely certain about a complete absence of bowel sounds. To be certain, listen for at least 3 to 5 minutes in each abdominal quadrant. This may seem like an excessively long time, but an absence of bowel sounds is significant and you must be certain before declaring that there are none.

Older adults may complain of not being able to control expulsion of flatus because the rectal sphincter loses some of its elasticity, thereby decreasing voluntary control. Intestinal peristalsis also slows, increasing the risk of constipation.

Next, palpate the four quadrants of the abdomen to determine whether the abdomen is soft, firm, or hard. (Box 21.4 lists contraindications to palpation.) Observe for flinching, grimacing, or guarding while palpating. **Guarding** is the defense

Box 21.4

Contraindications to Abdominal Palpation

There are certain situations and conditions when it may be contraindicated to palpate a patient's abdomen. Never palpate the abdomen of a patient who:

- Has a known or suspected abdominal aortic aneurysm
- Has had an organ transplant
- Is known or suspected to have a Wilms' tumor (more common in children than in adults), as palpation may cause seeding or spreading of the tumor into the abdomen

mechanism of tightening the abdominal muscles to prevent further compression of tender or inflamed areas. Ask the patient if the palpation elicits any pain or discomfort. Note any masses and/or pulsations that may be felt.

SUPRAPUBIC ASSESSMENT. The suprapubic region is proximal (above) to the pubic bone, which is where the urinary bladder is located. Assessment of this region is important to determine the retention (retaining) of urine in the bladder that can be the result of an adverse effect related to neurological or surgical procedures, or the adverse effects of medications.

Gently place your dominant hand over this region to lightly palpate the area to check if the bladder is distended (enlarged). Occasionally, with very thin patients, there will be a visible mound in this region. With obese patients who have bladder distention, light palpation may not be deep enough to determine retention.

Bladder scanning is used to determine the approximate amount of urine in the bladder. Please follow the manufacturer and facility policies regarding the use of the scanner. In Chapter 31, Figure 31.4 presents a bladder scan and Skill 31.4 provides information about performing a bladder scan.

Skin

Skin is assessed throughout the examination, as different areas of the body are exposed. The examination of the chest and abdomen is a particularly good time to further assess the skin. Assess for numbness or decreased sensation, known as **paresthesia;** if present, it indicates some type of nerve impairment, commonly seen as a complication of diabetes and as a result of a stroke or from a traumatic event.

COLOR. Skin color may vary from culture and ethnicity as well as from genetics. What color is the skin? Does it exhibit its normal pink, olive, tan, or brown tones? Or is it pale, lighter, or whiter than usual? As in the mucous membranes, pallor of the skin indicates decreased circulation or anemia. Individuals with dark skin usually have lips of a lighter color than the rest of the skin on the face. Although pallor can normally be detected on a dark-skinned person, the mucous membranes and nailbeds are the best indicator of circulation. Elderly patients often have numerous spots of yellowish-brown discoloration caused by years of sun exposure, known as **solar lentigines.** The older patient may refer to them as "liver spots." (Box 21.5 lists skin color descriptors.)

TEMPERATURE AND MOISTURE. Skin is normally warm and dry. When assessing skin temperature, use the dorsal side of the hand because it is more sensitive. Is the skin warm or cool? Is it dry or moist? Moisture that can be felt on the skin surface may be due to fever, exertion, or even anxiety. If the patient is perspiring, he or she is considered diaphoretic. If the skin is hot, further assessment is needed. Is the room temperature comfortable? Has the patient had too many blankets as covering? Does the patient have a fever? If the skin is too cool or cold, further assessment is again needed. Is it due to environmental temperature or poor circulation?

TURGOR. Evaluate the skin **turgor,** or elasticity, which is an indicator of hydration level in all ages of patients except elders. The skin of elderly patients loses its elasticity and is not a reliable assessment tool for hydration. Skin that has been exposed to the sun over the years is also considered not reliable because sunlight causes the skin to lose its elasticity. Gently pinch a fold of skin over the sternum or just below the clavicle between your index finger and thumb. Then release the skin; it should recoil immediately if the patient is well hydrated. If the skinfold remains tented for

Box 21.5

Skin Color Descriptors

Skin color provides you with data regarding multiple body system functions and is helpful in diagnosing certain conditions and disease processes. Skin color provides data related to the cardiovascular circulation as well as the efficiency of the respiratory system at providing adequate gas exchange of oxygen and carbon dioxide. It can serve as an indicator of liver disease and inflammation and infection. Below is a partial list of skin color descriptors and their possible *etiologies* (causes).

- **Pale:** a lighter color, more white than usual; if not the patient's normal "fair coloring," indicates poor circulation, anemia
- **Erythematous:** redness of a designated site; usually a sign of inflammation due to increased circulation to the inflamed site
- **Flushed:** widespread, diffuse red color of face; possibly includes the body; usually caused by fever, embarrassment, exertion, or sunburn
- **Jaundiced:** yellow or orange coloring of the skin and mucous membranes, easily detected in the sclera and palm of the hands; caused by liver impairment
- **Cyanotic:** bluish-gray color of the skin and mucous membranes due to hypoxia and extreme vasoconstriction
- **Ecchymotic:** caused by bruising of the skin (ecchymosis); fresh bruises are bluish-purple, and older bruises turn greenish-yellow as they begin to resolve
- **Bronzing:** bronze pigmentation of the skin due to disorders of iron metabolism; iron pigments are deposited in the body tissues

several seconds after release, it is considered to be nonelastic or to have slow recoil, a sign that may indicate a state of dehydration.

Integrity

Under normal conditions, the skin is intact without breaks or discontinuity. Assess whether the skin is intact, paying special attention to the pressure points as you continue to assess the rest of the body. Are there any areas of erythema and potential breakdown? Are there lesions or rashes? Older patients often have very thin and fragile skin, often so thin that it appears to be translucent and feels like tissue paper. Extra care must be taken during all aspects of nursing care for these individuals. It may take nothing more than a bump against a bed rail or wheelchair to cause a skin tear. Tape and bandage removal are frequent culprits causing skin tears in older adults. Care must be taken when removing tape; use of an adhesive remover is recommended. Any break in skin integrity, the first line of protection from microorganisms, will reduce the patient's ability to prevent infection.

BOWEL AND BLADDER STATUS. Is the patient continent or incontinent of urine? When performing an initial shift assessment, it is important to determine when the patient last voided or urinated because the maximum time the patient should be allowed to go without voiding is 8 hours. If it has been close to 8 hours since the patient voided, palpate just above the symphysis pubis to determine if the bladder is distended, which would require intervention. If the patient has a Foley catheter, assess its patency; whether it is secured properly to the thigh; and the amount, color, and clarity of the urine. The kidneys should produce a minimum of 30 mL of urine per hour. Amounts less than 30 mL per hour indicate that the patient is severely dehydrated and needs fluids or that the patient's kidneys are not functioning properly, as in renal failure. Ask the patient if there is any problem with urination, such as burning, urgency, or frequency. These assessments provide you information regarding renal system function as well as information related to level of hydration.

When assessing young children, especially infants, an inadequate urinary output is even more significant because young children normally have a higher body fluid ratio to maintain than do adults. This means that inadequate intake of fluids or smaller losses of fluid due to diarrhea or vomiting have a much higher and accelerated rate of dehydrating these patients to dangerous levels. Decreased urinary output may be severe enough to require IV fluids to prevent serious complications from dehydration. The older adult also dehydrates easier than the average adult and requires close observation of fluids taken in and urine output to maintain fluid and electrolyte balance.

Ask when the patient last had a bowel movement, and ask about the amount, color, and consistency of the stool. It is standard to make certain that each patient does not go longer than 3 days without having a bowel movement. The changes in dietary habits, source of drinking water, medications, and activity level that come with being hospitalized are enough to cause some patients to become constipated. Some elderly patients use laxatives on a daily basis and have become dependent on them to have bowel movements, thus making it important to be aware of their laxative habits. These elimination problems can be prevented with regular assessment followed by appropriate nursing interventions.

If the patient has a colostomy or ileostomy, assess the stoma for erythema, edema, and excoriation and assess for drainage bag intactness and content. You will learn more about stoma care in Chapter 30.

Unless the patient has a Foley catheter or some known problem of the perineal or anal area, these areas are normally not visualized until perineal care is provided or a bed bath is administered or unless the patient is incontinent. If the patient is bedridden or incontinent, the perineum, coccyx, and buttocks should be assessed for cleanliness, dryness, and integrity of the skin. Note any vaginal drainage, including color, amount, consistency, and odor.

Dressings and Equipment on the Chest or Abdomen

If the patient has telemetry electrodes, a chest tube, a surgical incision, a dressing, a drain, a binder, or any other piece of equipment attached to the chest or abdomen, assess it while you are in the vicinity for its status or proper function.

> **KNOWLEDGE CONNECTION**
>
> What is the order in which palpation, inspection, and auscultation should be performed on the abdomen? What are the four acronyms used to indicate the four sections of the abdomen? What is the longest period of time a patient should go without voiding? Without having a bowel movement?

Extremities

Assess the extremities for intact skin, erythema over pressure points, circulation, movement, coordination, strength, and joint flexibility.

Upper Extremities

Assess the peripheral pulses in both wrists for strength and equality. Are both RPs palpable? Do they both feel strong or weak, and is this strength equal on both the right and left sides? The strength of peripheral pulses is documented using a scale from 0 to 3 and should include whether the pulses are equal in strength (Box 21.6). This assessment provides you data about the circulatory system's function and fluid volume. A weak pulse may be a sign of decreased plasma volume as in hemorrhage or shock, decreased pumping ability of the heart, or problems with the heart's electrical conduction system. ***Safety: An absent pulse indicates some type of blockage or lack of blood perfusion to the extremity due to inadequate pumping capacity of the heart.*** A bounding RP can be related to hypertension or excess fluid volume.

Box 21.6

Peripheral Pulse Scale

Peripheral pulses are assessed to determine not only their presence, but also their strength. This provides you with data regarding the efficiency of the heart's pumping ability to deliver or *perfuse* blood to the farthest pulse sites from the heart. The following scale is commonly used to designate the strength of the peripheral pulses:

0	not able to palpate
1+	weak
2+	strong
3+	full, bounding

After assessing the RPs, assess the patient's ability to freely move both arms and flex all joints. Note if there is tightening and shortening of muscles that prevent full extension of joints, known as *contractures,* which provides data about the musculoskeletal system. Then hold out your hands with the index and middle finger extended on each hand, crossing your hands at the wrists. Ask the patient to squeeze your two fingers with each hand to test the grip strength. Note whether it is weak or strong and whether the grips are equal bilaterally. This assessment provides you with information regarding both the neurological and the musculoskeletal systems. It tells you whether the brain and the nerves are working together correctly to process your verbal instruction and deliver the impulse to the muscles, as well as the muscular strength of the hands.

Assess the color of the nailbeds. They should be pink if there is good circulation and if an ample supply of oxygen is being delivered to the tissues of the upper extremities. Cyanosis indicates hypoxia, and pallor signifies decreased blood flow to the extremity. This provides you with data regarding both the circulatory and the respiratory systems. Using the tip of your thumb, *gently* compress a nailbed on the patient's hand, emptying the capillaries of blood and causing the nailbed to turn white. Release the pressure and observe the length of time it takes the capillaries to refill with blood and turn the nailbed pink once again. Repeat the procedure on the other hand. The normal time for color return is 3 seconds or less in adults and 5 seconds or less in elderly individuals. This assessment is known as the *capillary refill time* and serves as one indicator of adequate arterial circulation to the periphery. The elderly patient frequently has thickened and yellowed nails that make it difficult or impossible to blanch the nail bed, but there is another way to check capillary refill time in these patients. Simply press on the tip of one of the patient's fingers until it blanches. Release the pressure and count how many seconds before the color returns to pink. Also assess for clubbing of the fingertips; this may be indicative of chronic respiratory disease (Fig. 21.17).

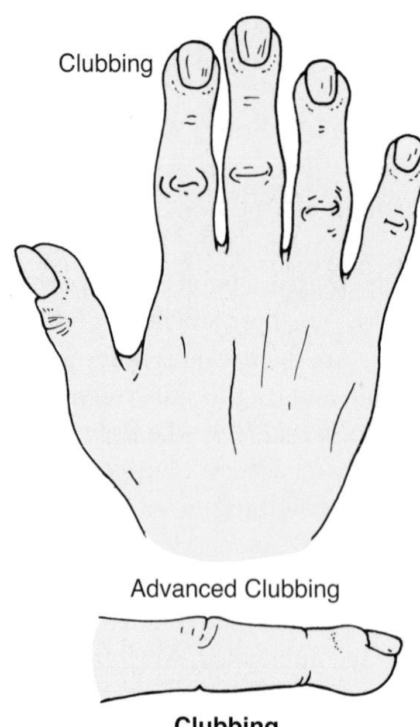

FIGURE 21.17 Clubbing of fingertips (from Venes D, ed. *Taber's Cyclopedic Medical Dictionary.* 22nd ed. Philadelphia, PA: FA Davis, 2013).

Lower Extremities

Now move to the legs and feet and assess for the presence of edema. Recall that edema is the result of excess fluid shifting out of the cardiovascular space into the interstitial space between the individual cells. It may be due to a number of factors, such as hypertension, fluid volume retention or overload, inadequate blood level of albumin to maintain enough osmotic pull to hold fluid within the vascular system, inflammation of the lower extremities, or inadequate pumping of the heart, which would allow fluid to back up in the venous side of the vascular system. As fluid backs up in the vasculature, it increases hydrostatic pressure and forces excessive fluid through the capillary walls into the interstitial spaces. If edema is present, how much is there? Is it pitting edema (Fig. 21.18)? (Box 21.7 presents a pitting edema scale.)

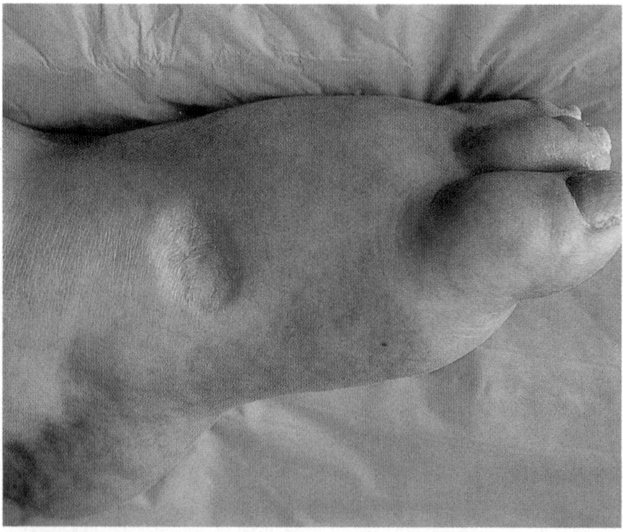

FIGURE 21.18 Pitting edema of the foot (from Williams LS, Hopper PD. *Understanding Medical-Surgical Nursing.* 5th ed. Philadelphia, PA: FA Davis; 2015).

Box 21.7

Pitting Edema

To assess for pitting edema, press the patient's skin over a bony prominence with your fingertip and hold for approximately 2 seconds, then release the pressure. Pitting edema will leave a fingerprint even after you remove your finger. The depth of the depression determines the amount of pitting edema present and can be measured using the following scale:

- **Trace pitting edema:** Minimal indention noted when pressure is applied; refills as soon as finger pressure is removed
- **1+ pitting edema:** Slight indention depth of 2 mm; lasts no longer than 15 seconds after removing finger pressure
- **2+ pitting edema:** Indention depth of 4 mm; lasts no longer than 15 seconds after removing finger pressure
- **3+ pitting edema:** Indention depth of 6 mm; lasts a full minute after removing finger pressure
- **4+ pitting edema:** Indention depth of 8 mm; lasts 2 minutes or longer after removing finger pressure

Where does the edema begin and end? Is it restricted to just the ankles, or does it extend from the toes to the midcalf or to the thigh?

Next assess the color of the legs and feet. Pallor of the legs and feet may be a sign of inadequate circulation to the lower extremities, which can be due to inadequate blood volume or vasoconstriction. A general erythema of the lower leg or foot may be indicative of inflammation or a blockage of the venous return, which can force an excessive volume of blood to remain in the lower extremity, making the extremity appear redder than normal. Cyanosis, or a bluish color, would be indicative of inadequate delivery of oxygen to the lower extremity. This could be the result of an arterial blockage, inadequate oxygen saturation of the blood's hemoglobin, inadequate blood volume due to hemorrhage or shock, or inadequate pumping of the heart, which fails to deliver sufficient oxygen-carrying blood to the feet. As you can see, these assessments for color and edema provide a large volume of data relating to the circulatory system's function.

Assess for the other signs for which you assessed in the hands. Further assess circulation to the feet by feeling for the skin temperature of the lower extremities. Apply the dorsal surface of your hands to the lower legs and feet, noting whether they are warm or cool. If they are cooler than the legs or if one foot is cooler than the other, assess further. Were the patient's feet uncovered? Does the patient have peripheral vascular disease, a disease that impairs circulation to the extremities?

Assess both pedal pulses for strength and equality. They normally are strong and equal bilaterally. If you are unable to palpate the pedal pulse in either one of the feet, move up the extremity to palpate the posterior tibialis. If the posterior tibialis is not palpable, move up the leg to assess for the popliteal pulse. If it is not detected, assess for a femoral pulse. Once you have identified the most distal pulse that you can palpate, obtain a Doppler ultrasound machine and assess the pulse sites at which you were not able to palpate a pulse to ensure that there is adequate arterial circulation to the foot. It is imperative, in the absence of pulse detection by palpation, that you can identify which peripheral pulses can be obtained with Doppler ultrasound before notifying the health-care provider.

Another assessment for circulation is the capillary refill time of the toenail beds. The normal refill time is the same as for the hands. In adults the capillaries should refill and turn pink again in 3 seconds or less, although in the elderly it may take up to 5 seconds. Any extremity with inadequate blood flow or oxygen delivery to the tissues has a reduced ability to prevent or fight infection.

To test neurological control and strength of the lower extremities, assess plantar flexion strength. Place the palms of your hands on the bottom or plantar side of the patient's feet. Ask the patient to press the soles of his or her feet against the palms of your hands. Note whether the movement is weak or strong or absent and whether it is equal bilaterally. Now, lay the palms of your hands over the dorsal aspects of both feet and apply firm pressure. Then direct the patient to pull the toes of both feet toward his or her head while you provide resistance. Again, assess for the strength of this dorsiflexion and whether the strength is equal bilaterally. As with the upper extremities, this assessment provides you with information regarding both the neurological and the musculoskeletal systems. It tells you whether the brain and the nerves are working together correctly to process your verbal instruction and deliver the impulse to the muscles, as well as the muscular strength of the feet. An example of one cause of either a weaker or absent flexion on one side is a cerebrovascular accident (stroke).

Dressings and Equipment Applied to the Upper or Lower Extremities

Assess any dressings, IV access, dialysis shunts, antiembolism stockings, elbow or heel protectors, alternating compression devices, casts, splints, and any other equipment or supplies attached to any of the extremities to determine their condition or status to ensure their proper function and to monitor for signs and symptoms indicating possible adverse reactions or complications. Also make note if the patient is on any type of specialty bed, such as an eggcrate mattress overlay or an air-fluidized bed. These beds represent interventions for preventing skin breakdown and increasing comfort.

KNOWLEDGE CONNECTION

What colors would be abnormal for the nailbeds? What would each abnormality signify? Compare the assessment of dorsiflexion to plantar flexion. Describe what to do if you are unable to palpate a pedal pulse. What supplies or equipment should also be assessed?

Visual Screening

Visual screening is most commonly performed in schools or public health settings but occasionally may be needed in a hospital setting. For this assessment, the most frequently used chart is the Snellen Standard Chart. A Snellen E Chart is used for nonreading patients, and a picture chart (Preliterate Chart) is used for small children (see Skill 21.8, page 420).

Needs and Comfort

A patient may have many and varied needs, and you will be responsible for meeting those needs. These needs are assessed as you perform the shift head-to-toe assessment (Box 21.8).

As you complete your assessment, give the patient one last opportunity to report any problems. Ask again if the patient is having any discomfort or pain. Inquire if the patient needs anything. If intake of fluid needs to be encouraged, ask the patient what fluids he or she likes. Provide one of the drinks of choice and remind the patient of the importance of adequate fluid intake. If the patient is on bedrest or requires assistance to get up, is on intake and output monitoring, or is NPO or on restricted oral fluids, remind the patient of these restrictions. Document any reinforcement or patient teaching that you provide along with the patient's response. ***Safety: Return the bed to its lowest level and raise the bed rails. Position the patient's call light, water carafe, telephone, tissues, and any other items the patient might need within easy reach.*** Inform the patient as to when you will return and encourage the patient to push the call light if there is anything you can provide or do.

Box 21.8 Needs Assessment

Each individual will have various needs that will impact his or her health status and ability to heal. It will be your responsibility to assess for all possible needs of each patient, including those needs that may not be medical.

Oxygen and Circulatory Needs

- Are respirations within normal ranges for rate, depth, effort, and pattern?
- Is SpO_2 adequate?
- Is there a need for supplemental oxygen?
- Is the patient alert and oriented?
- Is blood pressure within normal parameters?
- Is pulse within normal parameters for rate, rhythm, and strength?
- Are breath sounds clear to auscultation?
- Are heart sounds distinct?
- Is there jugular vein distention?
- Are peripheral pulses strong and equal bilaterally?
- Does the patient have a pacemaker or automatic defibrillator?
- Does the patient bruise easily?

Nutritional and Fluid Needs

- What is the patient's current weight? Has there been any weight gain or loss?
- Does the patient have any food preferences, including cultural considerations?
- Does the patient have an appetite?
- Does the patient have dentures or edentulous?
- Does the patient have food allergies?
- Is the patient on a prescribed special diet? Is the patient compliant with the diet?
- Is edema present?
- What is the volume of fluid drunk in last 24 hours?
- Does the patient need intake and output recorded?
- Is there any nausea, vomiting, diarrhea, or fluid losses?
- Does the patient have any special tubes, such as nasogastric or gastrostomy tubes, that may affect fluid losses?

Safety and Security Needs

- Is there a need for the side rails to be up?
- Does the patient use any assistive devices?
- Does the patient use a prosthesis?
- Does the patient have the ability to communicate? Is there a language barrier?
- Are there any cultural barriers restricting care?
- Is the patient disoriented?
- Does the patient have any sensory deficits, such as deafness, aphasia, blindness, or paresthesia?
- Is the patient in any pain?
- Does the patient have any paralysis?
- Does the patient have any anxiety relating to hospitalization, child care, job security while hospitalized, cost of hospitalization, or disease prognosis?

Psychosocial and Cultural Needs

- Does the patient have any fears or anxieties?
- Does the patient show any signs of depression?
- Is the patient in any pain?
- Does the patient have any coping strategies?
- Does the patient have a family or other support system?
- Does the patient have any social services needs?
- Does the patient have any cultural or religious differences needs?
- Does the patient need to contact a spiritual advisor?
- Is a psychological consult required?
- Does the patient have any concerns?
- Does the patient have a knowledge deficit?

Elimination Needs

- What is the amount and characteristics of urinary output?
- What is the amount, characteristics, and frequency of bowel movements?
- Are there any changes in bowel habits?
- Is the patient able to perform the act of elimination without assistance?

Box 21.8

Needs Assessment—cont'd

- Is the patient incontinent or continent?
- Does the patient have a Foley catheter? Suprapubic catheter?
- Does the patient have a colostomy or urostomy?
- Is the patient using diuretics or laxatives?

Rest and Activity Needs

- Does the patient have a tolerance for performance of activities of daily living, such as hygiene, toileting, feeding, and ambulation?
- Are the patient's balance and equilibrium okay?
- What is the number of hours of sleep that the patient requires?
- Is the patient using any sleeping aids?

Grooming Needs

- Is the patient able to perform activities of daily living, such as bathing; oral, skin, nail, and hair care; shaving; toileting; feeding; and ambulation?
- Does the patient have any preferences for bathing, including time of day and type of bath?

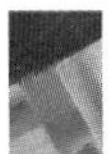

DOCUMENTATION OF ASSESSMENT FINDINGS

All assessment findings must be documented as soon as possible. Some hospitals use computerized documentation, while others still use handwritten documentation. Each facility will have a specific policy and procedures to follow. Whether or not the documentation is computerized, there will be designated forms to complete for initial head-to-toe shift assessments. Some facilities will use a form that requires narrative description (Fig. 21.19). Other facilities may use a flow sheet or checklist format (Fig. 21.20). An admission assessment form is normally 3 to 4 pages in length, with some checklists and some narrative sections. An example of this type of form may be found in the Student Workbook. (For further assistance with documentation of assessments, see Chapter 5.)

Date:	Progress Note
MM/DD/YYYY	0630 Lying supine with eyes closed. Snoring softly. Awakened
	to calling name. BP-116/68 T-99.6°F P-68 reg & strong
	R-15 reg & even. SpO_2 97% on room air. Complains of aching
	in lumbar area of back, a 3 on a scale of 0–10. Denies need of
	pain med. Alert & oriented to 4 spheres. States slept well
	last night. Pearla. Sclera white & clear. Conjunctival sacs
	pink & moist. Oral mucosa is pink and moist, without lesions.
	No neck vein distention. Skin is pink, warm, dry, with elastic
	turgor. Respirations regular & even, with equal chest
	excursion. Breath sounds auscultated, all lobes CTA except
	fine rales in RLL. Heart sounds auscultated, AP 68, reg. &
	distinct. Denies cough since yesterday morning. Abdominal
	dressing clean, dry, & intact. Bowel sounds active in RLQ,
	RUQ, LUQ, and hypoactive in LLQ. Abdomen flat & soft to
	palpation. Denies discomfort with palpation. Denies any
	further nausea since yesterday. States he is tolerating oral
	fluids without problems. Encouraged to drink at least 1200
	mL on this shift. Acknowledged verbally he would. States his
	last BM was 2 days ago, but feels as if he will have one this
	morning. Foley catheter intact, patent, & draining clear,
	medium yellow urine to gravity. Denies discomfort. Catheter
	secured to thigh. IV in right wrist, 1000 mL D51/2NS
	infusing per pump at 80 ml/hr. Site is clean, dry, without
	edema, erythema, or tenderness. 4 ext. warm, pink, dry. No
	edema noted. Peripheral pulses strong & bilaterally equal in
	all 4 ext. Has full ROM x4 ext. Strong & equal hand-grips
	bilaterally. Strong & equal dorsal & plantar flexion bilaterally.
	Cap refill less than 3 seconds in all 4 ext. ----------------------
	--W. Weaver, LPN

FIGURE 21.19 Initial head-to-toe shift assessment documented in a narrative format.

	PATIENT FLOW SHEET																								(PT STAMP)
	Date: MM/DD/YYYY	0700	0800	0900	1000	1100	1200	1300	1400	1500	1600	1700	1800	1900	2000	2100	2200	2300	2400	0100	0200	0300	0400	0500	0600
Care Given	Doctor's visit		✓																						
Care Given	Activity		CH	BB	AMB		CH		BR	AMB															
Care Given	Vital signs	✓				✓																			
Care Given	AM care			✓																					
Care Given	Turn R-right L-left S-supine P-prone	R		S		L		S		R															
Care Given	Dressing wound care	n/a																							
Care Given	IV therapy	n/a																							
Care Given	% of diet		90				100																		
Skin	Skin intact	✓																							
Skin	Warm-dry/ color WNL	✓																							
Skin	Comfort measures	HP						HP																	
Neuro/ Sensory	Alert & oriented	✓																							
Neuro/ Sensory	Denies pain	✓																							
Neuro/ Sensory	Denies anxiety	✓																							
Respiratory	O_2 therapy	n/a																							
Respiratory	Breath sounds clear & regular	✓																							
Respiratory	TC & DB/IS	n/a																							
CV	Pulse regular	P				P																			
CV	Heart tones	CL																							
CV	Telemetry # ___	n/a																							
GI	Abdomen soft	✓																							
GI	Bowel sounds present	✓					→																		
GI	BM								lg.																
Renal	Urine clear	✓					→																		
Renal	Foley patent	✓					→																		
M/S	Moves all extremities	✓																							
	Side rails up	✓		✓		✓		✓	✓																
Safety	Call light in reach	✓		✓		✓	✓	✓	✓																
Safety	Bed in low position	✓		✓		✓		✓	✓																
Other	Braden scale																								
Other																									

Nurse's initials/ signature	LL	L. Ludwig, RN			
Nurse's initials/ signature				RN assessment	
				Time	

CHARTING LEGEND
– = within normal limits
X = problem, see NN
→ = no change
p = exception is normal for patient
n/a = not applicable

ACTIVITY KEY (x1 or x2 = NURSES ASSISTING)
BED = bedrest
DAN = dangle
CH = chair
AMB = ambulate
BR = bathroom
TUB = tub
ASL = asleep
BP = bedpan
B/B = bedbath
AST = assist
SHR = shower
BSC = bedside commode

O_2 KEY
NC = nasal cannula
M = mask
NRB = non-rebreather mask

HEART TONES KEY
CL = clear
DIM = diminished

COMFORT MEASURES
EM = eggcrate mattress
HP = heel protectors

WOUND DRESSING KEY
– = dry and intact
D = dressing ▲
SLC = suture line care
I = irrigation

IV KEY
IP = patent
D = dressing ▲
TU = tubing ▲
HL = hep lock
C = central line

FIGURE 21.20 Assessment flow sheet or checklist form. (Courtesy of Kingfisher Regional Hospital, Kingfisher, OK.)

Skill 21.1 Measuring a Patient's Height

Assessment Steps

1. Assess whether the patient is able to stand unassisted.

Planning Steps

1. Obtain a platform scale or a wheelchair if the patient must be transported to the scale's location.

Implementation Steps

1. Follow the Initial Implementation Steps located on the inside back cover.
2. At the scale, remove the patient's shoes and have him or her step up on the scale with his or her back to the platform scale.

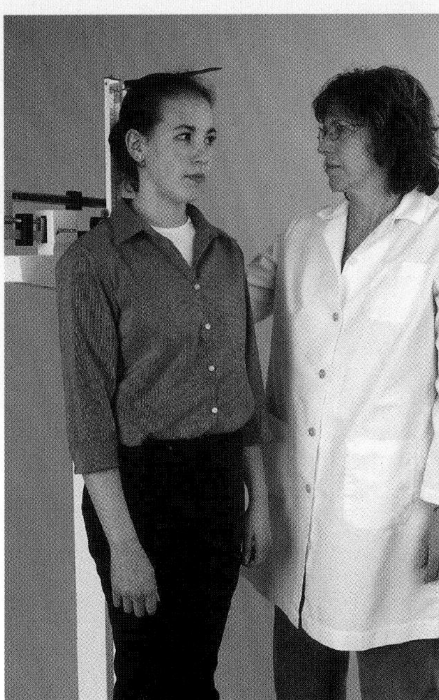

3. Raise the sliding ruler above the back of the patient's head and extend the height bar.
4. Carefully lower the height bar until it touches the highest point between the two parietal bones of the skull.
5. Have the patient step forward and off the scale without raising the height bar.
6. Read the height in feet and inches or centimeters according to facility policy.

Note: The height will not be read at the top of the sliding ruler but will be read at the point where the sliding ruler extends from its track.

7. Assist the patient back to bed as needed.
8. Follow the Ending Implementation Steps located on the inside back cover.

Evaluation Steps

1. Compare the patient's height to his or her weight, noting excessive or inadequate weight for the height.

Sample Documentation

04/04/22 1000 Ht. 5 ft 9 in. ____________ Nurse's signature and credentials

Skill 21.2 Measuring a Patient's Weight

Assessment Steps

1. Assess whether the patient's bed has built-in bed scales.
2. Assess the patient and the medical record ***to ensure that the patient is allowed out of bed and is able to stand alone if platform scales are to be used.***
3. Review the medical record to assess the patient's previous weight ***so that you can compare the current weight to determine whether there is a gain or loss.***

Planning Steps

1. Obtain a portable scale if necessary or a wheelchair if the patient must be transported to the scale's location.
2. If weight is to be assessed on a daily basis, plan to weigh the patient at the same time every day, such as before breakfast, ***so that the weights will more accurately reflect gains or losses.***
3. Plan to consistently weigh the patient wearing the same amount of clothing, such as gown or pajamas, and without shoes ***so that the weights will more accurately reflect gains or losses.***
4. Make certain the scale is balanced before use.

Implementation Steps

1. Follow the Initial Implementation Steps located on the inside back cover.
2. Place clean paper towels on the platform scale ***to keep the patient's feet clean.***

If Weighing an Adult or Child Who Can Stand Unassisted

3. Assist the patient as needed to get out of bed and stand, making certain that he or she is not experiencing dizziness. Assist in the removal of shoes.
4. Have the patient step up on the scale. *Safety: Place your hand just a couple of inches behind the patient's back in case the patient begins to lose his or her balance.*
5. Read the weight while the patient is freestanding, without holding on to anything.

(skill continues on page 416)

Skill 21.2 (continued)

6. Assist the patient as needed to step off the scale and return to bed.
7. Follow the Ending Implementation Steps located on the inside back cover.

If Using a Built-in Bed Scale

3. The patient may be weighed lying in the bed.
4. The patient must be wearing the same type of clothing and bedding consistently with this type of scale.
4. Follow the steps as listed in the manufacturer's instructions.
5. Follow the Ending Implementation Steps located at the back of the book.

Evaluation Steps

1. Compare the new weight with the previous weight, noting whether there is an increase or decrease.

Sample Documentation

02/02/22_0800_Wt. 156 lbs. per bed scales, a loss of 3 lbs. since yesterday._____
______________________Nurse's signature and credentials

Skill 21.3 Measuring an Infant's Weight and Length

Assessment Steps

1. Review the patient's medical record to see the previous weight ***so that you can compare the current weight to determine whether there is a gain or loss.***
2. Assess the room temperature where the scale is to be used, making certain that the environmental temperature is sufficiently warm ***to prevent chilling the infant after removal of clothing.***

Planning Steps

1. Gather needed equipment and supplies: tabletop scale; a separate tape measure if scale does not include a length ruler; and paper towels, lightweight cloth, or blanket.
2. Lay paper towels, cloth, or blanket in the scale cradle ***to provide a barrier between the infant and the cold surface of the metal scale surface to prevent chilling the infant.***
3. Balance the scale with the paper or cloth barrier on the scale ***to prevent inaccuracy.***

Implementation Steps

1. Follow the Initial Implementation Steps located on the inside back cover.
2. Remove all of the infant's clothing or leave on the diaper, according to facility policy.
3. Lay the infant supine on the paper or cloth barrier in the scale cradle.
4. Gently extend the infant's leg at the thigh and knee. Use the scale's length marker or place a measuring tape along the posterior aspect of the infant's body. Measure the infant's length from the top of the head to the plantar surface of the infant's heel, reading the length in inches or centimeters.

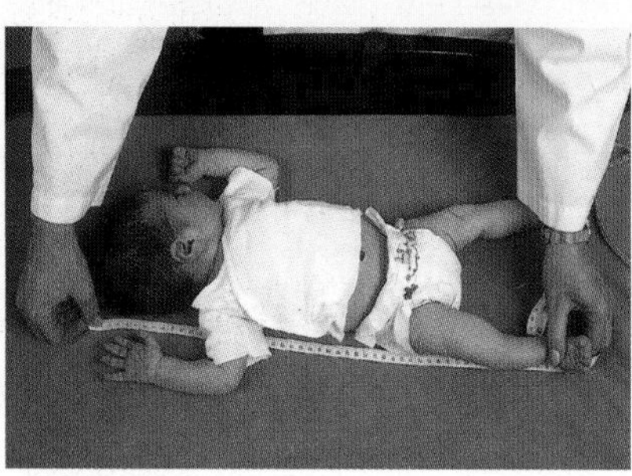

5. Next, weigh the infant. *Safety: Hold the palm of your hand 1 to 2 inches above the infant's abdomen to prevent the infant from falling. Even newborns can squirm and wiggle enough to present a fall risk. NEVER walk away and leave the infant unattended on the scale.*

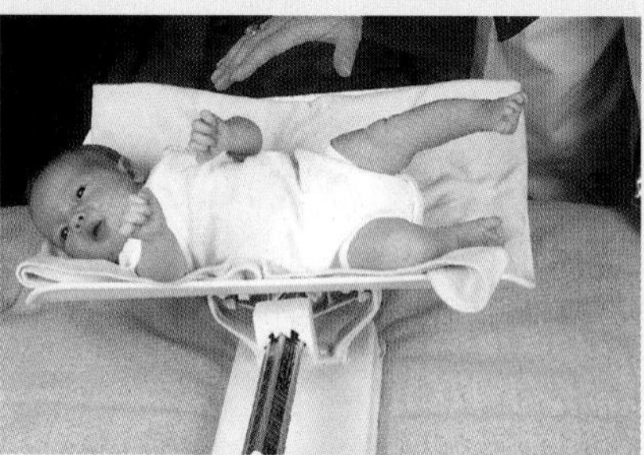

6. Read the weight in pounds and ounces or kilograms and grams, depending on facility policy.
7. Remove the infant from the scale and reapply clothing to prevent chilling.
8. Follow the Ending Implementation Steps located on the inside back cover.

Evaluation Steps

1. Compare the weight to the previously recorded weight, noting whether there is a gain or loss.

Sample Documentation

08/10/22_0930_Wt. 5 lbs. 2 oz. A loss of 1 oz. since yesterday._________ ____________________Nurse's signature and credentials

Skill 21.4 Performing a Shift Assessment

Assessment

1. Assess the patient's chart to determine gender, age, and ethnicity ***to assist you in planning size and type of sphygmomanometer and thermometer to use.***
2. Review the patient's chart to identify the patient's medical problems, including whether the patient can sit or stand. ***This helps you to plan techniques for assessment.***

Planning Steps

1. Gather needed equipment and supplies: sphygmomanometer, stethoscope, thermometer, pulse oximeter, penlight, tongue depressor, examination gloves, and scale if weight is needed. If body fluid samples are needed, include the appropriate specimen containers. Take a pen and an appropriate documentation form ***for recording assessment findings.***
2. Have the patient empty the bladder before beginning assessment. Remember to collect urine if a specimen is required.
3. Turn off the radio and television ***to provide a quiet environment in which to hear the heart, breath, and bowel sounds.***

Implementation Steps

1. Follow the Initial Implementation Steps located on the inside back cover.
2. Warm your hands before touching the patient ***to avoid discomfort.*** Limit use of examination gloves to portions of the examination that involve contact with body fluids.
3. Assess the patient's vital signs first ***to provide you with a baseline.*** Be certain to include SpO_2 and pain assessment, ***which can help to identify potential problem areas that may require extra assessment.***

   Safety: Inform the primary nurse and or instructor of any abnormal vital signs.
4. Obtain weight if needed (see Skill 21.2).

Head and Neck

5. Assess level of consciousness, orientation to the four spheres, and speech. Inquire whether the patient has any pain, nausea, or other discomforts before you begin the assessment.
6. Assess the pupils, including pupillary shape and response to light and accommodation.
7. Assess both sclera and conjunctiva for color and moisture.
8. Inspect the face for symmetry and skin color. Note affect and eye contact.
9. Assess the lips and oral mucous membranes for color, integrity, moisture, and lesions.
10. Assess the teeth and gums for dentures, missing teeth, decay, gum recession, bleeding, sordes, and lesions.
11. Assess the neck veins for distention.
12. Assess any tubes, equipment, or dressings of the head or neck ***to ensure patency and proper function.***

Chest and Abdomen

13. Inspect the chest for shape, symmetrical excursion, use of accessory respiratory muscles, and ease of breathing.
14. Assess skin turgor.
15. Auscultate the heart sounds for a full minute, noting the rate, rhythm, and strength. Compare the heart rate to the radial pulse (RP) to ensure there is not a pulse deficit.
16. Auscultate the breath sounds in all five lobes, listening anteriorly, posteriorly, and laterally. Note quality of sounds, adventitious sounds, and equality of left and right breath sounds.
17. Inquire about cough, sputum production, or shortness of breath upon exertion.
18. Inspect the abdomen for shape and size.
19. Auscultate for presence and activity level of bowel sounds in all four quadrants.
20. Palpate the abdomen for firmness and masses, noting if pain is elicited.
21. Inquire regarding nausea, vomiting, indigestion, and discomfort.
22. Inquire about the time of last voiding and bowel movement.
23. Inspect any tubes, equipment, or dressings of the chest and abdomen ***to ensure patency and proper function.***

Extremities

24. Palpate the RPs for strength and equality of both sides.
25. Palpate the hands for edema and warmth.
26. Assess the nailbeds for color and capillary refill time.
27. Assess range of motion of the arms and hands.
28. Assess hand grip for bilateral equality of strength.
29. Inspect any tubes, equipment, or dressings of the arms ***to ensure patency and proper function.***
30. Inspect the lower legs and feet for color.
31. Palpate the feet, ankles, and pretibial area for edema and skin temperature.
32. Palpate the pedal pulses for strength and equality.
33. Assess capillary refill time.
34. Assess for range of motion.
35. Assess for strength and equality of plantar flexion and dorsiflexion of both feet.
36. Inspect any tubes, equipment, or dressings of the legs ***to ensure patency and proper function.***
37. Follow the Ending Implementation Steps located on the inside back cover.

Evaluation Steps

1. Evaluate the normal and abnormal findings and whether there are further actions you should take.
2. Determine if all aspects of assessment pertinent to the diseases and conditions of the patient have been addressed.
3. Determine that the patient has remained safe and warm during assessment.
4. Allow the patient to ask questions.
5. Inquire whether the patient is comfortable or has any needs.
6. Compare your assessment with the previous assessment to determine if the patient's condition is the same, improved, or deteriorated.

Sample Documentation

An example of assessment documentation using a patient flow sheet is found in Figure 21.19. A sample using the narrative charting format can be found in Figure 21.20.

Skill 21.5 Performing a Basic Neurological Examination

Assessment Steps

1. Assess the patient's chart to determine gender, age, and ethnicity ***to assist you in planning size and type of sphygmomanometer and thermometer to use.***
2. Review the patient's chart to identify the patient's medical problems, including the responses noted during the last neurological examination. ***This helps you to plan techniques for assessment.***

Planning Steps

1. Gather needed equipment and supplies: sphygmomanometer, stethoscope, thermometer, pulse oximeter, penlight, and tongue depressor. Take a pen and an appropriate documentation form ***for recording neurological findings.***
2. Turn off the radio and television ***to provide a quiet environment.***

Implementation Steps

1. Follow the Initial Implementation Steps located on the inside back cover.
2. Explain to the patient what you are about to do even if you believe the patient is comatose. ***The hearing is thought to be the last sense to go.***
3. Try to arouse the patient by calling his or her name first in a normal tone of voice. If the patient does not respond, speak louder. If there still is no response, use tactile stimulus and gently touch the patient on the arm or hand. If there is no response, gently shake the patient. If no response, use an acceptable method of exerting mild pain, such as pressing moderately hard on a nailbed ***to determine if the patient responds to painful stimulus.***
4. Assess vital signs, making note of elevated blood pressure and decreased pulse rate.
5. If the patient is awake, ask the patient to identify his or her name and the place, time, and situation (the reason the patient is hospitalized) ***to determine orientation to the four spheres.***
6. Ask the patient first to smile, then to clench the teeth, protrude the tongue and then move it side to side, furrow the brow, raise the eyebrows, and finally squeeze both eyes shut at the same time ***so that you can observe for symmetry of muscle movement on both sides of the face.*** The tongue should protrude at the midline of the mouth and move equally from left to right. Both eyebrows should rise equally. As both eyes are squeezed shut, both cheeks should rise and the wrinkling/bunching of tissue around the orbital areas should appear equal.
7. Ask the patient to squeeze your fingers with each of his or her hands ***to test strength and equality of hand grip bilaterally.*** Note if the patient does not follow simple commands or if there is any difference in strength. If there is no response to your request, pick up the patient's arm. Raise it approximately 1 to 2 feet off the bed. Then release it and allow it to fall to the mattress. Note whether the arm falls flaccidly to the bed surface or if the patient offers any control of the muscles after releasing your hold on the arm.
8. Ask the patient to press the plantar side of the feet against the palms of your hands and then to pull the toes and feet toward his or her head as you provide resistance using the palms of your hands to pull against the dorsal surface of both the patient's feet. Note the strength and equality bilaterally. If there is no response to your request, raise one leg off the bed as you did the arms, and then release it. Allow it to fall to the bed surface. Note whether the leg falls limply or the patient offers some muscle control as it falls.
9. Follow the Ending Implementation Steps located on the inside back cover.

Evaluation Steps

1. Evaluate the normal and abnormal responses.
2. Compare to the previous neurological examination, noting any change in neurological response.
3. Determine whether further action is deemed necessary.

Sample Documentation

09/12/22 0745 T - 98.2°F, P - 73 reg & strong, R - 17. BP - 128/68, SpO_2 - 98%, denies any pain or discomfort. Does not respond to voice but awakens to tactile stimuli. Wife states he is hard of hearing. Alert and oriented to 4 spheres. PERRLA. Follows simple commands. No facial drooping. Symmetrical raising of eyebrows, smiling, clenching teeth, and tongue movement. Speech is clear and appropriate. Hand grips are strong and equal bilaterally. Dorsal plantar flexion is strong and equal bilaterally.__________
__________________ Nurse's signature and credentials

Skill 21.6 Auscultating Breath Sounds

Assessment Steps

1. Assess the patient's chart to determine gender and age ***to assist you in planning techniques to use.***
2. Review the patient's chart ***to identify the patient's medical problems, including whether the patient can sit up.***

Planning Steps

1. Obtain a stethoscope.
2. Turn off the radio and television ***to provide a quiet environment in which to hear the breath sounds.***

Implementation Steps

1. Follow the Initial Implementation Steps located on the inside back cover.
2. Warm your hands and the diaphragm of the stethoscope before touching the patient ***to avoid discomfort.***
3. Assist the patient into a sitting position or elevate the head of the bed between 45 and 90 degrees, if possible. If not, turn the patient to his or her left side.
4. Loosen the patient's gown and place the stethoscope diaphragm against the skin on the anterior chest wall and

Skill 21.6 (continued)

then the lateral aspects of the chest. Ask the patient to breathe in and out through an open mouth. Listen for a full breath at each location, moving the stethoscope from the apexes to the bases, in a zigzag pattern from left to right (refer to Fig. 21.13).

5. Place the stethoscope on the back and listen to the posterior aspects of the lungs in the same manner.
6. Follow the Ending Implementation Steps located on the inside back cover.

Evaluation Steps

1. Evaluate the normal and abnormal breath sounds heard.
2. Evaluate whether further action is needed.

Sample Documentation

05/27/22 1815 Breath sounds auscultated, coarse crackles noted in RUL, RML, RLL; LUL & LLL clear to auscultation. ________ Nurse's signature and credentials

Skill 21.7 Auscultating Heart Sounds

Assessment Steps

1. Assess the patient's chart to determine gender, age, and ethnicity ***to assist you in planning techniques to use.***
2. Review the patient's chart ***to identify the patient's medical problems, including whether the patient can sit up.***

Planning Steps

1. Obtain a stethoscope.
2. Turn off the radio and television ***to provide a quiet environment in which to hear the heart sounds.***

Implementation Steps

1. Follow the Initial Implementation Steps located on the inside back cover.
2. Warm your hands and the diaphragm of the stethoscope before touching the patient ***to avoid discomfort.***
3. Assist the patient into a sitting position or elevate the head of the bed between 45 and 90 degrees, if possible. If not, turn the patient to his or her left side.
4. Place the stethoscope diaphragm firmly against the patient's skin, not the gown, in the left midclavicular line at the fifth intercostal space. Adjust the stethoscope slightly until you can best hear the heart sounds (refer to Fig. 21.14).
5. Listen for a few seconds while you identify the S_1 and S_2. ***Remember that the heartbeat includes both the S_1 and the S_2.*** Then count the number of heartbeats in 1 minute while observing the second hand of your watch. Assess for rate, rhythm, and strength. Make note of any extra sounds heard.
6. Move the stethoscope to the second intercostal space just to the right of the sternum ***to listen to the right base heart sounds and the aortic valve.***
7. Move the stethoscope to the second intercostal space just to the left of the sternum ***to listen to the left base heart sound and the pulmonic valve.***
8. Move the stethoscope to the edge of the sternum, at the level of the fourth intercostal space just to the left of the sternum, ***to hear the left lateral sternal border heart sound and the tricuspid valve.***
9. Follow the Ending Implementation Steps located on the inside back cover.

Evaluation Steps

1. Evaluate the rate, rhythm, and strength of the heart sounds to determine normal and abnormal findings.
2. Determine that the patient has remained safe and warm during assessment.

Sample Documentation

05/26/22_2115_Heart sounds auscultated, S_1 & S_2 distinct and regular, rate equal to RP.________________
Nurse's signature and credentials

Skill 21.8 Assessing Visual Acuity Using a Snellen Standard Eye Chart, Snellen E Chart, or Preliterate Chart

Assessment Steps

1. Assess the patient's chart to determine gender, age, and ability to read ***to assist you in planning which chart should be used: a Snellen Standard Chart for those who can read, Snellen E for those who cannot read, or a Preliterate Chart for young children who cannot read.***

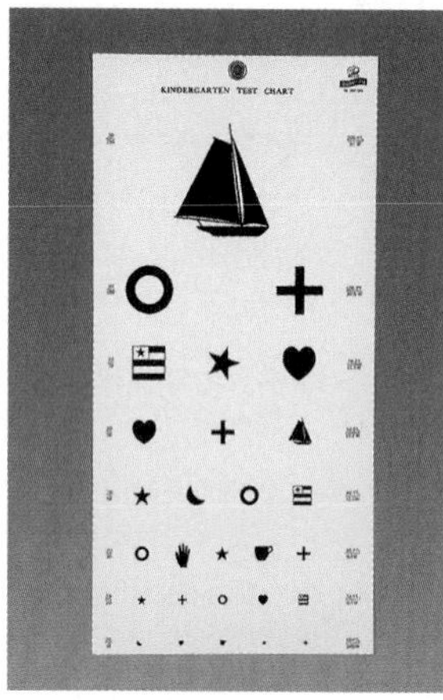

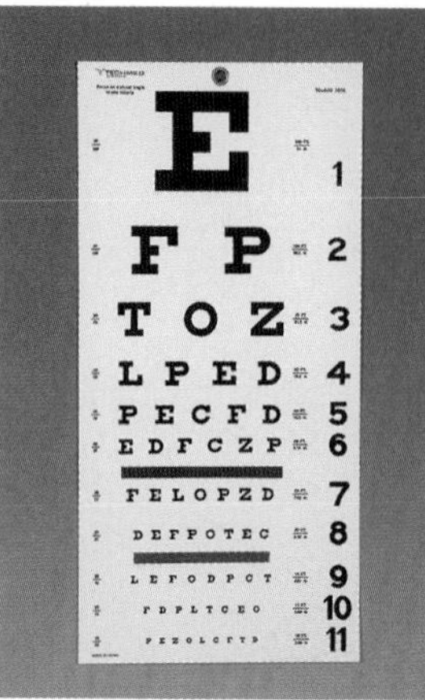

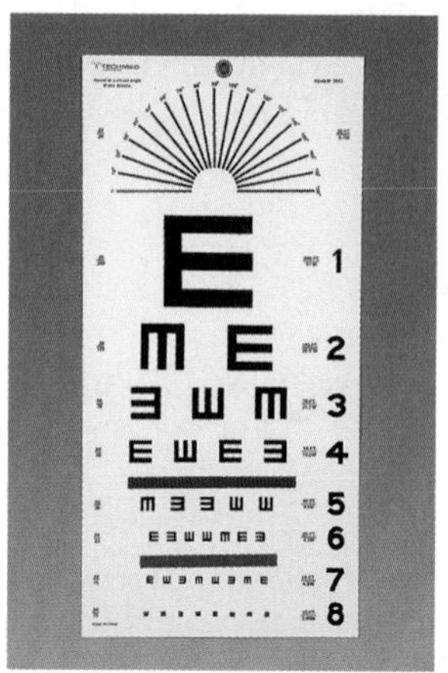

2. Review the patient's chart ***to identify the patient's medical problems, including whether the patient can stand up.***

Planning Steps

1. If the patient wears corrective lenses, they should be worn during the exam.
2. Pick a site where patient can sit or stand 20 feet away from the chart.
3. Gather the correct eye chart, a card to use to cover one eye, and pen and paper.

Implementation Steps

1. Follow the Initial Implementation Steps located on the inside front cover.
2. Have the patient sit or stand 20 feet from the eye chart.
3. Explain the process to the patient ***to decrease anxiety and increase compliance.***
4. Have the patient cover one eye with the card, keeping both eyes open. ***This allows for more accurate evaluation of vision in each eye.***
5. Ask patient to read the smallest line of print that he can distinguish. If it is a child or individual who cannot read, point to the line that you want him to identify the shapes or the direction the legs of the E points. Once you have determined the smallest line of print the patient can distinguish with NO MORE THAN 2 ERRORS, note the fraction at the end of the line, such as 20/20, 20/60, or 20/140. ***The top number denotes the distance the patient was standing from the chart. The bottom number denotes the distance at which a patient with normal vision would be able to read the chart.***
6. Have the patient cover the other eye and test the opposite eye in the same manner.
7. Uncover both eyes and test both eyes together.
8. Record each fraction, noting which is left, right, and both eyes together.
9. Follow the Ending Implementation Steps located on the inside back cover.

Evaluation Steps

1. Normal vision is 20/20. A smaller number on the bottom such as 20/15 indicates diminished close/near vision. A larger number on the bottom such as 20/180 indicates diminished far vision.
2. 20/20 vision does not usually develop in children before 6 years of age. Somewhere around 40 years of age, adults begin to lose some of their near vision.

Sample Documentation

08/09/22_Visual acuity tested using Snellen chart. Vision 20/20 in R eye, 20/40 in L eye, and 20/30 using both eyes. Health-care provider informed. ____________
____________________ Nurse's signature and credentials

POST CONFERENCE

At the end of the day, you feel good about the care you gave to this patient. After alerting your instructor to your patient's possibly worsening condition, you saw a thorough assessment in action. The staff nurse and your instructor showed you how to assess jugular vein distention, which was present in this patient. The patient's blood pressure continued to elevate as you monitored it every hour, eventually reaching 188/106. You learned the significance of sacral edema in a patient on bedrest. Your patient became more short of breath, even with increased oxygen. The staff nurse called the health-care provider, and the patient was moved to the intensive care unit with severe congestive heart failure. Your instructor credited you with observing and reporting assessments necessary for detecting the worsening of his condition.

Key Points

- Purposes of physical assessment include establishing a patient's current condition, establishing a baseline against which future changes may be measured, identifying problems the patient may have or may have the potential to develop, evaluating the effectiveness of nursing interventions, monitoring for changes in body function, and detecting specific body systems that need further assessment or testing.
- Techniques of assessment include interviewing, inspection, palpation, percussion, auscultation, percussion, and olfaction.
- Assessment is performed in a head-to-toe sequence, beginning with the head and neck, progressing to the chest and abdomen, and then to the four extremities.
- Components to be assessed during an initial shift assessment include the following systems: neurological, cardiovascular, respiratory, integumentary, gastrointestinal, genitourinary, and musculoskeletal. Also included in an initial shift assessment are vital signs, including pain and SpO_2; appearance; speech; safety risk factors; tubes and equipment; comfort or complaints; and a needs assessment.
- A comprehensive health assessment involves an in-depth assessment of the whole person, including the physical, mental, emotional, cultural, and spiritual aspects of the patient's health.
- You will begin your assessment with subjective data by interviewing and asking questions. The other five techniques involve objective data collected during your assessment. They include inspection or observation, palpation, percussion, auscultation, and olfaction. Percussion is typically performed by the health-care provider unless indicated for further evaluation.
- A focused assessment is less encompassing and involves an examination and an interview regarding a specific body system, such as examining solely the integumentary system or the respiratory system.
- An initial head-to-toe shift assessment provides you with a quick overall assessment of the patient's condition to establish a baseline against which you can compare later assessments.
- Ways to foster rapport and communication involve talking with a patient; it is important to establish a trusting, professional relationship.
- Various adaptations are necessary when assessing patients of different age groups.

Review Questions

Select the answer that is most appropriate for each of the following questions. Some questions may have more than one correct answer. Select all that apply.

1. Which of the following assessments would be included in a focused cardiovascular assessment?
   1. Radial pulse
   2. Range of motion of extremities
   3. Vital signs
   4. Pupillary reaction to light
   5. Edema of extremities
   6. Neck vein distention
   7. Heart sounds
   8. Bowel sounds
   9. Use of accessory respiratory muscles
   10. Last bowel movement
   11. Color and warmth of lower extremities

2. During an assessment, you noted two new findings in a patient: unable to palpate peripheral pulse in lower extremities and pupils that are not equal in size and rate of constriction. Which of these two findings provides you with information about the neurological system?
   1. Peripheral pulses
   2. Pupils
   3. Both findings

3. You have auscultated fine crackles in both the right and left lower lobes in a postoperative patient. What is the longest period of time you should allow to pass before you auscultate the breath sounds again?
   1. 1 hour
   2. 2 hours
   3. 3 hours
   4. 4 hours
   5. 5 hours
   6. 8 hours

4. When lightly palpating the abdomen, you notice a pulsation midline. What is the most important thing to do?
   1. Report it to the primary nurse or supervisor
   2. Document the findings
   3. Continue to palpate the abdomen using deep palpation
   4. Complete the physical assessment and document the findings
   5. Immediately discontinue the palpation

5. Which of the following are the most important respiratory findings on a postoperative patient several hours after she has returned to her room that need immediate attention?
   1. Crackles posteriorly
   2. Dyspnea
   3. Orthopnea
   4. Respiratory rate 24
   5. Pulse oximeter reading 92% on room air
   6. Pulse rate 88
   7. Cyanotic
   8. Capillary refill 4 seconds

6. Which of the following landmarks are used in anterior chest auscultation of the breath sounds?
   1. Right midscapular line
   2. Costovertebral angle
   3. Left midclavicular line
   4. Midsternal line
   5. Midspinal line

7. At which posterior intercostal space are the lung bases located during full inspiration?
   1. 1st
   2. 5th
   3. 8th
   4. 10th
   5. 12th

ANSWERS 1. 1, 3, 5, 6, 7, 11, 2. 2, 3. 4, 4. 1, 5, 5. 1, 2, 3, 4, 5, 7, 8, 6. 3, 7. 5

Critical Thinking Exercise

Answers available online.

1. How does the assessment of the cardiovascular system correlate with the assessment of the respiratory system?

Additional Resources

Use the scratch off code on the inside front cover of your book to access online quizzes that will help you to improve your scores on course exams and prepare for the NCLEX-PN®.

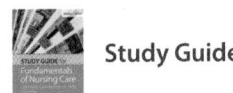

Study Guide

CHAPTER 22

Surgical Asepsis

KEY TERMS

Autoclaving (AW-toh-CLAY-ving)
Boiling (BOY-ling)
Chemical disinfection (KEM-i-kuhl DISS-in-FEK-shun)
Circulating nurse (SIR-kyoo-LAY-ting NERS)
Contamination (kon-TA-mi-NAY-shun)
Disinfection (DISS-in-FEK-shun)
Gaseous disinfection (GAS-ee-uss DISS-in-FEK-shun)
Ionizing radiation (EYE-on-EYE-zing RAY-dee-AY-shun)
Scrub nurse (SCRUHB NERS)
Sterile conscience (STAIR-ill KON-shuns)
Sterile field (STAIR-ill FEELD)
Sterile technique (STAIR-ill tek-NEEK)
Sterilization (STAIR-ill-eye-ZAY-shun)
Surgical asepsis (SER-ji-kuhl ay-SEP-siss)

CHAPTER CONCEPTS

Infection

LEARNING OUTCOMES

1. Define various terms associated with surgical asepsis.
2. Differentiate between medical asepsis and surgical asepsis.
3. Describe five methods of sterilization.
4. Explain how to tell if supplies are sterile.
5. Enumerate restricted settings in the hospital where aseptic surroundings are maintained.
6. Explain the necessity of developing a sterile conscience.
7. Identify guidelines for using sterile technique while opening sterile supplies, setting up and adding items to the sterile field, opening sterile packs, and working with a sterile field.
8. Determine when to use sterile technique.
9. Discuss information found in the Connection features of the chapter.
10. Identify safety issues related to surgical asepsis.
11. Answer questions about the skills in the chapter.

SKILLS

22.1 Setting up a Sterile Field, Opening Sterile Packs, and Pouring Sterile Liquids
22.2 Donning Sterile Gloves—Open Method
22.3 Performing a Surgical Hand Scrub
22.4 Donning a Sterile Gown and Sterile Gloves—Closed Method

CRITICAL THINKING CONNECTION

Clinical Assignment

During your clinical experience, you are asked to assist a health-care provider while he inserts a *central line,* a special type of IV catheter that is inserted through the subclavian vein near the patient's neck. Using sterile technique, the health-care provider makes a small incision, isolates the subclavian vein, and then inserts the narrow tube. You have very little time to think about what you will need to do as an assistant in this bedside procedure.

Critical Thinking Questions:

1. What are the principles of sterile technique?
2. How will you help without contaminating the sterile field or any of the supplies or equipment?
3. What will you need to obtain and have ready at the bedside for the health-care provider?

The use of medical asepsis and clean technique was discussed in Chapter 14, and by now you are very familiar with the principles of using medical asepsis as well as using standard precautions. But what about situations like the Critical Thinking Connection above? What about the times when you are assigned for clinical experience in the operating room or other areas of the hospital where invasive procedures occur? You need to know more than simple clean technique in those areas. You will be using **surgical asepsis,** or the **sterile technique,** which is the method used to prevent contamination during invasive procedures or procedures that involve entering body cavities. Surgical asepsis requires the use of sterile supplies and equipment that have been treated to kill all pathogens and spores.

DISINFECTION AND STERILIZATION

When you use surgical asepsis, you use supplies and equipment that have been disinfected by being cleaned with solutions to kill pathogens. **Disinfection** is the process used to kill bloodborne pathogens and the growth of organisms that cause infection. When disinfecting IV poles, pumps, and surfaces, most facilities utilize Clorox wipes or "Sani-wipes" to clean them. These products destroy many bloodborne pathogens and the growth of organisms such as HIV and hepatitis B, but they do not actually sterilize items. **Sterilization** uses steam under pressure, gas, or radiation to kill all pathogens and their spores. Sterile equipment and supplies are used during sterile procedures that may be done at the bedside or in the operating room.

Before being sterilized, instruments and equipment are cleaned. This may be done by first rinsing with cold or warm water and then washing them in warm soapy water, followed by rinsing in clear water, or through the use of ultrasound to loosen organic material from tiny crevices in the equipment. All instruments that are hinged are left open to prevent damage to the hinges when they are being prepared for sterilization.

Types of Sterilization

Equipment and supplies may be treated in a variety of ways to kill pathogens. Some of the most common treatments include the following:

- **Autoclaving:** This method delivers steam under pressure, with heat ranging from 250°F to 270°F, to sterilize instruments that will not be harmed by heat and water under pressure.
- **Boiling:** This method of boiling instruments and supplies in water for 10 minutes kills non–spore-forming organisms but does not kill spores.
- **Ionizing radiation:** This method kills pathogens on sutures, some plastics, and biological materials that cannot be boiled or autoclaved.
- **Chemical disinfection:** This method is used to kill pathogens on equipment and supplies that cannot be heated. An example of such a chemical is Cidex, which is used to sterilize rubber-based catheters used in urological procedures.
- **Gaseous disinfection:** This method kills pathogens on supplies and equipment that are heat sensitive or must remain dry.

Indications of Sterility

When you use supplies and equipment that have been disinfected or sterilized, you must ensure that they have not been contaminated in any way. Surgical instruments are often double-wrapped in a surgical towel and an outside wrapper and then sterilized in an autoclave. A piece of indicator tape is applied to the outer wrapper, across the final flap. Once the pack has been sterilized in an autoclave, the indicator tape shows black marks every half-inch (Fig. 22.1). The person who autoclaves the pack writes his or her initials, as well as the date and the expiration date, on the tape. Evidence that the wrapper has been wet appears as a discolored line at the level reached by the fluids. This is referred to as "strike-through." ***Safety: If you see strike-through, do not use the pack because the contents are no longer considered sterile.***

Single instruments or small items may be sterilized in individual peel-apart packs (Fig. 22.2). These packs are made of paper, with a clear cover so that the contents can be visualized. If they are commercially prepared, they are stamped with an expiration date. ***Safety: Always check the expiration date and examine the packaging to ensure that it remains intact. The item can no longer be considered sterile if the peel-apart pack is open anywhere or if the expiration date has passed.***

Sterile Settings

Although it is impossible to truly sterilize an entire unit in a hospital, some areas are considered restricted to help maintain surgical asepsis. In these areas, staff remove street clothes and dress in hospital-laundered scrubs upon entering the unit. This prevents contamination of the unit with lint, pet hair, or other potential pathogens from outside the area. If you do not keep a pair of shoes at the hospital to wear in the unit, you may be required to place shoe covers over your shoes to protect against outside contaminants. Examples of restricted areas in most hospitals include surgical suites, heart catheterization laboratories, delivery rooms, neonatal intensive care units, burn units, transplantation intensive care units, and oncology units.

To help maintain the aseptic surroundings in these types of units, you will be required to cover your scrubs with a lab

• WORD • BUILDING •

surgical asepsis: surgical – relating to surgery; a – without + sepsis – putrefaction
contamination: contamin – render impure + ation – action
disinfection: dis – opposite of + infection
sterilization: steriliz – barren + ation – action
autoclaving: auto – self + claving – key
gaseous disinfection: gaseous – relating to gas; dis – opposite of + infection – discoloration

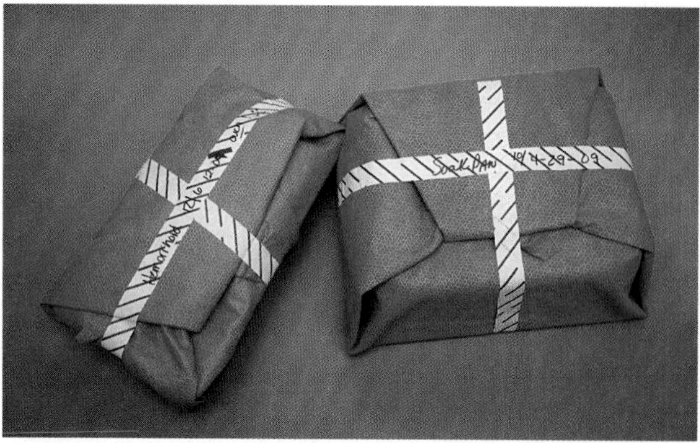

FIGURE 22.1 These sterilized packs show exposed indicator tape with dark hash marks.

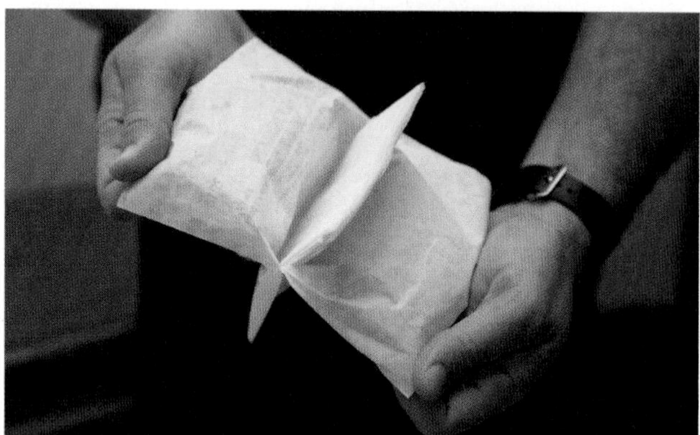

FIGURE 22.2 An example of a peel-apart pack being opened.

coat or cloth isolation gown when you leave the restricted unit to go to other areas of the hospital. When you return, you will remove the outer coverings before entering the patient care area of the unit. This helps keep pathogens from hospital areas outside the unit from entering the restricted area.

Using Sterile Technique in Other Settings

You may be called on to assist a health-care provider with a sterile procedure at the patient's bedside. Such a situation might include the insertion of chest tubes, insertion of an IV line into the subclavian vein, or performing a lumbar puncture. It is important that you know how to assist without contaminating the sterile field, are able to anticipate the health-care provider's needs, and know how to provide supplies and equipment using sterile technique.

Nurses use sterile technique frequently during patient care activities, such as when they give injections, start peripheral IV lines, flush intermittent access devices, insert urinary catheters, and suction deep airways. ***Safety: All of these procedures require meticulous use of surgical asepsis to prevent infection.***

During the insertion of these tubes or needles, the nurse is entering body tissues not normally exposed to pathogens. He or she is effectively bypassing some of the usual mechanisms for defending against invading pathogens.

KNOWLEDGE CONNECTION

Describe five types of sterilization. How can you tell that a wrapped pack has been sterilized? Give four examples of restricted areas in the hospital. List four situations in patient care that require sterile technique.

PRINCIPLES OF STERILE TECHNIQUE

When you perform skills requiring surgical asepsis, it is important to realize the consequences to the patient should contamination occur. **Contamination** refers to the potential presence of pathogens on a sterile field or sterile object due to contact with an unsterile surface. A **sterile field** is an area that is free from all microorganisms where additional sterile items can be placed until they are ready for use. Because skin cannot be sterilized, sterile gloves are used to touch sterile items on the sterile field. Skill 22.1 (page 430) presents the steps involved in setting up a sterile field, and Skill 22.2 (page 432) presents the steps needed to don sterile gloves.

Even if an object or surface is considered clean, pathogens are still present. Therefore, if the clean object touches the sterile field or a sterile object, transfer of pathogens could take place. An example of this would be when a nurse is preparing a sterile dressing to apply to an open wound and accidentally drops the dressing onto the bedside table, contaminating it. In this case, the nurse would need to obtain another sterile dressing rather than risk introducing pathogens from the bedside table into the patient's open wound. In many situations, it is up to the nurse to admit the error and correct it. Often others do not observe the contamination.

Sterile Conscience

As you learn about and practice sterile technique, you will need to develop a **sterile conscience.** This means always being aware of potential or certain contamination of the sterile field or sterile objects and taking appropriate steps to correct the situation, such as replacing the contaminated object or reassembling the sterile field with new supplies.

It is quite possible that no one other than you would be aware if contamination occurs. Therefore, you must be honest in admitting that such a thing did occur or could have occurred. ***Safety: You must always put the patient's safety above your own convenience and correct the error, starting the procedure over if necessary.*** When contamination occurs, you can no longer use the contaminated supplies. They must be replaced with new sterile supplies. Sometimes it is possible to have a second person open a sterile pack and add supplies to your sterile field or to open a sterile pack and allow you to use your sterile gloved fingers to lift the item from the pack without contamination. Box 22.1 provides additional information on opening sterile packs and adding sterile supplies.

Safety: Remember that you are responsible for your own sterile conscience and for the safety of your patients during sterile procedures, whether or not errors are observed by others.

Supervision/Delegation Connection

Sterile Technique and Assistive Personnel

In most situations, procedures requiring sterile technique are not delegated to assistive personnel but are performed by the licensed nurse. In some states, unlicensed assistive personnel are allowed to insert urinary catheters using sterile technique. No states allow certified nursing assistants to perform sterile procedures. Be sure you know your facility's policy and follow it carefully. If any task requiring sterile technique is permitted to be delegated, it is your responsibility to supervise and know that the UAP can correctly perform the task. It is also your responsibility to perform complicated procedures or perform skills requiring sterile technique if the patient is unstable. In these situations, the task should not be delegated to assistive personnel.

Guidelines for Using Sterile Technique

The principles of sterile technique are the same regardless of the setting. Whether you are assisting in the operating room or the emergency room or performing a sterile procedure at the patient's bedside on a nursing unit, the guidelines are the same. One clear guiding principle to remember is the following:

Sterile + sterile = sterile
Sterile + unsterile = contaminated
Unsterile + unsterile = contaminated

This means that anything sterile remains sterile as long as it only touches other sterile items. Anything sterile that touches anything unsterile must always be considered contaminated. Anything unsterile, no matter what it touches, is considered contaminated.

Opening Sterile Supplies

Before opening any sterile supplies, always be sure to do the following:

- Check the expiration date for sterility.
- Check the sterilization tape, if present, for color change—the hash marks should be dark.
- Check the packaging for any holes or tears, which would render the contents unsterile.

Setting Up the Sterile Field

When you are setting up a sterile field, keep the following guidelines in mind:

- The outer 1 inch of the sterile drape is considered contaminated because you must touch it as you set it up. Do not touch any other area of the sterile drape with your bare hands or any other nonsterile item (see Skill 22.1).
- Anything below the surface of the draped table is considered unsterile because you cannot see if it is touched by an unsterile surface.
- All parts of the sterile drape below the table surface are considered unsterile because they cannot be kept in your line of sight.
- Only sterile items can be placed on the sterile field.
- If the sterile field becomes damp or wet, it is no longer sterile because pathogens can be transmitted from the table through the drape when it is damp. The exception is a drape that is backed with moisture-proof material.

Box 22.1

Opening Sterile Packs and Adding Sterile Supplies

There are several rules to follow when you open sterile packs and when you add sterile supplies to a sterile field.

- When a person not wearing sterile gloves opens a peel-apart pack for a person wearing sterile gloves, he or she peels the pack apart with the opening toward the sterile person. The nonsterile person peels the packaging so that it covers his or her bare hands. The sterile person then grasps the item, touching only the sterile item and possibly the inside of the sterile pack.
- Use the same procedure if you are not wearing sterile gloves and are unwrapping a sterile item to hand off to a sterile person. Open the flaps in such a way that you are holding the item through the wrapper with one hand and holding the flaps out of the way with your other hand. This allows the sterile person to grasp the sterile item without contamination (see Fig. 22.5).
- When opening sterile supplies to add to the sterile field, open the peel pack away from you. Allow the item to drop onto the sterile field without reaching across the field. Come in from the side to drop the item onto the field, being careful that it lands in the middle of the field and does not touch the outer 1 inch of drape that is considered contaminated.

Adding Items to the Sterile Field

When you add items to an established sterile field, follow these guidelines to prevent contamination:

- Add sterile items to the field by opening peel-apart packs and dropping the item onto the field, staying away from the contaminated 1-inch outer border. As the sterile item drops from the package, do not allow the item to touch the edges of the package, as they are considered contaminated (see Skill 22.1).
- Add sterile liquids to a basin in a sterile field by holding the bottle so that the label is against the palm of your hand to prevent dripping onto the label, which could obscure the writing. Pour the liquid by holding the bottle approximately 4 to 6 inches above the basin. Pour slowly to avoid splashing, which could cause the sterile field to become

wet. (See Skill 22.1 for more information on pouring sterile liquids.)
- Only after you have donned sterile gloves can you touch the sterile field and the items in the sterile field (see Skill 22.2).

Opening Sterile Packs

While certain sterile supplies, such as gauze 4×4s or a pair of scissors, may be packaged individually, there are various supplies that may be sterilized together in a pack. A pack contains all, or most, of the supplies needed to perform a particular procedure, such as a circumcision, vaginal examination, or laceration suturing. Some commercially wrapped packs have a single-layer paper top that peels off to reveal a plastic tray of sterile supplies. The tray itself can serve as a mini sterile field if desired. Other commercially wrapped packs have an outer wrapper, somewhat like a plastic bag, that is removed to reveal an inner sterile wrapper that is used to set up the sterile field (Fig. 22.3).

If the sterile pack is sterilized by the facility, it will have both an outer and an inner wrapper. The outer wrapper is opened without touching the inside of it and serves as an additional barrier between the table and the sterile supplies inside the pack. The inner wrap, when opened, will serve as the actual sterile field surface upon which all sterile supplies are placed and arranged for use (Fig. 22.4). If you are not wearing sterile gloves and must hand a facility-sterilized pack to another person who is wearing sterile gloves, you will use the method demonstrated in Figure 22.5 and explained in Box 22.1.

When you open sterile packs to set up or add to a sterile field, it is important to follow these guidelines:

- Set the sterile pack on the clean surface positioned so that the first flap will open away from you.
- Open the flap that folds away from you first, and then open each of the side flaps. Open the flap that folds toward you last (Fig. 22.6). This prevents you from reaching across the sterile pack while you are opening it. If the pack is institutionally sterilized and has two wrappers, open each wrapper in the same manner, taking care to avoid touching the inner surface of the inner wrapper.

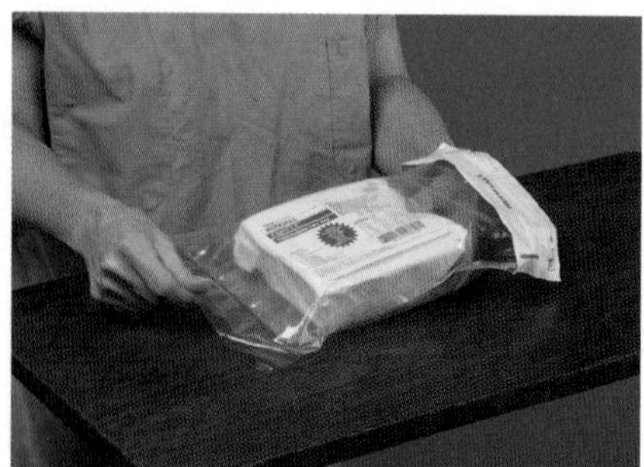

FIGURE 22.3 This nurse is removing the outer plastic bag wrap to access the inner sterile wrapper of a prepackaged kit (from Wilkinson JM, Treas LS. *Fundamentals of Nursing: Theory, Concepts & Applications*. Vol. 2. 3rd ed. Philadelphia, PA: FA Davis; 2016).

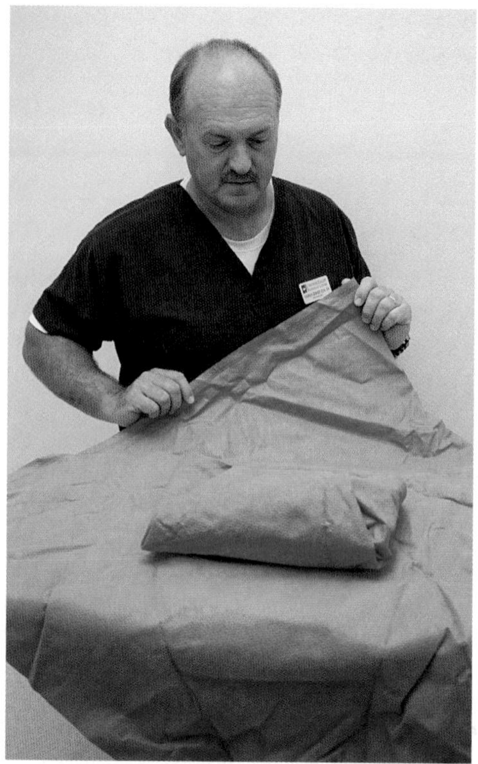

FIGURE 22.4 This nurse is opening an autoclaved, two-wrapper pack. The inner wrap remains sterile and rests on a sterile field created by the open outer wrapper.

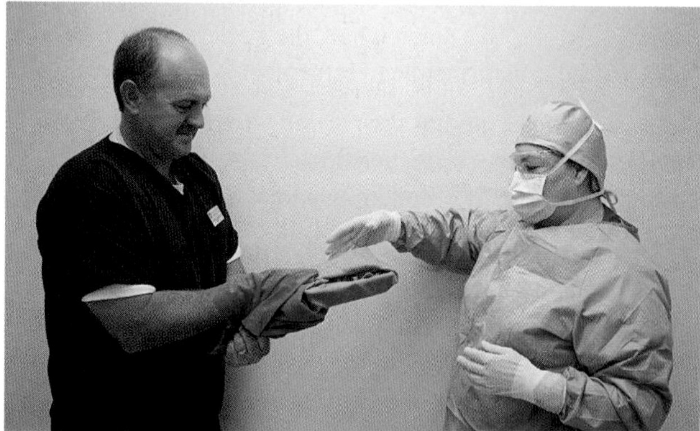

FIGURE 22.5 This unsterile nurse is handing off a sterile item by holding the outer wrapper gathered back around her unsterile hand. The nurse in sterile garb wearing sterile gloves can then grasp it without contamination.

Working With a Sterile Field

Once the sterile field has been established, follow these rules:

- Do not reach across the sterile field unless you are wearing a sterile gown and gloves. Your arms are not sterile, so you will contaminate the field by reaching across it.
- Keep the sterile field in view at all times to ensure that contamination does not occur.

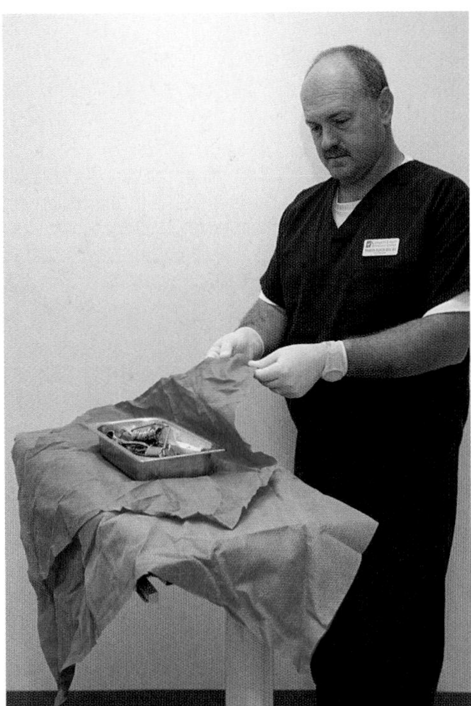

FIGURE 22.6 This nurse is opening the last flap of a sterile pack toward himself as he sets up a sterile field.

- Never turn your back on the sterile field, as you cannot see if it becomes contaminated.
- Once you have applied your sterile gloves, keep your gloved hands in the *safety zone,* which is above waist level, below eye level, and in front of your body at all times. If they fall below the waist, above eye level, or outside your peripheral vision, they are out of your line of vision, so they could accidentally brush against an unsterile surface, causing contamination. Any time they are outside of the safety zone, they must be considered contaminated, requiring you to apply a new pair of sterile gloves before continuing. For example, this means that you cannot reach behind you, nor can you reach below your waist to put anything in the trash can. You must learn to discard items by "dropping" the items from your hand and letting them fall to their intended target, while keeping your hand within the safety zone.
- When sterile objects are exposed to the air for a long period of time, they are no longer considered sterile. It is very important to wait to prepare the sterile field until just prior to its use.

KNOWLEDGE CONNECTION

What should you do if a sterile supply becomes contaminated? What is meant by "developing a sterile conscience"? What portion of a sterile drape is always considered unsterile?

When to Use Sterile Technique

Health-care providers' orders do not usually include directions to use sterile technique. Part of developing nursing judgment involves knowing when to use sterile technique and when clean technique is adequate. Use sterile technique in the following circumstances:

- When entering a sterile body cavity with a tube or other invasive equipment. Examples include inserting a catheter into the bladder, inserting an IV needle into the vein, and injecting medications into the muscles or subcutaneous tissue.
- When caring for patients whose skin is not intact, creating exposure to pathogens. An example is caring for patients with burns or open wounds.
- During procedures that expose body cavities or enter major blood vessels, such as surgery, heart catheterizations, and the delivery of babies.
- When handling needles, syringes, and lancets. Box 22.2 presents tips on using sterile technique when handling these items.

Real-World Connection

The Importance of Sterile Supplies

A group of nurses working in a coronary care unit noticed that several patients had developed infections at their IV insertion sites. One patient's infection spread to his bloodstream, causing septicemia, and even spread to his heart. He became quite ill and had to have emergency surgery. The nurses pressed for an investigation into the situation. Eventually, the infections were traced back to a batch of IV catheters that apparently had not been sterilized correctly, leading to these patients' infections.

Box 22.2
Tips for Handling Needles, Syringes, and Lancets

When you handle needles, syringes, and lancets, you must follow sterile technique to prevent contamination and potential for infection for your patient.

- Keep needles and lancing devices sterile at all times.
- The shaft, bevel, and hub of the needle and tip of syringe (Fig. 22.7) should be kept sterile.
- Do not touch the sharp portion of the lancet.
- After use, immediately put a used needle or lancet into a puncture-proof sharps container.
- Do not recap a used needle as the risk of puncturing yourself is too great.

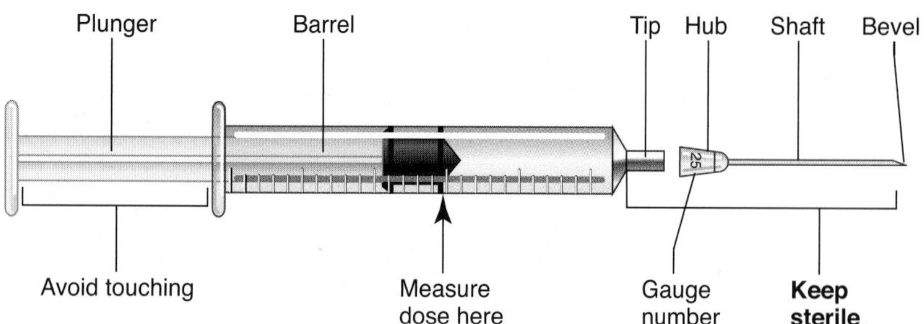

FIGURE 22.7 Areas of the needle and syringe that should remain sterile (from Wilkinson JM, Treas LS. *Fundamentals of Nursing: Theory, Concepts & Applications*. Vol. 1. 3rd ed. Philadelphia, PA: FA Davis; 2016).

Preparation for Entering the Operating Room

When you enter restricted areas, including the operating room (OR), you will be expected to perform a surgical hand scrub. This type of handwashing is more extensive than the skill you learned in Chapter 14. It involves cleaning the hands and arms up to the elbows to ensure that shedding skin cells and pathogens have been removed.

In the actual surgical area of the hospital, you will first change into hospital-laundered scrubs and then apply shoe covers, head cover, and mask before you begin the surgical hand scrub. Skill 22.3 (page 435) provides the steps needed to perform a surgical hand scrub.

You will then dry your hands with a sterile towel and proceed into the anteroom, where you will be assisted into a sterile gown by the circulating nurse. The **circulating nurse** is a registered nurse (RN) who assists in the OR by obtaining needed equipment and supplies. The circulating nurse is not "scrubbed in" on the case, so he or she may leave the operating suite to obtain needed items. The **scrub nurse** assists the health-care provider throughout the surgery by handing instruments, holding retractors, and performing other tasks that require sterile garb. This person, who may be a *surgical technologist* or a licensed practical nurse, does scrub in on the case. After donning your sterile gown with the assistance of the circulating nurse, you will don sterile gloves using the closed gloving method. Skill 22.4 (page 437) provides the steps involved in donning the sterile gown and performing closed gloving.

Settings Connection: Home Health

Nonsterile Technique May Be Used in the Home Setting

Some procedures that require sterile technique in the hospital setting may not be performed using sterile technique in the home setting. For example, patients with nerve damage that affects their ability to empty their bladder must catheterize the bladder several times a day to drain it. In that situation, a sterile catheter is used, but clean technique is used for the insertion. The reason for this is that the number and type of pathogens found in the hospital have a much greater risk of causing severe infection than the pathogens in the patient's home.

Settings Connection: Long-Term Care

Sterile Technique in the Nursing Facility

In the long-term care setting, the variety and number of pathogens are of concern as they are in hospitals. Because it is a more residential setting, sterile procedures may be performed infrequently. However, it is not uncommon for residents to have indwelling catheters or wounds requiring sterile treatment. Nurses in long-term care settings administer injections of insulin and other medications frequently. It is important to use meticulous sterile technique to prevent possible infections.

KNOWLEDGE CONNECTION

How will you know when to use sterile technique when you perform patient care procedures? What must you do before you enter the operating room? Which portions of the needle and syringe must always remain sterile?

Skill 22.1 Setting Up a Sterile Field, Opening Sterile Packs, and Pouring Sterile Liquids

Assessment Steps

1. Assess the room for a clean, dry, waist-high area to use for setting up the sterile field to ensure sterility when the field is established.
2. Assess the patient for any needs prior to the procedure, such as toileting or pain medication, to prevent interruptions during the sterile procedure.

Planning Steps

1. Gather needed equipment and supplies: sterile gloves in the correct size and sterile supplies needed for the procedure.
2. Determine where to place the over-bed table or other surface selected for establishing the sterile field.

Skill 22.1 (continued)

3. Determine where to place additional supplies so that they will be convenient but do not require that you reach over the sterile field to obtain them. Reaching over a sterile field causes contamination of the field.
4. Remember to choose a clean, dry surface that is waist-high ***to prevent potential contamination of the field.***

Implementation Steps

1. Follow the Initial Implementation Steps located on the inside back cover for procedures during which you will be working at the patient's bedside.
2. If you are establishing a sterile field with a wrapper:
   - Place the sterile pack on a clean and dry selected surface.

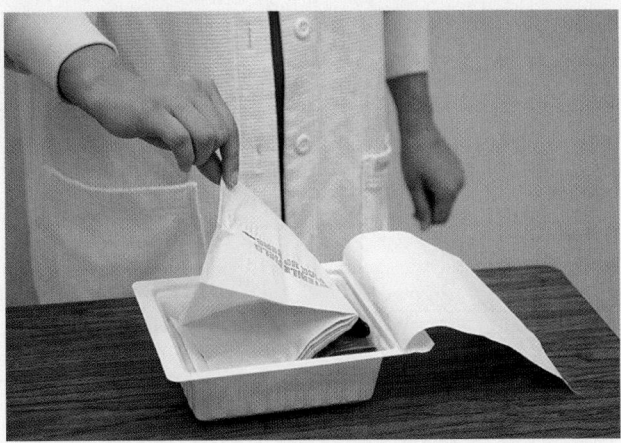

   - Open the first flap of the wrapper away from you, then open the side flaps. Open the last flap toward you to avoid reaching across the sterile field.

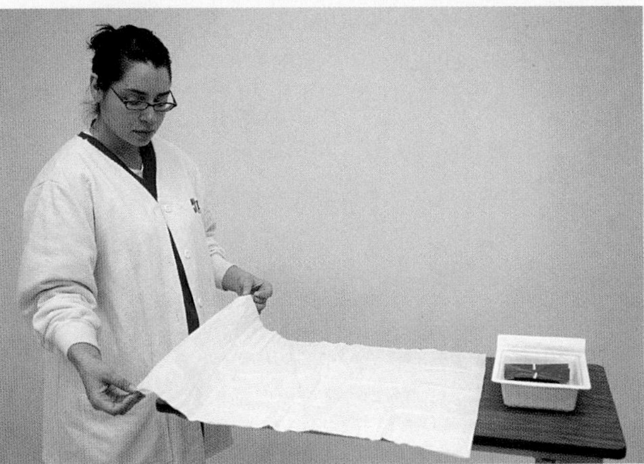

   If you are establishing a sterile field with a drape from a commercial pack:
   - Open the sterile container and remove the drape, touching only the outer 1-inch margin. Avoid touching any other items located in the pack, underneath the sterile drape.
   - Allow the drape to unfold and place it on the selected surface without contaminating the top working surface of the drape.
3. To add sterile items to the sterile field, open the peel-apart pack and drop the contents onto the drape, being careful not to touch the sterile items or the drape with your bare hands. The two inside surfaces of the peel-apart pack, which are sterile, should be the sides that are exposed to the sterile field as you drop the sterile item onto the field. Your nonsterile hands should be behind the sterile surface as the item is dropped. Avoid reaching over the sterile field to prevent contamination.

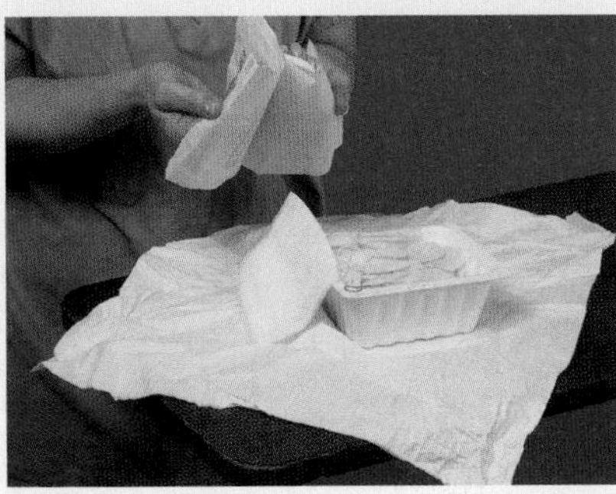

4. To add liquids to a sterile container such as a basin or bowl, follow these steps:
   - Check the container for the expiration date. If the container has been previously opened, follow facility policy for how long it can be used, generally 24 to 48 hours. Solutions are no longer sterile if they have been opened for too long or are past their expiration date. ***Safety: Write the date, time, and your initials on the label of the sterile solution when you open it for the first time.***
   - Hold the container with the label in your palm. This prevents any drips from the bottle from running onto the label and obscuring the printing on it.
   - Remove the lid from the solution bottle and place it with the edges up on a clean surface, but not on the sterile field. The outside of the lid is not sterile, but the inside is and should not touch unsterile surfaces.
   - Pour a small amount of solution across the lip of the bottle into a cup or trash can to remove dust or microorganisms that may be present to prevent them from being washed into the sterile basin. This is referred to as "lipping" the bottle.
   - Hold the bottle 4 to 6 inches above the sterile basin and pour in a gentle stream to avoid splashing. If you splash fluid on a sterile drape, your field becomes contaminated, unless you have used a barrier-style drape that has a plastic, moisture-proof backing on it. Moisture cannot permeate the backing and therefore the drape would still be considered sterile.
   - Carefully replace the lid on the container, touching only the outer surface. The inner surface of the lid is considered sterile.
5. Don sterile gloves according to Skill 22.2. Then you can touch the items on your sterile field and continue with the procedure.
6. Follow the Initial Implementation Steps located on the inside back cover for procedures during which you are working at the patient's bedside.

Evaluation Step

1. Evaluate whether the procedure was completed without contamination of the sterile field, sterile supplies, or sterile gloves.

Skill 22.2 Donning Sterile Gloves—Open Method

Assessment Steps

1. Determine the correct size of glove needed.

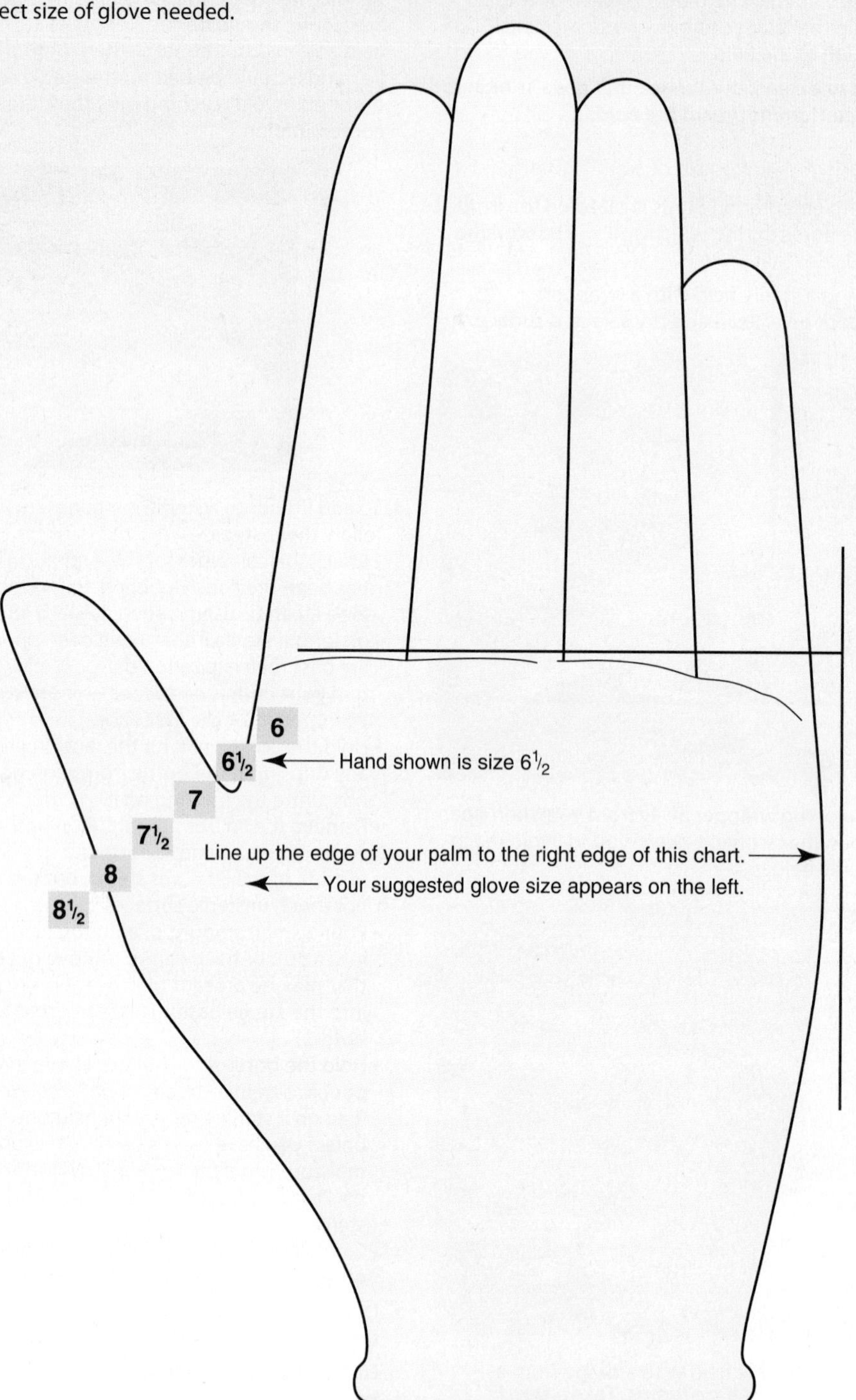
6
6½
Hand shown is size 6½
7
7½
Line up the edge of your palm to the right edge of this chart.
8
Your suggested glove size appears on the left.
8½

2. Assess the glove packaging for the expiration date and any holes or tears. Check to be sure the packaging is dry. ***Any open areas or wet areas would compromise sterility, and the gloves cannot be used.***

Planning Step

1. Determine where you will open the wrapper containing the sterile gloves, thereby establishing a mini sterile field. Remember to choose a clean, dry surface that is waist-high ***to prevent potential contamination of the field.***

Implementation Steps

1. Follow the Initial Implementation Steps located on the inside back cover for procedures during which you will be working at the patient's bedside.

Skill 22.2 (continued)

2. Open the outer wrapper and discard it. You may touch the outside of the inner wrapper with your bare hands. ***This part of the inner wrapper will be against the table and is considered unsterile.***
3. Position the inner wrapper so that the diagram on the wrapper indicates that the cuffs of the gloves are toward you. To open the inner wrapper, begin by unfolding the horizontal top and bottom 1-inch flaps, smoothing flat the fold creases in the paper wrapper to prevent the flaps from folding back down on themselves after you unfold them.

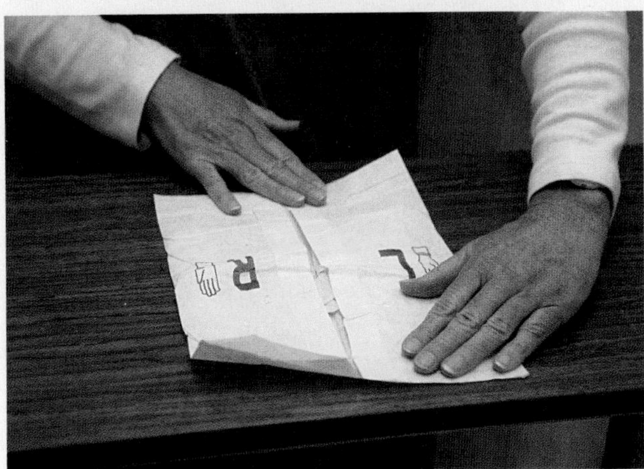

4. Then, to maintain sterility, touch only the 1-inch outer vertical flaps of the inside wrapper. Pull the flaps open until the wrapper lays flat. To prevent these two sides of the inner wrapper from closing again, you will probably have to gently pull the two flaps until they somewhat flatten out the fold creases in the paper wrapper.

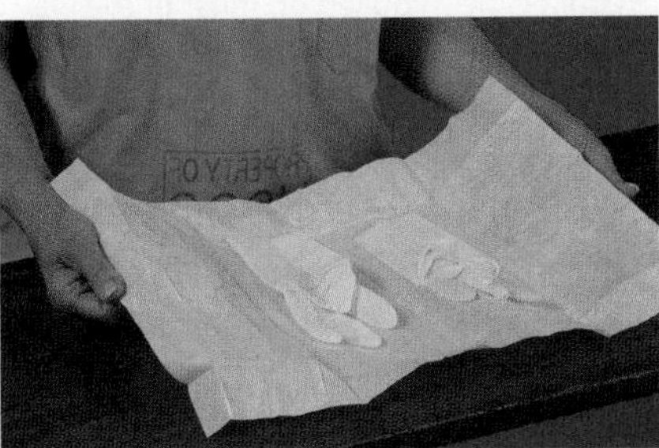

5. Use your nondominant hand to pick up the glove for your dominant hand. Pick up the glove by the folded cuff edge, making certain to lift the glove high enough so that the glove fingertips are at least 4 to 6 inches above the wrapper edges. ***The inside of the cuff and glove will not be considered sterile because they will touch your bare hands.*** Take a step back away from your package of sterile gloves. ***This provides you with extra room to help prevent contamination by touching the package or surface upon which it lies, while you apply the glove.***

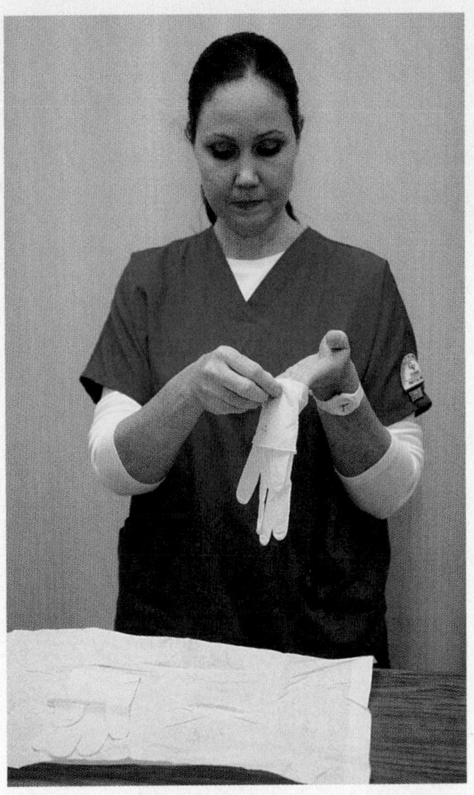

6. Align the thumb of the glove with your thumb before inserting your dominant hand into the glove. Pull the glove on until it fits snuggly over the dominant hand. Ensure that your hand and fingers remain above your waist while gloving. ***Items below waist level are considered contaminated.***

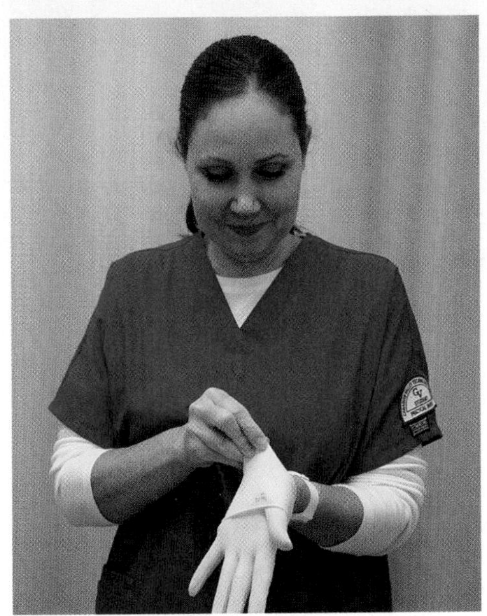

(skill continues on page 434)

Skill 22.2 (continued)

7. To pick up the second glove, slip your sterile gloved fingers underneath the cuff, between the cuff and the sterile palmar surface of the glove. ***In this way, your sterile gloved hand touches only sterile surfaces of the glove for the nondominant hand.***
   Remember to lift the glove above the package and take a step backward ***to allow yourself more room to prevent contamination.***

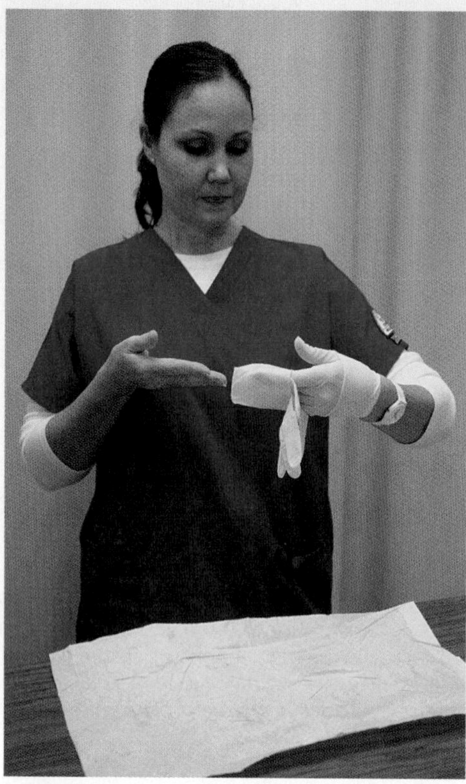

8. Slide your nondominant hand into the glove, being sure the thumb of the glove aligns with your thumb. Pull the glove on until it fits snuggly over the nondominant hand.
   Note: While donning the second glove, keep the thumb of your dominant hand abducted away from your nondominant hand to prevent possible contamination by accidental contact with bare skin.

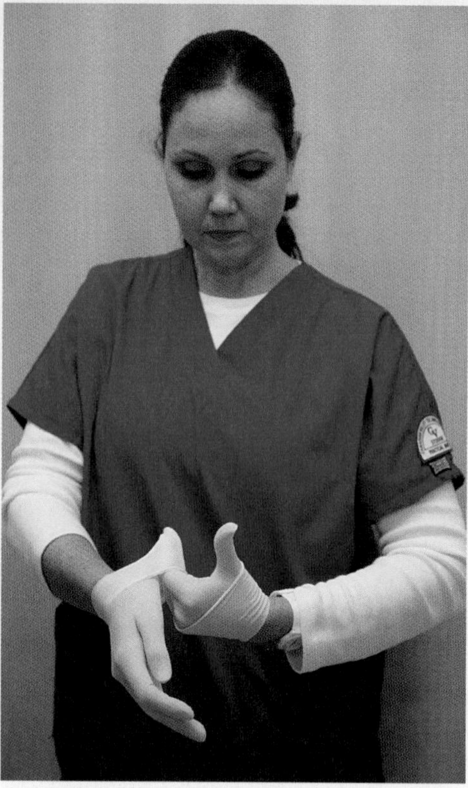

9. Now that gloves are on both hands, slip the gloved fingertips of your dominant hand underneath the cuff flap of the nondominant hand. Pull the cuff up using the gloved fingers only. Keep the dominant hand thumb abducted. ***Using the gloved thumb will likely cause contamination as the cuff unfolds.*** When the cuff has been pulled up most of the way on the forearm, remove your dominant hand fingers from underneath the cuff, allowing the cuff to recoil against the nonsterile surface of the forearm.

Skill 22.2 (continued)

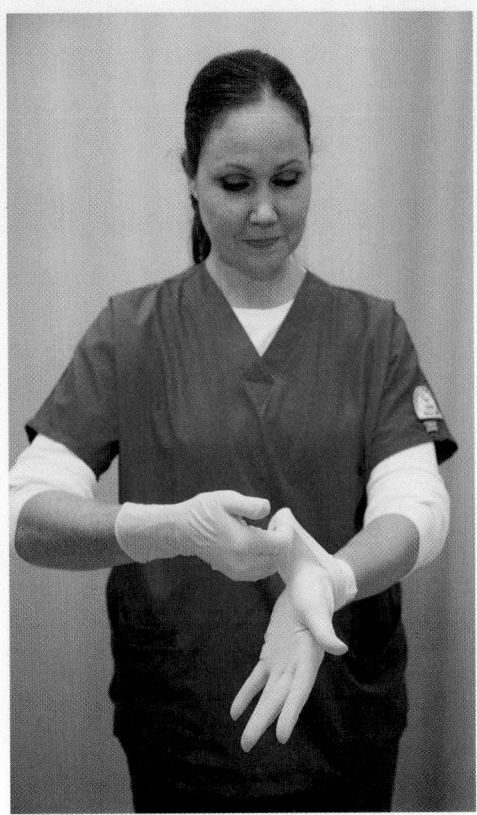

10. Slip the gloved fingertips of your nondominant hand underneath the cuff flap of the glove on your dominant hand, keeping your thumb abducted to prevent contamination. Using the gloved fingers only, pull the cuff up most of the way on the forearm, removing your nondominant hand fingers from underneath the cuff to allow the cuff to recoil against the nonsterile surface of the forearm.

11. Put your gloved hands together with your fingers interlaced to snug the fingers of the gloves against your fingertips so that no extra room remains at the fingertips.

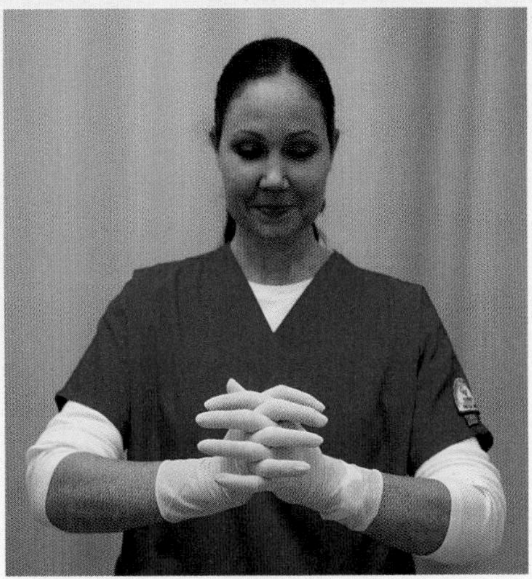

12. Follow the Initial Implementation Steps located on the inside back cover for procedures during which you are working at the patient's bedside.

Evaluation Steps

1. Determine that the procedure was completed without contaminating the sterile gloves or the sterile field.
2. Evaluate the fit of the gloves to determine if you have the correct size. They should fit closely without wrinkles, without excess material at the fingertips and without bowing due to tightness.

Skill 22.3 Performing a Surgical Hand Scrub

Assessment Step

1. Assess your readiness to perform the scrub:
   - You are wearing hospital-laundered scrubs.
   - You are wearing appropriate shoes or shoe covers.
   - You have a hair cover and mask in place.

Planning Steps

1. Determine that sterile supplies you will need after completing the hand scrub are available, including sterile towels, a sterile gown, and sterile gloves in the correct size.
2. Determine that needed supplies are available for the hand scrub: knee- or foot-controlled water source, antiseptic soap, and an orangewood stick or other tool for cleaning nails. ***Note: Brushes are NOT recommended for surgical hand scrubs due to the possibility of them causing microscopic abrasions on the skin. Alcohol hand rubs are preferred in some settings due to the possible contamination of rinse water after the scrub. In addition, the rapid antimicrobial action and wide spectrum antiseptic activity make the hand gels more effective.***
3. Remove all jewelry from your hands and arms, such as rings and watches. Remove nail polish if it is chipped.

Implementation Steps

1. Turn on the water to a comfortable warm temperature. ***Water that is too hot destroys natural oils and causes cracking of skin. Water that is too cold does not wash off soap or destroy bacteria and causes chapping.***
2. Rinse each hand and arm from the fingertips to the elbows. Keep your fingertips above your elbows as you wash and rinse ***to prevent water from your arms from running down over your clean hands.***
3. Obtain a palmful of antibacterial soap using a foot control. ***This prevents your rinsed hands from touching a dirty soap dispenser.***
4. For the first hand wash, lather your hands and up your arms to 2 inches above the elbow. ***This removes some micro-organisms before you begin the actual scrub.***

(skill continues on page 436)

Skill 22.3 (continued)

5. Under running water, use a clean orangewood stick or other tool, such as a single-use nail file, to clean beneath your nails and around the cuticles.

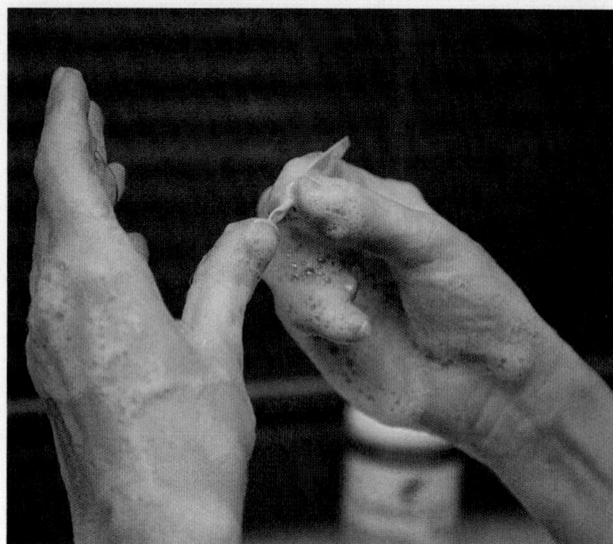

6. Rinse your hands and arms again from fingertips to elbows, with the hands kept above the elbows. ***Avoid touching the sink or dispensers with your hands as they are considered contaminated.***
7. Begin the hand scrub. **When scrubbing with an antimicrobial agent, follow these steps:**
   - Dispense the antimicrobial soap into your hand according to facility policy.
   - Apply to one hand and arm up to 2 inches above the elbow.
   - Divide each finger, hand, and arm into four surfaces in your mind: ventral (palm side of hand), dorsal (back of hand), and two lateral (sides of hand) surfaces.
   - Now divide your arm into the distal section, from the wrist to 4 inches up the forearm, and the proximal section, from 4 inches up the forearm to 2 inches above the elbow.
   - Rub the lather for at least 10 strokes on each surface, for a total of 40 strokes on each finger, 40 strokes on the hand, 40 strokes on the wrist and distal arm, and 40 strokes on the proximal arm and above the elbow. ***Note: The total scrub time is 2 to 6 minutes. Follow facility policy.***
   - Repeat for the other hand and arm.
   - Repeat the scrub process if directed by facility policy.
   - Rinse from the fingertips to the elbows, keeping the hands above the elbows ***so that contaminated water flows away from your hands.***

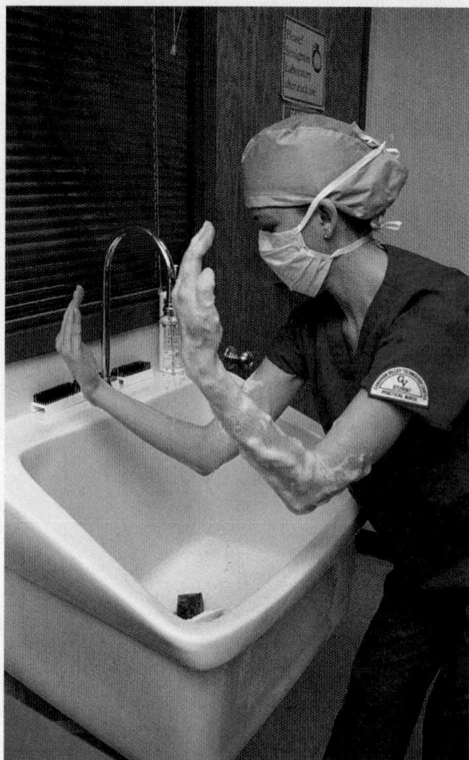

   - Dry your hands from the fingertips to the elbows using one sterile towel for each arm and hand. While drying, lean forward, bending from the waist, ***to prevent the sterile towel with which you are drying from coming in contact with your scrubs.***

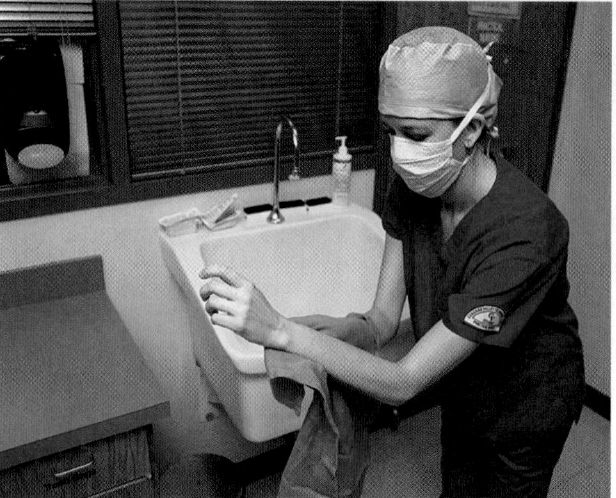

Skill 22.3 (continued)

When using an alcohol-based surgical hand gel, follow these steps:

- Dry hands thoroughly after the first hand wash with a paper towel.
- Obtain the recommended amount of surgical hand gel. Follow facility policy.
- Apply the product to completely cover your hands and forearms, rubbing until it is dry.
- Repeat the application of the product if that is what is recommended by the manufacturer. Again, follow facility policy.

8. Proceed to the anteroom of the operating room or other sterile area, keeping your cleansed hands raised above your elbows and positioned in front of you ***so that they remain within the "safe zone,"*** and don your sterile gown and gloves according to Skill 22.4.

Evaluation Steps

1. Determine if you completed the hand scrub according to facility policy, within the appropriate time frame and number of strokes recommended.
2. Evaluate whether you touched any contaminated surfaces during or after the surgical hand scrub. If this occurred, repeat the hand scrub.

Skill 22.4 Donning a Sterile Gown and Sterile Gloves—Closed Method

Assessment Step

1. Assess your readiness to gown and glove to enter the sterile area:
   - Are you dressed in appropriate scrubs, shoe covers, hair cover, and mask?
   - Have you determined if needed supplies of sterile towels, gown, and gloves are available before beginning the surgical hand scrub?
   - Have you completed a surgical hand scrub? (See Skill 22.3.)

Planning Step

1. Arrange for a circulating nurse to assist you.

Implementation Steps

1. Pick up the sterile gown at the inner neckline and allow it to unfold, keeping the gown away from unsterile surfaces ***to prevent contamination.***
2. Slip both of your arms into the arms of the gown and grasp the inside of the arms, leaving your hands within the cuffs of the gown.
3. Have the circulating nurse pull the neck area of the gown together, ***touching only the inside to prevent contamination.*** The circulating nurse will also tie the gown at the neck.
4. Do not push your hands through the gown sleeves. Keep them within the cuffs of the gown.

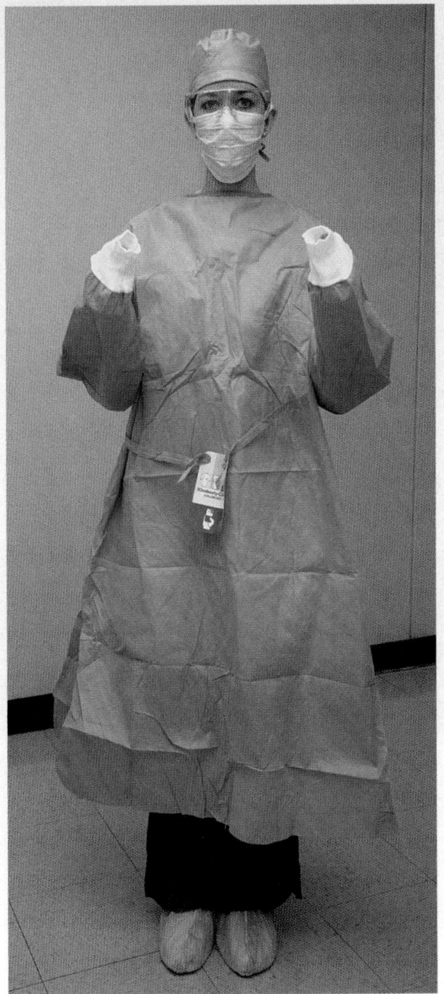

(skill continues on page 438)

Skill 22.4 (continued)

5. With your hands still inside the gown sleeves, open the sterile glove wrapper by grasping it through the gown material. ***Note: If the glove package is lying on a sterile field, the outer wrapper will already have been removed. If it is lying on a nonsterile field, the outer wrapper will have been opened and the sterile inner wrapper will be lying on the sterile inside surface of the outer wrapper. As you open this sterile inner wrapper, do not allow your sterile gown cuffs to touch anything other than the sterile inner wrapper and gloves.***
6. Pick up the glove for your dominant hand at the cuff with your nondominant hand, which is still inside the gown sleeve.

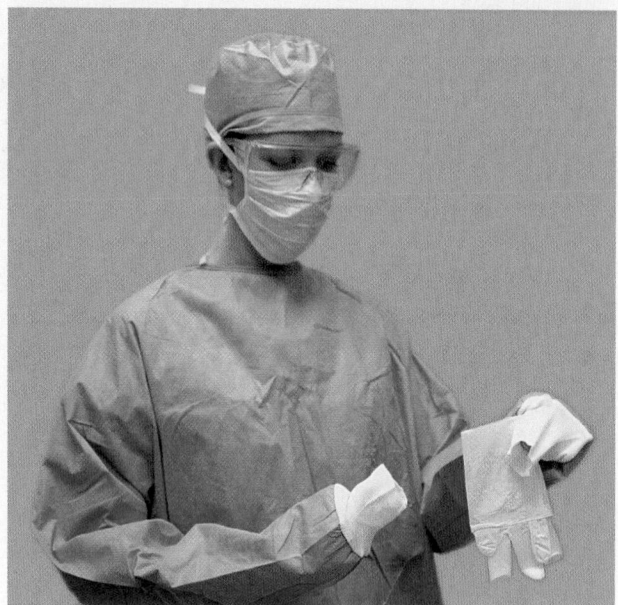

7. Place the glove on the forearm of your dominant hand, palm side down, with the glove fingers pointing toward your elbow and the glove thumb aligned with your thumb.

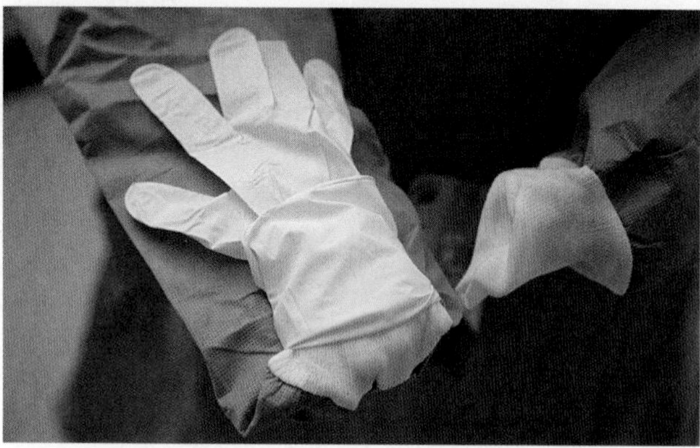

8. Grasp the inside of the cuff with the fingers of your dominant hand, which is still inside the gown sleeve.
9. Using your nondominant hand through the gown material, pull the dominant glove cuff over the gown cuff.

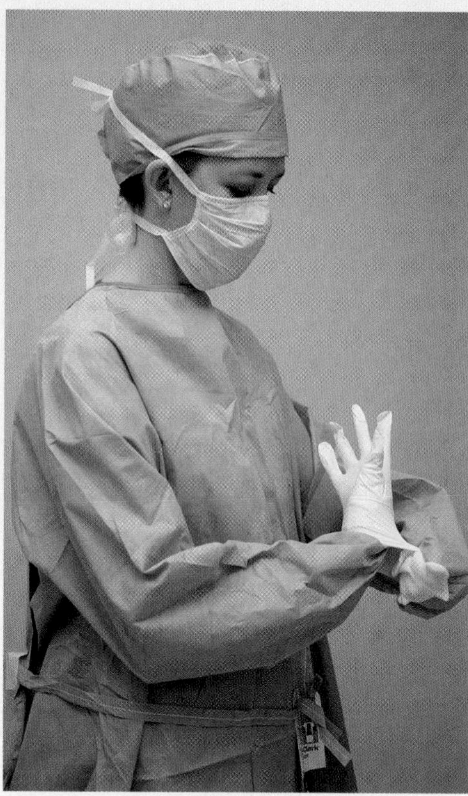

10. Slide your dominant hand into the glove as you pull up the glove cuff and gown cuff with your nondominant hand, which still remains within the gown sleeve.

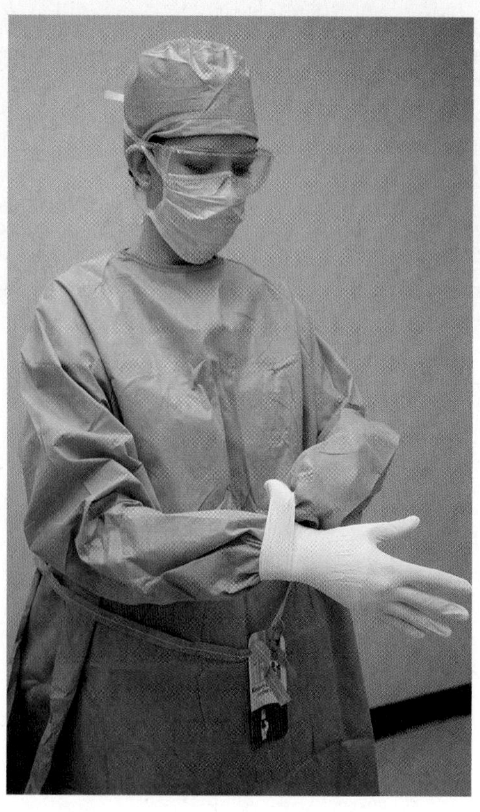

Skill 22.4 (continued)

11. Pick up the glove for your nondominant hand and place it on your forearm with the glove fingers pointing toward your elbow and the glove thumb aligned with your thumb.
12. Using your dominant gloved hand, pull the nondominant glove cuff over the gown cuff.
13. Slide your nondominant hand into the glove as you pull up the glove cuff and gown cuff with your gloved dominant hand.

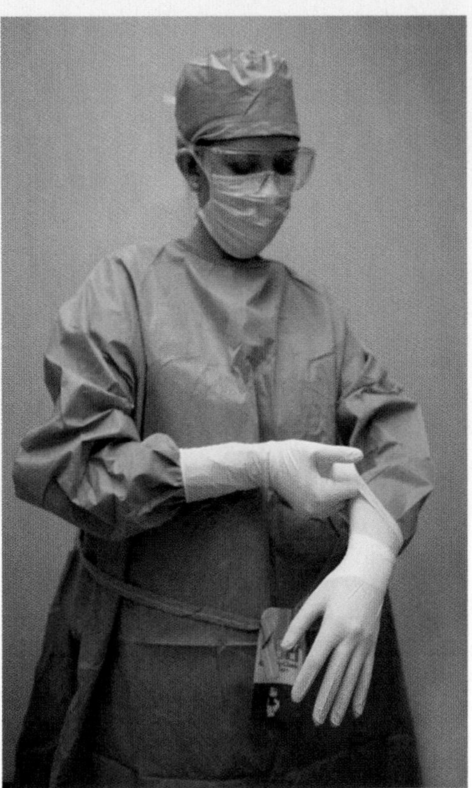

14 Adjust the fingers and smooth out any glove wrinkles. Ensure that the glove cuffs cover the gown cuffs so that no skin is exposed.
Note: Although your skin has been scrubbed, it cannot actually be sterile and therefore may still harbor some pathogens.
15. Keep your hands together and above your waist. Enter the operating room by backing through the swinging doors, using care to avoid touching the front and sleeves of your sterile gown, as well as your gloves, against any unsterile surface.

Evaluation Step

1. Evaluate whether you put on the sterile gown and sterile gloves with the closed method without contaminating them:
   - Did your bare hands touch any part of the sterile gown other than the inside?
   - Did your bare hands touch any part of the sterile gloves other than the inside?
   - Once the sterile gloves were donned, did they remain covering the cuffs of the sterile gown so that no bare skin was exposed at any time?

POST CONFERENCE

Your instructor asks you to share your experience with the other students during post conference. You tell them that, although you were very nervous, you were able to set up everything needed for the procedure. The staff nurse reminded you to obtain masks and goggles for the health-care provider, the nurse, and yourself. You remembered the principles of sterile technique while setting up the field and adding items to it. During the procedure, the health-care provider asked for more gauze 4×4s, which you had not opened but did have in the room. You remembered to peel apart the pack, with the opening toward the health-care provider. You kept your bare hands away from the sterile gauze, allowing the health-care provider to remove the 4×4s from the pack without contaminating his sterile gloves. The procedure went smoothly and safely for the patient with no breaches of sterile technique.

Key Points

- Disinfection is the process used to kill bloodborne pathogens and organisms.
- Common types of sterilization include autoclaving, boiling, ionizing radiation, chemical disinfection, and gaseous disinfection.
- To check the sterility of an item, look at the expiration date, check for black hash marks on the indicator tape, and examine the packaging for evidence that it has been wet (strike-through) or for holes or tears.
- Sterile technique is the method used for invasive procedures to prevent pathogens from entering the body by careful cleaning and sterilization of equipment and supplies, as well as the use of sterile gowns and gloves.
- A sterile conscience is the awareness of potential or certain contamination of a sterile field or items. It is up to you to admit that possible contamination occurred and to start the procedure again with fresh sterile supplies, even if no one else observed the contamination.
- When setting up a sterile field, anything below the table surface is considered contaminated, as is the outer 1 inch of the sterile drape. If it becomes damp or wet, it is no longer sterile.
- When opening sterile packs, always open the first flap away from you and the last flap toward you.
- When adding items to the sterile field, follow specific guidelines to avoid contamination with sterile liquids and avoid contamination of items you wish to add.
- Avoid reaching across a sterile field and keep it in view at all times, never turning your back to it. Set up the sterile field just before you are ready to use it.
- Contamination occurs when a sterile field or sterile object may be exposed to pathogens due to potential or full contact with a nonsterile surface or item. If in doubt, consider the sterile field to be unsterile.
- Sterile technique is used in restricted areas of the hospital as well as at the patient's bedside for invasive procedures.
- Use sterile technique when entering body cavities, veins, or arteries; when caring for patients with nonintact skin; and when handling needles, syringes, and lancets.

Review Questions

Select the answer that is most appropriate for each of the following questions. Some questions may have more than one correct answer. Select all that apply.

1. Your patient has been discharged from the hospital. Remaining in the room are an IV pump and a *hemostat,* a metal-hinged instrument used to clamp off tubes or blood vessels. Which actions will you take?
   1. Clean the pump with disinfectant and rinse the hemostat in cool or warm water before sending it to be sterilized.
   2. Take both items to the central supply area to be cleaned and then sterilized.
   3. Return the IV pump to the storage area on the nursing unit and throw away the hemostat.
   4. Call the housekeeping staff and ask them to dispose of the equipment when they clean the room.

2. You are preparing to use a sterile pack. Which of these findings would concern you the most?
   1. The expiration date is 2 weeks in the future.
   2. It is difficult to read the initials of the person who sterilized the pack.
   3. The hash marks on the indicator tape are the same color as the tape.
   4. There are no holes or tears and no evidence of strike-through.

3. As you prepare for a rotation in the heart catheterization laboratory, you will expect:
   1. to change into hospital-laundered scrubs.
   2. to wear street clothes covered by a lab coat in the patient care area.
   3. that it is a restricted area to maintain asepsis.
   4. to wear your regular scrubs covered by a gown, as well as wear a mask and goggles.

4. The nurse will use sterile technique when performing which of the following procedures?
   1. Insertion of a urinary catheter
   2. Emptying a catheter drainage bag
   3. Starting an IV line
   4. Assessing the IV drip rate
   5. Performing a bed bath
   6. Suctioning the trachea
   7. Administering an insulin injection

5. A nurse is attempting to insert a sterile catheter into a patient's bladder. The nurse accidentally brushes the tip of the catheter against the side rail of the bed. The patient is unaware of this incident. Which action will the nurse take?
   1. Clean the tip of the catheter with an alcohol swab and continue with the procedure.
   2. Discard the contaminated catheter and begin the procedure over again.
   3. Say nothing and use the catheter anyway, since no one saw what happened.
   4. Stop the procedure, leave the room to get a fresh catheter, and resume the procedure.

6. A nurse wearing sterile gloves pushes up his glasses with his gloved hand. The nurse's next action is to:
   1. wash his hands while wearing his sterile gloves.
   2. remove the sterile gloves and wash his hands.
   3. obtain and don a second pair of sterile gloves.
   4. Both 2 and 3

ANSWERS 1. 1, 2. 3, 3. 1, 3, 4. 1, 3, 6, 7, 5. 2, 6. 4

Critical Thinking Exercises

Answers available online.

1. You are a student assigned to observe in the operating room. During the preparations for the surgery, you notice that the health-care provider touches the sterile field before donning sterile gloves. What, if any, action will you take?

2. You are assigned to teach a patient with bladder problems how to perform self-catheterizations at home. The health-care provider tells you to teach the patient to do this using medical asepsis rather than surgical asepsis. What is the rationale for such an order?

3. You are preparing to enter the operating room for clinical observation. List, in order, the steps you will take to make yourself as sterile as possible before entering the operating suite.

Additional Resources

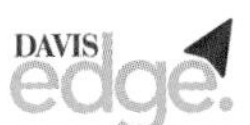

Use the scratch off code on the inside front cover of your book to access online quizzes that will help you to improve your scores on course exams and prepare for the NCLEX-PN®.

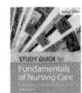

Study Guide

CHAPTER 23
Nutrition

KEY TERMS

Absorption (ab-ZORB-shun)
Anabolism (a-NAB-uh-lizm)
Antioxidant (AN-ti-OX-i-dent)
Body mass index (BAH-dee MASS IN-deks)
Catabolism (kuh-TAB-uh-lizm)
Complete proteins (kom-PLEET PRO-teenz)
Complex carbohydrates (KOM-pleks KAR-boh-HYE-drayts)
Digestion (dye-JES-chun)
Essential amino acids (e-SEN-shul ah-MEE-noh ASS-ids)
Incomplete proteins (IN-kom-PLEET PRO-teenz)
Nitrogen balance (NYE-troh-jen BA-lanss)
Nonessential amino acids (NON-e-SEN-shul ah-MEE-noh ASS-ids)
Simple carbohydrates (SIM-puhl KAR-boh-HYE-drayts)

CHAPTER CONCEPTS

Nutrition
Health Promotion
Patient-Centered Care

LEARNING OUTCOMES

1. Define various terms associated with nutrition.
2. Describe nutritional guidelines, including food label information, dietary guidelines for Americans, and My Plate recommendations.
3. Identify the six essential nutrients and the caloric value in 1 gram of each macronutrient.
4. Explain the types, functions, and digestion of proteins.
5. Discuss protein deficiency and excess disorders.
6. Explain the types, functions, and digestion of fats.
7. Discuss fat and lipid deficiency and excess disorders.
8. Explain the types, functions, and digestion of carbohydrates and fiber.
9. Discuss carbohydrate deficiency and excess disorders.
10. Differentiate between fat soluble and water soluble vitamins.
11. Identify sources and functions of vitamins, as well as symptoms of deficiencies and excesses of each.
12. Differentiate between major and trace minerals
13. Identify sources and functions of minerals, as well as symptoms of deficiencies and excesses of each.
14. Discuss the functions and importance of water in the body.
15. Discuss how nutritional needs vary over the life span, including the risks and prevention of being overweight or obese.
16. Discuss information found in the Connection features in this chapter.
17. Identify specific safety features.

CRITICAL THINKING CONNECTION

Clinical Assignment

You are caring for a 68-year-old male who has been hospitalized for extreme constipation. He is having bowel movements now, but he has had a poor diet that contributed to his constipation problems. His wife died 9 months ago. He eats mostly canned soups and processed lunch meats on white bread because he does not

CRITICAL THINKING CONNECTION—cont'd

cook much. He sometimes gets fast food, such as hamburgers or fried chicken. He likes meat but does not eat vegetables or fruits. He tells you they go bad before he can eat them all, so they are a waste of money. He mostly drinks soft drinks throughout the day.

Critical Thinking Questions:

1. How will you determine the effectiveness of the current treatment for constipation?
2. What nutritional concerns do you have for this patient?
3. How will you help him manage this issue?
4. How will you help this patient prevent rehospitalization for constipation in the future?

Good nutrition is a primary key to optimal health for each individual in any circumstance. Does it prevent or cure all diseases? Of course not, but it allows the body access to the nutrients needed to supply the energy for all body systems to work together for the good of the body. Energy is the product of *metabolism*, the chemical and physical processes in which body cells break down and utilize food, water, and other chemicals needed to maintain life and function of each body system. The breaking down phase of metabolism is known as **catabolism,** in which the body reduces complex substances down to the simpler substances and sometimes releases energy as a result. When the body uses components to build or reconstruct new components or tissue, it is called **anabolism.**

Proper nutrition is essential for a stronger immune system, less illness, and better health. Even a relatively small nutrient imbalance can cause severe health problems. This chapter will show you the importance of nutrition and specific nutrients pertinent for optimal health. You will learn how nutritional needs differ through the life span, sources of nutrients, and how culture influences individual food preferences.

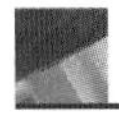

NUTRITIONAL GUIDELINES

Nutrients are provided through natural (food) and artificial (supplements) sources. Although each nutrient has its own specific functions, they all must work together to provide optimal functioning of the body systems.

Food provides energy, which is measured in kilocalories (kcal), and this energy can either be used instantly or stored to be utilized at a later time. The number of kilocalories that is required to function optimally varies depending on age, gender, and activity levels (Table 23.1).

KNOWLEDGE CONNECTION

How many calories does the average active adult male need per day? An active young child? Which would require intake of more calories: active adolescent male or female?

FDA Guidelines and Food Labels

The Food and Drug Administration (FDA) first established standards for the minimum amount of nutrients necessary to protect most individuals from disease. These standard guidelines are known as dietary reference intakes (DRIs) and contain recommendations for gender, age, pregnancy, and lactation. The DRIs for individuals and for various nutrients can be viewed on the government Web site at https://www.nal.usda.gov/fnic/dri-tables-and-application-reports. Various laws ensure that nutrition facts food labels are found on all processed food products. Each label provides an ingredient list and nutritional descriptions (Fig. 23.1). The New Nutrition Facts label went into effect in May 2016, with the goal of making it easier for consumers to make informed food choices. The differences from the previous food labeling requirements include the following:

- The amount of calories in a product is now printed in a large, bold font, making it easier to read.
- The serving size and servings per container are also easier to read, and serving sizes have been changed to reflect the amount people typically consume at one time.
- Labels now show "added sugars" in grams; these are sugars that were added during the processing of the food.
- The labeling breaks out vitamin D, calcium, iron, and potassium in actual amounts and gives the percentages of the daily recommended amounts provided in the product. They are different than previous micronutrients included on food labels; they were selected because Americans are typically deficient in these specific micronutrients.

Dietary Guidelines for Americans 2015–2020

To assist the public to eat nutritionally and reach optimal health, the United States Department of Agriculture (USDA) and the Department of Health and Human Services (DHHS) have jointly created and published recommended dietary guidelines. They review these guidelines every 5 years for currency and updating as necessary; the newest edition is the *Dietary Guidelines for Americans 2015–2020*. These guidelines may be viewed at the government Web site at: www.health.gov/dietaryguidelines/2015.

The key recommendations of these guidelines are that Americans should consume a healthy eating pattern that includes the following:

- A variety of vegetables, including dark green, red, and orange legumes (beans and peas), as well as starchy and other types of vegetables
- Fruits, especially whole fruits
- Grains (at least half of which are whole grains)

• **WORD • BUILDING •**

metabolism: metabol – change + ism – principle
catabolism: cata – down + bol – throw + ism – principle
anabolism: ana – up + bol – throw + ism – principle

Table 23.1

Estimated Calorie Requirements (in Kilocalories) for Each Gender and Age Group at Three Levels of Physical Activity

Gender	*Age (Years)*	*Activity Level*		
		Sedentary	*Moderately Active*	*Active*
Child, Female and Male	2–3	1,000	1,000–1,200	1,000–1,400
Female	4–8	1,200	1,400–1,600	1,400–1,600
	9–13	1,400–1,600	1,600–2,000	1,600–1,800
	14–18	1,800	2,000	2,400
	19–25	2,000	2,200	2,400
	26–50	1,800	2,000	2,200
	51+	1,600	1,800	2,000–2,200
Male	4–8	1,400	1,000–1,400	1,600–2,000
	9–13	1,800–2,000	1,800–2,200	2,000–2,600
	14–18	2,200–2,400	2,400–2,800	2,800–3,200
	19–25	2,400–2,600	2,800	3,000
	26–50	2,200–2,400	2,400–2,600	2,800–3,000
	51+	2,000–2,200	2,200–2,400	2,400–2,800

Source: United States Department of Agriculture and US Department of Health and Human Services. Dietary Guidelines for Americans 2015–2020, Appendix 2. Health.gov. https://health.gov/dietaryguidelines/2015/guidelines/appendix-2/. Accessed January 4, 2017.

Nutrition Facts

8 servings per container
Serving size 2/3 cup (55g)

Amount per serving
Calories 230

	% Daily Value*
Total Fat 8g	**10%**
Saturated Fat 1g	**5%**
Trans Fat 0g	
Cholesterol 0mg	**0%**
Sodium 160 mg	**7%**
Total Carbohydrate 37g	**13%**
Dietary Fiber 4g	**14%**
Total Sugars 12g	
Includes 10g Added Sugars	**20%**
Protein 3g	
Vitamin D 2mcg	10%
Calcium 260mg	20%
Iron 8mg	45%
Potassium 235mg	6%

* The % Daily Value (DV) tells you how much nutrient in a serving of food contributes to a daily diet. 2,000 calories a day is used for general nutrition advice.

FIGURE 23.1 Nutrition facts food labels (from Food and Drug Administration. Changes to the Nutritional Facts Label. Fda.gov. https://www.fda.gov/Food/GuidanceRegulation/ Guidance DocumentsRegulatoryInformation/LabelingNutrition/ucm385663.htm. Accessed January 6, 2017).

- Fat-free or low-fat dairy, such as milk, yogurt, cheese, and fortified soy beverages
- A variety of protein foods, such as seafood, lean meats, poultry, eggs, legumes, nuts, seeds, and soy products
- Oils

In addition, these guidelines recommend that Americans limit saturated fats, trans fats, added sugars, and sodium in their diets. Less than 10% of calories should come from added sugars, less than 10% should come from saturated fats, and sodium should be less than 2,300 mg per day. Alcohol may be consumed in moderation, which means one drink per day for women and two drinks per day for men. The Dietary Guidelines for Americans also provide healthy eating patterns for a Mediterranean diet and for a vegetarian diet.

Current eating patterns in the United States show that three-fourths of us do not consume enough vegetables, fruits, dairy, and oils. More than half of us meet or exceed the total grain and total protein recommendations but are not meeting the requirements for subgroups of proteins, such as seafood, legumes, nuts, and soy products. And most Americans exceed the recommendation for added sugars, saturated fats, and sodium. Two-thirds of all adults and nearly one-third of children and youth in the United States are overweight or obese.

Women of Child-Bearing Age

Safety: Because fetal development of the brain and spinal cord occurs within the first few weeks of pregnancy, one of the USDA and DHHS' key recommendations is that women of child-bearing age consume 200 mcg of synthetic folic acid daily from fortified foods and/or supplements in addition to the amounts of food folate contained in a healthy eating pattern. Food sources include all enriched grains, beans, peas, oranges, orange juice, and dark green leafy vegetables. These recommendations are intended to prevent neural tube defects, such as spina bifida, in the developing fetus. Box 23.1 provides nutrition recommendations for pregnant women.

KNOWLEDGE CONNECTION

Why are vitamin D, iron, calcium, and potassium included in the new food labels? What are "added sugars"? How much added sugar should be included in a healthy eating pattern? List sources of protein in addition to beef and chicken. What dietary recommendations are made for women who are of child-bearing age or who are pregnant?

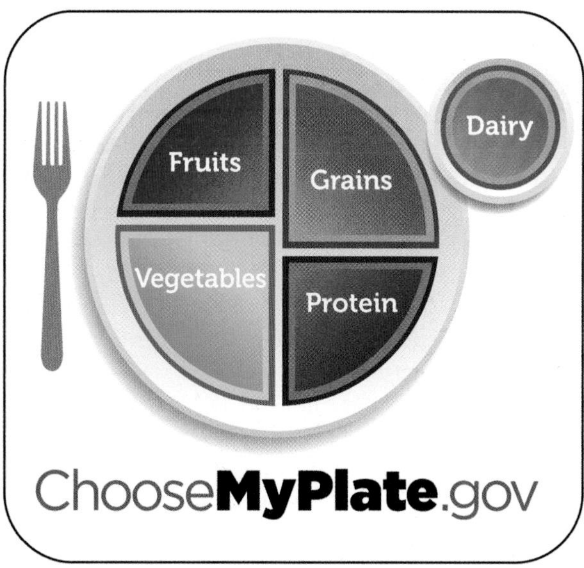

FIGURE 23.2 The USDA's MyPlate food management system (from U.S. Department of Agriculture. ChooseMyPlate. www.choosemyplate.gov. Accessed January 14, 2017).

MyPlate

The USDA's Center for Nutrition Policy and Promotion uses a visual symbol called MyPlate, along with numerous other materials to help guide Americans to healthier eating (Fig. 23.2). In essence, half of your plate of food should be fruits and vegetables, with veggies making up the greater portion of the two groups. Grains and protein should make up the other half of the plate, with the grains portion being the larger of the two groups. The dairy serving should be small and consist of low-fat or nonfat milk or small servings of other low-fat dairy products. Depending on the age of the individual, the entire daily intake of dairy should be restricted to a total of 2 to 3 cups of low-fat or nonfat milk, yogurt, or soymilk. (Refer to Box 23.2 for additional tips for healthy nutrition. To view all information associated with MyPlate, go to www.choosemyplate.gov.)

Box 23.2

ChooseMyPlate Nutrition Tips

- Make half of your plate fruits and vegetables
- Focus on whole fruits
- Vary your vegetables
- Make half of your grains whole grains
- Move to low-fat or fat-free milk or yogurt
- Vary the kinds of proteins you consume

Source: www:ChooseMyPlate.gov.

Box 23.1

Nutrition Recommendations During Pregnancy

The American College of Obstetricians and Gynecologists recommends that pregnant women double the amount of iron that they consumed prepregnancy. This is recommended because more iron is required to carry oxygen to the fetal tissues. Folic acid also must be increased to prevent birth defects of the nervous system. Most physicians recommend that pregnant women take prenatal vitamins to ensure the adequate intake of vital nutrients and to help provide these extra nutrients. The increased needs for iron and folic acid remain during lactation as well. During pregnancy, the only artificial sweeteners that the FDA has approved are aspartame, sucralose, and acesulfame-K. Other recommendations for pregnancy include an increase of 300 calories per day, and 500 calories daily for breastfeeding mothers.

The USDA ChooseMyPlate.gov has health and nutrition information for pregnant and breastfeeding mothers. They include a Daily Food Plan for Moms that calculates the increased nutritional needs for the mother and the mother-to-be based on data entered by the individual.

Anatomy and Physiology Connection

Digestion

Digestion is the process by which food is broken down in the gastrointestinal (GI) tract, releasing nutrients for the body to use. The process of digestion begins in the mouth, where a digestive enzyme called *salivary amylase* begins breaking down simple carbohydrates and fat. The mechanical motion of chewing breaks down starches into smaller products, with saliva moistening the foods. The esophagus transports foods from the mouth into the stomach but does not participate in chemical or mechanical digestion. Muscles and nerves work together to perform *peristalsis,* moving the food from the esophagus to the stomach, into the small intestine, into the large intestine, and finally to the rectum.

Once the food enters the stomach, the gastric juices of the stomach, which are acidic in nature, *hydrolyze* (adds water to break down) carbohydrates into maltose and sucrose. Proteolytic and lipolytic enzymes mix with food and break down small amounts of proteins and fat. The stomach gently contracts and expands to further break down food particles. Serving mostly as a reservoir for the food, little absorption occurs here except for alcohol. As peristalsis gently propels the food bolus from the stomach into the small intestine, the digestive processes in the small intestine are activated.

Most digestion occurs in the first several feet of the small intestine. Digestive enzymes are released from the liver, gallbladder, pancreas, and small intestine, resulting in the breakdown of starches and proteins. Dietary fats are reduced to free fatty acids and monoglycerides. Almost all macronutrients, minerals, and vitamins, along with some fluid, are absorbed at this point in the small intestine. **Absorption** is the process by which nutrients are taken from the end products of digestion into the villi (small projections of intestinal mucosa that line the walls of the small intestine) that contain capillaries. This is the point where the majority of nutrients are absorbed into the bloodstream.

The components of food, mostly cellulose, that are not absorbed in the small intestine are now moved by peristalsis into the large intestine. The colon and rectum absorb most of the fluid produced by the digestive process and some electrolytes into the bloodstream. The remaining bulk is expelled from the rectum as fecal material.

The nutrients absorbed from the GI tract travel through the portal vein to the liver, where they are released into circulation, transformed into other products, or stored. Once released into circulation, nutrients are delivered via the bloodstream or lymphatic system to areas of need. Certain nutrients, such as fatty acids, that are not immediately used are stored in the body as adipose tissue.

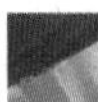

ESSENTIAL NUTRIENTS

Nutrients are divided into two major categories: macronutrients and micronutrients. Macronutrients are required in larger amounts on a daily basis and include the following:

- Protein
- Carbohydrates
- Fats
- Water

Micronutrients include the following:

- Vitamins
- Minerals (which are needed in smaller amounts, known as *trace minerals*)

For optimal health, it is important to ingest all the essential nutrients, including water, in a balanced ratio. ***Safety: Although most people understand that an inadequate intake of nutrients can lead to health problems and less-than-optimal body functioning, it is important to realize that too much of certain nutrients can be just as problematic.*** It will be your job to understand the problems of both nutrient deficiencies and excesses so that you will be prepared to educate your patients.

Protein

Protein is the primary building block of the body to make new cells and to help wounds heal. Most of the organs and muscular and integumentary systems are constructed of protein. A gram of protein contains 4 kcal, and in a well-balanced diet protein should provide between 10% and 35% of the total daily calories. Most adults require a daily intake of 50 to 60 g of protein.

Protein Functions

The functions of protein include the following:

- New tissue production
- Formation of antibodies, enzymes, and hormones
- Necessary component for heat and energy production
- Component to assist in maintaining fluid balance between cells and bloodstream
- Maintaining acid-base balance

Protein Types

The human body contains more than 100,000 types of protein. Approximately 50% of this protein is found in skeletal muscle tissue. These proteins are composed of three types of amino acids: (1) nonessential, (2) conditional, and (3) essential (there are nine of these, and they contain the nitrogen needed by the body to build new tissue). The body continuously breaks down these proteins into its smaller components (amino acids) using the process of catabolism. Then through anabolism, these amino acids are reorganized, or built, into tissue products.

Nonessential amino acids are produced by the liver and thus are not essential to be included in our diet. Conditional amino acids are those that become essential *only* when an individual is stressed or ill with certain conditions. Dietary-wise, **essential amino acids** are the most important: They must be obtained from food sources because the body is unable to produce them. The proteins that contain all nine of these essential amino acids (along with some of the nonessential amino acids) are known as **complete proteins.** They come from animal and plant sources such as eggs, cheese, milk, sesame, peanuts, whitefish, pork, and beef.

• **WORD • BUILDING** •

hydrolyze: hydro – water + lyze – dissolve
proteolytic: proteo – protein + lytic – able to dissolve
lipolytic: lipo – fat + lytic – able to dissolve

Soy protein is the only source of complete proteins that is not an animal source.

Proteins that do not contain all nine of the essential amino acids are termed **incomplete proteins** and come from plant sources. They include corn, wheat, seeds, beans, brown rice, and nuts. It is important to note, though, that eating *combinations* of incomplete proteins provides the body with all nine amino acids needed for complete protein synthesis. By consuming two or more of the incomplete protein sources, an individual can still meet his or her protein requirements. Commonly used combinations include the following:

- Red beans and brown rice
- Peanut butter and whole wheat bread
- Brown beans and cornbread

Protein Digestion

Although much of protein digestion occurs in the small intestine, it begins in the stomach, where hydrochloric acid breaks down large proteins into amino acids, which are partially digested by the enzyme pepsin. Once the food moves from the stomach into the duodenum, trypsin works to further digest the amino acids so that they can be absorbed into the small projections of the intestinal wall, known as *villi.* Networks of capillaries are found inside the villi, providing nutrients access to the bloodstream. Now the blood distributes the amino acids to the entire body so that they can be used for anabolism, with the goal of maintaining a balance of protein between the blood and tissues.

Protein Deficiency and Excess Disorders

Due to poverty, a lack of education, and a lack of farming resources, protein deficiencies are more commonly found in underdeveloped countries than here in the United States. When they are found in the United States, they are generally due to poverty, but they may be seen in the higher socioeconomic populations due to a simple failure to eat adequate protein. Severe protein deficiency results in a disease known as *kwashiorkor.* It causes severe emaciation, a grossly edematous (swollen) abdomen due to ascites (fluid collection in the peritoneal cavity) and liver enlargement, lethargy, failure to grow, and skin infections. If not treated early, limitations in mental development will also occur.

The consumption of excess protein does not result in additional muscle building. The excess protein is metabolized and stored as fat to be used at a later time when an additional energy source is required. Excess protein can play a role in worsening of kidney disease. Protein intake and the removal of nitrogen (a waste product of protein digestion) by the kidneys should be in balance in most situations. However, there are times when retained nitrogen needs to be more or less than at other times. (See Box 23.3 for information on nitrogen balance.)

Box 23.3

Nitrogen Balance

The amount of nitrogen that is ingested in the form of protein should balance with the level of nitrogen that is utilized by the body and excesses that are removed from the body by the kidneys. When these levels are equal, it is called ***nitrogen balance.*** When the intake of nitrogen is larger than the amounts excreted in the urine, there is nitrogen left over to build new tissue. This is known as a state of positive nitrogen balance and is necessary during the growth of a fetus during pregnancy, the quick growth spurts during childhood, and during times of repair, as in healing large burns or wounds.

Negative nitrogen balance occurs when excess nitrogen is excreted, with inadequate amounts of protein being consumed in the diet. Negative nitrogen balance occurs commonly in malnutrition. This condition can cause a loss of muscle tone, weight loss, failure to heal or repair tissue, and growth retardation. Nitrogen balance is measured in blood urea nitrogen in the blood and urea urine nitrogen levels in a 24-hour urine test.

KNOWLEDGE CONNECTION

How many calories are there in a gram of protein? How many grams of protein should the average adult ingest daily? What are the functions of protein? Explain the difference between complete and incomplete proteins. Which type of protein is found in animal sources? Plant sources? Give two examples of food combinations that will provide complete proteins.

Fats/Lipids

While fat may seem like something that we want to avoid, it is actually a necessary macronutrient needed for a variety of functions in the body. Unlike the other two macronutrients, fats provide 9 kcals per gram ingested, so they are twice as high in calories per gram as protein and carbohydrates. Knowing which fats are most beneficial and why will help you choose fat calories carefully.

Types of Fats and Lipids

Some fats and lipids are manufactured and stored by the body, and some are obtained through foods. Our livers manufacture a fat or lipid called *cholesterol.* It is a necessary component for good health, but it must be kept within certain limits or it can become a health hazard that leads to various disease processes.

Cholesterol is transported throughout the body by low-density lipoprotein (LDL) and high-density lipoprotein (HDL). The LDL is commonly known as *bad cholesterol* because it transports the cholesterol to the cells from the liver,

• WORD • BUILDING •

lipoprotein: lipo – fat + protein

and too much is a bad thing. If the cells do not use all of the cholesterol that is carried to them, the cholesterol can build up and lodge in artery walls. HDL is the transporter responsible for taking the excess cholesterol back to the liver from the cells, helping to maintain a proper balance. Thus, its common name is *good cholesterol.*

Triglycerides are a form of fat that is stored in the body but is also found in food. They are made from any combination of three fatty acids. Any time excess fats are ingested, they may be stored as triglyceride within the fat cells. An excessively high level of triglycerides contributes to coronary artery disease and other metabolic syndromes.

Laboratory values for total cholesterol, LDL, HDL, and triglycerides are grouped into a *lipid profile* (Table 23.2). A trick for remembering which cholesterol is desired at higher ranges and which one at lower ranges is that the *L*DL (bad cholesterol) should be *l*ow and the *H*DL (good cholesterol) should be *h*igh.

DIETARY FATS. When one hears the term *dietary fats* or *lipids*, it is commonly in connection with a negative perspective, but a healthy diet must include a certain amount of fat.

Dietary fat is broken down into several categories, including saturated, monounsaturated, polyunsaturated, and trans fats. Some fats are good for us, while others are implicated with cardiovascular disease because they raise cholesterol levels as well as being associated with type II diabetes. This makes it important that you learn the differences between them. The healthiest fats to include in the diet are the monounsaturated and the polyunsaturated fats.

MONOUNSATURATED AND POLYUNSATURATED FATS. Monounsaturated fats become solid when they are refrigerated but are liquid when they are kept at room temperature; they include olive oil, canola oil, and peanut oil. They are better for us because they help to lower our blood levels of the bad cholesterol, LDL.

Polyunsaturated fats are found in sources such as corn oil, soybean oil, sesame oil, and safflower oil. Two examples of essential polyunsaturated fats are the omega-3 and omega-6 fatty acids that are found in several types of fatty fish, walnuts, and flaxseed. These are known to decrease one's risk of type II diabetes and cardiovascular disease.

SATURATED FATS. *Saturated fats* come from animal sources, are solid at room temperature, and are implicated in cardiovascular disease because they raise blood cholesterol. Thus, these fats should be limited in a healthy diet. Although most saturated fats are found in animal sources such as meat, whole milk, and cheese, some are present in coconut and palm oils, hydrogenated vegetable oil, and cocoa butter, which are common ingredients in packaged foods such as cookies, cakes, and pies.

TRANS FATS. *Trans fats* are vegetable oils that have been partially hydrogenated, a process of adding hydrogen, which changes the unsaturated fat to saturated fat. Trans fats are used to keep foods fresh and are found mostly in processed and fast foods. They have been linked to increasing blood cholesterol levels and are being slowly removed from processed foods.

Functions of Fats

Cholesterol, which is manufactured by the body, is required to:

- Form each of the body cell membranes of every system
- Produce the adrenal and sex hormones as well as bile
- Protect our nerves
- Convert sunshine to vitamin D
- Help metabolize fat-soluble vitamins

Dietary fats that are ingested are needed by the body; they are an essential concentrated source of fatty acids and energy and are necessary for healthy skin. In addition, dietary fats are required to help the body absorb fat-soluble vitamins. They are stored as fatty (adipose) tissue, helping to support the internal organs and insulating the body from environmental temperature extremes.

Fat Digestion

Lingual lipase starts working on the fat in the mouth. Then food is swallowed and remains in the stomach longer than carbohydrates, which provides a longer sense of feeling full. Gastric lipase and gastric churning help to break down the fats before they move into the small intestine, where the bulk

Table 23.2
Lipid Panel Laboratory Value Ranges for Adults

Test Component	*Desired Level*	*Near Desired Level*	*Borderline*	*Health Risk*
Total cholesterol	less than 170 mg/dL	N/A	170–199 mg/dL	more than 200 mg/dL
Low-density lipoprotein (LDL) (bad)	less than 100 mg/dL	100–129 mg/dL	130–159 mg/dL	more than 159 mg/dL
High-density lipoprotein (HDL) (good)	more than 60 mg/dL	N/A	40–60 mg/dL	less than 40 mg/dL
Triglycerides	less than 150 mg/dL	N/A	150–199 mg/dL	more than 199 mg/dL

of fat digestion occurs. There the fats are emulsified, or broken down into tiny droplets, by bile acids from the gallbladder. Pancreatic lipase changes the fat molecules into fatty acids and monoglycerols, which are absorbed into the bloodstream through the intestinal villi for use throughout the body. Fatty acids and glycerol are utilized in the production of phospholipids, the primary component of cell membranes for all body systems. Any fats that are not used are stored as adipose (fatty) tissue.

Fat/Lipid Deficiency and Excess Disorders

Too little fat intake is rare in the United States. However, if a person is eating a severely fat-restricted diet for a long period of time, it is possible for him or her to become deficient in fat-soluble vitamins since they are stored in the body fat.

The American Heart Association recommends that no more than 25% to 35% of one's total daily intake of calories should come from fat to help prevent coronary artery disease and other metabolic syndromes. It is important to note that the majority of one's consumed fat should be the healthier fats rather than saturated fat. An overindulgence of saturated fats or eating more than 35% of the daily caloric intake in the form of fat is known to contribute to being overweight and obese. Remember that fat provides twice as many calories per gram ingested as protein and carbohydrates.

KNOWLEDGE CONNECTION

How many calories does a gram of fat provide? Which type of cholesterol is desired in higher ranges? Which of the types of fat are considered to contribute to cardiovascular disease? List several sources of trans fat, saturated fat, monounsaturated fat, and polyunsaturated fat. Which type of fat is known to decrease the bad cholesterol known as LDL? What are some food sources that a person might consume to help keep LDLs in the lower range?

Carbohydrates

Carbohydrates provide 4 kcal of energy per gram. As with fat, overindulgence in carbohydrates contributes to excessive weight gain and obesity.

Types of Carbohydrates

Carbohydrates are classified as either simple or complex. **Simple carbohydrates,** also known as *simple sugars,* are chemically made up of one or two sugar molecules that are absorbed rapidly. The following are four examples of simple sugars:

- ***Glucose:*** our primary energy source, the most common form
- ***Fructose:*** fruit sugar, the sweetest natural sugar
- ***Sucrose:*** table sugar
- ***Lactose:*** milk sugar, the least-sweet natural sugar

Box 23.4

Food Sources of Complex Carbohydrates

Potatoes, white and sweet	Oatmeal and rolled oats
Brown rice	Whole-grain wheat bread
Millet, buckwheat, and bulgur	Pasta
Broccoli	Whole fresh fruit
Beans and legumes	Peas and lentils
Whole-grain, high-fiber, low-sugar cereals	

Sources of simple carbohydrates include fruit juice, honey, milk, white bread, table sugar, syrup, candy, pastries, and colas. The starches and fiber (cellulose) make up **complex carbohydrates.** Chemically, they differ from the simple carbohydrates because they have long chains of three or more molecules of sugar, so they take a little longer to digest, absorb, and produce energy for the body. Food sources of complex carbohydrates can be found in Box 23.4.

One of the main differences between simple and complex carbohydrates is their effects on the blood glucose level. Simple carbohydrates, such as glucose and fructose, cause a rapid rise in the blood glucose level. The high blood glucose level then stimulates the pancreas to produce more insulin, which will rapidly decrease blood glucose and increase appetite, and thus increase eating. When this occurs excessively, we put on extra pounds. It is wiser to consume more complex carbohydrates than simple carbohydrates because they help us to feel full longer and provide a more stable blood glucose level.

Functions of Carbohydrates

Carbohydrates serve as the primary source of energy for the body, particularly the cardiovascular, musculoskeletal, and nervous systems. They are more quickly digested into a useable form for energy (glucose) than either proteins or fats.

The USDA recommends that 45% to 65% of one's total calorie consumption come from complex carbohydrates, but there is no actual recommendation for how much of the diet should come from simple carbohydrates, just that they should be limited. Excess glucose from carbohydrate breakdown normally is stored in the liver and skeletal muscles in the form of glycogen, to be used at a later time as an energy source. Without adequate consumption of complex carbohydrates, the readily available glucose and the stores of glycogen will be insufficient for energy production. Thus the body will resort to burning fat and protein for energy, reducing the available protein for repairing damaged tissue and growing new tissue.

Carbohydrate Digestion

As we just mentioned, the starchy carbohydrates are reduced to glucose during digestion. Salivary amylase in the mouth, along with amylase and maltase in the small intestine, break

• WORD • BUILDING •

phospholipids: phos – light + pho – carry + lipids – fat down the starches to glucose. Very little digestion of starch occurs while it is in the stomach. In the duodenum, absorption takes place through the intestinal wall villi into the bloodstream, where it is transported directly to the cells for immediate use, or to the liver for storage as glycogen.

Carbohydrate Deficiency and Excess Disorders

No known carbohydrate deficiency disease exists. However when a person does not eat enough glucose for the body's energy needs, the body burns stored fat. When this goes on for periods of time, it can cause a serious elevation in blood acid levels, called *ketosis.* This condition can be seen in people with type 1 diabetes mellitus whose bodies cannot access glucose to use for energy.

Excessive carbohydrate ingestion commonly leads to weight gain and obesity. Eating excessive carbohydrates raises the blood glucose; this in turn raises the insulin level, which then lowers blood glucose. A drop in one's glucose level results in hunger and food cravings, often for simple carbohydrates in the form of junk food. The more food that is consumed, especially simple carbohydrates, increases the amount of calories that must be burned to prevent weight gain.

Fiber

Fiber is included in our discussion of carbohydrates because it is a type of carbohydrate that the body cannot digest.

TYPES OF FIBER. Dietary fiber comes in two forms: soluble and insoluble. As soluble fiber is digested, it attracts water to form a gel-like substance, which remains in the stomach longer, providing the individual with a sense of feeling full for a longer period of time. The insoluble fiber is not digested but passes through the intestines, acting like a bulk laxative and drawing water into the intestines, helping to prevent constipation.

FUNCTIONS OF FIBER. A diet that includes adequate levels of fiber has numerous additional health benefits beyond the stabilization of blood glucose levels:

- A decrease in LDL cholesterol, which reduces the risk of coronary artery disease
- Promotion of normal bowel function and the prevention of constipation
- Increased absorption of minerals
- A lowered colon pH, which helps to discourage pathogen and cancer cell growth
- Support of GI tract normal flora by providing them with a food source
- Promotion of weight loss

For optimal health, the average adult needs 25 to 35 g of fiber every day, but few people in the United States consume more than half of this amount. This contributes to numerous health issues that are so easily prevented. Teach your patients about the health benefits of fiber, the food sources of fiber, and the amount to ingest daily. However, it is very important to explain that when increasing fiber intake, a person must do so gradually or he or she will suffer *extreme problems with flatus.* Explain that fiber should be increased slowly over 2 to 4 weeks to give the GI tract time to adjust to the sudden increase. Refer to Table 23.3 for food sources of soluble and insoluble fiber.

KNOWLEDGE CONNECTION

How many calories per gram are in carbohydrates compared to fats and protein? Explain the difference between simple carbohydrates and complex carbohydrates. What percentage of total daily caloric intake should come from carbohydrates? List at least four food sources of fiber. What is the recommended daily intake of fiber?

Vitamins

Safety: It is vital to consume an adequate amount of most vitamins in our daily diet (or through supplements) because the body cannot manufacture many of them. With exposure of the skin to sunlight 15 minutes twice per week, the body can synthesize a significant amount of the needed vitamin D. The normal flora of the intestines also helps by producing vitamin K, but most of our vitamins are obtained from plant sources and animal products. They are a crucial component for the body's metabolic processes, such as synthesis of hemoglobin, conduction of nerve impulses, bone and collagen development, and blood clotting. There are two categories of vitamins: water soluble and fat soluble.

Table 23.3
Food Sources of Fiber

Soluble	*Insoluble*
• Oat bran	• Brown rice
• Beans	• Whole wheat
• Rice bran	• Bran
• Oatmeal	• Dark green leafy vegetables
• Apples	• Nuts
• Strawberries	• Seeds
• Oranges	• Cucumbers
• Pears	• Cabbage
• Blueberries	• Tomatoes
• Dried peas	• Broccoli
• Celery	• Grapes/raisins
• Carrots	• Fruit

Water-soluble vitamins are dissolvable in water and therefore can be absorbed directly into the bloodstream from the GI tract. They cannot be stored in the body, and some of them are lost in the urine, thus the necessity of consuming them on a daily basis. Water-soluble vitamins include the following:

- B vitamins
  - B1 (thiamine)
  - B2 (riboflavin)
  - B3 (niacin)
  - B4 (adenine)
  - B5 (pantothenic acid)
  - B6 (pyridoxine)
  - B7 (biotin)
  - B8 (inositol)
  - B9 (folic acid)
  - B10 (para-aminobenzoic acid)
  - B11 (choline)
  - B12 (cyanocobalamin)
- Vitamin C (ascorbic acid)

Among other functions, the B vitamins serve as coenzymes for metabolism throughout the body, and they help to stimulate appetite, maintain healthy nervous and integumentary systems, and assist with growth. Vitamin C is essential in immune system functioning, helps the body absorb iron, and is vital for wound healing. Some vitamins are used to treat specific disease conditions. Vitamin B_3 (niacin) is used to treat hyperlipidemia, and vitamin B_6 (pyridoxine) is used to prevent peripheral neuropathy in patients taking the drug isoniazid (INH) for tuberculosis.

Fat-soluble vitamins A, D, E, and K are dissolvable only in fat, and, unlike water-soluble vitamins, they can be stored in body fat when there is more ingested than the body needs at that specific time. ***Safety: Because fat-soluble vitamins can be stored, they can become toxic when consumed in excessively large doses over a long period of time.***

Vitamin Deficiencies and Excesses

Vitamin deficiencies in the United States are generally due to malabsorption disorders that prevent the vitamins from being absorbed and used by the body. Examples of such disorders include Crohn's disease, celiac disease, and pancreatitis. Vitamin deficiencies may also be due to poor nutritional habits.

Vitamin excesses are usually due to overuse or inappropriate use of dietary supplements. Refer to Table 23.4 for information about deficiencies and excesses of vitamins.

Antioxidants

Physical and emotional stress and environmental factors such as poor diet, pollution, certain medications, and alcohol can cause body cells to react with molecules of oxygen in a way that produces unstable molecules called *free radicals.* These free radicals can cause damage to DNA and protein, which can lead to various diseases such as cancer. Vitamins A, C, and E are known as **antioxidants** because they have been identified as helping to deactivate these free radicals before they can cause damage. Ultimately, the antioxidants help to promote health and prevent disease. Table 23.4 provides information about vitamin functions, sources, deficiencies, and excesses.

KNOWLEDGE CONNECTION

Which vitamins are water soluble? Which are fat soluble? Which vitamins are toxic when consumed in excessive doses? Explain the function of antioxidants. Relate at least three functions of the B vitamins. Which vitamin is important for growing new tissue such as is required after surgery? Which vitamins are antioxidants?

Minerals

Minerals are inorganic compounds that come from the earth, and because they cannot be digested, they retain their original structure once ingested. They are classified as either major or trace minerals. Major minerals are those that we must ingest a minimum of 100 mg/d for optimal health, and trace minerals are those that we require less than 100 mg/d. The most abundant mineral in the body is calcium. Up to 99% of body calcium is stored in the bones, leaving only 1% to circulate in the bloodstream to be utilized by the rest of the body. Minerals are used by all body tissues for numerous functions, including the following:

- Forming the structure of the hard parts of the body (bones, teeth, nails)
- Assisting in water metabolism; fluid and electrolyte balance
- Activating enzymes and hormones
- Assisting in acid-base balance
- Nerve cell transmission
- Muscle contraction

For a breakdown of major and trace minerals, refer to Box 23.5. Major functions and sources of minerals are listed in Table 23.5.

Mineral Deficiencies and Excesses

Mineral deficiencies do not normally develop in people who routinely eat well-balanced diets. However, following a restrictive diet can result in a shortage of one or more minerals. Someone who does not use iodized salt and does not like any type of seafood will be at risk for developing an iodine deficiency. ***Safety: Vegetarians may be at risk for iron deficiency unless they are careful to ingest a higher level of iron-rich, nonmeat foods such as beans, dried fruit, whole grains, and molasses.***

• WORD • BUILDING •
hyperlipidemia: hyper – excessive + lipid – fat + emia – blood

Table 23.4
Vitamin Deficiencies and Excesses

Vitamin	*Source*	*Physiological Functions*	*Deficiency*	*Excess*
Fat-Soluble Vitamins				
A (two forms): retinol and beta-carotene	Liver, pumpkin, sweet potatoes, whole milk, cheese, carrots, egg yolk, cod, and cantaloupe	Beta-carotene is an antioxidant. Helps to form skin, bone, teeth, and mucous membranes and keeps them healthy. Promotes night vision.	Infections and vision problems	Nausea, dizziness, headache, dermatitis, coma, and death
D	Vitamin D–fortified dairy products, fortified margarine, fatty fish, beef liver, and eggs (The body can make vitamin D using the energy of sunlight on the skin.)	Helps to harden bones and teeth. Necessary to absorb calcium.	Rickets in children and bone softening and deformity in adults	Rare but serious, nausea, vomiting, anorexia, kidney stones and damage, and mental and physical growth retardation
E	Vegetable oils, fortified cereals, tomatoes, peanut butter, leafy vegetables, avocadoes, whole grains, sunflower seeds, nuts, and asparagus	Acts as an antioxidant, helping to slow down cell-damaging processes. Helps cells to communicate with each other. Helps protect skin from ultraviolet light damage.	Peripheral neuropathy and ataxia	Normally no side effects, but researchers differ in opinion; some feel it can act as an anticoagulant
K	Made by intestinal bacteria Food sources include spinach, meat, asparagus, beans, eggs, and strawberries	Helps blood to clot.	Excessive bleeding	No toxicity symptoms reported
Water-Soluble Vitamins				
B1 (thiamine)	Beef, liver, pork, whole grains, enriched breads and cereals, powdered milk, nuts, seeds, and dried peas and beans	Provides energy via carbohydrate metabolism. Promotes muscle function and nerve conduction.	Weakness, mental confusion, fatigue, heart problems, paralysis, edema, death, and beriberi and Wernicke's disease	No toxicity symptoms reported, excess eliminated in urine

Table 23.4
Vitamin Deficiencies and Excesses—cont'd

Vitamin	*Source*	*Physiological Functions*	*Deficiency*	*Excess*
B2 (riboflavin)	Eggs, milk and dairy products, broccoli, Brussels sprouts, spinach, mushrooms, and enriched breads and cereals	Antioxidant. Red blood cell production. Metabolism of carbohydrates into glucose.	Fatigue, GI problems, cracks at mouth corners, and swollen magenta-colored tongue *Uncommon:* dermatitis, light sensitivity, and anemia	No toxicity symptoms reported
B3 (niacin)	Meat, beets, yeast, fish, milk, sunflower seeds, and peanuts	Improves circulation. Helps break down fats and protein. Promotes healthy hair, skin, eyes, and liver. Assists adrenal gland to make hormones. Promotes healthy nervous system function.	Canker sores, indigestion, vomiting, and fatigue *Pellagra:* Four Ds • Dermatitis • Diarrhea • Dementia • Death	Flushing due to capillary dilation, liver damage, gastric ulcers, and nausea and vomiting
B6	Meat, fish, poultry, fruits (not citrus), potatoes, liver, and fortified cereals	Assists enzyme functions. Essential in protein metabolism. Promotes healthy nervous system and immune system function.	Can be asymptomatic Dermatitis, cracks at mouth corners, glossitis, weakened immune system, depression, and confusion	Peripheral neuropathy (numbness, pain, tingling of extremities)
B12	Sardines, salmon, cod, scallops, fortified breakfast cereals, yogurt, milk, and veal	Helps develop and maintain nervous system. Essential for red blood cell formation and DNA production. Assists with protein, carbohydrate, and fat metabolism.	Tongue soreness and erythema, dandruff, heart palpitations, pallor, nervousness, peripheral neuropathy, forgetfulness, and macrocytic anemia	No toxicity symptoms reported
C	Citrus fruits, papaya, strawberries, green and red peppers, parsley, turnip greens, Brussels sprouts, cauliflower, and broccoli	Antioxidant. Growth of collagen tissue, skin; especially wound healing. Helps to keep teeth and gums healthy.	*Scurvy:* bleeding gums, dry skin, petechia, poor wound healing, dry hair, and anemia	Rare but can cause diarrhea, abdominal cramping, and nausea

Box 23.5

Minerals

Six Major Minerals	Nine Trace Minerals
Calcium	Chromium
Chloride	Copper
Magnesium	Fluoride
Potassium	Iodine
Phosphorus	Iron
Sodium	Manganese
	Molybdenum
	Selenium
	Zinc

Note: Both major and trace minerals are equally important for optimal body functioning.

Mineral excesses may be due to improper use of supplements in adults. The accidental ingestion of iron supplements by infants and children can lead to serious iron toxicities. A genetic abnormality known as *hemochromatosis* is a disease in which the person absorbs and accumulates excessive stores of iron. Another genetic abnormality, Wilson's disease, causes the body to absorb an excess of copper from the intestine, which then accumulates in the corneas, brain, liver, and kidneys. Refer to Table 23.5 for information on the effects of mineral deficiencies and excesses.

Water

Next to oxygen, water is the most critical component to sustain life. Every cell, tissue, organ, and body system depends on adequate water intake to function properly. Water actually

Table 23.5

Functions and Sources of Minerals

Mineral	*Function*	*Sources*	*Effects of Deficiency and Excess*
Calcium	99% found in structure of bones and teeth, 1% in blood used for electrical conduction of nerve impulses in heart, and muscle contraction	Best sources are *dairy products (milk, cheese, cottage cheese, and yogurt), sardines, salmon, spinach, okra, broccoli, beans, almonds, oatmeal, and calcium-fortified juice	*Deficiency*: Tetany of muscles, bone and tooth loss; osteoporosis *Excess:* Constipation, flatus, and kidney stones
Chloride	Normal water distribution, electrical balance in cells, nerve impulse transmission	Beef, pork, cheese, *salt, lettuce, celery, and olives	*Deficiency*: Nausea, vomiting, and diarrhea
Chromium	Boosts metabolism, helps break down fat and glucose, promotes insulin balance	Green peppers, spinach, liver, beef, eggs, whole grains, bananas, and apples	*Deficiency*: May elevate blood glucose *Excess*: Liver damage
Copper	Assists with formation of red blood cells and bones, helps protect cells from damage, helps iron metabolism	Whole grains, mushrooms, beans, nuts, and oysters	*Deficiency:* Poor growth, fatigue, pallor, and anorexia
Fluoride	Promotes healthy bones and teeth	*Fluoridated drinking water, tea, coffee, and fish from salt water	*Deficiency:* Tooth decay *Excess:* Teeth staining and nausea
Iodine	Promotes thyroid function	Saltwater seafood and *iodized salt	*Deficiency:* Goiter, hypothyroidism, inhibited infant growth, mental sluggishness, and weight gain *Excess:* Nausea, burning of oral mucosa, diarrhea, inflammation of thyroid, and thyroid cancer

Table 23.5
Functions and Sources of Minerals—cont'd

Mineral	*Function*	*Sources*	*Effects of Deficiency and Excess*
Iron	Essential component of protein/hemoglobin that transports oxygen in the blood; serves as a component of enzymes	Red meats, fish, poultry, whole grains, molasses, dried fruits, lentils, and beans	*Deficiency:* Pallor, fatigue, shortness of breath, headache, increased irritability, anemia, and fainting *Excess:* Missed periods, discoloration of skin, and joint swelling and pain
Magnesium	Supports muscle contraction and nerve conduction, electrical conduction of heart, and energy production	Spinach, seafood, bran cereal, legumes, dairy products, and nuts and seeds	*Deficiency:* May cause elevated blood pressure (BP), agitation, restless leg syndrome, hypotension, muscle spasms, insomnia, and arrhythmias *Excess:* Increased calcium excretion, weakness, malaise, and GI symptoms
Manganese	Promotes bone formation and metabolism of carbohydrates, cholesterol, and amino acids	Whole grain products, beans, nuts, and tea	*Deficiency*: Fainting, hearing loss, dermatitis, ataxia, and slowed hair growth *Excess*: Shaking and tremors, stiff muscles, hypertension, impaired memory, and psychosis
Molybdenum	Assists in metabolism of amino acids	Nuts, grains and grain products, beans, and peas	*Deficiency*: Difficulty seeing at night, gum problems, tachypnea, and tachycardia *Excess*: Diarrhea, joint swelling, anemia
Phosphorus	Serves as a structural component of bone and cell membranes	Dairy products, eggs, poultry, red meat, and fish	*Deficiency*: Anorexia, fatigue, fragile bones, bone pain, bone loss, and increased irritability *Excess:* Muscle tetany, seizures, and hypocalcemia
Potassium	Needed for proper nerve conduction, especially the heart and muscles, helps to maintain healthy BP level	Bananas, cantaloupe, tomato sauce and puree, white and sweet potatoes, tuna, cod, skim milk, peas, and beans	*Deficiency:* Muscle weakness and cramping, malaise, fatigue, nausea, vomiting, cramping, numbness, tingling, and life-threatening arrhythmias and cardiac arrest *Excess:* Anorexia, fatigue, extreme muscle weakness, and life-threatening arrhythmias
Selenium	Antioxidant (reduces oxidation of certain molecules), promotes thyroid hormone function	Seafood and organ meats	*Deficiency*: Keshan disease *Excess*: Hair loss, nail problems, and increased irritability
Sodium	Regulates body compartment fluid levels, acid-base balance; needed for proper nerve conduction and muscle contraction	Salt, celery, beets, dairy products, pork, beef, and *processed foods (Americans' primary source)	*Deficiency:* Stomach cramps, nausea, vomiting, diarrhea, lethargy, headache, confusion, and seizures due to brain swelling *Excess:* Edema and fluid retention, thirst, dry sticky mucous membranes, and elevated BP
Zinc	Necessary for proper growth, supports immune system, serves as a component of over 50 enzymes, essential in wound healing, helps maintain senses of smell and taste	Pork, red meat, lamb, poultry, whole grains, yeast, fortified breakfast cereal, beans, and nuts	*Deficiency*: Hair loss, delayed wound healing, rashes, anorexia, hypogonadism in males, and difficulty with taste and smell *Excess*: Abdominal cramping and diarrhea

*Denotes primary source of specific nutrient.

comprises more than half of the body's weight: 55% to 60% in adult females, 60% to 65% in adult males, and 65% to 70% in full-term infants. Chapter 29 provides more information about the percentages of water found in individuals of different ages, as well as the water composition of the brain, lungs, and blood. Refer to Box 23.6 for a list of the functions of water in the body.

The Institute of Medicine recommends that the average male adult drink 14 to 15 8-ounce glasses of fluid per day and the average female adult approximately 11 glasses per day. There are other researchers who believe the average adult only needs a minimum of six to eight 8-ounce glasses, or 1,440 to 1,920 mL, of water per day. Amid the controversy surrounding the minimum volume of water and fluid required for optimal health, most tend to follow the lesser recommendations of eight 8-ounce glasses per day. We recommend following the latter guideline of six to eight glasses per day.

The volume required will also vary according to the level of activity, health status, age, size, and degree of body fat. Exercise and physical exertion will increase the body's water requirement due to the losses through increased metabolism and perspiration. When the environmental temperatures are hot, as in the summer, or when a person is working in a hot environment, their water requirements will naturally rise. An individual with congestive heart failure or renal failure may be more restricted in fluid volume intake. Someone with a bacterial or viral infection will need to drink more fluids to help flush the toxins from the body. Fever, vomiting, and diarrhea deplete fluid volumes, thus increasing the need for additional fluids. Those individuals who have a higher body fat content may require more fluids than lean individuals, as fat holds very little water compared to lean muscle. It is particularly pertinent that pregnant or nursing women drink more fluids than nonpregnant women.

KNOWLEDGE CONNECTION

Explain at least four functions of water. What is the commonly recommended volume of fluid intake per day? Which groups of people require more intake of water than the average person? How much water do you drink daily?

Box 23.6

Functions of Water

- Maintains body temperature
- Transports minerals, vitamins, and electrolytes
- Cushions the brain and spinal cord
- Lubricates joints
- Carries toxins and excreted waste products out of the body
- Moisturizes and lubricates the gastrointestinal tract to aid the passage of food through the intestines

Real-World Connection

If a Little Is Good, Is More Better?

A young registered nurse who had only been out of nursing school for 3 years was very health conscious and physically active. She exercised 5 to 6 days a week, participated in various sports, drank lots of water, took time to have fun and play regularly, worked to eat a balanced diet, and took a daily multiple vitamin. After having several bouts of colds and allergies, she decided to boost her immunity by taking a vitamin C supplement, adding up to 4,000 mg of vitamin C per day. After 7 months she got tired of taking so many pills every day and discontinued the supplement. A week or so later she noticed large areas of *petechiae,* pinpoint-size flat red spots due to capillary ruptures, over much of her body. The rash continued to spread for 4 days. Although the rash did not itch, it was a source of concern and she decided to seek medical attention. Ultimately, it was determined that even though she ate well and was in good nutritional condition, she was suffering from some of the symptoms of scurvy, a disease caused by inadequate intake of vitamin C. By ingesting such high levels of vitamin C supplements for several months and then stopping the supplements cold turkey rather than weaning herself off them slowly, she had subjected her body to a *faux* scurvy. Even though she was still getting adequate vitamin C in her diet, her body misinterpreted the sudden and dramatic drop in vitamin C intake to be a deficiency of vitamin C.

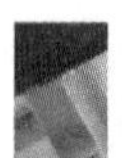

DIFFERING NUTRITIONAL NEEDS OVER THE LIFE SPAN

Nutritional requirements constantly change throughout one's life span. Certain factors such as age, gender, periods of high growth rate, activity level, illness and injuries, and pregnancy all will contribute to the changing needs of each individual.

Toddlers and Preschool-Age Children

After the age of 1 year, a child may be switched from breastfeeding or formula to cow's milk. Children need a serving of milk or another dairy product with each meal because their bones and teeth are growing rapidly. It is recommended that whole milk be used as opposed to reduced-fat milk because young children require a certain level of fat in their diets. Approximately 30% to 35% of caloric intake should come from fats, as dietary fats are vital to the formation of healthy nerves and brain.

Small children need to consume a wide variety of foods to meet their nutrient requirements for the rapid growth that occurs during this time. To meet needs for iron and protein, offer a peanut butter sandwich on whole-grain bread. Approximately one-fourth of each meal should come from whole grains, which contain more nutrients than refined grains. Whole wheat pasta and bread help provide these requirements.

To encourage small children to eat a wide variety of vegetables, offer "finger foods" such as the following:

- Raisins
- Grapes
- Sliced apples
- Sliced bananas
- Cut-up carrots
- Cherry tomatoes
- Broccoli, cauliflower, cucumbers, along with dip

Safety: For the very young child, it will be necessary to cut the fruits and veggies into smaller bite-size pieces to avoid choking. (See Table 23.6 for serving recommendations for children of this age.)

The American Academy of Pediatrics recommends that standard children's vitamin supplements are only necessary for children with poor appetites, those with health conditions that affect their nutritional intake, or those who eat restricted diets, such as a vegetarian diet. ***Safety: Mega doses of vitamins should never be given to children except under a pediatrician's direct order and care. Because many children's vitamins are made to take in the form of gummy bears or sweet treats, it is important to teach parents to keep all vitamins out of the child's reach to prevent accidental overdose.***

School-Age Children

It is important to gauge the quantities of food to be consumed according to the activity level of the child to prevent the child from becoming overweight and obese. However, school-age children will experience growth spurts at times that will increase their energy needs and thus their caloric intake.

School-age children need protein and calcium at higher rates than younger children. It is important to help children develop healthy eating habits that will generally last a lifetime. Encourage children to snack on healthier choices, such as the following:

- Dried fruits, nuts, and seeds (trail mix)
- Whole fruits and berries
- Raw vegetables with dip

In addition, encourage children to drink water more frequently than sugary beverages. Water flavored with slices of fruit such as strawberries, oranges, or melon may help it be more appealing to the school-age child. (See Table 23.6 for serving recommendations for children of this age.)

Adolescents

Adolescence brings additional periods of rapid growth, usually between 10 and 15 years of age for girls and between 12 and 14 years for boys. This is a period of great energy expenditure, which increases the need for nutrients, especially calcium, protein, iron, vitamins, and minerals.

Healthy eating patterns established in childhood are beneficial to adolescents. They may feel a great deal of pressure to be a certain body size or shape and to look a certain way. Such pressure may lead to anorexia nervosa or bulimia.

Teens are often very busy with many activities and are eating on the go. Fast foods are readily available but often lack the nutrition needed by this age group. Encourage foods that are high in calcium and other nutrients, such as the following:

- Milk, cheese sticks, and yogurt
- Green leafy vegetables and salads
- Calcium-fortified juices
- Cereals
- Soy products
- Enriched breads and bread products
- Vegetables and fruits

Some fast food restaurants and convenience foods are making an effort to offer healthier food items. Encourage adolescents to make better choices and eat more fruits and vegetables as half of their meal. (See Table 23.6 for serving recommendations for this age group.)

Table 23.6

Recommended Intake for Various Age Groups of Average Size and Activity Level

	Fruit	*Vegetables*	*Grains*	*Proteins*	*Dairy*	*Oils*
Toddlers and Preschoolers	1–1 1/2 c	1–1 1/2 c	3–5 oz	2–4 oz	2–2 1/2 c	3–4 tsp*
School-aged Children	1–1 1/2 c	1 1/2 –2 1/2 c	5–6 oz	4–6 1/2 oz	2 1/2–3 c	4–5 tsp*
Adolescents	1 1/2–2 c	2–3 c	5–8 oz	5–6 1/2 oz	3 c	5–6 tsp*
Adults	1 1/2–2 c	1 1/2–3 c	6–8 oz	5 1/2–6 oz	3 c	5–7 tsp*
Older Adults	1 1/2–2 c	2–2 1/2 c	5–6 oz	5–5 1/2 oz	3 c	5–6 tsp*

*If adequate amounts are not eaten in fish, nuts, etc.

Patient Teaching Connection

Pregnancy: Weight Gain and Diet

You are working with a group of pregnant teenagers at a local clinic. Many of the teens express concern about weight gain during pregnancy. ***Safety: It is essential to teach pregnant teens that weight gain and proper nutrition during pregnancy are important determinants of growth and proper development of the baby and that poor weight gain and abnormal development are directly associated with low calorie intake and inadequate intake of vital nutrients.*** This makes it pertinent that the young mothers eat adequate amounts of the essential nutrients in an effort to prevent low birth weights and unhealthy babies. Explain that weight gain is based on a person's prepregnancy BMI. Weight gain for a pregnant adolescent should total between 25 and 40 pounds (11.3 to 18.1 kg). During the second and third trimesters, adolescents should gain approximately 1 pound (2.2 kg) per week. Additional nutrient requirements, such as folic acid, iron, and vitamin C, should be emphasized. Explain to the teens that adequate calcium is also needed for healthy growth. The best way for a pregnant teenager to meet her dietary needs is to maintain a regular three-meal schedule with three nutritious snacks, keeping in mind that adequate servings from all five of the different food groups are important. A varied, balanced eating plan is the only way to provide enough nutrients and food energy during pregnancy and to allow for healthy development of the baby. Stress the importance of taking prenatal vitamins as directed throughout the pregnancy and lactation.

Adulthood

The nutritional needs of adults, as in every other age group, will vary somewhat depending on age, gender, height, weight, and level of activity, but they generally tend to decrease with age.

At the onset of adulthood, energy requirements usually reach a plateau that will last until one's mid-40s, after which they begin to decline, primarily because activity and the amount of muscle versus body fat both decline. So as activity level begins to slow, the total calories consumed each day should correspondingly decrease. To assist with weight maintenance and optimal adult health, a regular exercise program is considered vital. Weight gain in adulthood is closely associated with the development of cardiovascular disease and diabetes.

While total calories required by the adult decreases, there are some nutrient requirements for women that increase with age, and numerous nutrient needs increase with pregnancy and lactation. As women age and get closer to menopause, with a decrease in the occurrence of pregnancy, their need for iron decreases. However, there is a need to increase calcium intake due to the decreased calcium absorption and the increased risk for osteoporosis in postmenopausal females. (See Table 23.6 for serving recommendations for adults.)

Older Adults

Many factors, including decreased appetite, impaired digestion, decreased GI absorption and motility, decreased senses of smell and taste, less physical activity, and slower metabolism, affect the nutritional status of older adults. Bone and muscle mass decrease as a natural part of aging and becoming less active. More calories are stored as fat due to reduced energy needs.

As more fat is stored (commonly around the abdomen), more fatty acids are released into the bloodstream, raising lipid and glucose levels. Then insulin levels automatically rise in an effort to combat the elevated glucose levels in the blood, making the older adult at risk for development of diabetes and cardiovascular disease.

Weight-bearing exercise is necessary for calcium uptake into the bones, but this usually decreases with aging. Lack of weight-bearing exercise and menopause in women can lead to osteoporosis.

Sometimes when older adults are on a fixed income, they may find it difficult to afford the foods needed for healthy eating. However, this age group should be encouraged to eat different forms of protein and calcium if meat and dairy are too expensive. Elderly people who live alone may not enjoy preparing food for one person and may dislike eating alone. Meals served to senior citizens at various locations in the community can help mitigate this nutritional issue.

The older adult needs the same nutrients as he or she needed as a younger adult but may have increased needs for calcium and vitamin D for the absorption of calcium; increased fiber to combat the slowed GI motility that can cause constipation; adequate iron to prevent anemia; and adequate protein intake to help fight infection, restore muscle mass that is lost due to immobility, and to promote healing of fractures and wounds. (See Table 23.6 for serving recommendations for older adults.)

KNOWLEDGE CONNECTION

Describe at least two differences in nutritional needs for each age group through the life span. According to these recommendations, what might be lacking in your daily diet?

Obesity

Being overweight or obese results from eating more calories than you use each day. This affects all ages over the life span. The calories that are not burned are stored and add body weight. Obesity is measured by many scales, most commonly through measurement of the **body mass index** (BMI). This measurement uses a formula, along with an individual's weight and height, to calculate whether her or his level of fatness is within normal weight boundaries, or whether she or he is underweight, overweight, or obese. The BMI is a useful tool when evaluating a person's health risks. Individuals whose BMI falls under 18.5 are generally considered to be underweight, and those with a BMI between 18.5 and 24.9 are within the normal weight range. Those whose BMI is between 25 and 29.9 are considered to be overweight, and those with a BMI of 30 or greater are classified as obese.

However, athletes have more muscle mass weight than a nonathletic person, and pregnant women weigh more due to the pregnancy than they otherwise weigh. These examples show that the BMI number may be inaccurate. However, the BMI is still the best tool to use as an indicator of obesity in the general population. The BMI calculator tool may be found at: www.nhlbi.nih.gov/health/educational/lose_wt/BMI/bmicalc.htm. It is simple to use, and we recommend that you go to the Web site and play with the tool to get a better handle on the BMI.

KNOWLEDGE CONNECTION

What percentage of one's total daily caloric intake should come from fats? In which groups of people might the BMI calculation be inaccurate? Calculate your BMI. Do you need to modify your eating habits and weight?

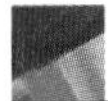

INFLUENCES ON NUTRITION

When discussing nutrition with your patients, take the time to ask about food restrictions. Many patients restrict their diets due to food preferences, intolerances, allergies, and cultural and religious influences. Providing healthy, nutritious meals that align with a patient's values and beliefs is an important part of caregiving.

POST CONFERENCE

At post conference, you talk about your patient and his misunderstandings about diet and how it affects constipation. He told you that he cannot eat fiber because it gives him gas. After you asked a few questions, you learned that he had tried only one time to increase the fiber in his diet, increasing his fiber intake from 14 to 15 g one day to 30 g the next day rather than gradually increasing fiber intake by a couple of grams per day. You know that such a large increase all at one time could cause flatus, and you were able to explain to him how to gradually increase fiber in his diet to prevent that from happening. You also helped him choose foods he likes and can easily prepare that have higher fiber content than what he has been eating. In addition, you were able to explain to him how drinking tea, coffee, or water would help increase the amount of fluid his body could use, while colas can cause the body to lose water.

Key Points

- The *Dietary Guidelines for Americans 2015–2020* encourage more variety of vegetable and protein sources, as well as increased intake for whole fruits and whole grains, while limiting added sugars, saturated fats, and sodium.
- Essential nutrients include macronutrients (protein, carbohydrates, fats, and water) and micronutrients (vitamins and minerals).
- Protein is the primary building block of the body to make new cells and help wounds heal. People must consume foods with all nine essential amino acids (called complete proteins) or a combination of foods that provide them.
- There are many types of dietary fats, including monounsaturated, polyunsaturated, saturated, and trans fats. Dietary fats are needed as a concentrated source of energy, to help absorb and store fat-soluble vitamins, and to support and insulate internal organs.
- Carbohydrates serve as the primary source for energy and are more quickly digested into a usable form than either proteins or fats. Carbohydrates may be simple or complex. Fiber is indigestible carbohydrate and is needed by the body.
- Fat-soluble vitamins are stored in body fat and include vitamins A, D, E, and K. Water-soluble vitamins are not stored and must be consumed daily. They include all of the B vitamins and vitamin C.
- Sources of vitamins vary greatly. The body cannot manufacture them so they must be consumed in the daily diet and by exposure to the sun (vitamin D). They are needed for a variety of metabolic processes.
- Minerals are inorganic compounds needed in small amounts by the body. Major minerals are those we need to ingest 100 mg per day for optimal health. Trace minerals are those we require less of each day.
- Water is a critical component to sustain life and is necessary for the whole body to function correctly.
- Different age groups need differing amounts of the food groups: vegetables, fruits, grain, protein, dairy, and oils. However, all age groups need all food groups. Healthy eating choices should be taught from an early age to help form a lifetime of better eating.
- Obesity is defined as a BMI of 30 or greater. Overweight is defined by a BMI between 25 and 29.9.

Review Questions

Select the answer that is most appropriate for each of the following questions. Some questions may have more than one correct answer. Select all that apply.

1. The primary function of carbohydrates as a food source is to:
   1. regulate metabolic processes.
   2. build body tissue.
   3. supply energy.
   4. provide bulk.

2. The primary function of protein in the body is to:
   1. supply energy.
   2. regulate metabolic processes.
   3. control muscle contractions.
   4. build tissue.

3. A characteristic of saturated fats is that they are:
   1. found primarily in animal products.
   2. liquid at room temperatures.
   3. composed of many double bonds.
   4. found primarily in vegetable products.

4. Rickets is caused by a deficiency of which vitamin?
   1. Vitamin A
   2. Cobalamin
   3. Niacin
   4. Vitamin D

5. Which foods are commonly fortified with vitamin D?
   1. Flour
   2. Cereal
   3. Milk
   4. Tuna
   5. Margarine

6. Which foods provide the most calcium per serving?
   1. Legumes
   2. Whole grains
   3. Dairy products
   4. Leafy vegetables

7. Which are recommendations for dietary changes during pregnancy?
   1. Double the amount of iron that was consumed prepregnancy
   2. Double the calorie intake since the woman is "eating for two" now
   3. Increase folic acid to prevent nervous system birth defects
   4. Increase calories by 300 per day during pregnancy
   5. Limit sugar and use any artificial sweeteners to prevent unnecessary weight gain

8. The vitamin that may help prevent fetal neural tube defects when consumed before pregnancy and through the early weeks of pregnancy is:
   1. vitamin B6.
   2. niacin.
   3. vitamin C.
   4. folic acid.

9. The largest source of sodium in the typical American diet is:
   1. processed foods.
   2. salt added at the table.
   3. salt added while cooking.
   4. foods naturally high in salt.

10. A patient with a BMI of 22 should be considered:
    1. overweight.
    2. at a healthy weight.
    3. underweight.
    4. obese.

ANSWERS 1. 3, 2. 4, 3. 1, 4. 4, 5. 3, 5, 6. 3, 7. 1, 3, 4, 8. 4, 9. 1, 10. 2

Critical Thinking Exercises

Answers available online.

1. Mr. Baze is 71 years old and is being seen in the clinic for hypertension. His primary care provider wants him to follow a low-sodium diet. He asks you about foods that he should avoid. What is your response?

2. Ms. Havner is concerned about her nutritional status. She has access to the Internet and has become confused about the many nutritional Web sites. What information can you give her to assess her current nutritional status?

Additional Resources

Use the scratch off code on the inside front cover of your book to access online quizzes that will help you to improve your scores on course exams and prepare for the NCLEX-PN®.

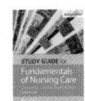

Study Guide

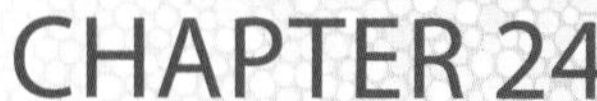

CHAPTER 24
Nutritional Care and Support

KEY TERMS

Anaphylaxis (AN-uh-fuh-LAK-siss)
Anorexia nervosa (AN-uh-REK-see-ah ner-VOH-sah)
Bolus feeding (BOH-lus FEE-ding)
Bulimia nervosa (buh-LEE-mee-ah ner-VOH-sah)
Clear liquid diet (KLEER LIK-wid DYE-uht)
Enteral nutrition (EN-ter-uhl new-TRISH-un)
Food intolerance (FOOD in-TALL-er-ens)
Full liquid diet (FUL LIK-wid DYE-uht)
Gastric decompression (GAS-trik DEE-kom-PRESH-un)
Hemoglobin A_{1C} (HEE-muh-GLOW-bin A_{1C})
Hyperglycemia (HYE-per-glye-SEE-mee-ah)
Hypoglycemia (HYE-poh-glye-SEE-mee-ah)
Jejunostomy tube (JAY-joo-NAWS-toh-mee TOOB)
Mechanical soft diet (muh-KAN-i-kuhl SOFT DYE-uht)
Nasogastric tube (NAY-zoh-GAS-trik TOOB)
NPO
Parenteral nutrition (pah-REN-tur-uhl new-TRISH-un)
Partial parenteral nutrition (PAR-shul pah-REN-tur-uhl new-TRISH-un)
Percutaneous endoscopic gastrostomy tube (PER-kyoo-TAY-nee-us EN-duh-SKOP-ik gas-TRAWS-toh-mee TOOB)
Pureed diet (PYOO-rayd DYE-uht)
Total parenteral nutrition (Toh-tuhl pah-REN-tur-uhl new-TRISH-un)

CHAPTER CONCEPTS

Nutrition
Patient-Centered Care
Safety

LEARNING OUTCOMES

1. Define various terms associated with nutritional care and support.
2. Discuss methods to assist with meals and improve the patient eating experience in the hospital.
3. Explain how to monitor intake and output and why it is important.
4. Describe NPO status, regular diets, and diets modified by consistency.
5. Describe diets modified for diseases and preferences.
6. Describe the nurse's responsibilities for patients on special diets, including diabetics and their specific needs.
7. List at least six guidelines to use in teaching patients with diabetes.
8. Identify common eating disorders.
9. Describe how drugs can affect food intake, absorption, metabolism, and excretion of nutrients.
10. Describe nasogastric and nasointestinal tubes, including size, length, and lumens.
11. Explain when and how nasogastric tubes are used for gastric decompression.
12. Discuss how feeding tubes are placed and used to provide nutrition.
13. Differentiate between intermittent and continuous tube feedings.
14. Describe the process for and importance of checking placement of nasogastric and nasointestinal tubes and checking residual gastric volume.
15. Identify nursing responsibilities for patients with feeding tubes, including the prevention of complications.
16. Discuss the use of partial and total parenteral nutrition to maintain nutritional status.
17. Discuss information found in the Connection features in this chapter.
18. Identify specific safety information.
19. Answer questions about the skills in this chapter.

SKILLS

24.1 Assisting a Patient With Feeding
24.2 Recording Intake and Output
24.3 Inserting a Nasogastric Tube
24.4 Irrigating a Nasogastric Tube
24.5 Removing a Nasogastric Tube
24.6 Administering Intermittent Bolus Enteral Feedings
24.7 Using a Feeding Pump

CRITICAL THINKING CONNECTION

Clinical Assignment

You are assigned to care for a 58-year-old male patient who has suffered a severe cerebrovascular accident (CVA). He is unable to swallow any food or fluids without choking and has been hydrated with IV fluids for the 2 days since the CVA occurred. The health-care provider has decided that the best course of action is to place a nasogastric (NG) tube and provide tube feedings for the next few weeks. After that, the patient may be able to regain his ability to swallow and can begin to eat soft foods again.

Critical Thinking Questions:

You will most likely be placing the NG tube for this patient.

1. What do you need to know before you perform the procedure?
2. What complications could occur?
3. How will you take measures to prevent them?

As you provide care to patients, you will encounter those who require nutritional support in the form of modified diets, nutritional restrictions, supplementation, or mechanical assistance with nutrition. In this chapter, you will learn about the nutritional needs of patients and different types of therapeutic diets, including diets modified for disease states. You will learn to assess a patient's ability to eat or need for alternative means of nutrition, as well as how to assist a patient with eating and how to make mealtimes pleasant. You will also learn to care for patients receiving enteral and parenteral nutrition, patients with feeding tubes, the different types of feeding formulas, and the care and management of feeding tubes.

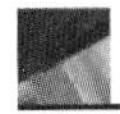

SUPPORTING NUTRITIONAL INTAKE

Hospitalized patients may experience a variety of factors related to illness or medication that impede their nutritional intake, such as anxiety, pain, fatigue, lack of appetite (called *anorexia*), or nausea and vomiting. Your role as the nurse in the nutritional care of the patient is to be supportive and ensure that he or she has adequate nutrient intake. This is more than just ensuring that the patient's meal is ordered or that the meal tray is delivered to the correct patient. Food and mealtimes in our society are often associated with social events or cultural or ethnic traditions, and most people have their own preferred routine for meals. For those patients receiving care in an institutional setting, individual patient needs may become secondary to the needs of the organization. Patient meal choices often are limited, and mealtimes are dictated by the needs of the various organizational services. Nursing intervention can improve the patient experience and optimize nutritional intake.

Assessment

When a patient is admitted to the hospital, it is important to assess his or her nutritional problems and needs. It is impossible to meet a patient's specific needs if you do not know what the patient's needs are. During the initial assessment, you should ask questions to identify specific allergies, special diets the patient may have been following at home, and dietary preferences the patient may have, including cultural or ethnic requirements or restrictions. You will also want to assess the patient's physical capabilities and identify any type of assistance with feeding that he or she may require. These may include cutting up foods, assisting in opening containers, or feeding the patient who is blind or too weak to feed himself or herself.

Another assessment you will perform is to determine what medications the patient has been taking at home, because many medications can create side effects such as nausea, diminished appetite, or altered sense taste. It often is possible to assist the patient to overcome medication side effects with simple interventions. These may include helping the patient to select foods or arranging meal and snack times that minimize nausea, thus helping to improve the patient's food intake.

Mealtime Preparation

It is sad to have to write this, but because it does happen, we feel that we should point it out. Sometimes "passing the meal trays" is treated as just that, a task to be completed and nothing more. It is not appropriate to walk down a hospital hallway and see meal trays setting on the over-bed table next to the bed, with dish covers still in place and no one eating the meal. This is a problem because it is difficult for the ill body to heal without adequate fluids and nutrition. It is your job as the nurse to do everything in your power to ensure all patients are prepared for each meal and are assisted as needed throughout the meal…not just to set the meal tray down and leave the room.

Odors

It is important to provide patients with a pleasant environment that is free of clutter and odors to enhance mealtimes. Odors can adversely affect the patient's desire to eat or may trigger nausea. Work to eliminate body excretion smells such as feces and infectious or bloody drainage. It is important for you to guard against breath odor (known as *halitosis*), body odor, and food odor on your hands, all of which can be a source of nausea, headache, or allergic reaction for the patient. Take care to eliminate these odors if they are present before mealtime.

Ill patients often are negatively affected by odors that normally would be pleasant or, at the very least, not offensive, such as perfume or aftershave, fragranced hair products, lotions, and strong fabric softeners. Avoid all personal care products that contain fragrance and laundry products that result in a strong residual fragrance on your clothing.

Environment

Plan to prepare the patient's room before the meal trays are delivered so that the over-bed table on which you will set the tray is ready. Make certain that the table is free of offensive items such as an emesis basin containing sputum, a urinal with or without urine in it, a roll of toilet tissue, a hair brush, or soiled tissues or washcloths. Remove anything that you would not want on your dining room table during mealtime. Wipe the table surface with a damp cloth or disinfectant if contaminated items have been on it.

Toileting

Inquire whether or not the patient needs to go to the bathroom, and, if so, assist the patient to the bathroom or with use of a bedpan. A patient who has a full bladder or needs to have a bowel movement probably will not eat as much as he or she would after toileting. If a patient has to interrupt a meal to attend to toileting, there is little likelihood that the patient will resume eating afterward.

Patient Comfort

Make certain the patient is comfortable because nausea, pain, or discomfort can inhibit eating. Make certain that the patient has slippers or socks on to keep the feet warm and either a robe or a second gown worn backward, with the opening in front similar to a robe. The patient may also need a blanket placed across the lap if he or she feels cold. If the patient wears dentures or glasses, obtain them and make sure that they are clean. Then assist the patient as needed to insert the dentures or put on the glasses.

Patient Positioning

If the patient is able to sit on the side of the bed or get up to sit in a chair, assist the patient to do so. An upright position is more conducive to eating. If not, make certain that the patient is positioned properly in the bed with good body alignment and then elevate the head of the bed between 60 and 90 degrees depending on the patient's condition and preference. Position the over-bed table over the patient's lap so that it is directly in front of the patient (Fig. 24.1). Adjust the height of the table according to the patient's needs.

Patient Cleanliness

To reduce the risk of bacterial contamination while eating, provide the patient with two warm wet washcloths (one with soap and one without soap for rinsing) to wash his or her face and hands before eating. If the patient is unable to perform this task independently, assist as needed. Also, make certain that you wash your hands before delivering and setting up the meal tray.

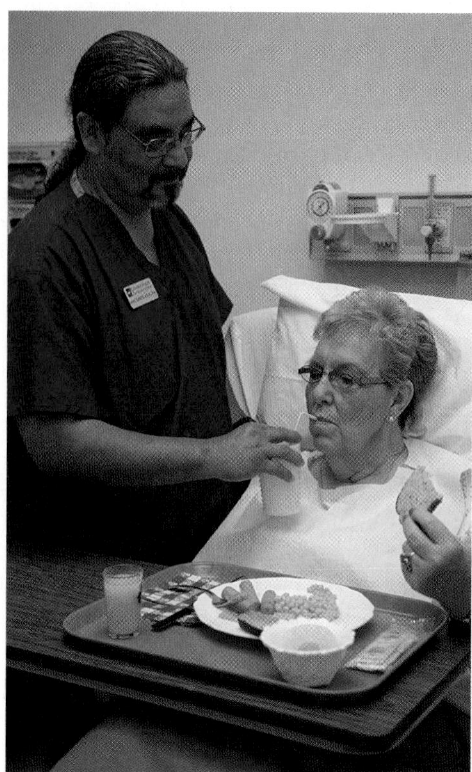

FIGURE 24.1 When feeding a patient, position the over-bed table in front of the patient, not off to the patient's side at the side of the bed.

> **KNOWLEDGE CONNECTION**
>
> Explain the importance of preparing the patient and the patient's environment before delivering meal trays. What specific steps should be taken to prepare the patient before meal trays arrive? Discuss patient comfort in relation to mealtimes. What are your responsibilities regarding cleanliness and sanitation for mealtimes? What is included in preparing the over-bed table to receive the meal tray?

Assistance With Eating

Your time spent assisting patients with meals can be used to learn more about your patients and to develop and enhance the nurse-patient relationship. Patients who require assistance often find themselves in a position that they are not used to, that of dependency on others to help them meet their needs. During mealtime, take time to talk with your patient and ask questions about his or her life situations and experiences. Probe to determine if the patient has anxiety, concerns, or questions that have not been answered or to gather insight into the dynamics of his or her life. Help to make mealtime more of a social event or at least a more pleasant interaction for the patient unless the patient's culture views it differently.

Mealtimes also offer an opportune time to educate patients regarding dietary changes they may need to make or the use of adaptive equipment. Box 24.1 offers tips on ways to assist patients with meal planning and eating. For more information regarding the steps of assisting a patient with feeding, see Skill 24.1 (page 492).

Assisting a patient with meals is a task that can be delegated to unlicensed assistive personnel (UAPs) or certified nursing assistants (CNAs). However, before delegating the task, make certain that the UAP or CNA understands the ethnic and cultural considerations related to different foods, nutrition, and mealtime. You may need to educate the UAP or CNA regarding ethnic and cultural beliefs and customs related to food and its consumption. It is also your responsibility to ensure that the UAP or CNA is knowledgeable about the patient's physiological status as it relates to impaired swallowing, which would require the patient to be fed slowly. He or she must know what to do if the patient chokes or aspirates.

Monitoring Intake and Output

Because fluid and electrolyte balance is critical to optimal health and recovery from illness and injury, ensuring adequate fluid intake is even more important than ensuring consumption of food. This should be a primary focus in your care of each patient. When there are concerns regarding a patient's fluid and electrolyte balance, it will be your responsibility to monitor the patient's intake and output, commonly called I&O. This simply means to measure and record all fluids taken in and all fluid volumes that are lost.

Intake includes fluids taken by mouth, those administered IV, and fluids administered by enteral or parenteral feedings, which will be discussed later in this chapter. A clear plastic drinking cup marked in increments of ounces and milliliters can be used to measure the amount of fluid that is drunk. It is also used to measure the remaining volume after the patient drinks only part of a container with a specified volume in it. For example, if a can of carbonated cola contained 360 mL and the patient drank only part of the cola, you would measure the remainder and subtract that from the 360 mL to determine the amount ingested. The cup should be held at approximately eye level to accurately read the volume (Fig. 24.2). Most hospitals have standardized volumes listed for their commonly used containers, making it easier to calculate intake. Box 24.2 provides a list of common container volumes.

Output includes all bodily fluids that are lost, including urine, emesis, liquid stool, blood, suctioned gastric contents, and drainage from drainage devices such as a Hemovac or Jackson-Pratt drain, which you will read about in Chapter 26. You will measure urine and emesis in clear containers that are larger than the one used to measure oral intake. The units of measurement will be the same: ounces and milliliters. You

Box 24.1

Tips for Assisting Patients With Meal Planning and Eating

Because good nutrition is so important to the healing process, it must be monitored and evaluated for adequacy. The patient commonly does not feel like eating much, so it is your responsibility to make it a priority to do everything you can to ensure optimal nutritional intake. Below are a few tips to help you to do this:

- Spend time getting to know the patient. Be warm and compassionate, letting the patient know you understand that his or her pain, anxiety, or other psychosocial factors are affecting appetite.
- If the patient is nauseated or hurting, provide appropriate medication before mealtime. You cannot expect a patient who is nauseated or having pain to eat adequately to meet his or her nutritional needs.
- Make certain the patient is prepared for mealtime by getting the patient comfortable in a bed or chair, providing a warm wet washcloth to wash the hands and face and clearing the over-bed table of clutter and unpleasantries to provide ample room for the meal tray. Think of how you would prepare your kitchen table for a meal at home. (Would you want to eat lunch with a roll of toilet tissue, a urinal, or an emesis basin containing green sputum next to your plate?) ***Safety: Wipe off the over-bed table with disinfectant if a urinal or other contaminated items have lain on it.*** This preparation should be carried out prior to tray arrival because it is impossible to do these tasks with a tray of food in one's hands.
- You and any assistive personnel should always wash your hands prior to passing out meal trays.
- Ensure that each meal tray is assessed for the correct diet and appropriate temperature of food.
- Many patients are elderly or frail, have poor eyesight or weakness due to illness or stroke, or have limited use of extremities related to IVs, dressings, and casts. Open all containers on the tray, such as milk carton, juice container, cellophane packaging for plastic utensils, and condiments. Many patients who are unable to accomplish these seemingly simple tasks will just not eat rather than have to ask for assistance.
- Take your time while feeding patients. Avoid rushing the patient.
- Be certain that assistive personnel know how to safely assist those patients who require assistance.
- Help the patient identify factors that would improve the eating experience, such as selecting foods he or she likes, creating a comfortable environment, arranging for early or later trays if the patient's normal routine is quite different from the hospital routine, or allowing friends and family to bring in foods from home provided there are no dietary restrictions.
- If the patient's appetite is limited, provide five to six smaller feedings per day rather than three larger ones. The health-care provider will generally write an order for this if you ask.
- Educate your patient as to the importance of nutritional intake and drinking adequate fluids in the healing process.
- Make rounds to your patients' rooms during mealtimes. Ask your patients if they have any needs or if they are satisfied with their meals; help facilitate a pleasant experience by being a problem-solver.

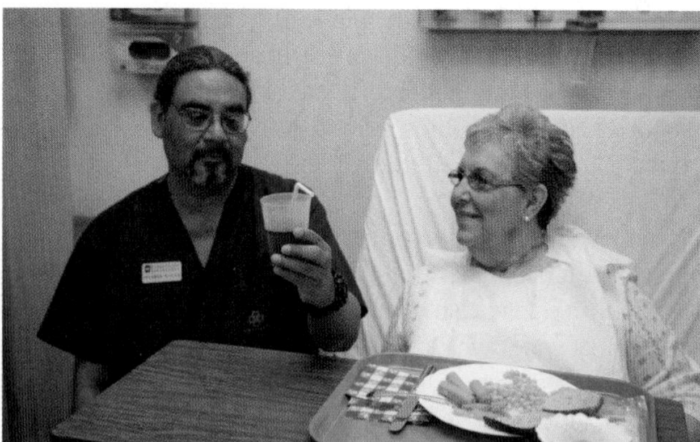

FIGURE 24.2 Use a graduated cup and hold up at eye level to accurately measure intake.

may hear the containers referred to as graduated containers or receptacles. When you measure any form of output, you will write it on the I&O sheet at the bedside, indicating the type of output, such as Hemovac drainage or gastric suction. Each category is totaled separately and documented on the I&O sheet or flow sheet in the patient's chart at the end of each shift. Then the total of all intake is calculated and compared with the calculated total of all output. The average adult requires between 1,500 and 2,500 mL of fluid intake per 24 hours depending on the patient's size and health status. The total urinary output should closely balance with the total intake, usually within 200 to 300 mL of the intake. Skill 24.2 (page 493) provides additional information regarding intake and output recording.

KNOWLEDGE CONNECTION

Describe how you can make mealtime more conducive to eating and more pleasant for the patient. What can you do to help increase nutritional intake for the patient with a limited appetite? Discuss at least five ways you can assist patients with meal planning and eating. Why is ensuring intake and output balance pertinent? How much fluid should the average adult take in over 24 hours?

Supporting Patients With Special Nutritional Needs

As you provide nursing care and nutritional support to patients, you will encounter patients who have special nutritional requirements. These patients may have an inability to tolerate certain nutrients or may have an actual eating disorder. Food allergies or intolerances present significant challenges. Food allergies are most commonly identified in infancy or early childhood. When identified in children, the patient and family have not had time to develop adaptive measures. Frequently, they are anxious and uncertain about their ability to effectively manage and meet their nutritional needs.

Box 24.2

Examples of Standard Container Volumes

Different facilities will use glasses, cups, and bowls of various sizes that will hold differing volumes of liquid. Each facility will have its own list of standard container volumes. Become familiar with the volumes where you work. The following is a list of common container volumes:

- **Popsicle:** 90 mL
- **Juice glass:** 120 mL
- **Individual ice cream cup:** 120 mL
- **Coffee cup:** 150 mL
- **Small gelatin cup:** 180 mL
- **Drinking glass:** 180 mL or 240 mL
- **Small soup bowl:** 180 mL
- **Large soup bowl:** 240 mL
- **Small carton of milk:** 240 mL

Food Allergies

A *food allergy* is a reaction by the patient's immune system to an allergen, which is a food protein that, once ingested, causes the immune system to develop antibodies. The following are the most common food allergies:

- Peanuts
- Wheat
- Dairy products
- Eggs

Typically, a patient with food allergy experiences symptoms such as skin, respiratory, and gastrointestinal (GI) reactions that get increasingly worse with repeated exposures to the offending agent. It is important that the nurse gather assessment data on the history of the allergy, when it was first identified, symptoms experienced, and interventions used in the event of a reaction. Allergic reactions can present as a rash or hives, or they can be severe and result in anaphylaxis, the most severe form of allergic reaction. **Anaphylaxis** is a life-threatening emergency; it involves swelling of the upper respiratory tract that can result in occlusion of the airway. The patient, the patient's family, and all persons involved with the care of the patient need to be aware of the signs and symptoms of anaphylaxis and the appropriate and immediate treatment of the reaction.

Food Intolerances

Food intolerance is not an allergic reaction; it is an adverse reaction to a food without activation of the immune response. The symptoms generated by the food intolerance can be triggered by distinct properties of the food, such as tyramine in aged cheese or wine, or by metabolic disorders, such as gluten intolerance. Food intolerance can stem from the body's lack of digestive enzymes or an inability to utilize

• WORD • BUILDING •

anaphylaxis: ana – against + phylaxis – protection

these enzymes. The resultant symptoms of intolerance are usually of a GI nature, such as bloating, flatulence, diarrhea, or nausea. Treatment of food intolerances requires identification of the offending agent; this can be accomplished by eliminating various foods from the diet over a period of time. Once the offending agent is identified, the patient will need to modify his or her diet to limit or eliminate the offending foods. Lactose intolerance, for example, would require that a patient limit milk intake. However, the patient also would have to evaluate other foods to determine if they contain lactose.

KNOWLEDGE CONNECTION

Discuss the differences between food allergy and food intolerance. Describe common symptoms of each.

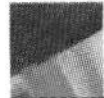

THERAPEUTIC DIETS

Many patients must follow a modified diet to help manage their illness or injury. Hospital food comes in a variety of regular and modified diets. Diets may be modified singularly, such as a 1,500-calorie diet, or may be modified in combinations, such as a 1,500-calorie, low-sodium, mechanical soft diet. Each facility will have a diet manual that contains details about each type of diet and the foods that are allowed. All patients must have a diet ordered by their health-care provider unless there is an order for the patient to remain NPO, which is explained below. Dietary modifications are made in collaboration with a hospital or institutional dietitian. The following represent the most commonly prescribed restrictions and modified diets.

NPO

NPO stands for "nothing per os," or mouth. It means the patient is restricted from oral intake of food or fluid, including water. This is frequently ordered before surgery, invasive procedures, and certain diagnostic studies to reduce the risk of aspiration. Common orders may be "NPO after midnight" or "NPO 8 hours prior to procedure." A patient who is vomiting may have an NPO order specified to be in effect until nausea and vomiting are no longer a problem.

Most patients who are nourished can tolerate brief periods without food or fluid; however, prolonged periods of NPO status, as when a procedure or surgery is delayed for 24 hours, should be avoided. During prolonged periods of NPO status, IV fluids may be given to maintain hydration and a minimally supportive caloric intake.

Any time a patient is NPO, the patient and family should be informed regarding the NPO status and the reason why it is ordered. This will help to increase compliance. An NPO sign should be placed on the door and on the wall over the patient's bed to serve as a reminder for staff and visitors. You should empty and remove the patient's water carafe and drinking glass from the bedside as a reminder that the patient is not to drink anything.

Regular Diet

A regular diet is appropriate for patients without special nutritional needs. This diet provides approximately 2,000 calories per day and offers a balanced meal plan. The nutritional value of this diet can vary widely depending on the food choices of the patient. Hospital meals offer the patient the opportunity to have adequate caloric intake but are not necessarily designed to be low in sodium, fat, or cholesterol. You may need to educate your patient to make nutritionally sound choices. Regular diets are adapted to meet the age-specific needs of patients, as the nutritional needs of a child differ from those of an elderly person and from those of a middle-aged adult.

For patients with specific cultural or ethnic needs, many facilities provide ethnic variances, such as Asian, kosher, or vegetarian. If a facility does not provide these variations, you may want to encourage the patient's family or friends to bring foods from home that will allow or encourage the patient to eat more.

Even though patients typically order their daily meals from a selection of menu choices, you may encounter patients with complaints related to the taste or texture of hospital food. They may complain of it being "bland and tasteless." This may be true because house diets must be prepared to meet the needs and tastes of a wide variety of patients. Usually foods available for selection on the hospital menu are limited to avoid unpopular food items such as turnips or those that are fatty, fried, or gas producing.

Diets Modified by Consistency

Patients with acute illnesses and those undergoing surgery or bowel procedures may need a diet that is modified in consistency to assist in the management of their illness. The health-care provider may order "Clear liquids, advance as tolerated." This means the patient is allowed to gradually progress from a diet of clear liquids to full liquids, then on to a soft diet, and finally to a regular diet as the patient is able to tolerate the increasing consistencies without nausea, vomiting, or distress.

For some elderly patients or those with chewing problems or dysphagia (difficulty swallowing), a long-term diet modification may be necessary. Common diets with consistency modifications include clear liquid, full liquid, mechanical soft, and pureed.

- A **clear liquid diet** is ordered to provide hydration and calories in the form of simple carbohydrates that help meet some of the body's energy needs. The defining characteristic that separates a clear liquid from a full liquid has to do with its clarity. Is the liquid, as is or diluted with water, clear enough that you can "read a newspaper" through it? For example, a dark carbonated cola that is diluted with water would become clear enough to see through it. If so, it may be considered a clear liquid. Examples of clear liquids include water, broth, and tea without milk. As clear liquid diets do not provide adequate calories, proteins, fats, vitamins, or minerals to meet the body's needs, a patient should be progressed as quickly as possible to a more nutritious diet.

Common examples of when a clear liquid diet might be appropriate include postoperatively or during recovery from GI disease such as vomiting and diarrhea, when the gut must be introduced slowly to food. When the clear liquids are tolerated, the patient may be advanced to a full liquid diet. It will be your responsibility to determine when to advance the diet by assessing how the patient tolerates each new level of diet.

- A **full liquid diet** consists of all the liquids found in a clear liquid diet with the addition of all other opaque liquids and food items that become liquid at room temperature. Examples of full liquids include milk, pudding, and ice cream. As is the case with the clear liquid diet, this diet also provides limited nutrients. Therefore, patients should remain on this plan for a limited period of time. Patients who need to remain on a liquid diet for an extended period of time should have the diet planned by a dietitian, who may recommend the addition of high-calorie, high-protein supplements.
- A **mechanical soft diet** is the diet of choice for patients with acute or chronic difficulties with chewing, such as those with jaw problems, missing teeth, poorly fitting dentures, or severe weakness or fatigue. This diet includes all of the items from the full liquid diet plus the addition of foods such as scrambled eggs and cottage cheese. Many items can be included in this diet by altering their texture through extensive cooking or use of a blender or food processor. Through the inclusion of a wide variety of foods, this diet is better able to meet a person's nutritional needs; however, it is quite low in fiber, so patients may be at risk for constipation.
- A **pureed diet** is one that is processed in a blender/food processor. Any food item can be included, but its consistency must be changed. Food items are placed in a blender while liquid is added to moisten them, creating a texture that is somewhat thicker than full liquid but that can still be swallowed easily.

Table 24.1 provides examples of foods for each of the four diets listed above.

KNOWLEDGE CONNECTION

What are the categories of diets modified by consistency? Describe the differences between a clear liquid and full liquid diet. Explain what "advance as tolerated" means in relation to a diet order. What assessments should you make before advancing the diet? What are the key nutrients these provide, and which may need to be supplemented?

Table 24.1 Partial List of Foods by Consistency

Clear Liquid	*Full Liquid*	*Mechanical Soft*	*Pureed*
• Water	• All clear liquids	• All liquids and pureed foods	• All liquids
• Broth/bouillon	• Cream soups	• All soups	• Scrambled eggs
• Black coffee	• Milk	• Ground/finely diced meats	• Pureed meats
• Tea	• Cream	• Finely diced/flaked fish	• Pureed vegetables
• Carbonated drinks	• Ice cream	• Cottage cheese	• Pureed fruits
• Clear fruit juices:	• Yogurt	• Soft cheeses	• Mashed potatoes
• Apple	• Milkshakes	• Mashed or riced potatoes	• Gravy
• Grape	• Sherbet	• Rice	• Applesauce
• Cranberry	• Custards/puddings	• Oatmeal	• Baby foods
• Gelatin	• Vegetable juices	• Grits	
• Popsicles	• Pureed vegetables	• Pancakes	
• Clear sports drinks:	• All fruit juices	• Soft breads	
• Gatorade	• Protein drinks	• Soda and graham crackers	
• Electrolyte drinks:	• Liquid supplements	• Cooked soft vegetables	
• Pedialyte™	• Refined cooked cereals:	• Cooked or canned fruits	
	• Cream of Wheat	• Bananas	
	• Malto-Meal	• Soft pastries	

Diets Modified for Disease

Certain patient conditions may require that the patient's diet be modified to either increase or restrict the intake of certain nutrients. The following will identify the most common of these diets:

- **Diabetic:** Used to manage calorie and carbohydrate intake for patients with diabetes mellitus, primarily those who are insulin dependent.
- **Calorie restricted:** Used for those patients who must lose weight.
- **Sodium restricted:** Used for those patients with hypertension, congestive heart failure, or kidney or liver failure, as well as those who require help to prevent or correct fluid retention. The degree of restriction is commensurate with disease severity, severity of symptoms, and the medication regimen prescribed. Typically sodium restrictions range from 2,000 to 3,000 mg per day. While many patients think that simply not adding salt to foods provides adequate sodium restriction, this is not actually the case. Most of the sodium that people ingest comes from processed foods, making it necessary to read labels for sodium content if the patient is sent home on this diet.
- **Fat restricted:** Used for patients who are experiencing problems with fat malabsorption, such as those with disorders affecting the gallbladder, liver, lymphatic system, pancreas, or intestines. It also may be used for those patients who have elevated triglyceride, lipid, or cholesterol levels, as well as for patients who need general weight loss.
- **Fiber restricted:** Used during the acute phase of intestinal disorders when the presence of fiber may exacerbate intestinal pain, produce diarrhea, or cause an intestinal blockage. This diet is often used before intestinal surgery to minimize fecal volume or after surgery to allow the GI system to transition gradually to a regular diet.
- **Renal:** Used to manage or limit fluids and electrolytes for patients with renal insufficiency or disease. The renal diet is complex, and the patient's nutritional needs change over the course of the disease. A dietitian specializing in renal disorders may guide the nutritional therapy.
- **Protein restricted:** Used to manage protein intake for those patients with liver or kidney disease.
- **High calorie, high protein:** Used to increase calorie and protein intake in those patients with increased need related to wound healing, growth promotion, and increasing or maintaining weight. High-fat foods also may be added to increase calories available for energy use.
- **Five to six small, frequent feedings:** A health-care provider may order any type of diet to be provided in several smaller feedings throughout the day rather than the traditional three meals per day. This is used with those patients who have difficulty tolerating larger meals or who simply are unable to eat more than a few bites at a time, as well as those who need to have food gradually reintroduced. Often elderly patients are only able to eat small amounts at a time. This makes it difficult for them to obtain the needed nutrients in the traditional three meals per day. By increasing the number of meal or snack times from three to five or six per day, the patient has a better chance of receiving the needed nutrients.

Diets Modified by Preference

Some patients are on certain diets by choice. Often they feel better if they restrict certain items in the usual diet. Alternately, they may feel strongly about the environmental impact of the food chain in the United States and therefore avoid eating foods that have a negative impact.

- **Gluten-free diets:** People with celiac disease must be on a gluten-free diet. However, other people may have a condition known as "nonceliac gluten sensitivity" and also need to avoid gluten. Still others may have a wheat allergy that requires them to avoid gluten-containing foods. Celiac disease is an autoimmune condition, and wheat allergy causes histamine release. Nonceliac gluten sensitivity is not an autoimmune response but has similar symptoms. Often the diagnosis is made if removing gluten from the diet causes symptoms to subside.

  Gluten is found in wheat, rice, and maize. It is present in foods like barley, flour, couscous, tabouli, and malt vinegar. Sometimes certain meat products and even some pharmaceuticals may contain gluten. There are now more "gluten-free" products available for purchase, but they may be actually lower in some nutrients than those that contain gluten. They may be higher in carbohydrates and fat and lower in fiber and iron, while still costing more than their counterparts. Foods such as buckwheat, lentils, garbanzo beans, and tapioca are all acceptable for a patient on a gluten-free diet.
- **Vegan diets:** People may choose to be vegan for a number of reasons. Some feel it is better for the environment, some feel that animals should not be food sources for people, and others may decide it is a healthier choice for them personally. Some studies have shown that eating a vegan diet has improved or reversed some diseases, particularly cardiovascular diseases.

  Those on a vegan diet eat plant-based only. They avoid all meat, including fish and poultry, and any other animal products or by-products. They do not consume eggs, dairy products, or honey. This diet is rich in fruits and vegetables, leafy greens, whole grains, nuts, seeds, legumes, and tofu (soy). Alternative products are often used to replace dairy, such as almond or soy milk and cashew cheese. This diet tends to be lower in saturated fat and cholesterol than vegetarian diets. Patients who follow a vegan diet may need supplementation for vitamins B12 and D, calcium, and omega-3 fatty acids.

KNOWLEDGE CONNECTION

Give an example of an illness or condition that might necessitate a high-protein diet. Identify one type of diet that might be ordered to help decrease swelling of a patient's hands and legs. For what type conditions might the health-care provider order a fat-restricted diet? What is the advantage of five to six small feedings over the routine three meals per day? High-calorie, high-protein diets might be ordered in what situations?

Nursing Responsibilities

You will be responsible for monitoring the diet type, percentage eaten, and whether or not the patient tolerated the meal. When the health-care provider has ordered "clear liquids, advance as tolerated," such as might be appropriate postoperatively or during recovery from GI illness, it will be your responsibility to determine when to advance the patient's diet. Utilizing the nursing process, you will assess how much the patient eats and record this as a percentage, record how the patient tolerates each meal, and evaluate whether he or she is ready to have the diet advanced to the next level of consistency. Factors indicating that the patient is not yet ready to advance the diet may include any of the following:

- Nausea
- Vomiting
- Abdominal distention
- Cramping
- Absent or hypoactive bowel sounds
- Complaints of indigestion
- Diarrhea

Once you evaluate how the patient is tolerating each level of increased consistency, you will notify the dietary service to advance the diet to the next level.

Diabetic Patients

If your patient is diabetic, you will be expected to monitor not only the amount eaten and the patient's tolerance of the meal, but most likely the patient's blood glucose level as well. Refer to the Laboratory and Diagnostic Connection and the Patient Teaching Connection. (The actual skill of performing the skin puncture for the finger stick blood sugar [FSBS] is taught in Chapter 34, Skill 34.4.)

An abnormally elevated blood glucose level is known as **hyperglycemia,** and an abnormally low level is **hypoglycemia.** Both of these conditions can have serious effects on the patient, including falls, loss of consciousness, and even death. Hypoglycemia signs and symptoms may develop rapidly once blood glucose begins to drop. Signs and symptoms of hypoglycemia for you to monitor include the following:

- Clammy skin
- Shakiness or nervousness
- Nausea
- Increased irritability
- Confusion
- Dizziness
- Headache
- Weakness/fatigue
- Seizures and unconsciousness (at a critically low level of blood glucose)

When you suspect a patient's glucose level is dropping, perform an FSBS. If it is below 70%, provide a small glass of juice or 8 ounces of low-fat milk (as long as the patient is conscious). The juice or milk will help to raise the glucose level quickly. Recheck the glucose level within 10 to 15 minutes to ensure it comes up to a safe level. If the next meal is not imminent (i.e., within the next half hour), administer a protein and complex carbohydrate snack to help maintain the glucose level until the next meal. A common snack used in this situation is peanut butter or cheese with a slice of whole-wheat bread. Continue to monitor the patient closely for hypoglycemia.

If the glucose level is low enough that the patient is at risk for or is having a seizure or is unconscious, the treatment is to administer dextrose 50% (D50W) intravenously. (Refer to your facility policy for specific glucose levels and treatment orders.)

Treatment for hyperglycemia is insulin administration, which will depend on the glucose level. If you suspect a patient's glucose level to be elevated, perform an FSBS to verify it. Signs and symptoms of hyperglycemia include the following:

- Increased thirst/dry mouth
- Hot, dry, flushed skin
- Headache
- Frequent urination
- Elevated blood glucose level
- Fruity-smelling breath
- Confusion
- Coma
- Death

Laboratory and Diagnostic Connection

Diabetes

In order to effectively manage insulin-dependent diabetes, also known as type 1 diabetes, it is imperative to maintain *glycemic control,* which refers to the blood glucose level. This is done by thorough monitoring of blood glucose levels on a prescribed basis, such as once daily or before meals and at bedtime. Blood glucose should remain within a prescribed range established by the patient's health-care provider. The 2016 American Diabetes Association guidelines state that

• WORD • BUILDING •

hyperglycemia: hyper – excessive + glyc – sugar + emia – blood
hypoglycemia: hypo – deficient + glyc – sugar + emia – blood
glycemic: glyc – sugar + emic – blood

the target range of 80 to 130 mg/dL before meals is acceptable for existing diabetics. Glucose testing provides valuable immediate information for patients to adjust their food intake, medications, or activity level and for preventing hypoglycemic and hyperglycemic events. Glucose in the blood freely enters red blood cells and attaches to hemoglobin molecules, producing glycated or glycosylated hemoglobin. Health-care providers evaluate a patient's long-term glycemic control by measuring glycated hemoglobin, with a laboratory test known as **hemoglobin A_{1c}** (Hb A_{1c}). A red blood cell has an average life span of 120 days, so the Hb A_{1c} measures the amount of glucose present over a period of 2 to 3 months, giving a better overall picture of glycemic control. In other words, the Hb A_{1c} monitors the long-term glucose level of the patient over the previous 90 days. In nondiabetics, Hb A_{1c} usually is less than 6% of the hemoglobin. The goal of diabetes treatment is to maintain an Hb A_{1c} less than 7%. For diabetics without adequate control, it can range as high as 12% to 20%.

Patient Teaching Connection

Diabetes

The diagnosis of diabetes can be overwhelming. It is a disease that requires new medications, development of an awareness of blood glucose levels, and modification of various aspects of the patient's lifestyle as well as nutritional habits. Eating a healthier diet is among the most significant modifications the patient with diabetes must make. It is important that the patient with diabetes understand his or her disease, how diet aids in symptom management, and the prevention of short- and long-term complications. Many patients with newly diagnosed diabetes erroneously believe that their disease is related to sugar intake and therefore should be alleviated by the diet.

Before discharge, you will need to teach the patient about effective meal planning and nutritional intake. Using the following patient instructions will help you emphasize the most important points about healthy eating:

1. Eat a well-balanced diet, which includes carbohydrates, moderate protein, and fat in sparing amounts.
2. Know the differences between simple and complex carbohydrates:
   - *Simple carbohydrates,* which are found primarily in fruits, fruit juices, processed baked goods, and sugar, are quickly converted to glucose and can be used to rapidly raise the blood glucose. There is no need to totally eliminate them from the diet, but simple carbohydrates should be ingested in moderation, and carbohydrate intake should be consistent from day to day to maintain better balanced blood glucose.
   - *Complex carbohydrates,* which are found in whole grains, vegetables high in fiber, and legumes such as dried peas and beans, require the body to work harder to break them down to use for energy. This helps to maintain a more consistent blood glucose level. The majority of ingested carbohydrates should be complex carbohydrates rather than simple carbohydrates.
3. Eat three meals and an evening snack daily. Some health-care providers may prefer you to eat an additional snack in midmorning and midafternoon. Each of these should contain some protein.
4. Do not skip meals.
5. Increase your fiber intake.
6. Reduce your fat intake by baking, broiling, or grilling foods.
7. Lose weight if you are overweight. Studies show that even a loss of 10% of total body weight is significant to help lower blood glucose.
8. Wear a diabetic identification bracelet or necklace for emergencies.

KNOWLEDGE CONNECTION

What are your responsibilities regarding monitoring dietary intake? What signs and symptoms might indicate that a postoperative patient's diet has been advanced too rapidly? What are the signs and symptoms of hypoglycemia? What is the first step you should take when hypoglycemia is suspected? Explain the significance of Hb A_{1C}.

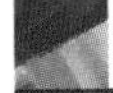

EATING DISORDERS

Eating disorders are evidenced by extreme disturbances in eating habits, to such a point that the patient's health can be severely affected or even result in death. The most common of these disorders are anorexia nervosa, bulimia nervosa, and binge eating disorder, all of which involve the patient's relationship with food and eating and her or his body image. Women and girls are more at risk for developing an eating disorder than are males. While most eating disorders occur during adolescence or early adulthood, it is becoming more common to see them in middle-aged women also. Eating disorders may result from either physical or psychological causes and result in both physical and psychological effects. These patients have an impaired perception of self and do not see their eating or lack of eating as problematic.

Anorexia Nervosa

Anorexia nervosa is characterized by an excessive leanness or wasting of the body, known as *emaciation.* There is relentless self-starvation in an effort to reduce the body weight below normal. These patients do not see themselves accurately and perceive that they are overweight even when they are at the point of physical starvation. Given the freedom to choose their meals, patients who are anorexic will continue to restrict their intake. They will exhibit obsessive thoughts related to their body shape and weight and will display an intense fear of obesity. The following are physical symptoms commonly seen in the severely underweight anorexic patient:

1. Brittle nails
2. Dull, dry, brittle hair
3. Amenorrhea
4. Severe constipation
5. Lethargy or fatigue
6. Below-normal vital signs
7. Muscle weakness
8. Muscle wasting
9. Anemia

A possible complication is electrolyte imbalances, such as abnormally low levels of calcium, magnesium, zinc, and phosphorus. Another complication can include dehydration and metabolic acidosis or alkalosis from overuse of diuretics and laxatives. Patients with anorexia may struggle with the disease for a decade or longer, resulting in death if medical treatment is not sought before the damage is too severe to reverse.

Anorexia nervosa is especially difficult to treat. Patients with this disorder are most effectively managed by an interdisciplinary team with very specialized knowledge and skills.

Bulimia Nervosa

Bulimia nervosa is a disorder of eating binges accompanied by some type of behavior that will help to get rid of some of the calories that were ingested while bingeing. These behaviors can include self- or medication-induced vomiting (known as *purging*), excessive exercise, fasting, or overuse of laxatives. Some patients will also abuse diuretics to reduce water weight. Psychologically, the bulimic patient is also obsessed with body shape and weight; the binge-purge cycles are triggered by stressful events or may be influenced by peer pressure in adolescents. The acts of bingeing and purging are generally hidden from friends and family. These patients may horde junk food and hide it for later bingeing. Physical symptoms that may be observed in a patient with bulimia nervosa include the following:

- Chronic inflammation or soreness of the throat due to retching and exposure to gastric acid during vomiting
- Diarrhea from laxative abuse
- Increasing dental decay from exposure to gastric acid when vomiting
- Indigestion
- Regurgitation of gastric fluids into the esophagus, known as *gastric reflux*
- Dehydration

Possible complications include renal damage, fluid and electrolyte imbalances, and gastroesophageal reflux disease. Patients with bulimia also may suffer from anorexia, increasing the extent and severity of damage, as well as the risk of death.

Patients with bulimia nervosa pose a significant challenge for the nurses working with them. They are most successfully managed by an interdisciplinary team with expert knowledge and skills in managing this disorder.

Binge Eating Disorder

A third type of eating disorder is characterized by episodes of eating large quantities of food at one time, with a loss of control while eating. The person with binge eating disorder may eat very quickly and be to a point of discomfort but continue to eat. This disorder is the most common eating disorder in the United States. According to the National Eating Disorders Association, it is seen in 3.5% of women, 2% of men, and 1.6% of adolescents. Feelings of shame, distress, and guilt accompany binges and are present after the binges. However, in binge eating disorder, the person does not purge. This disorder is often associated with being overweight or obese. It is considered a severe, life-threatening eating disorder, but it is treatable.

Patients with this disorder can benefit by treatment from the coordinated efforts of a team with expert knowledge and skills in managing binge eating.

KNOWLEDGE CONNECTION

Describe the common symptoms of the patient with anorexia nervosa and of the patient with bulimia nervosa.

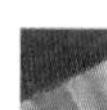

FOOD–DRUG INTERACTIONS

Certain drugs and foods can interact and alter the effects of medications. Some drug and food combinations result in less serious interactions and should simply be monitored. However, other food–drug combinations significantly change the drug's effect and can result in a serious adverse reaction, making it imperative to avoid the offending food while administration of the drug is necessary. Some of the general types of food–drug interactions include the following:

- Some medications can affect nutrient intake by inhibiting appetite, causing GI discomfort, or by causing some other reaction that inhibits food intake by making it unpleasant or painful. Other medications can stimulate appetite, increasing the quantity of food ingested.
- Certain medications can alter the absorption, metabolism, or excretion of nutrients. Alternatively, some nutrients can alter the absorption, metabolism, or excretion of medications.
- Other food–drug interactions can create medication toxicity.

• WORD • BUILDING •

gastroesophageal: gastro – stomach + esophageal – related to the esophagus

Prevention of these adverse events is possible with education. You have a primary responsibility to be aware of potential food–drug interactions and to educate your patients to be alert to these possibilities. There are numerous food–drug interactions, and as more medications are developed, the potential for new interactions increases. It would be impossible to memorize all of these adverse combinations, so you must faithfully research each new or unfamiliar drug in a drug book before you administer it. Many computer programs and smartphone apps can be used to look up medications that are new to you.

Drug Effects on Food Intake

The side effects of medication, such as nausea, vomiting, altered taste sensation, anorexia, decreased salivation, and sores or lesions in the mouth or the upper GI tract, can inhibit appetite or make food intake painful. Some medications can be very sedating or cause the patient to feel confused; this in turn will interfere with nutritional intake. These side effects may be monitored and managed when they occur on a short-term basis without causing significant weight loss. However, when the side effects are chronic, a plan of intervention must be developed to prevent weight loss and emaciation. For example, chemotherapy patients with severe nausea or vomiting probably would require the use of *antiemetics,* medications that help to prevent or reduce nausea and vomiting.

Many medications, such as corticosteroids, some antidepressants, and the atypical antipsychotics, can cause unintentional weight gain. For example, corticosteroids dramatically increase the appetite of some patients, resulting in increased consumption of food. These patients can gain large amounts of weight, often greater than 20 pounds, in a short period of time. It is important to teach patients about these potential problems and to devise strategies to manage them before the weight is gained. For some patients, such as those with *cachexia* (malnutrition and wasting associated with cancer), weight gain is desirable. These patients may be prescribed medications to increase their appetite.

Drug Effects on Absorption of Nutrients

Dietary effects that reduce medication absorption typically occur through the influence of increased gastric motility, conditions within the GI tract that are either too acidic or too alkaline, or direct interaction of food with a medication. Most medications are absorbed in the small intestine and may be absorbed more quickly if the stomach is empty during drug administration. It may be best that certain medications be given on an empty stomach to enhance absorption. However, there are other medications, such as ibuprofen or aspirin, that should be taken with food to decrease gastric irritation. Some medications are best absorbed in an acidic medium, but others may be damaged by acidity. Those that are damaged by acidity often are available in an enteric-coated formulation that dissolves in the small intestine, thereby promoting better absorption. High-fiber foods and diets may decrease the absorption of certain medications.

Medications also can influence the absorption of nutrients. Drugs that damage the intestinal mucosa, such as nonsteroidal anti-inflammatory drugs (NSAIDs) or antineoplastics (cancer drugs), and certain antibiotics can cause malabsorption. The binding of the drugs to nutrients impairs absorption of the drug and/or the nutrients. For example, some antibiotics bind to the calcium in foods or supplements, which reduces the absorption of both the antibiotic and the calcium. Certain medications, such as histamine$_2$ (H_2) blockers or proton pump inhibitors, can reduce stomach acidity and impede the absorption of vitamin B12, iron, and folate. Finally, medications can directly impede nutrient absorption by interfering with intestinal metabolism.

Drug Effects on Metabolism of Nutrients

Metabolism of food and medications occurs through the use of enzyme systems in the small intestine and liver. Some medications can inhibit or induce the activities of these enzyme systems, impairing the metabolism of nutrients. For example, the anticonvulsant phenytoin induces the liver system that metabolizes folate, vitamin D, and vitamin K. Patients taking this anticonvulsant will need additional supplements of these vitamins.

Many other medications can impact metabolism by mimicking the body's natural hormones, such as corticosteroid drugs that mimic the body-produced hormone cortisol. The human body, when exposed to these medications, acts as if it is experiencing an additional release of hormone. In the case of long-term treatment with corticosteroids, the patient may experience weight gain, rounding of the face shape called *moon facies,* hyperglycemia, bone loss, and muscle wasting.

Foods or their components can affect the enzyme systems as well and interfere with medication metabolism. Grapefruit juice, for example, has been found to inactivate or inhibit enzymes necessary for the metabolism of a number of medications. As a result, levels of the medication can be greatly increased, yielding a much stronger physiological effect. Another high-risk interaction occurs between many foods and herbs and the drug warfarin, an anticoagulant that is prescribed for patients with a history of blood clots. The patient taking warfarin should avoid eating foods containing moderate to high levels of vitamin K. Vitamin K can significantly weaken the anticoagulant effect of warfarin, increasing the risk of recurrent blood clots. In addition, the popular herbal supplements ginkgo, ginseng, St. John's wort, dong quai, and garlic, among others, contain compounds that enhance the effects of warfarin, which could possibly result in bleeding or hemorrhage. Patients who take warfarin should be educated to limit or avoid these foods and herbs. This education is your responsibility as well as that of the health-care provider and the pharmacist. Table 24.2 presents a sampling of foods and drugs that should not be administered at the same time and foods that should be completely avoided while taking a particular drug.

• **WORD** • **BUILDING** •

antiemetic: anti – against + emetic – vomit

Table 24.2
Selected Food–Drug Interactions

Food or Drink	*Drug*
Large amounts of potassium-rich foods: bananas, oranges, leafy green vegetables	Potassium-sparing diuretics: spironolactone, amiloride, triamterene
Foods high in vitamin K: broccoli, spinach, cauliflower, kale	Anticoagulant: warfarin
Grapefruit, grapefruit juice, alcohol	Statin drug for high cholesterol: Lipitor
Orange juice, large amounts of licorice	Beta blocker for angina and hypertension: Tenormin
Alcohol	Beta blocker for angina, hypertension, and migraine headaches: Inderal
Dairy products	Quinolone anti-infectives: Cipro, Levaquin Tetracycline anti-infectives: doxycycline Antifungals: Diflucan, Nizoral, Sporanox
Apple juice, orange juice, grapefruit juice	Antihistamine: Allegra

Drug Effects on Excretion of Nutrients

Excretion refers to the process of eliminating a medication or its metabolites or nutritional components from the body, a function usually performed by the kidneys. The length of time it takes to excrete a medication influences the extent of the medication's therapeutic effects. Slowed or inadequate excretion can raise the blood level of a medication and cause toxicity as successive scheduled doses are administered. Rapid or increased excretion can limit or greatly reduce the medication's therapeutic effect.

Certain medications can alter the kidney's excretion of nutrients such as minerals. Some diuretics, such as furosemide, can cause increased excretion of important minerals such as potassium, sodium, chloride, calcium, and magnesium. Long-term use of furosemide requires regular monitoring of the patient's fluid and electrolyte status and usually requires potassium supplementation. Similarly, isoniazid (INH), a medication used to treat tuberculosis, can lead to increased excretion of vitamin B6. Patients receiving INH therapy must be treated for more than 6 months, which can lead to vitamin B6 deficiency. To prevent the deficiency, patients are started on B6 as soon as INH is prescribed.

Many foods and nutrients can impact the excretion of medications. Lithium, a mood-stabilizing agent, is metabolized by the kidneys, where some of it is also reabsorbed and the remainder is excreted. This process is influenced by blood levels of sodium. Because lithium is similar in chemical structure to sodium, the kidneys often excrete lithium as if it were sodium. A person with a high level of sodium will excrete high levels of sodium and also of lithium, which can lead to subtherapeutic levels of the medication. Conversely, those with low sodium levels will retain extra lithium, leading to increased levels. Lithium is a medication that must be maintained in a specific therapeutic range, and increased levels can lead to adverse effects or even toxicity. This makes it extremely important to monitor the sodium levels in a patient taking lithium.

KNOWLEDGE CONNECTION

Which fruit juice is known to interfere with the metabolism of numerous medications? Patients taking warfarin should be educated to avoid foods with which vitamin? What side effects might you see in a patient taking long-term corticosteroids? Which vitamin must be supplemented in patients who are taking INH? Which electrolyte must be monitored in the patient taking lithium? Why is it important to educate patients about potential food–drug interactions?

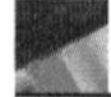

ENTERAL TUBES

Enteral tubes come in various styles and lengths and are used for multiple purposes. They may be used to decompress the stomach postoperatively, after abdominal injury, or as treatment for intestinal obstruction. These tubes may be inserted and used for nutritional support or medication administration. They may also be inserted to collect a specimen of stomach contents for diagnostic assessment of the GI tract, such as analyzing the gastric contents for pH or testing for blood.

• WORD • BUILDING •
subtherapeutic: sub – less than + therapeutic – treating

KNOWLEDGE CONNECTION

Explain four purposes for insertion of enteric tubes.

Anatomy and Physiology Connection

Gastrointestinal Tract

A review of the anatomy of the GI tract can help you to visualize the digestive organs and processes that occur as food moves through the body. The GI tract grows and changes through a person's life span, allowing greater digestion of food particles as it matures. This is part of the reason why solids are introduced to older infants, as the partially broken down food particles may contribute to a heightened allergic response.

The organs that comprise the GI tract include the mouth; pharynx; esophagus; stomach; small intestine, which is further divided into the duodenum, jejunum, and ileum; and large intestine. The accessory organs include the liver and the gallbladder (Fig. 24.3). Digestion begins as food enters the mouth, where enzymes begin to break down the food, and continues as it travels through the GI tract. Along the way, peristalsis and the musculature of the GI tract guide the mechanical digestion; enzymes and secretions are added by various organs for chemical digestion. Nutrient absorption primarily occurs in the small intestine. Absorption is the process by which nutrients pass through the walls of the small intestine and enter into the bloodstream in the capillaries. Absorption occurs by varying mechanisms, which include passive diffusion and osmosis, facilitated diffusion, and energy-dependent active transport. The process of *passive diffusion* occurs when the pressure on one side of the membrane is greater and the nutrients move from the area of greater pressure through the mucosa to the area of less pressure. At this point, the nutrients enter the circulatory system and are used for energy or stored for later use. While most nutrients are absorbed in the small intestine, most of the water absorption occurs within the large intestine, helping to maintain water and electrolyte balance and to solidify the remaining waste product into soft, formed feces to be expelled via the rectum.

Nasogastric and Nasointestinal Tubes

The **nasogastric tube** (NG tube) is shorter than the nasointestinal (NI) tube and is inserted through the nose, down the esophagus, and into the stomach. The longer NI tube is also inserted through the nose and continues through the stomach, into the duodenum, or even further into the jejunum. The terms *nasointestinal tube* and *nasoenteric tube* (NE tube) are often used interchangeably. The NI or NE tube usually is smaller in bore size and more flexible than an NG tube. Some of them are weighted on the tip to help pull the tube through

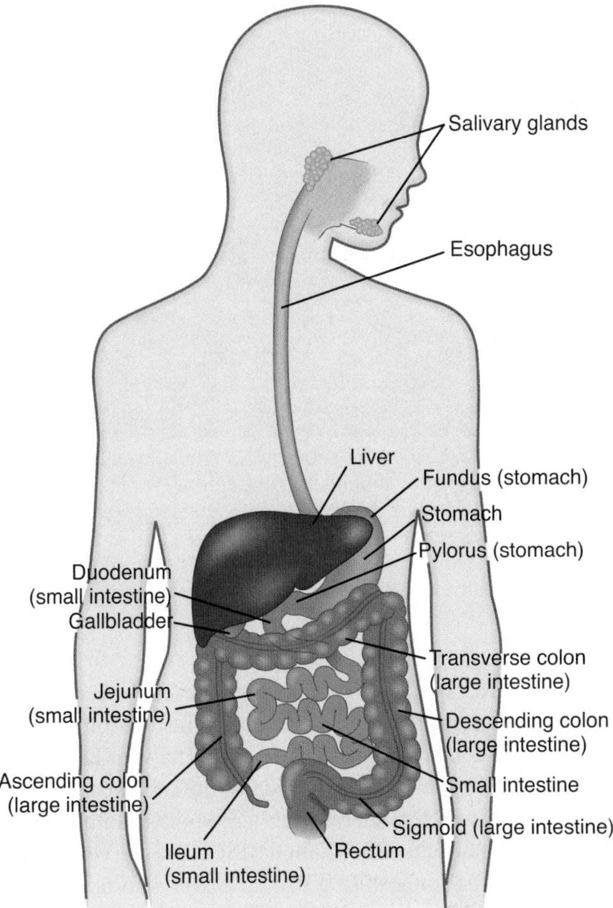

FIGURE 24.3 Organs of the digestive tract.

the stomach into the duodenum or jejunum; one commonly used NI tube is the Dobhoff (Fig. 24.4). It is mostly used for enteral feedings in patients who are at increased risk for aspiration, such as those with absent or diminished gag reflex or severe gastroesophageal reflux disease.

Tube Size and Length

The outside diameter of the NG or NI tube is measured using the French (Fr) scale: the larger the number, the larger the outside diameter of the tube. The most common sizes of feeding tubes measure 8 to 12 Fr with a length of 36 to 43 inches (90 to 108 cm). Larger-bore NG tubes, such as 16 or 18 Fr, are most commonly used for patients requiring gastric decompression or washing out of the stomach (termed *lavage*), obtaining gastric specimens, and instilling charcoal for the treatment of poisoning or drug overdose.

Single-Lumen Versus Double-Lumen

One style of NG tube is the Salem sump tube; it is a double-lumen tube, meaning that it has two separate channels inside

• WORD • BUILDING •

nasointestinal: naso – nose + intestinal – related to the intestine
nasoenteric: naso – nose + enteric – related to the small intestine

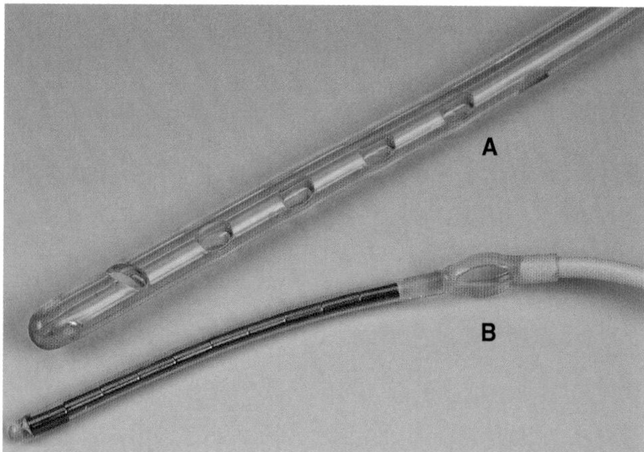

FIGURE 24.4 (a) Nasogastric tube: holes in the end of the tube allow contents to be suctioned from the stomach or fluid to be instilled into the stomach; (b) Weighted nasointestinal tube: smaller and more flexible than nasogastric tube, usually preferred for feeding (from Wilkinson JM, Treas LS. *Fundamentals of Nursing: Theory, Concepts & Applications.* Vol. 1. 3rd ed. Philadelphia, PA: FA Davis; 2016).

the tube. One lumen is an air vent; the other vent is for drainage of stomach contents, irrigation, instillation of medications, and obtaining gastric samples. The vent lumen extends like a "pigtail" from the side of the tube near the end that connects to the suction tubing. Some manufacturers make the pigtail blue to differentiate it as the *air vent.*

Several small holes are distributed over 3 to 6 inches of the end of the NG tube lumen that is inserted into the stomach (refer back to Fig. 24.4). Once the suction begins to pull a vacuum through these small openings, it can cause the end of the tube to adhere to the wall of the stomach, serving to irritate the mucosal lining. If it remains adhered to the same spot for an extended period of time, it can damage the mucosa. The smaller second lumen usually is blue to differentiate it from the primary lumen. It is designed to allow for atmospheric air to be drawn into the tube to equalize the vacuum pressure in the stomach caused by the suction, helping to prevent the tube from adhering to the gastric mucosa.

A second type of large-bore NG tube is Levin's tube, which has only one lumen. It can be used for the same purposes as the Salem sump tube, but it does not have the air vent lumen to allow equalization of vacuum pressure. Both the Salem sump and Levin's tube are intended for short-term use only. Leaving them in place for more than 10 to 14 days can result in necrosis of the nasal septum.

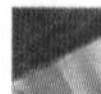 GASTRIC DECOMPRESSION

Gastric decompression is the process of reducing the pressure within the stomach by emptying it of its contents, including ingested food and liquids, gastric juices, and gas. It is often ordered when the patient is experiencing persistent vomiting. This may be accompanied by abdominal distention, which may be due to a partial or complete bowel obstruction. The appearance of the vomitus can often provide clues to the cause of persistent vomiting, so it is important for you to assess it and document your findings.

- Bright red blood indicates bleeding in the esophagus.
- Dark red blood indicates bleeding in the stomach.
- A coffee-ground appearance indicates blood that has been exposed to stomach acid; it has come from the esophagus and upper stomach and has reached the lower stomach and been mixed with stomach acid.
- Greenish-yellow liquid indicates bile. This usually means that the stomach is empty and the patient is vomiting the contents of the first part of the small intestine, the duodenum.

Insertion of an NG tube to low intermittent suction is part of the treatment for any of these conditions as well as for partial or complete bowel obstruction.

KNOWLEDGE CONNECTION

What does it mean to decompress the stomach? Describe the purpose of a double-lumen NG tube.

Insertion of NG Tube for Gastric Decompression

Placement of an NG tube requires a health-care provider's order, normally stating the type and size of tube and the purpose for the tube. If the health-care provider does not include this information, clarify all three pieces of information before inserting the tube. After reviewing the order on the medical record and clarifying it is necessary, review the record for conditions that might contraindicate insertion of the tube.

Preparing the Patient

Inquire of the patient whether he or she has ever experienced an NG tube insertion. Then explain the process to the patient, being honest but choosing your words carefully and observing the patient's responses. This helps you to know when the patient does not understand something, when he or she has a question, and when the patient begins to exhibit fear or anxiety. Your words and approach can have a dramatic impact on the patient's response. You can help a patient to better understand what you are about to do, gain the patient's confidence and cooperation, and alleviate some of his or her anxiety. However, if you fail to choose your words carefully, offer an incomplete explanation of what you are about to do, appear to be in a hurry, or display an apathetic or thoughtless attitude, you can raise his or her fear and anxiety level. This can result in a lack of patient cooperation that can make the insertion process much more uncomfortable for the patient and more difficult for you.

Preparing Supplies for Use

Gather your supplies, wash your hands, verify the patient's identity, provide for privacy, raise the bed to working height, and lower the rails. (See Skill 24.3, page 494, for a list of supplies and equipment that you will need.) Talk to the patient while you are preparing your work area and during the actual insertion of the tube. This will help to reduce the patient's anxiety and keep the patient focused on what you are saying rather than stressing as he or she watches you.

Arrange your supplies so that they are ready to use. Tear two pieces of 1-inch-wide silk tape, one piece approximately 1 inch long and the second piece 3 inches long. Beginning at one end of the 3-inch piece of tape, tear the tape lengthwise down the middle for approximately two-thirds of its length, leaving two 1/2-inch-wide tails that are about 2 inches long. The other end of the tape should still be 1 inch wide for about 1 inch of the tape's length. You will use the tape to secure the tube to the patient's nose; if your facility stocks them, you may obtain the adhesive securing device designed specifically for this purpose. Squeeze a small amount of water-soluble lubricant on a paper towel for lubricating the tip of the NG tube; place it within easy reach. Place your stethoscope on your neck so that it is ready for you to raise to your ears. Place a protective pad or towel over the patient's chest to prevent soiling his or her gown. Ask the patient to hold a finger against one side of his or her nose and exhale. Then have the patient repeat the action on the opposite side. Ask which side feels the most open. This will be the side you will want to use for inserting the NG tube.

Using the NG tube, measure the length from the tip of the patient's nose to the earlobe and then from the earlobe to the xiphoid process. Mark this spot on the tubing with a piece of tape, but do not wrap the tape around the tube so tightly that it is difficult to remove once the tube has been inserted. Obtain an irrigation syringe that:

- Will hold 50 or 60 mL,
- Has a plunger that is used to fill and empty the syringe, and
- Has a catheter tip or slip-tip so that the tip will fit into the NG tube opening.

Connect the irrigation syringe to the open end of the NG tube and pull the plunger about halfway back to allow room for gastric contents. Then lay the tube with attached syringe within easy reach. Connecting the irrigation syringe before insertion of the tube will prevent gastric juices from soiling the bed, requiring an extra linen change. Provide the patient with an emesis basin and tissue or washcloth to hold in the nondominant hand and a glass of ice water with a straw to hold in the dominant hand. Apply your clean examination gloves.

Inserting an NG Tube

Communicate to the patient some type of hand signal that he or she is to use if the procedure becomes too uncomfortable or the patient would like you to pause. Tell the patient that you will tell him or her when to take a drink and swallow. Explain that if he or she can do this each time you cue him or her, that it will make the tube go down much easier and faster.

Have the patient hyperextend the head just slightly. Gently insert the lubricated tip of the NG into the intended naris (Fig. 24.5). Remember that the nasal passageway begins to descend within a couple of centimeters. Avoid pushing the tip of the tube upward against the top side of the nasal passage, as it is quite painful and can damage tissue. Never force the tube. You should feel the tube begin to curve downward toward the nasopharynx. If not, gently lift the portion of the tube in your hand so that it directs the tip of the tube downward in the back of the patient's nasal passage. As soon as you reach the point of stimulating the patient's gag reflex, stop advancing the tube and pull it back just a tiny distance, about 1/8 inch (0.3 cm), *just to the point that the gag reflex is not being stimulated,* and instruct the patient to take a deep breath and relax. After giving the patient a couple seconds to relax, instruct the patient to begin drinking from the straw. Then, as the patient swallows, advance the tube, cueing the patient to "swallow…swallow." The advancement of the tube coordinated with swallowing allows normal peristalsis to help pull the NG tube along. Repeat this process until the tube is inserted to the tape marking. If the patient begins to gag or cough or gives you the designated hand signal to stop, pause and allow the patient to relax and breathe. Coax the patient along in this manner until the insertion is completed. ***Safety: If the patient gags or coughs continually and does not seem able to stop, the tube may be curled up in the back of the throat. Use a flashlight and tongue blade to view posterior pharynx to look for the tube. If the patient cannot speak, becomes cyanotic, or coughs incessantly, the tube likely is in the lungs. Immediately remove the tube.*** (Refer to Box 24.3 for more on what to do when an NG tube enters the lungs.)

SECURING THE NG TUBE. Once the tube is where you want it, remove the tape marker and apply the two pieces of tape you prepared to secure the tube to the patient's nose. There are various methods of taping the tube to the nose. Once you have managed several NG tubes, you probably will find that you prefer a particular method over the others. Here is one common way to apply the two pieces of tape. Apply the end of the 3-inch strip of silk tape (that you previously tore down

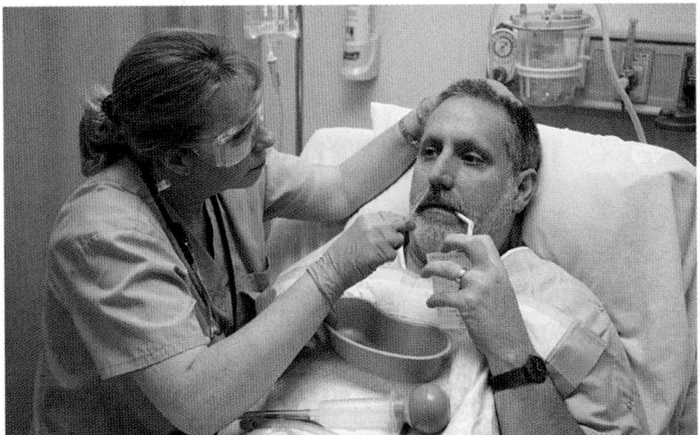

FIGURE 24.5 Gently insert the tip of the nasogastric tube into the most patent naris. As the tube begins to advance through the oropharynx, encourage the patient to sip water and swallow. This produces peristalsis, which helps to advance the tube into the stomach.

Box 24.3

Reacting When an NG Tube Enters the Lungs

When inserting an NG tube, it is important to know the signs and symptoms of the tube entering the lungs and the interventions to take if you believe the tube has entered the lungs. Signs and symptoms of a tube entering the lungs include the following:

- The patient becomes cyanotic
- The patient is unable to make a verbal sound
- The patient is coughing spasmodically and uncontrollably

If any of these signs and symptoms are present during NG tube insertion, the tube has likely entered the lungs. If this occurs, immediately and completely withdraw the NG tube. Once removed, the patient will most likely resume normal breathing and regain his or her proper coloring. However, if the patient continues to show signs of distress, take appropriate steps to restore his or her airway and breathing.

the middle) to the patient's nose with the two tails hanging down toward the NG tube. Then wrap one of the tails around the tube, spiraling tape down the tube until the entire tail of tape is secured to the tube. Then wrap the second tail in the opposite direction around the tube in the same manner. Finally, apply the other piece of tape that is 1 inch wide and 1 inch long directly across the end of the first piece of tape on the patient's nose. This helps to further secure the tape to reduce risk of the NG tube coming out unintentionally. ***Safety: Never let go of the tube until it is secured. It can come out in the blink of an eye, especially if the patient coughs, gags, or moves.*** The patient would be very upset if you allowed the tube to fall out and have put the patient through a repeat insertion. ***Safety: Be certain to tape the tube so that it is centered in the naris opening and does not press against any portion of the naris. If the tube presses against the nose, it can cause a pressure ulcer.***

VERIFYING PLACEMENT OF THE NG TUBE. In some hospitals, it may be policy to check the pH of the aspirated NG tube contents to determine placement. However, this is not a reliable method because the acidity of the gastric pH may be affected by certain medications and feedings. The most reliable way to check the placement of the tube is by x-ray. The tube has a radiopaque line that shows up on x-ray, confirming the location of the NG tube tip. ***Safety: X-ray confirmation of NG tube location should always be performed immediately after the insertion of any type of enteral tub, whether it is placed for gastric decompression, gastric analysis, or administration of medications or feedings.***

It is also recommended to use either a red or black indelible marker to mark the NG tube boldly at the point of insertion into the nose. This mark will be used as a point of reference for subsequent assessments of tube placement.

Skill 24.3 provides step-by-step instructions regarding how to insert an NG tube.

Attaching the NG Tube to Suction

Attach the primary lumen to a connecting tube that extends from the suction device. Set the suction on low continuous or intermittent suction according to health-care provider's orders. High suction is typically used only with intermittent suction.

Maintaining Patency of an NG Tube

To prevent an NG tube from clogging, it is important to assess the tube for *patency,* or the condition of being wide open, every 2 hours. Observe for the continual fluctuation and movement of gastric contents through the NG tube and connecting tube into the drainage container indicating patency. The health-care provider may write an "as needed" order for irrigation of the NG tube to maintain patency. Skill 24.4 (page 495) explains how to irrigate an NG tube.

Real-World Connection

Inserting an NG Tube

A patient presented to the emergency room with complaints of severe pain, nausea, and vomiting for more than 6 hours. After examining the patient and performing a couple of diagnostic procedures, it was determined the patient was suffering from an obstruction of the large intestine that was causing the portion of the bowel proximal to the obstruction to distend as it filled up with gastric juices and gas. Normal peristalsis was attempting to move the intestinal contents from the stomach through the small and large intestines but was unable to do so because of the obstruction, which explained why the patient was experiencing so much pain and nausea.

The patient was admitted, and orders were written to place the patient on NPO status, start IV fluids, and insert an NG tube connected to low intermittent suction. While the nurse was preparing to insert the NG tube, the patient vomited several hundred milliliters of brown semiliquid fecal material. Once the tube was successfully inserted, the extreme abdominal distention, pain, nausea, and vomiting began to improve immediately. With the administration of an analgesic and antiemetic, the patient got almost total relief by the time she had been there 1 hour. Within that first hour, a total of 2,000 mL of gastric contents and brown, foul-smelling, semiliquid stool were suctioned from the patient's GI tract. That particular patient later told the nurse that insertion of the NG tube was the best thing that had ever happened to her and she knew that it had saved her life.

Nursing Responsibilities for an NG Tube Connected to Suction

Your responsibilities when caring for an NG tube connected to suction include the following:

- Assess the tube every 2 to 4 hours to ensure patency.
- When necessary, irrigate a clogged tube according to the health-care provider's orders and facility policy.

- Monitor vacuum source settings for correct high or low suction and intermittent or continuous suction every 2 to 4 hours.
- Assess tubing connections to prevent accidental disconnection.
- Assess the color, amount, and consistency of gastric drainage.
- Assess the tube positioning and method of securing the tube so that the tube does not put pressure on the naris, which can result in a pressure ulcer.
- Manually clamp off the NG tube and auscultate bowel sounds every 4 hours, noting hyperactive, hypoactive, and absent sounds.
- Assess the abdomen for abdominal distention and palpate the abdomen, noting firmness.
- Assess the patient for reports of nausea, vomiting, pain, cramping, abdominal fullness, and discomfort every 2 hours.
- Assess for passage of rectal flatus, which may indicate the return of the bowel function known as *peristalsis.*
- Provide mouth care and apply lip moisturizer every 2 hours to prevent drying of the mucous membranes.
- Provide ice chips if allowed to keep the mouth moist.
- Monitor I&O to prevent fluid volume deficit or overload.
- ***Safety: Because the suction will deplete the potassium from the stomach, monitor the serum potassium level, noting a level below normal, known as hypokalemia.***

Removing an NG Tube

Once the health-care provider has ordered the NG tube to be discontinued, it will be your job to remove it. This procedure is not complicated and takes only a few minutes to accomplish. Explain the process to the patient to alleviate any anxiety and gain the patient's cooperation. Provide the patient with a tissue to wipe mucus from the nose. Wear protective gloves and position a waterproof pad across the patient's chest to prevent soiling of the patient's gown. Instill 10 to 20 mL of air into the NG tube's main lumen to empty the tube of any gastric contents. This prevents fluid from dripping onto the epiglottis during removal. Remove the tape securing the tube to the patient's nose, pinch off the tube, and ask the patient to hold his or her breath to close off the epiglottis. Twist the tube gently to loosen any dried secretions that may be making the tube stick to the lining of the nasal passage or throat, and quickly withdraw the tube from the patient's nose. Wrap it up in the waterproof pad you positioned on the patient's chest and dispose of it in a biohazard bag. You will want to remove it from the patient's view because it may be covered with unsightly mucus and secretions. Assist the patient to wash the face and perform mouth care. Document the procedure and the patient's tolerance of it. Skill 24.5 (page 496) presents more information on removing an NG tube.

KNOWLEDGE CONNECTION

Why is it so important to adequately explain what you are about to do prior to inserting an NG tube? Why should you insert the tip of the irrigating syringe into the distal end of the NG tube before insertion of the NG tube? Why should you cue the patient to "swallow…swallow…swallow" sips of water when you begin to advance the tube past the oropharynx? Why is x-ray confirmation of tube placement so important? Why must you monitor the potassium level of a patient with an NG tube connected to suction?

ENTERAL NUTRITION

Patients you care for are often too weak or too ill to take in sufficient nutrients by eating. Certain illnesses can interfere with eating, swallowing, digestion, or absorption of food to the degree that the body is not receiving adequate nourishment. In these cases, nutritional support, in the form of liquid formulations of nutrients, can be administered to meet a person's energy needs. The two types of nutritional support are enteral nutrition and parenteral nutrition.

Enteral nutrition uses the GI tract as a delivery system and involves tube feedings that usually replace all oral intake, but it also may be given as a supplement to oral ingestion of nutrients. Enteral nutrition is the preferred method for patients with high nutritional needs and an intact GI system, such as those with burns, trauma, severe malnutrition, or neurological problems that impair swallowing. Choosing an enteral feeding route depends on a number of factors. These include the patient's medical condition and stability, current nutritional status, and nutrient requirements for healing and recovery.

Feeding Tubes

As you read earlier, NG and NI tubes inserted for instillation of nutritional feedings are generally softer and smaller than those used for gastric decompression or lavage. They are inserted using basically the same method described previously; however, they tend to go down easier because they are smaller and softer.

Percutaneous Endoscopic Gastrostomy and Jejunostomy Tubes

Patients requiring long-term feedings have surgical endoscopic placement of a percutaneous feeding tube. *Percutaneous* means that an incision is made through the skin and abdominal wall, allowing the tube to extend from either the stomach or the jejunum to the external surface of the abdomen. If the tube is placed in the stomach, it is known as a **percutaneous endoscopic gastrostomy tube** (PEG tube) (Fig. 24.6). If the tube

• **WORD • BUILDING** •
percutaneous: per – through + cutaneous – skin

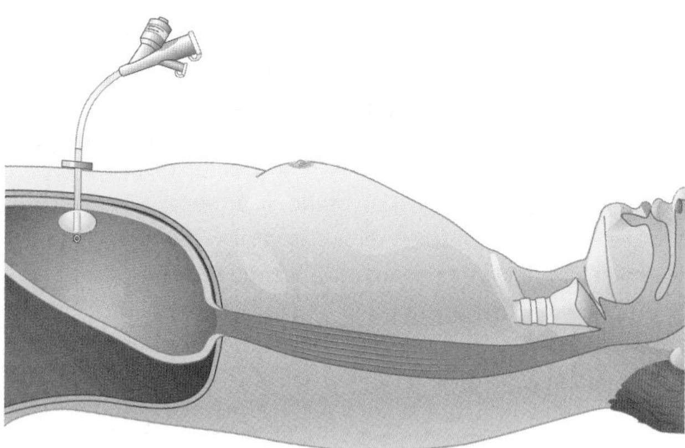

FIGURE 24.6 A percutaneous endoscopic gastrostomy tube (from Wilkinson JM, Treas LS. *Fundamentals of Nursing: Theory, Concepts & Applications.* Vol. 1. 3rd ed. Philadelphia, PA: FA Davis; 2016).

is inserted into the jejunum, it is called a **jejunostomy tube,** or J-tube. Figure 24.7 shows the insertion sites of different tubes. The tube is secured by tight suturing of the incision around the tube. This also helps to prevent leakage of formula during feedings. For patients with a newly inserted PEG tube or J-tube, the nurse must provide care for the surgical incision until it is completely healed. Of all the feeding tubes, the PEG tube is the most comfortable for the patient. Originally it was used for those patients needing long-term nutritional support. However, current trends in addressing patient comfort and improved technology have made this a good option for short-term therapy. The PEG tube or J-tube should also be marked at the point of insertion into the skin and measured from the point of insertion to the distal end of the tube. These two pieces of data should be recorded for use as a reference point when checking placement of the tube prior to instillations of feedings or medications.

Some gastrostomies and jejunostomies may not have a tube inserted. Instead, they have a button placed at skin level that goes through the abdominal wall into the stomach or intestine and is held in place with a balloon. The tubing to deliver the enteral feeding attaches to the button (see Fig. 24.8).

KNOWLEDGE CONNECTION

Discuss the various types of feeding tubes. When is enteral nutrition the preferred feeding method?

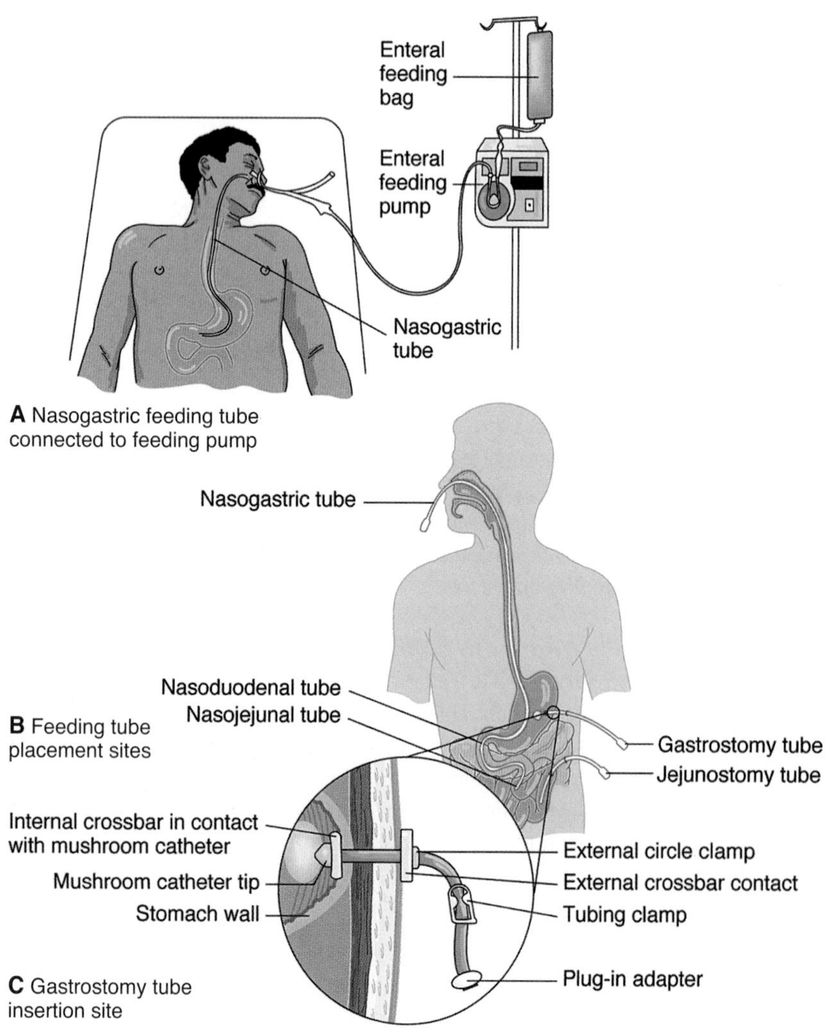

FIGURE 24.7 Feeding tubes: (a) Nasogastric tube connected to feeding pump; (b) Feeding tube placement sites: gastrostomy, jejunostomy; (c) View of gastrostomy tube insertion site showing the integument, subcutaneous, and muscle layers, as well as the stomach wall, which a percutaneous gastrostomy tube must go through before entering the stomach (from Williams LS, Hopper PD. *Understanding Medical-Surgical Nursing.* 5th ed. Philadelphia, PA: FA Davis; 2015).

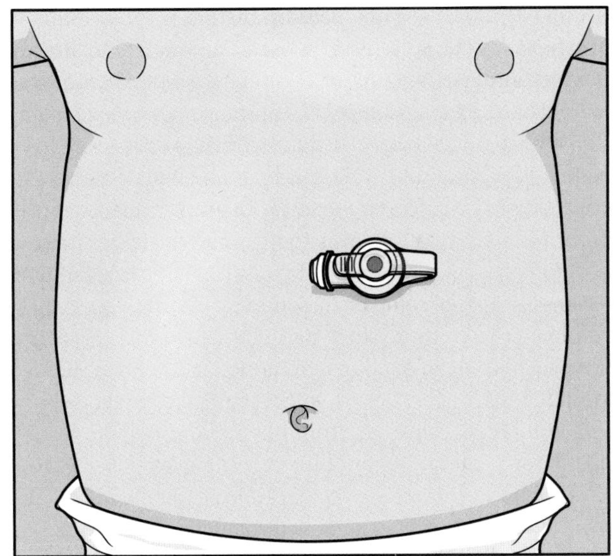

FIGURE 24.8 Gastrostomy button.

Tube Feeding Formulas

The selection of formula will be dependent on where the tube is placed and where formula will enter the GI tract. The patient's ability to digest and absorb nutrients will determine which type of formula is used. Table 24.3 describes the most common types of enteral feeding formulas.

Enteral Feeding Methods

The delivery method is chosen with consideration of a number of factors. These include the type and location of the feeding tube, the patient's medical condition and status of the digestive system, the type of formula being administered, and the length of time the patient has been on enteral feedings.

Feedings may be ordered for intermittent infusion and administered over 30 to 60 minutes or ordered continuously to be delivered over an 8-hour or even 24-hour period. The infusion rate will be regulated by either an infusion pump or gravity drip set according to the health-care provider's order.

Table 24.3
Types of Enteral Feeding Formulas

Type of Formula	*Formula Description*	*Use for Patient Diagnoses*
Standard formulas	Contain protein isolates from milk, soybeans, or a combination of purified proteins; provide 1 kcal/mL of solution and are proportionally balanced, delivering 12%–20% of kcal as protein, 45%–60% of kcal as carbohydrates, and 30%–40% of kcal as fats; also contain vitamins and minerals and meet the nutritional needs of most patients	Patients who can digest and absorb nutrients without difficulty but are unable to eat or swallow sufficiently Patients who need additional nutrition above their oral consumption
Hydrolyzed formulas	Contain macronutrients that are *predigested,* or have been partially or fully broken down to components that require little digestion before absorption; are often low in fat and may be enriched with medium-chain triglycerides to ease digestion and absorption	Patients who have compromised digestive or absorptive functions
High-protein formulas	Contain normal nutrients with additional protein	Burns Large open wounds Malnutrition
Diabetic formulas	Contain reduced levels of simple carbohydrates	Diabetes mellitus type 1 Diabetes mellitus type 2
Renal formulas	Contain reduced levels of potassium, sodium, and nitrogen	Renal insufficiency Renal failure
Pulmonary formulas	Provide 55% of the calories as fat so that less CO_2 is produced as oxygen is consumed	Lung cancer Chronic emphysema Chronic asthma Pulmonary fibrosis
Fiber-containing formulas	Contain higher levels of fiber	Diverticulosis Colon cancer Diabetes Heart disease Those in long-term care

New regulations by The Joint Commission require the use of new feeding tube, syringe, and feeding set (bag and tubing) connections, called ENFit connectors, for small-bore feeding tubes. This has been put in place after studies and surveys have shown that confusion existed between IV tubing and enteral feeding tubing and, when medications were drawn up in syringes that were compatible with IVs, the medications were sometimes accidentally given through the IV tubing instead of through the enteral feeding tubing. The requirement for using ENFit syringes, bags, and feeding tubes went into effect January 1, 2017. After that date, hospitals cannot use a connector for feeding tubes that would fit into any other tubes. These tubes will only connect with each other and will not connect with IV tubing, Luer lock syringes, or slip-tip syringes. Figure 24.9 shows an ENFit connection.

Intermittent Tube Feedings

Intermittent feedings are used in patients who are on long-term enteral feedings and are no longer acutely ill. These patients may be in a long-term health-care facility or at home. Intermittent feedings are administered in equal portions periodically throughout the day. The patient usually will receive 200 to 300 mL of formula every 4 to 6 hours. The formula is delivered by gravity via a bolus or drip set, or with a feeding pump, and administered over a 30- to 60-minute period. The amount of formula delivered per feeding will depend on the total quantity of formula the patient needs to receive in a 24-hour period. Feedings are divided into equal portions and scheduled over the course of the day or scheduled only during waking hours to provide patients with uninterrupted sleep time. This latter schedule is preferable for those patients on long-term feedings, as this allows the patient a schedule that more closely resembles normal.

Intermittent feedings are generally well tolerated; maintaining the formula at room temperature decreases the potential for gastric discomfort. ***Safety: Because of the high risk of aspiration with enteral feedings, the head of the bed should be elevated at least 30 to 45 degrees during the entire feeding and for 1 hour after the feeding to help reduce the risk of reflux and aspiration.***

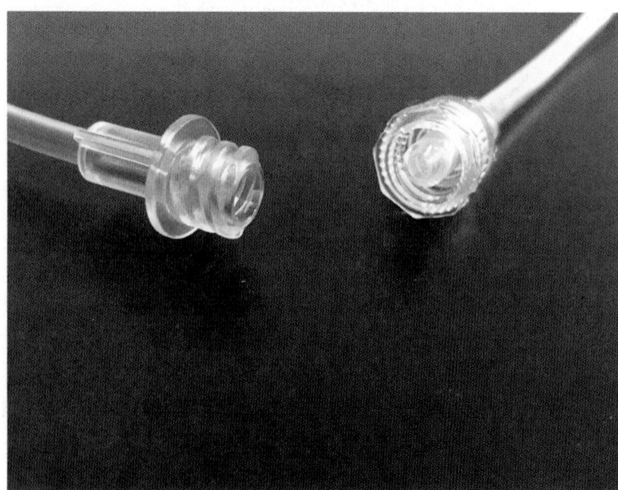

FIGURE 24.9 ENFit connector. (Borrowed with permission from the Global Enteral Device Supplier Association.)

BOLUS FEEDINGS. **Bolus feedings** are a type of intermittent tube feeding that is frequently used, in which a health-care provider–ordered volume of formula is administered at set intervals throughout the day. To administer a bolus feeding, a large irrigating syringe (50 mL or greater) is attached to the feeding tube. The size of the feeding tube will determine the size and type of syringe tip that can be used: a catheter-tipped 50- or 60-mL irrigation or piston syringe for larger tubes or a 20- to 30-mL slip-tipped injection syringe for smaller tubes. If using the larger catheter-tipped irrigation syringe, remove the plunger from the syringe barrel and then insert the tip of the syringe into the open lumen of the feeding tube. Bend or crimp the tubing just below where it attaches to the syringe. This will prevent formula from flowing through the feeding tube before you are ready. Flush the tube by pouring 30 to 60 mL of water into the syringe. Release the bend or crimp in the tube so that water can flow through the feeding tube and then recrimp the tube. Carefully begin to pour the formula into the syringe barrel until it is almost full. Then release the bend or crimp in the tubing, allowing formula to flow through the feeding tube until the syringe is almost empty (Fig. 24.10). At this time, you may stop the flow by bending the tubing again while you refill the syringe, or, if you are steady enough, you may continue pouring formula into the syringe as it is instilling until feeding is completed. Use whichever method works best for you, but *use caution to prevent air from entering the tube in between refilling the syringe.* Instilling air will increase gastric distress and should be avoided. This method should permit you to instill the feeding over a short period of time, generally 15 to 20 minutes, directly into the stomach or small intestine.

Feedings will be scheduled four to six times per day. ***Safety: Residuals should be checked before administering each feeding (see section on Checking Residual Gastric Volume below).*** Bolus feedings can be poorly tolerated, causing a number of problems such as cramping, gastric distention, diarrhea, and aspiration. For further information regarding administration of intermittent bolus enteral feedings, see Skill 24.6 (page 497).

Continuous Infusion Feedings

Continuous feedings are best administered via an infusion pump at a constant rate over an 8- to 24-hour period. The continuous infusion method promotes better tolerance of feedings and nutrient absorption. Use of the pump provides greater control of the rate and amount of feeding delivered. This method is used with critically ill patients because of the decrease in hypermetabolic response to stress, the risk for aspiration, and the incidence of diarrhea. Continuous feedings should be interrupted every 4 hours to check placement and residual volume, to administer water for hydration if ordered, and to flush the tube to prevent clogging. ***Safety: These patients must have the head of the bed raised at least 30 degrees continually to reduce the risk of aspiration.***

Tube feedings are typically initiated at full strength but at a slower rate to allow the intestinal tract time to adapt. You will

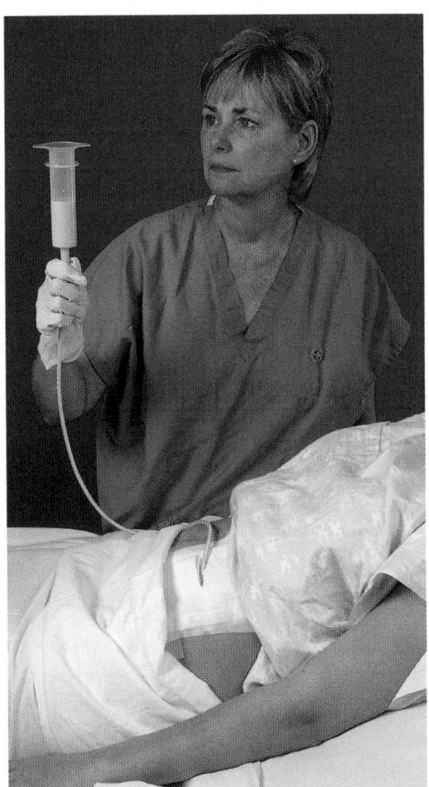

FIGURE 24.10 Nurse administering intermittent bolus percutaneous endoscopic gastrostomy feeding (from Wilkinson JM, Treas LS. *Fundamentals of Nursing: Theory, Concepts & Applications*. Vol. 1. 3rd ed. Philadelphia, PA: FA Davis; 2016).

monitor the patients for symptoms indicating poor tolerance, such as nausea, diarrhea, abdominal cramping, vomiting, or high gastric residuals. Once the patient exhibits tolerance of the feeding, the hourly rate can be increased every 8 to 12 hours until the desired rate of infusion is achieved. Feeding by the enteral route has been shown to improve nutritional status, strengthen immune response and reduce sepsis, minimize the hypermetabolic response to trauma, and maintain the function of the intestinal tract. Skill 24.7 (page 498) provides information on how to use a feeding pump.

Checking Placement of a Feeding Tube

You read earlier in the chapter that you must assess placement of any type of NG or NI tube prior to instillation of medication, irrigant, or feedings. It is so important that we want to emphasize it once more. ***Safety: If the placement of a tube is not confirmed prior to administering a feeding or medication, there is a risk of instilling the formula or medication directly into the lungs via an NG tube or into the sterile peritoneal cavity via a PEG tube or J-tube.*** Some patients have developed pneumonia—and other patients have actually died—from failure to confirm tube placement prior to instillations.

Checking Residual Gastric Volume

Before you can safely administer a tube feeding, not only must you check tube placement but you also must assess the *residual gastric volume*, or the amount of formula that still remains in the stomach from the previous feeding. If the previous feeding has not been absorbed and remains within the stomach and you proceed to instill another formula feeding, the additional formula can fill the stomach, which increases the risk of reflux via the cardiac sphincter into the esophagus. The esophagus lies in the immediate vicinity of the opening to the larynx at the superior end of the trachea, allowing refluxed formula to be aspirated into the lungs. Aspiration of fluids can initiate laryngeal spasms and/or result in pneumonia. ***Safety: It is vital that you check the residual volume as well as tube placement before instilling each tube feeding.***

The process of checking residual volume is not complicated. Aspirate contents through the tube until the stomach is empty. If residual amount is greater than the syringe can hold, measure the aspirate volume using a graduated container. Do not discard the residual aspirate, as it is rich in electrolytes and should be reinstilled into the stomach to prevent an electrolyte imbalance unless health-care provider's orders state otherwise. Determine whether the residual volume exceeds the health-care provider's order for the amount at which to withhold the feeding. If the health-care provider does not write specific orders for handling residuals, then follow the facility's policy and procedure. However, if the health-care provider fails to provide specific instructions and the facility's policy and procedure manual does not specify a residual volume at which to withhold the feeding, then you must rely on what you learned as a student. Checking residual volume should also be documented (Fig. 24.11).

For intermittent feedings, check to see if the residual volume is 150 mL or less. If so, you should reinstill the aspirated contents and continue with the tube feeding. If the amount is greater than 250 mL, follow the directions for the patient receiving continuous tube feedings.

If the patient is receiving continuous tube feedings, determine the amount of residual volume and check the patient for any distention or abdominal pain. If the residual is less than the flow rate for 1 hour or less than 150 mL, proceed with the continuous feeding. If the residual is greater than 250 mL and there are no symptoms, reinstill the residual and check the patient again in 1 hour. If the residual is still greater than 250 mL, stop the infusion for 4 hours and recheck. If the residual is still greater than 250 mL, call the health-care provider. If it is less than 250 mL, restart the infusion at 50% of the original rate. *Note: Always follow any health-care provider orders or facility policy for amounts of gastric residual volume. Use these guidelines only if no other guidelines exist.*

Nursing Care of the PEG Tube or J-Tube Insertion Site

Inspect the insertion site each day, noting any redness, tenderness, irritation, or drainage that might indicate infection. A new PEG tube or J-tube site should be cleaned daily with gauze and sterile saline. Using a circular motion, cleanse from the inner aspects of the site to the outer aspects. Ensure that the site is thoroughly dry and then cover it with a split-gauze dressing, also known as a *drain gauze,* which fits around the tube. For existing

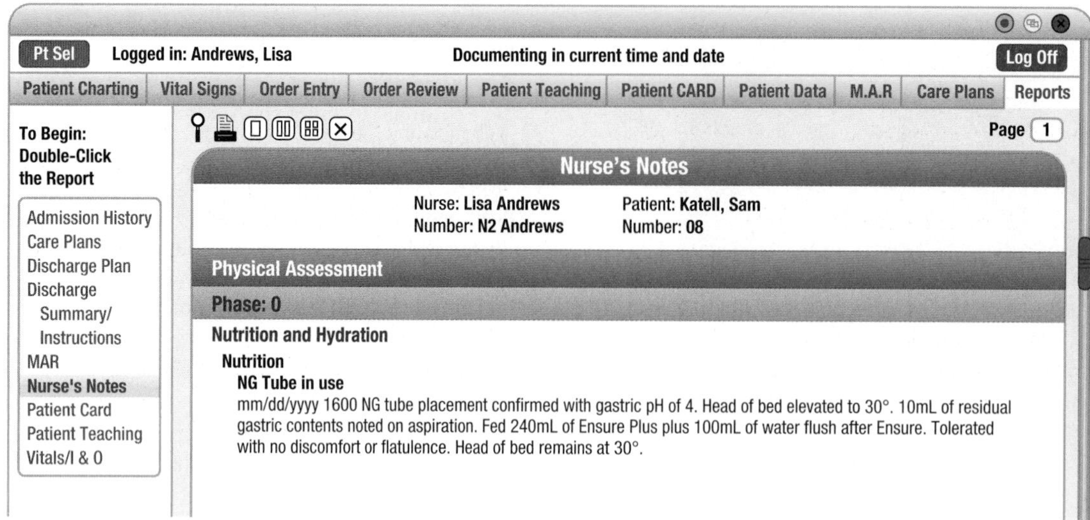

FIGURE 24.11 Sample electronic health record documentation.

mature sites, cleansing should occur daily with a clean washcloth, warm water, and soap. The inner aspects of the site should be cleaned with a cotton swab to remove any drainage or leakage. Allow the site to dry thoroughly and leave it uncovered.

Nursing Responsibilities for a Patient with a PEG Tube or J-Tube

Your responsibilities for a PEG tube or J-tube include the following:

- Assessing tube placement by checking the tube markings to determine that the tube has not shifted or dislodged prior to each instillation
- Maintaining patency of the tube
- Performing daily assessment of skin integrity surrounding the tube
- Performing daily cleansing of the tube insertion site as appropriate
- Assessing bowel sounds daily, noting absent, hypoactive, or hyperactive sounds
- Assessing the abdomen, noting distention
- Assessing for gastric residual prior to instillation of medications or formula
- Elevating the head of the bed during feedings and for 30 to 60 minutes afterward
- Monitoring intake and output to ensure proper balance
- Monitoring weight, noting any loss
- Monitoring for diarrhea or constipation that might result from certain feeding formulas

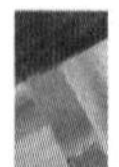

COMPLICATIONS ASSOCIATED WITH TUBE FEEDINGS

Tube feedings are an artificial means of feeding a patient, and complications can arise. Common complications such as nausea and diarrhea are related to the patient's inability to tolerate the type of formula. The problem usually can be resolved by changing to a different formula.

Clogged feeding tubes are a problem that can stem from the processes associated with the feedings. It is important to prevent clogging by flushing the tube before and after instillations. If the feeding tube does clog, obtain a health-care provider's order to irrigate the tube to restore patency.

Patients receiving tube feedings may have impaired swallowing ability due to stroke or debilitation from chronic illness, or they may be unconscious. *Aspiration* is an adverse event that places these patients at risk for additional serious illness. Aspirated material can include oropharyngeal bacteria, particulate matter, and acidified gastric contents. Aspiration of bacteria can cause aspiration pneumonia. Aspirated particulates can cause severe laryngospasm and bronchial constriction, wheezing, chest pain, and even respiratory failure. Aspiration of acidified gastric contents produces a chemical burn to the alveolar walls, causing rapid movement of protein and fluids into the alveoli. This results in a decline in lung compliance, with respiratory failure ensuing. The nurse can undertake a number of preventative measures to avoid aspiration (Box 24.4).

Metabolic problems are also potential complications: hyperglycemia, dehydration, fluid overload, or electrolyte imbalances can occur in patients receiving tube feedings. The proper choice of formula, a slow rate of infusion, and ensuring adequate hydration with water can help minimize and eliminate these complications.

Another serious complication associated with tube feedings is contamination of formula. Feeding formulas should be kept refrigerated until you are ready to use them. Contaminated formula can cause severe GI problems, including cramping, vomiting, and diarrhea, or food poisoning. Your patients receiving enteral feedings are already seriously medically compromised, and contaminated formula can lead to serious adverse consequences. Patients tolerate room-temperature formula better than cold formula, so you will need to plan to take formula out of the refrigerator and allow it to warm to room temperature approximately 1 hour before administering it. Box 24.5 presents key points related to managing formula.

Box 24.4

Techniques to Prevent Aspiration

Because aspiration may be life-threatening, you are responsible for implementing interventions to reduce the risk of aspiration. This is a partial list of interventions that you should implement.

- Use the smallest diameter feeding tube possible.
- Confirm tube placement with x-ray immediately after insertion and prior to initiating tube feeding.
- Confirm tube placement prior to each instillation of medication, water, or formula.
- Make certain that active bowel sounds are present prior to instillations.
- Assess for abdominal distention before feedings.
- Elevate the head of the patient's bed to 30 to 45 degrees during intermittent feedings and at least 1 hour afterward; for continual feedings, the head of the bed must remain elevated at 30 to 45 degrees.
- Check gastric residual volumes prior to intermittent feedings and every 4 hours during continuous feedings.

KNOWLEDGE CONNECTION

When is enteral nutrition the preferred feeding method? Why cannot all medications be administered via an enteral tube?

Supervision/Delegation Connection

Tube Feedings

UAPs work under the supervision of the registered nurse (RN) or licensed practical/vocational nurse (LPN/LVN). Tasks that may be delegated include administration of enteral tube feedings via an NG tube, NI tube, PEG tube, or J-tube. The delegation of feeding can occur only after verification of the feeding tube placement. You are responsible for this assessment and cannot delegate performance of tube placement verification. You also are responsible for supervising the UAP in preparing and positioning the patient to receive the tube feeding. The UAP can document the intake and output and report these data. Remember that the rules governing delegation are dictated by each state's Nurse Practice Act. It is your responsibility to know the role and scope of practice for both yourself and the UAPs whom you supervise, as well as delegating nursing care appropriately.

Box 24.5

Tips for Managing Tube Feeding Formulas

Tube feeding formulas should be carefully managed to prevent spoilage, just as you protect the food you serve to patients as well as your own family. Patients receiving tube feedings may have compromised immunity, making it an even higher priority to prevent bacterial contamination of the formula. Here are some basic tips to remember.

- Wash hands thoroughly before handling formula or the feeding system.
- Rinse and wipe the top of the can before opening.
- Label all opened formula with the patient's name, date, and time when opened; follow the label instructions regarding the length of time you may use the formula once opened.
- Make sure all open cans are covered and stored in the refrigerator when not in use.
- Do not use and discard all unlabeled formula and out-of-date formula.
- Rinse the feeding bag and tubing with clean water before adding new formula.
- Flush the tube with water before and after each use.
- Hang only the amount of formula that can be administered in 6 hours; discard formula that hangs for more than 6 hours.
- Never add new formula to old.
- Change the feeding bag and syringe every 24 hours.

PARENTERAL NUTRITION

Parenteral nutrition is administered directly into the bloodstream via a central venous catheter, bypassing the GI tract. Parenteral nutrition can supply complete nutrition, including amino acids, dextrose, emulsified fats, vitamins, minerals, and trace elements, to the patient who cannot meet his or her nutritional needs via the oral route. ***Safety: Aseptic technique is required, and the bag of solution must be changed every 24 hours.*** It is used for patients with one or more problems that are complicated by malnutrition and low protein levels. These patients generally do not have a functioning GI tract or are unable to absorb adequate nutrients through enteral feedings. Box 24.6 presents a partial list of conditions in which parenteral nutrition might be appropriate.

The administration of parenteral nutrition depends on the patient's nutritional needs and the expected length of time parenteral feedings will be required. **Partial parenteral nutrition** (PPN) may be administered through a peripherally inserted central catheter inserted into a smaller peripheral vein. **Total parenteral nutrition** (TPN) may be administered through a central venous catheter (CVC) placed in a larger central vein. The core differences between TPN and PPN are the vessel selected to receive the nutrition and the concentration of solution infused. Only the "least hypertonic" solutions may be infused into the peripheral veins, whereas it is possible to deliver higher concentrations through the larger central veins.

Partial Parenteral Nutrition

PPN is used for those patients who are able to meet some of their nutritional needs orally but require additional calories or nutrients for a limited period of time because of their illness. PPN does not meet the patient's total nutritional needs without concurrent ingestion of food via the GI tract. Patients

Box 24.6

Conditions That Might Require Parenteral Feeding

There are many medical conditions for which parenteral feeding may be required. Here is a partial list of conditions that may be treated with parenteral feeding.

- Burns or trauma, severe
- Cancer
- Chemotherapy
- Hepatic failure
- Intestinal obstruction
- Intractable vomiting or diarrhea
- Malabsorption disorders
- Necrotizing enterocolitis
- Paralytic ileus, unrelenting
- Renal failure
- Short bowel syndrome

with short bowel syndrome or malabsorption syndromes often require PPN in addition to oral intake. Solutions infused into peripheral veins must be isotonic or only mildly hypertonic to prevent phlebitis and decrease the risk of thrombus. Parenteral nutrition solutions include a mixture of dextrose, amino acids, lipid emulsions, electrolytes, vitamins, and trace minerals in sterile water. The Infusion Nurses Society states that peripherally administered PPN solution cannot contain a concentration that exceeds 10% dextrose and 5% amino acids. Due to these restrictions, PPN will provide a limited amount of calories, necessitating oral supplementation for the patient to have adequate daily caloric intake.

Total Parenteral Nutrition

TPN is a hypertonic, nutritionally complete solution that is delivered via a large-diameter central vein. It provides calories, essential vitamins, minerals, and electrolytes and restores nitrogen balance, promoting tissue growth and wound healing, which makes it useful in patients who are nutritionally depleted. Infusion into a large vein allows for the TPN solution to be diluted quickly. TPN is used when a patient's nutritional requirements are high, and it is anticipated that the need will be long term. Patients for whom it may be used are those being treated for extensive trauma, burns, or sepsis; those undergoing aggressive cancer treatment; or those with GI illnesses that interfere with metabolism and absorption of nutrients.

The CVC that is used for TPN can have two, three, or four separate lumens, or channels (Fig. 24.12). It must be inserted surgically into one of the larger central veins, such as the subclavian vein or internal jugular vein, and advanced until the catheter tip is positioned in the superior vena cava (Fig. 24.13). The insertion site where the catheter perforates the cutaneous layer must be continually covered with a sterile dressing, usually a transparent occlusive dressing. Often the patient who is a candidate for insertion of a central line for TPN already has a suppressed or impaired immune system. Because this

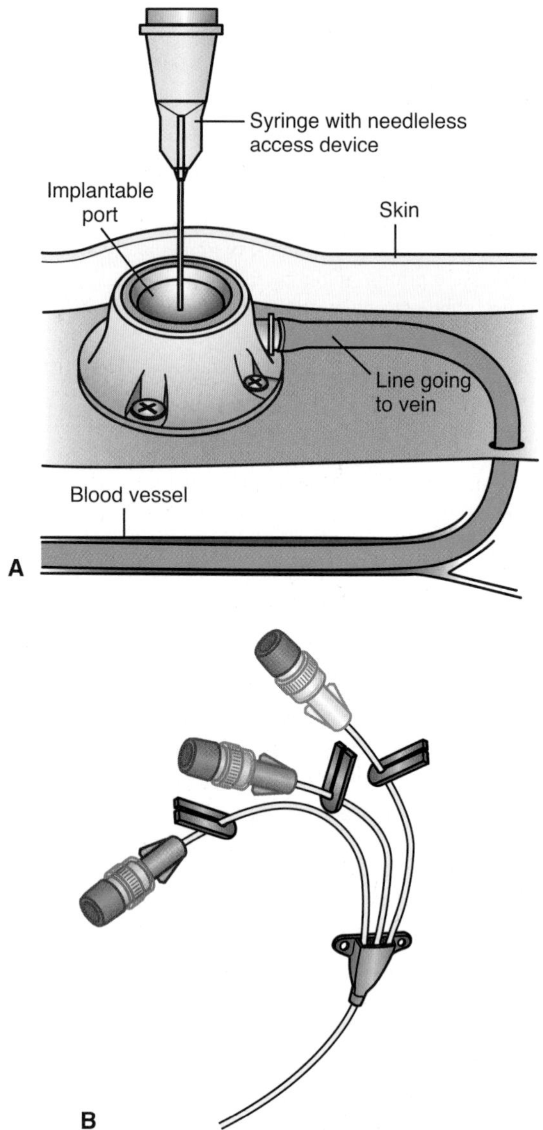

FIGURE 24.12 Triple-lumen central venous catheter injection ports (from Wilkinson JM, Treas LS. *Fundamentals of Nursing: Theory, Concepts & Applications.* Vol. 1. 3rd ed. Philadelphia, PA: FA Davis; 2016).

extremely invasive procedure places the patient at risk for infection, you should receive specific training before providing nursing care for a central line. Some facilities limit care of central lines to RNs only, while others permit LPN/LVNs once they have been trained. It is your responsibility to know the facility policies and procedures where you are employed, as well as knowing what is allowed by the Nurse Practice Act in your state.

Patients receiving TPN may receive their medications mixed into their solution or intravenously infused into the designated lumen or a port linked to the central line. They often receive insulin to help control serum glucose, as the TPN solution has a high glucose concentration. In general, due to the potential for incompatibilities, the addition of medications to TPN solution should be limited, and compatibility must be ensured. TPN is expensive, administration requires

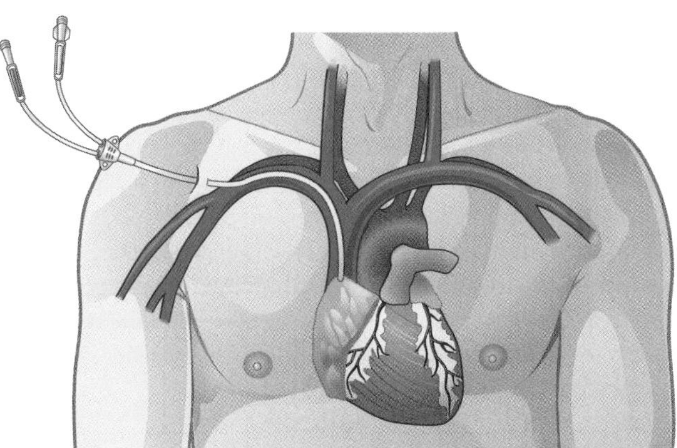

FIGURE 24.13 Central venous catheters are typically inserted into larger central veins such as the subclavian or jugular veins and threaded into the superior vena cava (from Wilkinson JM, Treas LS. *Fundamentals of Nursing: Theory, Concepts & Applications*. Vol. 1. 3rd ed. Philadelphia, PA: FA Davis; 2016).

that the patient be continually monitored while receiving TPN, and TPN increases the risk for the development of infection or mechanical or metabolic problems. Therefore, TPN is discontinued as soon as the patient's nutritional needs have been met or the patient can tolerate enteral or oral feedings.

TPN Infusion

Initially, TPN is infused slowly to give the body time to adapt to the infusion of a highly concentrated glucose solution. It is increased in increments of 25 mL per hour until the desired rate of infusion is achieved. It is administered via a continuous drip infusion on a pump to ensure a controlled rate of infusion. It is essential that infusion be slow and controlled, as a rapid infusion of TPN solution can cause severe hyperglycemia or hypoglycemia, with the potential for further complications such as coma or death. Initially, a patient will receive 1 liter of solution infused over 24 hours, with the rate being increased by 1 liter per day until the desired volume delivery is reached.

When caring for a patient receiving parenteral nutrition, it is important that you monitor laboratory values closely to assess for fluid or electrolyte imbalance until the patient is fully stable on a parenteral formula. Before you can discontinue a patient's TPN, the patient must be gradually weaned from TPN to either enteral or oral feedings in order to prevent metabolic complications.

> **KNOWLEDGE CONNECTION**
> What is the difference between TPN and PPN? Why is TPN administered via a central line catheter? What laboratory values should be monitored in patients receiving TPN?

Monitoring Nutritional Status

Patients receiving parenteral nutrition should be monitored closely for nutritional status. This includes monitoring daily weights until stable and certain laboratory results. Electrolyte levels should be monitored daily for 1 week before decreasing to twice a week. Prealbumin, albumin, and total protein should be monitored, but they do not have to be monitored as frequently as the electrolyte levels. The glucose level should be monitored at least twice daily, usually four times, in order to determine how often the patient requires insulin, and how much, to maintain a stable blood glucose level.

Prealbumin is produced primarily by cells in the liver, but it also is produced by GI mucosa and the pancreas. It is quite sensitive to changes in nutritional status, has a relatively short half-life, and is rapidly responsive to protein depletion. These characteristics make prealbumin a good indicator of acute changes, while albumin remains the standard for monitoring chronic malnutrition. Normal prealbumin levels are 15 to 35 mg/dL. FSBS should be assessed every hour during the initial TPN infusion and then every 4 to 6 hours thereafter to provide a reference for insulin administration.

> **KNOWLEDGE CONNECTION**
> Why do you need to monitor prealbumin in patients receiving parenteral nutrition? Why is it important to perform FSBS every hour initially and then every 4 to 6 hours afterwards?

Settings Connection: Home Health

Enteral and Parenteral Therapy in the Home

Patients receiving enteral or parenteral therapy may be on these feedings for long periods of time. Many patients will not require lengthy hospital stays and will be discharged home on feedings. The home health nurse's role in management of the patient requiring nutritional support is one of patient/family advocate, coordinator, and educator. A key factor in the success of enteral or parenteral nutrition will be family or caregiver involvement. This should begin early in the process, ideally as soon as parenteral nutrition is implemented in the hospital setting. Caregivers should be involved in discussions regarding site selection, nutrient delivery method, and formula selection, with consideration given to their ability to manage the care and the affordability of the feeding formula. The nurse will educate the patient and caregiver regarding care of the feeding tube, tube placement site, flushing the tube, administering feedings, safety issues, and managing complications that may arise, such as a clogged tube. Safety in the administration of enteral and parenteral feedings is important. Caregivers must be taught how to verify the tube placement, how to minimize risk for aspiration, and how to manage air in the PPN or TPN line. The nurse will also teach the caregiver how to safely store formula and minimize the risk of contamination. Signs and symptoms of problems for which the patient should be monitored must be taught and made available in printed format for later referral.

The home health nurse will follow the patient to assist with management of feedings as the patient transitions to home. However, the nurse will gradually assume a more supportive role as he or she teaches the caregiver to assume responsibility for the feedings and care and management of the tube. Once the caregiver has assumed full responsibility, the nurse will remain involved and continue to follow the patient, assessing for adequate nutrition as evidenced by maintenance of weight and normal laboratory values, including glucose and albumin levels. The nurse will also perform physical assessments regularly, monitoring skin integrity by looking for areas of pressure ulceration or risk for breakdown, checking for signs of muscle wasting, monitoring the lungs for signs indicating aspiration of particulates and evolving pneumonia, and monitoring for signs of difficulty tolerating tube feedings, such as increased abdominal discomfort, bloating, or diarrhea. The nurse will serve as the primary communicator with the health-care provider and assist to coordinate care as the patient's condition changes.

Nursing Care Plan for a Patient Post CVA With a PEG Tube

You have been assigned to provide care for 56-year-old Mr. Ayala, who has now had a PEG tube placed. He was admitted earlier in the week and is 5 days post CVA, more commonly called a "stroke." He had an NG feeding tube placed first, but now has a new PEG tube. What do you need to know before you begin planning his nursing care? What questions might you want to ask yourself as you collect data? What are the areas in which the patient might have problems or be at high risk for developing problems? For Mr. Ayala, you would probably seek to answer the following questions:

- What is the status of his neurological and cardiovascular systems?
- What residual deficits from the stroke does he have?
- How is he coping with those deficits?
- Does he have impaired mobility?
- Is he at risk for injury?
- Is he at risk for aspiration?
- Is he continent of bowel and bladder?
- Is he able to communicate?

Assessment

Now that you have an idea of what data you need to collect, your initial step will be to review the current medical record. Specifically, you need to review the patient's medical history, noting medical conditions that alter the patient's nutritional needs and influence the type of feeding formula selected. While reviewing the patient's chart, observe for data that indicate possible complications or that may influence the timing of administration or formula selection, such as the following:

- Height and weight
- Aspiration risk
- Diarrhea or constipation
- Fluid or electrolyte imbalance
- Nausea and vomiting
- Skin breakdown

Your next step will be to review the patient's laboratory results for the following tests:

- Hemoglobin and hematocrit levels
- Blood glucose levels
- Protein level
- Fluid and electrolyte status

Review of the patient's vital signs show that they are stable: blood pressure – 136/82 mm Hg; temperature – 99°F; pulse – 70; respirations – 16. His serum albumin is 34 g/L, and his electrolyte panel indicates normal results. Parts of his blood count, the hematocrit and hemoglobin, are within normal range, indicating no anemia, but there was no order to check his protein level. A continuous enteral feeding was initiated today, infusing at 20 mL per hour via a feeding pump. You noted in the chart that he is unable to speak, known as *dysphasia,* but he is able to answer questions by nodding or shaking his head.

Next you will need to review the patient's medication record, checking listed medications for incompatibility with feeding formulas; for example, those that may in some way affect GI tract functions, such as increasing or decreasing peristalsis. When you enter Mr. Ayala's room he is awake and alert and makes eye contact as you introduce yourself. He also attempts to smile; however, only the left side of his face moves. He reaches out with his right hand to shake your hand. He can use the urinal but requires assistance to get up to the bedside commode. You know that he has difficulty swallowing since the stroke, and a PEG tube was surgically placed yesterday. He shakes his head when you inquire if he is experiencing any pain or discomfort. He writes that he would like to be bathed and get up in a chair as soon as someone can help him. You explain that part of your nursing care will be to check his PEG tube and site to ensure that healing has begun, assess the security of the PEG tube, and check for signs of infection. You check the site and note an approximately 1/4-inch ring of mild erythema but no signs of purulent drainage or leakage of gastric contents. The tube is secured to the patient's abdomen with tape and the feeding system is connected, infusing formula at 20 mL per hour. He shakes his head to indicate that he has had no nausea, vomiting, or diarrhea. You auscultate active bowel sounds in all four quadrants.

You previously noted health-care provider orders to advance the feeding to 30 mL per hour by 3 p.m. You end the assessment with an evaluation of his skin, noting a slight reddening of intact skin over the coccyx. The rest of the initial shift assessment findings are within normal limits.

Nursing Care Plan for a Patient Post CVA With a PEG Tube—cont'd

Prior to leaving the room, you say good-bye to Mr. Ayala. You also lower the bed to its lowest position, raise the head of the bed to 30 degrees, confirm that its wheels are locked and side rails are up, and position his call light and tissues where he can easily reach them.

The new PEG insertion site, located on the left upper quadrant of his abdomen, exhibits no signs of infection or bleeding. His PEG tube is intact and patent, with a continuous infusion of formula at 20 mL per hour that needs to be increased to 30 mL per hour over the next 6 hours. He is continent of both bowel and bladder. He has a 2-cm reddened area on the coccyx that blanches and returns to normal color after repositioning. The data tell you that your patient is status post CVA with stable cardiovascular status, vital signs, and glucose level. Thus far, he is tolerating his enteral feedings, he has had adequate I&O, and his fluid and electrolyte panels indicate adequate hydration and nutritional status.

Nursing Diagnoses

After analyzing the data, you determine that Mr. Ayala has a few high-risk and problem areas. Your first priority is his safety, as he has right-sided hemiparesis and has difficulty swallowing. The appropriate nursing diagnoses for these problems include the following:

- Impaired swallowing
- Impaired physical mobility

The patient has two actual problems that place him at risk to develop additional problems. When there is evidence that a problem could develop, that is known as a *potential* problem. For example, the impaired swallowing places the patient in danger of aspirating, resulting in the additional nursing diagnosis "Risk for aspiration." Because the patient actually suffers impaired physical mobility, this problem places him at risk for developing additional problems. Also, because he already has a new incision, he also has impaired skin integrity.

Assessment of the coccyx found the skin reddened, further data reinforcing his risk for impaired skin integrity in the form of a pressure ulcer. This potential problem requires that action be taken to prevent its occurrence. He already has one site of impaired skin integrity—the new incision made to insert his PEG tube.

Planning

Your nursing care plan will include your role and that of the UAPs, CNAs, and other health-care providers working with you. Your plan of care will be tailored to meet Mr. Ayala's needs; therefore, the interventions will be specific to him. Your first priority will be his safety, then his nutrition, and next his activities of daily living. You must remain aware of his psychosocial needs, as he is experiencing role change, isolation, and impaired verbal communication. You need to provide care that will help him adapt to his body changes while preventing problems that are directly related to mobility impairments.

Because the top priority is impaired swallowing, your plan must ensure that the patient is identified as high risk for aspiration.

The patient also has impaired mobility, and because of this he is at risk for falls and for constipation.

The patient also has impaired skin integrity related to the newly inserted PEG tube and is at risk for infection at the site.

Implementation

Now that you have developed a plan, you need to put it into action. See below for the nursing interventions needed to help prevent possible problems and deal with his existing problems.

Evaluation

Now that you have enacted the patient's care plan, you will want to evaluate its effectiveness and your patient's progress toward health. You want to see if the interventions you have chosen and implemented have helped prevent further skin breakdown, promoted healing of his PEG site, and prevented him from aspirating. His problems are improving or resolving, and your plan of care has helped him improve.

Nursing Diagnosis: Impaired swallowing
Expected Outcomes: Will maintain patent airway. No aspiration.

Interventions	Evaluations
Note in the care plan that patient is NPO with only occasional ice chips. Post NPO sign on the door and above the bed.	Day 1: Eats ice chips sparingly. Remains NPO. Day 3: No change.
Keep the head of the bed elevated a minimum of 30 degrees at all times.	Day 1: HOB maintained at 30 degrees. No signs of aspiration. Day 4: No aspiration.
Reinforce NPO status, elevation of bed, and risk of providing oral fluids with the patient and family members.	Day 1: Verbally instructed patient, wife, grown daughter regarding importance of NPO status and risk of aspiration. Family verbally acknowledged understanding. Patient nodded agreement. Day 2: Following instructions.
Assist the patient with mouth care to prevent dryness four times per day. Apply lip moisturizer to lips prn.	Day 2: Mucous membranes pink, moist, and intact. Able to apply lip balm unassisted. Day 5: Mucous membranes remain pink, intact, and moist.

(nursing care plan continues on page 490)

Nursing Care Plan for a Patient Post CVA With a PEG Tube—cont'd

Interventions	Evaluations
Keep suction equipment at the bedside ready for use at all times. Discontinued Day 7	Day 1: Suction not needed. Day 2: No choking or aspiration. Day 3: Working to relearn swallowing technique with therapists. Day 6: Makes effort to swallow melted ice chips without problems. No suction needed. Day 7: Suction removed from room.
Keep the call light within reach at all times.	Day 1: Uses call light when assistance is needed. Day 5: Calls staff as needed.
Infuse Jevity per PEG tube with pump at 30 mL/hr. If tolerated for 24 hours without GI distress, increase to 50 mL/hr. If tolerated for 24 hours, increase to 75 mL/hr.	Day 1: Tolerated 30 mL/hr without nausea or distention; bowel sounds active in all quads except RLQ, which was hyperactive. Day 2: Tolerated 50 mL/hr. No distention, nausea, or diarrhea. Day 3: Rate increased to 75 mL/hr. Day 4: Active bowel sounds throughout; no reports of gastric distress.
Check PEG tube placement and residual volume every 4 hours. Follow health-care provider orders, hospital policy, or protocol in chapter for gastric residual volume.	Day 1: Placement confirmed; residuals 30 mL and less. Day 2: Placement confirmed; residuals 40 mL, 50 mL, 35 mL. Day 4: Residuals less than 50 mL consistently. Day 6: Residuals and placement checks unchanged.
Monitor I/O closely for 2 weeks; report variances.	Day 1: In – 880 mL; Out – 630 mL. Day 3: In – 1,925 mL; Out – 1,475 mL. Day 7: I/O balanced.
Record daily weights at 8:00 a.m.; report losses. Discontinued 08/10	Day 1: Admission: 179 lbs. Day 2: 177 lbs. Day 4: 177 lbs. Day 7: 177.5 lbs.

Nursing Diagnosis: Impaired physical mobility
Expected Outcomes: During hospitalization: (1) Skin integrity will remain intact. (2) No development of contractures. (3) Will remain injury-free. (4) No development of constipation. Maintain bowel elimination with a BM at least every 3 days.

Interventions	Evaluations
Assist the patient to get up into a chair a minimum of three times per day and to a bedside commode as needed.	Day 1: Requires 2 assists to stand and pivot to chair; reported fatigue afterward. Day 4: Assists with right arm; can bear weight on unaffected leg with 2 assists to balance. Day 5: Still unable to move left leg voluntarily; no longer reports fatigue after up. Day 7: Able to transfer to bedside commode with retractable arms, using short slide board.
Cue the patient to reposition every 2 hours; teach him the importance of activity. Discontinued Day 7	Day 1: Cued every 2 hr. Requires 2 assists to turn to either side. Day 3: Continues to require 2 assists to turn to right side, but can turn to left side unassisted; needs help to position support pillows. Day 5: Continues to help reposition self and do a little more each day. Day 7: Moves about unassisted in bed; no longer requires staff to cue or assist.

Nursing Care Plan for a Patient Post CVA With a PEG Tube—cont'd

Interventions	Evaluations
Encourage and assist the patient as needed to perform active/passive ROM to all extremities twice a day.	Day 1: Active ROM exercises performed; 5 sets of each movement. Day 3: Active-passive ROM today; able to move unaffected joints and use right hand to move left arm and hand; states he feels so much better after exercises. Day 5: Reported sleeping better at night; believes it is due to ROM; working hard to move left leg; some left shoulder lift performed independently. Day 7: Increasing strength; slight movement of left arm.
Assess pressure points for erythema and apply lotion to back and all pressure points three times per day. Day 9: Modified to twice per day, during bath and p.m. care.	Day 1: Skin over pressure points intact; mild redness over coccyx, 2-inch circle, resolves 15 min after repositioning. Day 4: No redness noted on pressure points except pale pink area on right elbow where patient leans on elbow to sit up; gel-filled elbow pads applied. Day 6: No further redness of elbows or other pressure points. Day 7: Able to sit up without leaning on elbow; removed elbow pads; skin intact; no redness.
Keep a hand roll positioned in the left hand.	Day 1: States the hand roll keeps the left hand from sweating so badly. Day 3: Left fingers still flaccid; hand roll replaced daily. Day 7: No signs of contractures in left hand. Day 8: Exercises his left hand 8 to 10 times/day, even while watching TV and visiting; only places hand roll during sleep hours.
Keep the bed in its lowest position with the wheels locked.	Day 1: Bed kept in low position and brakes locked; does not attempt to get up unassisted. Day 5: Calls for assistance when he needs to get up.
Raise both bed rails continually.	Day 1: 2 rails up; doesn't try to get out of bed alone. Day 4: Pulls on bed rail with right hand to help turn him.
Assess bowel sounds with each tube placement check, noting hyper- or hypoactivity.	Day 1: Active bowel sounds in RLQ, RUQ, LUQ, and hyperactive in LLQ. Day 5: Active times 4 quadrants. Day 8: Hypoactive.
Monitor and document bowel movements for frequency, consistency, color, and amount.	Day 1: Chart shows last BM 2 days prior. Day 2: Continent of small, brown, soft BM. Day 3: None. Day 4: Large, soft dark brown BM. Day 5: 3 semi-soft BMs. Day 7: None in 2 days. Day 8: Moderate amount soft brown BM.
Administer a laxative of choice, if there is no BM after 2 days.	Day 5: Having BMs without difficulty. Day 7: Laxative requested and given.

Skill 24.1 Assisting a Patient With Feeding

Assessment Steps

1. Review the patient's medical record ***to determine diet orders.*** Review the chart for problems that might impair the patient's ability to self-feed.
2. Assess the patient for risk of aspiration. ***Patients at high risk are those with dysphagia, decreased gag or cough reflex, or decreased level of consciousness, as well as those with difficulty managing saliva. If the patient is at high risk, ensure that suction is available at the bedside.***
3. Assess the patient's intake and output, weights, and laboratory values. ***This helps to evaluate nutritional status.***

Planning Steps

1. Gather needed equipment and supplies: a protective barrier to protect the patient's gown and assistive devices. ***Being prepared saves you time and effort and increases efficiency.***
2. Provide the patient an opportunity to use the bathroom. ***This helps to reduce mealtime interruptions.***
3. Clean the over-bed table of clutter and unpleasantries such as a urinal, toilet tissue, or emesis basin containing sputum. ***A clean and neat table is more conducive to eating.***

Implementation Steps

1. Follow the Initial Implementation Steps located on the inside back cover.
2. Assist the patient to a chair or elevate the head of bed to the high Fowler's position. ***This positions the patient for eating and decreases risk of aspiration.***
3. Provide a warm, wet washcloth to wash the face and hands ***to reduce microorganisms.***
4. Place a protective barrier beneath the patient's chin so that it covers the patient's gown, ***to prevent the gown from becoming soiled.***
5. Provide as much assistance as the patient needs while encouraging optimal independent feeding. ***It is important to encourage optimal independence for the patient's self-esteem but to still ensure that adequate assistance is provided to optimize nutritional intake.***
6. Position the over-bed table directly in front of the patient so that food is in front of the patient, as it is at one's own dining room table. ***This helps to make it more like mealtimes at home and is more conducive to eating.***
7. If the patient is able to feed himself or herself, assist with tray setup as needed: open containers, cut up meat, butter bread, and open condiments and apply them if the patient desires. If the patient is unable to feed himself or herself, proceed with feeding the patient. ***It is important to do everything possible to encourage nutritional intake.***
8. If possible, sit down while feeding the patient. ***This shows the patient that you are not in a hurry, which encourages the patient to eat more.***
   If the patient is blind:
   - First identify whether the sight impairment is long-standing or a new loss. If the patient is not used to being blind, you probably will need to feed the patient or assist the patient in feeding himself or herself. If the patient has been blind for a long time, you will need to ask the patient if you can help feed him or her.
   - Be certain to approach the subject judiciously and compassionately, as the patient may be very sensitive about the inability to do certain things and the loss of independence.

   If a blind patient is able to self-feed:
   - Open containers and cellophane-wrapped flatware or condiments, cut meat, butter bread, and season food if the patient desires.
   - Verbally inform the patient where each food item is located on the plate using the numbers on the face of a clock and the relationship of plates, bowls, glasses, and flatware for identifiers. For example: "Your meatloaf is at 12 o'clock, mashed potatoes are at 3 o'clock, green beans are at 6 o'clock, a glass of iced tea is on the right above your fork and spoon, a bowl of peaches is on the left above your knife, and apple cobbler is to the far left of the bowl of peaches. Here is your napkin."
   - It is helpful to gently guide the patient's hands to feel the sides of the dinner plate as you begin to tell where the food contained on the plate is located. Also guide the patient's hand to feel the glass, flatware, and extra bowls. ***These things will encourage more intake.***
9. Allow the patient to determine the order in which he or she will eat foods ***to allow the patient more control.***
10. Encourage the patient to handle easy-to-eat foods such as bread or small pieces of fruit ***to promote independence.***
11. Keep food bits small and allow the patient adequate time to chew and swallow food ***to reduce the risk of choking.***
12. Make mealtime a pleasant social occasion, engaging in conversation while feeding and encouraging the patient to talk about his or her life, children, or favorite hobbies. Smile during the meal. ***This makes mealtime more conducive to eating.***
13. Follow the Ending Implementation Steps located on the inside back cover.

Evaluation Steps

1. Observe the level of independence and amount of assistance required ***to determine if additional assistance is needed.***
2. Observe for signs of difficulty swallowing, such as gagging, choking, or significant coughing, during oral intake ***to prevent aspiration.***
3. Measure the amount of oral fluid intake each meal. Estimate the percentage of the solid foods eaten. Measure liquids in milliliters. Document this in the appropriate location in the chart.
4. Observe the patient's ability to tolerate his or her diet, monitoring for signs such as abdominal distention and complaints of cramping, nausea or vomiting, or indigestion, and document in the chart. ***This helps to determine whether or not the diet should be changed.***

Sample Documentation

05/25/22 1230 Required total assistance with soft diet. Consumed 50% of potatoes, green beans, & chicken without swallowing problems. No complaints of GI distress. ——
—————— Nurse's signature and credentials

Skill 24.2 Recording Intake and Output

Assessment Steps

1. Review the patient's medical record for previous intake and output (I&O) to see if there are imbalances. ***This helps you to know if you need to encourage fluids or not.***
2. Introduce yourself to the patient and explain the procedure. Review the rationale for the monitoring of I&O so that the patient and family understand the importance of measuring. ***This results in better compliance.***

Planning Steps

1. Gather needed equipment and supplies: paper and pen, specimen pan, urinal, graduated receptacle, and drinking glass with increments marked in milliliters. ***Being prepared saves you time and effort and increases efficiency.***
2. Instruct the unlicensed assistive personnel (UAP) who will be assisting in the patient's care. ***It is your responsibility to communicate the needs of the patient to the UAP.***
3. Place paper and pen at the bedside for recording I&O ***to increase compliance.***

Implementation Steps

1. Follow the Initial Implementation Steps located on the inside back cover.
2. Measure, do not estimate, the volume of liquid consumed, except when the exact volume of an empty container is known, such as a milk carton that holds 240 mL. If only part of the liquid was consumed, measure what is left and record the difference *to increase accuracy.*
3. Document on the I&O sheet in the room; at the end of the shift, transcribe the total to the flow sheet. ***Documenting at the bedside increases accuracy.***
4. If intake volumes are less than desired, encourage the patient to drink more. Find out the patient's likes and dislikes and provide the preferred items as long as they are not contraindicated by his or her diet order. If necessary, offer a few ounces every hour to get adequate fluid in the patient. ***Don't wait until the end of the shift to become concerned about inadequate intake. Be proactive. This helps to more accurately determine fluid balance.***
5. Measure the amount of urine and other sources of output, such as the amount emptied from drainage devices, stomach aspirate, emesis, or diarrhea excreted by the patient, and document on the flow sheet in the chart. ***This helps to more accurately determine fluid balance.***
6. Document all output in the room immediately after measurement. Avoid trying to remember totals until the end of the shift. At the end of the shift, transcribe the totals to the flow sheet in the chart ***to increase accuracy.***
7. Follow the Ending Implementation Steps located on the inside back cover.

Evaluation Step

1. Compare the I&O amounts, noting any significant imbalance. ***The output total should be within 300 to 500 mL of the intake, allowing the difference for the insensible losses.***

Sample Documentation

At the bedside:

Date Jan 1 *Shift* 3/11

Intake	*Output* — *Urine*	*Emesis*
240 mL	255 ml	130 mL
70 mL	155 mL	
240 mL	530 mL	
85 mL	940 mL	
90 mL		
725 mL		

Then, the end-of-shift totals are transcribed to the I&O sheet in the chart as follows:

Date	*Shift*	*Oral*	*IV*	*Irrig*	*Total Shift Intake*	*Urine*	*Emesis*	*NG*	*Drains*	*Total Shift Output*
10/1	7a-7p	1,050 mL	240 mL		1,290 mL	1,115 mL	275 mL			1,390 mL
	7p-7a	725 mL	240 mL		965 mL	940 mL	130 mL			1,070 mL
	24-hour Total									

Skill 24.3 Inserting a Nasogastric Tube

Assessment Step

1. Review the medical record for medical history, current diagnoses and problems, and conditions that might limit the patient's ability to cooperate during the procedure or that contraindicate insertion of an NG tube.

Planning Steps

1. Gather needed equipment and supplies: correct type and size of ENFit NG tube if for feeding, ENFit irrigation syringe, container of water, emesis basin, washcloth towel or waterproof pad, examination gloves, lubricating jelly, tape or device to secure tubing to nose, glass of ice water and straw, stethoscope, flashlight, tongue blade, suction setup with a long connector tube or ENfit feeding setup, indelible marker, and tape measure. ***Being prepared saves time and effort and increases efficiency.***
2. Explain the procedure to the patient, discussing it fully and instructing the patient in ways in which he or she can assist to make the procedure go smoothly. ***This reduces anxiety and increases patient compliance during the procedure.***
3. **If the NG tube is to be connected to suction:** Set up the suction apparatus, including a canister and connector tube that connects to the NG tube adaptor.
4. Measure the length of the NG tube by measuring from the tip of the patient's nose to the earlobe and then to the xiphoid process. Mark this length on the tube with a small piece of tape, but do not wrap the tape so tightly around the tube that it is difficult to remove once the tube has been inserted. ***This determines the approximate length to insert the NG tube.***

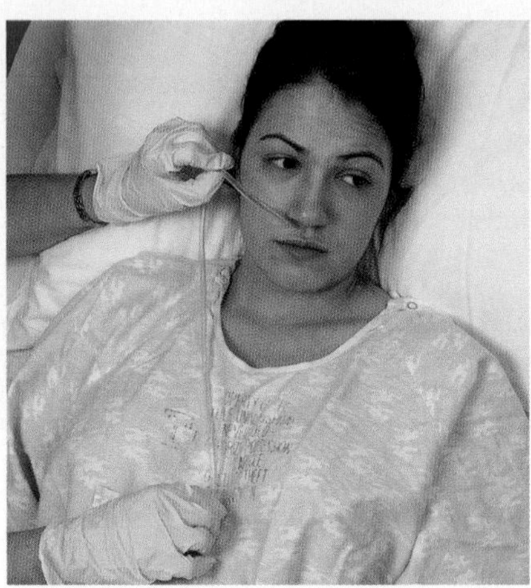

5. Determine the patency of the patient's nares before selecting an acceptable naris. Select the nostril with the greatest airflow. Have patient blow his or her nose.

Implementation Steps

1. Follow the Initial Implementation Steps located on the inside back cover.
2. Wearing clean examination gloves ***to protect yourself from potential contact with body fluids,*** pull the plunger back on the irrigation syringe ***to make room for gastric contents to drain into the syringe.*** Snugly insert the tip of the irrigation syringe into the open end of the NG tube. ***This will prevent soiling the bed with gastric contents as the NG tube reaches the stomach, which saves you from having to change linens.***
3. Lubricate 3 to 4 inches of the tip of the NG tube with a small amount of water-soluble lubricant. ***This reduces friction and increases ease of passage of the tube.*** *Safety: Avoid using petroleum-based lubricants because they increase the risk of pneumonia due to inhaling petrolatum products.*
4. Repeat the instructions for the patient and ask if he or she has further questions. ***Because this procedure frightens many patients, repeating the instructions is sometimes helpful to alleviate anxiety.***
5. Have the patient hyperextend the neck. Insert the tube through the patient's naris, slowly advancing the tube downward into the nasopharynx. You may feel slight resistance as the tube enters the nasopharynx; gentle rotation or changing the angle of the tube typically overcomes this. *Safety: Never force the tube if there is more than the slightest resistance. Forcing the tube can result in serious damage to the nasal mucosa. If you meet resistance, remove the tube, relubricate the end of the tube, and attempt insertion in the opposite naris.* It is typical for the patient's eyes to water during tube insertion. ***Remember to be gentle and reassure the patient.***

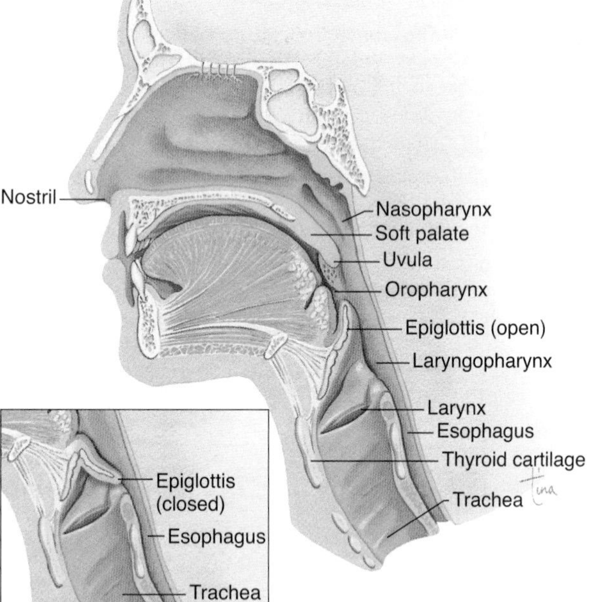

6. When the patient begins to gag, you know that the tube is in the posterior nasopharynx; stop advancing the tube and withdraw it a very short distance (about 1/8 inch), ***just enough to stop the gagging.*** Encourage the patient to take a couple of deep breaths and relax. Then instruct the patient to flex his or her head forward slightly, drink a sip of water, and swallow. ***This position aids passage of the tube through the posterior pharynx and esophagus rather than the larynx.***
   - Continue to cue the patient to "swallow…swallow…swallow." Continue to gently advance the tube each time the patient swallows. After two to three advancements, allow the patient brief rest periods (if needed) before resuming cues and advancement of the NG tube. If the patient continues to gag and cough, use a penlight and

Skill 24.3 (continued)

tongue blade ***to make certain the tube has not curled up in the back of the patient's throat.*** *Safety: If the patient exhibits symptoms of respiratory distress or cyanosis, stop the procedure and withdraw the tube immediately.*

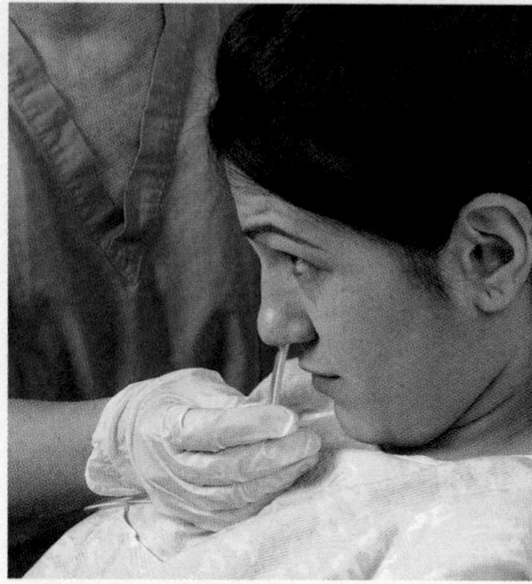

- Monitor the depth of tube insertion, noting when you reach the tape-marked level. Observe for return of stomach contents into tube and attached syringe.
- Once the tube is in place, secure the end by taping it to the patient's nose. As you tape the tube, make certain to avoid positioning the tube where it is pressing against the naris ***to prevent accidental dislodgment of the tube.***

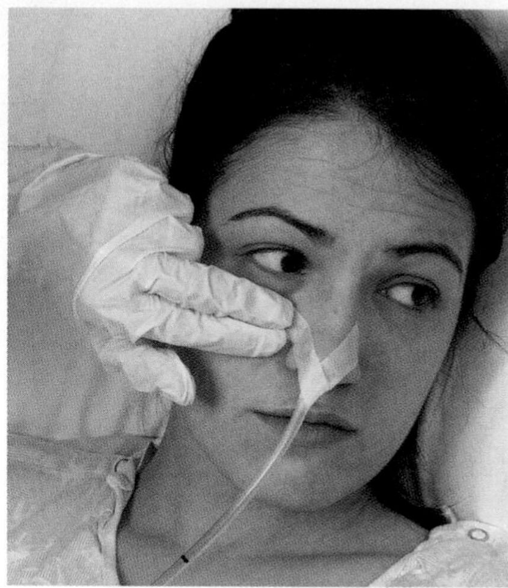

7. Apply a tubing clamp or insert a plug. *Safety: Until placement has been verified by x-ray, nothing can be instilled into the NG tube, including a normal saline flush, water, medications, and formula.*
8. Using an indelible marker, boldly mark the tube at the point of insertion and measure the length of tube extending from the body. Record this measurement ***for comparison at future placement checks.*** Notify radiology and transport the patient to the radiology department for an x-ray. After tube placement has been verified, return the patient to his or her room and connect the NG tube to suction or feeding as ordered.
9. Follow the Ending Implementation Steps located on the inside back cover.
10. Document the procedure, time it was performed, patient's tolerance of the procedure, length of tube extending from insertion site, method used to determine correct placement and findings, characteristics of any drainage, and patient's current respiratory status.

Evaluation Steps

1. Confirm tube placement by x-ray ***to ensure proper placement.***
2. Assess the patient's level of comfort ***to enable you to provide optimal comfort.***
3. Assess the characteristics of any aspirate or drainage: color, consistency, and amount.

Sample Documentation

05/31/22 1015 Explained procedure. States she has had an NG tube previously and understands the process. Inserted 18 Fr Salem sump NG tube into Rt. naris without resistance or difficulty, per health-care provider's order. 17.5-in NG tube extending from insertion site. Obtained 450 mL thick, dark green gastric contents within a few minutes. Denies discomfort. ——————

—————— Nurse's signature and credentials

05/31/22 1035 To x-ray per W/C accompanied by UAP. Tube placement confirmed in the stomach. Returned to room per W/C. NG tube attached to low intermittent suction per health-care provider's order. ——————

—————— Nurse's signature and credentials

Skill 24.4 Irrigating a Nasogastric Tube

Assessment Steps

1. Check the patient's medical record for orders and a radiographic report verifying correct placement of the NG tube. ***This helps to prevent instilling irrigant into a displaced tube.***
2. Observe the NG tube and assess for secure placement ***to prevent accidental dislodgment of the tube.***

Planning Step

1. Gather needed equipment and supplies: catheter-tipped irrigating syringe or a 50-mL syringe with a smaller slip-tip if required to fit the NG tube to suction or ENFit catheter for a feeding tube, normal saline (NS), pH paper and color chart, tape measure, emesis basin or bag, towel or waterproof pad, examination gloves, lubricating jelly, and tape or a device to secure tubing to nose. ***Being prepared saves time and effort and increases efficiency.***

Implementation Steps

1. Follow the Initial Implementation Steps located on the inside back cover.

(skill continues on page 496)

Skill 24.4 (continued)

2. Place the patient in a sitting or high Fowler's position ***to help reduce reflux and aspiration.***
3. Position waterproof pad under the end of the NG tube and unclamp the end of the NG tube if clamped. Otherwise, disconnect the tube from suction or the feeding setup. ***This protects linens from soiling and allows access to the tube.***
4. To verify placement, assess whether the insertion mark is still positioned at the point of entry and measure the length of tube extending from the insertion site, comparing it with the recorded length. If your hospital uses the pH method for checking placement, use a syringe to withdraw 5 to 10 mL of gastric residual volume, observe the color of the contents, and measure the pH.
   Patients who have been fasting at least 4 hours have a pH of 1 to 4; those on continuous feedings will have a slightly higher pH. ***This ensures that the irrigant enters the stomach.***
5. Reinstill aspirated gastric contents ***to prevent electrolyte imbalance*** and disconnect the syringe from the NG tube.
6. Draw up the ordered volume of normal saline (usually 30 to 60 mL) into the syringe and reconnect the syringe to the NG tube.
7. Gently instill the normal saline into the tube. ***Excessive force increases risk of reflux and aspiration. Saline helps clear debris that may clog the tube and prevent it from draining effectively.***
8. Lower the end of the NG tube and gently aspirate the irrigant back into the syringe. ***Excessive suction can damage the gastric mucosa.*** Repeat steps 7 and 8 as needed until the saline flows freely into and out of the tube.
   For a Double-Lumen (Salem Sump) Tube:
   Draw up 30 mL of air into the syringe and inject it into the blue "pigtail." Always follow facility policy. ***This helps clear the air vent of secretions that could cause it not to function properly.***
9. Remove the syringe from the tube; clamp or plug the proximal end of the tube or reconnect it to suction. Secure the tube to the patient's gown.
10. Follow the Ending Implementation Steps located on the inside back cover.

Evaluation Steps

1. Assess the patient's tolerance of the procedure.
2. If the NG tube was connected to a suction source, observe for fluid movement through tube ***to verify patency.***

Sample Documentation

06/04/22 0920 NG tube irrigated with 30 mL NS according to health-care provider's orders. Irrigated without difficulty. NG tube patent. Reconnected to low intermittent suction. No C/O discomfort during irrigation.
____________ Nurse's signature and credentials

Skill 24.5 Removing a Nasogastric Tube

Assessment Step

1. Review the patient's intake and output *to determine fluid imbalances.*

Planning Step

1. Gather needed equipment and supplies: towel or protective pad; washcloth; tissues; examination gloves; irrigation syringe; and the patient's toothbrush, toothpaste, and mouthwash. ***Being prepared saves time and effort and increases efficiency.***

Implementation Steps

1. Follow the Initial Implementation Steps located on the inside back cover.
2. Place the patient in the high Fowler's position and hand the patient some tissues.
3. Clear the tube of any secretions by using an irrigation syringe to inject 10 mL of air through the main lumen. ***This reduces the risk of fluid dripping into the airway as the tube is withdrawn.***
4. Remove all tape from the patient's nose and the NG tube ***so that the tube can be removed.***
5. Have the patient hold his or her breath and then gently but quickly withdraw the tube, immediately wrapping it in the disposable protective pad to remove it from the patient's line of vision. ***This reduces the risk of aspiration during removal of the tube.***
6. Discard all contaminated supplies in the appropriate biohazard waste receptacle.
7. Provide the patient with a warm, wet washcloth to wash the face.
8. Assist the patient as needed to brush the teeth and rinse the mouth with mouthwash ***to rid the mouth of debris, mucus, and bad taste from the tube removal.***
9. Offer a glass of cold water to drink, if the patient is not NPO, ***to soothe a dry throat.***
10. Follow the Ending Implementation Steps located on the inside back cover.

Evaluation Steps

1. Determine if the patient is experiencing any discomfort or pain related to the procedure and medicate accordingly. ***This provides for patient comfort.***
2. Assess for active bowel sounds and repeat in 4 hours, while observing for abdominal distention, nausea, or vomiting. ***This helps to determine GI tract tolerance of tube removal.***

Sample Documentation

11/21/22 0930 NG tube removed without difficulty per Dr's orders. Abdomen flat and soft; no complaints of nausea. Bowel sounds active in all 4 quadrants. Instructed to eat no more than 1 tsp of ice every 30 min and to report any nausea or bloating to staff. ____________
____________ Nurse's signature and credentials

Skill 24.6 Administering Intermittent Bolus Enteral Feedings

Assessment Steps

1. Review the patient's medical record and health-care provider's order to determine the rate, route, and type of formula to be administered and ***to reduce the risk of error.***
2. Evaluate the patient's current nutritional status. Review the laboratory data and other available diagnostic data, such as FSBS readings. Assess for fluid volume excess or deficit and metabolic or electrolyte imbalances. ***This helps to determine patient's nutritional needs.***
3. Assess whether the patient has impaired swallowing or has had facial trauma or surgeries of the alimentary canal, head, or neck. ***These conditions indicate the patient's need for enteral tube feedings.***
4. Obtain a baseline weight to determine increases or decreases after initiation of feedings. ***This provides for later comparisons to help evaluate the effectiveness of feedings.***
5. Assess for active bowel sounds; if absent, withhold feeding until you check with the health-care provider.

Planning Step

1. Gather needed equipment and supplies: clean gloves; pH paper strips; prescribed enteral formula; an irrigation syringe or a 30-mL or larger syringe with a smaller slip-tip catheter tip if required for a snug fit into the NG, NI, or PEG tube for a large-bore feeding tube or an ENFit irrigation syringe for a small-bore feeding tube; a tape measure; and a cup of water. ***Being prepared saves time and effort and increases efficiency.***

Implementation Steps

1. Follow the Initial Implementation Steps located on the inside back cover.
2. Raise the head of the bed 30 to 45 degrees ***to reduce the risk of reflux and aspiration.***
3. Have the tube feeding formula at room temperature ***to reduce intestinal cramping.***
4. Check the expiration date of the formula and the integrity of its container ***to determine the safety of the formula.***
5. Arrange supplies on the over-bed table within easy reach.
6. Check for correct tube placement and gastric content residual volume by assessing whether the insertion mark is still located at the insertion point, measuring the length of the tube from the point of insertion to the distal end, comparing it with the recorded measurement, and using the irrigation syringe to aspirate all stomach contents. *Safety: If the tube is a Salem sump tube, do not insert the syringe tip into the blue air vent.* Measure the amount of residual aspirate and check the pH with pH paper if your facility uses pH to determine placement. Reinstill aspirate ***unless*** the amount is 250 mL or greater, in which case you will check for abdominal distention. If there are no such symptoms, you will:
   - Reinstill the aspirate and wait an hour. Then repeat assessment of residual gastric volume. If it is still 250 mL or greater, call the doctor. If it is less than 250 mL, restart the infusion at 50% of the original rate or follow facility policy. ***This helps to prevent electrolyte imbalance and prevent overfeeding the patient.***

   With a J-Tube: Proceed as above; however, you will aspirate intestinal secretions. Intestinal residuals tend to be small in amount and more alkaline. Residuals of more than 10 mL with an acidic pH may indicate that the tube has dislodged and is displaced to the stomach.
7. Shake the feeding formula to ensure that it is mixed well.
8. Remove the plunger from the irrigation syringe barrel and attach the tip to the feeding tube for a large-bore feeding tube. For a small-bore feeding tube, use an ENFit syringe and remove the plunger from the barrel.
9. Bend or crimp the feeding tube just below the connection to the tip of the irrigation syringe ***to prevent the flow of formula as you fill the syringe.***
10. Carefully pour the formula into the syringe barrel.
11. Release the bent or crimped tube, allowing formula to begin to flow. Do not raise the syringe more than 15 to 18 inches above the tube insertion site, ***which can cause discomfort due to excessive pressure and too rapid instillation.*** Recrimp the tube before the syringe runs completely dry ***to prevent air from filling the line and infusing, as added formula pushes the air in front of it.***
12. When the syringe is nearly empty refill it in the same manner until the feeding is completed. Monitor the patient throughout the feeding, ***observing for any signs of respiratory distress.***
13. Flush the tube with 30 to 60 mL of water to clear formula from the line and ensure that the tube is patent. ***This will reduce clogging and bacterial growth.***
14. Administer water via the feeding tube between feedings or as ordered.
15. Maintain the patient in a semi-Fowler's position or with the head of bed elevated at least 30 degrees for 1 hour ***to promote gastric emptying and prevent vomiting or aspiration.***
16. Follow the Ending Implementation Steps located on the inside back cover.

Evaluation Steps

1. Observe and assess the patient's respiratory status post feeding because changes such as increased rate, wheezing, increased coughing, or sudden decrease in O_2 saturation ***can indicate aspiration.***
2. Auscultate breath sounds at least once every 8 hours ***to detect adventitious sounds that may indicate aspiration.***
3. Measure aspirate every 4 hours ***to evaluate the patient's tolerance of feedings.***
4. Monitor laboratory values, including albumin, prealbumin, and transferrin. Notify the health-care provider of significant changes. ***This provides information to determine if the patient's nutritional status is stable, improving, or worsening.***
5. Monitor intake and output every shift and calculate 24-hour totals, ***noting if there is an imbalance.***

(skill continues on page 498)

Skill 24.6 (continued)

6. Weigh the patient daily, at the same time of day and with the same scale to maintain consistency, until the tube feeding maximum rate has been reached; then weigh three times per week or per the health-care provider's order, noting if weight begins to decline. ***Evaluate the effectiveness of feedings.***
7. For patients with tubes placed through the abdominal wall, inspect the insertion site for erythema, edema, increased warmth, and drainage ***to detect signs and symptoms of infection.***

Sample Documentation

06/02/22 0645 Awake and alert, lying supine. NG tube placement checked by aspirating residual gastric contents, obtained 75 mL of yellowish-brown gastric contents, pH - 3. Insertion mark remains at point of entry. C/O of mild discomfort in left nostril, no erythema noted, skin intact. Replaced tape securing NG tube to nose. States it feels better. Head of bed elevated 45 degrees. Tube flushed with 30 mL of water, and 250 mL of Jevity instilled per gravity. Tube flushed with 30 mL water. No signs of gastric or respiratory distress noted. ——————————————————— Nurse's signature and credentials

Skill 24.7 Using a Feeding Pump

Assessment Steps

1. Review the patient's medical record and health-care provider's order to determine the rate, route, and type of formula to be administered ***to reduce the risk of error.***
2. Evaluate the patient's current nutritional status. Review the laboratory data and other available diagnostic data, such as finger stick blood sugar readings. Assess for fluid volume excess or deficit and metabolic or electrolyte imbalances.
3. Assess whether the patient has impaired swallowing or has had facial trauma or surgeries of the alimentary canal, head, or neck. ***These conditions indicate the patient's need for enteral tube feedings.***
4. Obtain a baseline weight to determine increases or decreases after initiation of feedings. ***This provides for later comparisons to help evaluate effectiveness of feedings.***
5. For PEG tubes or J-tubes, inspect the skin around the tube for irritation, signs of skin breakdown, infection, or drainage.
6. Auscultate bowel sounds before feeding. If no bowel sounds are heard, consult the health-care provider before initiating feeding.

Planning Step

1. Gather needed equipment and supplies: clean gloves, stethoscope, pH strips, tape measure, prescribed enteral formula, disposable feeding bag and tubing or a ready-to-hang system with ENFit connections, ENFit syringe for small-bore feeding tube, and feeding pump. ***Being prepared saves time and effort and increases efficiency.*** *Safety: Note that a feeding pump is not the same as an IV pump.*
2. Plan to change the bag every 24 hours or according to facility policy. Bags should be flagged with the date and time they are hung ***so it is easy to tell when to change them.***

Implementation Steps

1. Follow the Initial Implementation Steps located on the inside back cover.
2. Have the tube feeding formula at room temperature ***to reduce intestinal cramping.***
3. Check the expiration date of the formula and the integrity of its container ***to prevent using outdated or spoiled formula.***
4. Prepare a ready-to-hang system or pour formula into a disposable feeding bag with clamped tubing. Hang the formula bag on the IV pole.
5. Place the patient in the high Fowler's position or elevate the head of the bed 30 to 45 degrees ***to reduce the risk of reflux and aspiration.***
6. Prime the tubing from the formula bag by opening the clamp and allowing formula to flow until all air in the tubing is displaced with formula. ***Instillation of air can cause discomfort, belching, and reflux.***
7. Position a waterproof pad under the distal end of the NG tube, PEG tube, or J-tube ***to protect the bed from soiling.***
8. Put on clean gloves and proceed to verify tube placement. Assess the location of the insertion mark to determine that it is still at the point of entry. Measure the length of the tube extending from the insertion site to the distal end of the tube. Use an irrigation syringe to aspirate residual gastric contents. If your facility uses pH to check placement, ensure that it is between 1 and 4. ***This reduces the risk of instillation into a displaced tube.***
9. Return the entire aspirate to the stomach ***to prevent electrolyte imbalance.*** If the residual is 250 mL or greater and the patient has no symptoms of abdominal pain or a distended abdomen and no nausea or vomiting, withhold the feeding and reassess the residual in 1 hour. Once the residual volume is within acceptable parameters, you may proceed with the feeding process.
10. Flush the tube with 30 mL of water ***to ensure that the tube is clear and patent.***
11. Connect the feeding setup tubing to the patient's feeding tube, thread it through the feeding pump, set the volume and rate, and initiate the feeding.

Skill 24.7 (continued)

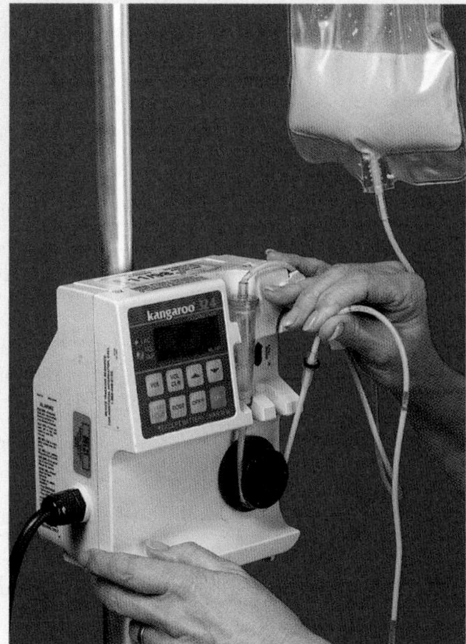

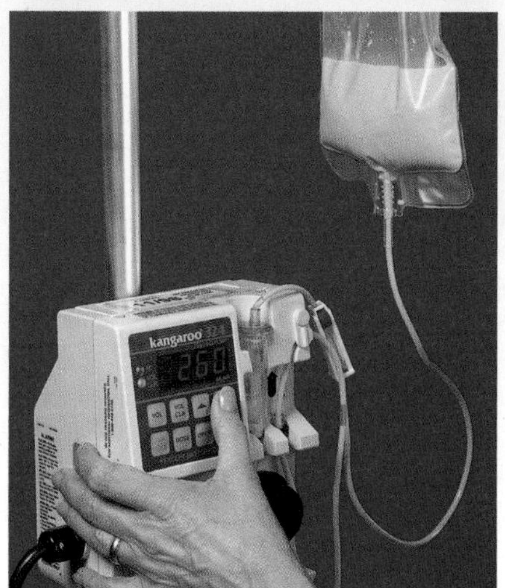

12. Maintain the patient in the semi-Fowler's position or with the head of the bed elevated continuously ***to promote gastric emptying and prevent vomiting or aspiration.***
13. Follow the Ending Implementation Steps located on the inside back cover.

Evaluation Steps

1. Measure aspirate every 4 hours ***to evaluate the patient's tolerance of feedings.***
2. Monitor all laboratory values regularly: Albumin, prealbumin, and transferrin indicate stable, improving, or worsening nutritional status. Notify the health-care provider of significant changes. ***This evaluates nutritional status and effectiveness of feedings.***
3. Observe and assess the patient's respiratory status post feeding because changes such as increased rate, wheezing, increased coughing, or sudden decrease in O_2 saturation ***can indicate aspiration.***
4. Monitor intake and output every shift and calculate 24-hour totals, ***noting imbalance.***
5. Weigh the patient daily, at the same time of day and with same scale to maintain consistency, for the first 2 weeks of continuous feeding, noting any decrease. Then weigh three times per week or per the health-care provider's order, noting if weight begins to decline. ***This evaluates the effectiveness of feedings.***

Sample Documentation

03/24/22 1130 NG tube placement verified by x-ray. Jevity 500-mL tube feeding initiated per feeding pump 50 mL/hr. Hob elevated 45 degrees. ————
———— Nurse's signature and credentials

POST CONFERENCE

After caring for your patient for 2 days, you feel much more comfortable around NG tubes. You inserted his tube on the first day, and placement was verified by aspirating greenish stomach contents, which had a pH of 3, and also by x-ray before instilling anything into the tube. You were still nervous, though, when you first attached the feeding pump and started the feedings. You kept watching the patient and checking for any signs of aspiration. On the second day, the patient pulled out his tube, and you had to insert a new one. This time it went even more smoothly, and you began to feel confidence about this skill. Now you are glad that you were the student assigned to this patient.

Key Points

- Methods for assisting with meals for patients in the hospital include preparing the environment and preparing the patient, as well as assisting the patient with eating, if needed.
- It is important to carefully measure and record all fluids taken in as intake, whether they are taken in by mouth, are given via IV, or are administered as enteral or parenteral fluids. It is also important to measure and record all bodily fluids that are lost as output, including urine, emesis, liquid stool, blood, gastric contents, and drainage. These measures give valuable information about the patient's fluid balance.
- NPO status means *nothing by mouth* and is usually ordered for a limited time as preparation for procedures or tests. Regular diets are ordered for patients without special nutritional needs. Diets that are modified by consistency include clear liquid, full liquid, mechanical soft, and pureed.
- Some common diets modified for disease are diabetic, sodium-restricted, fat-restricted, and renal diets. Diets that may be modified by preference include gluten-free and vegan.
- Nurses are responsible for monitoring the type of diet, percentage eaten, and whether or not the patient tolerated the meal. They are also responsible for advancing the patient's diet when "Advance as tolerated" is ordered. Diabetic patients have many special needs, and the nurse is responsible for teaching as well as assessing the patient for complications such as hypoglycemia and hyperglycemia.
- Common eating disorders include anorexia nervosa, bulimia nervosa, and binge eating disorder.
- Some drugs can affect appetite or digestion due to side effects. Some drugs can alter the absorption, metabolism, and excretion of nutrients by affecting GI and liver function. Some drugs affect the kidneys and interfere with the excretion of nutrients.
- NG tubes are shorter than NI tubes because they go only to the stomach. NI tubes are usually smaller in diameter and more flexible than NG tubes. The double lumen tube, also called a Salem sump, is used strictly for gastric decompression.
- Gastric decompression is the process of reducing the pressure within the stomach by emptying it of its contents. An NG tube is inserted into the stomach and connected to low intermittent suction to accomplish this.
- Patients with difficulties tolerating oral intake may receive enteral feedings. Tube feedings can be NG or NI or via the lower GI tract via a PEG tube or J-tube.
- Small-bore feeding tubes now require the use of ENFit tubes, bags with tubing, and syringes. These will only connect to one another and will not connect to IV tubing to prevent misconnection errors.
- Tube feedings can be continuous or intermittent bolus. Continuous feedings should be administered with a feeding pump.
- Verification of NG/NI tube placement by radiography is the most accurate method. Aspiration of gastric contents and assessment of the pH are used to verify continued presence of the tube in the proper location of the GI tract.
- Complications can arise with enteral tube feeding, such as clogged tubes, aspiration, electrolyte imbalance, hyperglycemia, and severe diarrhea.
- There are two types of parenteral nutrition: PPN and TPN. PPN solutions contain a lower concentration of dextrose than TPN. When administering any type of parenteral nutrition, the nurse must adhere strictly to sterile technique; contamination can lead to serious infection and septicemia.

Review Questions

Select the answer that is most appropriate for each of the following questions. Some questions may have more than one correct answer. Select all that apply.

1. You are caring for an 80-year-old female who has poorly fitting dentures and significant difficulty chewing food. Which diet would be most appropriate for her?
   1. Full liquid diet
   2. Regular diet
   3. Pureed, low-residue diet
   4. Mechanical soft diet
   5. Clear liquid diet

2. You are caring for a patient receiving intermittent bolus feedings, and it is time for the next feeding. Which of these interventions will you perform first?
   1. Total the intake and output for the shift.
   2. Have the patient move from the chair to the bed to lie down.
   3. Aspirate the residual gastric contents, test the pH, and measure it.
   4. Flush the tube with 30 mL of water.
   5. Measure the length of the tube extending from the insertion site.

3. A patient is receiving TPN via a central venous catheter. The patient's wife is concerned about his care and wants to know why the TPN bag is not changed as often as a regular IV bag of solution would be. You respond by telling her the standard for changing the TPN bag is every:
   1. 6 hours.
   2. 8 hours.
   3. 12 hours.
   4. 24 hours.

4. You are caring for a patient who is scheduled for surgery. Your teaching will include information about nutrition and healing. You will tell the patient which of the following macronutrients is required for tissue repair?
   1. Carbohydrates
   2. Fat
   3. Vitamin E
   4. Protein
   5. Vitamin K

5. As a home health nurse, you will be caring for the patients noted below. Which patient is at greatest risk for experiencing inadequate nutrition?
   1. A 60-year-old white male recently diagnosed with type 2 diabetes
   2. A 72-year-old widow who had a mild CVA 3 days ago
   3. A 25-year-old mother with two preschoolers who is recovering from a tonsillectomy
   4. A 55-year-old black male recovering at home following coronary artery bypass surgery

6. Critically ill, tube-fed patients should have the head of the bed raised to ________ during feedings and for up to 1 hour after feedings.
   1. 5 to 10 degrees
   2. 15 to 25 degrees
   3. 30 to 45 degrees
   4. 50 to 60 degrees
   5. 90 degrees

7. What intervention(s) should you prepare for when caring for a patient who is 6 hours post burn with 30% second-degree burns and absent bowel sounds?
   1. Withholding oral intake
   2. Insertion of an NG tube to low intermittent suction
   3. Starting a diet of clear liquids only
   4. Inserting a feeding tube for nutrition
   5. Feeding the patient a soft diet

8. Which actions are taken to verify the correct placement of a small-bore NG tube immediately after insertion? (Rank your answers in the correct order.)
   1. Aspirate the gastric contents, check the pH of contents, and observe the color
   2. Confirm the size of the feeding tube after taping
   3. Place the distal end of the tube in a glass of water and observe for bubbles indicating air exchange
   4. Take an x-ray
   5. Flush the tube with 15 to 30 mL of water to ensure its correct placement

9. You are working in a pediatric clinic when the mother of a 15-year-old female patient calls with concerns about her daughter. Which behaviors she describes would alert you to a possible eating disorder?
   1. She constantly worries about her weight.
   2. She talks about various foods and their nutritional quality.
   3. She exercises 2 to 3 hours daily.
   4. She often complains of a sore throat and indigestion.
   5. She talks frequently with friends about school activities.

ANSWERS 1. 4, 2. 3, 3. 4, 4. 4, 5. 2, 6. 3, 7. 1, 2, 8. 1 = first, 4 = second, 9. 1, 4

Critical Thinking Exercises

Answers available online.

1. You are working on a cardiovascular unit and are assigned to care for a 68-year-old black female who is being admitted. She has advanced multiple sclerosis, virtually no motor function from the neck down, and significant dysphagia. What are your nursing priorities for this patient? Develop a plan of care to assist her in meeting her nutritional needs.

2. A 75-year-old white male has been ill with nausea, vomiting, and diarrhea for the last 4 days. He transferred from his long-term care (LTC) facility to your hospital. His weight 1 week ago at the LTC was 165 lbs. (75 kg); today it is 156 lbs. (70.9 kg). Your assessment reveals hyperactive bowel sounds, a soft and slightly tender abdomen in all four quadrants, and continued nausea and diarrhea but no vomiting in the last 8 hours. He is afebrile with normal electrolyte values. What type of diet order would be the best choice for him? What nursing interventions should you perform during your 7-to-3 shift?

3. You are caring for a patient receiving 250 mL of formula via intermittent enteral feedings. You withdraw 50 mL of residual gastric content when you check his NG tube's placement, patency, and residual. Should you return the gastric aspirate to the patient's stomach or discard it? Provide a rationale for your response.

Additional Resources

Use the scratch off code on the inside front cover of your book to access online quizzes that will help you to improve your scores on course exams and prepare for the NCLEX-PN®.

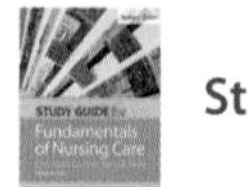

Study Guide

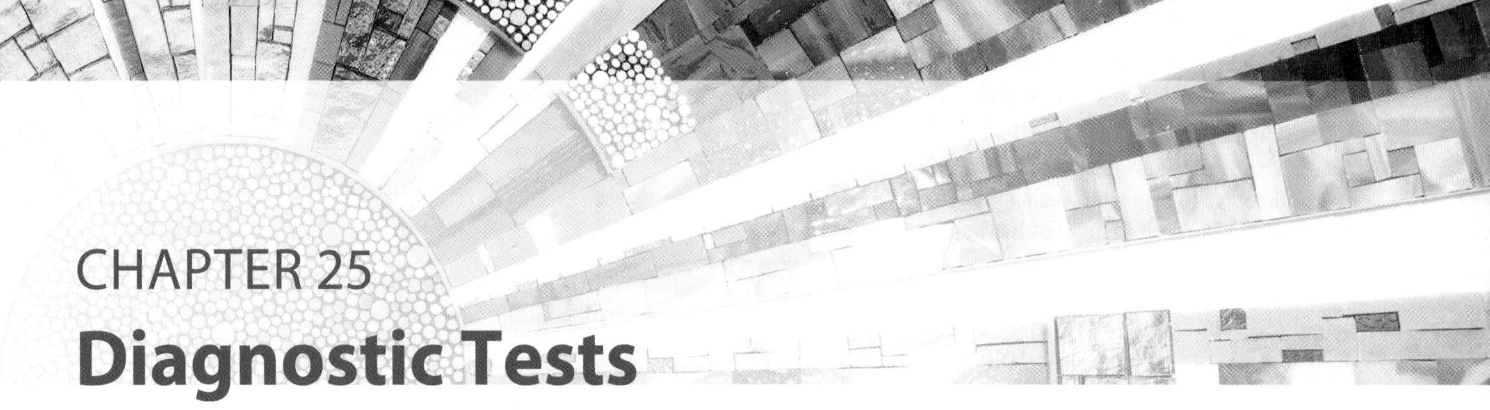

CHAPTER 25
Diagnostic Tests

KEY TERMS

Arteriography (ar-TEER-ee-AWG-ruh-fee)
Barium enema (BA-ree-um EN-e-muh)
Bone marrow aspiration (BOWN MA-roh ASS-pi-RAY-shun)
Chest x-ray (CHEST EKS-ray)
Colonoscopy (KOH-lun-AWS-kuh-pee)
Complete blood cell count (kom-PLEET BLUHD SELL KOWNT)
Complete metabolic panel (kom-PLEET MET-uh-BAH-lik PAN-uhl)
Computed tomography (kom-PEW-ted toh-MAWG-ruh-fee)
Differential (dif-uh-REN-shul)
Echocardiogram (EK-oh-KAR-dee-oh-GRAM)
Electrocardiography (ee-LEK-troh-KAR-dee-AWG-ruh-fee)
Electroencephalography (ee-LEK-troh-en-SEF-uh-LAWG-ruh-fee)
Esophagogastroduodenoscopy (eh-SOF-ah-goh-GAS-troh-doo-AW-den-AWS-kuh-pee)
Glomerular filtration rate (gloh-MER-yoo-ler fill-TRAY-shun RAYT)
Glycosylated hemoglobin (GLY-koh-sye-LAYT-uhd HEE-muh-GLOW-bin)
Intravenous pyelogram (IN-trah-VEE-nus PIE-eh-loh-GRAM)
KUB
Left shift (LEFT SHIFT)
Lumbar puncture (LUM-bar PUNK-chur)
Magnetic resonance imaging (mag-NET-ik REZ-uh-nanss IM-uh-jing)
Oral glucose tolerance test (OR-uhl GLOO-kohss TALL-er-ens TEST)
Paracentesis (PAR-ah-sen-TEE-siss)
Right shift (RIGHT SHIFT)
Thoracentesis (THOR-uh-sen-TEE-siss)
Ultrasonography (UHL-truh-son-AWG-ruh-fee)
Venography (vee-NAWG-ruh-fee)

CHAPTER CONCEPTS

Patient-Centered Care

LEARNING OUTCOMES

1. Define various terms associated with diagnostic tests, as well as the five types of diagnostic tests.
2. Explain the nurse's role and responsibilities regarding preparation for tests and posttest nursing care.
3. Discuss all the components of a complete blood cell count, including normal ranges for each.
4. Identify the components of a white cell count with differential, including possible causes for abnormal values.
5. Explain components of blood chemistry testing and their significance.
6. Determine the purposes of testing cardiac enzymes, B-type natriuretic peptide, lipase, and glycosylated hemoglobin.
7. Contrast the normal and abnormal findings of a urinalysis and their significance.
8. Explain how the glomerular filtration rate is determined, along with its significance.
9. Describe radiology and imaging tests, including computed tomography and magnetic resonance imaging, along with the nursing care of each.
10. Discuss arteriography, venography, computed tomography angiography, and magnetic resonance angiography, as well as the nursing care for each.
11. Explain the preparation for, purpose of, and nursing care after endoscopic exams.
12. Identify allergies for which the nurse should assess prior to procedures and tests requiring use of contrast medium.
13. Discuss the purposes of graphic recording tests, including telemetry, and the nursing care required.
14. Explain the purposes for lumbar puncture, bone marrow aspiration, paracentesis, and thoracentesis, including how to position a patient for each procedure.
15. Discuss information found in the Connection features in this chapter.
16. Identify specific safety information.
17. Answer questions about the skills in this chapter.

SKILLS

25.1 Assisting With Aspiration Procedures: Bone Marrow, Lumbar Puncture, Paracentesis, and Thoracentesis
25.2 Performing a 12-Lead Electrocardiogram

CRITICAL THINKING CONNECTION

Clinical Assignment

You are caring for a 37-year-old female who has been hospitalized with abdominal pain, nausea, and vomiting of an unknown origin. The health-care provider has ordered an esophagogastroduodenoscopy; an ultrasound of the gallbladder and pancreas; and blood work to include a blood chemistry, electrolyte panel, alkaline phosphatase, glomerular filtration rate, and creatinine. Your patient tells you that she hopes they do it all quickly because she hates needles and has no idea what the other tests are like.

Critical Thinking Questions:

1. How will you prepare your patient for her tests?
2. What will you assess for after the tests are completed?
3. Why is it important for you to know normal ranges for diagnostic tests?

It is important that you know the purpose of each test and the normal findings so that you can notify the health-care provider of abnormal results.

Diagnostic tests are those tests and examinations that help to make a medical diagnosis by ruling out other possible diagnoses or by specifically pinpointing the disease process or injury afflicting the patient. This chapter will assist you to identify your role as a nurse in relation to diagnostic tests and to familiarize you with some of the more commonly used examinations.

Please note that this chapter does not provide a comprehensive review of diagnostic testing; rather, the focus is on routine tests that you will likely see on a daily basis. As you will find out throughout the course of your schooling and even as you start your career, the number of diagnostic tests available to health-care professionals cannot be covered in a single chapter. We encourage you to utilize books dedicated solely to this specialized subject to further your knowledge.

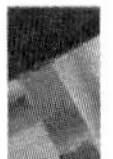

NURSING'S ROLE IN DIAGNOSTIC TESTING

As the nurse, you will not be performing many of the tests discussed in this chapter, but you will have numerous responsibilities relating to health-care provider–ordered diagnostic tests and procedures. Depending on the test, your responsibilities before the test may include the following:

- Noting the health-care provider's order.
- Occasionally scheduling the test or procedure.
- Educating the patient regarding the process.
- ***Safety: Determine that the patient is not allergic to any dyes or preparations that may be used for the test, including allergies to iodine, shellfish, and contrast medium.***
- Administering laxatives or enemas to remove fecal material from the intestinal tract, which allows for better visualization of the intestine for various imaging tests.
- Making certain written consent is obtained, if the procedure requires it; the health-care provider is responsible for explaining the diagnostic tests and answering the patient's questions prior to the consent being signed.
- Knowing when to withhold food and fluids (Box 25.1).
- Preparing the patient.
- Assisting the examiner with performance of the test or procedure.

Your responsibilities after the diagnostic tests may include the following:

- Obtaining specimens or delivering specimens to the laboratory.
- Monitoring and assessing the patient's condition after the test.
- Reassuring or supporting the patient as needed.
- Notifying the health-care provider of significant abnormal results.
- Monitoring for complications.
- Providing necessary postprocedure nursing care.
- Being able to relate the significance of the test findings to the patient's condition.

With all of these responsibilities, you can easily see that understanding the purposes, preparation for, and processes of commonly administered diagnostic tests is paramount to your role as a nurse. Table 25.1 details the preparation and posttest nursing care for selected tests.

Settings Connection: Medical Office

Diagnostic Testing and Results

Many times licensed practical/vocational nurses working in medical offices or clinics will be the staff member who sees the results of diagnostic tests first. Or they may be the person who gets the telephone call about abnormal blood tests. It is very important that you recognize values that are severely abnormal and let the health-care provider know about them right away.

If you are working in an office or clinic, you may also be responsible for scheduling diagnostic testing for your patients, as well as giving them preparation instructions. Your knowledge about the diagnostic tests, their purposes, preparation, and normal results will be very important in this setting.

Patient Teaching Connection

Diagnostic Tests

Prepare the patient for upcoming tests or procedures to alleviate the patient's anxiety and increase compliance. Using terminology that the patient will understand, explain the purpose of the test or procedure, as well as the test's benefits and dangers. The physician will explain the purpose and risks for the procedure. Describe what will occur, including any preparatory steps that must be performed prior to the test. If a specimen such as urine or sputum is required, explain how to correctly obtain the specimen. Avoid using acronyms for the name of the test or procedure; instead, use the complete name; for example, use "white blood cell count" rather than "WBC." Remember that the average patient is not familiar with medical terminology. However, this does not mean that you should talk down to the patient as if he or she is ignorant.

It is generally helpful to provide the patient with a written pamphlet or brochure about the procedure. Some patients prefer to read about it before you verbally explain it, while others would rather discuss it with you first and then relax and read the pamphlet to reinforce your teaching. If written consent must be obtained to perform the procedure, be certain that all patient teaching is completed before the consent is signed.

KNOWLEDGE CONNECTION

Discuss at least eight responsibilities you will have regarding diagnostic testing. What types of preparations are common prior to diagnostic procedures?

Box 25.1
When to Withhold Food and Fluids

Withholding food and fluids, or permitting "nothing by mouth," is known as keeping the patient NPO. Many tests require that the patient be kept NPO prior to the test, but there are no hard and fast rules for which tests require this. Each facility will have its own policies for diagnostic tests and whether or not preparation includes being kept NPO. Which blood chemistry tests include being kept NPO vary in different facilities. Some of the tests that commonly require the patient to be kept NPO for 6 to 8 hours include the following:

- Any type of endoscopy, such as EGD and colonoscopy
- Cardiac catheterization
- Any CT with contrast medium or dye
- Any test reflecting glucose levels, such as the glucose tolerance test and fasting blood glucose
- Lung and brain scans if contrast medium is used
- Cholesterol and lipid tests

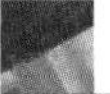

CATEGORIES OF DIAGNOSTIC TESTS

There are five general categories of diagnostic tests that we will discuss in this chapter:

1. Laboratory tests
2. Radiology and imaging tests and procedures
3. Ultrasonography
4. Endoscopic examinations
5. Graphic recording tests

Laboratory Tests

Laboratory test is a broad classification for numerous types of examinations performed on some type of body fluid, such as whole blood or the serum portion of the blood, spinal fluid, sputum, urine, gastric contents, feces, and bone marrow.

Anatomy and Physiology Connection

Blood

Let's briefly review the production of blood cells. In adults, *red blood cells* (RBCs) are produced by the bone marrow within the sternum, vertebrae, ribs, and pelvis. The kidneys release a protein known as erythropoietin, which acts on stem cells in the bone marrow to produce more RBCs. The RBC has a relatively short life span of approximately 120 days, after which it is destroyed by the reticuloendothelial system. *White blood cells* (WBCs) are mostly produced in the bone marrow, with limited production in the lymphoid tissues. *Platelets* (PLTs) are produced from large bone marrow cells known as *megakaryocytes.*

Hematology

Hematology is the study of blood cells and the blood-forming tissues (the bone marrow). It includes different types of blood counts.

COMPLETE BLOOD COUNT. The most common test ordered is the **complete blood cell count** (CBC), which measures the number of leukocytes, or WBCs; erythrocytes, or RBCs; and thrombocytes, also called platelets and abbreviated as PLTs. It also differentiates the percentages of the five types of WBCs (lymphocytes, neutrophils, eosinophils, basophils, and monocytes); measures the *hemoglobin* (Hgb), or iron pigment; and the *hematocrit* (Hct), which is the measurement of the percentage of packed RBCs compared to the whole blood

• WORD • BUILDING •

radiology: radio – radiant energy + logy – study of

ultrasonography: ultra – extreme + sono – sound + graphy – writing

hematology: hemato – blood + logy – study of

Table 25.1
Preparation and Posttest Nursing Care for Selected Tests

Test	*Description*	*Purpose*	*Preparation*	*Posttest Nursing Care*
Barium enema	Rectal instillation of barium (a contrast medium) provides for radiographic visualization of the large intestine, to see its shape and any abnormalities that might be present.	To detect cancerous tumors, obstructions, polyps, inflammatory disease, or diverticula in the colon.	Explain the procedure. Offer assurance and support. The day before, perform bowel prep of laxatives and enemas according to facility or physician orders. Clear liquid diet. NPO after midnight.	Administer milk of magnesia or laxative of choice to remove barium before it hardens. Monitor for constipation. Explain that stools will be white until barium is eliminated. Provide fluids and physician-ordered diet.
Bone marrow aspiration (See Skill 25.1, page 517, for more information on assisting with bone marrow aspiration.)	Under local anesthetic, a sample of marrow is removed from the sternum, tibia, or iliac crest by needle aspiration for evaluation of blood cell production.	To diagnose some serious anemias, thrombocytopenia, and cancerous tumors, and to stage Hodgkin's disease.	Describe the procedure and explain that it only takes 10 to 20 minutes to perform. Assess for allergy to local anesthetic to be used. Explain there will be a feeling of pressure and a brief period of discomfort when the marrow is actually aspirated. Offer reassurance and support. Make certain written consent has been obtained. Administer sedative or analgesic 60 to 90 minutes prior to test. Assess vital signs for baseline.	Hold pressure to puncture site and observe for bleeding at site. Apply dressing. Monitor vital signs for shock: ↓BP, ↑P. Monitor for signs of infection: ↑T, ↑P.
Intravenous pyelogram (also known as excretory urogram)	An iodine-based contrast dye is injected intravenously. X-rays are taken for visualization of the kidney parenchyma, pelvis, calyces, ureters, and bladder.	Evaluation of renal structure and function; aids in detection of kidney stones, obstruction, tumors, urinary tract disease, and trauma.	Explain the procedure. Assess for allergy to iodine, shellfish, and contrast medium dyes. Keep the patient NPO for 8 hours prior to test. Make certain a consent form has been signed.	Observe for hematoma at the injection site. Observe for delayed reaction to the contrast dye. Assess for adequate urination. Encourage PO fluids to rehydrate the patient and flush dye from body. Provide physician-ordered diet.
Lumbar puncture (See Skill 25.1, page 517, for more information on	A spinal needle is inserted between vertebral spinous processes into the lumbar section of the arachnoid space to obtain a cerebrospinal fluid (CSF)	To diagnose meningitis, subarachnoid hemorrhage, tumors, and other infections of the	Explain the procedure and that it takes 10 to 15 minutes. Make certain written consent has been obtained. Assess allergy to iodine prep and local anesthetic.	Keep the patient flat in bed for 8 hours. May turn from side to side but may not raise head. Encourage plenty of PO fluids to reduce risk of spinal headache.

assisting with lumbar puncture.)	sample to culture for organisms and measure CSF pressure.	central nervous system.	When ready for the procedure, position the patient on his or her side at the edge of the bed. Have the patient draw knees up to abdomen and tuck chin down to chest to flex the spine for ease of needle insertion. Help to hold the patient in this position for duration of test.	Provide a flexible straw for drinking. Monitor needle insertion site for bleeding or drainage of CSF hourly for 4 hours and then every 4 hours for a period of 24 hours. Perform neurological status checks as ordered by physician. Assess for numbness and tingling of extremities, fever, neck rigidity, change in level of consciousness, BP changes, widening pulse pressure, ↓P, or irregular respirations for the first 24 hours.
Oral glucose tolerance test	Patient drinks concentrated glucose syrup to stimulate pancreatic production of insulin. Blood and urine samples are collected at five to six intervals over a 3- to 6-hour span to evaluate glucose levels.	To diagnose diabetes mellitus or hypoglycemia.	Explain the procedure. Keep the patient NPO for 12 hours, except for water, which must be drunk for production of urine samples.	Provide physician-ordered diet and fluids. Observe for hypoglycemia and hyperglycemia.
Paracentesis (See Skill 25.1, page 517, for more information on assisting with paracentesis.)	Under local anesthetic, a needle is inserted through the abdominal wall into the peritoneal cavity to remove free fluid from within the cavity (ascites).	To relieve discomfort of the pressure of ascites, common in abdominal organ cancers and liver disease.	Explain the procedure. Assess for allergy to local anesthetic to be used. Offer assurance and support. Make certain written consent has been obtained. Weigh the patient. Measure abdominal girth. Have the patient empty bladder. Assess baseline vital signs.	Document amount of fluid removed. Monitor vital signs. Assess for *syncope* (fainting). Encourage rest for several hours. Observe the needle insertion site for hematoma. Weigh the patient and compare to pretest weight. Measure abdominal girth and compare to pretest girth.
Thoracentesis (See Skill 25.1, page 517, for more information on assisting with thoracentesis.)	Under local anesthetic, a needle is inserted through the chest wall into the pleural space to remove excess fluid.	To remove fluid for diagnostic purposes or to decrease respiratory distress resulting from excess fluid because of lung disease or cancer.	Explain the procedure. Assess for allergy to local anesthetic to be used. Offer assurance and support. Make certain written consent has been obtained. Weigh the patient. Assess vital signs. Apply cardiac monitor and supplemental O_2.	Document amount of fluid removed. Monitor vital signs, especially SpO_2. Auscultate breath sounds. Assess for dyspnea and arrhythmias. Encourage rest for several hours. Observe needle insertion site for hematoma. Weigh the patient and compare to pretest weight.

volume. Each of these tests may be ordered as a stand-alone test as well as components of a CBC. *Even as a new nursing student attending clinical experiences, it is important to comprehend the different components of a CBC because it is performed on every patient upon admission to a hospital.* Table 25.2 lists the normal CBC values.

WHITE CELL COUNT AND DIFFERENTIAL. When the WBC count is elevated above normal, it is termed *leukocytosis;* when it is below normal, it is called *leukopenia.* WBCs, especially the neutrophils, function primarily to protect the body from infection. Once a bacterial infection begins, the bone marrow increases the production of WBCs, specifically the neutrophils, monocytes, and a few lymphocytes. The lymph tissue produces the majority of lymphocytes. A **differential** is the breakdown of the total WBC into percentages of the five types of white cells, each of which becomes elevated in response to different situations:

- *Neutrophils elevate* with infection. Slightly immature neutrophils are called *bands.* When their level is elevated, as opposed to the more mature segmented neutrophils, it is known as a **left shift**, which generally indicates bacterial infection.
- *Eosinophils* elevate in response to allergic reactions and parasites.
- *Basophils* contain large amounts of histamine and elevate in hypersensitivity reactions, such as reactions to stings, iodine, or medications. These reactions, known as *anaphylactic reactions,* are life-threatening allergic reactions.
- *Monocyte* levels rise as a second line of defense against bacterial infections.
- *Lymphocytes* increase with viral infections and allergic conditions. When their level is elevated, it is known as a **right shift,** a typical indicator of viral infection.

As shown above, a differential can help to discern whether there is a bacterial or viral infection, an allergic or hypersensitivity reaction, a parasitic invasion, or a disease of the blood-forming organs.

RED BLOOD CELL COUNT, HEMOGLOBIN, AND HEMATOCRIT LEVELS. An RBC count provides the number of RBCs in a cubic millimeter (mm^3) of whole blood, whose function is to carry the Hgb, which binds with oxygen to be delivered to cells throughout the body. When the RBC count is lower than normal, it is known as *erythropenia* or *erythrocytopenia.* A lower-than-normal level of RBCs can help to diagnose hemorrhage beyond 24 hours, fluid overload, or anemia. *Anemia* is a condition in which there is a reduction in the delivery of oxygen to the tissues; it is usually indicated by depressed RBC and Hgb levels. *Polycythemia* describes an elevated RBC count.

Closely related to the RBC count—and part of a CBC—is the Hgb test. This test helps to determine the presence and severity of the different types of anemia. When Hgb is decreased, the body's oxygen-carrying capacity is reduced, which interferes with the ability of different body tissues and systems to function at optimal level.

The RBC, Hgb, and Hct levels are closely related and are useful in diagnosing dehydration, anemia, and polycythemia. As well as being ordered as a stand-alone Hct or as part of a CBC, the Hgb and Hct are often ordered as an *H&H.*

PLATELET COUNT. PLTs are the blood cells that aid in the blood *clotting* process to prevent hemorrhage and help to protect vascular surfaces. If a patient has too many PLTs, the patient has *thrombocytosis,* which can result in abnormal clotting. If a patient has too few PLTs, *thrombocytopenia* develops, which hinders the body's hemostatic ability, or the ability to stop bleeding.

Table 25.2 Complete Blood Count Normal Values

Blood Component	*Normal Range*
WBC, total	Adults older than 10 years: 4.5–11.1 mm^3
WBC, differential total neutrophils	40%-75% of total WBC
(Bands)*	(3%–5%)
Lymphocytes†	12%-44% of total WBC
Monocytes	4%–9% of total WBC
Eosinophils	0%–5.5% of total WBC
Basophils	0%–1% of total WBC
RBCs	Adult males: 4.21–5.81 mm^3 Adult females: 3.61–5.11 mm^3
Hemoglobin	Adult males: 14–17.3 g/dL Adult females: 11.7–15.5 g/dL
Hematocrit	Adult males: 42%–52% Adult females: 36%–48%
PLTs	140,000–400,000/mm^3

*When bands elevate to higher percentage levels, called a left shift, this indicates bacterial infection.

†When lymphocytes elevate to higher percentage levels, called a right shift, this indicates viral infection.

KNOWLEDGE CONNECTION

Differentiate between the five types of WBCs, including possible etiologies of their elevations. What are the medical terms for the different types of blood cells, including RBCs, WBCs, and PLTs? Describe the components of a complete WBC count. List three ways an Hgb level may be ordered. Describe what is meant by a *left shift.*

• WORD • BUILDING •

leukocytosis: leuko – white + cyt – cell + osis – condition

leukopenia: leuko – white + pen – lack + ia – condition

Blood Chemistry Tests

Blood chemistry tests may be performed on whole blood, plasma, or serum. They are generally performed to detect changes in the biological chemical reactions in the body. They may be used to rule out certain conditions as well as to diagnose a disease or syndrome. The following are some of the more common chemistry tests:

- **Blood glucose:** When carbohydrates are digested by the body, they are broken down to glucose (see Chapter 23). Elevated blood glucose levels can be indicative of diabetes mellitus, which is a disorder of carbohydrate digestion and insulin production and use. Blood glucose is also known to elevate when an individual is under stress, such as with hospitalization. Some health-care providers routinely monitor glucose levels of patients admitted to the hospital, even if they are not diagnosed with diabetes mellitus.
- **Electrolyte levels:** Potassium (K^+), chloride (Cl^-), sodium (Na^+), magnesium (Mg^{2+}), calcium (Ca^{2+}), and phosphate (PO_4^-) levels are obtained to evaluate fluid and electrolyte balance and acid-base balance, which you will learn more about in Chapter 29.
- **Enzymes and isoenzymes:** These substances are released into the blood from specific tissue cells when those cells are injured; the enzymes and isoenzymes present help identify damage to specific organs. Cardiac cells release troponin, creatine kinase-MB, and lactate dehydrogenase types 1 and 2. Damaged liver cells release aspartate aminotransferase, alanine aminotransferase, and alkaline phosphatase.
- **Blood urea nitrogen:** Nitrogen is an end product of protein breakdown, excreted by the kidneys into the urine. Some common medications can cause elevation of the blood urea nitrogen (BUN) level, such as aspirin and certain antibiotics, as well as a high protein diet. Elevated blood levels occur with dehydration, heart failure, urinary tract obstruction, recent heart attack, or gastrointestinal bleeding. For these reasons, BUN alone is not indicative of kidney damage, but is considered along with creatinine and the *estimated glomerular filtration rate* (eGFR) in evaluating kidney function.
- **Serum creatinine:** Creatinine is a product of metabolism, removed from blood by the kidneys. Elevated levels indicate impairment of kidney function.
- **Total protein:** Total protein is used to evaluate many conditions, such as malnutrition, dehydration, severe burns, gastrointestinal disease, renal disease, liver disease, and diabetes mellitus. It measures serum levels of albumin and globulins, which are vital to numerous body functions. These proteins:
  - Serve as a buffer in the acid-base balance;
  - Help to maintain osmolarity of body fluids;
  - Act as carrier transporters of iron, copper, and other ions;
  - Perform as enzymes and antibodies;
  - Help to bind and detoxify medications; and
  - Serve as a resource for tissue nutrition.
- **Total bilirubin:** Total bilirubin measures the blood level of *bilirubin*, which is an orange pigment that is released during the destruction or breakdown of Hgb. Once an RBC's normal life span is over, the RBC is destroyed, releasing the Hgb and, eventually, the bilirubin. Normally, Kupffer cells in the liver transform the bilirubin into bile, which aids in digestion and is excreted in the feces. Certain disease processes can interfere with this process, resulting in excessive blood levels of bilirubin that stain the skin and tissues a yellowish-orange color, a condition known as *jaundice*. The bilirubin test is performed to evaluate liver function and to help in the diagnosis of certain anemias and biliary obstruction.

Most facilities have designated names for specific clusters or groups of blood chemistry tests. For example, some facilities use terms such as *basic metabolic panel* or **complete metabolic panel,** each representing a specific grouping of tests in which 8 or 14 respective tests are to be done. Box 25.2 provides a list of the tests included in a complete metabolic panel.

Box 25.2

Complete Metabolic Panel

A complete, or comprehensive, metabolic panel (CMP) is the name for a group of 14 separate tests that provide an overview of some of the functions of the liver, kidneys, and pancreas. The following are the tests included in a CMP:

- **Albumin:** a protein produced by the liver
- **Alkaline phosphatase (ALP):** an enzyme produced by the liver
- **Alanine aminotransferase (ALT),** also known as **SGPT:** an enzyme produced by the liver
- **Aspartate aminotransferase (AST),** also known as **SGOT:** an enzyme produced by the liver
- **Bilirubin:** a waste product remaining after the liver destroys old RBCs
- **Blood urea nitrogen:** a waste product filtered from the blood by the kidneys
- **Calcium:** an electrolyte; excess levels are removed from the blood by the kidneys
- **Chloride:** an electrolyte; excess levels are removed from the blood by the kidneys
- **Creatinine:** a waste product filtered from the blood by the kidneys
- **Glucose:** a simple sugar fuel source for cellular energy; needs insulin (from the pancreas) to transport glucose into the cells
- **Potassium:** an electrolyte; excess levels are removed from the blood by the kidneys
- **Sodium:** an electrolyte; excess levels are removed from the blood by the kidneys
- **Total protein:** measures all serum proteins, including albumin and globulins
- **Total serum CO_2:** measures serum level of bicarbonate (HCO_3^-), which provides data about serum CO_2 level because 95% of serum CO_2 is carried as part of HCO_3^-

Other Blood Tests

- **B-type natriuretic peptide**: The B-type natriuretic peptide (BNP) is secreted by the heart ventricles. When the pressure and blood volume in the ventricles rise, as occurs with congestive heart failure, production of BNP increases. This makes the BNP a valuable tool to diagnose congestive heart failure.
- **Cardiac enzymes:** Tests for three enzymes called *myoglobin, troponin*, and *creatine kinase* (CK) are done to determine if a myocardial infarction (heart attack) has occurred. You may hear these terms often when patients experience chest pain or are admitted with chest pain. Myoglobin is released with any muscle damage; however, if the patient has chest pain and no other muscle injury, this test is very helpful because myoglobin levels elevate within 30 minutes after an injury. Troponin actually includes two enzymes: troponin 1 and troponin T, which are released 3 to 4 hours after a myocardial infarction and will remain elevated for 10 days. CK includes three isoenzymes. However, the MB fraction is the one released with myocardial injury. The CK level begins to rise 3 to 4 hours after a myocardial infarction and stays elevated for 3 to 4 days.
- **Lipase:** Lipase is a group of digestive enzymes that are secreted by the pancreas into the duodenum. Elevated levels of lipase in the bloodstream are generally indicative of pancreatic disease, such as pancreatitis or pancreatic cancer. Although elevated lipase levels are most helpful in diagnosing pancreatic disease, they also may be elevated with acute inflammation of the biliary tract and during kidney failure, which is due to impaired renal excretion of the enzyme.
- **Glycosylated or glycated hemoglobin (Hbg A_{1c}): Glycosylated hemoglobin** is the measurement of the Hgb that has become bound with glucose. It provides a method of calculating the average blood glucose for the previous 3-month period of time, giving the health-care provider a picture of how well controlled the patient's diabetes is. Normally an A_{1c} should range from 4.0% to 5.5%. If the A_{1c} is between 5.7% and 6.4%, it is considered *prediabetes*. The American Diabetes Association recommends that diabetic patients be maintained at 6.5% or less for optimal disease control. There is no preparation for this test. The patient does not have to be NPO.

NURSING CARE FOR BLOOD TESTS. The patient should be informed that a blood sample will have to be drawn for any of the tests mentioned above. Most laboratories do not place restrictions on food or fluid for the tests listed here. However, many other tests do require the patient be kept NPO. Please refer to a laboratory diagnostic text book as you learn more about other diagnostic tests during your nurse's training and actual patient care. It will be your responsibility to know when to keep a patient NPO.

KNOWLEDGE CONNECTION

Describe at least four common laboratory tests and their purposes. Name two tests that evaluate renal function. Identify three diagnostic tests that would provide you with information relating to nutrition. Name three diagnostic tests that would be useful in evaluating liver function. Name three enzymes that would be used to diagnose myocardial infarction. Identify a test useful in diagnosing congestive heart failure. What blood test provides a 90-day average of the patient's blood glucose level?

Urine Tests

Urine tests may be performed on voided or catheterized urine specimens; urine also may be collected over 24 hours for examination (see Chapter 31). Analysis of the urine and its contents provides you with much useful information.

URINALYSIS. Routine urinalysis tests are ordered frequently in medical clinics and are routinely ordered on admission to hospitals. Normal findings in a routine urinalysis include the following:

- **Color:** straw to dark yellow
- **Odor:** slightly aromatic
- **Appearance:** clear
- **Specific gravity:** 1.001 to 1.029
- **pH:** 5 to 9
- **Glucose:** none
- **Protein:** less than 20 mg/dL
- **Ketones:** none
- **Nitrites:** none
- **Bilirubin:** none
- **Urobilinogen**: up to 1 mg/dL
- **RBCs:** less than 5 per high-power field
- **WBCs:** less than 5 per high-power field
- **Transitional/epithelial cells:** none
- **Casts:** none
- **Bacteria:** none
- **Yeast:** none
- **Parasites:** none

A basic urinalysis is simple to perform but can provide you with valuable information about the patient's health status, not just about the renal system. For example, the urine of a dehydrated patient may be a darker color, even amber. Color changes and abnormal pH values can be due to different diseases, medications, or dietary habits. The appearance may be cloudy due to the presence of bacteria or WBCs, often indicating infection of the urinary system. The specific gravity, which is the weight of the urine, will increase as dehydration increases the urine's ratio of solutes to water; it also may cause the odor to become stronger, even to the point that it smells like ammonia. Other systemic diseases and conditions that can affect the specific gravity are diabetes insipidus, congestive heart failure, and shock. Protein in the urine, known as *proteinuria,* usually is related to some type of renal disease. The presence of ketones in the urine, known as *ketonuria,* is generally related to diabetes mellitus, indicating that adequate blood glucose is not being delivered to individual cells throughout the body. Therefore, it is to your benefit, as well as important to your patients' well-being, to become familiar with the components normally present in the urine and the significance of elevated or decreased amounts. It also is important to know the significance of abnormal components present in the urine.

Glomerular Filtration Rate

Now considered the most accurate test for evaluating kidney function, the **glomerular filtration rate** (GFR) measures the volume of urine, in milliliters, that is filtered by the kidney in 1 minute. The test involves a 24-hour collection of urine and determination of a blood creatinine level; however, more commonly an eGFR is performed. Using a formula and the creatinine results, the eGFR is calculated without waiting to collect a 24-hour urine sample. Anything below 60 mL/min is considered to be significant renal impairment (Table 25.3).

Radiology and Imaging Tests

Radiography or *x-ray* provides an image of the bones without any preparation and is the most common test performed on the skeletal system. It is useful in detecting bone fractures and displacement of bone structures.

Table 25.3
Glomerular Filtration Rate

Glomerular Filtration Rate (mL/min)	*Level of Kidney Impairment*	*Description*
100–120	None	Normal function
90–99	1	Slight kidney impairment with adequate glomerular filtration rate
60–89	2	Mild kidney impairment
30–59	3	Moderate kidney impairment
15–29	4	Severe kidney impairment
Less than 15	5	Complete kidney failure

Chest X-Ray

Chest x-ray (CXR) not only will allow you to see the bony structures of the thorax; it also will allow you to visualize the following:

- The heart's position and size
- The lungs and whether they are fully expanded or have collapsed lobes (known as *atelectasis*) and whether they are clear or congested
- Densities that may indicate malignant tumors or tuberculosis

Flat Plate of Abdomen or KUB X-Ray

A flat plate or **KUB** (which stands for kidneys, ureters, and bladder) is an x-ray of the abdomen that shows the structures and positions of the abdominal organs. It can provide information such as obstruction of, or excessive gas accumulation in, the intestines, tumors, kidney stones, or fluid collection in the peritoneal cavity, known as *ascites.* The abdominal flat plate or KUB is often the initial diagnostic tool used when an abdominal organ disease is suspected.

NURSING CARE FOR CHEST X-RAY OR KUB. Little nursing care is necessary for a CXR. Explain to the patient that painless x-ray pictures will be taken, requiring removal of jewelry, bras, and shirts or blouses with buttons, zippers, or snaps. A hospital gown will be used to protect modesty.

Magnetic Resonance Imaging

Magnetic resonance imaging (MRI) is a form of radiology that uses a magnetic scanner to detect the magnetic properties of atoms, usually hydrogen, while radiofrequency energy produces images of body tissues. It produces slices of the site, similar to computed tomography scans, allowing the examiner to view organs and tissues at all depths. MRI is useful in evaluation of the brain, spinal cord, bone, organs, and vessels in motion, as well as other fluid-filled soft tissues. It aids in diagnosing hemorrhagic and embolic cerebrovascular accidents, more commonly known as strokes; tumors; multiple sclerosis; spinal cord aberrations; and other fluid-filled soft tissue disorders. MRI can be done with or without contrast medium or dye.

The patient is placed in a tunnel opening within the scanner, which is not very large. Some patients become claustrophobic and require sedation, while others are unable to tolerate the procedure. These patients usually are better able to tolerate the procedure if it is performed in an open-style MRI machine.

NURSING CARE FOR MAGNETIC RESONANCE IMAGING. When an MRI is ordered, you will need to verify if contrast

• WORD • BUILDING •
proteinuria: protein – protein + ur – urine + ia – condition
ketonuria: keton – ketone + ur – urine + ia – condition
radiography: radio – radiant energy + graphy – writing

is to be used for enhanced visualization. The patient may need to be kept NPO depending on the organs to be scanned, whether or not contrast dye will be used, and the facility's policy. The contrast dye used in MRI is not iodine based as with computed tomography.

It is important to educate the patient regarding an impending MRI, making certain to inquire if the patient has claustrophobia. You should inform the patient of the limited space inside the scanner tunnel and of the loud knocking and clicking sounds that will be emitted from the scanner throughout the test. Ear plugs, music, and sound-reducing headphones are routinely used to muffle the noise. Inform the patient that even though the MRI is painless the noise can be annoying and that the scan generally takes from 30 to 90 minutes to complete. For patients with severe claustrophobia, a mild sedative or antianxiety medication may be ordered preprocedure. Most facilities require that a consent form be signed. ***Safety: Ask the patient if he or she has any metal implants, aneurysm clips, residual buckshot from gunshot wounds, or a pacemaker. MRI is contraindicated for patients with any type of internal ferrous metal due to the strong magnetic pull of the scanner. Also assist the patient to remove any ferrous metal from body piercings. If the patient is unsure what kind of metal is in the piercing jewelry, remove it to be safe.***

Computed Tomography

Computed tomography (CT), also known as computed axial tomography (CAT) scanning, is an x-ray procedure that takes many x-ray images of body parts from different angles. It then uses a computer to combine all the images to generate cross-sectional pictures and three-dimensional images of the internal organs and structures of the body. In other words, a CT scan helps to visualize slices of the organ or structure being imaged or scanned. This form of imaging can be used to detect normal and abnormal structures in the body, such as tumors. A contrast medium or dye may be ingested or injected prior to the procedure to better differentiate certain structures.

NURSING CARE FOR COMPUTED TOMOGRAPHY. As with an MRI, it is pertinent to assess whether or not the patient has claustrophobia and to explain the types of things that may be used to combat or decrease these feelings. ***Safety: Be certain to ask the patient if he or she is allergic to iodine, shellfish, radiopaque dye, or any contrast medium.*** Allergic reactions to iodine-based products may be more serious than just a "typical rash." This type of allergy can often result in systemic anaphylaxis, a life-threatening reaction causing bronchospasm, laryngeal edema, and peripheral vasodilation, which drops the blood pressure.

If contrast medium is to be administered, assess the patient's kidney function tests to confirm adequate kidney function to handle the contrast medium. This would include the creatinine, BUN, and GFR. An elevated creatinine or BUN should be reported to the health-care provider before proceeding with contrast medium administration. Poorly functioning kidneys are indicated by a lower GFR and should also be reported to the physician. ***Safety: If the patient is currently taking metformin (a drug for diabetes), it should be withheld the day of the CT scan and for an additional 2 days to prevent lactic acidosis problems.*** To assist with the elimination of contrast dye after the procedure, encourage fluids.

Arteriography and Venography

Arteriography, also known as *angiography,* and **venography** are forms of radiology that require a contrast medium be instilled into designated arteries in the case of arteriography or into veins in the case of venography. In arteriography, this contrast medium is instilled through a long catheter inserted into the artery and floated through the circulatory system to the desired organ or structure. This allows examination of the vessel to assess for abnormalities such as *thrombosis* (blood clots) or tumors. It will also show constrictions, occlusions, and *aneurysms,* which are areas of weakening or dilations in a vessel wall that are at risk for rupturing. These studies are commonly used to examine vessels in the heart, brain, lungs, and lower extremities.

NURSING CARE FOR ARTERIOGRAPHY AND VENOGRAPHY. Nursing care is dependent on the vessels accessed during the procedure. For example, when arterial access is performed, such as on the femoral artery, written consent must be obtained and allergy to the dye must be assessed. ***Safety: You must assess whether the patient has been taking anticoagulants, and you must monitor bleeding and coagulation test results prior to the test and make certain they are within normal ranges. An IV line is established prior to the procedure for administration of any needed sedatives or emergency drugs.*** Vital signs are monitored prior to, during, and after the procedure. After completion of the femoral arteriogram, pressure must be maintained on the needle insertion site. A vascular closure device, or plug, is used to prevent bleeding from the puncture site, along with a pressure dressing. The patient must be kept on bedrest for 6 to 8 hours, keeping the involved leg straight. Distal pulses, capillary refill, color, and temperature of the lower extremity must be assessed hourly. The radial artery is sometimes used for cardiac arteriography. An inflated band is placed over the radial artery to maintain pressure after the catheter is removed. This approach does not require bedrest after the procedure.

Computed Tomography Angiography and Magnetic Resonance Angiography

CTA and MRA are noninvasive imaging studies of the arteries and veins, but they do involve the injection of contrast

• WORD • BUILDING •
angiography: angio - lymph or blood vessels + graphy – writing

media. They show information about blood vessels in great detail, including blood flow through the vessels and the connections of the vessels to other organs. This testing shows a three-dimensional view of diseased blood vessels. ***Safety: As with an MRI, any implanted metal is contraindicated for the MRA, such as pacemakers, implanted defibrillators, spinal stimulators, and insulin pumps. Ferrous metal in piercings should be removed before an MRA.***

NURSING CARE AFTER CTA AND MRA. Assess for any allergic reaction to the contrast media used. If the patient has kidney disease or is pregnant, the tests are usually done without contrast.

> **KNOWLEDGE CONNECTION**
> Name three purposes for performing a CXR. Why would femoral arteriography require more assessment than the radial approach after the catheter is removed? What safety concern must you address with a patient prior to an MRI?

Ultrasonography

In **ultrasonography,** ultrasound waves are used to produce images of organs and tissues that can be recorded and printed. It is painless and easy to use, and it can show motion of the organ. Some situations in which ultrasound has been found beneficial include determining the size and position of the fetus or placenta, determining function of cardiac valves, identifying arterial blockages, detecting abscesses and cancerous tumors, and visualizing female reproductive organs. Generally, there is no preparation for ultrasound except for obstetrics, when the patient may be required to drink several glasses of water to provide a full urinary bladder for the test. However, it is important to educate the patient regarding the ease of the test to decrease anxiety and increase patient compliance.

Ultrasonography of the heart is known as an **echocardiogram** and is commonly used because it is noninvasive, quick, easy, and reliable. It can detect problems in heart wall motion, defective heart valves, volume of blood that is pumped from the heart with each heartbeat, and enlargement of the heart wall muscles, which happens with heart failure.

Endoscopic Examinations

Endoscopic examinations use a flexible scope with optical capability that allows visualization of body cavities and hollow organs, such as the colon or urinary bladder. Most endoscopies are performed using light sedation to alleviate patient discomfort during the procedure. Some of the more common endoscopies include esophagogastroduodenoscopy and colonoscopy.

Esophagogastroduodenoscopy

In **esophagogastroduodenoscopy** (EGD), the mouth and throat are sprayed with a local anesthetic and mild sedation is administered. Then a flexible scope is inserted through the mouth, down the esophagus, through the stomach, and into the upper duodenum, allowing visualization of the lining of each. It is useful in detection and biopsy of polyps, ulcers, tumors, gastric reflux, and constrictions, as well as evaluation of chemical burns after ingestion of poisons.

NURSING CARE FOR ESOPHAGOGASTRODUODENOSCOPY. The only preparation for EGD is placing the patient on NPO status for 8 to 12 hours prior to the test or as ordered by the health-care provider. The patient needs to be educated regarding the procedure and that there is minimal or no discomfort associated with the test. Assess vital signs prior to the procedure for a baseline, during the procedure, every 15 minutes for 1 hour, and then every hour for 4 hours after the procedure. Cardiac, neurological, respiratory, and gastrointestinal assessments should be performed on arrival back to the floor to make certain the patient is stable. Be certain the patient's gag reflex has returned postprocedure prior to giving fluids and food. ***Safety: Observe the patient for possible perforation.*** Signs of perforation might include severe pain or difficulty swallowing; epigastric, abdominal, shoulder, or back pain that increases with torso movement; and dyspnea or cyanosis. ***Safety: Check for the gag reflex to return after an EGD before allowing the patient to eat or drink anything, usually 2 to 4 hours after the procedure.***

Colonoscopy

In **colonoscopy,** once the patient is sedated, a flexible endoscope is inserted via the rectum into the colon and terminal ileum, allowing the physician to visualize the lining for abnormalities such as polyps, ulcerations, and tumors and to biopsy tissue as needed. The patient usually feels no discomfort during the examination and is unable to remember anything about the procedure after awakening. This examination should be performed at least every 5 to 10 years after the age of 50 years, and more often if there is a familial history of colon cancer. This exam helps detect cancerous and precancerous lesions early so they can be removed before spreading in the colon.

NURSING CARE FOR COLONOSCOPY. The colon must be prepared so that it is empty and clean for visualization. This preparation begins with limiting the patient's intake to clear liquids for 24 hours before the examination, with avoidance of ingestion of anything "red" such as red Jell-O, popsicles, or soda. Laxatives of the physician's choice are administered, usually beginning about 2 p.m. the day before the examination to evacuate the bowel. This may or may not be followed by

• WORD • BUILDING •

esophagogastroduodenoscopy: esophago – esophagus + gastro – stomach + duodeno – duodenum + scopy – examination

one to three enemas the evening before the test to completely clean out the bowel. Again, it is important to explain to the patient that there is minimal or no discomfort with the procedure. Often, the patient is concerned about the embarrassment of being exposed. Explain that the patient will be covered with drapes. Establish an IV line to be used to administer the conscious sedation medication. Assess vital signs prior to the procedure for a baseline, during the procedure, and every 15 minutes for 1 hour and then every hour for 4 hours after the procedure. Cardiac, neurological, respiratory, and gastrointestinal assessments should be performed on arrival back to the floor to make certain the patient is stable. ***Safety: Observe the patient for signs of possible bowel perforation, such as abdominal distention and rigidity or rectal bleeding.*** Remember to reassure the patient that sedation will be administered, causing him or her to sleep during the procedure.

Capsule Endoscopy

For this procedure, the patient swallows a tiny capsule that contains a camera. The patient also wears a recorder on a belt around his or her waist. The camera takes thousands of pictures of the digestive tract as it travels through it and transmits them to the recorder.

This test is used for several reasons:

- To determine the location of gastrointestinal bleeding
- To visualize the small intestine, which cannot be seen by EGD or colonoscopy
- To diagnose cancer, celiac disease, irritable bowel disorder, and Crohn's disease

After the capsule travels throughout the entire GI system, the pictures are downloaded from the recorder and examined for abnormalities in the digestive tract.

NURSING CARE FOR CAPSULE ENDOSCOPY. The patient will be NPO for 12 hours prior to the test and may have to take a laxative the night before the procedure. The nurse should ensure that medications are given 2 hours before or 2 hours after swallowing the camera capsule. The patient can have clear liquids 2 hours after swallowing the camera capsule and then a light meal 4 hours after swallowing it. The patient and the nurse need to watch for the camera capsule to be expelled in the toilet, which occurs 8 or more hours after it was swallowed. ***Safety: It is important to know that it has been expelled. Rarely a capsule remains in the body, but when it does, it must be removed surgically.***

> **KNOWLEDGE CONNECTION**
> Why would it be pertinent to have the large intestine clean and free of feces prior to a colonoscopy? What preparation is required for an EGD? What type of problems might be detected during an EGD? Name one major risk of EGD and colonoscopy. What type of problems could be discerned during a colonoscopy? What signs and symptoms would you observe for after an EGD? Why might a capsule endoscopy be ordered?

Graphic Recording Tests

Numerous graphic recording tests are performed to detect abnormalities in the electrical activity of the heart, skeletal muscles, and brain. Two of the more common are electrocardiography and electroencephalography.

Electrocardiography

Electrocardiography (ECG) uses six electrodes applied to specific locations on the chest wall and four electrodes applied to the four extremities to graphically record the electrical activity through the heart's electrical conduction pathway. It analyzes the heart's electrical activity from 12 different angles or views, detecting any abnormalities. The printout indicates how long it takes for the electrical impulse to travel from the sinoatrial node through the intra-atrial pathways to the atrioventricular node, and then through the bundle of His and the Purkinje fibers. This time span is demonstrated by deflections of the baseline known as P waves, QRS complexes, and T waves, as well as the P-R interval and the S-T interval (Fig. 25.1). Aberrations from normal time spans and complexes that are altered in shape indicate injury or malfunction of the heart. Skill 25.2 (page 518) provides more information on performing a 12-lead ECG.

Although an ECG can be beneficial in diagnosing heart attacks and *myocardial ischemia,* which is a lack of adequate blood flow and oxygen to the heart muscle itself, a normal ECG does not always rule out a heart problem. If you work in a cardiac unit, clinic, or hospital setting where you perform or view ECGs regularly, you will acquire a better working knowledge of how to interpret ECG waveforms.

NURSING CARE FOR ELECTROCARDIOGRAPHY. Inform the patient that an ECG helps to assess cardiac function and takes about 10 to 15 minutes. Describe the procedure and inform the patient that there should be no discomfort related to the ECG. Obtain a list of medications that the patient is currently taking, as well as a history of the patient's cardiovascular system symptoms if they have not already been documented in the medical record. Ask the patient to remove any jewelry that may interfere with electrode placement. Preserve the patient's modesty as much as possible while attaching the chest electrodes and during the procedure. Ask the patient to lie as still as possible during the actual ECG.

• WORD • BUILDING •

electrocardiography: electro – electricity + cardio – heart + graphy – writing

electroencephalography: electro – electricity + encephalo – brain + graphy – writing

Real-World Connection

ECG Imperfection

A 44-year-old female had not been feeling well for 3 to 4 weeks. She visited her family practitioner on several occasions, but her complaints were vague and hard to describe. She said that she was tired and "just did not feel right." Various blood tests were run, producing normal results. After discussing her case with her physician during one of her visits, they mutually decided she should start taking a good multiple vitamin, pay more attention to her eating habits, drink plenty of water, and get plenty of rest and regular exercise.

The physician ran a routine ECG before increasing the patient's exercise level. The ECG was the first one the patient had ever had, and the results appeared normal with no areas of concern. However, a couple days later she was at work when she suddenly stood up and grabbed her chest. Before she could utter a word, she fell to the floor, unresponsive and without pulse or respiration. One of her employees called 911, and an ambulance was dispatched. She was pronounced dead on arrival at the local hospital emergency room. Autopsy results indicated that she had died of a massive myocardial infarction (MI) and that she had experienced numerous MIs previously that had gone undetected.

This real-life example demonstrates the fact that ECGs *cannot* rule out heart disease or a past or current MI. Although an ECG *may* be helpful and sometimes does detect *cardiac ischemia,* which is a lack of blood to the heart muscle, and an active MI, it is not 100% assured that a patient is not having heart problems, especially in women, whose cardiac signs and symptoms present differently than they do in men.

Exercise Stress Test

Because a regular ECG cannot conclusively rule out cardiac problems, it is sometimes feasible to perform an exercise stress test to assist in the detection of reduced blood flow to the heart. The heart function is monitored by continuous ECG while the patient exercises on a treadmill. The patient is also monitored for blood pressure changes, chest pain, and shortness of breath. The patient exercises until the heart rate is 80% to 90% of the maximum rate for age and gender. If symptoms develop, the test is stopped before the symptoms become too extreme.

To be of even further value, this test may also be done in conjunction with a tiny amount of radioactive tracer that is injected intravenously. Scans are then done to provide imaging of the coronary vessels to detect narrowing, known as *radionuclide scanning.*

Chemical Stress Test

A chemical stress test may be ordered if the patient is unable to physically exercise while the heart is tested during exertion. The patient must refrain from eating or drinking anything containing caffeine for 24 hours prior to the test. For this test, the patient is attached to an ECG monitor while he or she is given an IV medication that causes the coronary arteries to dilate quickly, which is what happens in exercise. The ECG is monitored for changes that would indicate narrowing of the coronary arteries and lack of blood flow to the left ventricle. The patient may experience shortness of breath or chest discomfort during the test. This test may also be done in conjunction with a nuclear scan of the heart.

TELEMETRY MONITORING. A telemetry monitor is a portable heart monitor. Wires (also called leads) attached to the battery pack connect to electrodes placed on the patient's chest. The electrodes are disposable foam circles with a connection in the middle that transmit the electrical activity of the heart as a waveform. The patient can then get up and move around without being hardwired to a bedside monitor while his or her heart rhythm is being continuously monitored. At a remote monitoring station, monitor technicians will watch the continuous waveform on a screen. Any abnormalities in the heart's activity are detected by the computerized equipment and printed out as an ECG strip. The monitor technician notifies the nurse caring for the patient of any abnormal rhythms. (Refer to Fig. 25.2 for a sample electronic documentation of a patient with a telemetry monitor.)

You may get a call to check the telemetry unit on a patient if the monitor technician is not able to clearly see the waveform. Go to the patient's room promptly and check each wire to be sure it is firmly inserted in the battery pack as well as firmly attached to the electrode. Check each electrode to be sure it is firmly stuck to the chest wall. If you need to change the battery, open the sliding cover at the bottom of the battery pack, replace the old battery with a fresh one, and close the cover. Telephone the monitor station from the patient's room to verify that a clearer picture has been obtained.

Safety: When you remove a telemetry unit for any reason, such as to give a bath or shower, you MUST first call the monitor station and tell the technician that you are going to remove the unit. The monitor technician will flag the patient's display with the reason the telemetry unit is off. Replace the unit immediately after completing the bath or shower and then telephone the monitor station from the patient's room to be sure the display is clear. It is also important to call the monitor technician prior to removing the unit when the health-care provider has discontinued the order for it.

The disposable electrodes usually are changed after the bath or when they no longer stick to the chest well. Replace the electrodes according to your facility's policy. Return the battery pack to the gown pocket or pouch. Be sure the pouch is clean and comfortable for the patient.

The electrodes and wires may be placed on the chest in a variety of patterns to transmit the heart's electrical activity. The right and left upper chest near the shoulders are used for the arm lead placements. The lower limb leads usually are placed on the lower ribs toward the patient's sides. A ground wire may

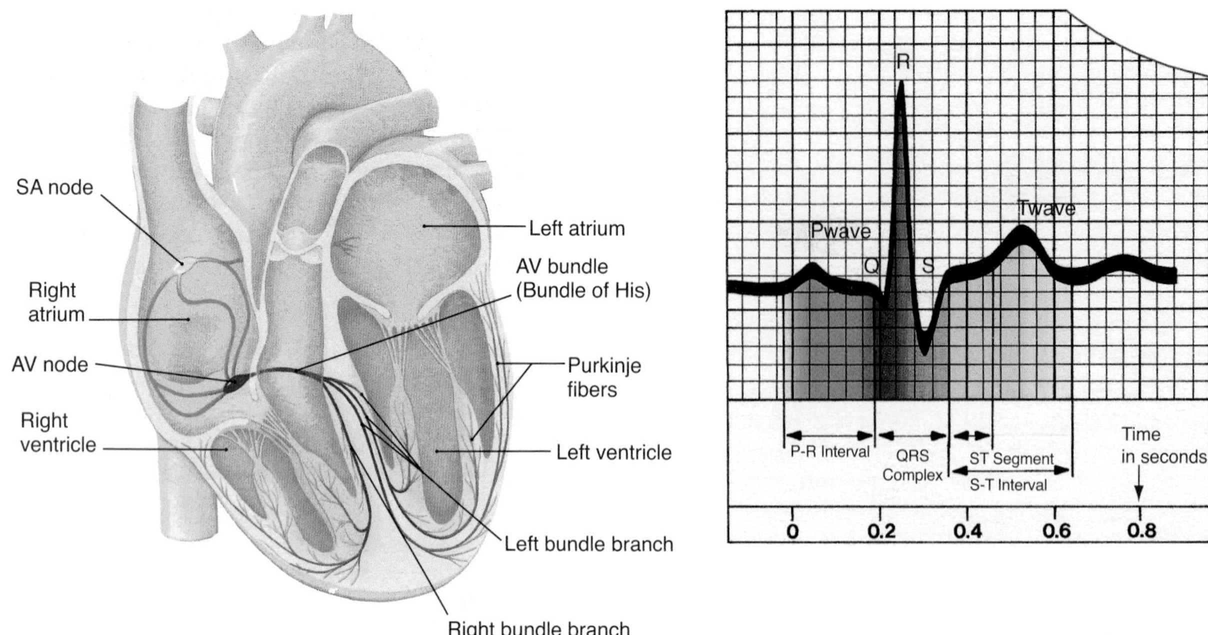

FIGURE 25.1 The electrical impulse initiating contraction of the heart muscle (heartbeat) begins in the sinoatrial node and is conveyed through the rest of the electrical conduction pathway. The P wave represents the depolarization of the atria, the result of which is contraction of the atria. The QRS complex represents the depolarization of the ventricles, resulting in contraction of the ventricles. The T wave represents the repolarization of the ventricles, during which the ventricles relax in preparation for the next depolarization. Each of the boxes on the ECG strip represents the length of time that it takes for the impulse to travel through the designated sections of the conduction pathway (from Scanlon V, Sanders T. *Essentials of Anatomy and Physiology.* 7th ed. Philadelphia, PA: FA Davis; 2015).

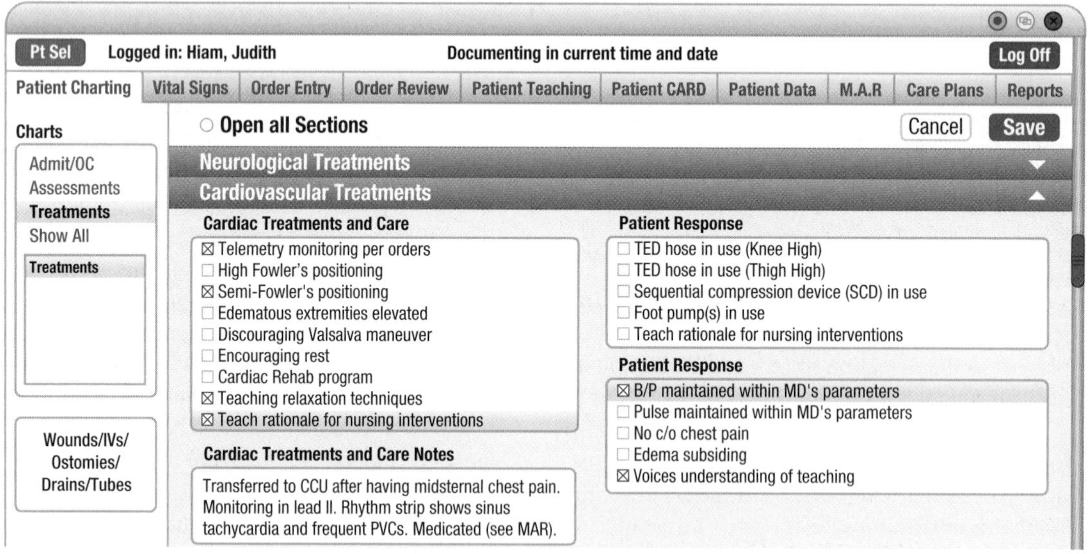

FIGURE 25.2 A sample electronic documentation of a patient with telemetry.

be placed on the center of the chest when five wires are used. The wires are color-coded for placement. For example, the white wire is placed on the right upper chest to represent the right arm. Follow your facility's policy for electrode placement.

One way to remember electrode placement is to follow this guide:

- **White to the right:** White goes on right upper chest
- **Clouds over grass:** White on right upper chest, green on right lower chest
- **Smoke over fire:** Black on left upper chest, red on left lower chest
- **Brown is ground:** Brown goes in the middle of the chest

HOLTER MONITORS. A Holter monitor is an even more portable electrocardiograph than the telemetry unit. This type of monitoring device can be worn by the patient at home. It usually is ordered for a 24- to 48-hour period. It weighs about 2 pounds and is placed in a harness that the patient wears on his or her back. Again, electrodes are placed on the patient's chest with lead wires attached. The Holter monitor records the patient's ECG for the entire period that the monitor is worn. The patient is asked to keep a diary of his or her activities during the 24- to 48-hour period. If the patient feels symptoms, such as chest discomfort, pain, or palpitations, he or she will push the "event" button, which marks the ECG recording for later analysis by the physician. This type of monitoring works well for patients who have cardiac symptoms that occur with activity or at widely spaced intervals.

Electroencephalography

In **electroencephalography** (EEG), electrodes are placed strategically on the scalp and record the electrical activity of the brain, known as *brain waves.* This study is beneficial in detecting epilepsy, diseases of the central nervous system, and tumors, as well as to confirm brain death.

NURSING CARE FOR ELECTROENCEPHALOGRAPHY. Explain the procedure to the patient and family, being careful to include that the test is painless. Wash the patient's hair to remove all hair spray and styling products. After the patient returns to his or her room, it may be necessary to shampoo the hair to remove the electrode paste. If the EEG confirms brain death, be prepared to support the family in this difficult time. It may be helpful to offer to telephone a spiritual advisor or other support person for the family if they wish.

> **KNOWLEDGE CONNECTION**
> What is the purpose of an ECG? Does a normal ECG always prove that the patient does not have heart problems? Give three purposes for which an EEG might be performed.

Skill 25.1 Assisting With Aspiration Procedures: Bone Marrow, Lumbar Puncture, Paracentesis, and Thoracentesis

Assessment Steps

1. Verify the patient's understanding of preprocedure teaching.
2. Verify that written consent has been obtained for the procedure.
3. *Safety: Assess for patient allergies to local anesthetic, as well as iodine and shellfish, if an iodine-based cleanser is to be used for the preparation.*

Planning Steps

1. Gather needed equipment and supplies:
   - **Bone marrow aspiration:** Bone marrow aspiration tray, sterile gloves, local anesthetic, prep cleansing solution, labels for laboratory specimens, and dressing supplies (sterile gauze and tape or bandage)
   - **Lumbar puncture:** Lumbar puncture tray, extra spinal needle, sterile gloves, local anesthetic, prep cleansing solution, labels for laboratory specimens, vital sign equipment, and dressing supplies (sterile gauze and tape, bandage, or small occlusive pressure dressing)
   - **Paracentesis:** Paracentesis tray, sterile gloves, large calibrated container, local anesthetic, prep cleansing solution, labels for laboratory specimens, vital sign equipment, and dressing supplies (sterile gauze and tape or bandage)
   - **Thoracentesis:** Thoracentesis tray, sterile gloves, large calibrated container, local anesthetic, prep cleansing solution, labels for laboratory specimens, vital sign equipment, and dressing supplies (sterile gauze and tape or bandage)

Implementation Steps

1. Follow the Initial Implementation Steps located on the inside back cover.
2. **Paracentesis:** Weigh the patient. Have the patient empty his or her bladder. Measure abdominal girth. Assess vital signs. **Thoracentesis:** Weigh the patient. Assess vital signs. Auscultate breath sounds. Apply supplemental O_2 and cardiac monitor.
3. Set up the sterile field ***to prevent contamination.***
4. Position the patient for the procedure:
   - **Bone marrow aspiration:** Supine for tibial or sternal aspiration, side-lying for iliac crest aspiration
   - **Lumbar puncture:** Side-lying with knees flexed onto abdomen and chin tucked against chest, close to the edge of the bed

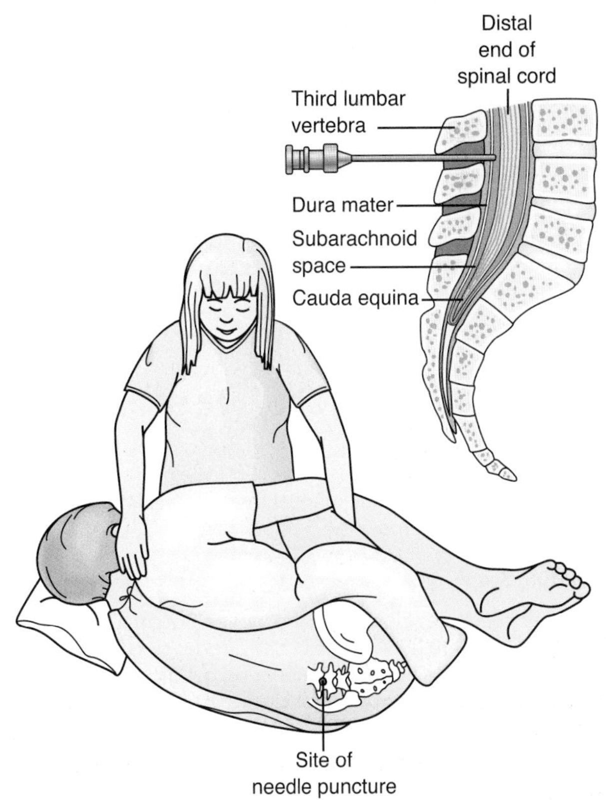

(skill continues on page 518)

Skill 25.1 (continued)

- **Paracentesis:** Semi-Fowler's position or sitting, as directed by physician

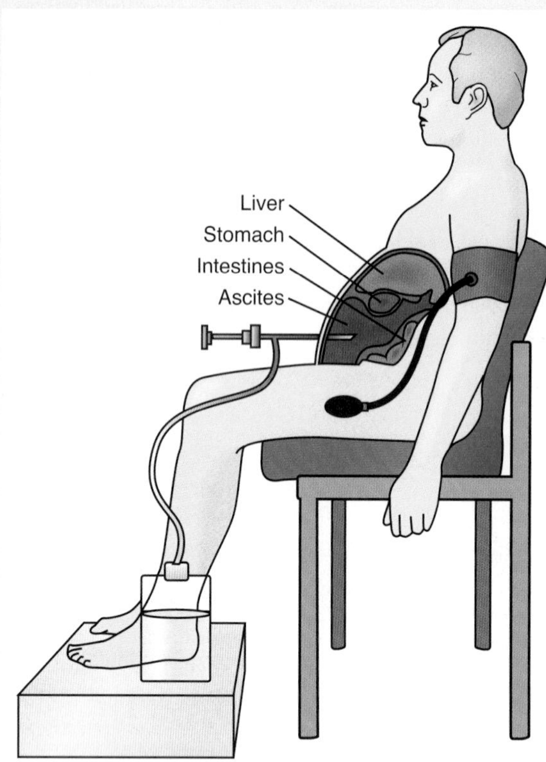

- **Thoracentesis:** Orthopneic position (sitting upright with head and raised arms resting on over-bed table)

5. Assist the physician as needed with cleansing prep of injection site and drawing up of local anesthetic.
6. Reassure the patient and assist him or her to remain in the proper position throughout the procedure.
7. After completion of the procedure, hold pressure on the puncture site for at least 5 minutes ***to prevent bleeding.*** Once you are certain that bleeding has stopped, apply a bandage, small dressing, or occlusive pressure dressing as appropriate.
8. Apply labels to specimens before sending them to the laboratory.
9. Follow the Ending Implementation Steps located on the inside back cover.
10. Document the procedure and the patient's tolerance of it.

Evaluation Steps

1. Assess vital signs, noting any signs of hypotension or shock.
   Paracentesis: Weigh patient. Measure abdominal girth and compare to previous measurement.
   Thoracentesis: Weigh patient. Assess vital signs. Observe for dyspnea, arrhythmias.
2. Assess the puncture site for bleeding or drainage.
3. Position the patient for comfort.
4. Send laboratory specimens to the laboratory.

Sample Documentation

12/01/22 0900 Procedure explained to patient by Dr. Evans; permit signed. Weight 189 lbs. Voided. Placed in supine position. Baseline VS: BP - 132/68, T - 98.6, P - 68 reg & strong, R - 14 reg & even, SpO_2 - 95%. Denies pain. Abdominal girth 49 inches. Abdomen cleansing prep performed using Betadine. 1% lidocaine injected at intended puncture site just above the umbilicus. Paracentesis performed by Dr. Holsted with 750 mL cloudy, yellow fluid returned. Pressure held on injection site for 5 minutes. No signs of bleeding noted. Abdominal girth now 45 inches. Postprocedure weight 186.5 lbs. No problems noted during procedure. No complaints of discomfort.
———— Nurse's signature and credentials

0925 VS: BP - 138/74, P - 74 reg & strong, R - 17 reg & even. SpO_2 96%. Denies pain. No bleeding at injection site.
———— Nurse's signature and credentials

Skill 25.2 Performing a 12-Lead Electrocardiogram

Assessment Step

1. Review the ECG machine manual for the specifics of operating that particular model.

Planning Step

1. Gather needed equipment and supplies: ECG machine with 10 lead wires, 10 new pre-gelled electrodes or 10 non-gelled electrodes with a bottle of conduction gel, alcohol sponges, razor, and washcloth.

Implementation Steps

1. Follow the Initial Implementation Steps located on the inside back cover.
2. Position the patient in the semi-Fowler's or supine position, making him or her as comfortable as possible. Remove the patient's shirt or blouse and bra. Cover with a patient gown that opens in the front ***to help preserve modesty.*** Remove necklaces, bracelets, and watches ***to prevent interference with the electrical tracing.***
3. If necessary, shave small areas on the chest at the sites for application of electrodes. If shaving is not necessary, remove body oil at the sites using alcohol sponges ***so that electrodes will make good contact with the skin.***
4. Enter appropriate data into the ECG machine ***to allow for proper identification and interpretation of results on the ECG printout.***

Skill 25.2 (continued)

5. Apply 10 electrodes. Either the electrodes will be pre-gelled, or you may have to apply a small amount of conduction gel ***to ensure adequate conduction of electrical impulses.*** Apply four electrodes to the medial or inner aspects of both wrists and ankles, ensuring good contact with skin. Then apply six electrodes to the chest:
   - V_1 at the right sternal border in the fourth intercostal space
   - V_2 at the left sternal border in the fourth intercostal space
   - V_4 in the fifth intercostal space in the midclavicular line
   - V_3 halfway between V_2 and V_4
   - V_5 to the left of the V_4 electrode in the anterior axillary line
   - V_6 to the left of the V_5 electrode in the midaxillary line

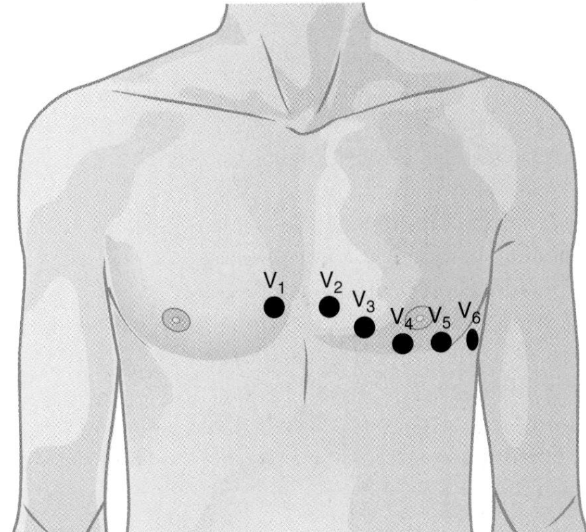

Ensure good contact with skin. ***If the electrodes are not placed correctly, the tracing will not be reliable.***

6. Attach the lead wires to the electrodes. The six chest lead wires will be marked V_1, V_2, V_3, V_4, V_5, and V_6. Attach the lead wires to the electrodes at the corresponding sites on the patient's chest.

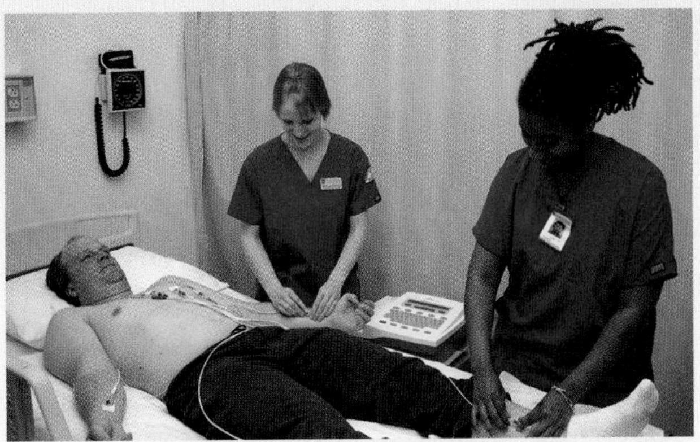

7. Request that the patient hold completely still ***to prevent interference during the ECG.***
8. Following the manual instructions, press the run button.
9. After reviewing the ECG printout for correct appearance, turn off the machine.
10. Remove the electrodes and clean the skin with alcohol wipes or a damp cloth ***to remove any residue from the conduction gel.*** Assist the patient to dress if necessary.
11. Follow the Ending Implementation Steps located on the inside back cover.

Evaluation Step

1. Review the ECG printout and notify the physician of pertinent findings.

Sample Documentation

03/12/22 1415 12-lead ECG performed without difficulty. Results phoned to Dr. Heart. ———— Nurse's signature and credentials

POST CONFERENCE

When you enter the conference room for post conference, another student says, "I bet you had an easy day. Your patient was just having tests, right?" You respond, "She had quite a time of it. She was terrified of having her blood drawn, vomited while she was in the radiology department, and had abdominal pains during the ultrasound." Your patient benefited from your teaching and was relieved to know that although four vials of blood were drawn, the technician only had to stick her once with the needle, not once for each test. She knew what to expect when she was sedated for the EGD, and she was glad you were there when she had the ultrasound, which turned out to be painful because of her extreme abdominal tenderness. By the end of your shift, the physician was feeling confident about a diagnosis of pancreatitis. And you would never have the attitude that a patient was "just having tests," having seen firsthand what was involved in her care.

Key Points

- Nurses have key responsibilities in preparing patients for diagnostic tests and caring for them after the tests.
- The five categories of diagnostic tests are laboratory tests, radiology and imaging tests, ultrasonography, endoscopic examinations, and graphic recording tests.
- Hematology tests include the CBC, WBC count with differential, RBC count with Hgb and Hct, and PLT count.
- A WBC count with differential involves the number and type of cells: neutrophils, eosinophils, basophils, monocytes, and lymphocytes. An elevation of young neutrophils, called bands, causes a left shift which indicates bacterial infection. An elevation of lymphocytes causes a right shift which indicates viral infection.
- A blood chemistry test includes a number of components including electrolytes, enzymes and isoenzymes, BUN, serum creatinine, protein, and bilirubin.
- Blood testing to diagnose and monitor specific illnesses include BNP, cardiac enzymes, lipase, and A_{1c}.
- Urine testing provides information about the patient's overall health status, not just the condition of the urinary system.
- The eGFR and GFR indicate kidney function and are measured by creatinine level in the blood and other calculations. The GFR requires 24-hour urine collection. The eGFR is calculated using a formula. If either one is below 60, it indicates significant renal impairment.
- Radiology and imaging testing, including MRI and CT, give information about structures in the body without having to invade the body. Arteriography, venography, MRA, and CTA give information about blood vessels and circulation to various organs.
- Ultrasonography is used to visualize a number of internal structures such as a fetus, placenta, female pelvic organs, and function of the heart valves and wall movement.
- Endoscopy is used to look inside the digestive system. An EGD allows the physician to see the esophagus, stomach, and duodenum, as well as the sphincters between each structure. Colonoscopy provides visual examination of the full colon. The small intestine can be visualized by using camera capsule endoscopy. Nursing care is needed after each of these tests.
- Assess your patients for allergies to iodine, shellfish, radiopaque dye, or any previous reactions to contrast medium before they undergo tests using contrast media.
- Graphic recording tests include ECG and EEG. An exercise stress test involves recording heart activity during the stress of exercise or after injection of a medication to mimic the effect of exercise on the heart. Telemetry is a portable heart monitor that allows ECG tracings at all times while still allowing the patient to be mobile in the hospital.

Review Questions

Select the answer that is most appropriate for each of the following questions. Some questions may have more than one correct answer. Select all that apply.

1. Which of the following urinalysis findings would you need to report to the physician?
   1. Protein: 30 mg/dL
   2. Bacteria: 0
   3. WBCs: 3 to 4 per high-power field
   4. pH: 4.1
   5. Specific gravity: 1.025
   6. RBCs: 10 per high-power field

2. Which of the following preparatory steps would you be likely to perform prior to a barium enema?
   1. Start an IV line the day prior to the test
   2. Keep the patient NPO 48 hours prior to the test
   3. Administer a laxative the day before the test
   4. Place the patient on a clear liquid diet for 24 hours prior to the test
   5. Administer an enema the evening before the test

3. Which of the following tests would be helpful for evaluating the large intestine?
   1. Colonoscopy
   2. EGD
   3. Barium enema
   4. ECG
   5. Intravenous pyelogram
   6. Hgb and Hct

4. Which of the following findings indicate a left shift and bacterial infection in an adult?
   1. WBC: 13,900/mm^3; total neutrophils: 76% (bands: 30%, segmented: 46%); eosinophils: 2.5%; basophils: 0.5%; monocytes: 4%; lymphocytes: 17%
   2. WBC: 4,600/mm^3; total neutrophils: 59% (bands: 3%, segmented: 56%); eosinophils: 4%; basophils: 1%; monocytes: 6%; lymphocytes: 30%
   3. WBC: 11,350/mm^3; total neutrophils: 55% (bands: 3%, segmented: 52%); eosinophils: 12 %; basophils: 2%; monocytes: 8%; lymphocytes: 23%
   4. WBC: 9,450/mm^3; total neutrophils: 61% (bands: 5%, segmented: 65%); eosinophils: 4%; basophils: 1%; monocytes: 3%; lymphocytes: 28%

5. Which of the following tests or procedures is (are) beneficial in evaluation of the kidneys?
   1. IV pyelogram
   2. 24-hour urine
   3. Oral glucose tolerance test
   4. Urinalysis
   5. Glomerular filtration rate
   6. Creatinine

6. You are to provide nursing care for a patient who just had a femoral arteriogram. Which of the following actions would take priority?
   1. Assessment of vital signs
   2. Assessment of puncture site for bleeding
   3. Assessment of temperature of lower extremity on the affected side
   4. Keeping the affected leg straight
   5. Assessment of ability to void
   6. Providing PO fluids

7. You should measure the abdominal girth and weight of a patient who is about to undergo:
   1. a glucose tolerance test.
   2. a CT scan of the cerebrum.
   3. an alkaline phosphatase test.
   4. a paracentesis.
   5. a lumbar puncture.

8. When performing a 12-lead ECG, you know that you will apply:
   1. 12 lead wires.
   2. 10 lead wires.
   3. 6 lead wires.
   4. 4 lead wires.

ANSWERS 1. 1, 4, 6, 2. 3, 4, 5, 3. 1, 3, 4, 4. 1, 5. 1, 2, 4, 5, 6, 6. 2, 7. 4, 8. 2

Critical Thinking Exercises

Answers available online.

1. You are assigned to provide nursing care for a patient who is scheduled for a colonoscopy tomorrow morning. In report, you are told that she is extremely nervous and frightened regarding the procedure. What can you do to help this patient?

2. Why is it so important that you provide thorough patient teaching regarding any upcoming tests or procedures?

Additional Resources

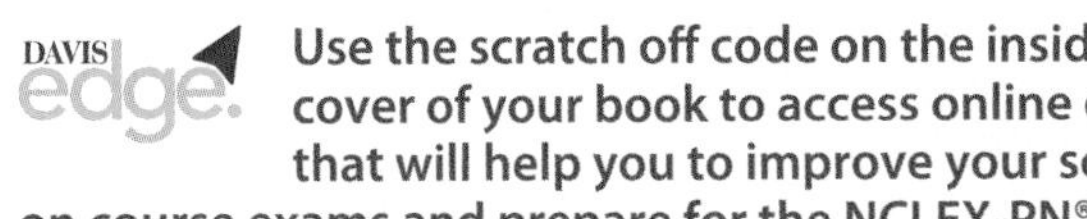

DAVIS
edge
Use the scratch off code on the inside front cover of your book to access online quizzes that will help you to improve your scores on course exams and prepare for the NCLEX-PN®.

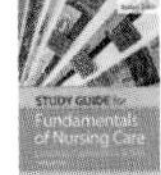

Study Guide

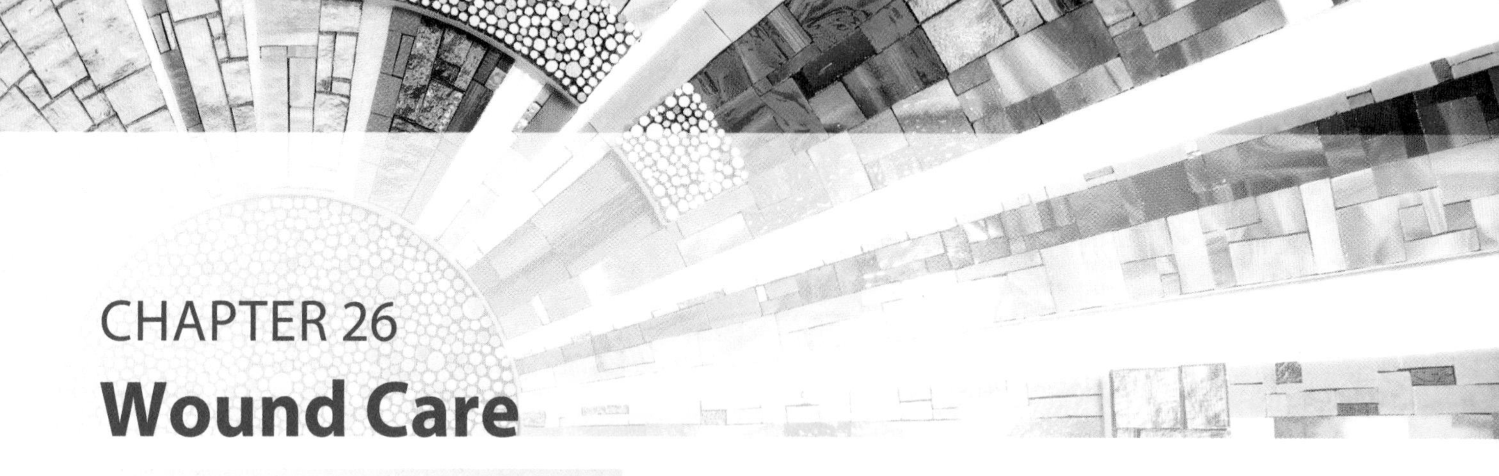

CHAPTER 26

Wound Care

KEY TERMS

Abrasion (ah-BRAY-zhun)
Débridement (day-BREED-ment)
Dehiscence (deh-HISS-ents)
Erythema (ER-ih-THEE-mah)
Eschar (ESS-kar)
Evisceration (ee-VIS-sir-AY-shun)
Granulation tissue (GRAN-yoo-LAY-shun TISH-yoo)
Hemorrhage (HEM-o-rahj)
Ischemia (iss-KEE-mee-ah)
Laceration (lass-er-RAY-shun)
Methicillin-resistant *Staphylococcus aureus* (METH-ih-SIL-in ree-ZIS-tint STAF-ih-loh-KOK-us AW-ree-us)
Necrotic (nek-ROT-ik)
Pressure injury (PREH-shur IN-juh-ree)
Purulent (PYOO-ru-lent)
Sanguineous (sang-GWIN-ee-uss)
Serosanguineous (SEER-oh-sang-GWIN-ee-uss)
Serous (SEER-us)
Sinus tract (SIGH-nuss TRAKT)

CHAPTER CONCEPTS

Tissue Integrity
Infection

LEARNING OUTCOME

1. Define various terms related to wound care.
2. Contrast contusion, abrasion, puncture, penetrating, and laceration wounds, as well as pressure injuries.
3. Differentiate between clean, clean-contaminated, contaminated, infected, colonized, open, and closed wounds.
4. Identify risk factors for pressure injuries.
5. Correctly stage pressure injuries.
6. Outline nursing interventions to prevent pressure injuries.
7. Describe other types of wounds, such as stasis ulcers, sinus tracts, and surgical incisions.
8. Explain the three phases of healing.
9. Compare first-, second-, and third-intention wound closures.
10. Explain how different factors affect wound healing.
11. Describe possible complications of wound healing and appropriate nursing care for each.
12. Discuss wound treatments and the nursing responsibilities for each.
13. Accurately assess a wound and wound drainage.
14. Describe types of dressings and their uses.
15. Identify information to document concerning wounds.
16. Develop a care plan for a patient with an infected pressure injury.
17. Discuss information found in the Connection features of the chapter.
18. Identify safety issues related to wound care.
19. Answer questions about the skills in the chapter.

SKILLS

26.1 Removing Sutures and Staples
26.2 Caring for Drainage Devices
26.3 Irrigating a Wound
26.4 Obtaining a Wound Culture
26.5 Changing Sterile Dressings and Wet-to-Damp Dressings
26.6 Applying Transparent and Hydrocolloid Dressings
26.7 Changing a Negative Pressure Wound Therapy Dressing (Wound VAC)

CRITICAL THINKING CONNECTION

Clinical Assignment

You are assigned to care for a 74-year-old male patient with a stage 3 pressure injury on his coccyx that is infected with methicillin-resistant *Staphylococcus aureus* (MRSA). You will need to irrigate the injury and apply a wet-to-damp dressing. You will also need to take the proper transmission-based precautions for MRSA in a wound.

Critical Thinking Questions:

1. What makes a pressure injury classified as stage 3?
2. How will you assess it for increasing or decreasing infection?
3. What is MRSA, and how will it impact the wound care you provide? (You can review transmission-based precautions in Chapter 14.)
4. How will you document the size and appearance of the wound?
5. How will you apply the correct dressing for this wound?

As you care for patients, you will encounter a variety of wounds requiring various treatments. In this chapter, you will learn about different types of wounds, injuries, ulcers, drains, drainage, and dressings. You will be able to determine the likelihood of infection by assessing a wound. You will learn to measure and describe a wound, as well as to evaluate healing in a wound. You will be prepared and confident that you will not miss anything.

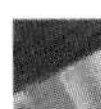

TYPES OF WOUNDS

Wounds are categorized as either open or closed. A wound in which the skin remains intact is considered a *closed wound.* A wound in which the skin integrity has been breached is an *open wound.* In addition to being categorized as open or closed, wounds may be classified as contusions, abrasions, puncture wounds, penetrating wounds, lacerations, or pressure injuries.

Contusions

A contusion is a closed discolored wound caused by blunt trauma, better known as a *bruise.* Although the skin is intact, there is injury to the tissues underneath the epidermis, which may swell as blood leaks from broken blood vessels into the *interstitial spaces* (the spaces between cells). This extra fluid in the interstitial space causes pressure on the nerve endings, resulting in pain or tenderness. The leakage of blood causes the skin to be discolored, generally a bright red or purple color that fades over a period of days to blue, bluish-green, and finally to yellow as the contusion heals (Fig. 26.1).

Abrasions

An **abrasion** is a superficial open wound. Abrasions include scrapes, scratches, or rub-type wounds where the skin is broken, such as a carpet burn or a skinned knee. These wounds are generally superficial and heal well if they are kept clean (see Fig. 26.1).

Puncture Wounds

A puncture wound is an open wound that results when a sharp item, such as a needle, nail, or piece of wire, pierces the skin. The resulting wound is a round hole in the skin that extends down into the deeper tissues, according to the diameter and length of the offending sharp item (see Fig. 26.1).

Penetrating Wounds

A penetrating wound is similar to a puncture wound; the difference is that the offending object remains embedded in the tissue. The degree of damage depends on the size of the object and the tissues or organs affected by the penetration (see Fig. 26.1).

Lacerations

A **laceration** is an open wound made by the accidental cutting or tearing of tissue. Common sources of lacerations include knives and pieces of glass and metal. Unlike a surgical incision, it has jagged edges, often making closure of the wound more difficult and less aesthetically pleasing (see Fig. 26.1).

Pressure Injuries

A **pressure injury** is a wound resulting from pressure and friction. The skin may be intact and *erythemic* (reddened), or the skin may be nonintact with open areas. If the skin is not intact, the ulcer may be superficial or very deep. The injury may develop over a bony prominence or related to a medical device.

CONTAMINATION OF WOUNDS

Wounds fall into one of the following categories:

- **Clean:** A wound that is not infected.
- **Clean-contaminated:** A wound that was surgically made and is not infected, but it has direct contact with the normal flora in either the respiratory tract, urinary tract, or gastrointestinal tract. It has more potential to become infected.
- **Contaminated:** This can be a surgical wound or a wound caused by trauma that has been grossly contaminated by breaking asepsis.
- **Infected:** An infected wound is one in which the infectious process is already established, as evidenced by high numbers of microorganisms and either **purulent** (containing pus) drainage or **necrotic** (dead) tissue. The classic signs of infection include **erythema** (redness), increased warmth, edema (swelling), pain, odor, and drainage.
- **Colonized:** A colonized wound differs from an infected wound in that it has a high number of microorganisms present but is without signs of infection.

• WORD • BUILDING •

interstitial: inter – between + stitial – place
erythemic: eruthema – red
purulent: pur – pus + ulent – full of
necrotic: necr – corpse + otic – condition

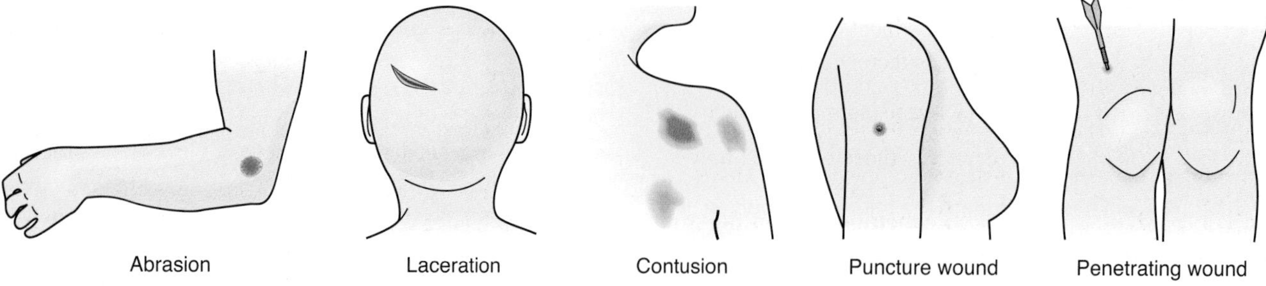

FIGURE 26.1 Types of wounds: abrasion, laceration, contusion, puncture, and penetrating.

KNOWLEDGE CONNECTION

Which types of wounds are considered *open?* Which types of wounds are considered *closed?* List the classic signs and symptoms of an infected wound.

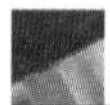

PRESSURE INJURIES

The National Pressure Ulcer Advisory Panel (NPUAP) changed the name from *pressure ulcer* to *pressure injury* in 2016 because some of the stages do not involve ulcers. Instead, they suggest using the terms *intact skin* and *nonintact skin.* The NPUAP emphasizes, however, that by calling these areas *injuries*, it does not at all imply that they are caused by health-care staff.

A pressure injury is also called a *pressure ulcer, decubitus ulcer,* or *bedsore* and occurs when external pressure is exerted on soft tissues, especially over bony prominences, for a prolonged period of time. Tissues and capillaries are compressed, resulting in reduced blood flow to the area, known as **ischemia.** Under normal conditions, blood delivers the vital oxygen and nutrients that cells require to stay alive. Ischemia deprives the involved tissues of adequate oxygen and nutrients, and, if this state persists, the cells will eventually *necrose* (die).

Pressure injuries also can develop as a direct result of friction or shearing force. Shearing force occurs when the patient's skin and another item, such as bed linens or the surface of a chair, move in opposite directions while they are being pressed together by the weight of the body. This movement results in friction that can pull the tissue apart, or shear it from the body. ***Safety: Avoid pulling or dragging a patient across the bed rather than lifting him or her because the shearing force to the patient's skin can result in destruction of the epidermis and dermis.***

The most common sites for development of pressure injuries are over bony prominences, such as the sacrum, buttocks, greater trochanters, elbows, heels, ankles, occiput (back of the head), and scapulae (Fig. 26.2). The longer the pressure is maintained on the area, the worse the extent of necrosis that occurs.

KNOWLEDGE CONNECTION

What is the main cause of pressure injuries? Where are the most common sites for them to develop?

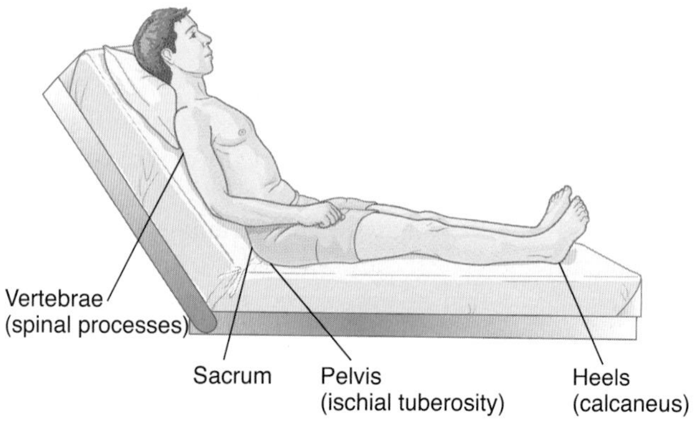

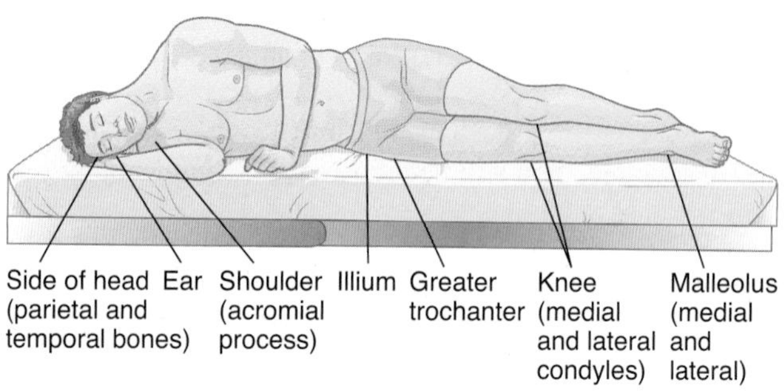

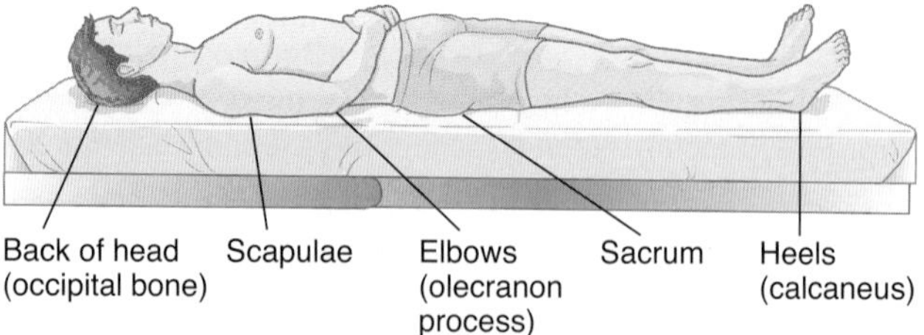

FIGURE 26.2 Pressure points in the Fowler's, lateral, and supine positions (from Wilkinson JM, Treas LM. *Fundamentals of Nursing: Theory, Concepts & Applications.* Vol. 1. 3rd ed. Philadelphia, PA: FA Davis; 2016).

Risk Factors for Pressure Injuries

Patients who are prone to development of pressure injuries include patients who are:

- **Elderly:** The skin of elderly individuals is thinner and less elastic, making the skin more susceptible to friction and shearing force.
- **Emaciated or malnourished:** *Emaciation* is the state of being very lean or having very little muscle.

- **Incontinent of bowel or bladder:** With incontinence of bowel or bladder, the skin of the perineal area tends to be wet much of the time, leading it to become *macerated,* or softened.
- **Immobile:** This includes patients who are paralyzed or who have casts or splints, as well as those restricted to a bed or chair.
- **Impaired circulation or chronic metabolic conditions:** Chronic metabolic conditions such as diabetes result in impairment of circulation, which can increase the risk of ischemic tissue.

Staging Pressure Injuries

Pressure injuries can range in appearance from a reddened area to deep craters that involve muscle and even bone. They are *staged,* or classified, according to the extent and depth of damage. This staging scale is used solely for pressure injuries (Fig. 26.3).

The NPUAP also instituted a change in how pressure injury stages are numbered. Now, instead of using Roman numerals, they recommend using Arabic numerals for the first four stages. In addition, they have added two other pressure injury diagnoses: medical device related pressure injury and mucosal membrane pressure injury.

Stage 1

A stage 1 pressure injury is indicated by erythema of intact skin, generally over a bony prominence, that will not *blanch,* or turn white, when you gently touch it with your fingertip. In a darker-skinned individual, the skin may appear darkened rather than red. The color will not, however, be purple or maroon, which indicates a deep tissue pressure injury (DTPI). The area may feel warm and firm, soft, or boggy. ***Safety: Avoid massaging the erythematous area as this may cause further tissue damage.*** The patient may complain of burning or tingling at the site. Further damage and progression of the pressure injury can be prevented at this stage if appropriate measures are taken.

Stage 2

A stage 2 pressure injury occurs when there is a partial-thickness loss and exposed dermis. This includes intact serum-filled blisters and broken blisters that reveal a shallow, pink or

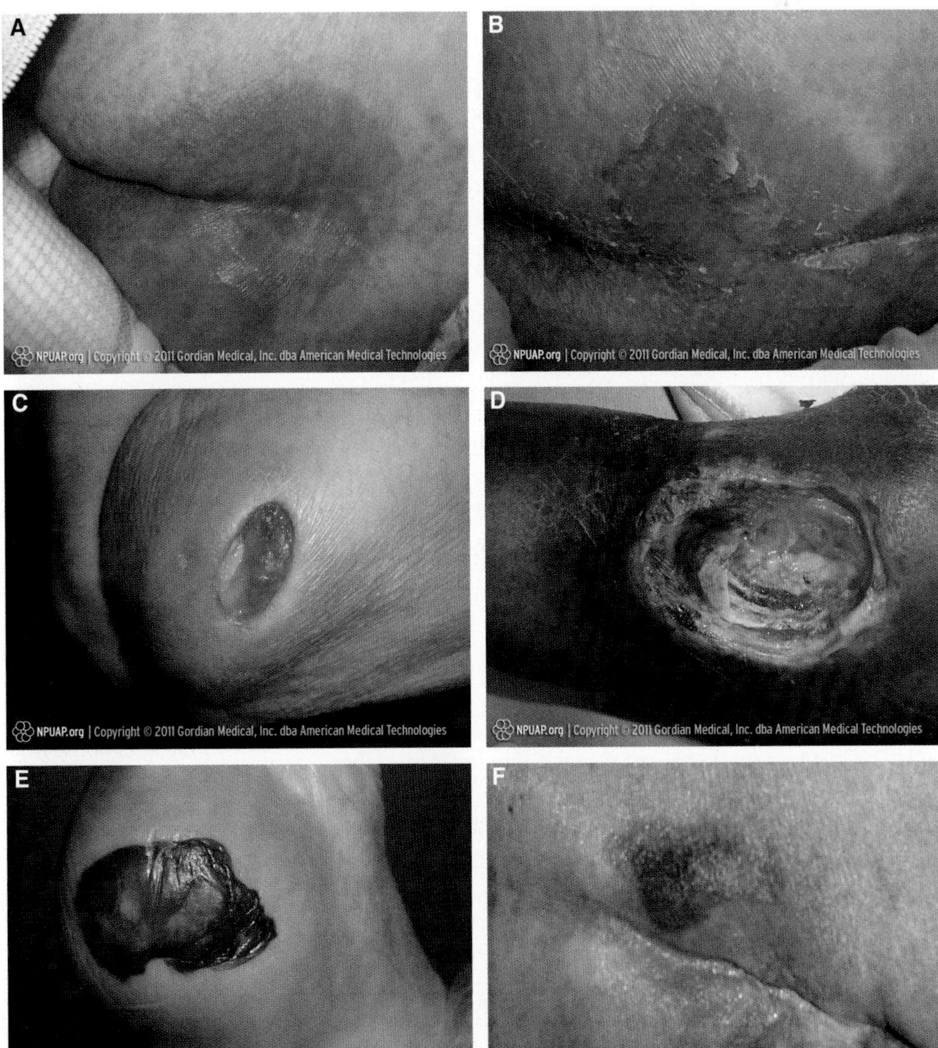

FIGURE 26.3 The stages of pressure ulcers: (a) Stage 1 pressure injury; (b) Stage 2 pressure injury; (c) Stage 3 pressure injury; (d) Stage 4 pressure injury; (e) Unstageable pressure injury; (f) Deep tissue pressure injury (from Wilkinson JM, Treas LM. *Fundamentals of Nursing: Theory, Concepts & Applications.* Vol. 1. 3rd ed. Philadelphia, PA: FA Davis; 2016).

red ulceration that is moist. Generally there is erythema surrounding the skin break. The erythematous area may feel warmer than the surrounding skin due to the increased blood flow. Subcutaneous tissue is not visible.

A stage 2 injury is harder to heal than a stage 1 injury and may allow microorganisms to enter and multiply so that an infection is possible. It is not due to incontinence or traumatic wounds, nor is it an adhesive-related skin injury such as a tape allergy.

Stage 3

The stage 3 pressure injury is a full-thickness loss involving damage to the epidermis, dermis, and subcutaneous tissue but not involving muscle or bone. Undermining and tunneling may be seen in this stage. These wounds tend to be infected, may produce drainage, and take longer to heal than a stage 1 or 2 pressure injury because a great deal of granulation tissue must be produced to fill the wound and repair the damage. Often, rolled wound edges are present at this stage.

Stage 4

The stage 4 pressure injury is also a full-thickness skin and tissue loss, only it involves deep tissue necrosis of muscle, fascia, tendon, joint capsule, and sometimes bone. As in a stage 3 injury, there may be tunneling and undermining. Infection in a stage 4 injury can involve deeper tissues such as the bone, a condition known as *osteomyelitis.* Due to the massive tissue destruction, this injury may be extremely slow to completely heal depending on the patient's health status.

Unstageable

These pressure injuries also involve full-thickness tissue loss but are impossible to accurately stage due to the wound bed being obscured by eschar or excessive slough. **Eschar** is hard, dry, dead tissue that has a leathery appearance. It can be black, brown, or tan. If eschar remains intact and stable, completely covering a site such as the heel, it should not be removed. It should be left alone to cover and protect the damaged tissue underneath it. If the eschar comes off, it reveals a stage 3 or stage 4 pressure injury.

Deep Tissue Pressure Injury

A DTPI may be intact or nonintact skin. It is deep red, maroon, or purple in color and does not blanch. It may form a blood-filled blister or a thin blister that overlies a dark wound bed. The blister may break and reveal a thin layer of eschar underneath. This injury results from prolonged pressure and/or shear force. It may get worse rapidly and open, or it may resolve without opening.

A *medical device–related pressure injury* occurs due to the use of a diagnostic or therapeutic device and often appears in the shape or pattern of that device. These injuries are staged using the above staging pressure injury system. An example is injury caused by splints, braces, or oxygen tubing pressing against the patient's skin. A *mucosal membrane pressure injury* occurs due to the use of a medical device in the area of mucous membranes. These injuries cannot be staged. Examples of this type of injury include damage to the tongue or lips from the pressure of an endotracheal tube.

KNOWLEDGE CONNECTION

Describe the differences between the six classifications of pressure injuries. How do you explain the fact that eschar must be removed before an injury can be accurately staged?

Real-World Connection

How Deep Can a Pressure Injury Be?

In a skilled nursing facility, a 29-year-old male patient was admitted from a distant hospital. The patient was a paraplegic and had no feeling from the waist down, with bilateral above-the-knee amputations and severe uncontrolled diabetes. It was noted in the records that the patient had a pressure injury on the sacral-coccyx area and a Foley catheter to drain his bladder of urine. While admitting the patient and making him comfortable in the bed, the nursing staff noted that the linens under his hips were wet with urine, thought to be from a leaking catheter. As the assessment continued, the nursing staff rolled the patient to one side to assess the pressure injury. When the dressing was removed, the nurses discovered that the inflated Foley catheter balloon was visible deep in the base of the wound. The pressure injury was so large and deep that it extended through the subcutaneous layers, fascia, and muscular layers all the way through the posterior wall of his bladder. Most of the urine was leaking directly from the bladder onto the dressing and bed.

This is why it is important to take appropriate measures to prevent the development of pressure injuries before they begin and to treat even mild stage 1 pressure injuries as soon as they are identified. Otherwise, they can progress to unbelievable extents very quickly.

Prevention of Pressure Injuries

The majority of pressure injuries can be prevented with good nursing care, which starts with thorough assessment of the skin and pressure points. Many facilities use standardized scales of assessment, such as the Braden scale (Fig. 26.4).

Skin assessment should be done on a daily basis. If the patient is restricted in mobility to any degree, assess the skin every 8 hours at a minimum. If the patient is bedfast, assess the pressure points every 2 hours. In an individual with multiple risk factors for skin breakdown, it is possible for pressure injury to occur in 2 to 3 hours. Look for excessively dry skin as evidenced by flaking or peeling. Look for areas where the skin is broken, excoriated, or blistered. Assess the color of the skin, noting any:

- **Pallor:** related to impaired circulation, which is a major risk factor for skin breakdown

BRADEN SCALE FOR PREDICTING PRESSURE SORE RISK

Patient's Name ______________ Evaluator's Name______________ Date of Assessment

SENSORY PERCEPTION ability to respond meaningfully to pressure-related discomfort	**1. Completely Limited** Unresponsive (does not moan, flinch, or grasp) to painful stimuli, due to diminished level of consciousness or sedation. OR limited ability to feel pain over most of body.	**2. Very Limited** Responds only to painful stimuli. Cannot communicate discomfort except by moaning or restlessness OR has a sensory impairment which limits the ability to feel pain or discomfort over 1/2 of body.	**3. Slightly Limited** Responds to verbal commands, but cannot always communicate discomfort or the need to be turned. OR has some sensory impairment which limits ability to feel pain or discomfort in 1 or 2 extremities.	**4. No Impairment** Responds to verbal commands. Has no sensory deficit which would limit ability to feel or voice pain or discomfort.				
MOISTURE degree to which skin is exposed to moisture	**1. Constantly Moist** Skin is kept moist almost constantly by perspiration, urine, etc. Dampness is detected every time patient is moved or turned.	**2. Very Moist** Skin is often, but not always moist. Linen must be changed at least once a shift.	**3. Occasionally Moist:** Skin is occasionally moist, requiring an extra linen change approximately once a day.	**4. Rarely Moist** Skin is usually dry, linen only requires changing at routine intervals.				
ACTIVITY degree of physical activity	**1. Bedfast** Confined to bed.	**2. Chairfast** Ability to walk severely limited or non-existent. Cannot bear own weight and/or must be assisted into chair or wheelchair.	**3. Walks Occasionally** Walks occasionally during day, but for very short distances, with or without assistance. Spends majority of each shift in bed or chair.	**4. Walks Frequently** Walks outside room at least twice a day and inside room at least once every two hours during waking hours.				
MOBILITY ability to change and control body position	**1. Completely Immobile** Does not make even slight changes in body or extremity position without assistance.	**2. Very Limited** Makes occasional slight changes in body or extremity position but unable to make frequent or significant changes independently.	**3. Slightly Limited** Makes frequent though slight changes in body or extremity position independently.	**4. No Limitation** Makes major and frequent changes in position without assistance.				
NUTRITION <u>usual</u> food intake pattern	**1. Very Poor** Never eats a complete meal. Rarely eats more than 1/2 of any food offered. Eats 2 servings or less of protein (meat or dairy products) per day. Takes fluids poorly. Does not take a liquid dietary supplement OR is NPO and/or maintained on clear liquids or IVs for more than 5 days.	**2. Probably Inadequate** Rarely eats a complete meal and generally eats only about 1/2 of any food offered. Protein intake includes only 3 servings of meat or dairy products per day. Occasionally will take a dietary supplement. OR receives less than optimum amount of liquid diet or tube feeding.	**3. Adequate** Eats over half of most meals. Eats a total of 4 servings of protein (meat, dairy products) per day. Occasionally will refuse a meal, but will usually take a supplement when offered OR is on a tube feeding or TPN regimen which probably meets most of nutritional needs.	**4. Excellent** Eats most of every meal. Never refuses a meal. Usually eats a total of 4 or more servings of meat and dairy products. Occasionally eats between meals. Does not require supplementation.				
FRICTION & SHEAR	**1. Problem** Requires moderate to maximum assistance in moving. Complete lifting without sliding against sheets is impossible. Frequently slides down in bed or chair, requiring frequent repositioning with maximum assistance. Spasticity, contractures or agitation leads to almost constant friction.	**2. Potential Problem** Moves feebly or requires minimum assistance. During a move skin probably slides to some extent against sheets, chair, restraints or other devices. Maintains relatively good position in chair or bed most of the time but occasionally slides down.	**3. No Apparent Problem** Moves in bed and in chair independently and has sufficient muscle strength to lift up completely during move. Maintains good position in bed or chair.					
				Total Score				

FIGURE 26.4 Braden scale for predicting pressure sore risk (from Wilkinson JM, Treas LM. *Fundamentals of Nursing: Theory, Concepts & Applications.* Vol. 1. 3rd ed. Philadelphia, PA: FA Davis; 2016).

- **Erythema:** indicates the increased capillary blood flow associated with inflammation
- **Jaundice:** also known as yellowing of the skin; is a sign of an abnormally high serum level of bilirubin, which can make skin itch and be more susceptible to loss of integrity
- **Bruising:** discolored areas; make notations of any such areas that are found so that it will be easy to determine if new breakdown occurs

Determine if skin turgor is elastic or nonelastic. This helps you determine whether the patient's hydration is adequate, another important factor for healthy skin. A patient who is dehydrated or edematous from overhydration will have increased risk for skin breakdown.

Box 26.1 provides nursing interventions to prevent pressure injuries.

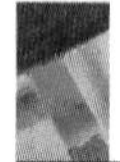

OTHER WOUNDS FOUND IN HOSPITALIZED PATIENTS

Pressure injuries are only one kind of wound found in hospitalized patients. Other wounds include stasis ulcers, draining sinus tracts, and surgical incisions.

Box 26.1

Nursing Interventions to Prevent Pressure Injuries

To prevent pressure injuries from occurring, take the following nursing actions:

- Reposition the patient at least every 2 hours to prevent pressure and compromise of circulation to the area. ***Safety: The longer a patient lies in one position, the more necrosis can occur in the area of pressure.***
- Keep the skin clean and dry.
- Assess an incontinent patient's incontinence pads or linens every hour.
- Keep linens free of wrinkles, which can cause further areas of increased pressure.
- For immobile patients, apply lotion to dry skin and assess pressure points for erythema every 1 to 2 hours.
- Lift patients who cannot move themselves with a draw sheet or mechanical lift rather than pulling them across the bed or chair.
- Remove linens from underneath a patient by rolling him or her to one side and folding the linens to the center of the bed. Then the patient is rolled to the other side and linens are removed to prevent shearing.
- Encourage adequate fluids and nutrition. Protein, mineral, and vitamin drink supplements may be given when patients fail to consume adequate meats, fruits, and vegetables at mealtimes.
- Use specialty beds and devices to help decrease pressure injuries, such as foam eggcrate mattresses, gel-filled pads and mattresses, air-filled mattresses and overlays, and beds that pump air through mattresses filled with tiny beads, known as air-fluidized beds. (These devices are discussed in Chapter 16.) For extremities, use foam, sheepskin, or inflatable protectors made to fit elbows and heels (Fig. 26.5).

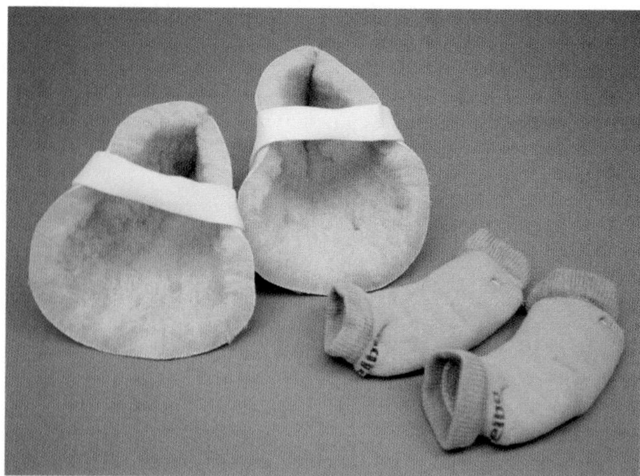

FIGURE 26.5 Heel protectors are lined with soft material and are strapped onto the foot. Elbow protectors slip over the patient's arms to prevent pressure on the bony prominences of the elbows.

Stasis Ulcers

Stasis ulcers develop when venous blood flow is sluggish, generally in the lower extremities, allowing deoxygenated blood to pool in the veins. These ulcers develop from chronic valve problems, blood clots, and other conditions that interrupt venous blood flow, such as chronic venous insufficiency. The resulting edema damages surrounding tissues and causes ulcers to develop. This chronic condition is very difficult to heal.

Sinus Tracts

A **sinus tract** is a channel or tunnel that develops between two cavities or between an infected cavity and the surface of the skin, sometimes known as a *fistula* (Fig. 26.6). A sinus tract that forms due to infection usually produces purulent

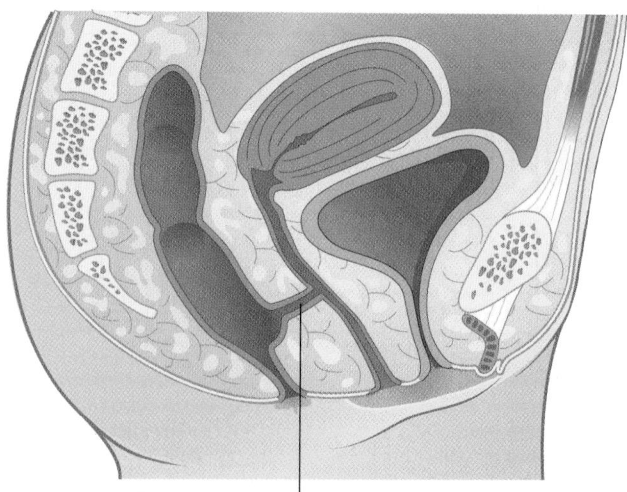

FIGURE 26.6 A fistula or sinus tract can connect two body cavities or can tunnel from a body cavity or wound to the skin. This fistula connects the vagina and the rectum (from Wilkinson JM and Treas LM. *Fundamentals of Nursing: Theory, Concepts & Applications.* Vol. 1. 3rd ed. Philadelphia, PA: FA Davis; 2016).

drainage that is thick and yellow or green. If the sinus tract opens onto the skin's surface, it usually has to be irrigated and packed with strips of tiny gauzelike material to absorb the drainage until the infection clears and the tract can be allowed to heal.

Surgical Incisions

Surgical incisions, intentionally made with sharp instruments, are linear with more sharply defined edges than most wounds. The two edges of an incision should have good *approximation,* meaning they should be close together (see Fig. 26.7 for an illustration of an incision with areas of poor approximation). An incision may be closed with sutures, staples, Steri-Strips, or skin adhesive.

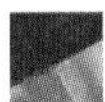

WOUND HEALING

To accurately assess a wound, you must know how a wound heals. Whether the wound is a surgical incision or a pressure injury or is due to trauma, the steps in the healing process are the same and occur in three phases.

Phases of the Healing Process

Inflammatory Phase

This phase occurs when the wound is fresh and includes both hemostasis and phagocytosis. During *hemostasis,* the body stops the bleeding associated with the fresh wound. The damaged blood vessels constrict and retract to decrease blood flow. A clot begins to form as fibrin is deposited in the wound. Eventually, a scab forms over the wound, protecting it from contamination. During *phagocytosis,* specialized white blood cells (WBCs) called macrophages engulf and digest invading microorganisms and the remaining fragments of damaged cells.

Signs of inflammation include warmth, redness, pain, and edema. These are due to increased blood supply to the wound so that hemostasis and phagocytosis can occur. It is not always a wise choice to medicate with drugs that block inflammation, such as anti-inflammatories and steroids, because they interfere with the body's natural processes and therefore delay healing.

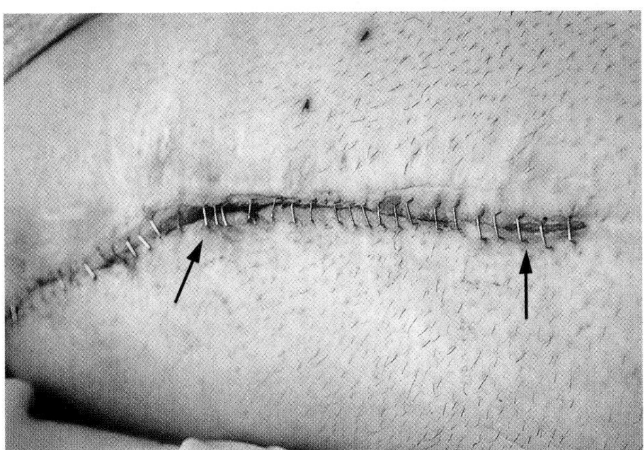

FIGURE 26.7 The wound edges of this surgical incision are not well approximated. The *arrows* point to areas where the skin edges do not meet (from Williams LS, Hopper PD. *Understanding Medical-Surgical Nursing.* 5th ed. Philadelphia, PA: FA Davis; 2015).

Reconstruction Phase

This phase occurs when the wound begins to heal and lasts for about 21 days after the injury. It is also referred to as the *proliferation phase.* The process of initiating healing begins with the presence of fibroblasts in the wound. These fibroblasts produce collagen, which is a tough protein material that forms scar tissue and helps strengthen the wound. The capillaries produce new networks so that the wound is supplied with oxygenated blood and nutrients. As new tissue begins to grow and fill in the wound, it looks red and semitransparent. This new tissue, called **granulation tissue,** is extremely fragile. If it is irritated or abraded, it bleeds easily. When you measure a wound and find that it is getting smaller, filling with deep pink to light red tissue, you know that the wound is healing, or "granulating."

Maturation Phase

This phase, also known as the *remodeling phase,* occurs when the wound contracts and the scar strengthens. Initially, a healing ridge develops just beneath the incision and approximately 1 cm on either side. Depending on the size of the wound and other factors, this phase can last 1 to 2 years. The macrophages continue to produce refined collagen to give the scar strength. As the scar thins and lightens in color, it also becomes firm and less elastic than the skin around it. This gives the area extra support to prevent reopening of the wound. Overproduction of collagen results in a thick, raised scar called a *keloid.* Keloids can form on any type of skin but are most common on darkly pigmented skin.

Types of Wound Closures for Healing

When a wound must be closed to promote healing, one of three methods will be used: first, second, or third intention closure (Fig. 26.8).

First Intention

When the wound is clean with little tissue loss, such as a surgical incision, the edges are approximated and the wound is sutured closed. This helps prevent pathogens from entering the wound and allows healing to occur quickly. Box 26.2 describes the typical progression of healing in a healthy individual with a new surgical incision.

Second Intention

When there is greater tissue loss and the wound edges are irregular, the edges cannot be brought together. Examples of this are a pressure injury or a traumatic wound. In these situations,

• WORD • BUILDING •
hemostasis: hemo – blood + stasis – stoppage

Primary intention

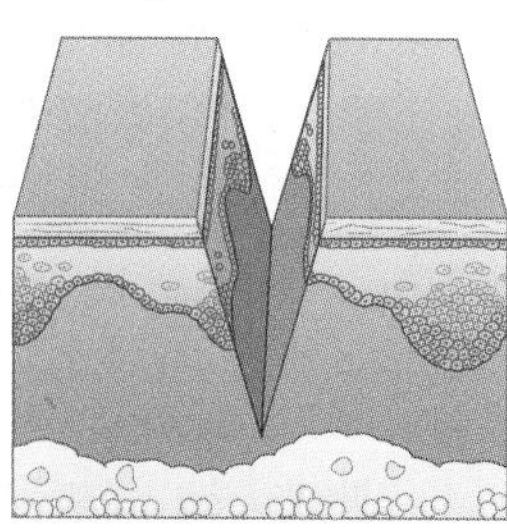

A Clean wound

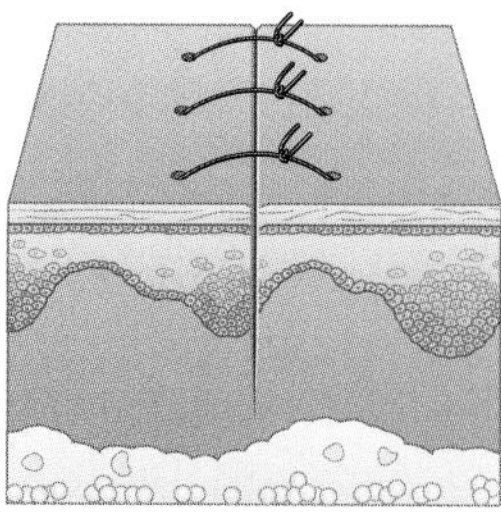

Sutured early

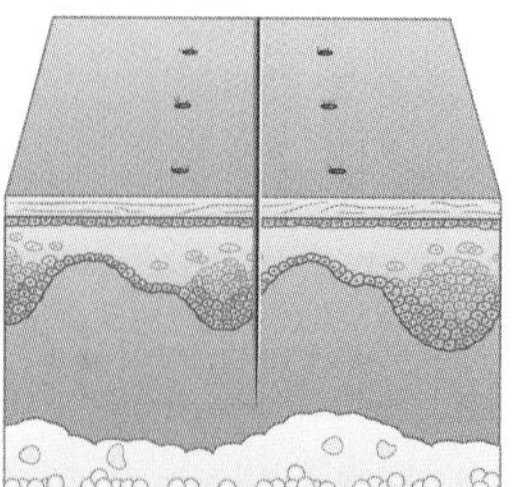

Results in hairline scar

Secondary intention

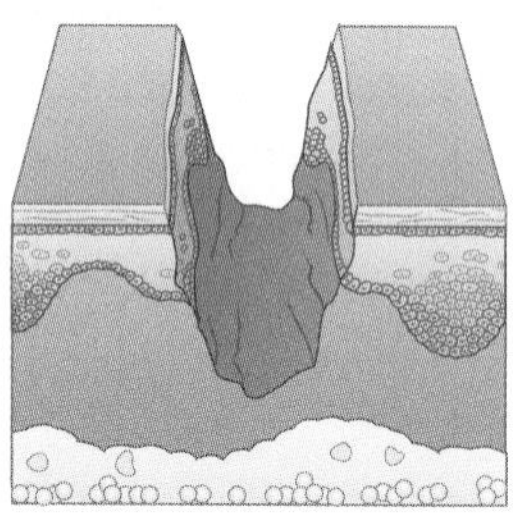

B Wound gaping and irregular

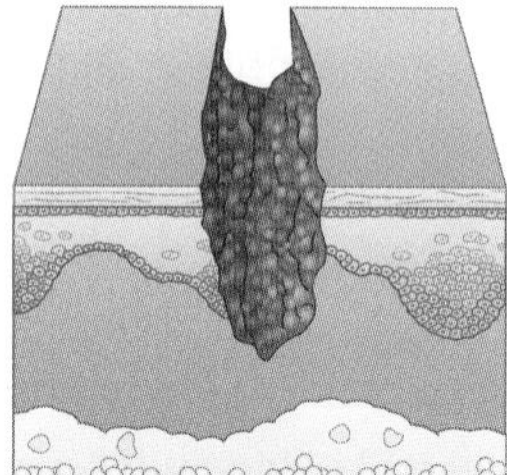

Granulation occurring

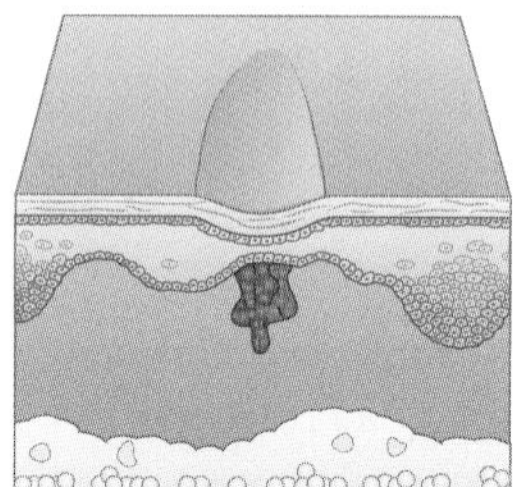

Epithelium fills in scar

Tertiary intention

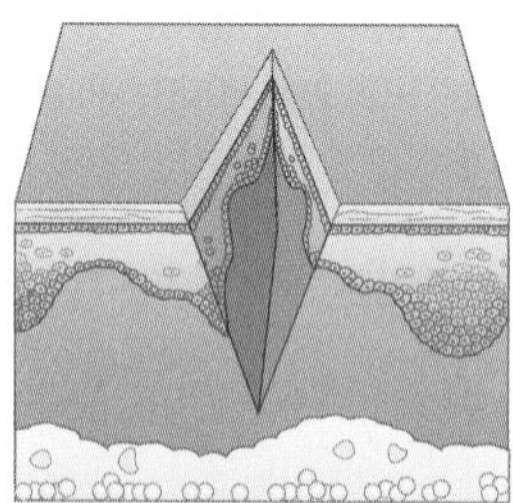

C Wound not sutured

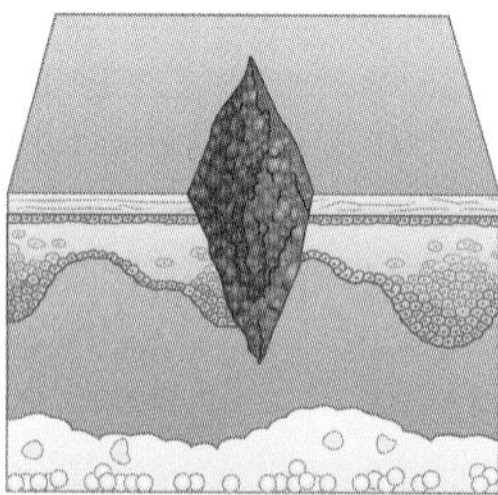

Granulation partially fills in wound

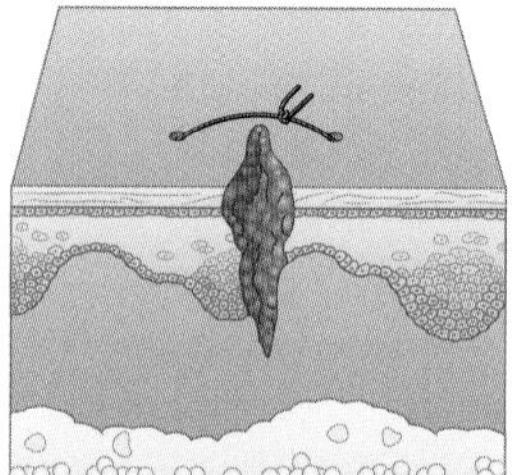

Granulating tissue sutured together

FIGURE 26.8 The three different types of closure: (a) Primary intention healing with a clean wound sutured closed and well healed; (b) Secondary intention healing with an irregular wound, unsutured for granulation to occur, and scar formation; (c) Third intention healing with an unsutured wound, partially filled with granulation tissue, then closed with suture (from Wilkinson JM, Treas LM. *Fundamentals of Nursing: Theory, Concepts & Applications.* Vol. 1. 3rd ed. Philadelphia: FA Davis; 2016).

Box 26.2

Typical Healing of Surgical Incisions

Surgical incisions typically heal in the following manner:

- Within 48 hours after surgery, the incision begins to bind together.
- Due to the normal inflammatory reaction, you will observe slight swelling around staples or sutures and mild erythema of the incision in the first day or two.
- Most incisions have scant or no drainage at all, but some have a scant to moderate amount of sanguineous or serosanguineous drainage. It will change from sanguineous to serosanguineous to serous and will decrease in amount over the first 5 postoperative days.
- By the fifth day postoperatively, you will be able to feel a ridge of granulation tissue directly below the incision. This ridge may extend to both sides of the incision for about a centimeter. Some patients become alarmed if they discover this ridge, but it is part of the normal healing process.

the wound must be left open to gradually heal by filling in with granulation tissue, which will leave a wide scar. Open wounds must be packed with moist gauze to absorb drainage and allow tissue to grow. They are covered with additional dressings to help prevent microorganisms from entering the wound. Strict sterile technique must be used when applying dressings to open wounds in order to prevent infection.

Third Intention

When third intention healing is used, the wound is left open for a time to allow granulation tissue to form, and then it is sutured closed. An example of this is a draining wound, which is left open until the drainage ceases and then is sutured closed.

Factors Affecting Wound Healing

For optimum wound healing, conditions must be favorable for new tissue growth. A number of factors can delay the healing process, including the age and lifestyle of the patient, additional illness and wounds, nutritional status, oxygenation, medications, and tension on the edges of the wound (Table 26.1).

Table 26.1
Factors Affecting Wound Healing

Factor	*Effect on Wound Healing*	*Example*
Age	Wounds contract more slowly. Strength of scarred area is decreased. Skin is less elastic as people age. Collagen replacement is impaired.	An elderly patient with skin tears may heal slowly due to lack of collagen and elasticity.
Chronic illness	Illnesses affecting major body systems, such as heart, lung, and kidney disease, as well as neurological deficits affect optimal functioning of those systems. In turn, healing of wounds is negatively affected by impairment of other body systems.	A patient with chronic lung disease and congestive heart failure experiences very slow healing of an operative wound.
Diabetes mellitus	Causes decreased circulation due to narrowed peripheral blood vessels. Increased blood glucose interferes with the healing process.	A patient with diabetes whose blood glucose levels are poorly controlled could be expected to have slow wound healing.
Hypoxemia	Decreased oxygen delivered to the wound by the bloodstream causes impaired healing; oxygen is necessary for wounds to heal properly.	A patient with anemia or chronic lung disease may have hypoxemia, leading to impaired wound healing.
Lifestyle choices	Smoking decreases the oxygen content of the blood and constricts blood vessels, impeding circulation to wounds. Excessive alcohol intake can lead to poor nutrition, which affects wound healing. Obesity puts patients at risk for wound complications such as infection and dehiscence.	An obese patient who smokes and consumes alcohol in large amounts is at high risk for impaired wound healing and wound complications.
Lymphedema	When the area around a wound is edematous, circulation to and from the wound is impaired. Lack of efficient circulation decreases wound healing.	A patient with stasis ulcers on his or her leg experiences swelling in the area. Without compression applied by using leg wraps or support hose, the patient will be at risk for impaired healing of the leg ulcers.
Medications	Certain prescription medications delay the healing process and can mask symptoms of inflammation and infection.	A patient taking steroids or cytotoxic medications, such as chemotherapy, will be at risk for delayed or impaired wound healing.
Multiple wounds	Each wound competes for the available protein and substrates needed for tissue repair, resulting in delayed wound healing for all the wounds.	A patient injured in a motorcycle accident has multiple wounds and abrasions. It can be expected that all of them will be slow to heal.
Nutrition and hydration	Lack of calories and adequate protein impairs tissue growth. Deficiency in intake of vitamins A and C and zinc in the diet interferes with wound repair. Inadequate fluid intake causes the wound to be dry, restricting granulation of tissue.	A patient who is tube fed often receives a nominal amount of calories and protein, which delays wound healing.

Continued

Table 26.1
Factors Affecting Wound Healing—cont'd

Factor	*Effect on Wound Healing*	*Example*
Radiation exposure	Cancer treatments involving radiation can cause breakdown of underlying connective tissue, affecting repair capabilities.	A patient receiving radiation treatments for lung cancer after surgery on the lung is at risk for impaired wound healing of the surgical site or reopening of the surgical site.
Wound tension	Extra tension placed on the wound edges can lead to *ischemia* (lack of blood supply to the area) and *necrosis* (death of tissue due to lack of blood supply). Tension on wound edges may be due to activities such as coughing, sneezing, lifting, and vomiting.	A patient who is vomiting repeatedly causes increased tension on the sutures of an abdominal wound, pulling the edges apart and interfering with normal healing.

Anatomy and Physiology Connection

The Inflammatory Process

The skin, consisting of the *epidermis* (outermost layer) and the *dermis* (innermost layer or true skin), serves as the first line of defense against microorganisms and foreign bodies. Whenever this first barrier is broken, the inflammatory process is initiated. The damaged cells release histamine and other chemicals, which cause the capillaries to *dilate*, or widen, and increase permeability of the capillary walls. The dilation allows increased blood flow to the site, causing erythema and increased warmth. More leukocytes are delivered to the site to help guard against infection. The increased permeability allows leukocytes to leave the vascular space and enter into the interstitial space and attack microorganisms directly, while red blood cells deliver more oxygen and nutrients to aid the healing process. This increase of fluid in the interstitial space results in edema. The edema causes pressure on nerve endings, producing discomfort and pain.

Complications of Wound Healing

Several types of complications can occur as a wound heals. It will be your responsibility to differentiate between normal healing and the presence of complications. You will be expected to assess your patients' wounds for signs and symptoms of these complications and to know what to do if they occur. Some complications of wound healing are considered medical emergencies, and your fast action can mean the difference between a good outcome and a poor one.

Infection

One of the most common wound complications is infection. A patient who has just undergone a surgical procedure or who has an open wound will have impaired defenses against infection. The most common microbial pathogen associated with wound infections is *Staphylococcus aureus.* This bacterium is present on the skin of all people, so it easily enters wounds unless special precautions are followed. In the operating room, strict sterile technique must be enforced. Surgical instruments, equipment, and personnel are all potential sources of infection.

Laboratory and Diagnostic Connection

Testing to Determine If a Wound Is Infected

In order to effectively treat an infected wound, you must identify the microorganism that is causing the infection and determine which antibiotics will be effective against the microorganism and kill it. This test is known as a wound *culture and sensitivity*. Some microorganisms have mutated so that they are no longer sensitive to certain antibiotics. These strains are labeled as resistant to the specific antibiotics. After the offending microorganism is identified, tiny disks, each saturated with a different antibiotic, are placed on the agar plate to observe whether or not the antibiotic kills the microorganism. If the antibiotic successfully kills the microorganism, the microorganism is sensitive to that specific drug. If it does not kill the microorganism, the microorganism is considered resistant to that antibiotic.

Another laboratory test valuable in the treatment of wounds is the WBC count and differential. A WBC count is a microscopic examination of the total number of WBCs that are present in the patient's blood. The normal range is 4,500 to 11,100/mm^3, while infection may cause an increased level of WBCs. A differential shows the percentage of each of the five types of WBCs: neutrophils, lymphocytes, basophils, eosinophils, and monocytes. An increase in percentage of lymphocytes may be seen with chronic bacterial infections. An increased percentage of neutrophils may be seen with acute infections and a decreased percentage in widespread bacterial infections.

METHICILLIN-RESISTANT *STAPHYLOCOCCUS AUREUS*. A resistant strain of *S. aureus*, identified as **methicillin-resistant *S. aureus*** (MRSA), is an extremely serious issue. Like other staph microorganisms, this resistant form can live on the skin of healthy people without causing illness. However, when a wound becomes infected with MRSA, the health-care provider has little choice in effective antibiotics for treatment. Although vancomycin is the current antibiotic of choice to treat MRSA, an even more resistant strain is now making an appearance. This strain, vancomycin-intermediate *S. aureus*, is developing resistance even to vancomycin.

***ESCHERICHIA COLI*.** Another common infective pathogen appears in wounds after surgery on the gastrointestinal system. Bacteria normally found in the bowel are referred to as enterococci. One specific bacterium from this group, *E. coli,* helps to break down food for digestion. When the intestines are opened during surgery, the bacteria from the bowel, including *E. coli,* can easily infect the surgical wound. Special preparation before bowel surgery helps decrease the chances of such an infection. When emergency surgery is performed on the gastrointestinal tract, especially when perforation or rupture has occurred, infection is quite likely.

CLOSTRIDIA. When a wound is infected with bacteria called *clostridia,* the result is a condition known as *gas gangrene.* This pathogen grows only in the absence of oxygen and is called an *anaerobe.* As the bacteria multiply in the wound, poisonous toxins and gases are emitted.

Gangrene most often occurs due to poor circulation to a body part, especially a digit or limb, or as a complication of an untreated infection in a wound. Essentially, a portion of the body dies while it is still attached to living tissue in the body. The area may become black due to tissue death and produce a characteristic foul odor associated with decaying tissue. When the affected area is pressed, a crackling sensation will be felt due to the gas produced by the bacteria.

This infection is treated with antibiotics and surgical removal of the dead tissue, a process known as **débridement.** If the condition is due to impaired circulation, the patient will be evaluated for revascularization surgery. Infected wounds are débrided and may be treated in a *hyperbaric chamber.* Such a chamber delivers oxygen under high pressure to help kill anaerobic bacteria and promote wound healing. Aggressive antibiotic therapy is necessary to prevent the spread of toxins into the bloodstream. If other treatment fails, the affected limb may have to be amputated.

STAT NURSING RESPONSE TO WOUND INFECTION. You are responsible for assessing surgical and open wounds for any signs of infection. Be sure to differentiate normal wound healing from the early onset of infection. Inspect and assess surgical incisions and other wounds at least every 8 hours. When you assess an infected wound, you will see pronounced erythema around the staples or sutures and on the edges of the incision. Drainage may increase in amount with each successive day rather than decrease. The drainage may be purulent and *malodorous* (bad smelling). The by-products of the bacteria infecting the wound emit a strong odor. The incision itself may begin to open between sutures or staples. The patient's vital signs usually reflect infection: Elevated temperature and heart rate may be noted. Laboratory results often show an elevated WBC count, and the patient will often complain of increasing incisional pain, rather than decreasing pain, with each postoperative day.

When you observe possible signs of infection in a wound, notify the health-care provider of your findings immediately. Before calling, be sure to have all of the following appropriate information at hand:

- Vital sign readings
- Laboratory results
- Amount and type of drainage
- Description of the wound, including observed signs of infection
- Patient's rating of incisional pain

If the patient is already on an oral or IV antibiotic, have the name and dosage of the medication available when you call the health-care provider. Be prepared to obtain a specimen of wound drainage for culture and sensitivity.

KNOWLEDGE CONNECTION

What will you expect the health-care provider to order when you call to report signs of infection in a surgical wound? Which microorganism is the most resistant to antibiotics?

Patient Teaching Connection

Wound Care

Before discharging a patient with a wound from the hospital, teach the patient the signs and symptoms of wound infection using layperson's terminology:

- Redness or increased warmth of the wound
- Swelling
- Wound drainage
- Wound has an unpleasant smell
- Pain around the wound
- Fever above 100°F

Explain that the health-care provider should be notified if any of these signs or symptoms occurs. If antibiotics are prescribed, instruct the patient regarding the importance of taking antibiotics until they are gone. If the patient or family member will be changing the dressing at home, give detailed instructions, both verbally and in writing, and then demonstrate how to change the dressing. Have the patient or family member return to demonstrate the procedure to evaluate their understanding.

• WORD • BUILDING •

malodorous: mal – bad + odorous – smelling

Wound Dehiscence and Evisceration

Wound **dehiscence** is not a common complication of wound healing, but it is an extremely serious one. It occurs when there is a partial or complete separation of the outer layers of a wound (Fig. 26.9). Dehiscence occurs in about 3% of abdominal surgery patients, with a mortality rate between 14% and 50%. This condition occurs most often between the 5th and 12th postoperative days.

Several reasons for wound separation exist, and many occur in surgery. If sutures or staples are placed too far apart or too close to the edges of the incision, the edges do not meet together for optimum healing. Anything that can lead to necrosis of the wound edges, such as wound infection, extremely tight sutures, or impaired blood supply, can result in wound dehiscence. If the wound edges are separating between sutures or if sutures are removed too soon, the wound may reopen (see Fig. 26.7). It is best not to remove sutures until the ridge of granulation tissue can be felt. ***Safety: Be sure to help your patient splint his or her incision with a pillow before he or she coughs or sneezes to help prevent extra stress on wound edges.*** Provide patients with medications as ordered for nausea and stool softeners to prevent tension on the wound from vomiting or straining to have a bowel movement.

As you might imagine, if an abdominal wound reopens, the abdominal contents may protrude through the opening (Fig. 26.10). This condition is referred to as **evisceration** and is a life-threatening situation. Exposure of abdominal contents can lead to necrosis of the intestines or overwhelming sepsis. If a patient tells you, "I feel like something just split open," be ready to act quickly.

STAT NURSING RESPONSE TO WOUND DEHISCENCE AND EVISCERATION. This situation usually occurs suddenly; often the only warning is a pronounced increase in serosanguineous drainage from the wound. Should dehiscence occur, reassure your patient and assist him or her to a supine position. Stay with your patient and notify the health-care provider immediately. Request that sterile supplies be brought to the room, including a basin, normal saline, abdominal dressings, a 60-mL syringe, masks, gowns, gloves, and drapes. A suture removal kit may be necessary. Sterile adhesive strips also should be on hand.

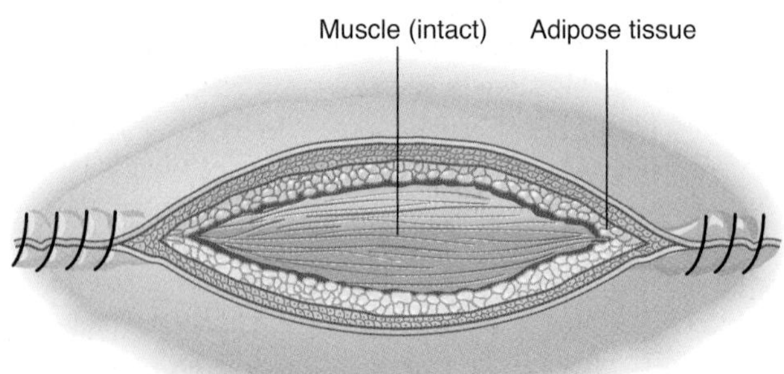

FIGURE 26.9 This wound has separated, and the muscle layer is visible beneath. It is an example of wound dehiscence (from Wilkinson JM, Treas LM. *Fundamentals of Nursing: Theory, Concepts & Applications.* Vol. 1. 3rd ed. Philadelphia, PA: FA Davis; 2016).

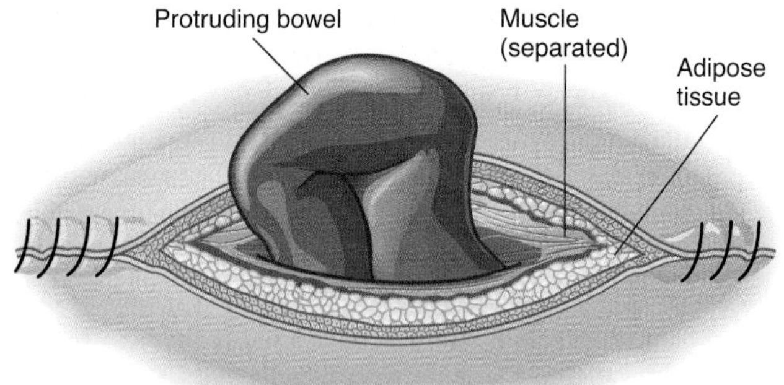

FIGURE 26.10 This wound and the muscle layer beneath have separated, allowing the intestine to protrude outward through the wound. It is an example of wound evisceration (from Wilkinson JM, Treas LM. *Fundamentals of Nursing: Theory, Concepts & Applications.* Vol. 1. 3rd ed. Philadelphia, PA: FA Davis; 2016).

If the wound is completely separated or a large portion of it has reopened, be prepared to send the patient to the operating room as soon as possible. If only a small portion of the wound has reopened, the health-care provider may use sterile adhesive strip closures.

If evisceration has occurred as well, you must act immediately. ***Safety: Do not attempt to replace the organs into the abdominal cavity.*** Cover the exposed organs with sterile dressings soaked in normal saline. Keep the dressings moist by adding sterile saline using the sterile syringe. When you moisten the dressings, assess the exposed organs for signs of necrosis, such as a color change to blue, purple, or black. Position the patient in the low Fowler's position with the knees flexed to reduce strain on the abdominal wound. Do not give your patient anything by mouth (keep the patient NPO) because surgery will have to be performed. Be sure that you have a patent IV line and administer fluids and medications as ordered through it. Monitor vital signs at least every 15 minutes to detect signs of shock. Be calm and continue to reassure your patient.

> **KNOWLEDGE CONNECTION**
> What is the difference between wound dehiscence and evisceration? How are they treated similarly? How are they treated differently?

Hemorrhage

Rarely, a surgical wound may **hemorrhage,** or bleed profusely. This is also a medical emergency. When you check for bleeding postoperatively, always look and feel beneath

• WORD • BUILDING •

dehiscence: dehisc – burst open + ence – action

serosanguineous: sero – serum + sanguin – blood + eous – resembling

the patient for blood that might have pooled there rather than being absorbed into the dressing. Hemorrhage may be due to a slipped suture, displaced blood clot, or trauma to the incision. A large amount of bright red blood indicates bleeding from an artery. Patients taking anticoagulant medications (blood thinners) and those with clotting disorders are at risk for hemorrhage postoperatively.

Hemorrhage may also occur internally. No discharge of blood will be present, but symptoms of blood loss are the same. As blood gathers in the abdominal cavity, the abdomen becomes distended and taut. This is a cardinal sign of potential postoperative hemorrhage, and the patient should be evaluated immediately for that complication. Pale mucous membranes; a rapid and thready pulse; hypotension; diaphoresis; and cool, clammy skin are later signs of hemorrhage. This condition can lead to death if not detected and treated without delay. ***Safety: Act immediately if you suspect a patient may be hemorrhaging internally or externally.***

STAT NURSING RESPONSE TO HEMORRHAGE. External or internal hemorrhage is a medical emergency. Notify the health-care provider immediately. Position the patient in the low Fowler's position with the knees flexed. If you can see the source of the bleeding, put on gloves and apply firm pressure over the area. Administer oxygen via mask or nasal cannula. Monitor vital signs at least every 15 minutes and be prepared for the patient to return to the operating room as soon as possible. Ensure a patent IV line and administer fluids as ordered to help prevent circulatory collapse.

KNOWLEDGE CONNECTION
What are possible causes of wound hemorrhage?

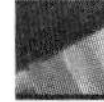

WOUND TREATMENT

You will provide wound care as ordered by the health-care provider. Treatments will differ for each wound, depending on the type and extent of the wound, whether it is an open or closed wound, the level of contamination, and the health-care provider's personal preferences.

Closure

Surgical wounds and traumatic wounds with intact tissue are generally closed using some type of closure material. Most common are sutures, staples, surgical adhesive, and sterile adhesive strips, sometimes referred to by the brand name Steri-Strips. A surgical wound is closed from the inner layers to the outer layers of tissue. Absorbable sutures are used in the inner tissue layers. The outer skin layers are approximated and held in place using one of several closure methods. Nonabsorbable sutures or staples are used on the outer layers of tissue and are removed after 7 to 14 days. Surgical adhesive can only be used on the outer skin layers and "glues" the wound together. No removal is necessary, and the edges of the wound remain approximated during the healing process. Sterile adhesive strips are used to close small wounds, or wounds that are healing. For example, you may apply sterile adhesive strips to an incision after you remove the sutures or staples, to give the incision support as it continues to heal. Sterile adhesive strips are narrow reinforced tape strips that eventually will peel free of the skin.

Nursing Responsibilities for Suture/Staple Care

Your responsibilities include assessment of the suture line each time you inspect an incision. This may be when you perform a dressing change or when you assess your patient at the beginning of your shift. Note any sign of loosening sutures, gaps in the incision, or redness around the staples or sutures that indicates infection. Assess incisions every 8 hours to detect changes that may occur. You also may be responsible for removing sutures and staples when the wound has healed. Skill 26.1 (page 545) shows how to remove sutures and staples.

Drains and Drainage

After traumatic injury or surgery, wounds generally produce drainage. At first, this drainage looks like blood (**sanguineous**); then it looks pink (**serosanguineous**); and finally, as the wound heals, the drainage becomes clearer to slightly yellow fluid (**serous**). This is a predictable pattern as a wound heals; deviations from this pattern indicate some type of wound complication. Box 26.3 describes types of wound drainage.

When a wound is expected to produce significant drainage, the surgeon will place a drain in the wound before closure. A tube then extends through the skin and to the outside of the body, ending in some type of collection receptacle. If drainage is allowed to remain in the tissues, it will prevent granulation from occurring and impede wound healing.

Closed drains attach to a device that, when compressed, causes gentle suction, allowing fluid to be drawn from the wound into the collection container. The Hemovac and Jackson-Pratt, also called J-P, are both active drains that operate on the suction principle (Fig. 26.11). A T-tube is a passive drain. It is placed in the common bile duct after gallbladder surgery to drain excess bile from the area via gravity. It connects to a small collection bag but does not cause suction within the wound.

A Penrose drain is an open drain (see Fig. 26.11). A flat tube is inserted in the wound during surgery and then is brought out through a "stab wound" or slit in the skin. A sterile safety pin is fastened through the flat tube to keep it from sliding into the wound. Drainage from the wound exits through the Penrose drain and is absorbed by the dressing. Several sterile gauze 4×4s are layered over and under the end of the drain to absorb the exudate. Open drains are used less frequently than in the past because they provide a pathway for pathogens to reach the wound. Closed drains are seen most frequently.

• WORD • BUILDING •
sanguineous: sanguin – blood + eous – resembling

Box 26.3

Types of Wound Drainage

It is important to describe wound drainage accurately so that other health-care workers can compare your findings with theirs.

- **Sanguineous:** Comes from the Latin word for "bloody" and means "containing blood." It refers to red, bloody drainage.
- **Serous:** Comes from the Latin word for "serum," the clear liquid portion of the blood. It refers to clear to pale yellow drainage that looks like serum.
- **Purulent:** Comes from the Latin word meaning "full of pus," and means "containing pus." It is thick yellow or green drainage and is a sign of infection.
- **Bilious:** Comes from the word "bile," which is made by the body to help break down fats for digestion. It is a dark greenish color and is often present in wound drainage after gallbladder surgery.

Sometimes more than one type of drainage is present. These words are then combined to indicate the two types of drainage from the wound:

- **Serosanguineous:** Both blood and clear drainage are present. Combined, they turn dressing materials a pink color.
- **Seropurulent:** Both clear drainage and drainage with pus are present.

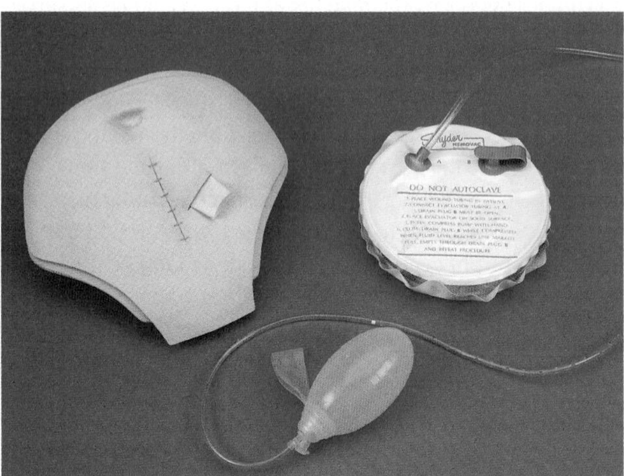

FIGURE 26.11 These are different types of wound drains: Penrose on the left, Jackson-Pratt in the center, and Hemovac on the right (from Wilkinson JM, Treas LM. *Fundamentals of Nursing: Theory, Concepts & Applications.* Vol. 1. 3rd ed. Philadelphia, PA: FA Davis; 2016).

Nursing Responsibilities for Drain Care

You will be responsible for any drains that your patients have. Empty drains every 8 hours or when they become one-half to two-thirds full. If the bulb on the Jackson-Pratt drain or the round receptacle on the Hemovac drain is no longer compressed, the container is full and must be emptied. When compression is absent, no suction is present. Skill 26.2 (page 546) shows the steps required to care for and empty drainage devices.

Measure drainage in a calibrated container and record the amount on the intake and output record. Note the type of drainage. Report a significant increase in the amount of drainage and the presence of purulent drainage to the health-care provider immediately because these could indicate impaired healing and infection.

If a Penrose drain is in use, change the dressings around the drain carefully to prevent dislodging the tube. The health-care provider may order the drain to be shortened a specified length, for example, 2 inches. This involves removing the safety pin and pulling the specified length of tubing out of the wound, cutting off the excess tubing, and reattaching the safety pin. This procedure may not be in the entry-level nurse's scope of practice, so be sure to check facility policy before performing it.

KNOWLEDGE CONNECTION

What are four ways wounds are closed? What is the purpose of a wound drain? When should wound drains be emptied?

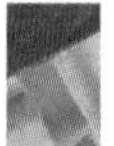

MEASUREMENT OF WOUNDS AND OBSERVATION OF DRAINAGE

Assessing a wound is the only way to determine whether the wound is healing or complications such as infection are occurring, so it is pertinent that you be skilled in wound assessment (Box 26.4). One of the first things you will note is the amount of drainage on the old dressing, which is generally referred to as a scant, small, moderate, or large amount. You also must describe the color of the drainage.

In some situations, the health-care provider may not want the dressing to be changed for 24 or 48 hours, even though it contains drainage. If that is the case, nurses mark

Box 26.4

Wound Assessment Summary

When you assess a wound, be sure to include all of the following aspects of the wound.

- **Site:** anatomical location
- **Wound type:** open or closed
- **Wound closure:** sutures, staples, Steri-Strips, approximation
- **Size:** width, length, depth
- **Condition of wound bed:** color, texture, eschar, sloughing, presence of granulation tissue, undermining, sinus tracts
- **Condition of skin surrounding wound:** color, texture, maceration
- **Pain:** rate discomfort/tenderness using pain scale
- **Drainage:** amount, type/color, odor

the drainage on the dressing to show increases over time. For example, a patient who has just returned from surgery has an abdominal dressing with a quarter-sized amount of drainage visible on the outside dressing. Draw around the drainage with a pen, then write the date, time, and your initials next to it. When the nurse on the next shift cares for this patient, he or she will be able to tell if the drainage has increased since that time.

If large amounts of drainage occur and the dressing is not to be changed for 24 hours, reinforce the dressing with additional abdominal dressings to absorb additional drainage. Notify the health-care provider of the excessive drainage because it is not normally expected after most surgeries.

You will need to assess the size of a wound: its length, width, and depth. Use a ruler or a disposable paper wound measurement ruler. Without touching the paper or ruler to the skin, measure the width of the wound at its widest point. Do the same for the length of the wound. If the wound is completely round, you can measure the width and consider it the diameter of the wound. To measure depth, use a sterile cotton-tipped swab. Carefully insert the swab at the deepest area of the wound and mark skin level with your gloved finger against the handle portion of the swab. Then carefully hold the swab near the ruler or paper ruler to determine depth. It is common to measure wounds in centimeters or millimeters, rather than inches. If the wound has a sinus tract connected with it, the swab can be used to determine the length of the tract as well. Insert the swab as far as it will go, mark the handle portion with your finger, and then measure the length of the tract.

If the wound is open, assess the base or bed of the wound for color of tissue, texture of tissue, granulation tissue, eschar, sinus tracts, and undermining. If the wound has been surgically closed, assess the number of staples, sutures, or Steri-Strips that are intact. To help you describe the appearance of different areas of the wound, visualize a clock face. Make notes using the clock face as a reference. For example, there may be eschar at 12 o'clock and granulation tissue at 6 o'clock. Once you have completed your wound and drainage assessment, you are ready to clean the wound.

CLEANING WOUNDS

Some wounds contain dissolved necrotic tissue and pus; others may hold tissue fluid and blood (*exudate*). In these situations, you will anticipate health-care provider's orders to clean the wound with dressing changes. Cleaning of wounds may be accomplished in the physical therapy department of some hospitals, especially if vigorous cleansing in a whirlpool bath is ordered to remove dead tissue or wound contaminants. Irrigation is the more gentle method of wound cleansing and is ordered when fragile granulation tissue is present. Wounds also can be cleaned with soft gauze moistened with sterile saline, using a light patting movement. Use care to prevent damaging healthy tissue.

To clean around a drain exiting from a wound, use a sterile antiseptic swab such as chlorhexidine gluconate, forceps and cotton balls soaked in normal saline, or another ordered solution. Clean in a circular motion on the skin, starting as close as possible to the drain. Move outward in enlarging circles, overlapping slightly to be sure no gaps are left and all skin is cleansed. Make one circle with a swab or cotton ball and then dispose of it. Make the next slightly larger circle with a new swab or cotton ball.

To clean a long incision that is sutured or stapled closed with approximated edges, again use sterile antiseptic swabs or forceps and cotton balls soaked in normal saline or other ordered solution. Clean from the superior end of the incision to the inferior end. The superior portion of the wound is considered less contaminated than the inferior portion because drainage usually flows downward. ***Safety: Do not go back over an area that has already been cleansed. If you do so, you can contaminate the cleansed area with pathogens from an unclean area.*** If the incision itself is contaminated, clean from the superior to the inferior end of the wound with one swab or cotton ball, then dispose of it. Continue cleaning using long strokes from superior to inferior along the incision, using a new swab or cotton ball for each stroke. Alternate cleaning one side of the incision and then cleaning the opposite side until an area of several inches on either side has been cleansed. Dispose of each swab or cotton ball after every stroke.

Nursing Responsibilities for Cleaning Wounds

When wound irrigation is ordered, the purpose is to remove surface debris without injuring granulation tissue. This is best accomplished by using mild pressure of 8 pounds per square inch. To deliver the correct amount of pressure, you will use a 35-mL syringe with a 19-gauge Angiocath attached. As you spray normal saline through the Angiocath, it will gently remove surface debris without causing damage to the wound. Hold a basin below the inferior margin of the wound to catch the irrigant. Skill 26.3 (page 547) presents the steps for performing a wound irrigation.

The most commonly used irrigant is sterile normal saline because it is isotonic to the body. If a different fluid is to be used, the health-care provider will order it. Be sure to assess the amount, color, and consistency of debris removed by the irrigation and document this information in the patient's chart.

Obtaining a Wound Culture

The health-care provider may order a specimen of the wound drainage to be tested for culture and sensitivity to see which pathogens might be growing in the wound and determine the appropriate antibiotics for treatment. You will obtain the wound culture during the dressing change. If a wound irrigation is ordered, perform the irrigation first and then obtain the specimen of wound drainage for culture.

Skill 26.4 (page 548) lists the steps for obtaining a wound culture specimen.

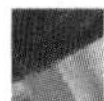

DRESSINGS

Dressings serve several purposes. In the case of a surgical incision, dressings protect the incision and absorb drainage as the wound heals. In the case of chronic wounds, such as pressure injuries and vascular ulcers, the dressings also protect from further injury, provide the moist environment required for healing, and fill the open space within the wound. Because healing of these ulcers must occur from the inside out, open spaces need to be packed until they fill with granulation tissue. Without packing, the pooling debris and exudate would cause the wound to become larger.

Wounds cannot heal without the appropriate amount of moisture. When a wound is covered and moisture is maintained within it, the epidermal cells can move freely through the moisture to promote healing. When wounds are dry, the cells must first tunnel below the surface to a moist area where they secrete enzymes. The enzymes help dissolve the scab so the epidermal cells can begin healing. The purpose of many dressings is to preserve a moist wound environment so healing can occur.

Many different types of dressings exist. Some are designed simply to cover the wound. Others are intended to be packed into the wound. Still others have been developed specifically to maintain a moist wound bed. The health-care provider will order the type of dressing to be used for each patient. However, you will be expected to know the appropriate use of each type of dressing and to assess wound healing response. Table 26.2 shows a comparison of common dressings and their uses.

Eye dressings must be applied carefully without putting pressure on the eye itself. The dressing must remain sterile. It is placed over the closed eye and secured with only one or two pieces of tape. It is important not to apply the tape to the patient's eyebrow or hair.

Wet-to-Damp Dressings

Wet-to-damp wound dressings are ordered to maintain a moist wound bed and to wick out drainage from the wound. They are changed frequently to prevent the gauze in the wound from drying out completely. Removing the gauze in the wound helps to gently debride necrotic tissue. Skill 26.5 (page 549) gives the steps required to change a sterile dressing and a wet-to-damp dressing.

You may also apply other dressings, such as those listed in Table 26.2. Two of the most common dressings you will apply are transparent film dressings and hydrocolloid dressings. Skill 26.6 (page 552) provides directions for applying transparent and hydrocolloid dressings. Skill 26.7 (page 553) gives the steps for applying negative pressure wound therapy.

Table 26.2
Types and Purposes of Dressings

Type	*Purpose*	*Composition*	*Examples*
Antimicrobial impregnated with silver or cadexomer iodine	Used with infected wounds or those at high risk for infection and for wounds with heavy drainage; absorbs exudates Avoid using silver if the patient is allergic or sensitive to silver	Available as gel, film, mesh, foam, paste, or ointment; provides controlled release of silver or iodine to inhibit bacterial growth	Acticoat Allevyn Ag Aquacel Ag Iodosorb
Alginate	Loosely packed or layered in wounds and sinus tracts; used for wounds with moderate to large amounts of drainage and clinically infected pressure injuries; also comes in "ropes" that are cut to fit in the wound; wound is covered with absorbent dressing	Derived from seaweed; when it absorbs drainage, it turns into a soft gel that does not adhere to the wound; absorbs up to 20 times its own weight	Algisite Curasorb Kaltogel Sorbsan Tegagel
Collagen Matrix	Indicated for partial and full-thickness pressure injuries, venous stasis ulcers, surgical wounds, and diabetic ulcers Usually requires a secondary dressing to keep it in place	Contains collagen from animal sources and a microbial agent to prevent infection; some form a gel in the wound when they mix with exudate; collagen helps promote the growth of new human collagen to fill the wound	Biostep Mucograft Endoform Helix 3 Naturin Viscofan

Table 26.2
Types and Purposes of Dressings—cont'd

Type	*Purpose*	*Composition*	*Examples*
Foam dressings	Used to cover wounds with heavy exudates, especially during inflammatory phase; highly absorbent; used in stage 2 and shallow stage 3 pressure injuries	Made from hydrophilic poly urethane foam; some have adhesive borders to stay in place	Flexzan Curafoam Mepilex
Gauze	Used to loosely pack large wounds in wet-to-damp dressings for débridement, then covered with a thicker dressing to absorb drainage May require irrigation with dressing change to remove all fibers from wound Used when other forms of moisture-retentive dressings are not available	Cotton, polyester, or rayon fibers, loosely or tightly woven; filled dressings include absorbent material; unfilled are composed of woven threads only; Telfa pads are coated to prevent sticking	ABD (abdominal dressing) Curity gauze sponge Gauze 4×4s Kerlix gauze fluff Telfa
Honey-impregnated dressings	Used in stage 2 or stage 3 pressure injuries as an antimicrobial and to increase rate of healing; avoid using if patient is allergic to honey	Available as gel, paste, in alginate, hydrocolloid, and other dressing forms	Medihoney Apinate
Hydrocolloid	Used on wounds with minimal wound drainage and on dry, clean wounds; used on body areas where the dressings won't melt or roll Recommended for stage 2 pressure injuries; not recommended for infected wounds	Made of water-attracting gelling agents such as pectin or gelatin; absorbs excess fluid from the wound while still holding in moisture	CombiDERM Comfeel DuoDERM Tegasorb
Hydrogels	Provides moist wound environment; aids in wound débridement by supplying moisture to dry wound beds Recommended for shallow, minimally exuding pressure injuries and painful pressure injuries	Water or glycerin-based gels, impregnated gauze, or sheet dressings	Hypergel CarraSorb Nu-gel Curafil
Negative pressure wound therapy (NPWT)	Used in deep open wounds and covered with transparent polyvinyl dressing; uses gentle negative pressure to remove drainage and contaminants Allows new growth of blood vessels and increased circulation to promote healing; maintains a moist environment	Sterile foam dressing that is packed loosely into the wound or injury; an adhesive drape is applied over it to form an airtight seal; a vacuum source attaches to the motor unit and causes negative pressure	Wound VAC

Continued

Table 26.2 Types and Purposes of Dressings—cont'd

Type	*Purpose*	*Composition*	*Examples*
Silicone	Used as a dressing layer that contacts the wound bed to prevent damage when dressings changed; silicone layers do not absorb exudate, rather it passes through to a secondary absorbent dressing Recommended for skin tears and superficial burns	Soft and tacky dressing that conforms well to dry surfaces; should not be placed in a moist wound bed	Askina DresSil Mepitel Adaptic Touch Comfitel
Transparent films	Used on clean wounds without drainage; can be used to hold other dressings or IVs in place; can be used as a secondary dressing for pressure injuries treated with alginates or other filler that will remain in place several days	Transparent adhesive that is semipermeable; keeps oxygen and moisture in but bacteria out	Bioclusive Opsite Skintact Tegaderm

KNOWLEDGE CONNECTION

When would you expect to see wound irrigation ordered for your patient? Why is moisture necessary for wounds to heal?

Securing Dressings

Once dressings are in place, they must be secured well enough to keep the outer dressing fixed and to keep any additional dressings beneath it from becoming dislodged. Tape is one option for holding dressings in place. Several types of tapes are available, including foam tape, silk tape, and paper tape. Foam tape is thicker than the other types and anchors well. Paper tape is a good choice for those with thin, fragile skin, such as elderly individuals as well as patients who are allergic to other types of tape.

In addition to tape, dressings may be held in place with Montgomery straps or abdominal binders. Montgomery straps attach to the skin with adhesive on either side of the wound. The slotted flaps lay over the dressing and lace up with narrow gauze strips that are then tied together. They are used when frequent dressing changes are necessary so that tape does not have to be removed frequently from the skin. Figure 26.12 shows Montgomery straps in use.

Abdominal binders can also be used to hold abdominal dressings in place. Because they are made of elastic and held in place with Velcro, they tend to apply some pressure to the incision, which may be uncomfortable for the patient. They are often used when the incision needs extra support.

Taping Dressings

When taping a dressing to a joint, place the tape across the joint, allowing movement without dislodging the dressing (Fig. 26.13). When taping dressings to other areas, place the tape at the top and bottom edges, catching both dressing and skin, and then add one or two pieces of tape across the middle. Use enough tape to overlap the dressing by 1 ½ to 2 inches on either side. Avoid allowing the edges of the dressing to curl down over the tape at the top or bottom because that can contaminate the wound.

KNOWLEDGE CONNECTION

When would you consider using Montgomery straps? How would you tape a dressing to a patient's elbow area?

Nursing Responsibilities for Applying Dressings

Applying dressings to an open wound is considered a sterile procedure in most situations. Gloves should always be worn, and a gown, goggles, and mask are worn when there is danger of splashing. You must keep a good "sterile conscience"; that is, you must admit to any breaks in technique and start over to protect your patient from possible infection.

You are also responsible for assessing the wound during a dressing change. Measure the length, width, and depth of the wound. Inspect the wound for dark pink or red granulation tissue, as well as yellow or black tissue. Note the location

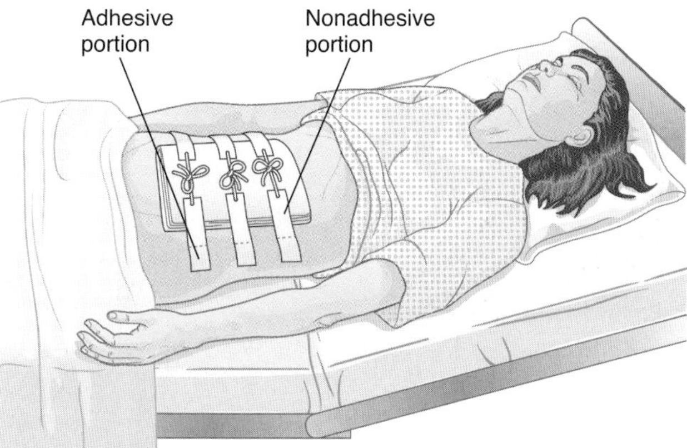

FIGURE 26.12 Montgomery straps may be used to hold an abdominal dressing in place to prevent the need to remove tape with each dressing change (from Wilkinson JM, Treas LM. *Fundamentals of Nursing: Theory, Concepts & Applications.* Vol. 1. 3rd ed. Philadelphia, PA: FA Davis; 2016).

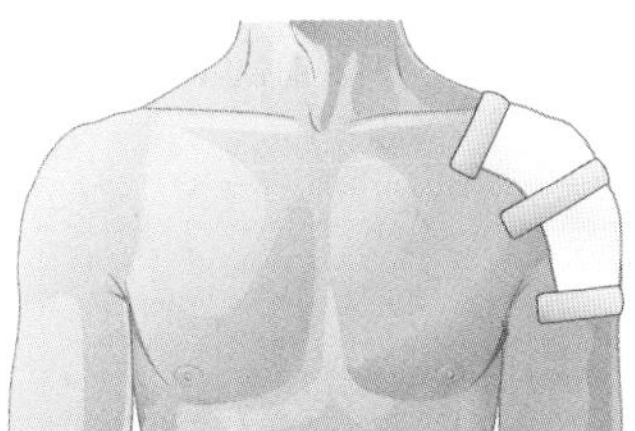

FIGURE 26.13 The correct placement of tape to secure a dressing over a joint.

and length of sinus tracts connected with the wound. Assess the type of drainage on the old dressing for color and amount. Remove your gloves and wash your hands before applying a new dressing. Follow orders for irrigation or cleansing of the wound. Apply the new dressing carefully, following orders for the type of dressing. Write the date, time, and your initials on the new dressing.

Elder Care Connection

Wound Care of Elderly Patients

Elderly patients with wounds can be a challenge. Because of physiological factors, wounds in elders heal more slowly. In addition, the elderly may not see well enough to observe changes in wounds, so infection may occur without the patients realizing it. It may be difficult for elderly patients to change their own dressings with good technique. The cost of supplies for wound care may deter them from getting care they need. Decreased circulation to extremities may prevent elderly patients from experiencing the degree of pain normally associated with a stasis ulcer or extremity wound, therefore leading to a delay in seeking treatment.

Settings Connection: Home Health

Wound Care

Often nurses make visits in the home health-care setting to perform dressing changes. The case manager generally opens the case, formulates the care plan, and manages the care. Field nurses make daily visits to change the dressing and observe the wound. In home health care, different nurses may make visits on different days. A "weekend nurse" may make the Saturday and Sunday visits. So, it is very important that each nurse document thoroughly his or her observations about the size, shape, and color of the wound, as well as the nature of the wound drainage. The nurses' description of the wound and how it is healing is the only information used to determine Medicare reimbursement, so it is important to show progress in wound healing or a change in the plan of care if the wound is not healing.

Supervision/Delegation Connection

Wound Care and Unlicensed Assistive Personnel

In some states the registered nurse or licensed practical/vocational nurse (LPN/LVN) can delegate certain tasks to unlicensed assistive personnel (UAPs), including applying a simple dressing such as a bandage or gauze and tape. Under no circumstances should the packing or assessment of a wound be delegated. In some states, UAPs may be allowed to obtain a wound specimen or empty a wound drainage container. Be sure you know the laws and rules in your state. When in doubt, do not delegate.

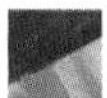 DOCUMENTING WOUND CARE

Accurate documentation of wound care is extremely important. Describe the amount and color of drainage on the old dressing. Document the length, width or diameter, and depth of the wound. Refer to a clock face to describe the interior of the wound, including sinus tracts and their length. Describe the color of the wound and appearance of the surrounding skin. Document the type of dressing applied. It is helpful to say how many gauze 4×4s you used, for example, in a wet-to-damp dressing, so that the next nurse knows exactly what to prepare.

Review documentation to be sure that the wound is getting smaller, not larger. This is essential for third-party payers to continue to pay for care. If the wound is not getting smaller over several days or a week, notify the health-care provider. Different orders may be necessary to promote healing. (See Figure 26.14 for an example of electronic documentation of wound care.)

5 Right Buttocks

☐ Wound Healed

Cancel Save

Charts

☐ Surgical
☒ Lesions
☐ Decubitus
☐ Burns
☐ Body Modifications

Wound Category:

☒ Open Wound
☐ Skin Tear
☐ Abrasion
☐ Laceration
☐ Bruising (Contusion)
☐ Puncture

Length 3.0 cm
Width 2.0 cm
Depth 2.0 cm

Wound Area:

☒ Open wound with subcutaneous tissue exposed
☐ Open wound with subcutaneous tissue and muscle exposed
☐ Open wound with subcutaneous tissue and muscle/bone exposed
☐ Skin graft intact
☐ Skin graft not intact
☐ Wound edges are attached
☒ Undermining at wound edges

Wound Drainage/Exudate:

☐ No drainage
☐ Scant drainage/exudates
☐ Minimal drainage/exudates
☐ Moderate drainage/exudates
☐ Copious drainage/exudates
☒ Draining serous fluid
☐ Draining serosanguinous fluid

Peri-Wound Area:

☒ Red
☐ Pink
☐ Excoriation
☐ Maceration
☐ Warm to touch
☐ Swollen
☒ Painful

Dressing and Wound Care:

☐ Occlusive dressing
☐ Dressing clean, dry and intact
☐ Wound cleansing & dressing change per MD orders
☒ Wound cleansing & dressing change per hospital protocol
☐ Cleansed with soap and water
☐ Wet to damp dressing change
☒ Aseptic technique during the wound care

Dressing and Wound Care:

☐ None
☒ Normal saline
☐ Betadine
☐ Hydrogen peroxide
☐ Iodine
☐ Alcohol
☐ Dakin's Solution

Interventions:

☒ Increasing nutrition and hydration
☐ Keeping skin clean and dry
☐ Using paper tape
☐ Tape removal done slowly
☒ Using absorbent dressings to absorb exudates
☐ Using debriding products
☐ Packing wound to increase proper healing

Patient Response:

☐ No complaints at this time
☐ Tolerated procedure well
☒ Reports procedural pain
☐ Refused dressing change
☐ Complaints with rushing regimen
☐ Non-compliant with nursing regimen
☐ Voices understanding of teaching

Notes:

mm/dd/yyyy 0900 Patient reported pain of 5 on a scale of 1 to 10. Administered analgesic 30 minutes prior to dressing change. See MAR. Two pieces of black foam removed. Two pieces of black foam replaced to obliterate undermining using modified sterile technique. Activated negative pressure wound therapy unit to 125 mmHg.

Cancel Save

FIGURE 26.14 Sample EHR documentation.

Nursing Care Plan for a Patient With an Infected Stage 2 Pressure Injury

Assessment

You are assigned to care for Ms. Moreau. The patient is an 81-year-old female with no circulatory diseases. She has a stage 2 pressure injury on her left heel.

Your first step in planning care for her is to gather all the available data. An assessment of the injury must be made so it can be staged, including the location, size, depth, color, condition of the surrounding skin, drainage, odor, and discomfort level.

- **Location:** The injury is over a bony prominence. Will pressure be exerted on it while the patient is sitting or lying in the supine, prone, or lateral position?
- **Size:** What is the width? Length? Measure both.
- **Depth:** How deep is the injury? Which layers of tissue are involved? If it goes beyond a shallow crater, you may use a long-handled sterile cotton-tipped swab to mark the depth. Insert it into the deepest part of the crater and mark the height of the skin surface with your thumb. Then hold the swab next to a measuring device to determine the actual measurement. Is there undermining? Are there any sinus tracts?
- **Color:** What color is the skin around the injury? What color is the base of the injury? Is there granulation tissue (grains of soft, fragile pinkish-red tissue)? Eschar tissue (firm, brown or black)?
- **Condition of surrounding skin:** Is the skin around the injury sloughing? Intact? Are the edges of the wound rolled?
- **Drainage:** Is there drainage? Is it serous, serosanguineous, sanguineous, or purulent? How much drainage is there?
- **Odor:** Does the wound or drainage have a foul odor?
- **Discomfort level:** Is there tenderness or pain? What number on a pain scale from 0 to 10?

It is also important to note if the patient's WBC is elevated.

Nursing Care Plan for a Patient With an Infected Stage 2 Pressure Injury—cont'd

You must assess nutritional factors and risk factors relating to the development and treatment of a pressure injury, including diet, hydration, and lab work such as hemoglobin and serum protein levels. What risk factors does this patient have?

After your assessment, you determine that the pressure injury on Ms. Moreau's left heel measures 1.5 by 2.5 cm, with a depth of 0.5 cm. The skin around the injury is erythemic and slightly warmer than the surrounding skin. The injury bed is bright red with tiny red bumpy tissue across most of the injury. There is a moderate amount of yellow purulent drainage on the dressing. The drainage has no odor, and the patient denies any discomfort. The patient can no longer walk, but she is able to sit in a chair with assistance. She spends several hours per day in bed. Her appetite is fair, but she eats little meat because of poorly-fitting dentures. Her lab work is normal except for slightly lowered hemoglobin and serum protein levels. She has lost 6 pounds in the past 2 weeks.

Nursing Diagnoses

Review what you have learned about this particular patient.

Ms. Moreau has good circulation to her feet and has no history of an injury to her heel. Her mobility is limited, and she spends most of her time in the bed or a wheelchair. Without any evidence to indicate another cause, it probably is safe to assume the wound on her heel is a pressure injury with infection due to the purulent drainage and erythema. Her weight loss, difficulty eating meat, and lab results are indicative of nutritional problems.

By grouping the information this way, you can identify that this patient has a problem with skin integrity that seems to be related to direct pressure on the heel. The injury is not healing well, and that may be a direct result of poor nutrition and continued pressure on the heel. The two priority nursing diagnoses given for this patient are:

- Impaired skin integrity (a stage 2 pressure injury that is infected)
- Inadequate nutrition (less than her body demands)

Now you can begin planning how to care for these problems (see the nursing diagnoses in the Care Plan below).

Planning

For this patient, appropriate interventions begin with reducing pressure on the patient's left heel while she is in bed and sitting up in a chair.

Because a pressure injury is already present, heel protectors will not be appropriate. A gel pad is a possibility, but the patient has other pressure points that have to be protected from developing further pressure injuries. Consider a gel-filled mattress overlay. Also, the patient said that she prefers to be up several times a day, so the plan should be to get her into a chair at least three times daily.

Plan to relieve heel pressure by elevating the lower legs on pillows and allow the patient's heels to overhang the pillows. When the patient is in a chair, plan to use a combination of a stool and pillows to prop her left leg so that the heel does not rest on the stool. Plan to assess the wound frequently for signs and symptoms of worsening or improving infection and wound healing.

Identify high-protein foods and supplements that she likes and notify the dietary department as well as other staff of her preferences. Determine if she has difficulty chewing meat and, if so, ask the dietary service to grind it for her.

To determine if these interventions are working, plan to monitor the patient's laboratory results to see if her hemoglobin and serum protein levels begin to rise after the dietary changes and to take daily weights.

Implementation

At this stage of the nursing process, you can now implement the interventions that you have planned (see interventions in the Care Plan below).

Evaluation

The last step in the nursing process is to evaluate whether the interventions you have been implementing are helping (see evaluations in the Care Plan below). It appears that the injury is indeed healing, and the patient's blood levels of protein are slowly coming up toward normal.

Nursing Diagnosis: Impaired skin integrity, related to infected pressure injury on left heel, as evidenced by tissue destruction of stage 2 pressure injury

Expected Outcomes: Patient will have no evidence of infection at discharge: normal WBC, no fever, wound bed pink and moist.

Patient will show no evidence of new skin breakdown or extension of current wound dimensions at discharge.

Interventions	Evaluations
Keep a gel-filled overlay pad on top of the mattress.	Day 2: No new skin breakdown. States she sleeps better on the gel overlay. Day 5: No new skin breakdown. Day 6: No new skin breakdown.
Reposition the patient every 2 hours when in bed.	Day 2: Requires no assist to reposition but has to be cued. Cap. refill brisk × 4 extremities. Day 4: Now turns self without cueing except while sleeping. Turning schedule maintained by staff at night. Cap. refill brisk bilaterally × 4 extremities.

(nursing care plan continues on page 544)

Nursing Care Plan for a Patient With an Infected Stage 2 Pressure Injury—cont'd

Interventions	Evaluations
Elevate both lower legs on a small pillow to keep the heels off the bed.	Day 2: Prefers to let heels overhang the end of the bed to avoid contact with bed. Skin around wound intact, pink, dry. Day 4: Skin on Rt. heel intact. Day 6: Rt. heel without erythema.
Keep pillows between the knees and ankles when the patient is lying in the lateral position.	Day 2: Body alignment maintained. States the support feels better than letting bony places rub together. Day 4: No erythema on knees or ankles. Day 6: Skin on knees and ankles intact.
Assist the patient out of bed to sit in a chair for 1–2 hours at mealtimes and at least one other time during the day that patient would like to be out of bed.	Day 2: States enjoys being up more. Often sits up most of evening. Day 4: Sits up most of evening and 2–2.5 hours in a.m. Day 6: Continues to voice enjoyment of time out of bed.
When the patient is up in a chair, elevate the feet on a footstool using a pillow to keep the left heel off the surface of the stool.	Day 2: Compliant, keeps feet elevated and heels off stool. Slight edema of Lt. heel. Day 4: Edema decreased, nearly gone. Day 6: No edema.
Change Mepilex foam dressing every other day as ordered. Assess injury and drainage, documenting in the nurse's notes daily.	Day 2: Continues w/ sm. amt. serous drainage. No change in size. Day 4: Scant serous drainage. Beginning to granulate. Day 6: Injury improving, granulating well, pink & moist. Measures 0.5 cm × 1.5 cm, depth 3–4 mm. No drainage for past 7 days.
Monitor WBC counts and signs and symptoms of infection in the wound.	Day 1: WBC 11,350/mm³. Day 4: WBC 7,900/mm³. Day 6: Healing well. See above assessment. Continue to use sterile technique. No fever. WBC 7,500/mm³ (within normal limits).

Nursing Diagnosis: Imbalanced nutrition, less than body requirements, related to inability to chew meat as evidenced by recent loss of 6 pounds (2.72 kg)
Expected Outcome: Patient will increase high-protein foods in diet, including protein supplements, and will increase weight by 5 pounds (2.27 kg) within 10 days.

Interventions	Evaluations
Provide brand Z high-calorie, high-protein drink between meals and at bedtime.	Day 2: Consumes 100% of supplement consistently. Likes chocolate better than vanilla. Day 6: Consumes 100% of supplement most days.
Provide a high-protein diet. The patient likes peanut butter, beans, cheese, and eggs. Grind meat for ease of chewing.	Day 2: Eats 80%–100% of meals consistently. Frequently requests & eats peanut butter & crackers. Eats eggs for breakfast daily. Eating ground meat without problems. Day 6: Eats more than 80% of meals & snacks.
Monitor laboratory results—hemoglobin, serum protein—noting drops or failure to increase.	Serum protein @ admission: 5.8 g/dL (below normal). Day 4: 6.2 g/dL (WNL). Day 6: 6.4 g/dL. Hgb @ admission: 11.9 g/dL (little low). Day 6: 12.1 g/dL (low normal).
Record daily weights, noting losses.	Admit: 129 lbs. Day 2: 129.5 lbs. Day 4: 131 lbs. Day 6: 132 lbs.

Skill 26.1 Removing Sutures and Staples

Assessment Steps

1. Review the health-care provider's order for specific instructions, such as orders to remove alternating staples rather than all staples. In orthopedic surgeries, orders are often written to remove alternating staples one day and any remaining staples the next day.
2. Assess the patient's pain level and medicate if needed. Discomfort associated with suture or staple removal usually is mild and brief. However, ***if the patient is already experiencing significant pain, removal of closures may exacerbate it.***

Planning Step

1. Gather needed equipment and supplies: clean gloves; a suture removal kit or staple removal kit; and reinforced adhesive strips, such as Steri-Strips.

Intervention Steps

1. Follow the Initial Implementation Steps located on the inside back cover.
2. Open the peel pack containing the suture removal set or staple remover.

Removing Sutures

3. Using the forceps in the removal kit, grasp the knot of the suture with your nondominant hand and lift the suture away from the skin.
4. Using the notched scissors from the removal kit in your dominant hand, slide the notched blade under the suture. Cut the suture next to the skin, adjacent to the knot.
5. As soon as the suture is clipped, pull smoothly and firmly with your nondominant hand. The suture will slide out, and ***the contaminated portion of the suture will not be pulled through the skin.***
6. Remove every other suture and observe the wound edges for any signs of separation. ***This helps prevent the possibility of dehiscence when all sutures are removed.***
7. Remove the remaining sutures, unless otherwise ordered.

Removing Staples

3. Hold the staple remover in your dominant hand.
4. Slide the lower hooked jaw under the middle of the staple.
5. Gently squeeze the handles together. The staple ends will slide upward out of the skin.
6. Remove alternating staples while continually assessing wound edges for evidence of separation. *Safety: If there is any indication that edges might be separating, stop and do not remove any more staples. Apply Steri-Strips and notify the health-care provider.*

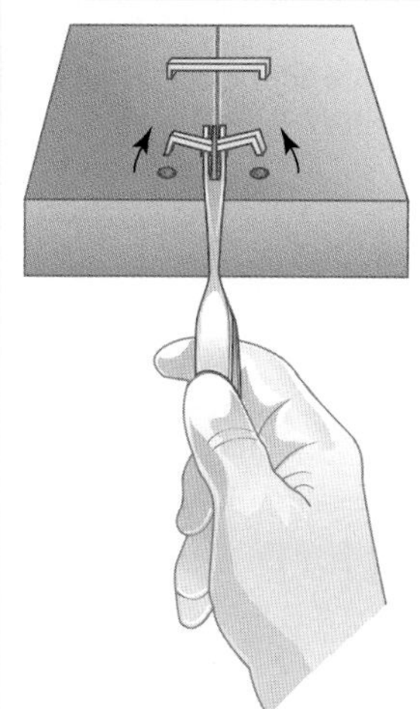

7. If wound edges remain approximated, continue to remove the rest of the staples as ordered.

Cleaning and Dressing the Wound

8. Gently wipe the area with an alcohol pad or saline-soaked gauze 4×4 ***to remove debris and dried blood, which could become a medium for bacteria growth. Note: Follow facility policy because some facilities may require the use of alcohol or chlorhexidine gluconate swabs rather than saline.***
9. Place Steri-Strips across the incision area. ***This provides extra support to wound edges as healing continues.***
10. If desired by the patient, cover the incision with a gauze 4×4 ***to protect the wound from irritation by clothing.***
11. Follow the Ending Implementation Steps located on the inside back cover.
12. Document the procedure and appearance of the wound.

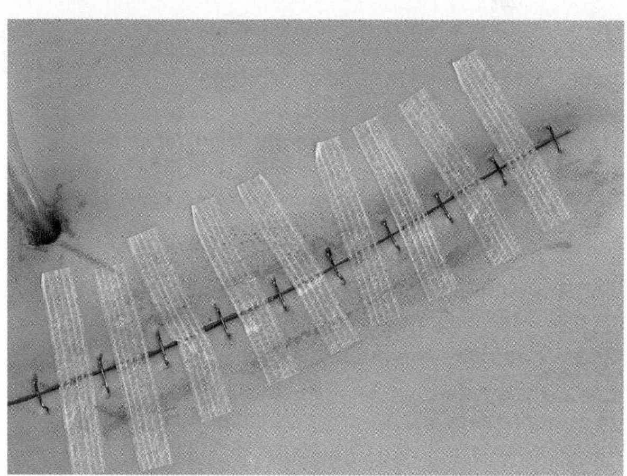

(skill continues on page 546)

Skill 26.1 (continued)

Evaluation Step

1. Check the incision line after a few hours ***to be sure the incision edges remain approximated after patient activity.***

Sample Documentation

05/31/22 1120 Rt. hip incision well approximated, without erythema, edema, or drainage. Every other staple (6 staples) removed and Steri-Strips applied (7 staples remaining). Incision integrity remains intact. Denies incisional discomfort.
——————— Nurse's signature and credentials

Skill 26.2 Caring for Drainage Devices

Assessment Steps

1. Review the health-care provider's order for frequency to empty the drainage device. It should be emptied at the end of the shift or when it is one-half to two-thirds full unless otherwise indicated in the order.
2. Assess the amount and characteristics of the drainage in the drain container.

Planning Step

1. Gather needed equipment and supplies: water-repellant drape, graduated container, clean gloves, two alcohol sponges, and goggles if splashing is possible.

Implementation Steps

1. Follow the Initial Implementation Steps located on the inside back cover.
2. Don clean gloves and apply goggles ***to follow standard precautions when handling the drainage device.*** Unpin the drain from the patient's gown.
3. Place the water-repellant drape under the drainage device ***to prevent soiling linens.***
4. Assess the drain insertion site for erythema, edema, and drainage ***to detect any signs of infection.***
5. Wipe the drain spout with an alcohol sponge ***to prevent introducing microorganisms into the drain.*** Avoid raising the drainage device above the insertion site. ***This prevents reflux of contents into the wound bed, which decreases the risk of infection.***
6. Pointing the spout away from your face, open the spout and pour the contents into the graduated container so that it can be measured, taking care to avoid splashing.
7. Clean around the drain spout with a new alcohol sponge.
8. Compress the drainage device with it pointed away from you ***to establish suction*** (known as ***reactivating*** the drain) and close the spout without contaminating it. Pin the drain tubing back to the patient's gown.
9. Note the amount, color, and other characteristics of the drainage before pouring the contents down the toilet.

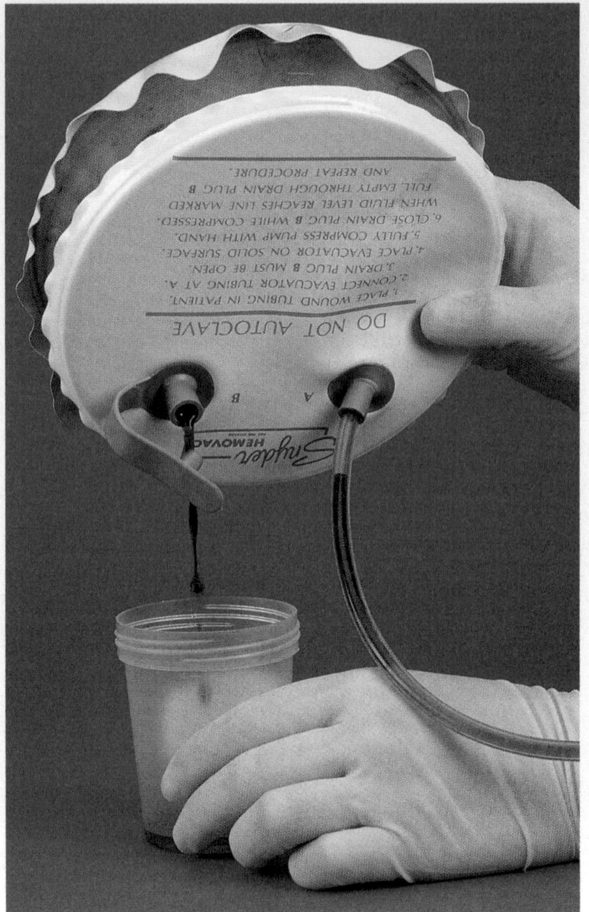

10. Follow the Ending Implementation Steps located on the inside back cover.
11. Document the volume and characteristics of the drainage emptied as well as the assessment of the drain insertion site.

Skill 26.2 (continued)

Evaluation Steps

1. Compare the amount and appearance of the drainage with previous descriptions for evidence of decreasing drainage production.
2. Make certain the drainage system is draining and remains below wound height.

Sample Documentation

10/08/22 1100 J-P drain emptied of 110 mL serosanguineous drainage. Drain insertion site in RUQ abdomen without erythema, drainage, or edema. JP reactivated and secured to gown below level of wound site. ——————————————— Nurse's signature and credentials

Skill 26.3 Irrigating a Wound

Assessment Steps

1. Review the health-care provider's orders ***to determine the type of solution and frequency of irrigation.***
2. Assess the patient's pain level and medicate if needed. ***Irrigation usually is part of a dressing change, which may be uncomfortable for the patient.***

Planning Steps

1. Gather needed equipment and supplies: emesis basin, sterile saline or other ordered solution, sterile irrigation kit or basin, 35-mL syringe and 19-gauge Angiocath for correct pressure, bed protector, gown, goggles, mask, and clean gloves.
2. Obtain sterile drape for setting up a sterile field. ***Note: Some nurses find it helpful to obtain a sterile towel or drape to use to prepare a small sterile field upon which to place sterile items.*** Some irrigation kits have a sterile drape that may also be used as a mini sterile field.
3. Prepare for dressing change as well with a biohazard bag, sterile dressings, and sterile gloves ***because irrigation usually is performed during a dressing change.***
4. Enlist assistance if needed ***to keep the patient in the correct position during the procedure.***

Intervention Steps

1. Follow the Initial Implementation Steps located on the inside back cover. Don a gown, goggles, and mask ***to protect yourself from splashing.***
2. Set up the sterile field for your supplies. Remember to include any dressing supplies that you may need to redress the wound.
3. Don clean gloves.
4. Remove old dressing and place in the biohazard bag.
5. Remove contaminated gloves and sanitize your hands.
6. Pour sterile saline into a sterile basin or irrigation kit.
7. Open the Angiocath and the syringe packages without contaminating the sterile items and drop them onto the sterile field.
8. Position the patient in a manner that will best allow the irrigation solution to drain from the wound into the emesis basin that will be positioned at the wound's edge.
9. Place the bed protector on the bed ***to prevent the irrigant from soaking the bed.***
10. Position the emesis basin underneath the bottom edge of the wound and prop it with a towel or washcloth ***to catch the irrigant as it flows from the wound.*** If the patient is able to assist you, he or she may be able to hold the basin in place.
11. Don sterile gloves.
12. Carefully remove the Angiocath sheath from the needle, laying the needle back on the sterile field. Touch the hub of the Angiocath only. Do not touch the sheath. Attach the hub of the 19-gauge Angiocath sheath to the 35-mL syringe. ***These sizes ensure the ideal amount of pressure to remove debris without damaging any granulation tissue that may be present.*** *Safety: Leave the needle on the sterile field until you are done with the procedure so that you can open the lid to the wall-mounted sharps container without contaminating your sterile gloves.*
13. Draw up 25 to 30 mL of irrigating solution into the syringe.

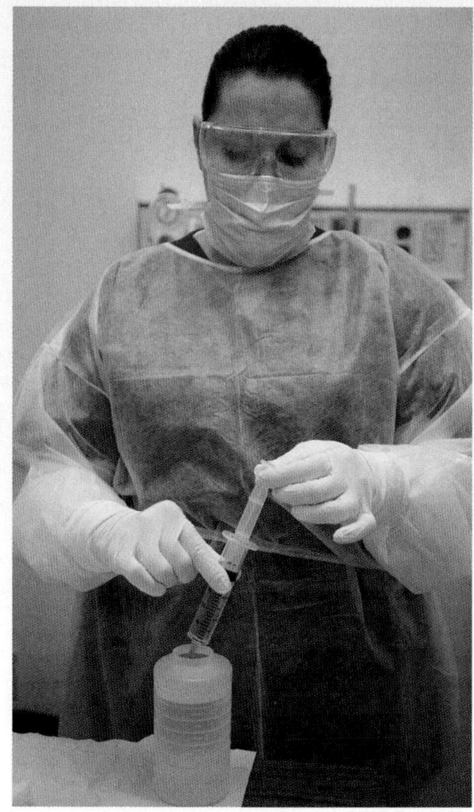

14. Hold the syringe so that the Angiocath is approximately 1 inch (2.5 cm) from the wound surface, starting at the

(skill continues on page 548)

Skill 26.3 (continued)

superior edge of the wound. Depress the syringe plunger to cause a steady spray of fluid into the wound ***to wash away debris.*** Spray using a back-and-forth motion, moving from one side of the wound to the opposite side, and gradually working your way from the top of the wound to the bottom wound edge. ***This prevents rinsing debris back into previously cleansed areas.***

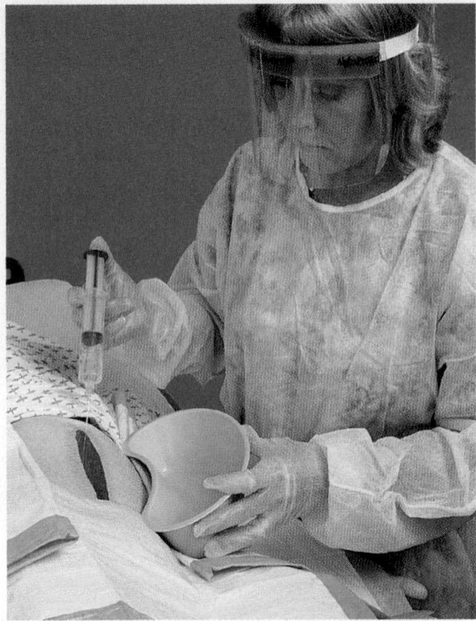

15. Continue filling the syringe and irrigating the wound until the fluid leaving the wound is clear. ***This ensures that all debris has been removed.*** Remove the basin.
16. Using a sterile gauze 4×4 with the four corners bunched up between your fingers, dry the skin around the outside perimeter of the wound. Avoid touching the interior of the wound ***to prevent cross-contamination.***
17. Inspect the wound and note the size, depth, and color. Note the amount and color of any necrotic tissue.
18. Dispose of the contaminated irrigation fluid according to facility policy.
19. Apply a new dressing following the steps in Skill 26.5.
20. Follow the Ending Implementation Steps located on the inside back cover.
21. Document the procedure, including the type and amount of solution used, the appearance of the return fluid, an assessment of the wound, and the type of dressing applied.

Evaluation Step

1. Determine the effectiveness of wound cleansing using irrigation. Note whether any loose, necrotic tissue is mostly removed after irrigation. Notify the health-care provider if irrigation is not effective.

Sample Documentation

01/25/22 0930 States no wound discomfort and does not desire pain med before irrigation. 4×4 dressing removed with 2-cm spot of dried serous drainage. Puncture wound edges mildly pink. Wound measures 1/2 cm across and 4 cm deep. Irrigated with sterile NS 100 mL using 19-g Angiocath and 35-mL syringe, using sterile technique. Wound covered with five sterile gauze 4×4s. No c/o discomfort at any time.
———————— Nurse's signature and credentials

Skill 26.4 Obtaining a Wound Culture

Assessment Steps

1. Review the health-care provider's order for an aerobic or anaerobic culture.
2. Assess the wound and the type of dressing, if there is one, ***to determine supplies you will need to replace the dressing.***

Planning Steps

1. If the patient already has a dressing change scheduled, ***performing the culture at the same time as the dressing change will save time.***
2. Gather needed equipment and supplies for the dressing change and supplies for the wound culture: clean gloves and a sterile Culturette tube with cotton-tipped swab.

Implementation Steps

1. Follow the Initial Implementation Steps located on the inside back cover.
2. Irrigate or cleanse the wound first ***to remove exudate. Surface pathogens are not necessarily the cause of the wound infection.***
3. Don clean gloves and remove the old dressing if present.
4. Holding the Culturette container in your nondominant hand, loosen the cap and remove the Culturette swab from container with your dominant hand. ***Use caution to avoid contaminating the distal cotton-tipped end of the swab.***
5. Holding only the proximal tip of the Culturette swab, swirl the distal cotton-tipped end only on the granulation tissue in the wound bed. Avoid touching the cotton tip to the outer edges of the wound ***because normal flora (microorganisms that live on the patient's skin) can contaminate the culture.*** Do not swab areas where slough or eschar are present or roll the swab in a pool of exudate ***because the culture will not reflect microorganisms only present in the wound.***

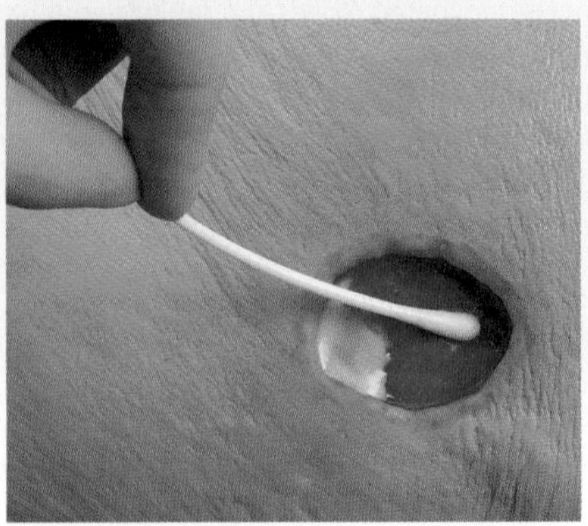

Skill 26.4 (continued)

6. Quickly place the distal cotton-tipped end of the swab back into the Culturette container, ***using care to avoid touching it to the outside edges of the container.*** Push the cap tightly onto the container. Crush the ampule in the bottom of the tube, if present. ***This releases culture medium and moisture to keep the microorganisms alive.***
7. If a dressing was present, replace it using sterile technique.
8. Label the container with the patient's name, room number, ID number, and birthdate, as well as the physician's name, the date and time, and the name of the test to be performed.
9. Arrange for transport to the lab. Do not refrigerate.
10. Follow the Ending Implementation Steps located on the inside back cover.

Evaluation Steps

1. Evaluate the patient's pain level during and after obtaining the culture.
2. Assess laboratory results of the culture after 48 and 72 hours.

Sample Documentation

08/13/22 0730 Surgical incision on RLQ abdomen with poor approximation on lateral aspect. 1.5-cm open area. 0.5-cm deep, oozing moderate amount thick yellow purulent drainage. Wound irrigated per order. Wound culture obtained and sent to lab. C/o incisional tenderness using scale of 0 to 10, a 1 before performing culture, a 2 during, and a 1 afterward. ——————

—————— Nurse's signature and credentials

Skill 26.5 Changing Sterile Dressings and Wet-to-Damp Dressings

Assessment Steps

1. Review the health-care provider's order and previous nurses' notes on the dressing change. ***This will help you know how many dressings and what type you will need.***
2. Assess the patient's pain level. Medicate at least 30 minutes prior to performing the dressing change. ***This will help keep the patient comfortable during a potentially uncomfortable procedure.***

Planning Steps

1. Gather needed equipment and supplies: dressings (sterile gauze 4×4s and abdominal dressings), tape, clean gloves, a biohazard discard bag, sterile cotton-tipped swabs, a paper wound ruler, and sterile gloves. ***For the wet-to-damp dressing change,*** you will also need a sterile basin or a dressing change kit and a pour-top bottle of sterile normal saline.
2. Enlist assistance, if needed, to keep the patient positioned off of the wound during the dressing change ***to prevent possible contamination of the wound during the procedure.***

Implementation Steps

1. Follow the Initial Implementation Steps located on the inside back cover.
2. Wash hands and follow standard precautions ***to prevent transmission of blood-borne pathogens.***
3. Set up a sterile field, adding all additional sterile supplies that you will need. ***Note: If you will be pouring sterile liquids, drape a sterile barrier with a moisture-proof backing over the clean over-bed table. This will keep your field sterile even if you splash sterile solution onto it.***
   If Applying a Wet-to-Damp Dressing: Additional supplies must be prepared as part of the sterile field:
   - Check the label on the bottle of sterile normal saline three times ***to make certain you have the right solution.*** Check the manufacturer's date of expiration ***to ensure it is still in date.*** If the bottle has been previously opened, also check the date and time the nurse has written on the label. ***If bottle has been open for longer than 24 hours, it can no longer be considered sterile. Dispose of it and obtain a new bottle.***
   - If the bottle has never been opened, write the date, time, and your initials on the label. ***This tells the next nurse who will change the dressing when the normal saline was opened.***
   - Remove the cap from the bottle and place it on the table next to the sterile field drape with the open rim pointing upward.
   - ***Note: If the bottle has been previously opened and is still within the 24-hour window, hold the bottle over the trash can and pour out a small amount of saline. The liquid pouring over the lip of the bottle helps to wash away any microorganisms that might be present. This process is known as "lipping" the bottle.***
   - Pour saline into the sterile basin or the well of the dressing change kit to use in preparing the wet-to-damp dressings. **Alternative:** If bulk sterile gauze 4×4s are supplied in a separate plastic tub or tray, you can pour the saline directly over the gauze 4×4s without taking them out of the sterile tray. It can serve as a mini sterile field.
4. Open and position the biohazard bag ***to receive contaminated waste.***

Remove Old Dressing

5. Don clean gloves ***to follow standard precautions when handling the old dressing.***
6. Loosen the tape on the old dressing by gently pulling it from each side toward the wound. ***This prevents tension on wound edges.***
7. Remove the old dressing and inspect the color and amount of the drainage present.

(skill continues on page 550)

Skill 26.5 (continued)

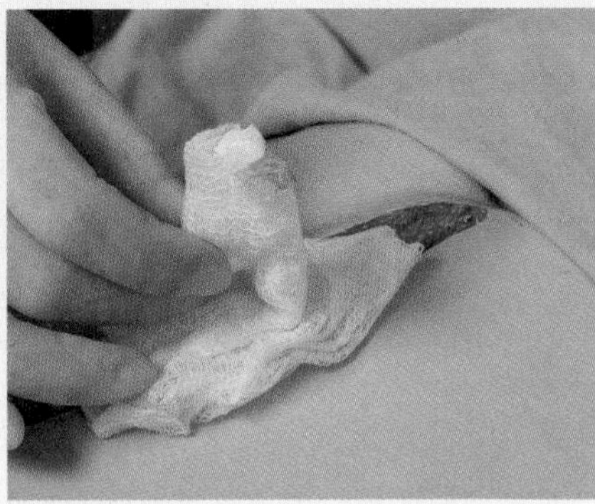

Assess the Wound

8. Inspect the wound and assess the color, odor, and presence of sinus tracts. Also assess for the presence of granulation tissue.
9. Measure the length, width, and depth of the wound ***to determine degree of healing.*** To measure the wound length and width, use either a paper wound ruler or a transparent cellophane wound-sizing device. Hold the measuring device above the wound without touching the wound surface. ***Hint: Use a sterile cotton-tipped swab to measure the depth of the wound and of any sinus tracts.***
   - Information obtained in Steps 7, 8, and 9 is important for accurate documentation and may indicate complications to wound healing.

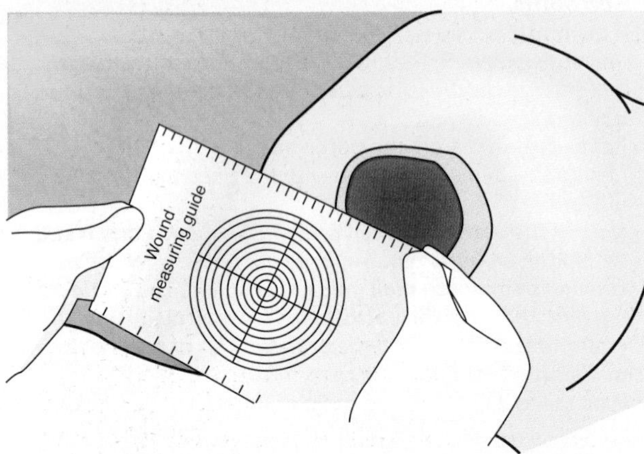

10. If a drain is present, assess the drain insertion site for erythema and edema.

Cleanse the Wound

11. Remove contaminated gloves.
12. Apply sterile gloves, taking care to maintain sterility of the gloves and sterile field.
13. Clean wound as ordered ***to remove exudates and to promote granulation.*** **Alternative:** If wound irrigation has been ordered, it should be done at this time (see Skill 26.3).
14. If a drain is present, clean around it as well.

Apply a Sterile Dressing

15. Apply a new sterile dressing to the wound.

    For a Wet-to-Damp Dressing:
   - Unfold the sterile gauze 4×4s completely and place them in the sterile saline you poured into the basin or well of the kit. **Alternative:** If the bulk gauze 4×4s came in a sterile plastic tub or tray, you can pour saline directly on the gauze 4×4s in their tray.

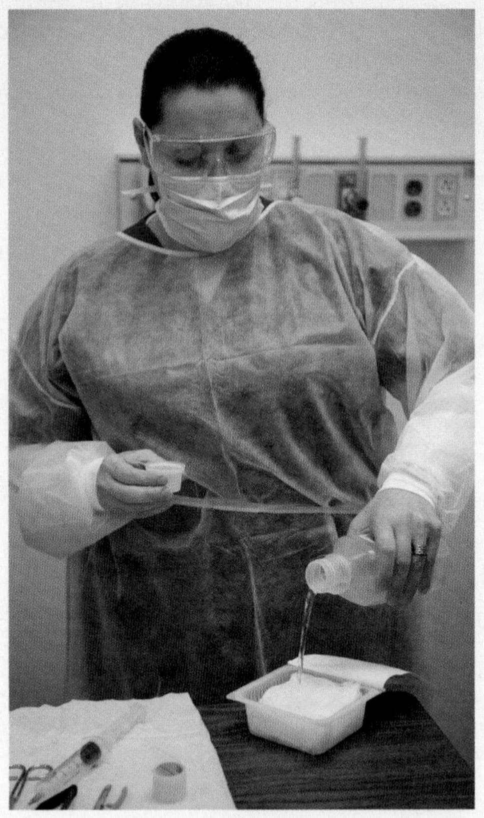

   - Press the excess saline out of a gauze 4×4 until it is moist but not dripping. ***Excessive moisture in the wound may cause maceration (softening) of the skin.***
   - Fluff the gauze 4×4 ***to increase the surface area of the gauze for contact with the wound.***

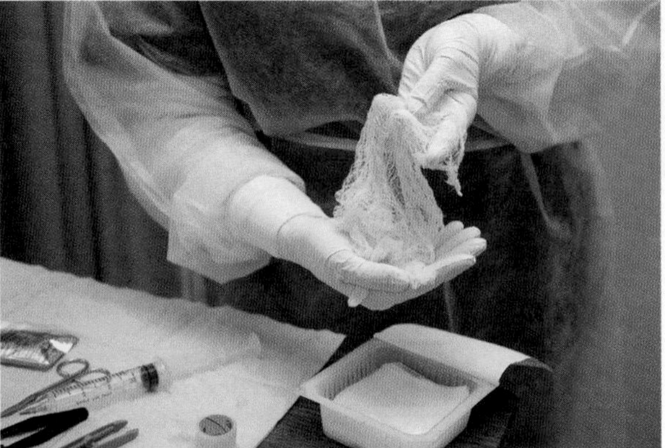

   - Carefully hold the moist gauze 4×4 in your hand, and using sterile forceps from the kit or a sterile swab, gently pack the fluffed gauze 4×4 into the wound. *Safety: Avoid pressing gauze tightly under any overhanging edges of the wound because this will interfere with granulation tissue formation.*

Skill 26.5 (continued)

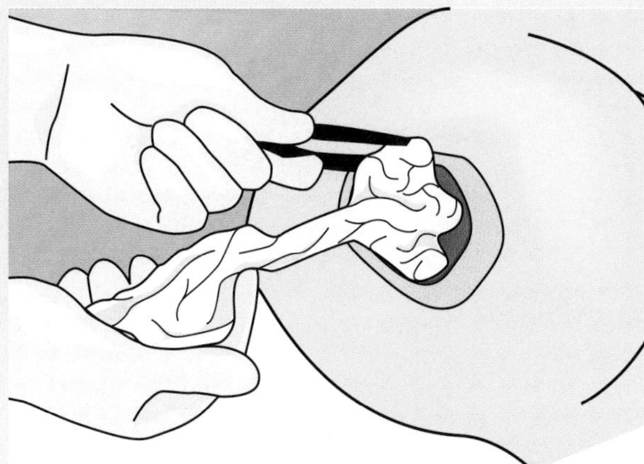

- Do not allow the gauze to touch the skin surface outside the wound. ***This could cause contamination of the wound with surface microbes.***
- Completely fill the wound with fluffed, saline-moistened gauze 4×4s ***to keep all surfaces of the wound moist and promote healing.***

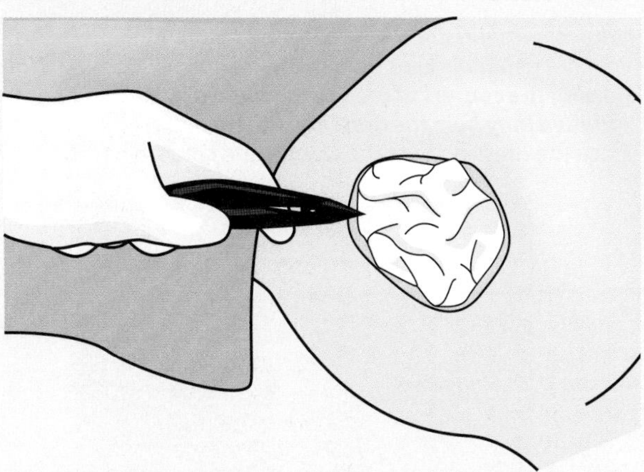

- Cover the filled wound with damp, unfluffed gauze 4×4s ***to help maintain moisture.***
- Cover the unfluffed gauze 4×4s with an abdominal dressing pad, with the stripe on the pad facing outward so that it is visible after the dressing is in place. ***This will hold moisture in the wound, protect it from contaminants, and absorb drainage.***

For a Dry Dressing:

- Cover the wound with enough sterile gauze 4×4s for adequate absorption of drainage. If there is a wound drain, place a split gauze 4×4 around it to prevent maceration of the skin.
- Cover the gauze 4×4s with an abdominal dressing pad. The stripe on the abdominal dressing should be facing outward so that it is visible after the dressing is in place. Use the correct size of abdominal dressing so that it completely covers the gauze 4×4s and drain.

Secure Dressing

16. Tape the superior and inferior edges of the dressing to the skin, taping from one lateral side to the opposite lateral side of the dressing. Then place another piece or two of tape across the middle of the dressing. Make strips of tape long enough to extend beyond dressing edges by 1 ½ to 2 inches.

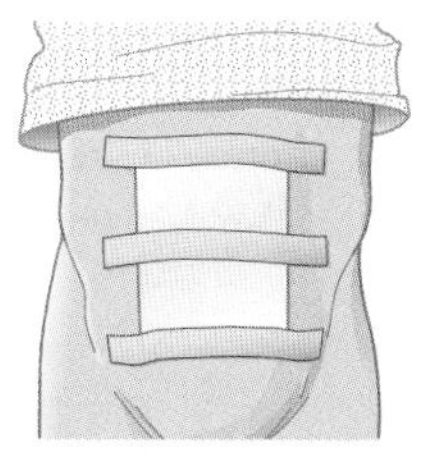

Less length will not adequately secure the dressing. More will result in unnecessary discomfort on removal.

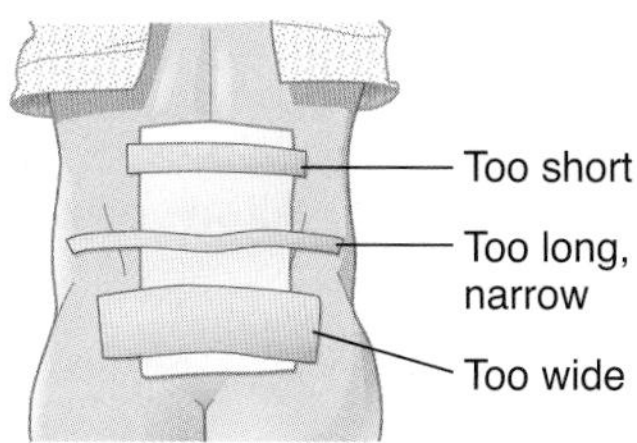

Complete the Dressing Change

17. Remove gloves and wash hands.
18. Write the date, time, and your initials on the edge of the dressing.
19. Dispose of the biohazard bag and used supplies according to facility policy.
20. Follow the Ending Implementation Steps located on the inside back cover.
21. Document the date and time; wound appearance, including size, depth, color, and presence of granulation tissue; amount and type of drainage; dressing change procedure; and your signature and credentials.

Evaluation Steps

1. Compare measurements and appearance of the wound with previous descriptions for evidence of healing.
2. Determine the patient's comfort level during the dressing change ***to ensure adequate pain control with prescribed medications.***
3. Review any laboratory reports, such as wound culture and sensitivity results or WBC counts, for evidence of improving infection indicators.

Sample Documentation

07/19/22 0920 States pain med has reduced pain level from a 6 to a 1 on 0–10 scale. Removed 5 1/2 in. × 9 in. ABD dressing from suprapubic incision. Removed damp packing with moderate amount green purulent drainage. Incision open end-to-end. 15 cm × 2 cm × 2.5 cm deep. Wound bed bright red and some pallor noted on medial aspect. Moderate amount granulation tissue on lateral aspect of wound bed. No erythema or edema of surrounding skin. Wound irrigated with 250 mL St. NS using 19-g Angiocath and 35-mL syringe, using sterile technique. Repacked wound with sterile moist gauze packing. Covered with ABD dressing. C/o pain @ 3 during irrigation and @ 1 on completion of dressing change. ————

———— *Nurse's signature and credentials*

Skill 26.6 Applying Transparent and Hydrocolloid Dressings

Assessment Steps

1. Review the health-care provider's order for dressing change.
2. Determine the need for change of dressing. Has the barrier been in place 3 to 5 days? Is the barrier loosening, leaking, or developing an odor?

Planning Steps

1. Obtain needed equipment and supplies: clean gloves, scissors, a biohazard bag, sterile saline and gauze 4×4s if the wound is to be cleansed, transparent or hydrocolloid dressing as ordered, tape, a disposable paper ruler, and alcohol swabs.
2. Ensure that the size of the dressing is appropriate. Transparent dressings should overlap the wound onto the skin for a 1-inch margin around the wound. For a hydrocolloid dressing, the overlap should be a 1 ¼-inch to 1 ½-inch margin around the wound. ***This helps the dressing adhere to the skin and remain in place.***

Implementation Steps

1. Follow the Initial Implementation Steps located on the inside back cover.
2. Wash hands and don clean gloves ***to follow standard precautions.***

Remove Old Dressing

3. Gently loosen the edges of the dressing and pull it toward the wound ***to prevent tension on the wound edges.***
4. Dispose of the dressing in the biohazard bag ***because it is contaminated with blood and body fluids.***
5. Inspect the wound for amount and type of drainage, odor, and color.
6. Measure the size of the wound using a disposable paper ruler, being careful not to touch the wound. ***This information is needed for documentation.***
7. Remove gloves and wash hands.

Apply New Dressing

8. Apply clean gloves.
9. Clean the wound if ordered. Use sterile saline and sterile gauze 4×4s to gently clean the area. Gather the four corners of a gauze 4×4 together and hold them with your fingers, forming a puff ball with the central portion of the gauze 4×4. Take care to avoid touching the central portion of the gauze 4×4's sterile surface that is used to clean the wound. Pour a small amount of sterile normal saline over the central portion of the gauze 4×4. Cleanse the wound from the center to the outer edges. Repeat the process using additional gauze 4×4s as needed.
10. Use a final gauze 4×4 to dry the surrounding skin thoroughly.

Transparent Dressings:

- You may need to clean the skin around the wound with an alcohol pad to remove skin oils ***so that the dressing will adhere better.***
- Apply the transparent dressing to one side of the wound. Remove the paper backing from the adhesive side of the dressing, carefully pulling away while holding the dressing against the wound. *Safety: Do not stretch the transparent dressing tightly against the wound or it will impair movement and comfort.*

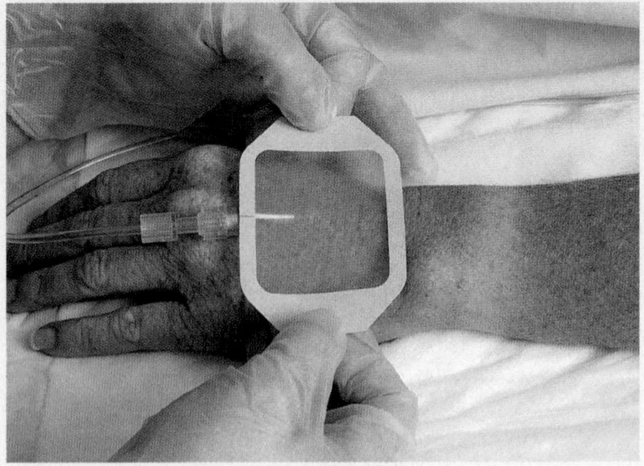

- Remove the surface film from the top of the transparent dressing, if present.
- Remove the edge pieces of the paper backing that remain on the adhesive side of the dressing.
- Write the date, time, and your initials on the edge of the transparent dressing.

Hydrocolloid Dressings:

- Peel the paper backing from the hydrocolloid dressing. ***Note: Cutting the corners of the hydrocolloid dressing so they are rounded may help the dressing adhere better.***
- Place the dressing over the wound and smooth gently.

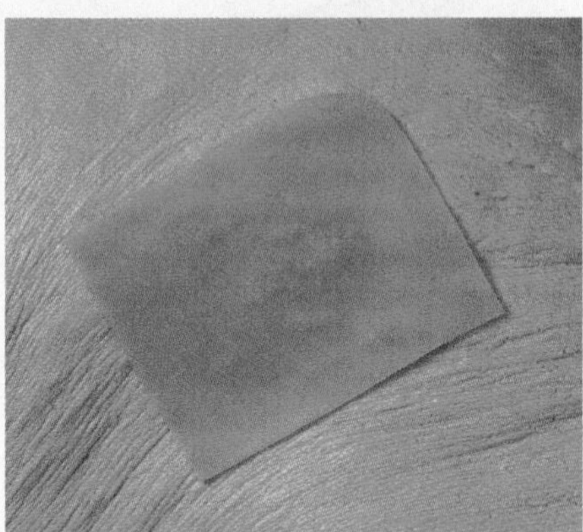

- Remove the surface paper from the hydrocolloid dressing, if present. ***Hint: Hold your hand on the applied dressing for a few seconds. The warmth of your hand will help mold it to the skin and promote better adherence.***
- Write the date, time, and your initials on the edge of the hydrocolloid dressing.

Complete the Dressing Change

11. Inspect the dressing for any wrinkles and smooth them out ***to prevent access to the wound by contaminants.***
12. Follow the Ending Implementation Steps located on the inside back cover.
13. Document the date and time, appearance of wound, size of wound, and type and amount of drainage.

Evaluation Steps

1. Apply tape to the edges of the dressings if they start to lift or roll up.

Skill 26.6 (continued)

2. Inspect the wound through the transparent dressing daily. Inspect the hydrocolloid dressing daily for drainage escaping under the dressing, wrinkling, or excessive exudate absorption.
3. Evaluate appropriate use of the barrier dressing. These dressings are not indicated if excessive drainage occurs or if the wound is infected. Notify the health-care provider if either of these situations occurs.

Sample Documentation

06/04/22 1415 States no wound pain. Denies need for pain med prior to dressing change. Hydrocolloid dressing removed from sacrum. 3 cm × 3.5 cm erythema, skin intact. No blistering. Cleansed with sterile NS using clean technique. New 5 cm × 8 cm hydrocolloid dressing applied. No c/o discomfort during or after dressing change. ———— ———— Nurse's signature and credentials

Skill 26.7 Changing a Negative Pressure Wound Therapy Dressing (Wound VAC)

Assessment Steps

1. Review the health-care provider's order for wound vac therapy.
2. Check orders for pain medication and administer prior to changing the wound vac dressing ***to allow the patient to be medicated during the procedure, which may cause pain or discomfort.***

Planning Step

1. Obtain needed equipment and supplies: clean gloves, sterile gloves, sterile field, scissors, biohazard bag, sterile saline and irrigation supplies if the wound is to be irrigated, appropriate foam dressing, transparent film, and suction track tubing. Ensure that the size of the foam dressing is appropriate. It will be cut to fit inside the wound without causing stretching.

Implementation Steps

1. Follow the Initial Implementation Steps located on the inside back cover.
2. Wash hands and don clean gloves ***to follow standard precautions.***

Remove Old Dressing

3. Don clean gloves, gently loosen the edges of the transparent dressing, and pull it toward the wound ***to prevent tension on the wound edges.***
4. Gently lift out the foam dressing and dispose of it in the biohazard bag ***because it is contaminated with blood and body fluids.***
5. Inspect the wound for amount and type of drainage, odor, and color. Also inspect for any foam debris left in the wound ***because this can lead to irritation.***
6. Measure the size of the wound using a disposable paper ruler, being careful not to touch the wound. ***This information is needed for documentation.***
7. Remove gloves and wash hands. ***Note: The wound may be irrigated here if irrigation is ordered (see Skill 26.3).***

Apply New Dressing

3. Set up sterile field with scissors, foam pad, and tubing and connectors and don sterile gloves. ***Note: Sterile technique is required unless the wound is colonized without signs of infection. Follow your facility's policy.***
4. Cut foam dressing to the correct size to fit inside the wound and fill it without being forced. *Safety: Cut foam away from the wound to avoid causing small pieces to fall into the wound. Remove any loose pieces from the edges of the foam for the same reason.*

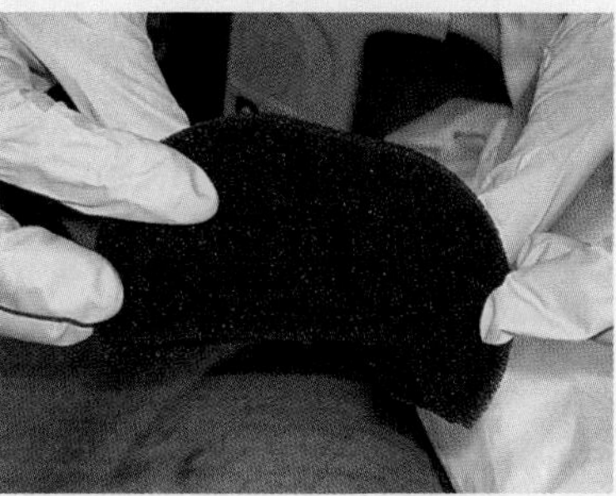

5. Insert the foam dressing into the wound without contaminating it ***by touching it to the skin's surface, which would allow microorganisms from the skin to enter the wound.***
6. If the foam is too large to fit without being forced or without stretching the wound, trim the edges for a better fit. *Safety: If the wound is stretched by a piece of foam that is too large, it will affect the negative pressure in the wound and possibly leave exudates in the wound.*
7. Cover the wound and the foam dressing with a large piece of transparent film, ensuring that the film extends 1 to 2 inches from the wound edges ***to create a seal for negative pressure to occur. Safety: Avoid stretching or wrinkling the transparent film because the excess pressure on the foam dressing can cause injury to the wound bed.***
8. Locate the area of the film where you will attach the suction track tubing ***to prevent pulling on the film.***
9. Carefully lift up the film at this point and cut a round hole approximately 1 inch in diameter. *Safety: Avoid cutting the foam dressing because this can result in debris in the wound and interfere with suction.*
10. Place the round suction area of the track tubing directly over the hole you have cut and press gently in place against the transparent film ***to allow for the negative pressure to pull exudate from the wound.***

(skill continues on page 554)

Skill 26.7 (continued)

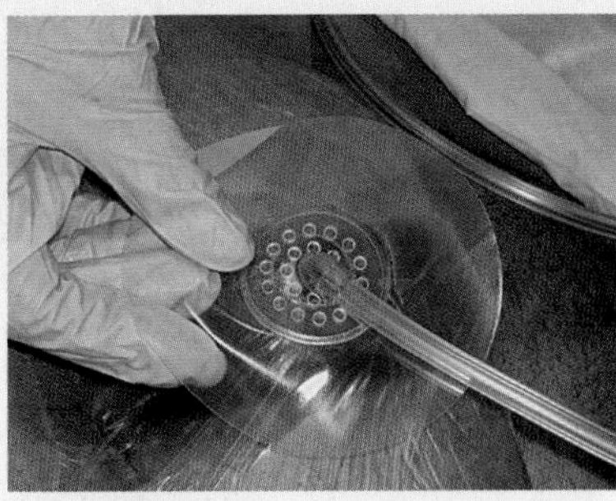

11. Connect the tubing to the canister on the suction pump and open the clamps on the tubing.
12. Place the pump and suction tubing in such a way that there is no tension on the transparent film and the tubing is not causing pressure on the skin ***to maximize the negative pressure and avoid pressure injuries.***

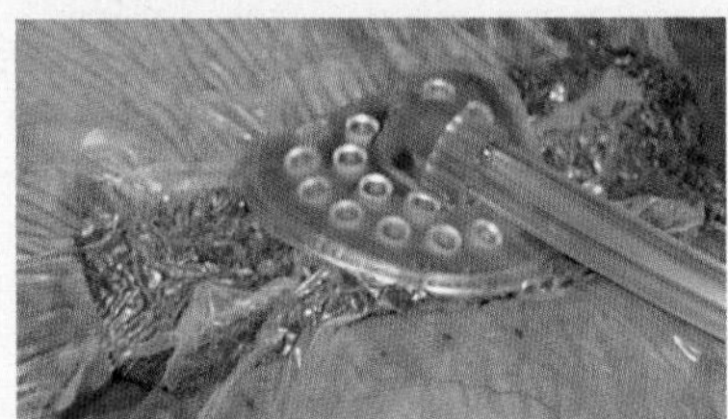

13. Set negative pressure to ordered amount (between -5 and -125 mm Hg) and to intermittent or continuous suction as ordered. ***Different settings for pressure and intermittent or continuous suction will be ordered for different types of wounds.*** Ensure that all clamps on the tubing are open.
14. Turn on the pump and watch for the foam dressing to collapse in response to the vacuum. *Safety: If this does not occur, check all connections for leaks.*

Complete the Dressing Change

15. Follow the Ending Implementation Steps located on the inside back cover.
16. Document the date, time, appearance of wound, size of wound, application of foam dressing or transparent dressing, and settings on pump, as well as the patient's response to the procedure. *Safety: Include the number of foam dressings used so that all will be removed when the dressing is changed again.*

Evaluation Steps

1. Inspect the wound edges through the transparent dressing daily.
2. Evaluate for air leaks whenever you are in the room. Check the output in the suction canister each shift.
3. Change the canister at least once per week or when it is full ***to maintain adequate suction at all times.***

Sample Documentation

*06/04/22 1415 Rated pain at 6 prior to dressing change. Medicated with IV analgesic per order (See MAR).
———————— Nurse's signature and credentials*

*06/04/22 1440 Transparent dressing and one 3 cm × 4 cm piece of foam removed from wound. Wound is 3.2 cm × 4.1 cm and 2 cm deep. Wound bed is dark pink with bits of tan tissue at sides. Irrigated with 50 mL normal saline with small amt of tan tissue obtained. 3 cm × 4 cm foam dressing inserted in wound and covered with transparent dressing. Attached to intermittent suction at -7 mm Hg as ordered. C/o pain during procedure only when foam dressing inserted. Resting comfortably without c/o discomfort. ————
———————— Nurse's signature and credentials*

POST CONFERENCE

After your clinical experience, you have an opportunity to evaluate the care you gave. As you discuss your day with your classmates, you realize how much you have learned and accomplished. You were able to maintain contact precautions as you cared for your patient with MRSA. You observed your patient for any reactions to the vancomycin he was taking to treat the MRSA. You changed the dressing very carefully, removing the old dressing and measuring the wound. You were able to identify granulation tissue and the location of infected tissue. Although it took some practice, you were able to fluff the wet gauze 4×4s and place them inside the wound without contaminating it; then you covered the wound with damp gauze 4×4s and covered the entire area with an abdominal dressing pad that you taped in place. Your instructor was very pleased with your accurate and detailed documentation of the procedure.

Key Points

- Types of wounds include contusions, abrasions, lacerations, puncture wounds, penetrating wounds, and pressure injuries.
- Wounds fall into one of these contamination categories: clean, clean-contaminated, contaminated, infected, and colonized.
- Pressure injuries are the result of pressure and/or shear and are preventable with good nursing care. Many risk factors predispose patients to developing pressure injuries.
- Pressure injuries are identified by stages, based on tissues involved and intact or nonintact skin. They are identified by one of the following: stages 1 to 4, unstageable, and DTPI. In addition, they may be determined to be medical device related (which can be staged) or a mucosal membrane pressure injury (which cannot be staged).
- A variety of nursing interventions are needed to prevent pressure injuries. These include turning, positioning, pressure relief devices, assessment of bony prominences, and keeping skin clean.
- Other wounds that occur in hospitalized patients include stasis ulcers, sinus tracts, and surgical incisions.
- Wound healing involves the inflammatory phase, reconstruction phase, and maturation phase. Wounds may be closed by one of three methods to promote healing. Wounds may not heal well due to a variety of factors.
- Complications of wound healing include infection, dehiscence, evisceration, and hemorrhage. Each of these requires immediate nursing responses.
- Wounds may be closed with sutures, staples, or glue. They may have drains in place after surgery. Wounds must be assessed and measured carefully.
- Wound treatments include irrigation to remove necrotic tissue. After irrigation, a wound culture may be obtained to determine which microorganisms are causing infection and which antibiotics will kill them.
- Many types of dressings may be used to help heal wounds. They are secured in a way to prevent damage to the skin and still keep the dressing in place. Dressing changes are often done using sterile technique.
- Accurate documentation of wound care is important so that nurses will know what supplies they need, how many gauze 4×4s are in the wound to be removed, and for purposes of reimbursement.

Review Questions

Select the answer that is most appropriate for each of the following questions. Some questions may have more than one correct answer. Select all that apply.

1. A patient's J-P drain should be emptied:
   1. every 2 hours.
   2. every 8 hours.
   3. when one-half to two-thirds full.
   4. only when it needs to be reactivated.
   5. when the container is full.

2. Which one of the following assessment findings makes it impossible to stage a pressure injury?
   1. Purulent drainage
   2. Eschar
   3. Sloughing tissue
   4. Erythema
   5. Drainage
   6. Signs of infection
   7. Undermining

3. The phase of healing during which granulation tissue forms in a wound is the:
   1. inflammatory phase.
   2. reconstruction phase.
   3. maturation phase.
   4. remodeling phase.

4. You observe pink drainage from a patient's wound. You would describe this as:
   1. sanguineous.
   2. serous.
   3. purulent.
   4. seropurulent.
   5. serosanguineous.

5. Your patient has a large abdominal wound with copious drainage and many layers of gauze 4×4s in the dressing. The patient develops a skin reaction to the tape due to frequent dressing changes. What might you recommend for this patient?
   1. Change to surgical adhesive instead of tape to hold dressings in place.
   2. Call the doctor and ask for an order to decrease dressing change frequency.
   3. Ask the charge nurse about using Montgomery straps or an abdominal binder instead of tape.
   4. Wrap gauze around the patient's trunk to hold the dressings in place.

6. A patient returns from surgery with a left shoulder dressing. A 3-inch diameter spot of red drainage is visible on the anterior portion of the dressing. The health-care provider does not want the dressing disturbed for 24 hours. What will you do?
   1. Call the health-care provider to report the drainage and request a change in orders.
   2. Reinforce the dressing by adding several gauze 4×4s over the area.
   3. Draw a line on the dressing outlining the drainage, with the date, time, and your initials.
   4. Document the drainage in the chart and observe for further drainage over the next several hours.

7. A patient has signs of infection in his left shoulder incision—erythema, warmth, and a small amount of purulent drainage. You prepare to report this to the health-care provider. Which information will you have ready when you call?
   1. Vital signs
   2. Name and dosage of pain medication currently ordered
   3. Appropriate laboratory results
   4. Patient's rating of incisional pain
   5. Description of the wound and drainage
   6. Names of all staff who have changed his dressing since surgery
   7. Signs of infection you observe
   8. Name and dosage of antibiotics currently ordered, if any

8. You are caring for a 67-year-old male who had a cerebrovascular accident 3 weeks ago. In addition, he has developed a pressure injury on his right hip. Which of the following data that you collected will be useful in developing a care plan that will address his pressure ulcer?
   1. Last week he weighed 165.5 pounds, and today he weighs 161.8 pounds.
   2. The pressure injury is a stage 3.
   3. He has 250 mL of clear yellow urine in his Foley catheter.
   4. He is not able to sit up in a chair for longer than 15 minutes at a time.
   5. He dislikes cheese, beans, chicken, and fish, but loves steak, eggs, all kinds of nuts, and peanut butter.
   6. His affect is flat.
   7. He has been on an eggcrate mattress while in the hospital.

9. Which one of the following interventions would you rate as the most important for care of his pressure injury?
   1. Change the wet-to-damp dressing on his right hip wound qid using sterile technique.
   2. Tell dietary service about his food likes and dislikes.
   3. Reposition the patient every 2 hours around the clock, avoiding the right lateral position.
   4. Assess the condition of the pressure injury once daily.
   5. Provide Foley care every shift.
   6. Work to increase the length of time the patient can tolerate sitting in a chair.

ANSWERS 1. 2, 3, 2. 2, 3. 2, 4. 5, 5. 3, 6. 3, 7. 1, 3, 4, 5, 7, 8, 8. 1, 2, 4, 5, 7, 9. 1

Critical Thinking Exercises

Answers available online.

1. Create and describe a scenario of a patient with a wound in whom there are *at least four indicators* that a wound culture would be beneficial.

2. Describe a scenario when it would not be wise to remove all the staples in a surgical incision.

Additional Resources

Use the scratch off code on the inside front cover of your book to access online quizzes that will help you to improve your scores on course exams and prepare for the NCLEX-PN®.

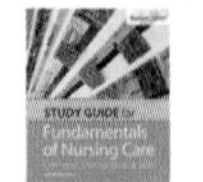

Study Guide

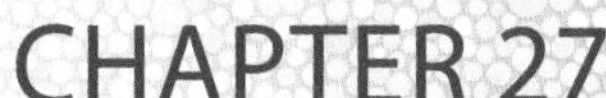

CHAPTER 27
Musculoskeletal Care

KEY TERMS

Amputate (AMP-yoo-tayt)
Continuous passive motion machine (kon-TIN-yoo-us PASS-iv MOH-shun muh-SHEEN)
External fixator (eks-TER-nuhl fiks-AY-ter)
Fracture (FRAK-chuhr)
Joint replacement (arthroplasty) (JOYNT ree-PLAYSS-ment (AR-throh-PLAS-tee))
Osteoarthritis (OSS-tee-oh-arth-RYE-tiss)
Physical therapist (FIZ-ih-kuhl THER-ah-pist)
Prosthesis (pross-THEE-siss)
Skeletal traction (SKEL-uh-tuhl TRAK-shun)
Skin traction (SKIN TRAK-shun)
Spica (SPYE-kah)
Sprain (SPRAYN)
Stump (STUMP)

CHAPTER CONCEPTS

Comfort
Mobility
Patient-Centered Care

LEARNING OUTCOMES

1. Define various terms associated with musculoskeletal care.
2. Describe common musculoskeletal conditions that result in limited mobility.
3. Discuss the role of the physical therapist in the health-care team.
4. Differentiate between indications for use of x-rays, computed tomography scans, and magnetic resonance imaging to diagnose musculoskeletal conditions.
5. Enumerate six types of immobilizing devices used for musculoskeletal disorders.
6. Describe nursing care of patients with musculoskeletal conditions, including casts, traction, joint replacement, and amputation.
7. Discuss guidelines for patients using assistive devices for ambulation.
8. Describe the steps necessary to develop a plan of care for a patient with impaired mobility related to a musculoskeletal condition.
9. Discuss information found in the Connection features of the chapter.
10. Identify safety issues related to musculoskeletal care.
11. Answer questions about the skills in the chapter.

SKILLS

27.1 Performing Neurovascular Checks
27.2 Setting Up a Continuous Passive Motion Machine
27.3 Applying Elastic Bandages

CRITICAL THINKING CONNECTION

Clinical Assignment

You have been assigned to care for a patient who is having a right total knee replacement due to osteoarthritis. She is scheduled to go to the operating room at 7:30 a.m. You will be assisting with her preoperative care and performing postoperative care when she returns to her room on the patient unit.

Continued

CRITICAL THINKING CONNECTION—cont'd

Critical Thinking Questions:

- What do you know about a total knee replacement?
- Are there any special concerns during preoperative care?
- How will you care for someone immediately following this surgery?
- What care will you need to provide postoperatively in addition to taking routine postoperative vital signs and managing pain after surgery?
- What is a continuous passive motion machine and what will you do with it?
- How soon will this patient be able to get up in a chair?
- What special care will the replaced joint require?

When you care for patients who have musculoskeletal disorders, they often will have at least some degree of restricted mobility. As you recall from Chapter 16, immobility can place patients at risk for a number of complications, in addition to potential complications from surgery or other procedures. You will study more details about different types of musculoskeletal disorders, their treatment, and their prognoses when you study medical-surgical nursing. The purpose of this chapter is to prepare you to care for patients with limited mobility related to musculoskeletal conditions.

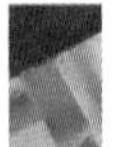

MUSCULOSKELETAL CONDITIONS RESULTING IN LIMITED MOBILITY

A variety of musculoskeletal conditions can result in immobilization of a joint, a limb, or the entire body. Some of the most common conditions are fractures, joint replacements, and lower limb amputations.

Common Musculoskeletal Conditions

A **sprain** is an injury to a joint that results in damage to muscles and ligaments. Severe sprains may cause ligaments to be completely torn. Mild sprains often cause only minor muscle and ligament damage. The ankle is the joint that is most often sprained, but a sprain can occur in other joints as well. The sprained joint must be supported and rested in order to heal. The acronym RICE is used to help you remember treatment for a sprain:

- **R**est: The joint must be rested and should not bear weight until it can do so without pain.
- **I**ce: Apply ice to the joint during the first 48 hours after the injury occurs to help decrease swelling and pain.
- **C**ompression: Apply an elastic bandage or compression stocking or sleeve to compress the joint and prevent further swelling.
- **E**levation: Keep the joint elevated above the heart, again to help decrease swelling and pain.

Fractures are breaks in the bone. They may range from a narrow crack, called a *hairline fracture,* to a bone that is broken into many small pieces, called a *comminuted fracture.* To promote healing of a fracture, the broken ends of the bones must be supported in close proximity to one another for 4 to 8 weeks or longer to allow the bone to grow together. This may require the insertion of pins, wires, or screws to hold the bone pieces together. Generally, a cast or immobilizer is placed on a limb to accomplish this. If the fractured bones are in the trunk of the body, support may be provided in other ways, such as a thoracolumbarsacral orthosis, also called a "turtle shell brace." A **joint replacement** (arthroplasty) is a surgery to remove damaged articular bone surfaces and replace them with metal and plastic surfaces. It is performed when a joint has severe degenerative changes, usually due to advanced **osteoarthritis.** This disease causes degeneration and inflammation of joints over time. The most commonly replaced joints are the knees and the hips. Because these joints bear the body's weight, they often become stressed over time. If the joint has been injured in the past, osteoarthritis is more likely to develop in later life.

When a limb is so damaged by trauma that it cannot be saved, it will be **amputated,** or surgically removed. Other reasons for amputation include cancerous tumors, severely decreased blood flow to the limb, and *gangrene* (death of tissue) in a limb. The remaining portion of a limb after amputation is referred to as a **stump.** While the stump is not immobilized after surgery, it requires specialized nursing care, discussed later in this chapter. When a lower limb is amputated, the patient will be dealing with mobility issues as well.

As a result of immobilization, the patient will need assistance to regain muscle strength and ambulation ability. The **physical therapist** is the member of the health-care team who is responsible for assessing musculoskeletal deficiencies and developing the plan of care to strengthen muscles and restore mobility. The health-care provider and physical therapist may order that the patient be ambulated a specific number of times per day or a specific distance at each walk. It is your nursing responsibility to be sure that such orders are carried out so that the patient can gain strength and be prepared for discharge. Sometimes nurses may feel that they are too busy to get the patient up and assist with ambulation, but these activity orders are very important and must be carried out.

KNOWLEDGE CONNECTION

List four musculoskeletal conditions that result in limited mobility. What is the role of the physical therapist on the health-care team?

• WORD • BUILDING •

mobility: mobil – able to move + ity – condition
immobility: im – not + mobil – able to move + ity – condition
thoracolumbarsacral orthosis: thoraco – chest + lumbar – loin + sacral – related to sacral bone; orthosis – straightening
osteoarthritis: osteo – bone + arthr – joint + itis – inflammation
ambulation: ambulat – move about + ion – action

Laboratory and Diagnostic Connection

Testing for Musculoskeletal Conditions

Different types of diagnostic tests are used to diagnose different types of musculoskeletal conditions. X-rays typically are ordered for suspected fractures or significant trauma. Computed tomography scans are most helpful to further identify fractures that may be difficult to see on x-rays, as well to view congenital abnormalities of the musculoskeletal system. They can be used when magnetic resonance imaging (MRI) would be contraindicated because of metal implants, pacemakers, or claustrophobia. MRI is used when pathological fractures occur because these fractures usually are associated with bone tumors. MRI is also used to examine congenital problems of the spine. MRIs are generally ordered to view soft tissue conditions such as injuries to joints, and ligament, tendon, or muscle tears. Bone scans are ordered when there is suspected widespread disease of the bones, as in a metabolic condition or cancer.

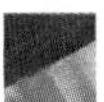

TYPES OF IMMOBILIZATION

When a bone or joint has to be immobilized, the health-care provider chooses the appropriate device for the situation. The devices used for immobilization are varied, depending on the condition and the time needed for healing. Sometimes when students think about musculoskeletal conditions and immobilization, they think only of fractures and casts. However, you will see that there are many such conditions and devices. Table 27.1 contains descriptions of various types of immobilization devices used to treat musculoskeletal disorders.

External fixators are the wires, pins, tongs, and rods that may be used in skeletal traction. These devices are found on the outside of the limb but are also fixed to the bone of the limb (Fig. 27.1). They may help hold the bone in place while healing occurs, or they may be used for attaching weight to move bones in traction.

An additional type of external fixator is the *Ilizarov frame,* named for the Russian doctor who developed it. This frame is composed of metal rings on the outside of the limb, with rods and wires that attach to those rings. The rods and wires also penetrate the skin and insert into the bone. This fixator is used to stabilize small bone pieces, such as in a comminuted fracture, keeping the fragments aligned while bone growth occurs. It is also used in situations in which one leg has been left shorter than the other after trauma. By turning screws in the frame, the rings separate slightly; over time, the bone grows to fill in the gap. This allows for a very gradual increase in bone length to help the legs become more even.

KNOWLEDGE CONNECTION

What are the purposes of traction? When might an Ilizarov frame be used?

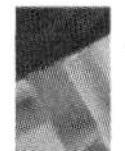

CARING FOR PATIENTS WITH MUSCULOSKELETAL IMMOBILIZATION

As a nurse, you will be expected to know how to care for patients with musculoskeletal immobilization devices. You will be responsible for delivering appropriate care to the patient regardless of the type of device being used. Cast care and traction care will be discussed here as fundamental nursing skills. If you care for a patient with a different type of device, be sure you look up information about the device in a medical-surgical textbook or you are instructed in the appropriate care by nursing staff.

Caring for a Patient in a Cast

Casts may be made of plaster of Paris, fiberglass, or other types of polymers. Plaster casts or splints are often applied initially after a fracture or surgery because they mold easily to a more precise shape. Plaster is the material of choice when bone realignment is necessary to keep the bone in place. A fiberglass cast is often applied a week or two after injury because it is more durable once the bone starts healing. Fiberglass casting may also be used if the fractured bone is not out of position. It allows for better air circulation, is lighter in weight, and is penetrated better by x-rays for clearer visualization of the healing bone. A **spica** cast encases the hips and one or both legs. There is an open area for the perineum, and an abductor bar keeps the legs and hips a specific distance apart. These casts are often used to correct hip dysplasia in young children. It is very important that you move the patient in a spica cast carefully and do not use the abductor bar to lift the patient. It is not designed for that purpose, and doing so can damage the spica cast.

When a plaster cast is applied, it takes many hours for it to dry. If you are caring for a patient in a plaster cast that is not yet dry, follow these guidelines:

- Support the limb on pillows in such a way that air circulates all around the cast for even drying.
- Avoid touching the wet or damp cast with your fingers because they can leave dents in the cast that will remain after it dries, causing pressure points on the skin beneath the cast.
- If it is necessary to touch the cast, use only the palms of your hands.

• WORD • BUILDING •

fixator: fix – fasten + ator – a thing performing an action

Table 27.1
Immobilization Devices

Device	*Description and Use*
Abductor pillow	Wedge-shaped foam pillow, often with Velcro straps, placed between the legs of patients who have had total hip replacement surgery; keeps hips abducted while patient is in bed; straps keep the pillow in place and prevent shifting
Cast	Hard plaster or fiberglass encasement for a limb; used to immobilize joints, usually to stabilize fractures until they heal; sometimes used to immobilize severely sprained joints until healing can occur; often used after musculoskeletal surgeries to stabilize the joint and surgical sites
Elastic bandages	Woven bandage containing elastic to stretch as it is wrapped around an injured area; elastic helps compress the area to decrease edema
Amputee compression sock	Also called a "shrinker sock"; elastic sock or sleeve that fits snugly over a stump to help decrease edema and help it heal in a shape to fit in the prosthesis
Immobilizer	Soft fabric with firm internal stays; opens and closes with Velcro fasteners; used to protect an injured limb and to keep its joints from flexing; often a "boot" for foot and ankle injuries
Splint	Firm plastic molded form used to keep a joint or joints from flexing; may be applied to a limb and wrapped in place with gauze or an elastic bandage; sometimes "air splints" are used when transporting injured patients; can be slipped beneath the injured limb, wrapped around it, then inflated to immobilize the joint
Traction	*Skin traction:* Involves the use of ropes, pulleys, and weights to align bone ends after a fracture; weights are attached to a frame held in place with elastic bandages or other wrap on the skin; may be used to prevent severe muscle spasm due to displaced bones until surgery can be performed *Skeletal traction:* Uses wires, rods, or tongs that penetrate the skin and subcutaneous tissue and are inserted into the bone; these are then attached to a frame with weights or only to a frame to hold the bone in place or move the bone with the weights

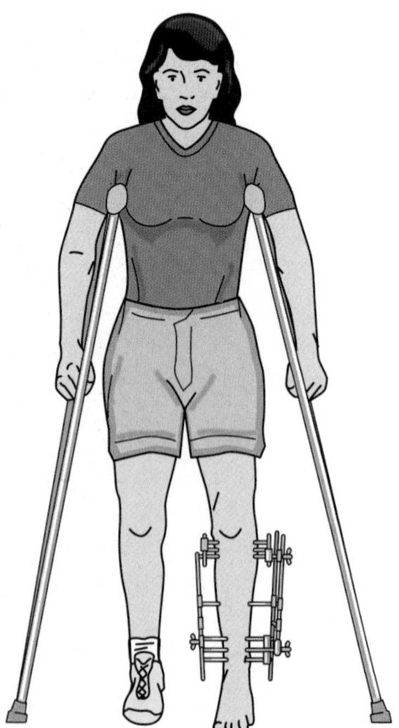

FIGURE 27.1 This patient has an external fixator in place on the lower leg (from Williams LS, Hopper PD. *Understanding Medical-Surgical Nursing*. 5th ed. Philadelphia, PA: FA Davis; 2015).

Fiberglass casts are more lightweight and dry very quickly compared to plaster casts. A special light may be used to promote drying of the fiberglass cast.

When you care for patients with dry casts, whether plaster or fiberglass, follow these guidelines:

- Teach the patient to avoid putting anything between the cast and the skin beneath it, especially for the purpose of scratching. Skin sheds outer epidermal cells, but when the cast is in place, the cells that have been shed tend to pile up rather than flake off, causing intense itching at times. If the patient uses an implement such as an ink pen or straightened coat hanger to scratch beneath the cast, it can abrade the skin. The warm, dark, moist area beneath the cast is a perfect medium for bacterial growth, leading to severe infection. One alternative is to use a portable hair dryer to blow cool air down the cast to relieve the itching.
- Observe for any drainage staining the cast or any malodorous discharge, which would indicate infection beneath the cast. Report such observations to the health-care provider.
- Assess circulation to the casted limb. If swelling occurs, the cast may cause restricted circulation, which can lead to tissue necrosis or nerve damage. To assess circulation,

perform neurovascular checks every 2 hours for the first 24 hours after the cast is applied or surgery is performed. The neurovascular checks then may be decreased to every 4 hours or according to facility policy (see Skill 27.1, page 570).
- Place tape "petals" over the edges of the cast if they begin to crack or crumble over time. To reinforce the edges of the cast with tape, also called "petaling" a cast, cut 3- to 4-inch strips of tape. On one end of each strip, cut the tape in a point. Place the square end of the tape against the cast between the patient's skin and the cast. Fold the pointed edge of the tape over to the outside of the cast. This technique also can be used to cover rough edges of the cast that may irritate the skin and cause breakdown.
- Casts of all materials are being used less frequently now, with removable walking boots and splints favored more by health-care provider and patients alike. These types of immobilizers can be removed at night and therefore do not cause pressure on the injured limb. They also allow better for swelling and often are more comfortable for patients.

Caring for a Patient in Traction

Two types of traction may be used: skin traction and skeletal traction. When **skin traction** is used, the limb is wrapped with an elastic bandage or fitted with a Velcro wrap to which a frame is attached. One or more ropes are attached to the frame; on the other end of each rope, a weight is attached. An overhead frame is affixed to the bed, with a *trapeze bar,* or triangular piece, attached for the patient to use as a hand grip when moving in bed. Figure 27.2 shows a patient in skin traction with the overhead frame and trapeze bar in place.

When **skeletal traction** is used, pins, screws, or tongs are surgically inserted into the bone. These devices, referred to as *external fixators,* require meticulous nursing care. Because these fixators penetrate the skin and enter the bone, they provide a pathway for pathogens to enter the body. Infections of the bone are very serious and sometimes quite difficult to treat. It is the nurse's responsibility to prevent such infections by performing pin-site care as ordered. Generally, orders for this care include cleansing the skin insertion sites using sterile gauze saturated with normal saline or hydrogen peroxide. In addition, you need to assess the pin sites for signs of infection. Small amounts of serous or serosanguineous drainage at the insertion site is a normal finding. Immediately report to the health-care provider any purulent drainage because this is indicative of infection. Also report increasing redness of the skin around the insertion site. Most physicians do not order ointment at pin sites because the moisture can promote bacterial growth.

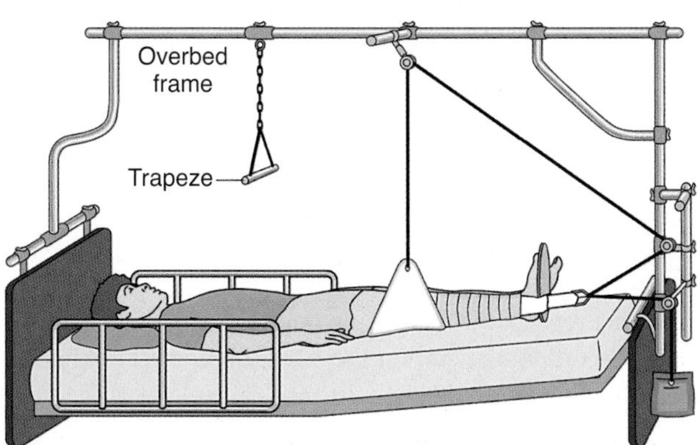

FIGURE 27.2 This patient is in skin traction but can use the trapeze bar attached to the over-bed frame to assist with movement. Note that the weight is hanging freely off of the end of the bed (from Williams LS, Hopper PD. *Understanding Medical-Surgical Nursing.* 5th ed. Philadelphia, PA: FA Davis; 2015).

Tongs are used on the skull to provide cervical traction after surgery or fracture to the cervical vertebrae. The tong insertion sites are located on either side of the skull. The hair in the area usually has been shaved to decrease the chances of infection. Again, you will clean the insertion sites according to orders and make the same assessments as for pin sites.

In addition to pin-site care, nurses are responsible for monitoring traction to ensure that no complications occur:

- Ensure that the weights hang freely and do not rest on the floor.
- Ensure that the ropes pull in a straight line without crossing one another.
- Assess for skin breakdown beneath the external traction devices.
- When turning a patient in traction, have another person lift up on the weights, causing slack in the ropes while the patient is turned. After the patient is supported and aligned, the second person then gently and slowly releases the weights to hang freely.
- Ensure that the patient's body is in proper alignment so that the traction pulls correctly.

KNOWLEDGE CONNECTION

Why does itching occur beneath a cast? How can it be safely relieved? What is the difference between skin traction and skeletal traction? When might tongs be used for traction? What do you need to do when turning a patient in traction?

Caring for a Patient After Joint Replacement

When a joint is replaced, specialized nursing care is needed to avoid postoperative dislocation or other complications. It is very important that you know the appropriate nursing care for joint replacements, during both your practice as a student and your practice as a nurse.

• WORD • BUILDING •

dislocation: dis – opposite of + locat – place + ion – action

Total Hip Replacement (Total Hip Arthroplasty)

It is necessary to review the normal anatomy of the hip joint to understand how a total hip replacement is performed.

Anatomy and Physiology Connection

The Hip Joint

The normal hip joint consists of the head of the femur, which fits into the acetabulum of the pelvis, forming a ball-and-socket joint (Fig. 27.3). The acetabulum is lined with smooth cartilage, and the rounded head of the femur rotates freely and smoothly in the socket. A small amount of fluid, called *synovial fluid,* is also found in the joint to lubricate that movement.

When a hip joint is replaced, the head and neck of the femur are removed and replaced with a titanium implant that is bonded into the top of the femur. It is in the shape of the head and neck of the femur. The acetabulum is revised, and a titanium acetabular cup lined with smooth plastic is cemented into the pelvic bone. Now the new femur head fits exactly into the new acetabular cup and moves smoothly and easily. However, the muscles that had attached to the head of the femur do not attach to the artificial femur immediately, so muscular support for the joint is absent. Eventually, the muscles repair and support the new joint, but that takes several months.

A somewhat newer approach to performing this surgery is called the *direct anterior approach*, which involves a 3- to 4-inch incision in the front of the hip instead of a longer one along the side of the hip. In this approach, the muscles and tendons are not detached from the bone so it causes less muscle damage and less risk of dislocation due to crossing the legs or adducting the leg. The patient does not have to avoid adducting the leg, and there is no need to use the abduction pillow.

For a lateral approach hip arthroplasty, the patient must avoid adducting the operative leg to the midpoint of the body or beyond beginning immediately after surgery and continuing for several more months. In addition, the patient must not flex the hip joint more than 90 degrees. Both of these actions could cause the new femur head to pop out of the acetabular cup, which would require treatment for a joint dislocation, often involving a return to surgery.

A wedge-shaped abductor pillow is used to keep the patient from accidentally moving the affected leg to or beyond the midline (Fig. 27.4). When you turn the patient to the unaffected side or the back, the abductor pillow must be kept in place. Generally, you will have orders not to turn the patient on the operative side during the immediate postoperative period.

When you assist the patient to get out of bed, to sit in a chair, or to use the bedside commode, you must be very careful that the patient does not lean forward at any time because that would flex the hip beyond 90 degrees and possibly cause hip dislocation. Figure 27.5 illustrates the angle that occurs when a patient leans forward. After discharge, patients are encouraged to use an extension gripper to pick up any dropped items so that they do not flex the hip too far. Box 27.1 contains guidelines to follow when caring for patients who have had total hip replacements.

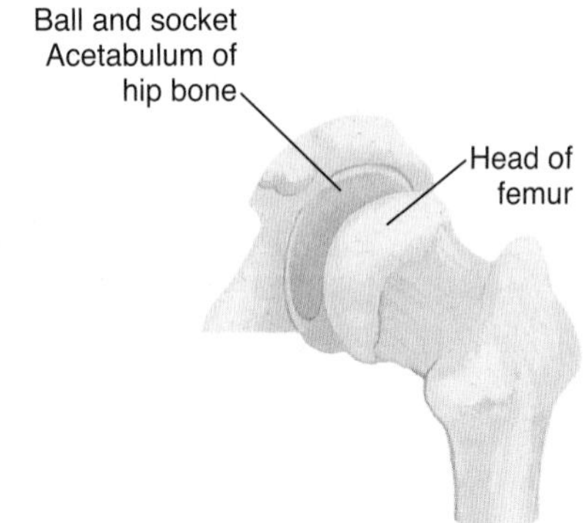

FIGURE 27.3 The hip joint includes the acetabulum and the head of the femur (from Scanlon V, Sanders T. *Essentials of Anatomy and Physiology*. 7th ed. Philadelphia, PA: FA Davis; 2015).

Real-World Connection

Researching the Right Condition

A nursing student was assigned to care for a patient who was 1 day postoperative with a lateral approach total hip replacement. The student researched how to care for a patient with a fractured hip repaired with open reduction and internal fixation, rather than researching care for a patient who had a total hip replacement. During clinicals, the student turned the patient onto her operative side (contraindicated in either situation) and flexed the unaffected leg at the knee, bringing it over the operated leg. No abductor pillow was in use. This had the effect of adducting the operated leg beyond the midpoint of the body. The patient began to cry out in pain because the hip replacement had dislocated. It required a return trip to surgery to relocate the replaced joint.

Knee Replacement (Knee Arthroplasty)

Another commonly replaced joint is the knee. When the knee is totally replaced, the top of the tibia and lower end of the femur are replaced with titanium or other metal implants. The femoral component sits on the tibial component, which is topped with a durable plastic surface. The metal of the tibial component articulates against the plastic surface to allow smooth movement of the two surfaces. The patella may be completely replaced with a rounded piece of polyethylene or durable plastic. Sometimes plastic is affixed to the back of the existing patella to provide a smooth articular surface when the knee is flexed.

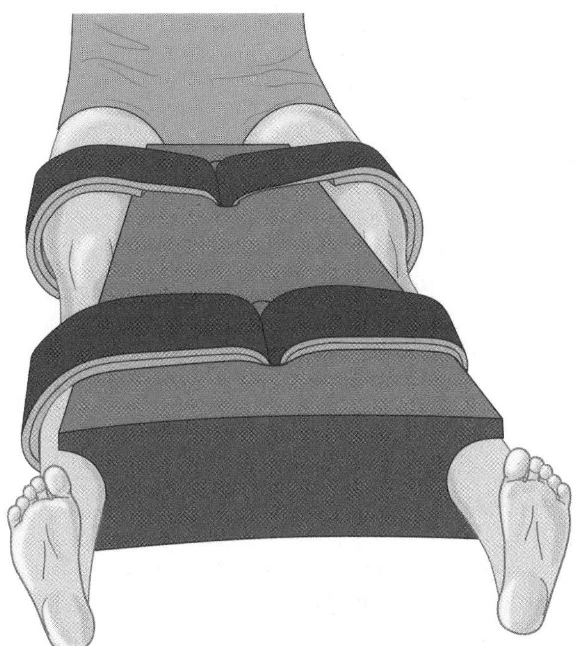

FIGURE 27.4 This patient has an abductor pillow in place to prevent adduction of the prosthetic right hip joint, causing possible dislocation (from Nugent PM, Vitale B. *Davis Essential Nursing Content + Practice Questions Fundamentals*. 2nd ed. Philadelphia, PA: FA Davis; 2017).

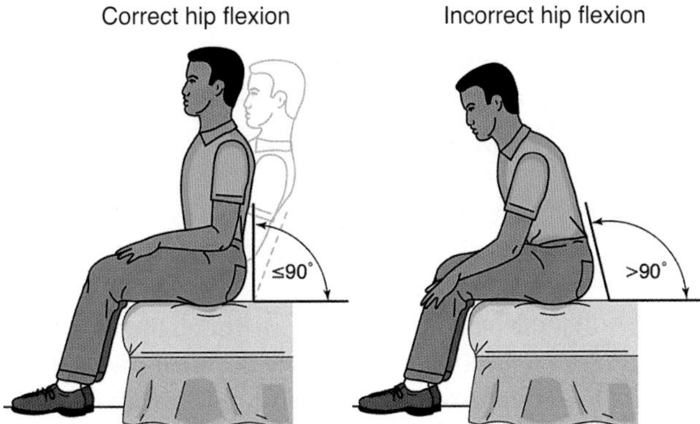

FIGURE 27.5 If the patient with a lateral approach total hip replacement leans forward, the hip angle is greater than 90 degrees, which can cause dislocation of the head of the femur (from Williams LS, Hopper PD. *Understanding Medical-Surgical Nursing*. 5th ed. Philadelphia, PA: FA Davis; 2015).

A partial knee replacement, also called a *unicompartmental knee replacement,* is performed when only one side of the knee, either medial or lateral, is severely damaged by arthritis. In this surgery, only one side of the end of the femur and one side of the top of the tibia are replaced with metal implants. The advantages of a partial knee replacement include a quicker recovery, less postoperative pain, and less blood loss. A disadvantage of having a partial knee replacement is that more surgery may be needed in the future if arthritis develops on the other side.

Some nursing concerns after a total knee replacement are different than those after a total hip replacement. Very soon after surgery, flexion of the new knee joint begins, in both the total and partial knee replacement. To accomplish this, a

Box 27.1

Mobility Guidelines for Patients With Lateral Approach Total Hip Replacements

To prevent dislocation of a new total hip replacement, the patient and nursing staff must be careful to avoid hip flexion beyond 90 degrees. The following guidelines will help you keep the patient's hip prosthesis in place:

- Keep the abductor pillow in place while the patient is in bed.
- Avoid turning the patient on the operative side, according to physician's orders.
- Assist the patient out of bed carefully to prevent flexion of the hip more than 90 degrees.
- Ensure that the patient calls for help if any items are dropped and that the patient does not lean forward, which would flex the hip beyond 90 degrees.
- Assist the patient to get up from the chair or bedside commode without leaning forward.

continuous passive motion machine (CPM machine) is used. This machine is designed to gently flex the patient's knee according to the number of degrees of flexion on the setting and then to gently extend the knee. The leg is supported on a platform that gently bends and straightens the knee as it moves. The patient will require effective pain management in order to tolerate the passive exercise.

The CPM machine sits on the patient's bed and is connected to a power source. The platform where the patient's leg rests is lined with sheepskin to prevent skin breakdown. It is important that you line up the machine so that the break in the platform is centered beneath the patient's knee. It also is important to ensure that the CPM machine is positioned so that the supported leg is maintained in correct body alignment with the hips and the rest of the body. The only way to verify this positioning is to stand at the foot of the bed and inspect the visual alignment of the CPM machine with the hips and torso. Place the machine so that the patient's leg rests comfortably on the platform, set the dial to the degrees of flexion and speed of flexion ordered by the physician, and turn on the machine. Remain with the patient for 10 to 20 repetitions to ensure that he or she is tolerating the passive exercise. The physician will order the length of time the CPM machine is to be on during a 24-hour period, as well as when to increase the degrees of flexion to improve joint function. Skill 27.2 (page 570) presents more information on setting up a CPM machine.

During the first 24 hours postoperatively, even with adequate pain medication, the patient may experience much discomfort when the machine first begins to flex the knee. The more the patient tenses the affected leg muscles, the more pain he or she will experience. This is a good time to teach and assist your patient to use relaxation breathing. Box 27.2 contains guidelines to follow when caring for patients with total knee replacements.

• WORD • BUILDING •

unicompartmental: uni – one + compartment – division + al – relating to

Box 27.2

Guidelines for Caring for Patients With Partial and Total Knee Replacements

When a patient has had a total knee replacement, it is important that the CPM therapy be performed correctly to prevent limited range of motion in the prosthetic knee joint. These guidelines will be useful when caring for a patient with a total knee replacement:

- Ensure that the patient's pain is managed so that he or she can tolerate passive exercise.
- Set the degrees of flexion on the CPM machine according to the physician's orders.
- Follow orders exactly regarding the length of time the CPM machine is to be in use and advancing the degrees of flexion.
- Assist the patient in and out of bed using a walker or other assistive device.
- Follow the physician's orders regarding the amount of weight bearing allowed on the operative knee.

KNOWLEDGE CONNECTION

Why must a patient with a new total hip replacement refrain from adducting the leg or flexing the hip more than 90 degrees? What is the function of a CPM machine after a total knee replacement?

Caring for a Patient After Amputation

Amputation of a body part is an emotionally traumatic event. Not only does the patient need physical care, but he or she requires emotional support as well. Physical care of the patient with an amputation is focused on rehabilitation, even immediately after surgery. It is important that the limb stump heal well and be shaped correctly to fit into a **prosthesis,** or artificial limb, such as an arm or a leg.

Initially, observe the sutures or staples in the stump to ensure that all edges of the wound are approximated and growing together well. If the incision does not heal well, it may break open or the skin may break down with the pressure of a prosthesis. If left to heal on its own, the stump will have a squared-off shape. However, in order to fit into the socket of a prosthetic limb, the stump must have a smooth, rounded shape. That is the reason for wrapping the stump with an elastic bandage in the postoperative healing phase, so it will heal in the correct shape to fit into the prosthesis. Skill 27.3 (page 571) provides information about wrapping extremities with elastic bandages. In many situations, a compression sock is used to shape the stump rather than elastic bandage.

In addition, the patient with an amputation is dealing with a disturbed body image and all the possible life changes that accompany it. It is important for you to be accepting of the patient and not communicate rejection of the altered body image, even nonverbally. You need to listen when the patient wants to talk about his or her feelings and lifestyle changes as a result of the amputation. It is not unusual for the patient to be angry and perhaps direct that anger at you. These patients are mourning a loss and often go through some or all of the stages of grieving discussed in Chapter 10.

KNOWLEDGE CONNECTION

What is the purpose of wrapping a stump? How can you help a patient with an amputation adjust to body image changes?

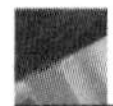

ASSISTIVE DEVICES FOR AMBULATION

Various types of assistive devices are available for people who are unable to ambulate independently. In most acute care settings, a physical therapist will fit the assistive device to the patient and instruct him or her on its proper use. You may be responsible for reinforcing the therapist's teaching. The following information will help you do so.

Crutches

Crutches are used when a patient is unable to bear full weight on a lower limb. The patient may be restricted to no weight bearing or partial weight bearing. Crutches fit correctly when there are three fingerbreadths of space between the axillary pad and the patient's axilla when the patient is standing with the crutch tips 4 to 6 inches (10 to 15 cm) to the side of the heel.

Guidelines for assisting patients using crutches include the following:

- Ensure that the patient is bearing weight on the hands and wrists, not on the axillary pads. ***Safety: Bearing weight on the axilla can cause compression of nerves and can lead to nerve damage affecting the arm and hand.***
- Instruct the patient that when walking upstairs on crutches, he or she should place the unaffected leg on the step first and then move up the crutches and the affected leg.
- Instruct the patient that when walking downstairs on crutches, he or she should place the crutches and affected leg on the downward step first and then bring down the unaffected leg. If a handrail is available, the patient may hold onto it and put both crutches on the opposite side.
- Assist the patient, if needed, to use the appropriate crutch-walking gait. (Table 27.2 describes common gaits.)
- Remind the patient to keep the affected foot slightly forward rather than bending the knee and holding the foot behind the crutches. ***Safety: If the knee is flexed and the foot is held behind the crutches, it can affect the patient's balance, causing him or her to fall backward.***

Table 27.2
Common Crutch-Walking Gaits

Type	*Description*
Two-point gait	For patients who are able to bear partial weight on the affected limb; patient moves one foot and the opposite crutch forward at the same time, and then moves remaining foot and crutch forward.
Three-point gait	For patients who are unable to bear weight on the affected limb; patient moves both crutches and the affected foot forward at the same time without touching down or placing weight on it, and then brings the unaffected foot forward.
Four-point gait	For patients able to bear weight on the affected limb; patient moves the first crutch forward and then the opposite foot forward; patient then moves remaining crutch forward and then remaining affected foot forward.
Swing-to gait	For patients able to bear weight on the affected limb; patient stands on both feet and moves both crutches forward at the same time; patient then swings both feet forward to the level of the crutches.
Swing-through gait	This is the same as the swing-to gait except that the patient swings both feet forward beyond the level of the crutches.

Canes

A cane is used when a patient can bear weight on the affected leg but needs extra support while ambulating. Several styles of canes exist, but they generally fall into two categories: single pronged and multipronged.

A single-pronged cane has one tip and may have a variety of handles (Fig. 27.6). A multipronged cane generally has three or four tips. A three-pronged tip may be called a tripod cane, and a four-pronged tip may be called a quad cane. In many situations, the multipronged cane is preferred because there is less chance that the cane could slide or slip as the patient leans on it. A cane is the correct height when the top of it is even with the patient's hip joint as the tip is positioned 4 inches (10 cm) away from the side of the foot.

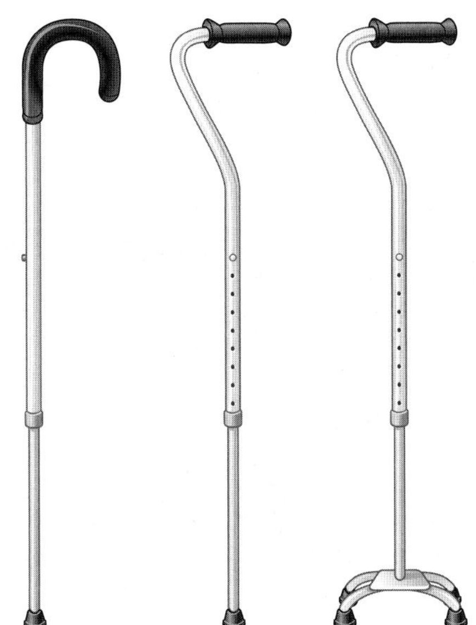

FIGURE 27.6 Two styles of single-tipped canes and a quad cane (from Wilkinson JM, Treas LS, Barnett KL, Smith MH. *Fundamentals of Nursing: Theory, Concepts & Applications*. Vol. 1. 3rd ed. Philadelphia, PA: FA Davis; 2016).

Guidelines for assisting patients using a cane include the following:

- Ensure that the patient holds the cane on the unaffected side.
- Remind the patient to remain erect rather than leaning over the cane.
- Ensure that the patient moves the affected leg and the cane forward together and then moves the unaffected leg forward.

Walkers

Walkers are used by patients who can bear full weight on both legs but need assistance to maintain balance. Several styles of walkers are available. The most common style is a metal frame with four legs and one open side so that the patient moves behind the walker and steps into the frame. Other styles include the type with two legs and two wheels. The wheels are located on the front of the walker, allowing the patient to push the walker rather than having to pick up the whole frame to advance it forward. A walker style popular for home use has four wheels with hand brakes and a seat where the person can sit to rest when the brakes are secured (Fig. 27.7). A walker that is the correct fit will come up to the patient's hip joint. When the patient grips the handles, his or her elbows should be bent at a 30-degree angle.

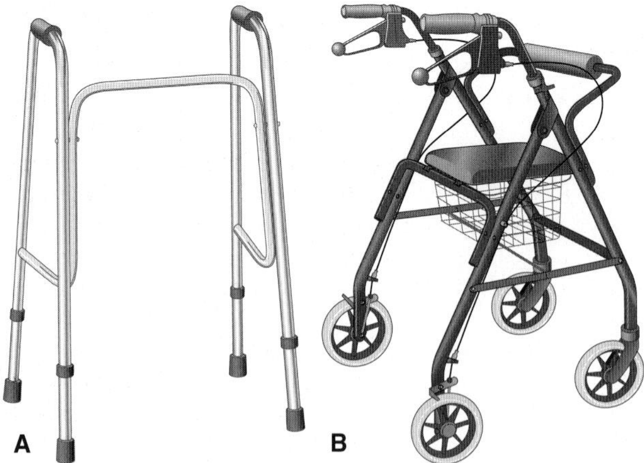

FIGURE 27.7 (a) Standard walker that the patient must lift and advance; (b) Rolling walker with brakes and a seat (from Wilkinson JM, Treas LS, Barnett KL, Smith MH. *Fundamentals of Nursing: Theory, Concepts & Applications*. Vol. 1. 3rd ed. Philadelphia, PA: FA Davis; 2016).

Guidelines for assisting patients using walkers include the following:

- Ensure that the patient stands between the back legs of the walker. ***Safety: Standing too far behind the walker can affect balance and lead to falls.***
- If the walker is the type that the patient must pick up and move forward, ensure that the patient sets the walker down and steps forward into it rather than simply carrying it.
- If the walker is the rolling style with hand brakes, ensure that the brakes are set (handles pulled downward) before the patient attempts to sit on the walker seat.
- If one leg is weak, instruct the patient to move the affected leg forward with the walker and then move the unaffected leg forward.

Settings Connection: Medical Office

Instructing a Patient to Use Ambulation Devices

When you work in a medical office, you may find that you are the person instructing a patient on how to correctly use crutches, a cane, or a walker. It is not unusual for patients to purchase or rent such equipment for themselves after an injury or trauma when they have little or no instruction on how to correctly use it. Observe patients with canes and walkers to be sure they come to the right height and are being used correctly. You may need to demonstrate correct crutch-walking gait for patients on crutches.

KNOWLEDGE CONNECTION

How should a patient using crutches bear his or her body weight? What is a quad cane? How do you instruct a patient to ambulate with a walker if he or she is weak on the left side?

Knee Walkers

Knee walkers, also called *knee scooters*, consist of a platform for the knee or the knee and lower leg, a front post with handlebars for steering, and three or four wheels. They are helpful for patients who cannot bear weight on a foot or ankle, such as after a surgery or due to sprains, fractures, gout, or a below-the-knee amputation. The affected leg rests on the platform, while the unaffected leg and foot are used to propel the person forward. There are hand brakes on the steerable handlebars. The front post folds down to fit better when getting it in and out of a car. It is not suitable for patients with knee injuries or knee surgeries because the person's weight rests on the knee and anterior surface of the lower leg.

Research studies have shown that the knee walker helps improve patients' mobility and decreases energy requirements compared to using crutches. Some patients feel more secure with the knee walker as well.

Settings Connection: Home Health

Promoting Mobility in the Home

When you care for patients in their homes, be sure that you evaluate the need for physical therapy if it is not already being given. Many times patients are weak from hospital stays and are unable to ambulate safely in the home as they did before their illness. If you see the need for physical therapy, let your nursing supervisor know so that orders can be obtained from the physician.

Settings Connection: Long-Term Care

Promoting Resident's Mobility

In the long-term care setting, it is so important that residents remain mobile for as long as possible. In order to help preserve the residents' mobility, be sure that you follow activity orders, such as assisting with ambulation and increasing time in sitting up in a chair.

Nursing Care Plan for a Patient With Total Left Knee Replacement

When you plan care for a patient with impaired mobility, protection from injury and restoring mobility are two prominent concerns. If you were going to develop a care plan for the patient that you were assigned in the Clinical Connection of this chapter, you would need a little more information. Here is what you find from reading the chart:

The patient is a 66-year-old female with a history of severe osteoarthritis in her left knee. She is overweight at 160 pounds (72.5 kg) and is 64 inches (162.5 cm) tall. Her right knee is arthritic as well, but the left knee is worse, so the decision has been made to replace the left knee first. She is a widow and lives alone. Her daughter is here from out of state and can stay with her for 2 weeks.

When your patient returns to her room after surgery, she has been medicated for pain and is very sleepy. Once she is moved from the stretcher to the bed, she becomes your responsibility. Figure 27.8 presents a concept map care plan for a patient with a total left knee replacement. Begin with your immediate postoperative assessment.

Assessment

One of the first assessments you will make is that of vital signs. Watch for changes that could indicate shock, such as decreasing blood pressure and increasing pulse, or changes that could indicate increasing pain, such as elevated blood pressure and pulse.

Next, assess the incision. It will most likely have a dressing in place. Look for drainage on the dressing. If any is present, draw a line around it and write the time, date, and your initials. This way, you can tell if and when the drainage increases. Check beneath the patient's knee for pooling blood or drainage.

Assess the patient's pain level. Although the patient was medicated in the recovery room, movement and transfer to the bed may exacerbate knee pain. Evaluate the pain using a scale from 0 to10 and assess the pain level frequently. Chapter 19 contains more information about managing pain and promoting rest and sleep.

The patient has one IV line connected to a pump. Note the quantity and solution of the IV fluids, and note the setting on the pump, which usually is the number of milliliters per hour at which the fluid is infusing.

Assess the patient's circulation distal to the surgery site. It is important to detect any compromise as quickly as possible. Assess posttibial and pedal pulses bilaterally. When you compare the operative side with the unaffected side, the pulses should be equal in strength. Check the foot for warmth, color,

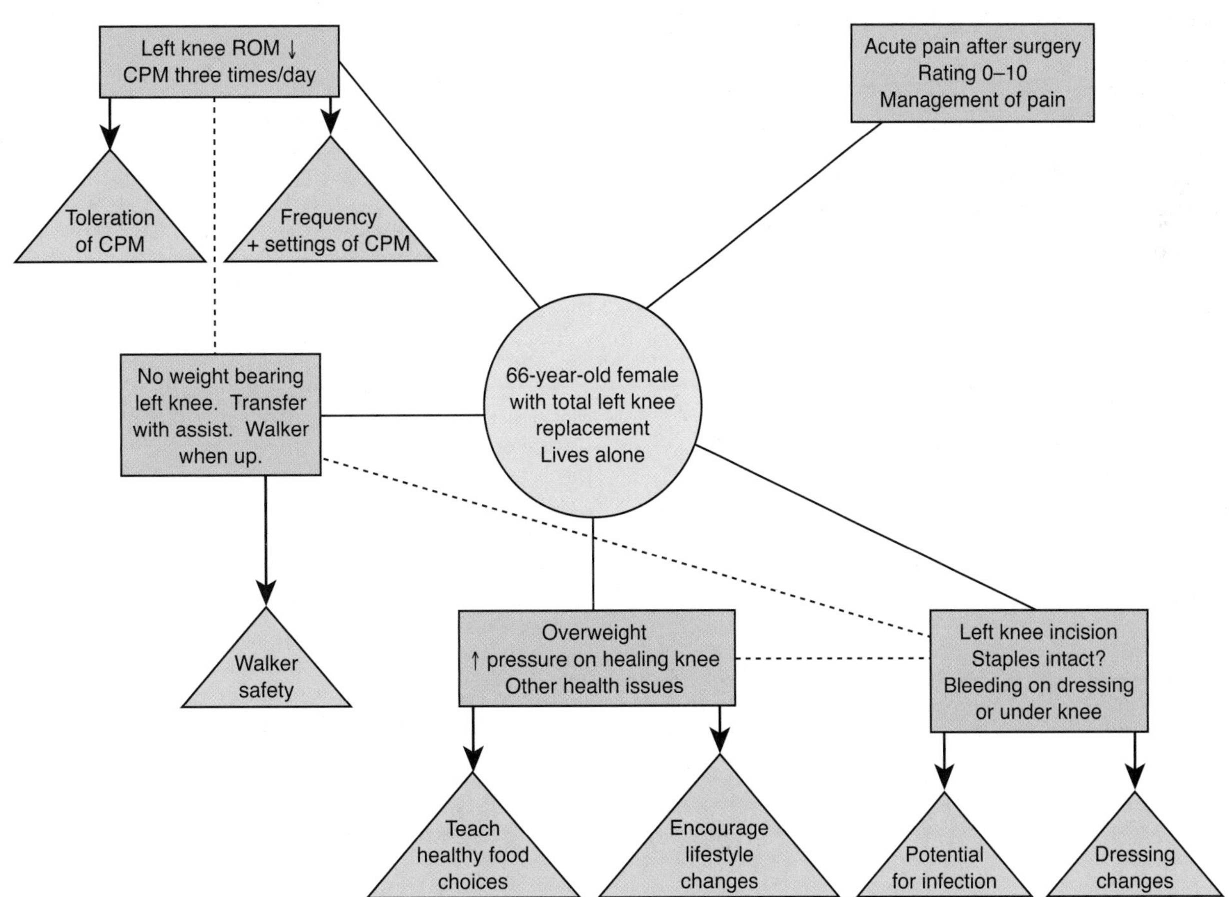

FIGURE 27.8 Concept map care plan for a patient with total left knee replacement.

(nursing care plan continues on page 568)

Nursing Care Plan for a Patient With Total Left Knee Replacement—cont'd

and capillary refill. (See Skill 27.1, page 570, for more details on neurovascular checks.)

Follow the additional assessment guidelines in Chapter 21.

Nursing Diagnoses

A concern for this patient will be her postoperative pain and her pain management. Another will be the incision and its healing. Another will be her limited mobility after surgery. In addition, she needs to be mobile enough to perform self-care by the time her daughter leaves. The nursing diagnoses given for this patient include the following:

- Acute pain related to physical injury as evidenced by restlessness and verbal reports of pain
- Impaired skin integrity related to knee surgery as evidenced by incision into body structures
- Impaired physical mobility related to the loss of integrity of bone structures as evidenced by limited range of motion

There may be additional possible nursing diagnoses for this patient, but in this chapter we will focus on these three as priorities.

Planning

When you plan care, you not only are planning what you need to do for the patient, you also are planning what outcomes or goals you want your patient to meet. Your obvious goal is to keep her comfortable; as it may be impossible for her to be totally pain free in the first few days after surgery, a good goal is keeping the pain at a 4 or below.

You must also plan to assess her left knee incision and to provide care as ordered by the health-care provider. First, you plan how to assess drainage and hemorrhage while the dressing is in place. Then, when the dressing is removed, generally about the second day postoperatively, you will assess the incision itself. Your goal for her incision is for it to heal without infection or other problems.

Your patient will definitely need help to get out of bed to use the bedside commode or bedpan and to obtain items that are not within reach. Your goals for her mobility are that she will be safe using the walker when she is up and that she will call for help when she needs to get out of bed.

Implementation

You are now at the stage of the nursing process to implement, or actually perform, the interventions that you have planned. Refer to the interventions listed below.

Evaluation

Once the interventions, or nursing actions, have been performed, you will want to evaluate whether or not they were effective. Did they accomplish what you intended? Did they help the patient's problems?

Nursing Diagnosis: Acute pain related to physical injury as evidenced by restlessness and verbal reports of pain
Expected Outcome: Patient will report that pain is consistently rated 4 or below before discharge from the hospital.

Interventions	Evaluations
Use a pain scale of 0–10 to assess for pain and discomfort several times per shift.	Day 1: Initial c/o pain @ 8. Day 2: C/o pain @ 6. Day 3: C/o pain @ 4.
Encourage the patient to ask for pain medication before pain becomes severe.	Day 1: Waited until pain was 7 before asking for meds, reminded to call earlier to try to keep pain below 5. Day 3: Called for meds at level 5 pain.
Provide distraction and other nonpharmacological interventions for pain (see Chapter 19).	Day 2: Distracted from pain and CPM machine while visitors were present and while watching a movie on TV. Day 3: Laughing with family and able to wait longer between pain medication requests when family present.
Medicate for pain before starting the CPM machine.	Day 1: Medicated every 4 hours for pain. CPM on 1 hr × 3. Day 2: Medicated every 4–6 hours for pain, always within 1 hr of using CPM. Day 3: Able to tolerate CPM with lower strength pain med.

Care Plan for a Patient With a Total Left Knee Replacement—cont'd

Nursing Diagnosis: Impaired skin integrity related to knee surgery as evidenced by incision into body structures
Expected Outcome: Patient will display healing incision with edges approximated and without signs of infection by discharge from hospital. Patient will verbalize signs of infection and criteria for contacting the health-care provider prior to discharge.

Interventions	Evaluations
Assess dressing for drainage and beneath the knee for bleeding postoperatively, then every 4 hours for the first 24 hours; reinforce dressing as needed.	Day 1: Quarter-size drainage on dressing during first 8 hr after surgery. 8 hr later had increased to 4 inches in diameter. Day 2: Dressing removed by health-care provider.
Change the left knee dressing every shift using 2 gauze 4×4s to protect the incision.	Day 1: Dressing changed every shift, quarter-sized amount serosanguineous drainage on old dressing. Day 2: Dressing changed each shift; quarter-sized amount serous drainage on old dressing. Day 3: Dressing changed each shift; dime-sized amount serous drainage on old dressing.
Assess the incision for approximated edges, signs of infection, and bleeding.	Day 1: Edges approximated, redness around all staples, no drainage or bleeding. Day 2: Less redness present, edges remain approximated, no drainage or bleeding. Day 3: Sl. redness around staples, 1-cm open area between staple #2 and #3 with sm. amount serous drainage present.
Teach the patient signs of infection (redness, heat, increasing pain, purulent drainage, elevated temperature) and wound dehiscence to report to the health-care provider prior to discharge.	Day 1: Able to verbalize two signs of infection. Day 2: Able to verbalize signs of wound dehiscence, including gaping of wound or small deep openings with or without drainage. Day 3: Able to verbalize four signs of infection and signs of wound dehiscence.

Nursing Diagnosis: Impaired physical mobility related to loss of integrity of bone structures as evidenced by limited range of motion
Expected Outcome: Patient will demonstrate increased range of motion in knee to 80 degrees by discharge from the hospital. Patient will be able to participate in activities of daily living and desired activities using touch-down weight bearing within 5 days of surgery.

Interventions	Evaluations
Follow the physician's orders for the CPM machine: 1–2 hours tid; settings of 40 degrees of flexion at 10 degrees per minute to start and advance to 80 degrees of flexion at 30 degrees per minute as tolerated.	Day 1: CPM machine set at lowest setting tid. Day 2: CPM advanced to 50 degrees of flexion at 20 degrees per minute tid; tolerated with minor c/o discomfort. Day 3: CPM advanced to 60 degrees of flexion at 30 degrees per minute tid; pt. complained of increased discomfort on second session; decreased flexion by 5 degrees for third session and tolerated without complaints.
Assist the patient when out of bed; instruct the patient not to get out of bed without assistance.	Day 1: Assisted to BSC × 3; pivoted well on right leg. Day 2: Assisted to BR with walker × 4 on 7–3 shift with toe touch-down only. Day 3: Ambulated with walker in room and hallway with minimal weight bearing on left leg.
Reinforce the teaching by the physical therapist.	Day 1: Reminded to pivot on right leg only and not to bear weight on left leg; instructed in active range of motion for other joints. Day 2: Instructed to amb to BR; touch-down with foot only when using walker. Day 3: Instructed in minimal weight-bearing techniques while amb with walker in hallway.

Skill 27.1 Performing Neurovascular Checks

Assessment Step

1. Determine the area of the limb distal to the surgical site or cast that is to be evaluated.

Planning Step

1. Determine when the last neurovascular check was done. Perform checks every 2 hours for the first 24 hours after surgery or application of a cast unless otherwise ordered.

Implementation Steps

1. Follow the Initial Implementation Steps located on the inside back cover.
2. Ask the patient if he or she is experiencing numbness, burning, or tingling in the affected limb. Test sensation of the affected and unaffected limbs by touching each with a paper clip and asking the patient to tell you when he or she feels the sensation of the paper clip touching the limb. ***A decreased sensation in the affected limb may indicate impairment of sensory nerve function.***
3. Assess for edema at the surgical site and distal to the site or cast. Compare the size of the distal aspect of the extremity to the unaffected extremity. ***Edema indicates impairment of circulation and should be monitored closely to determine if it increases.***
4. Touch the patient's skin distal to the surgical site or cast with the back of your hand. Assess for warmth and compare to the warmth of the same area on the unaffected limb. ***Cooler temperature of the affected limb may indicate impairment of circulation.***
5. Assess the color of the skin and nailbeds in the distal portion of the affected limb. These should be the same as in the unaffected limb; nailbeds should be pink. ***Pallor or cyanosis indicates impairment of circulation.***
6. Test capillary refill in the nailbeds of the fingers or toes distal to the surgical site or cast. Compare it to that in the unaffected limb. ***Slower refill time in the affected limb or refill longer than 5 seconds indicates that circulation is impaired.***
7. Ask the patient to move the fingers or toes of the affected extremity. ***Movement should be free of discomfort if motor nerves are unimpaired.***
8. Palpate distal pulses if possible and compare with the pulses on the unaffected limb. ***Each should be present and equal if no circulatory impairment is present.***
9. Ask the patient to describe his or her pain in the affected limb, including the type of pain and its intensity. Ask him or her to rate it on a scale of 0 to 10. ***Pain should gradually decrease in intensity as healing occurs. A sudden increase in pain could indicate infection or compression.***
10. Follow the Ending Implementation Steps located on the inside back cover.

Evaluation Steps

1. Determine deviations from normal during neurovascular checks and report them to the health-care provider.
2. Evaluate the patient's pain level and report complaints of increasing pain, which could indicate impaired circulation.

Sample Documentation

01/22/22 0900 Casted Lt. arm elevated on 2 pillows. Lt. fingers exhibit moderate edema with no increase from 0700, pink, warm, good motion & sensation, cap. refill less than 3 seconds. No C/O pain. ———
——— Nurse's signature and credentials

Skill 27.2 Setting Up a Continuous Passive Motion Machine

Assessment Steps

1. Review the physician's order. Note the degrees of flexion and the speed ordered, as well as the length of time the machine is to be in use.
2. Assess the patient's pain level. Determine the need for and administer pain medication before beginning CPM treatment.
3. Determine patient comfort needs before starting CPM treatment: assist to the bathroom or bedside commode if needed and place desired items within reach.

Planning Step

1. Obtain needed equipment: CPM machine and sheepskin for the platform. Follow the facility policy for charging out the equipment.

Implementation Steps

1. Follow the Initial Implementation Steps located on the inside back cover.
2. Place the CPM machine on the bed and connect it to the power source.
3. Place the sheepskin on the platform where the patient's leg will rest, especially at the end near the gluteal fold ***to prevent pressure on the patient's skin, which could lead to a pressure ulcer.***
4. Position the CPM machine so that the break in the platform is centered beneath the patient's knee. Align the machine and the patient's leg with the hips and torso of the patient's body ***to prevent injury or muscle spasms.***
5. Carefully assist the patient to place the affected leg on the CPM platform.

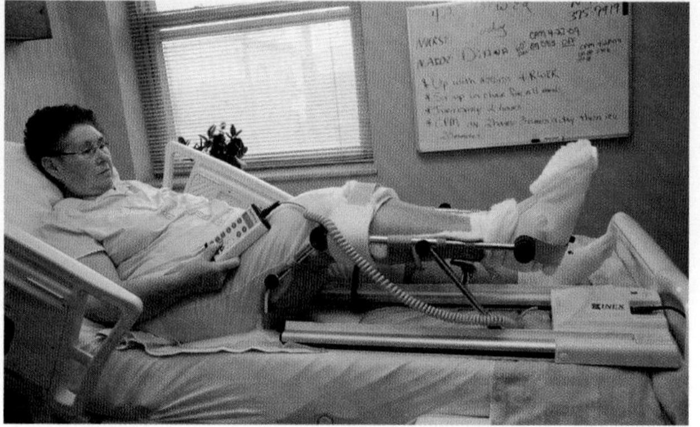

Skill 27.2 (continued)

6. Set the degrees of flexion and speed as ordered by the physician.
7. Turn on the CPM machine.
8. Observe the machine as it flexes and extends the patient's knee and ensure that the passive exercise is being well tolerated by the patient. ***Gentle passive exercise should not cause pain.***
9. Follow the Ending Implementation Steps located on the inside back cover.

Evaluation Steps

1. Evaluate the movement of the patient's knee for appropriate degrees of flexion and extension.
2. Evaluate the patient's pain level while using the CPM machine.
3. Ensure that the CPM therapy is in use for the length of time ordered.

Sample Documentation

08/12/22 1430 CPM machine in place and on. Set at 90-degree flexion at speed of 30 degrees per minute per physician's order. States knee feels stiff but passive motion is not painful. ——— Nurse's signature and credentials ———

08/12/22 1530 CPM off per physician's order. No edema noted. States pain is at a 4 after treatment. ——— Nurse's signature and credentials ———

Skill 27.3 Applying Elastic Bandages

Assessment Steps

1. Check the physician's order for placement and purpose of the elastic bandage.
2. Assess the patient's limb or stump for skin breakdown or wounds.
3. Assess for edema in the limb or stump.

Planning Steps

1. Obtain the correct width of elastic bandage. ***Use wider widths to cover larger areas, such as for stump wrapping.***
2. Obtain metal closures, safety pins, or tape ***to hold wrap in place.***

Implementation Steps

1. Follow the Initial Implementation Steps located on the inside back cover.

For Figure-of-Eight Wrap on the Ankle

2. Wrap two turns around the instep of the foot to secure the end of the wrap.
3. Bring the bandage around the inner ankle and behind the lower leg.
4. Bring the bandage around the outer ankle, across the top of the foot, and back to the instep.
5. Bring the bandage under the foot, then across the top of the foot to the inner ankle.
6. Bring the bandage around the inner ankle and behind the lower leg.

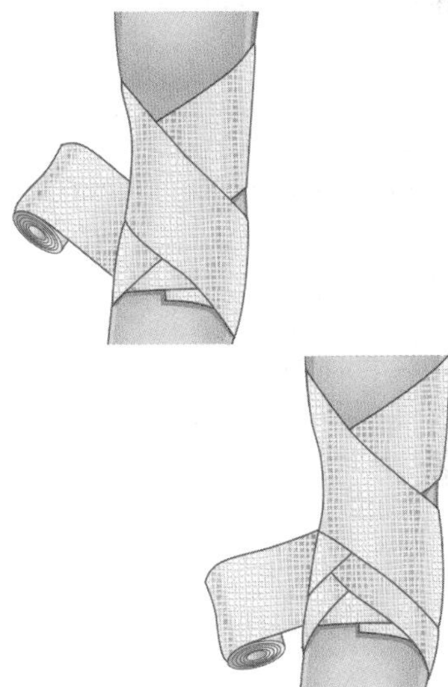

7. Repeat the above steps until bandaging is complete. Each additional wrap should be approximately 1/4 to 1/2 inch (0.51 to 1.3 cm) more proximal than the previous wrap, making an evenly distributed crisscross pattern across the dorsal surface of the foot and ankle.
8. Secure the bandage end with tape, safety pins, or metal clasps.
9. Follow the Ending Implementation Steps located on the inside back cover.

(skill continues on page 572)

Skill 27.3 (continued)

For Spiral Turn on the Forearm or Leg

2. Start at the narrower area of the lower leg or wrist area of the forearm.
3. Wrap two turns to anchor the wrap.
4. Wrap the bandage around the arm or leg, progressing up the limb with each turn at a 30-degree angle, overlapping the elastic bandage with each turn.

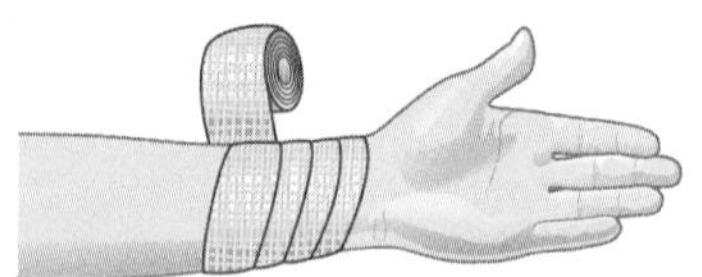

5. Repeat the above steps until bandaging is complete.
6. Secure the bandage end with tape, safety pins, or metal clasps.
7. Follow the Ending Implementation Steps located on the inside back cover.

Evaluation Steps

1. Make certain the wrap is not too tight by ensuring that you can slip two fingers underneath the bandage at its proximal end. Ask the patient if it is painful or causing numbness or tingling in the limb. If so, remove and rewrap more loosely.
2. Assess fingers and toes for edema, warmth, capillary refill, sensation, movement, and color. If circulation is impaired, remove and rewrap more loosely.
3. Determine if wrap is too loose such that it sags or comes loose as the patient moves. If so, remove and rewrap more tightly.

Sample Documentation

08/18/22 1207 Elastic bandage applied to left ankle using figure eight. States it is comfortable. Left toes pink, warm, with cap. refill less than 3 seconds, and without edema or numbness. Able to wiggle toes. Left ankle elevated on pillow. ______________ Nurse's signature and credentials ______________

POST CONFERENCE

You followed this patient from her return from the recovery room to her third postoperative day, and you found it amazing how mobile she was by that last day. She went from being nearly immobile to ambulating the length of the hall using a walker. She insisted that the surgical pain was less uncomfortable than the previous arthritic pain she experienced with every step. You learned how effective the CPM machine was at keeping the knee mobile and flexing it without the patient having to intentionally do so. She slept through the CPM use, even as it flexed her knee up to 60 degrees, more than she has been able to flex it in 20 years.

Key Points

- Sprains, fractures, joint replacements, and amputations are common musculoskeletal conditions that limit mobility.
- The physical therapist is the member of the health-care team who is responsible for assessing deficiencies in musculoskeletal function and developing a plan of care. It is very important to follow the orders of the health-care provider and the recommendations of the physical therapist regarding patient activity and mobility.
- A variety of immobilization devices are used to promote healing of musculoskeletal disorders. These include casts, traction, splints, immobilizers, and abductor pillows.
- When a plaster cast is drying, handle it only with the palms of your hands because using your fingers may cause dents in the cast that can lead to pressure ulcers under the cast.
- When caring for patients with dry casts, observe carefully for drainage or discharge on or under the cast. Teach patients how to relieve itching under the cast without causing skin abrasions.
- Perform neurovascular checks every 2 hours in the first 24 hours after a cast is applied or surgery is performed on a limb and then every 4 hours or according to facility policy.
- When caring for a patient in traction, keep all ropes straight without kinks and aligned in pulleys, with weights hanging freely. Assess for skin breakdown beneath the traction boot or elastic bandage.
- When caring for a patient in skeletal traction, clean the pin sites using sterile technique with the solution ordered. Observe them carefully for signs of infection because any infection at the pin site can easily invade the bone.

- When caring for a patient with a lateral total hip replacement, keep the abductor pillow in place while the patient is in bed. When the patient transfers from the bed to a chair and while he or she is sitting in the chair, prevent him or her from flexing the hip more than 90 degrees. Adduction of the leg or flexion of the hip can cause dislocation of the hip prosthesis.
- When caring for a patient with a knee replacement, a CPM machine will be ordered. This passively exercises the knee with flexion and extension and must be set at the speed and degree of flexion ordered by the physician.
- When caring for a patient with an amputated limb, it is important to give emotional as well as physical support. It also is important to constantly plan toward rehabilitation and the use of a prosthetic limb. Assess the incision for healing and apply a compression "shrinker sock" as ordered to form the proper shape for fitting into the socket of the prosthesis.
- Assistive devices for ambulation include crutches, canes, and walkers. It is important to ensure the correct fit of each device and then reinforce the teaching of the physical therapist on the use of each.
- When planning care for patients with impaired mobility, it is important to address pain before expecting the patient to exercise the affected limb or to ambulate.

Review Questions

Select the answer that is most appropriate for each of the following questions. Some questions may have more than one correct answer. Select all that apply.

1. A coworker twisted her ankle going down the stairs. It is swollen and is painful when she bears weight on it. Which intervention would be the least helpful for healing this sprain?
   1. Avoiding bearing weight on her ankle
   2. Wrapping her ankle with an elastic bandage
   3. Applying heat to her ankle for 20 minutes at a time
   4. Elevating her ankle on a pillow while she is lying down

2. The purpose of which of the following devices is to prevent flexion of an affected joint?
   1. Cast
   2. Immobilizer
   3. Splint
   4. Elastic bandages
   5. Traction
   6. Abductor pillow
   7. Ilizarov frame

3. A patient comes into the clinic with his arm in a cast. You notice a small amount of thick, light yellow drainage coming from under the cast, and it has an unpleasant odor. There is no drainage staining the cast, and no open areas of skin are visible at the edge of the cast. Which question is most appropriate to ask this patient?
   1. "Have you inserted anything under the cast to scratch your arm?"
   2. "Have you had an upper respiratory infection recently?"
   3. "Do you have a skin rash anywhere on your body?"
   4. "Is the edge of the cast irritating your skin?"

4. A patient is in skeletal traction for a comminuted fracture of the tibia. While giving pin care, you notice a small amount of serous drainage around each pin site. Which observation is most accurate?
   1. The drainage is a symptom of skin infection.
   2. This finding is normal for skeletal traction.
   3. This is an indication of pin dislocation.
   4. The drainage is an indication of a bone infection.

5. Which surfaces are replaced when a patient has a total hip replacement?
   1. The articular surfaces of the femur and the tibia
   2. The posterior surface of the patella and the tibia
   3. The acetabular cup and head of the tibia and fibula
   4. The head and neck of the femur and the acetabular cup

6. You are caring for a patient with a fresh total hip replacement. Which statement would indicate that your patient needs more teaching?
   1. "I will sleep with the abductor pillow between my legs every night for several months."
   2. "I can cross my legs when I am sitting in a chair as long as my feet are elevated on a footstool."
   3. "I need to use an extension gripper to pick up anything I drop."
   4. "I will sit in the recliner with the back slightly reclined when I am out of bed."

7. The purpose of the CPM machine is to provide:
   1. active abduction and adduction.
   2. active range of motion to all joints.
   3. passive flexion and extension.
   4. passive internal and external rotation.

8. A patient has had his hand and part of his forearm amputated due to a traumatic injury. What would be the result if he refused to have his stump wrapped continuously with an elastic bandage or wear a compression sock?
   1. The incision on the end of the stump will not heal.
   2. There will be excessive bruising and swelling of the stump.
   3. The stump will not heal in a shape to fit inside the prosthesis well.
   4. He can wait a few weeks after surgery before wrapping the stump or wearing the compression sock.

ANSWERS 1. 3, 2. 1, 2, 3, 3. 1, 4. 2, 5. 4, 6. 2, 7. 3, 8. 3

Critical Thinking Exercises

Answers available online.

1. Why does a dislocated hip prosthesis cause pain to a patient since the socket is not made of the patient's bones?

2. A patient with a left fractured ankle was put in an immobilizing boot and told to use crutches 2 days ago. She fell this morning and is complaining of left arm pain when she arrives at the clinic where you work. What would you ask her about her use of crutches?

Additional Resources

DAVIS edge. **Use the scratch off code on the inside front cover of your book to access online quizzes that will help you to improve your scores on course exams and prepare for the NCLEX-PN®.**

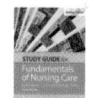

Study Guide

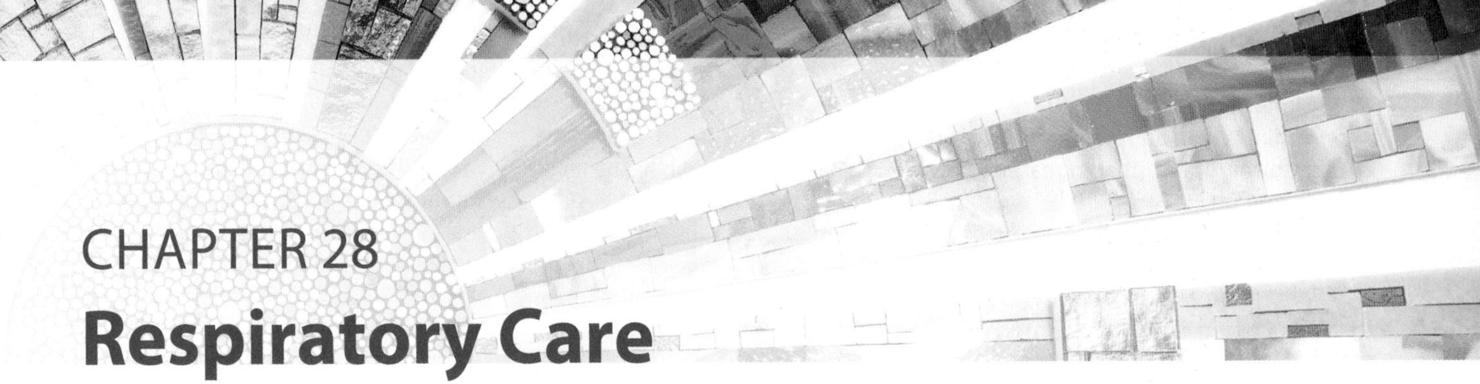

CHAPTER 28
Respiratory Care

KEY TERMS

Crepitus (KREP-ih-tuss)
Cyanosis (SYE-uh-NOH-siss)
Endotracheal tube (EN-doh-TRAY-kee-uhl TOOB)
Exhalation (EKS-ha-LAY-shun)
Hemothorax (HEE-moh-THAW-raks)
Hypoxemia (HYE-pok-SEE-mee-ah)
Hypoxia (hye-POK-see-ah)
Incentive spirometer (in-SEN-tiv spye-ROM-uh-tur)
Inhalation (IN-hah-LAY-shun)
Nebulizer (NEB-yoo-LYE-zer)
Parietal pleura (pah-RYE-et-uhl PLOO-rah)
Pleural effusion (PLOOR-uhl ef-YOO-zhun)
Pneumothorax (NEW-moh-THAW-raks)
Sputum (SPYOO-tum)
Tension pneumothorax (TEN-shun NEW-moh-THAW-raks)
Tracheostomy (TRAY-kee-AWS-tuh-mee)
Visceral pleura (VISS-uh-ruhl PLOO-rah)

CHAPTER CONCEPTS

Acid-Base Balance
Oxygenation
Patient-Centered Care
Safety

LEARNING OUTCOMES

1. Define various terms associated with respiratory care.
2. Explain the mechanics of inhalation and exhalation.
3. Describe chemical and nervous regulation of respirations.
4. Explain the changes in physiological regulation of respiration in patients with chronic lung disease.
5. Differentiate between internal and external respiration.
6. Contrast hypoxia and hypoxemia.
7. Identify causes of impaired oxygenation.
8. List inspection points in the assessment of a patient with impaired oxygenation.
9. Describe palpation, auscultation, and other assessment findings that could indicate impaired oxygenation.
10. Discuss the significance of selected diagnostic tests when caring for patients with impaired oxygenation.
11. Explain nursing interventions to use for patients with impaired oxygenation.
12. Discuss safety measures to enforce when the patient is receiving supplemental oxygen.
13. Identify types of oxygen sources and delivery devices used for supplemental oxygen.
14. List tips for conservation of energy for patients with chronic lung disease.
15. Describe various artificial airways and how to suction the patient with the airway in place.
16. Describe a tracheostomy tube and the nursing care needed to keep it patent.
17. Illustrate chest tube placement and how the chest drainage system works.
18. Discuss nursing care of patients with chest tubes.
19. Plan care for a patient with a respiratory disorder.
20. Discuss information found in the Connection features of the chapter.
21. Identify safety issues related to respiratory care.
22. Answer questions about skills in the chapter.

SKILLS

28.1 Obtaining a Sputum Specimen
28.2 Obtaining a Throat Culture Specimen
28.3 Assisting With Incentive Spirometry

Continued

SKILLS—cont'd

28.4 Administering a Nebulizer Treatment
28.5 Administering Supplemental Oxygen
28.6 Performing Nasopharyngeal and Oropharyngeal Suctioning
28.7 Performing Endotracheal and Tracheostomy Suctioning
28.8 Performing Tracheostomy Care
28.9 Maintaining Chest Tubes

CRITICAL THINKING CONNECTION

Clinical Assignment

You are assigned to care for a hospitalized patient tomorrow in clinical who has a tracheostomy. He was injured in a car accident and was on a ventilator for several weeks. He is breathing on his own now, but he still has the tracheostomy in place. In addition, he has recently developed pneumonia in his right lung. He has a large amount of secretions and requires suctioning every 2 to 3 hours. The tracheostomy will have to be cleaned on your shift and a new inner cannula put in place. He has humidified oxygen at 4 L/min via a tracheostomy collar.

Critical Thinking Questions:

1. Why is a tracheostomy done?
2. How does a tracheostomy work?
3. How will you suction it?
4. How will you clean it and replace the inner cannula?
5. What is a tracheostomy collar?

It can be alarming to see a patient struggle to breathe or to have to assist a patient who must be suctioned to be able to breathe. As the patient becomes more anxious, it is easy for your anxiety to increase as well. This chapter will help you prepare to care for patients who have respiratory problems, assisting them to improve oxygenation and breathe more easily.

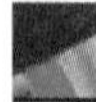

NORMAL OXYGENATION

The term *airway* refers to the path that air takes as it enters and exits the lungs. The normal pathway is through the nostrils into the pharynx, into the trachea, and then to either the right or the left bronchus, which branches into the bronchioles that terminate into the alveoli. When this pathway is unblocked and air is moving freely, it is referred to as a *patent airway*.

The Mechanics of Breathing

When the airway is patent, air is inhaled and follows the pathway to the alveoli, where oxygen is absorbed into the blood and carbon dioxide leaves the blood to be exhaled. Oxygen and carbon dioxide move across the alveolar cell membranes and the cell membranes of the capillaries surrounding the alveoli by the process of *diffusion*.

This process occurs involuntarily, meaning that no conscious thought is given to it. It is important to understand the mechanics of how breathing occurs so that you can grasp the treatments for respiratory disorders affecting those mechanics, such as chest tubes, endotracheal tubes, and mechanical ventilation.

The diaphragm and the intercostals are the muscles required for breathing to occur. When the diaphragm contracts in response to stimulus from the phrenic nerves, it moves downward, which increases the size of the chest cavity. Intercostal muscles then contract, moving the ribs up and out, which also enlarges the chest cavity from side to side and from front to back. When the chest cavity size increases, it causes the lungs to expand. The pressure within the lungs then drops below atmospheric pressure, or becomes negative pressure. This causes a sort of vacuum; air is pulled into the lungs until the pressure in the lungs equals the pressure outside the body. The term used to describe this is **inhalation,** also known as *inspiration.*

As these muscles relax, again in response to nerve stimulus, the size of the chest cavity decreases. The ribs come inward, the diaphragm rises upward, and the lungs are then compressed, forcing the air to go out. This is referred to as **exhalation,** also known as *expiration.*

Regulation of Respiration

Nerves and a chemical control mechanism both contribute to the regulation of respirations. The respiratory center is in the medulla, located in the brainstem. This brain function automatically controls inhalation by sending impulses to the phrenic nerve, which causes contraction of the diaphragm and intercostal muscles.

Chemical regulation of respirations is influenced by chemoreceptors located in the carotid and aortic bodies and in the medulla of the brain. When these chemoreceptors detect a decrease in the oxygen level of the blood or a change in blood pH, they send a message to the medulla, which in turn causes an increase in the rate and depth of respirations. When carbon dioxide increases above normal amounts, it causes the blood to become more acidic. The chemoreceptors respond by sending the message to the medulla, which in turn causes the respiratory rate to increase to "blow off" or remove excess carbon dioxide, returning the blood pH to normal levels. (See Chapter 29 for more information about acid-base balance and the role of the lungs in maintaining blood pH.)

Rising carbon dioxide levels that in turn cause the blood to become more acidic provide the brain's stimulus to breathe.

• WORD • BUILDING •

inhalation: in – in + hala – breath + tion – action
exhalation: ex – out + hala – breath + tion – action

That is why you cannot hold your breath for long periods of time—not because your oxygen level is falling, but because you are trapping carbon dioxide in your blood, causing a buildup of carbonic acid, which in turn prompts the medulla to make you breathe.

REGULATION OF RESPIRATION IN CHRONIC LUNG DISEASE. People who have severe chronic lung disease gradually develop a different stimulus to breathe. Unlike the situation in persons with healthy lung tissue, in people with severe chronic lung disease air is trapped in the alveoli for long periods of time because oxygen and carbon dioxide are unable to diffuse freely across the stiff, nonelastic alveolar membrane. This raises the blood's level of carbon dioxide and lowers the oxygen level. The body gradually acclimates to the higher carbon dioxide level because it cannot continue to increase the respiratory rate higher and higher to blow it off. Thus, the high carbon dioxide level no longer stimulates respiration, and the body begins to respond to the lower level of oxygen, which now becomes its stimulus to breathe. Then, if the oxygen level is raised too high, it can impair the message from the medulla that instructs the body to breathe. It will be important to remember this later in the chapter when we discuss oxygen flow rates for patients with chronic lung disease.

Internal and External Respiration

External respiration occurs between the alveoli and the capillaries. The alveoli are air sacs encircled by tiny capillaries. Oxygen moves via diffusion from an area of higher concentration to an area of lower concentration. When you inhale, the inspired air contains more oxygen, so it passes from the alveoli into the capillaries.

Internal respiration occurs between the bloodstream and the body cells. When fresh oxygen enters the bloodstream, it is carried by the hemoglobin on the red blood cells through the arteries and arterioles to the capillaries. In the tiny capillaries, where the walls are just one cell thick, the oxygen diffuses to the tissue cells where the concentration is lower. At the same time, carbon dioxide and other waste products diffuse into the blood from the tissue cells for the same reason. The blood then returns to the heart and lungs through the venules and veins. Once the blood is pumped back to the lungs by the right side of the heart, the carbon dioxide and waste products leave the blood and enter the alveoli to leave the body with exhalation.

Anatomy and Physiology Connection

The Pleura

The chest cavity is lined with a thin membrane that also covers each lung, similar to a sac within a sac. This membrane is called the *pleura.* The portion of the pleura that lines the chest cavity is called the **parietal pleura.** This continuous membrane then covers the lungs, and that portion is called the **visceral pleura.** There is a very narrow space between the two layers, referred to as the *pleural space,* in which a negative pressure, or vacuum, must be maintained so that expansion of the chest wall will cause the lung to expand as the chest wall expands. If this vacuum is lost and air or fluid enters into the pleural space, the lung will collapse rather than expand. This space contains a small amount of fluid that helps hold the two layers together but also allows them to glide smoothly against one another with each inhalation and exhalation. A similar situation occurs when you add a drop of water to a microscope slide, then place the coverslip over it. The water forms a film that holds the coverslip on the slide but allows it to glide against the slide for correct placement.

KNOWLEDGE CONNECTION

What role do muscles, nerves, and chemicals play in respiration? What are the similarities and differences between internal and external respiration?

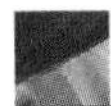

IMPAIRED OXYGENATION

If a blockage occurs in the airway or oxygen cannot pass into the blood in the alveolar capillaries, the patient is unable to obtain needed oxygen from room air. If oxygen cannot cross into the tissue cells in the peripheral capillaries, the patient is unable to provide oxygen to body cells. Each of these situations can lead to impaired oxygenation.

It is very important to recognize the signs and symptoms of decreased oxygen in the blood and tissues because oxygen is necessary for brain and organ function. Often the symptoms do not become noticeable until the oxygen level has dropped considerably.

When oxygen levels in the blood drop below normal range, it is referred to as **hypoxemia.** In the event of hypoxemia, the blood cannot take adequate amounts of oxygen to the tissues during internal respiration, causing **hypoxia.** Without enough oxygen in the tissues, you will see changes in mental function, in the color of the skin and mucous membranes, and in respiratory rate and rhythm. Box 28.1 lists the signs and symptoms of hypoxia.

• WORD • BUILDING •

parietal pleura: parietal – forming wall of a cavity; pleura – pleural membrane

visceral pleura: visceral – body organs; pleura – pleural membranes

hypoxemia: hypo – deficient + ox – oxygen + em – blood + ia – condition

hypoxia: hypo – deficient + ox – oxygen + ia – condition

Box 28.1

Signs and Symptoms of Hypoxia

When patients become hypoxic, the early symptoms may be missed if you are not aware of them. By the time the later symptoms are evident, the patient is severely hypoxic. It is important to assess your patients for the early subtle signs as well as the more apparent ones.

Early

- Agitation
- Anxiety
- Changes in level of consciousness
- Disorientation
- Headache
- Irritability
- Restlessness
- Tachypnea

Late

- Bradycardia
- Cardiac dysrhythmias
- Cyanosis
- Decreased respiratory rate (bradypnea)
- Retractions

Real-World Connection

Effects of Hypoxia on Thinking

Hypoxia to the brain can cause changes in mental function, including affecting judgment. A home health nurse went to visit a patient with chronic lung disease who had recently been hospitalized with respiratory failure. When the nurse arrived, she found that the patient had recently discharged his gun in his home. He had seen his reflection in a mirror, and his hypoxic brain had misinterpreted the face as that of a stranger; he thought that someone was looking in the window of his home. After discharging the gun, he realized that he had shot at his own reflection. His oxygen saturation was very low at 66%, and he was readmitted to the hospital.

Causes of Impaired Oxygenation

A variety of situations can contribute to impaired oxygen exchange. It may be due to some type of obstruction in the pharynx, trachea, or bronchi causing a decrease in inspired air. If the nose is blocked due to mucus congestion, the body utilizes an alternate path and mouth breathing occurs. If the trachea is blocked by secretions, coughing clears them. If the trachea becomes blocked by a foreign body, such as a piece of food, and coughing is either impossible or not sufficient to remove the blockage, the Heimlich maneuver can be performed to clear the airway. If the bronchi or bronchioles are blocked by thick mucus or secretions, deep coughs and possibly mucus-thinning agents are required to clear it.

Another cause of impaired oxygenation may be secretions in the alveoli or damage to the alveoli caused by chronic lung disease. When the alveoli are not fully functional, less oxygen can cross into the blood and less carbon dioxide is able to leave the blood. Low oxygen in the blood may also be due to a situation in which the patient is unable to fully expand the lungs due to fluid or pus in the chest cavity or a blood clot in the lung preventing circulation to the alveoli. Patients who have had surgery or chest trauma may have hypoxemia due to pain that prevents them from taking a deep breath.

Chronic lung disease is also a cause of hypoxemia. Over time, the alveoli and airways are damaged, making them unable to expand and move air in and out, so oxygen does not cross into the alveolar capillaries to be taken to the body tissues.

Damage or trauma to the lung itself also can cause hypoxemia. If a lung collapses, called *atelectasis,* expansion does not occur, so air is not pulled into the lungs. This may be the result of trauma such as a bullet or knife wound to the chest. It also may be due to blockage of the airway to the lung, preventing expansion of the lung. For example, if a large tumor is blocking the air path in the right main bronchus, inhaled air is unable to fill the lung.

Be aware that a patient can have a normal pulse oximetry reading and still suffer from hypoxia. If the blood is carrying adequate amounts of oxygen, the pulse oximetry reading will be normal. However, the oxygen may not be crossing the capillary wall and entering the tissue cells. Box 28.2 summarizes the causes of hypoxia and hypoxemia.

Caring for Patients With Impaired Oxygenation

You will care for many patients with impaired oxygenation. Generally, these patients are anxious and frightened; being unable to get your breath is a terrifying experience. As the patient's nurse, it is very important for you to remain calm. Speak in a normal tone of voice, without sounding excited or upset. Tell the patient what you need him or her to do. Help

Box 28.2

Causes of Hypoxia and Hypoxemia

A variety of conditions can lead to hypoxia and hypoxemia. These may be due to a mechanical problem that interferes with air entering the body, blood conditions interfering with the blood's ability to transport oxygen, side effects of medications, or environmental situations. Causes include the following:

- Airway obstruction due to a tumor, choking on a foreign body, thick mucus, or swollen airways
- Anemia
- Atelectasis (collapsed lung)
- Chronic lung disease
- Decreased cardiac output
- High altitude
- Hypoventilation due to anesthetics, sedatives, or coma
- Poor peripheral circulation
- Pulmonary embolus

him or her slow down breathing by repeating "Breath in, breath out" at the tempo at which you want the patient to breathe. It is important that you reassure the patient that help is present. Do not leave the patient in acute respiratory distress alone, even if you think that the patient is "just anxious."

Assessing Respiratory Status

As you perform a respiratory assessment, you will inspect, palpate, and auscultate the patient. As you enter the room and interact with the patient, note the following:

- Color of skin and mucous membranes
- Respiratory effort
- Cough
- Chest appearance
- Oxygenation status
- Oxygen saturation

COLOR OF SKIN AND MUCOUS MEMBRANES. When oxygen levels in the tissues decrease, the lips take on a bluish color, called **cyanosis**. This color change may also be observed on the tip of the nose, on tops of the ears, and in the nailbeds. When the patient has dark skin, the color may appear more ashen than cyanotic and you will depend more on the color of the mucous membranes. Check the palms of the hands and soles of the feet for color changes as well. ***Safety: Cyanosis is a late sign of hypoxia. Take action immediately and notify the health-care provider immediately.***

RESPIRATORY EFFORT. When the patient is having difficulty moving air in and out of the lungs, it is referred to as *dyspnea.* Notice if the patient is having difficulty breathing while at rest and also if he or she becomes short of breath when ambulating a short distance, such as to the bathroom and back. If the patient has to stop to rest or catch his or her breath when ambulating a brief distance, then the patient is short of breath, known as *exertional dyspnea.* Patients with impaired oxygenation often assume a position of sitting upright and leaning slightly forward with arms and head over a table. This is the *orthopneic* position. It increases the intrathoracic area, allowing the patient to inhale more air. Watch for gasping respirations, or "air hunger," and expressions of grimacing or fear on the patient's face.

COUGH. If the patient is bringing up **sputum**, or mucus, from the lungs when coughing, it is referred to as a *productive cough.* If the cough is dry, it is referred to as a *nonproductive cough.* It is important to notice the color, consistency, and amount of any sputum the patient produces. Sputum that is clear or white may indicate a viral infection; if it is yellow or green, it may be indicative of a bacterial infection. Rust-colored sputum indicates the presence of blood and may be seen in some pneumonia infections and tuberculosis. When sputum is gray or black, it usually indicates that the patient has inhaled smoke or soot. Pink and frothy, or bubbly, sputum is indicative of fluid and blood mixed together and is seen in a life-threatening condition called *pulmonary edema.*

In addition to the color of sputum, the consistency of the sputum is an important observation. Thick, tenacious, sticky mucus is difficult to cough out. It tends to remain in the lungs and provides a good medium for bacteria growth. If you observe this in your patient, encourage him or her to drink more fluids to help thin the mucus and make it easier to cough out.

CHEST ASSESSMENT. ***Inspection.*** Look for muscular retractions between the ribs, substernally, and around the neck, evidenced by muscles and skin pulling inward as the patient inhales. ***Safety: This is also a late sign of hypoxia and hypoxemia. Notify the health-care provider immediately.*** Observe the patient for use of the accessory muscles in the neck and shoulders while breathing, indicating excessive muscular effort to breathe (Fig. 28.1).

Palpation. To begin palpating the chest, place your hands on either side of the chest. As the patient inhales and exhales, determine if each side of the chest is moving equally, called excursion. Differences in chest wall movement, along with shortness of breath, can indicate a serious problem, such as airway obstruction, pneumothorax, or **pleural effusion** (fluid in the chest cavity). A **pneumothorax** occurs when a hole allows air to enter the pleural space, also termed the pleural cavity, where there is supposed to be negative pressure. A life-threatening type of pneumothorax is a **tension pneumothorax.** When this occurs, air is trapped in the pleural cavity surrounding the lungs, which not only compresses and collapses the lungs, but also causes pressure on the heart and major blood vessels, causing them to shift within the thorax. ***Safety: Tension pneumothorax is a medical emergency. Notify the health-care provider immediately.***

Feel for **crepitus,** or air in the subcutaneous tissues, in the chest wall, face, and neck. When you gently press your fingertips on the patient's skin, you will feel a crackling sensation, much like the feeling of crispy rice cereal being crushed beneath the patient's skin. Crepitus is usually felt beneath an area of edema. ***Safety: Air in the subcutaneous tissues, also called subcutaneous emphysema, indicates that air that should be in the lungs is in the tissues. Notify the physician immediately.***

Auscultation. Now use your stethoscope to auscultate the lungs, as you learned in Chapter 21. As you listen to respirations, both with and without the stethoscope, observe the rate, character, and quality of respirations. Note if the rate is outside the normal range of 12 to 20 breaths per minute. As you assess quality, determine if the respirations are shallow or deep, or if the patient is struggling to breathe. Determine the pattern of respirations. (Refer to Table 21.3 in Chapter 21 to refresh yourself on patterns of respirations, including tachypnea, bradypnea, eupnea, Kussmaul's, Cheyne-Stokes, Biot's, and apnea.) As you listen with the stethoscope to both the anterior and

• WORD • BUILDING •

cyanosis: cyan – blue + osis – condition
orthopneic: ortho – straight + pneic – breathing
pleural effusion: pleural – pleural membrane; effusion – pouring out
pneumothorax: pneumo – air + thorax – chest

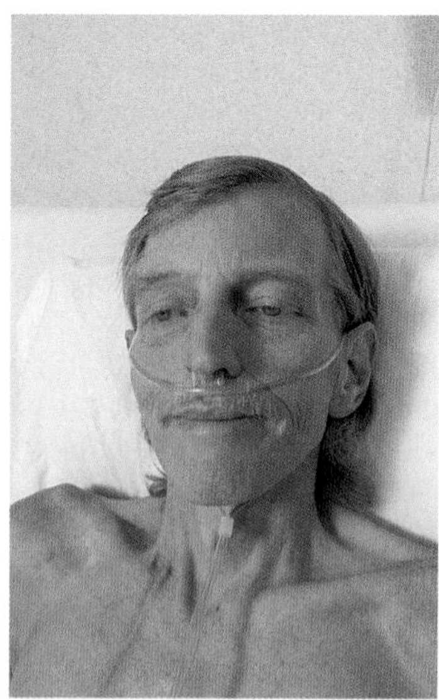

FIGURE 28.1 This patient shows evidence of retractions in the neck and shoulders as he inhales (from Williams LS, Hopper PD. *Understanding Medical-Surgical Nursing*. 5th ed. Philadelphia, PA: FA Davis; 2015).

posterior chest, assess for adventitious breath sounds. If the patient has fluid in the lungs or airways, the sound is described as crackles. It is similar to the sound a soft drink makes after you pour it into a glass because it is the sound of air moving through fluid. Refer to Chapter 21 for a review of adventitious lung sounds. To listen to adventitious lung sounds, go to DavisPlus, located at http://davisplus.fadavis.com.

OXYGENATION STATUS. When beginning to assess the patient's oxygenation status, determine the patient's orientation to time, place, and person. Note restlessness and unusual irritability or confusion. Even minor changes can indicate hypoxia. ***Safety: Remember that changes in level of consciousness can indicate decreased oxygen reaching the brain.***

OXYGEN SATURATION. Determine oxygen saturation using a pulse oximeter. (Refer to Chapter 17 for the procedure for using pulse oximetry.) The pulse oximeter is used to measure the oxygen saturation of capillary blood (SaO_2). The normal range for SAO_2 is 95% to 100%. In healthy people, a saturation of 94% or below is cause for concern. ***Safety: Remember that nail polish, especially a dark color, and artificial nails will cause inaccurate pulse oximetry results.*** Remove nail polish or use an alternative site such as the earlobe or forehead. You can check a patient's oxygen saturation without a health-care provider's order. Be alert to subtle signs and symptoms of hypoxemia, and check the oxygen saturation when indicated.

> **KNOWLEDGE CONNECTION**
>
> What areas will you inspect when assessing a patient with impaired oxygenation? When you palpate, what two evaluations are you making? How can you tell if the patient is becoming hypoxic or hypoxemic?

Diagnostic Tests

In addition to your assessment, certain diagnostic tests help clearly explain the patient's oxygenation status. Table 28.1 lists the types of diagnostic tests and the significance of abnormal results. Obtain sputum specimens and throat culture specimens when ordered by the health-care provider to help diagnose respiratory conditions.

SPUTUM SPECIMENS. When you obtain a sputum specimen, keep in mind that the best time to do this is first thing in the morning. Patients may have mucus that has pooled during the night, making it easier to obtain a specimen. There are two ways to obtain a sputum specimen:

1. The patient coughs and brings up mucus from the lungs and expectorates it into a sterile specimen container.
2. You suction the throat or trachea and trap the mucus in a specimen container attached to the suctioning tubing.

The results of sputum testing help diagnose infection, tuberculosis, bleeding, and fluids in the lungs. Skill 28.1 (page 594) gives the steps needed to obtain a sputum specimen.

THROAT CULTURE SPECIMENS. Specimens from the throat for culture and sensitivity are frequently obtained by nurses in health-care providers' offices and clinics, but sometimes they are ordered in home health care and hospitals as well. Generally a throat culture is ordered to detect a *Streptococcus* infection in the throat, commonly referred to as *strep throat,* so that it may be treated promptly. If such an infection is present and is not treated, it can lead to other illnesses, including rheumatic fever and rheumatic heart disease. Skill 28.2 (page 595) gives the steps in obtaining a throat culture specimen.

> **Laboratory and Diagnostic Connection**
>
> **Arterial Blood Gases**
>
> Arterial blood gases (ABGs) are drawn from an artery rather than a vein as are other blood tests. The most commonly used arteries are the radial, femoral, and brachial. A glass or plastic syringe is used; the syringe has a small amount of heparin added, which is an anticoagulant to prevent the blood from clotting.
>
> After testing for collateral circulation, the health-care professional inserts the needle into the artery at a 90-degree angle. Unlike other blood samples, no vacuum tube is used for ABGs. Instead, the pressure of the blood in the artery causes the plunger of the syringe to rise as blood enters the syringe.
>
> After the needle is withdrawn from the artery, the health-care professional inserts it into a cork to prevent additional air from entering the syringe or uses a special

needle that will not allow air to enter the syringe after the blood is drawn. The syringe is then transported to the laboratory in a bag or cup containing ice to keep it cold.

ABGs measure the pH, the partial pressures of oxygen (PaO_2) and carbon dioxide ($PaCO_2$), the bicarbonate level (HCO_3^-), and the oxygen saturation (SaO_2) of arterial blood. Information from ABGs will help you know your patient's pH status. If the pH is above 7.45, the patient is in alkalosis. If the pH is below 7.35, the patient is in acidosis. Both of these conditions require immediate action by the health-care provider to correct.

Blood gases also show if the cause of the acidosis or alkalosis is a respiratory problem, which would cause the $PaCO_2$ to be increased or decreased, or a metabolic problem as a result of kidney regulation of bicarbonate. In that case, the patient's HCO_3^- levels would be above or below normal. Normal ranges for ABGs, along with the significance of findings above and below normal, can be found in Table 28.2.

ABGs usually are drawn by respiratory therapists or specially trained nurses or laboratory technicians. Registered nurses also may take a sample of arterial blood for ABGs from an arterial line in a critical care setting.

Nursing Interventions for Patients With Impaired Oxygenation

You will use a variety of nursing interventions to help prevent decreased oxygenation in your patients who have undergone surgery or who must remain in bed. In addition, there are a number of actions for you to take to improve oxygenation in your patients with lung disorders.

Turn, Cough, and Deep Breathe

Patients who have undergone surgery or are on bedrest must be turned every 2 hours to prevent respiratory complications due to immobility. (See Chapter 16 for a review of complications of immobility.) In addition to assisting patients to turn from side to side, you must encourage patients to take three deep breaths and then cough to remove secretions from the lungs and airways. ***Safety: You need to assist the patient to turn, cough, and deep breathe every 2 hours to help prevent hypostatic pneumonia.*** If the patient has an incision or is weak, he or she may find this task difficult to perform. If the patient has an abdominal or chest incision, encourage him or her to hold a pillow against the incision while taking deep breaths and coughing. The pillow will splint the incision, making it less uncomfortable for the patient to comply with coughing and deep breathing.

Table 28.1
Respiratory Diagnostic Tests and Their Purposes

Diagnostic Test	*Purpose*	*Significance of Abnormal Results*
Pulmonary function tests	To determine lung capacity, volume, and flow rates.	Used to diagnose obstructive or restrictive lung diseases such as COPD and asthma.
Peak flow	Measures the amount of air that can be exhaled with force using a peak flowmeter.	Used to determine dosage and frequency of some respiratory medications. Can be used by patient to monitor the effectiveness of medications.
Chest x-ray	Used to visualize lung fields; air appears dark so it can be determined if all lobes are filling with air. Fluid, dense tissue, and infiltrate appear white.	Used to determine lung filling and size of cardiac silhouette, as well as to identify tumors, pneumonia, infiltrate, and effusions.
Tuberculin skin test	To determine reaction to presence of tuberculin bacillus in skin layers.	If skin over and around injection site elevates and *indurates* (gets hard) with or without redness, the result is positive. This indicates past exposure to the disease or current disease. Must be followed up with chest x-ray for confirmation. False positives are caused by the malaria vaccine given in many African countries.
Bronchoscopy	To visualize trachea and bronchii; to obtain biopsies of abnormal tissue; and to obtain samples of lung cells, fluids, and other material inside the air sacs.	Used to diagnose lung conditions such as interstitial disease, infection, airway blockage and cancer; also used to dilate narrowed airways.

Table 28.2
Normal Ranges for Arterial Blood Gases and the Significance of Abnormal Levels

Blood Gas Component	*Normal Range*	*Significance of Levels Above Normal*	*Significance of Levels Below Normal*
pH	7.35–7.45	Alkalosis	Acidosis
PaO_2	80–100 mm Hg	Hyperventilation	Hypoxemia
$PaCO_2$	35–45 mm Hg	Converts to carbonic acid and causes acidosis	Lack of carbonic acid causes alkalosis
HCO_3^-	22–26	Excess of alkalinity causes alkalosis	Lack of alkalinity leads to acidosis
SaO_2	95%–99%	Hyperventilation or excess supplemental oxygen	Hypoxemia and hypoxia

After the pillow is in place, have the patient follow these steps:

1. Breathe in through the nose and hold your breath for 3 to 5 seconds.
2. Slowly exhale through your mouth with the lips in the "whistle position." This is called pursed-lip breathing.
3. Repeat deep breathing in this manner three times.
4. On the fourth inhalation, cough during the exhalation. To be most effective, you should cough three times during one exhalation. This helps bring the mucus up from deep in the airways and move it up and out. This is referred to as "huff coughing."
5. Repeat the deep breathing and coughing exercise two or three times, until the cough no longer produces sputum.

Incentive Spirometry

One way to encourage patients to take frequent deep breaths is through the use of an **incentive spirometer,** which is a device with one or more chambers and a mouthpiece. As the patient inhales, a set of balls or a piston with a platform top rises, showing the patient the volume of the inhalation. The patient continues to try to improve the volume of inhalations to raise the balls or piston higher, which helps to expand the lungs fully and prevent atelectasis. Instruct the patient to use the incentive spirometer every hour and to repeat the inhalations 10 times. Skill 28.3 (page 596) provides more information on assisting with incentive spirometry.

Patient Teaching Connection

Incentive Spirometry

When you instruct the patient to use an incentive spirometer, it is important to give clear directions. Often, patients think they should blow into the device using a forceful exhalation, which could cause lung injury. Explain that the purpose of the incentive spirometer is to increase the amount of air inhaled, which expands the air sacs in the lungs. This decreases the patient's risk for developing pneumonia and atelectasis, or a collapsed lung.

Instruct the patient to breathe in slowly and deeply, trying to raise the platform above the piston to the preset slide pointer. Alternately, if you are using a three-chamber device, the patient tries to inhale slowly and deeply enough to raise all three balls in the chambers.

Instruct the patient to use the incentive spirometer 10 times each hour to expand the lungs fully. However, your responsibility does not end with those instructions. Follow up with your patient several times during your shift to ensure that he or she is using the incentive spirometer. Ask the patient to demonstrate using it for you so that you can be sure that he or she is performing the procedure correctly and you can see the volume of air the patient is inhaling. Enlist the assistance of family or friends if necessary to help remind the patient to use the incentive spirometer.

Nebulizer Treatments

A **nebulizer** is a medication delivery system containing an air compressor and a mask or handheld mouthpiece. Liquid medication, usually a bronchodilator, is ordered by the health-care provider and is placed in a small cup that attaches to the air compressor via tubing. The medication may be ordered to be mixed with saline. ***Safety: Follow orders carefully because failing to mix the medication as ordered could lead to an overdose.*** Saline without medication may also be used to provide moisture to the airways in order to thin tenacious mucus. The compressed air travels through the liquid medication or saline, converting it into a fine mist that the patient inhales directly into the airways and lungs. A health-care provider's order is required for all nebulizer treatments.

Once you add the liquid medication, medication with saline, or saline alone to the cup, you will assemble the remaining apparatus for medication delivery. When the compressor is turned on, you will see vapor in the mask or from the spacer on the back side of the handheld mouthpiece. The patient then breathes the vapor in, slowly and deeply. If the patient is using the mouthpiece, he or she must close the lips around it and breathe in through the mouth and out through the nose. If the patient is unable to breathe in this manner during the nebulizer treatment, you will want to use the mask apparatus rather than the mouthpiece. The patient can then breathe in and out through the nose or mouth and still inhale the medication effectively. Skill 28.4 (page 597) gives the steps for preparing a nebulizer and administering a nebulizer treatment.

Chest Physical Therapy

To help drain mucus from the lobes of the lungs, chest physical therapy (CPT) may be ordered. This involves assisting the patient into different positions to encourage the drainage of mucus out of the lungs. It also involves using percussion to help loosen pooled mucus. In most hospitals, this will be performed by respiratory therapists. However, it is possible that in home health care and long-term care settings, a licensed practical/vocational nurse might need to assist with CPT.

Postural drainage refers to positioning the patient in ways to specifically drain each lobe of the lungs. The right and left upper lobes are best drained with the patient in the orthopneic and high Fowler's positions. To drain the middle lobes, place the bed in the Trendelenburg position and have the patient lie in the right lateral position and then the left lateral position. To drain the lower lobes, continue to keep the bed in the Trendelenburg position and assist the patient to lie in the Sims' position on the right and left sides and then to lie in the prone position. Keep in mind that not all patients who have respiratory illnesses can tolerate remaining in all of these positions.

Percussion refers to cupping or clapping over the lung fields to loosen mucus and help it drain. This is done with the hands cupped, clapping against the rib cage, and pausing to let the patient cough as needed.

Supplemental Oxygen

When a patient is hypoxemic, the health-care provider orders supplemental oxygen. It is important to understand the purpose of this; remember that room air contains 21% oxygen, so it is always available as we breathe. However, in the presence of lung disease or other conditions that interfere with external respiration, supplemental oxygen increases the amount of available oxygen with each inhalation.

Oxygen is not without its risks, however. ***Safety: Oxygen supports combustion, meaning that its presence will cause any fire to burn faster and hotter.*** Whenever oxygen is in use, you must ensure that safety precautions are followed:

- Ensure that "No Smoking" signs are posted on the doors and above the bed. In hospitals, smoking is no longer allowed anywhere. However, in home health care and some long-term care or assisted living facilities, smoking could still be an issue. In those settings, be sure the signs are in place and the restrictions on smoking are enforced.
- Ensure that no open flames are in the same room as an oxygen source. In home health care, this refers to open-flame heaters, candles, and fireplaces. The oxygen source must be in another room away from any flame.
- Check electrical devices such as electric razors to ensure that there are no frayed wires that could cause sparks, which could lead to a fire.
- Eliminate the possibility of static electricity, which could spark a fire. Use cotton gowns and linens, not synthetics.
- Avoid using petroleum-based products such as petroleum jelly on the lips of patients using supplemental oxygen. Use a water-soluble or non–petroleum-based product instead.

Oxygen can cause toxicity in some situations. If a person breathes a high concentration of oxygen for long periods, it can cause central nervous system damage. If a high-liter flow of oxygen is given to patients with chronic lung disease, it can cause severe respiratory problems. Remember that the patient's stimulus to breathe is low oxygen in the blood rather than higher-than-normal carbon dioxide levels. During a severe exacerbation, such as an acute worsening of chronic lung disease, higher levels of oxygen may be used *short term only* to help get the patient through the crisis. If the patient receives supplemental oxygen at a liter flow above 2 to 3 L/min beyond the acute crisis, it can cause respiratory depression and even death. ***Safety: Always keep routine supplemental oxygen liter flow for patients with chronic obstructive lung disease below 3 L/min.***

OXYGEN DELIVERY. Supplemental oxygen can be delivered in a variety of ways. The health-care provider will order the specific device. However, it is important for you to evaluate the effectiveness of such orders and to suggest a change if it is appropriate. It also is important for you to understand how oxygen is delivered by each device. For example, if a patient who is using a nasal cannula, which delivers oxygen via nasal prongs, is breathing mostly through his or her mouth, a mask may be more appropriate for oxygen delivery.

Oxygen may be derived from different types of sources. For example, in the hospital setting, oxygen is piped in through the walls and accessed by inserting a flowmeter into a valve. The oxygen then flows through tubing to the patient (Fig. 28.2). When the patient leaves the hospital room, a portable oxygen tank, called an E-cylinder, is used to provide continuous oxygen. This is a small portable tank on a wheeled cart (Fig. 28.3). You will need to know how to switch the patient from one type of source to another when you ambulate a patient in the hallway of the hospital.

Patients at home may use liquid oxygen or oxygen concentrators. When they leave home or move about the house, they can use a portable container called a stroller, which is light enough to be carried by the patient (Fig. 28.4). A portable oxygen concentrator runs on batteries and can be taken on airplanes. The patient can use continuous oxygen or

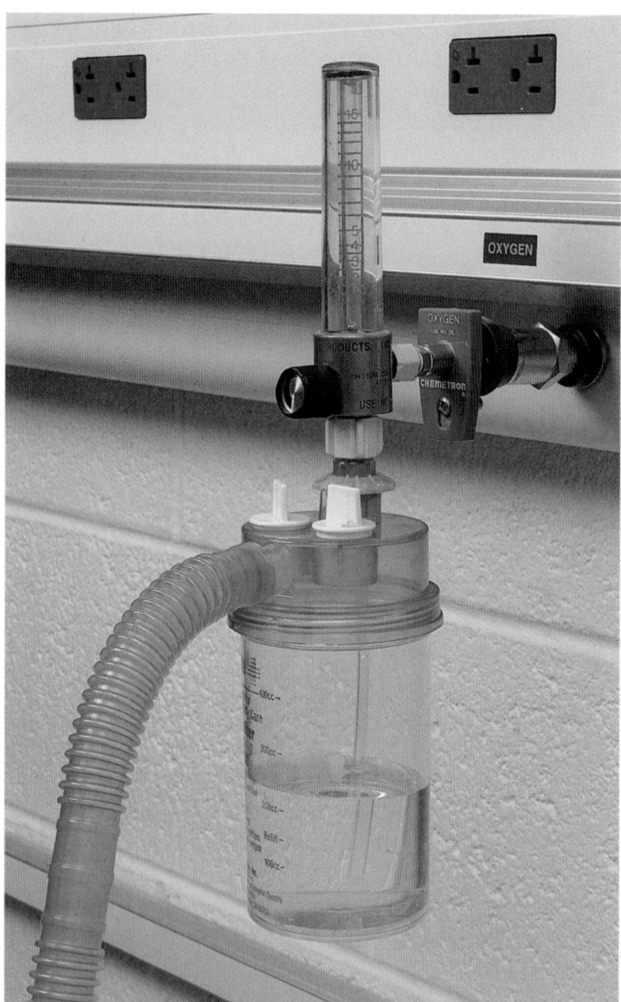

FIGURE 28.2 An oxygen flowmeter connected to piped-in oxygen (from Wilkinson JM, Treas LS, Barnett, KL, Smith MH. *Fundamentals of Nursing: Theory, Concepts & Applications*. Vol. 2. 3rd ed. Philadelphia, PA: FA Davis; 2016).

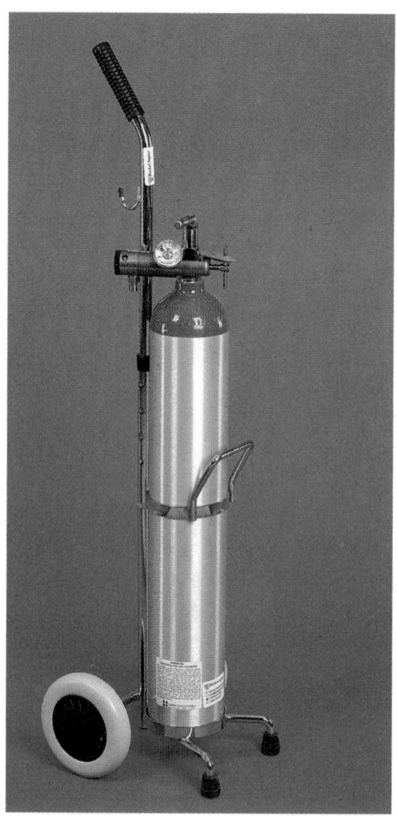

FIGURE 28.3 This is an example of an E-cylinder (from Wilkinson JM, Treas LS, Barnett, KL, Smith MH. *Fundamentals of Nursing: Theory, Concepts & Applications*. Vol. 2. 3rd ed. Philadelphia, PA: FA Davis; 2016).

something called *pulse flow,* which only delivers oxygen when the patient breathes in through his or her nose. The pulse flow is delivered in "equivalent liter flow" because it is not continuous. The number on the portable oxygen concentrator for pulse flow is a setting, not a liter flow measurement. These types of strollers are not recommended for patients who need high-flow oxygen (greater than 4 L/min). It is also recommended that the patient carry an extra battery with him or her because the portable oxygen concentrator batteries only last 2 to 4 hours. Table 28.3 lists the types of oxygen sources along with a description of each.

Oxygen is supplied from the source to the patient in a variety of ways. The nasal cannula, which has short curved prongs designed to fit inside the nostrils, interferes the least with eating and talking. It works best for patients who breathe through the nose. Masks of various types are used for different needs. Table 28.4 describes the different oxygen delivery devices, their liter flows, and the purposes of each. Skill 28.5 (page 597) gives the steps in administering supplemental oxygen.

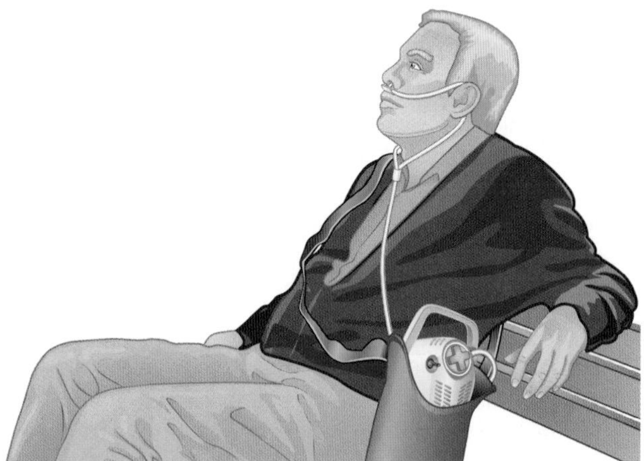

FIGURE 28.4 This patient is using a liquid oxygen stroller (from Wilkinson JM, Treas LS, Barnett, KL, Smith MH. *Fundamentals of Nursing: Theory, Concepts & Applications*. Vol. 1. 3rd ed. Philadelphia, PA: FA Davis; 2016).

Conservation of Energy

Patients with chronic lung disease often must use the accessory muscles in the neck and shoulders to move air in and out of their lungs. When this is the case, the patient cannot use the same muscles to perform tasks such as bathing and eating. The patient must then make a choice between bathing and breathing or eating and breathing. That is why you often

Table 28.3 Types of Oxygen Sources

Type	*Description*
Piped-in oxygen	Found in health-care facilities with a wall outlet above the bed. The flowmeter is inserted into the wall to access oxygen within the pipe (see Fig. 28.2). When the patient ambulates in the hall or is taken to other departments in the hospital, an E-cylinder is used.
Oxygen tank	Large, green, heavy tanks that hold oxygen gas and must be exchanged for a full tank when empty. They usually are delivered by an oxygen supply or medical equipment company. The patient is connected to the tank with extension tubing, allowing for a limited area for ambulation.
Oxygen E-cylinder	Small green tank that holds oxygen gas and sits on a wheeled holder, allowing patient mobility (see Fig. 28.3). It can be used when the patient leaves the hospital room, the home, or a facility and is wheeled alongside as he or she walks. When empty, it must be exchanged for a full tank.
Oxygen concentrator	Removes some oxygen from room air and concentrates it for oxygen delivery of up to 4 L/min. Requires electricity to work and may increase the cost of the patient's electric bill. Looks similar to a piece of furniture. If the patient leaves home or a facility, a portable concentrator may be used. These run on batteries and can deliver either a continuous flow of oxygen or a pulse flow.
Liquid oxygen	Oxygen that is kept cold so that it is a liquid rather than a gas. A larger barrel-shaped tank contains the oxygen supply. A smaller stroller is filled from the large tank (see Fig. 28.4). It is lightweight and easy to carry with a shoulder strap. The contents of the stroller last up to 10 hours set on 2 L/min. Can be refilled from the main tank by the patient.

Table 28.4 Oxygen Delivery Devices

Delivery Device	*Liter Flow*	*Description*	*Tips for Use*
Nasal cannula	1–6 L/min	Delivers oxygen into the nares; patient can more easily eat and talk with it in place; patient must breathe mostly through the nose for full benefit.	Apply correctly. Nasal prongs curve inward when inserted into the nares, and tubing slips over the ears. The slider fits under the chin.
Simple face mask	5–10 L/min	Delivers oxygen directly to the nose and mouth; patient may breathe through nose or mouth; flow rate less than 5 L/min will cause carbon dioxide to accumulate in the mask.	May cause patient to feel claustrophobic and hot; elastic straps hold mask in place and may irritate skin above the ears, causing pressure. Pad with gauze 4×4s if needed.

Continued

Table 28.4
Oxygen Delivery Devices—cont'd

Delivery Device	*Liter Flow*	*Description*	*Tips for Use* 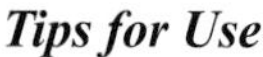
Partial rebreathing mask	6–15 L/min 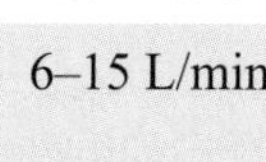	Mask with bag attached that traps carbon dioxide for rebreathing to lower pH levels; ports on the side of the mask allow most exhaled air to discharge.	When used correctly, rebreathing bag will not collapse during inhalation; if collapse occurs, increase flow rate according to prescriber's orders.
Nonrebreathing mask 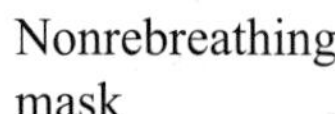 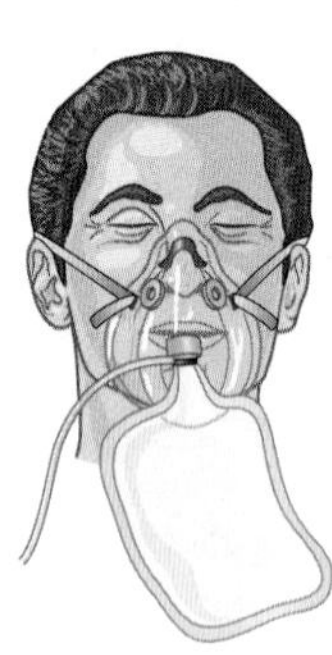	6–15 L/min	Prevents the patient from rebreathing any exhaled air; it escapes through a one-way valve that does not allow room air to enter. The bag traps oxygen as a reservoir for inhalation; only delivery device that can provide 100% oxygen when set at 15 L/min.	When used correctly, rebreathing bag will not collapse during inhalation; it should remain at least half full. If it does not, increase the oxygen flow rate according to prescriber's orders.
Venturi mask 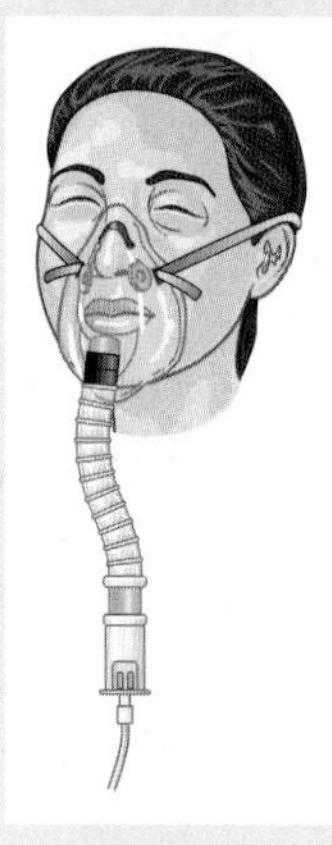	24%–80%	Contains a plastic valve between the tubing from the oxygen source and the mask, which allows a precise mix of room air and oxygen to equal a specific percentage of oxygen. The dial on the valve (or interchangeable adapter) indicates the liter flow to use to equal a specific percentage of oxygen. This gives more exact control of inspired oxygen, especially for patients with COPD.	The physician orders percentage of oxygen, not liter flow. You must check the dial or adapter to determine the liter flow necessary to equal the oxygen percentage and set the flowmeter accordingly.
Face tent 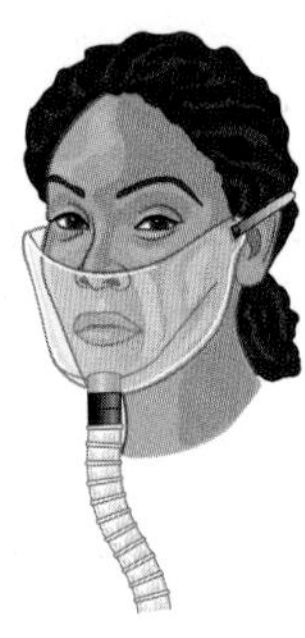	8–12 L/min	Used for patients who feel claustrophobic with other masks because the top is open; allows for high amounts of humidity to be used due to open top.	Oxygen delivery is not as precise, so it is important to assess oxygen saturation and signs and symptoms of hypoxia in your patient using this device.

Table 28.4
Oxygen Delivery Devices—cont'd

Delivery Device	*Liter Flow*	*Description*	*Tips for Use*
Tracheostomy collar	4–10 L/min	Delivers highly humidified oxygen through large tubing; rests over the tracheostomy with an elastic band that goes around the neck and can be tightened at the sides.	Due to high humidity, condensation builds up in the large tubing. Be cautious when turning or moving the patient so that pooled water does not migrate into the tracheostomy and cause choking.
T-piece	4–10 L/min	Attaches to the flange of the tracheostomy; oxygen flows from one side of the T-piece to the trachea. During exhalation, air exits through the open end of the T-piece.	Keep the connection to the tracheostomy intact, being careful not to allow tension on it to pull out the inner cannula.

Source: Adapted from Wilkinson JM, Treas LS, Barnett, KL, Smith MH. *Fundamentals of Nursing: Theory, Concepts & Applications.* Vol. 2. 3rd ed. Philadelphia, PA: FA Davis; 2016.

see patients with chronic lung disease who are very thin and have poor nutritional status.

You can help these patients conserve their energy so that they can use those accessory muscles to breathe but still are able to obtain nourishment and perform some activities of daily living (ADLs). Some tips for assisting them include the following:

- For bathing assistance, encourage the patient to place a nonrusting chair or bench in the shower and to get a terrycloth robe. During the shower, the patient can sit while applying soap and rinsing the body. After the shower, the patient can slip on the robe and sit and rest outside the shower. The robe will absorb water, and the patient will not have to use the shoulder and neck muscles to dry off with a towel. Often just the activity of taking a shower is exhausting for the patient with chronic lung disease.
- For nutritional assistance, encourage the patient to use Pulmocare or a similar meal supplement to increase protein and calories without high carbohydrate intake. Metabolism of carbohydrates produces carbonic acid, which in turn can contribute to acidosis in the patient with chronic lung disease.

  Encourage the patient to eat frequent, small meals several times per day rather than three larger meals. This will help him or her get in more calories before tiring. The patient may become weary after eating only a few bites of a meal because he or she is using the accessory muscles to eat instead of breathe.
- For other ADLs, encourage the patient to take frequent rest periods during these activities. When you care for a patient with chronic lung disease in the hospital setting, plan to take a longer time than usual for bathing, dressing, grooming, and oral care. The patient will require frequent breaks to rest and breathe with those accessory muscles rather than using them for daily care.

Be patient and kind. Rushing the patient causes more stress for both of you. The patient cannot go any faster and needs your understanding and patience regarding the pace required to complete activities.

Bilateral Positive Airway Pressure Machine

In a few situations, a patient may be placed on a bilateral positive airway pressure (BIPAP) machine, which delivers oxygen and air into the lungs through pressure. This machine may help prevent the patient from having to be connected to a ventilator via an endotracheal tube or tracheostomy tube,

• WORD • BUILDING •
tracheostomy: trachea – windpipe + stomy – surgical opening

at least for a short time. It is also used at night for some people who have severe sleep apnea. (See Chapter 19 for more information about BIPAP.)

> **KNOWLEDGE CONNECTION**
> How often should patients be turned and asked to deep breathe and cough? What is the purpose of delivering a medication via a nebulizer? Why is conservation of energy important for patients with chronic lung disease? What safety issues are of concern to home health-care patients with supplemental oxygen?

Nursing Interventions for Patients Needing Airway Assistance

In some situations, the patient cannot maintain his or her own open airway because of decreased level of consciousness, recent surgery, or other situations. An *artificial airway* is used to assist in maintaining a patent airway. It usually is made of hard plastic or soft rubber and may be placed in the oropharynx, in the nasopharynx, or within the trachea. An endotracheal airway may be inserted through the nose or mouth.

Pharyngeal Airways

An *oropharyngeal airway* is made of hard plastic in a slightly curved shape and is designed to hold the tongue in place so that it cannot obstruct the airway of an unconscious patient (Fig. 28.5). They come in a variety of sizes, from infant through adult. This type of airway is not used for conscious patients because it can cause gagging or vomiting.

A *nasopharyngeal airway* is made of pliable rubber and is designed to be inserted through the nose into the pharynx. This type of airway is also referred to as a nasal trumpet because of its shape (see Fig. 28.5).

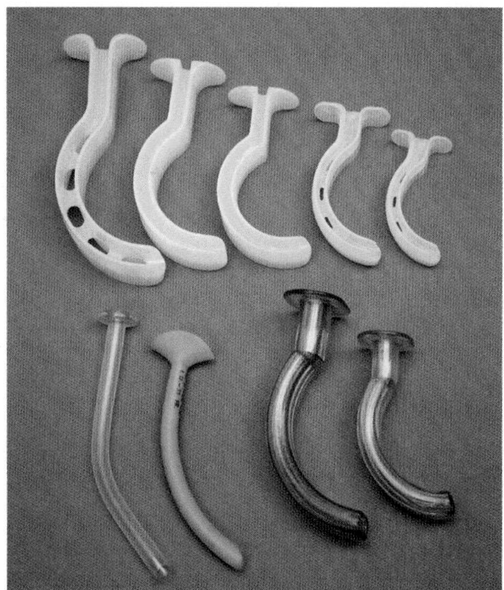

FIGURE 28.5 A variety of airway sizes and types.

SUCTIONING WITH PHARYNGEAL AIRWAYS IN PLACE. The patient may be unable to clear the airway for a variety of reasons, including a weak cough, decreased level of consciousness, or postoperative pain. It is important to be aware of signs that the patient needs to be suctioned, such as rattling sounds in the throat, shortness of breath, ineffective cough, and crackles on auscultating the lungs.

You will use a *suction catheter,* a thin pliable tube with holes in the end, to remove secretions from the patient's nose, throat, and mouth. If an oropharyngeal airway is in place, you will pass the suction catheter along the grooves in the sides of the airway. If a nasopharyngeal airway is in place, you can pass the suction catheter through the airway to the throat. If no airway is in place, you can use the pliable suction catheter to suction through the nose and down the throat. Skill 28.6 (page 599) gives the steps in performing nasopharyngeal and oropharyngeal suctioning. Then you can switch to a hard plastic tube with a larger diameter to suction the mouth. This type of suction device is referred to as a Yankauer suction catheter or tonsil tip suction tube (Fig. 28.6). If the patient reacts to the presence of the tube in his or her mouth by biting down, it will not damage the tonsil tip, and you will still be able to suction. If that reaction occurs with the softer type of suction catheter, it will impede suction and damage the catheter. Skill 28.6 also discusses the steps of using a tonsil-tip suction device.

Endotracheal Airways

Some airways are designed to enter the trachea, not the pharynx. These airways are used when the patient is unable to breathe independently due to airway obstruction or respiratory arrest. An **endotracheal tube** is a firm but flexible plastic tube that may be inserted through the nose or the mouth. The tube usually is inserted by a physician or specially trained respiratory therapist. These tubes are often placed in the surgery suite to support ventilation during surgery. Their purpose is to connect the patient to the ventilator so that oxygen and air are delivered directly to the lungs. The positive pressure of the ventilator causes the air to go into the lungs.

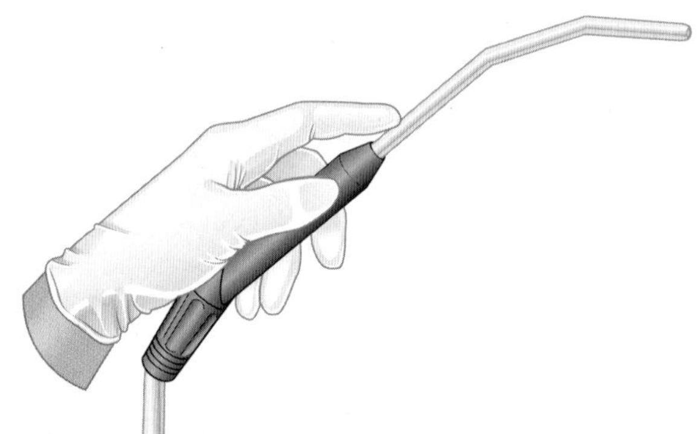

FIGURE 28.6 A Yankauer or tonsil-tip suction tube (from Wilkinson JM, Treas LS, Barnett, KL, Smith MH. *Fundamentals of Nursing: Theory, Concepts & Applications*. Vol. 1. 3rd ed. Philadelphia, PA: FA Davis; 2016).

To ensure that air does not exit through the trachea around the tube, the endotracheal tube contains an inflatable cuff located near the distal end. When the cuff is inflated, air cannot leak around the tube but goes completely into the lungs for full ventilation (Fig. 28.7).

SUCTIONING AN ENDOTRACHEAL TUBE. Patients with endotracheal tubes are cared for in critical care settings. Suctioning the tube is considered a sterile procedure because it goes deep into the trachea, and poor technique could introduce pathogens into the lungs. The sterile suction catheter is inserted using sterile technique through the endotracheal tube, and suction is applied as the catheter is pulled outward. Some suction catheters are inside a sleeve of clear plastic, keeping the catheter itself sterile but allowing you to touch the outside of the sleeve without the need to put on sterile gloves. Skill 28.7 (page 601) gives the steps in performing endotracheal suctioning using a sleeved catheter.

Tracheostomy

A **tracheostomy,** an incision into the trachea that is held open with a tube to promote breathing, may be performed for several reasons. If a patient has had an endotracheal tube in place for 7 to 10 days and will require longer-term ventilator support, a tracheostomy usually is performed. A tracheostomy is also performed when the airway is obstructed, either temporarily or permanently. In many cases, the obstruction is due to cancerous tumors in the laryngeal area.

Because the endotracheal tube can erode the trachea after being in place longer than 2 weeks, the tracheostomy is necessary. First, an incision is made into the trachea, called a *tracheotomy.* Then the shorter tracheostomy tube is inserted directly into the trachea and anchored in place. The ventilator is then attached to the tracheostomy tube.

A tracheostomy tube has three parts (Fig. 28.8):

1. The *outer cannula,* with or without a cuff. The cuff is inflated to prevent air leakage when the patient is on a ventilator, just as it is on the endotracheal tube. The cuff on the tracheostomy tube should remain inflated while the patient eats to prevent aspiration of food or fluids. Most hospitals have a policy for deflating the cuff periodically to prevent erosion of the trachea due to pressure. You can tell if the cuff is inflated or deflated by checking the "pillow" on the tracheostomy. If it is inflated, the cuff is inflated.
2. The *obturator,* which fits inside the outer cannula and forms a smooth end for inserting the tracheostomy tube into the tracheotomy. The obturator is removed once the tube is in place and kept at the bedside in case the tube comes out and must be reinserted. The blunt edge of the open tube could not easily be inserted into the trachea. The obturator fills the blunt edge with a smooth, rounded end for ease of insertion.
3. The *inner cannula* is inserted after the obturator is removed. It may be a disposable tube, or it may be designed to be cleaned and replaced every 8 hours. Mucus collects in the inner cannula and can block the patient's airway if it is not suctioned frequently and cleaned or replaced regularly.

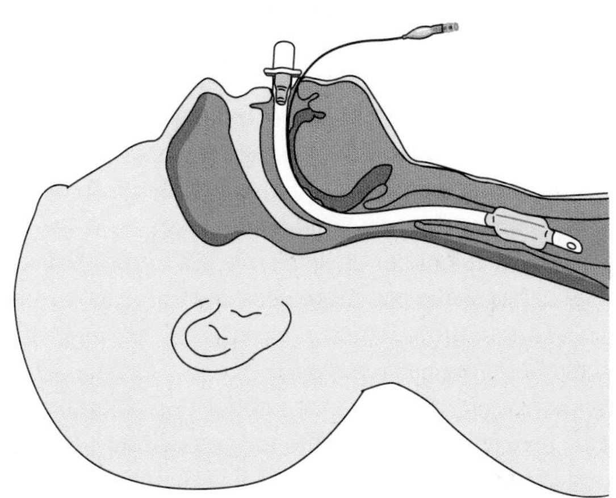

FIGURE 28.7 An endotracheal tube placed through the mouth and into the trachea with the cuff inflated to prevent air leaks (from Wilkinson JM, Treas LS. *Fundamentals of Nursing: Theory, Concepts & Applications.* Vol. 1. 3rd ed. Philadelphia, PA: FA Davis; 2016).

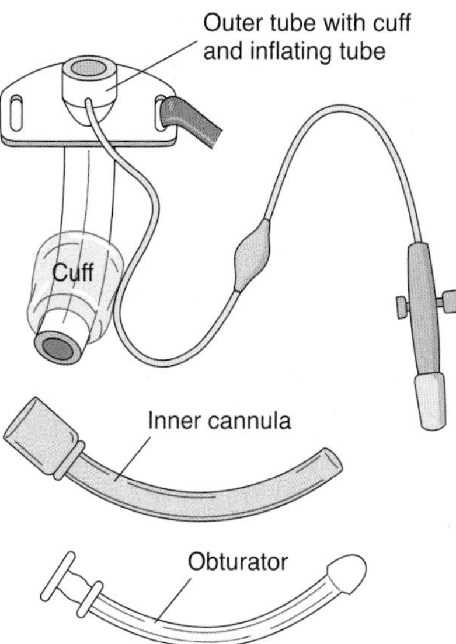

FIGURE 28.8 A tracheostomy tube with inflatable cuff and "pillow," inner cannula, and obturator (from Williams LS, Hopper PD. *Understanding Medical-Surgical Nursing.* 5th ed. Philadelphia, PA: FA Davis; 2015).

Because the tracheostomy diverts airflow from going past the vocal cords, the patient with a tracheostomy is unable to make vocal sounds. A *fenestrated tracheostomy tube* has two cannulas with an opening in the outer cannula, on the posterior side, just above the cuff. When the inner cannula is removed, the patient can breathe through the mouth and nose and can vocalize. The inner cannula must be in place to suction a fenestrated tracheostomy tube.

A Passy-Muir valve is placed on the hub of the tracheostomy and allows air to move into the trachea and past the vocal cords when the patient inhales, enabling speech.

The remainder of the time the valve is in a closed position, which prevents air leaks.

SUCTIONING AND CLEANING A TRACHEOSTOMY. To clear a tracheostomy tube, you will use aseptic technique to insert a suction catheter into the inner cannula and apply suction as you withdraw it. When you are applying suction, you are also removing oxygen as you remove mucus. Therefore, this procedure should be done quickly and effectively. The suction catheter may be sheathed or unsheathed. As with the sheathed catheter for suctioning an endotracheal tube, you do not have to wear sterile gloves to touch the sheath because the sterile catheter remains protected inside it. Skill 28.7 explains the process of suctioning a tracheostomy.

When you clean a tracheostomy, you will remove the inner cannula and clean it in hydrogen peroxide mixed half-strength with saline and then rinse it in saline, dry it, and reinsert it. This is done every 8 hours using sterile technique to prevent introducing pathogens into the trachea and lungs. If the inner cannula is disposable, you will remove it and reinsert a new one rather than cleaning and reinserting. When a patient has a permanent tracheostomy and is caring for it at home, the technique used may be a clean procedure rather than a sterile one.

Tracheostomy ties are generally changed at this time. ***Safety: If possible, have an assistant hold the tracheostomy tube in place while you change the ties or holders. If you are performing this procedure alone, do NOT loosen and remove the old ties until the new ties are in place and secured. The patient can easily cough the tube completely out of the trachea if it does not remain secured in place.*** You may use foam tracheostomy tube holders that are held in place by Velcro or twill ties that you thread through the slots on the tracheostomy tube and tie. Skill 28.8 (page 603) gives the steps for cleaning a tracheostomy tube and changing tracheostomy ties.

KNOWLEDGE CONNECTION

What is the difference between an oropharyngeal airway and a nasopharyngeal airway? What is the purpose of an endotracheal tube? What is an obturator, and how is it used?

Chest Tubes

If the negative pressure in the pleural cavity is disrupted, the lungs can no longer fully expand. This causes dyspnea, chest pain, hypoxia, and respiratory distress. It may be due to secretions obstructing the airways or traumatic injuries that penetrate the chest wall, for example, gunshot or stab wounds. This disruption also occurs after surgery that involves opening the chest, such as surgery on the lungs or heart. To reestablish the negative pressure within the pleural space, also known as the *pleural cavity,* the physician will insert chest tubes.

Placement of Chest Tubes

When air enters the pleural space, it rises to the top of the cavity. As you learned earlier, this is referred to as a *pneumothorax.* A chest tube is inserted into the pleural space through an incision in the anterior superior surface of the chest in the second to fourth intercostal space to release this air. When blood and drainage are present in the pleural space, they pool in the lower portion of the cavity; this is called a **hemothorax.** The chest tube to drain this fluid is inserted in the anterior inferior area of the chest, between the eighth and ninth intercostal space, and enters the pleural space. In situations in which both air and blood are in the pleural cavity, two tubes are placed, one higher and one lower, joined by a Y-connector, and then attached to tubing leading to a drainage system.

Chest tubes may be inserted at the bedside or in the emergency department. They also may be placed in surgery during a thoracic procedure. When chest tubes are placed outside of surgery, a nurse must immediately connect them to the drainage system and tape all connections thoroughly to prevent leaks.

Chest Drainage System

The drainage system for chest tubes is most commonly a single molded plastic unit containing three chambers (Fig. 28.9).

CHAMBER ONE. The chamber on the left (chamber one) is for wet suction. This is used when drainage needs to be gently pulled out of the pleural space. While the drainage unit may be connected to wall suction, the amount of suction is actually controlled by the amount of water in this chamber. Follow the physician's order for the amount of water to add. You will generally fill the chamber to the line marked -20 cm with sterile water. When the suction source is attached, bubbles will be present in this chamber, which you will be able to see and hear. Set the suction so that gentle bubbling occurs. Rapid bubbling will just cause the water to evaporate faster; it will not change the amount of suction.

In systems with dry suction, a dial on the drainage unit is set to the suction ordered by the physician, then the unit is connected to wall suction. The same amount of suction, -20 cm, is operating, but there is no continuous bubbling and no fluid that can evaporate. ***Safety: Be sure you know how to use and evaluate the chest drainage system used in your facility.***

CHAMBER TWO. The middle chamber (chamber two) is for the water seal. This is required to reestablish negative pressure in the pleural space and to prevent air from entering the cavity through the chest tube. It is standard to establish a 2-cm water seal, which means that you will add sterile water up to the 2-cm mark on the middle chamber.

Observe this chamber closely. It is not unusual to see the water level rise as the patient inhales and to fall as the patient exhales. This motion, which is referred to as *tidaling,* will stop when the lung has reinflated.

Another observation to make about this chamber is that when the patient has a pneumothorax, you will see the air leave the chest cavity and make bubbles in this chamber. Some types of drainage systems have a scale from 1 to 7 measuring the

• WORD • BUILDING •

hemothorax: hemo – blood + thorax – chest

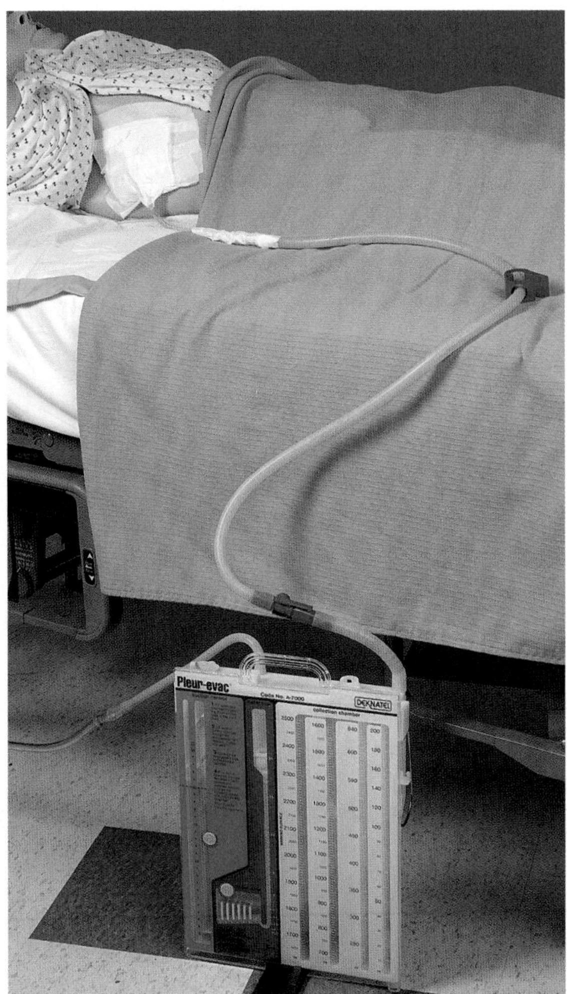

FIGURE 28.9 A chest drainage system with the tubes in the correct position for gravity drainage. Note the taped connections and the three sections of the drainage system. The blue area is the suction chamber, the red area is the water-seal chamber, and the white area is the collection chamber (from Wilkinson JM, Treas LM, Barnett, KL, Smith MH. *Fundamentals of Nursing: Theory, Concepts & Applications.* Vol. 2. 3rd ed., Philadelphia, PA: FA Davis; 2016).

amount of escaping air. This allows you to document the resolution of the pneumothorax.

Once the air is removed and the pneumothorax is resolved, you should not see bubbles in the water-seal chamber; if you do see bubbles in the water-seal chamber, there is an air leak in the system. ***Safety: At the first sign of bubbles in the water-seal chamber of a patient with a resolved pneumothorax, check all tubing connections and the dressings at the insertion site for possible air leaks.***

CHAMBER THREE. The remaining chamber (chamber three) on the right is the collection chamber. This is where blood and other fluids from the pleural cavity are trapped and measured. Because this is a closed system that reestablishes negative pressure within the pleural space, the drainage is never emptied. Rather, you will mark the level of drainage on the writable surface adjacent to the collection chamber. You will also write the date and time, along with your initials, next to the amount of drainage. Then you will determine the amount of output for an 8-hour period. Take the following scenario as an example:

> When you come on shift, you find the collection chamber contains 325 mL of output counted by the previous shift. Eight hours later, the collection chamber contains 440 mL. To determine the amount of output for your shift, subtract 325 from 440 and record 115 mL as the chest tube output.

You should expect the amount of drainage to gradually decrease each day until the pleural space has been drained and the physician removes the chest tube. It is important for you to assess the color and amount of chest tube drainage several times during your shift. ***Safety: If a sudden increase in total output or a sudden increase in bright red output occurs in the chest tube drainage unit, notify the physician immediately because this could indicate hemorrhage.***

Nursing Interventions for Patients With Chest Tubes

Patients with chest tubes may be in critical care units, but they also may be on regular nursing units, which is why it is important for you to know how to care for them. Your responsibilities include assessing the patient's respiratory status every 2 hours to ensure that no complications occur. The patient should have audible breath sounds in all lung fields as the pneumothorax and/or hemothorax resolves. It is possible that you will hear a friction rub because of the presence of the chest tube in the pleural space.

It is important for you to assess for clots that might occlude the tubing, preventing the suction from maintaining the "vacuum" necessary to restore the negative pressure within the pleural space. An increase of positive pressure can build up within the pleural space and, if it is not resolved, can cause a tension pneumothorax. This condition can eventually shift the entire mediastinal area, which includes the heart, bronchial trees, and major blood vessels, from the center to one side, causing compression of the heart. This shift can prevent the previously unaffected lung from optimally exchanging gases, further adding to the problem. If clots are noted, follow your facility's policy and your health-care provider's orders. The previous practice of "stripping" the tubes that lead to the drainage unit (pinching the tubing closed and sliding your fingers down the tubing to pull clots toward the drainage unit) is no longer recommended because it increases positive pressure within the pleural space. However, a clot that occludes the tubing can have the same result. "Milking" chest tubes refers to pinching the tube above the clot briefly and repeating this action to work the clot gently toward the drainage unit. ***Safety: Know your facility's policy for intervening when clots are present in the tubing from the chest tube to the drainage unit.*** In many situations, the response to a blood clot in chest tubing lies with the physician's preference.

It is also important to know what to do if a chest tube comes out. A special dressing impregnated with petroleum jelly makes an occlusive barrier to cover the opening and prevent air from entering. It is the policy at some hospitals to keep such a dressing at the bedside of the patient with chest tubes. However, if the patient has an unresolved pneumothorax, placing petroleum gauze over the opening could cause a tension pneumothorax because of air trapped in the chest. In that case, some researchers recommend placing regular gauze over the opening and preparing for reinsertion. ***Safety: Notify the physician immediately if a chest tube comes out. Follow facility policy regarding the use of petroleum gauze.***

If the chest tube becomes disconnected from the drainage unit, place the end of the tube in a bottle of sterile saline or sterile water so that it is 2 cm below the surface of the fluid to reestablish the water seal. You can then connect the tube to a new drainage system. It is no longer recommended that chest tubes be clamped with padded hemostats except for very short periods in specific circumstances, such as to change the drainage unit or to test the patient's ability to tolerate the removal of the chest tube.

If the drainage unit is a wet suction setup, it must be kept upright at all times. Inspect tubing to be sure that there are no kinks and that the fluids are draining to gravity. Eliminate any loops that would require drainage to run uphill. Always check for leaks. Keep all connections securely taped. Keep all dressings around the insertion site intact. These are petroleum gauze dressings covered with regular gauze. Check the patient for *subcutaneous emphysema,* the feeling of crepitus under the skin, to detect any air leaks into the tissue. Skill 28.9 (page 605) gives the steps for maintaining chest tubes.

KNOWLEDGE CONNECTION

Why is the chest tube for a pneumothorax placed in the upper area of the chest? List the three chambers of a standard chest tube drainage system. What might indicate hemorrhage in a patient with chest tubes?

Nursing Care Plan for a Patient With COPD and Pneumonia

You are planning care for a 60-year-old male patient with a diagnosis of bilateral pneumonia and chronic obstructive pulmonary disease (COPD). He lives with his wife, who is also having health problems, but she is his primary caregiver. He has had pneumonia several times in the past 2 years, but this is the most severe case. The following are questions you might ask yourself as you assess him and collect data:

- What are his lung sounds like?
- Is he hypoxemic?
- Does he have a productive cough?
- What is the amount, color, and consistency of the sputum?

Figure 28.10 presents a concept map care plan for a patient with COPD and pneumonia.

Assessment

When you research his chart and perform your assessment, you discover that your patient is 5 feet 10 inches (177.6 cm) tall and weighs 135 pounds (61.2 kg). His skin color is pale, with a bluish tinge to his lips and nailbeds. His temperature is elevated at 102.2°F (39°C), his pulse is 108, respirations are 26, and blood pressure is 144/86. His SaO_2 using a pulse oximeter is 89%. He is short of breath with any movement and has oxygen on at 2 L/min per nasal cannula (2L/NC).

He has a history of smoking two packs per day for 20 years. He has a weak cough that often is nonproductive. When he does expectorate sputum, it is a small amount of rust-colored sputum. He appears anxious and is sitting in the high Fowler's position in bed. His activity orders are for bedrest with bathroom privileges. When you assist him to the bathroom, he is extremely short of breath with exertion. When you auscultate his lungs, you hear coarse crackles in the lower lobes bilaterally that do not clear with coughing.

Nursing Diagnoses

The highest-priority nursing diagnoses given for this patient are the following:

- Ineffective airway clearance related to secretions in the airways as evidenced by ineffective cough and adventitious breath sounds
- Impaired gas exchange related to chronic lung changes as evidenced by dyspnea and decreased oxygen saturation
- Activity intolerance related to imbalance between oxygen supply and demand as evidenced by dyspnea with exertion

Planning

You will now plan your interventions and the outcomes for this patient. You decide that the outcomes for him will be that he will cough more effectively to remove secretions before discharge, that his gas exchange will then improve when the secretions are removed, and therefore his oxygen saturation will also improve. You determine that his activity tolerance can be increased when his oxygenation improves. You begin to think of a number of nursing interventions to help him accomplish these outcomes, including ways to help him conserve his energy, as well as ways to help him expectorate sputum and keep his lungs expanded.

Implementation

You are now at the stage of the nursing process to implement, or actually perform, the interventions that you have planned. Refer to the interventions listed below.

Evaluation

Once the interventions, or nursing actions, have been performed, you will need to evaluate whether or not they were effective. Did they accomplish what you intended? Did they help the patient's problems? Refer to the evaluations below.

Nursing Care Plan for a Patient With COPD and Pneumonia—cont'd

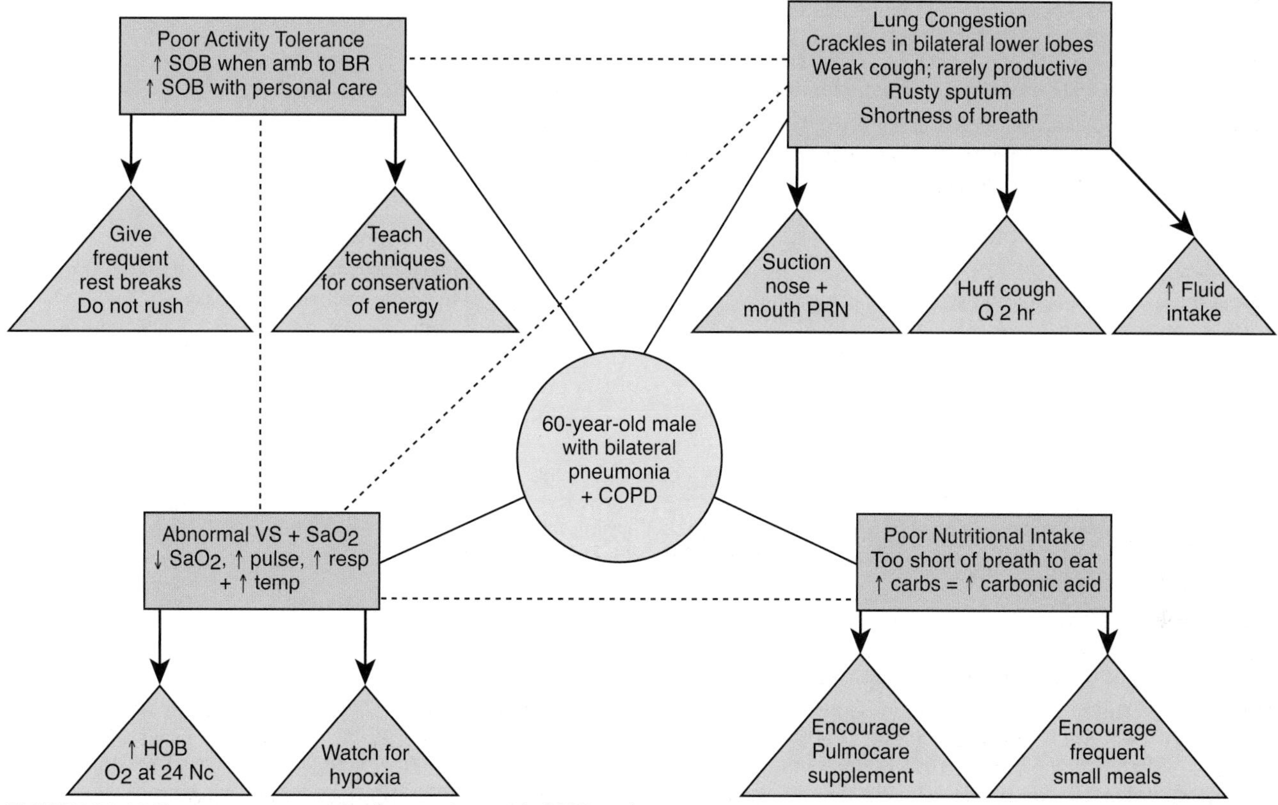

FIGURE 28.10 Concept map care plan for a patient with COPD and pneumonia.

Nursing Diagnosis: Ineffective airway clearance related to secretions in the airways as evidenced by ineffective cough and adventitious breath sounds
Expected Outcomes: Patient will demonstrate effective huff coughing prior to discharge. Patient will verbalize the importance of drinking 8 ounces of fluid every 2 hours while awake to thin mucus by discharge.

Interventions	Evaluations
Encourage fluid intake to help thin mucus, making it easier to cough up and expectorate. Find out what liquids the patient prefers to drink and offer 8 ounces every 2 hours. Obtain an order to perform oropharyngeal and nasopharyngeal suctioning as needed until the patient can cough more effectively. Use a Yankauer catheter for oral suctioning. Teach the patient how to huff cough and encourage him to do so every 2 hours.	Day 1: Likes to drink apple juice and iced tea. Taking fluids every 2 hours. Suctioned and obtained thick rust-colored secretions from the nasopharynx. Instructed on huff coughing, but effort still weak. Day 2: Coughing better, able to bring up some sputum that is now a greenish-yellow color. Continues to take fluids well. Doing better with huff coughing. Day 3: Breath sounds clearer, fewer coarse crackles in the bases of the lungs. Huff coughing well, without being prompted.

(nursing care plan continues on page 594)

Nursing Care Plan for a Patient With COPD and Pneumonia—cont'd

Nursing Diagnosis: Impaired gas exchange related to chronic lung changes as evidenced by dyspnea and decreased oxygen saturation
Expected Outcome: Patient will be able to ambulate to bathroom without dyspnea before discharge. Patient will maintain oxygen saturation of 92% or above before discharge.

Interventions	Evaluations
Maintain supplemental oxygen as ordered at 2 L per nasal cannula. Assess pulse oximetry every 4 hours to determine effective oxygenation. Assess the patient for signs and symptoms of hypoxia, including confusion, restlessness, and irritability. Assess color and circulation by evaluating the nailbeds, lips, and mucous membranes every 2 hours.	Day 1: Oxygen maintained as ordered. SaO_2 still low at 90%. Mild restlessness, but no other signs of hypoxia. Lips and mucous membranes dusky. Day 2: Lung sounds improving. SaO_2 now at 91%. No signs or symptoms of hypoxia. Nailbeds less dusky. Day 3: Oxygen continued as ordered. SaO_2 at 92%, which is very good for his situation. Cough more effective and lung sounds clearer. Nailbeds and mucous membranes remain slightly dusky.

Nursing Diagnosis: Activity intolerance related to imbalance between oxygen supply and demand as evidenced by dyspnea with exertion
Expected Outcome: Patient will be able to participate in ADLs with minimal dyspnea by discharge. Patient will verbalize ways to conserve energy when performing ADLs at home prior to discharge.

Interventions	Evaluations
Assist the patient with conservation-of-energy techniques: • Decrease activities that require use of accessory muscles. Use a bench or chair in the shower; use a terrycloth robe instead of drying after a shower when home. • Take frequent rest breaks during activities. Do not rush the patient; plan for extra time when assisting with ADLs.	Day 1: Refused bed bath due to shortness of breath. Allowed nurse to sponge off perineal area and armpits only. Day 2: Able to tolerate full bed bath with assistance. Became short of breath after washing arms and face. Took a 10-minute break, then able to assist by washing own perineal area. Day 3: Able to ambulate to bathroom. Had to rest on chair once at the sink. Waited for him to regain energy, then assisted with sponge bath at sink. Verbalizes plans to try chair in shower at home and using a terrycloth robe instead of drying after shower.

Skill 28.1 Obtaining a Sputum Specimen

Assessment Steps

1. Verify the health-care provider's order for the sputum specimen.
2. Determine the frequency and type of cough the patient is experiencing. If it is frequent and productive, you may be able to get the specimen at any time. If not, plan to obtain the specimen in the early morning ***when the most sputum is available for expectoration.***
3. Determine the patient's pain level and medicate if necessary. ***The patient may be unable to give good cough effort if he or she is in pain.***

Planning Step

1. Gather needed equipment and supplies: a sterile sputum specimen container with a lid and clean gloves. If obtaining a suctioned specimen, you will need a sterile suction catheter kit and a sputum trap that attaches to the suction tubing. You will also need a preprinted label for the specimen container, a biohazard specimen bag for transport, and protective eyewear.

Implementation Steps

1. Follow the Initial Implementation Steps located on the inside front cover.

For Obtaining a Sputum Specimen by Coughing and Expectoration

2. Assist the patient to sit upright ***to facilitate lung expansion*** and have the patient rinse his or her mouth ***to prevent food particles or other debris from being in the sputum specimen.***
3. Splint the abdominal or chest incisions with a pillow ***to help prevent incisional pain.***
4. Instruct the patient to inhale deeply two times and then take a third deep breath and cough while exhaling. ***This expands the lungs and opens the airways to allow mucus production with cough.***
5. Instruct the patient to expectorate the mucus into a sterile specimen container. Ask the patient to avoid touching the inside of the container with his or her mouth or tongue, and avoid touching the inside with your hands ***to prevent cross-contamination.***

Skill 28.1 (continued)

6. Repeat Steps 4 and 5 until approximately 30 mL of sputum has been obtained. ***This is the minimum amount needed for laboratory testing.***
7. Follow the Ending Implementation Steps located on the inside back cover.

For Obtaining a Sputum Specimen by Suction

2. Follow the steps for suctioning the nasopharynx in Skill 28.6 except that when you assemble the suction tubing and suction catheter, you will attach a sputum trap between them. When you suction the nasopharynx, you will go deep into the trachea and obtain sputum that will be suctioned into the sputum trap for testing.

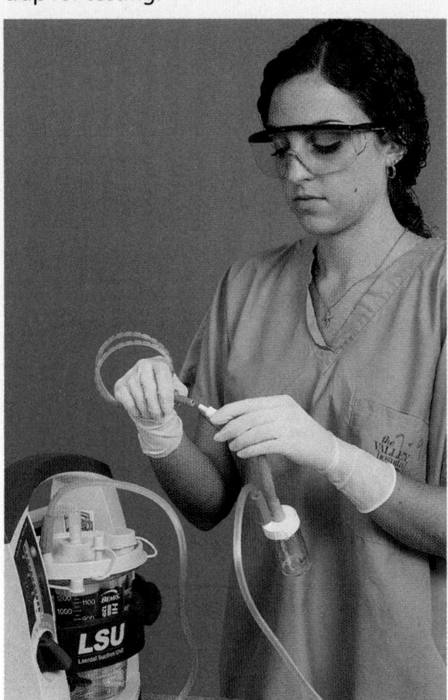

3. After obtaining the specimen, remove the suction tubing from the connection and attach the rubber tubing on the specimen trap to the port where the suction tubing was attached.
4. Follow the Ending Implementation Steps located on the inside back cover.

Evaluation Steps

1. Ensure that you have at least 30 mL of sputum in the container.
2. Determine the patient's response to the procedure.
3. Ensure that the specimen is labeled and placed in the appropriate biohazard specimen bag with the requisition.
4. Ensure that the specimen is taken to the laboratory promptly or refrigerated until it can be transported.

Sample Documentation

10/10/22 1330 Sputum spec of 30 mL of thick yellow mucus obtained. C/o fatigue after coughing effort. Resp increased to 26/min. Assisted to Fowler's position to rest. Sputum spec labeled and delivered to lab. ———— ———— Nurse's signature and credentials

Skill 28.2 Obtaining a Throat Culture Specimen

Assessment Step

1. Verify the health-care provider's order for throat culture.

Planning Step

1. Gather needed equipment and supplies: throat culture swab, tongue blade, clean gloves, and examination light if needed.

Implementation Steps

1. Follow the Initial Implementation Steps located on the inside front cover.
2. Assist the patient to an upright position in the bed or chair ***to allow better visualization of the throat.*** If the room is dark, use an examination light ***to make it easier to visualize the throat.***
3. Ask the patient to open his or her mouth widely and say "Ah" ***to allow access to the back of the throat.*** Place the tongue blade on the tongue ***to hold it down during the procedure.*** Tell the patient to breathe through the mouth. ***This helps prevent gagging.***
4. Remove the swab from the tube without touching any part of the swab itself. Hold onto the cap into which the swab handle is inserted. ***Touching any part of the swab, even while wearing clean gloves, can contaminate the specimen.***
5. Insert the swab into the patient's mouth without touching the teeth, cheeks, lips, or gums, ***which would cause contamination of the specimen.***
6. Using one side of the swab, slide it against the back of the throat and tonsils to the right of the uvula. Target reddened areas or patches of white or yellow exudate ***to ensure that pathogens are obtained.***
7. Using the other side of the swab, slide it against the back of the throat and tonsils to the left of the uvula, targeting the same type of areas. ***This allows collection of specimens from different areas of the throat to more easily identify pathogens.***

(skill continues on page 596)

Skill 28.2 (continued)

8. Carefully replace the swab into the sterile tube. ***Contamination of the swab or tube can lead to misdiagnosis and inappropriate treatment for the patient.***
9. Crush the capsule in the end of the tube ***to provide a moist environment for the pathogens until the culture is done.***
10. Label the tube according to facility policy.
11. Follow the Ending Implementation Steps located on the inside back cover.

Evaluation Steps

1. Ensure that an adequate specimen has been taken ***so that the culture will grow any pathogens present in the patient's throat.***
2. Evaluate the patient's tolerance of the procedure. Did it cause gagging or throat discomfort?
3. Ensure that the throat culture tube is placed in the appropriate biohazard specimen bag with the requisition and taken to the laboratory.

Sample Documentation

10/10/22 1330 Throat culture obtained per order and delivered to the lab. Pharynx red with yellowish-white patches noted on tonsils bilaterally. Culture taken from these areas. C/o sore throat before and after procedure. ———— Nurse's signature and credentials

Skill 28.3 Assisting With Incentive Spirometry

Assessment Steps

1. Verify the health-care provider's order for incentive spirometry. ***Note: Some hospitals do not require a health-care provider's order for this because it is considered a nursing or respiratory therapy order. Always follow your facility's policy.***
2. Determine the patient's pain level, availability, and willingness to perform the procedure. It may be necessary to medicate the patient for pain before beginning the procedure.

Planning Steps

1. Obtain an incentive spirometer.
2. Plan for appropriate time for incentive spirometry; avoid mealtimes.

Implementation Steps

1. Follow the Initial Implementation Steps located on the inside front cover.
2. Assist the patient to an upright position in the bed or chair ***to enlarge the rib cage and allow for maximum lung expansion.***
3. Splint abdominal or chest incisions with a pillow ***to prevent pain during deep inhalation and exhalation.***
4. Place the mouthpiece of the incentive spirometer between the patient's lips ***to prevent air from escaping around it during inhalation.***
5. Instruct the patient to take a deep breath through the mouth, then exhale through the nose. ***This helps the patient understand that the focus is on deep inhalation, not exhalation.***

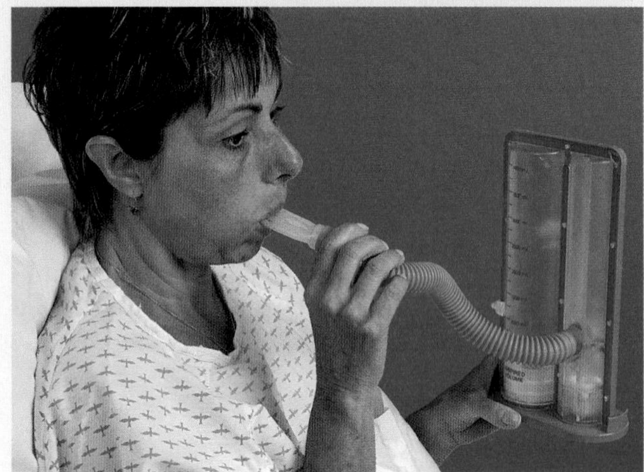

6. Show the patient how far the platform or balls moved. Identify the goal for the patient to work toward. Set the slide pointer to the goal volume on the spirometer.
7. Instruct the patient to repeat the inhalations 10 times every hour while awake ***to prevent respiratory complications of immobility such as pneumonia and atelectasis.***
8. Follow the Ending Implementation Steps located on the inside back cover.

Evaluation Steps

1. Ask the patient to demonstrate the use of the incentive spirometer without verbal cues ***to ensure that he or she understands how to correctly use it.***
2. Check back frequently ***to be sure the patient is using the incentive spirometer as ordered.***

Sample Documentation

10/10/22 1100 Assisted with incentive spirometry. Able to raise 2 out of 3 balls in unit. Instructed to repeat 10 times each hour. ———— Nurse's signature and credentials

Skill 28.4 Administering a Nebulizer Treatment

Assessment Steps

1. Verify the health-care provider's order for nebulizer treatment and medication. Determine if the medication is to be diluted with saline or administered full strength.
2. Research the medication if you are unfamiliar with it. Know the expected effects, side effects, and contraindications before administering any medication. (See Chapter 35 for more information on researching medications.)
3. Assess the patient's lungs for adventitious breath sounds and the patient for dyspnea.

Planning Steps

1. Obtain a nebulizer if one is not already in place at the bedside. Obtain ordered respiratory medications according to facility policy.
2. Determine if the patient can use a handheld mouthpiece or needs a mask for treatment. Use a mask if the patient is unable to hold the mouthpiece or to breathe in through the mouth and out through the nose during the treatment.
3. Pour the ordered medication and saline into the medication cup, checking the medication three times (see Chapter 35).
4. Assemble the mouthpiece parts or mask parts and attach the compressor tubing to the medication cup.

Implementation Steps

1. Follow the Initial Implementation Steps located on the inside front cover.
2. Assist the patient to an upright position in the bed or chair to enlarge the rib cage and allow for maximum lung expansion.
3. Check the patient's pulse. *Safety: Bronchodilators, if ordered, will increase the pulse rate. If the pulse is above 100, you may want to consult with the health-care provider before administering a bronchodilator.*
4. Place the mouthpiece between the patient's teeth and have him or her close the lips about it to prevent escape of medication around the mouthpiece. If using a mask, place it over the nose and mouth and tighten the elastic straps to keep it in place.
5. Turn on the air compressor. This causes the medication to be converted to a fine mist for inhalation.
6. Instruct the patient to breathe slowly and deeply to inhale the medication into the small airways and lungs.
7. Instruct the patient to continue the treatment until the vapor is no longer visible from the spacer on the mouthpiece or in the mask. This indicates that the medication has been completely inhaled.
8. Remain with the patient if necessary to ensure that the treatment is completed correctly.
9. Turn off the air compressor when the vapor is gone and the medication cup is empty.
10. Check the patient's pulse again to determine the effect of the medication. Expect an increase of approximately 20 beats per minute. *Safety: If the pulse rate is significantly higher than expected, notify the health-care provider.*
11. Disassemble the parts of the mouthpiece or mask and rinse them in warm water to remove any remnants of medication or saline that could crust in openings and affect function.
12. Allow the parts to drain on a clean paper towel and air dry to be ready for the patient's next treatment.
13. Follow the Ending Implementation Steps located on the inside back cover.

Evaluation Steps

1. Determine the effectiveness of the treatment. Auscultate the lungs to evaluate for decreased adventitious sounds.
2. Determine how the patient tolerated the treatment. Did it cause exhaustion? Was the patient able to follow directions? Did the patient inhale all the medication? Does the patient feel relief of dyspnea after treatment?

Sample Documentation

10/10/22 1340 C/o tightness in chest with inhalation. Lungs auscultated. Bilateral wheezes and coarse crackles noted bilaterally throughout lung fields. ———————— Nurse's signature and credentials

10/10/22 1400 Nebulizer treatment with 2 mL DuoNeb administered per order. Able to use mouthpiece with deep inhalations. Tolerated without c/o discomfort or fatigue. States "breathing easier" afterward. Lungs auscultated. Scattered coarse crackles heard in bilateral lower lobes. ———————— Nurse's signature and credentials

Skill 28.5 Administering Supplemental Oxygen

Assessment Steps

1. Verify the health-care provider's order for oxygen. Be certain of liter flow and type of delivery device ordered ***because some types are contraindicated in certain lung diseases.***
2. Assess the patient's respiratory status, including pulse oximetry, ***to document improved SaO_2 with oxygen.***

Planning Steps

1. Gather needed equipment and supplies: oxygen flowmeter, humidifier bottle, and ordered delivery device with tubing.
2. Obtain appropriate safety signs regarding smoking and open flames and post them in the home setting.

Implementation Steps

1. Follow the Initial Implementation Steps located on the inside front cover.
2. Connect the oxygen flowmeter to the oxygen source. For piped-in oxygen, follow facility guidelines. The flowmeter may have to be positioned in a certain way to enter the valve, or a release button may have to be pressed for the flowmeter to enter.
3. Fill the oxygen humidifier with sterile water so that the level is between the minimum and maximum lines, if not using a prefilled humidifier bottle. *Safety: Oxygen at low flow rates (below 3 L/min) does not have to be humidified. Any flow rate of*

(skill continues on page 598)

Skill 28.5 (continued)

about 3 L/min or higher must be humidified to prevent excessive drying of the mucous membranes.

4. Attach the humidifier to the flowmeter by screwing it onto the connector completely.
5. Attach the tubing from the oxygen device to the humidifier.
6. Set the ordered liter flow. Turn the dial on the flowmeter so that the silver ball rises to the ordered liters per minute. The line of the selected liter number should cross the middle of the silver ball for correct flow.
7. Place the oxygen delivery device on the patient:
   - **Nasal cannula:** Place the prongs so that the curve is toward the nares and loop the tubing over the ears. Push the slider up under the patient's chin ***to hold it securely in place.***

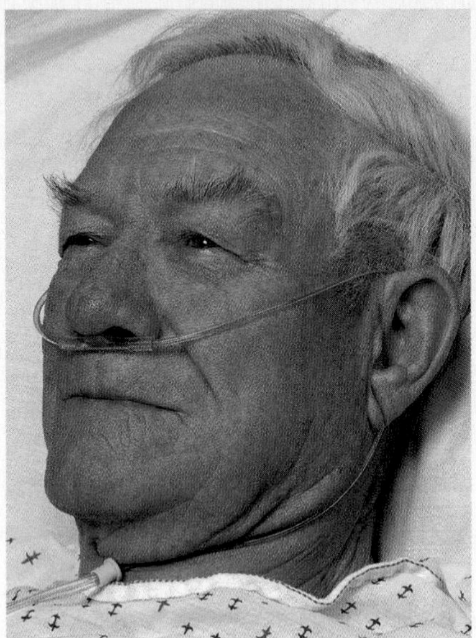

   - **Simple, rebreathing, and nonrebreathing masks:** Place the mask over the patient's nose and mouth and the elastic strip around the head, above the ears. Pull the strap at the sides of the mask to tighten ***so that the mask fits snugly over the face.*** Bend the metal nosepiece ***to conform to the bridge of the nose.***

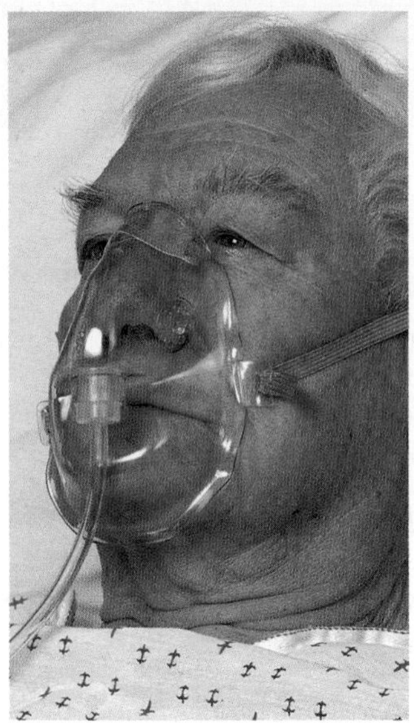

   - **Venturi mask:** Ensure that the dial or interchangeable valve between the mask and the oxygen source is correct ***to deliver the ordered percentage of oxygen.*** Apply the mask the same as the other masks.

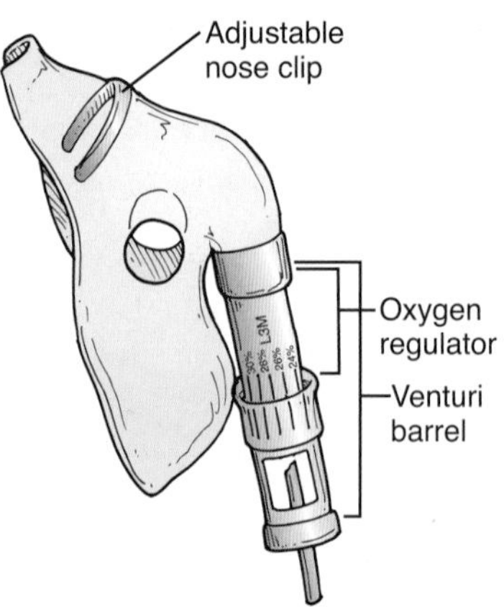

   - **Face tent:** Fit the tent under the patient's chin with the elastic strap around the head. Tighten at sides as needed ***for a snug chin fit.***

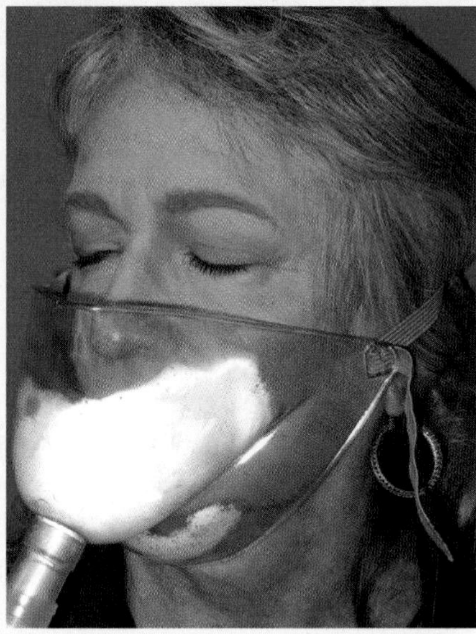

   - **Tracheostomy collar:** Place the collar loosely over the tracheostomy tube with the elastic strap around the patient's neck. Tighten at the sides as needed ***to keep the collar in place.***
   - **T-piece:** Attach to the tracheostomy tube and ensure that it is arranged so that any condensation within the tubing drains away from the patient.
8. Follow the Ending Implementation Steps located on the inside back cover.

Skill 28.5 (continued)

Evaluation Steps

1. Ensure that oxygen is flowing through the delivery device. There should be bubbles in the humidifier, ***indicating the flow of oxygen through it.*** To check low liter flow through an unhumidified cannula, place the cannula in a cup of water. ***If you see bubbles, the oxygen is flowing.***
2. Measure pulse oximetry after 30 minutes ***to evaluate improvement of SaO_2 due to supplemental oxygen.***
3. Evaluate the patient's comfort with oxygen. Does he or she complain of feeling claustrophobic? Is he or she mouth-breathing? It may be necessary to consider a change of delivery device with the health-care provider's approval.

Sample Documentation

10/10/22 1440 SaO_2 on room air was 90%. O_2 started per order at 2L/NC. ——— Nurse's signature and credentials

10/10/22 1520 SaO_2 94%. Tolerating cannula without c/o discomfort. States, "easier to breathe now." ——— Nurse's signature and credentials

Sample of Electronic Documentation

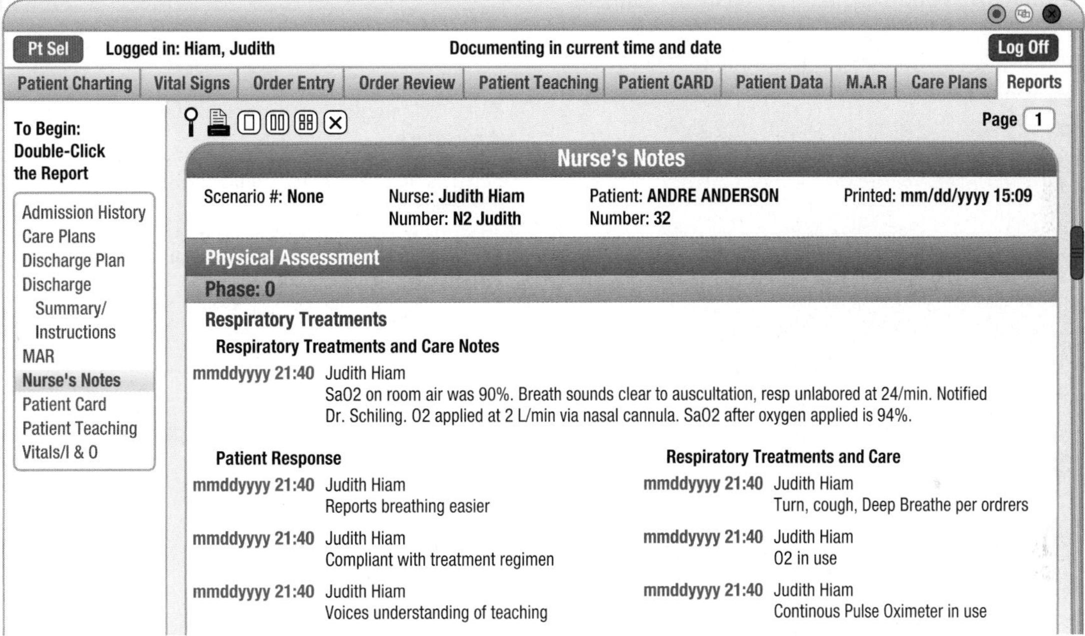
Pt Sel | Logged in: Hiam, Judith | Documenting in current time and date | Log Off

Patient Charting | Vital Signs | Order Entry | Order Review | Patient Teaching | Patient CARD | Patient Data | M.A.R | Care Plans | Reports

To Begin: Double-Click the Report

Admission History
Care Plans
Discharge Plan
Discharge Summary/ Instructions
MAR
Nurse's Notes
Patient Card
Patient Teaching
Vitals/I & O

Page 1

Nurse's Notes

Scenario #: None | Nurse: Judith Hiam Number: N2 Judith | Patient: ANDRE ANDERSON Number: 32 | Printed: mm/dd/yyyy 15:09

Physical Assessment

Phase: 0

Respiratory Treatments

Respiratory Treatments and Care Notes

mmddyyyy 21:40 Judith Hiam
Sa02 on room air was 90%. Breath sounds clear to auscultation, resp unlabored at 24/min. Notified Dr. Schiling. 02 applied at 2 L/min via nasal cannula. Sa02 after oxygen applied is 94%.

Patient Response

mmddyyyy 21:40 Judith Hiam
Reports breathing easier

mmddyyyy 21:40 Judith Hiam
Compliant with treatment regimen

mmddyyyy 21:40 Judith Hiam
Voices understanding of teaching

Respiratory Treatments and Care

mmddyyyy 21:40 Judith Hiam
Turn, cough, Deep Breathe per ordrers

mmddyyyy 21:40 Judith Hiam
02 in use

mmddyyyy 21:40 Judith Hiam
Continous Pulse Oximeter in use

Skill 28.6 Performing Nasopharyngeal and Oropharyngeal Suctioning

Assessment Steps

1. Verify the health-care provider's order for nasopharyngeal or oropharyngeal suctioning. ***Note: In some hospital settings, a health-care provider's order may not be required for suctioning. Follow facility's policy.***
2. Assess the patient and the need for suctioning. Auscultate the lungs and listen for rattling or moist sounds in the airways as the patient breathes, as well as oxygen saturation readings, color, and respiratory rate and rhythm.

Planning Step

1. Gather needed equipment and supplies: sterile suction catheter and glove kit; saline; a sterile basin or cup to hold the saline; water-soluble lubricant; goggles and a mask; or a mask, face shield, and gown. For oropharyngeal suctioning, obtain a Yankauer or tonsil-tip suction device and clean gloves.

Intervention Steps

1. Follow the Initial Implementation Steps located on the inside front cover and assist the patient to semi- or high Fowler's position.

For Nasopharyngeal Suctioning

2. Ensure that the connection tubing is attached to the suction catheter on the wall and set the regulator at 80 to 120 mm Hg. Test the suction by placing your thumb over the tubing ***to determine that it is working correctly.***
3. Open the sterile saline and mark it with the date and time if it is a multiuse container ***to ensure that it is not used beyond 24 hours or hospital policy.***
4. Pour some saline into the sterile basin or cup. ***This will be used to moisten and rinse the suction catheter between suctioning.***
5. Open the water-soluble lubricant.

(skill continues on page 600)

Skill 28.6 (continued)

6. Put a clean glove on your nondominant hand for controlling the suction.
7. Open the sterile catheter and glove kit. Put the sterile glove in the kit on your dominant hand ***because this is the hand that will hold and manipulate the suction catheter.*** If two gloves come in the kit, put them both on, but consider your nondominant hand as not sterile.
8. Hold the sterile suction catheter in your sterilely gloved dominant hand, being careful to keep the tip within your grasp ***to prevent it from becoming contaminated.***
9. Hold the nonsterile connection tubing connected to the suction canister in your nondominant hand.
10. Hold the proximal end of the sterile suction catheter in your dominant hand and connect it to the nonsterile connection tubing without contaminating your dominant hand.
11. Place the thumb-valve portion of the sterile suction catheter in your nondominant hand.
12. Lubricate the first 3 to 4 inches of the suction catheter with the water-soluble lubricant.

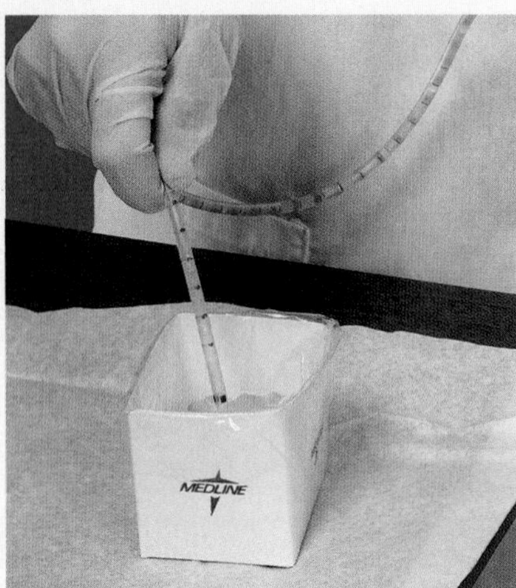

13. Insert the sterile catheter into the right nostril. *Safety: Do not apply your thumb while entering the nose and throat to prevent causing hypoxia.*
14. Continue inserting the catheter through the nose to the back of the throat.
15. Apply your thumb to the valve as you gently but quickly pull the catheter out of the throat and nose. *Safety: Use intermittent suction by lifting your thumb periodically. Suction for no longer than 10 to 15 seconds at a time to prevent hypoxia.*

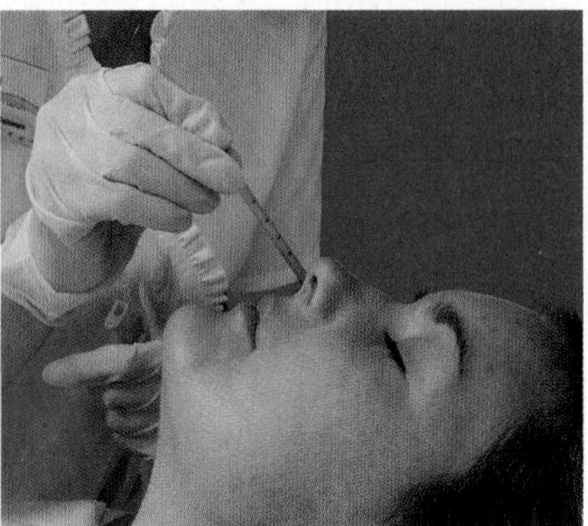

16. Insert the catheter into the basin or cup of saline and apply your thumb to the valve ***to rinse the inside and outside of the catheter.***
17. Repeat Steps 11 through 14 going through the left nostril.
18. The suction catheter can now be used to suction the patient's mouth, which has a higher number of bacteria and pathogens present, so it is suctioned last. However, some patients may find this objectionable. Also, the patient may bite down on the suction catheter if it is inserted into the mouth. It is appropriate to change to a Yankauer, or tonsil-tip, suction device at this time.

For Oropharyngeal Suctioning

2. Disconnect the suction catheter from the suction tubing. Hold the catheter in the palm of your dominant hand and remove the glove over the catheter. ***This contains the catheter for disposal and prevents contamination of the hands.***
3. Remove the glove from your nondominant hand and wash or sanitize your hands ***to prevent cross-contamination.***
4. Put on clean gloves ***because oral suctioning is not a sterile procedure.***
5. Attach the Yankauer, or tonsil-tip, suction device to the suction tubing.
6. Insert the tonsil tip into the patient's mouth to the back of the throat and then cover the opening with your thumb or finger ***to create suction.***

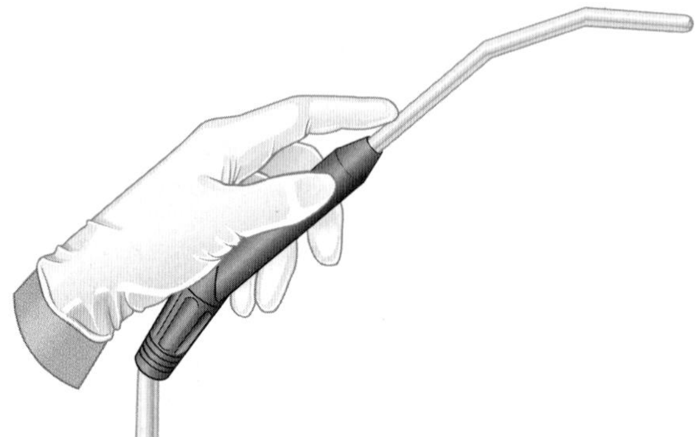

7. Suction each side of the throat, in the cheek pouches, and around the tongue ***to remove mucus.***
8. Insert the tonsil tip into the saline in the basin or cup and place your thumb or finger over the valve ***to rinse the inside and outside of the tonsil tip.*** Repeat as necessary during suctioning of the mouth.
9. Disconnect the rinsed tonsil tip and replace it in the wrapper for reuse. Follow facility's policy for the length of time it can be used.
10. Follow the Ending Implementation Steps located on the inside back cover.

Skill 28.6 (continued)

Evaluation Steps

1. Auscultate the patient's lungs and listen to the patient breathe to determine that the airways are clearer after suctioning.
2. Evaluate the patient's response to the procedure. Did he or she complain of shortness of breath? Pain or discomfort? Fatigue?

Sample Documentation

10/11/22 1730 Respirations moist sounding, with rattling in throat. Coarse crackles heard in bilateral upper lobes. ——— *Nurse's signature and credentials*

10/11/22 1745 Nasopharyngeal suctioning performed. Lrg amt of thick white mucus obtained. Suctioned orally for sm amt of yellow mucus. Lung sounds clear bilaterally. Resp quiet and even at 20/min. ——— *Nurse's signature and credentials*

Skill 28.7 Performing Endotracheal and Tracheostomy Suctioning

Assessment Steps

1. Verify the health-care provider's order for endotracheal or tracheostomy suctioning.
2. Assess the patient for the need for suctioning. Auscultate the lungs and listen for moist respirations through the tracheostomy. If the patient is on a ventilator, you may hear the pressure alarm go off, indicating the need for suctioning.

Planning Step

1. Gather needed equipment and supplies: sterile suction catheter kit (which contains gloves, a catheter, and a cup for saline), sterile saline, goggles and a mask or a mask and face shield, a gown if indicated, and an Ambu bag for tracheostomy suctioning.

Intervention Steps

1. Follow the Initial Implementation Steps located on the inside front cover.

Suctioning an Endotracheal Tube When Patient Is Connected to a Ventilator

2. Turn the suction on between 100 and 150 mm Hg.
3. Put on the sterile gloves and prepare the sterile suction catheter and saline as you did in Skill 28.6, keeping in mind that your nondominant hand is not sterile.
4. Lubricate the suction catheter in the sterile saline by placing the first 3 to 4 inches in the container of sterile saline and placing your thumb over the valve to suction up some of the liquid.
5. Push the button on the ventilator to give 100% oxygen. ***This gives 100% oxygen to the patient for 2 minutes while you perform suctioning to help prevent hypoxia.***
6. Insert the catheter into the endotracheal tube until you meet resistance, which is the carina of the trachea. *Safety: Do not apply suction while inserting the catheter to prevent hypoxia.*
7. Apply suction with your thumb as you withdraw the catheter. Use a circular motion and rotate the catheter between your thumb and first finger as you withdraw it ***to ensure that you suction all areas inside the endotracheal tube.***
8. Perform suctioning quickly. *Safety: Suctioning for longer than 10 to 15 seconds at a time can cause hypoxia.*
9. Rinse the suction catheter by placing it in the cup of sterile saline and using your thumb on the valve to create suction.
10. Repeat Steps 5 through 9 as needed to clear the endotracheal tube of secretions. *Safety: Wait 30 seconds between suctioning passes to allow the patient time to rest. Limit the total time to 5 minutes or less.*
11. Disconnect the suction catheter from the suction tubing. Hold the catheter in the palm of your dominant hand and remove the glove over the catheter. ***This contains the catheter for disposal and prevents contamination of the hands.***
12. Remove the glove from your nondominant hand and wash or sanitize your hands ***to prevent cross-contamination.***
13. Follow the Ending Implementation Steps located on the inside back cover.

For In-Line Suction of an Endotracheal Tube

2. Turn the suction on between 100 and 150 mm Hg.
3. It is unnecessary to use sterile gloves for in-line suction because the suction catheter is contained inside a sterile sleeve, which is connected to the endotracheal tube.
4. Push the button on the ventilator to give 100% oxygen. ***This gives 100% oxygen to the patient for 2 minutes while you perform suctioning to help prevent hypoxia.***
5. Wearing clean gloves, gently insert the suction catheter into the endotracheal tube until you meet resistance.
6. Apply suction by pressing the button over the suction port as you withdraw the catheter. Again, apply suction for no longer than 10 to 15 seconds at a time. Repeat suctioning as needed to clear the endotracheal tube of secretions.

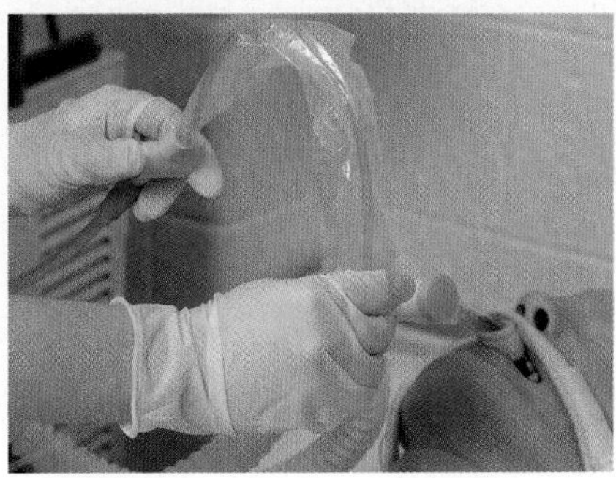

(skill continues on page 602)

Skill 28.7 (continued)

7. Rather than placing the suction catheter in saline to clear it, squeeze a 10-mL plastic container of saline into the port located on the in-line setup. As you insert the saline, apply suction so that it will clear the suction catheter.
8. Follow the Ending Implementation Steps located on the inside back cover.

For Suctioning a Tracheostomy When Patient Is Not Connected to a Ventilator

2. Turn the suction on between 80 and 120 mm Hg.
3. Attach the Ambu bag to 100% oxygen from the piped-in oxygen.
4. Enlist the assistance of another health-care worker. *Safety: It is very difficult to attach the Ambu bag to the tracheostomy and squeeze the bag to hyperoxygenate the patient using only one hand because you will be keeping your other hand sterile.*
5. Put on the sterile gloves and prepare the sterile suction catheter and saline as you did in Skill 28.6, keeping in mind that your nondominant hand is not sterile.
6. Lubricate the suction catheter in the sterile saline as in Step 4 earlier in this skill.
7. Have your assistant attach the Ambu bag to the tracheostomy tubing, give the patient three to five breaths, and then disconnect it from the tracheostomy tube. If you have no assistant, you must do this while keeping your dominant hand sterile and holding the sterile suction catheter.

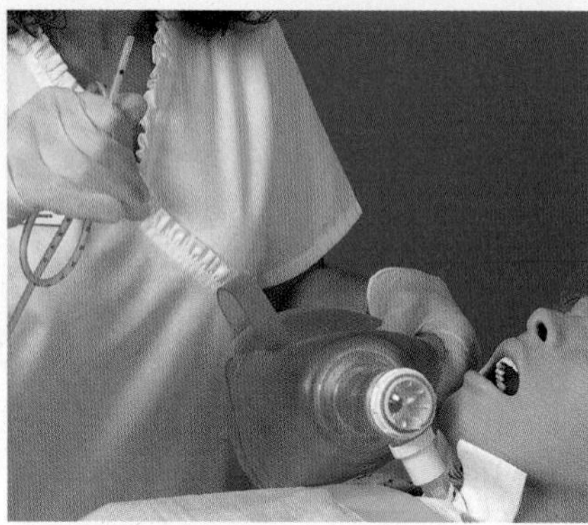

8. Insert the catheter into the tracheostomy tube until you meet resistance, which is at the carina of the trachea. *Safety: Do not apply suction while inserting the catheter to prevent hypoxia.*
9. Apply suction with your thumb as you withdraw the catheter. Use a circular motion and rotate the catheter between your thumb and first finger as you withdraw it ***to ensure that you suction all areas inside the tracheostomy tube.***
10. Lift your thumb off the valve after a few seconds and then return it to the valve. ***This helps prevent the suction catheter from sticking against tracheal tissue and causing trauma to it.***
11. Perform suctioning quickly. *Safety: Suctioning for longer than 10 to 15 seconds at a time can cause hypoxia.*
12. Rinse the suction catheter by placing it in the cup of sterile saline and using your thumb on the valve to create suction.
13. Repeat Steps 7 to 12 as needed to clear the tracheostomy tube of secretions. Wait at least 30 seconds between suctionings ***to allow the patient to breathe easily.*** Reoxygenate with Ambu bag between suctionings. Avoid suctioning for more than a total of 5 minutes ***to prevent fatigue, trauma, and hypoxia.*** *Safety: It is a good idea to hold your breath while you are suctioning a patient with a tracheostomy because this will remind you that the patient cannot breathe while the suction catheter is in the tracheostomy.*
14. Disconnect the suction catheter from the suction tubing. Hold the catheter in the palm of your dominant hand and remove the glove over the catheter. ***This contains the catheter for disposal and prevents contamination of the hands.***
15. Remove the glove from your nondominant hand and wash or sanitize your hands ***to prevent cross-contamination.***
16. Follow the Ending Implementation Steps located on the inside back cover.

Evaluation Steps

1. Evaluate the patient's ease of respirations after suctioning. Is the ventilator working properly without pressure alarms? Can the patient with a tracheostomy breathe without mucus bubbling or rattling?
2. Determine how the patient tolerated the procedure. Was he or she frightened? Anxious? Did he or she complain of fatigue or discomfort afterward?

Sample Documentation

10/11/22 2010 Respirations moist with rattling noted in trach. Suctioned for mod amt of light yellow mucus. Coughed repeatedly during procedure and c/o fatigue after suctioning complete. Resp quiet and even at 22/min. ——— ——— Nurse's signature and credentials

Skill 28.7 (continued)

Sample of Electronic Documentation

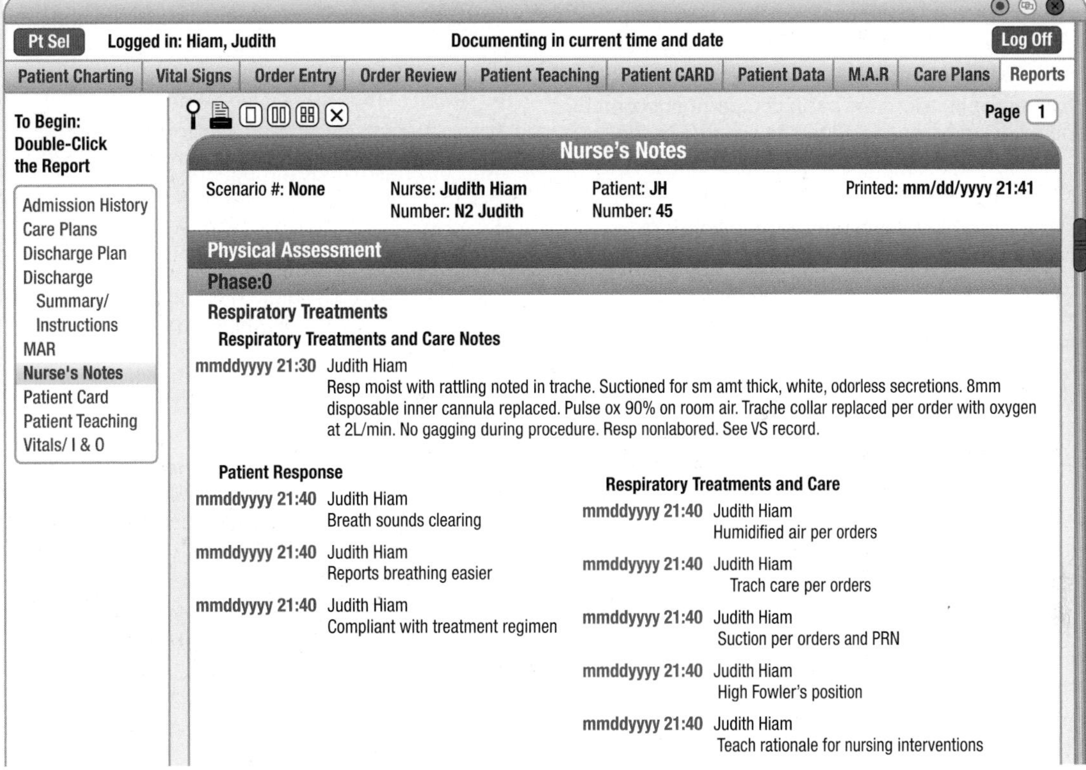

Pt Sel
Logged in: Hiam, Judith
Documenting in current time and date
Log Off
Patient Charting
Vital Signs
Order Entry
Order Review
Patient Teaching
Patient CARD
Patient Data
M.A.R
Care Plans
Reports
To Begin: Double-Click the Report
Page 1
Nurse's Notes
Admission History
Care Plans
Discharge Plan
Discharge Summary/ Instructions
MAR
Nurse's Notes
Patient Card
Patient Teaching
Vitals/ I & O
Scenario #: None
Nurse: Judith Hiam
Number: N2 Judith
Patient: JH
Number: 45
Printed: mm/dd/yyyy 21:41
Physical Assessment
Phase:0
Respiratory Treatments
Respiratory Treatments and Care Notes
mmddyyyy 21:30 Judith Hiam
Resp moist with rattling noted in trache. Suctioned for sm amt thick, white, odorless secretions. 8mm disposable inner cannula replaced. Pulse ox 90% on room air. Trache collar replaced per order with oxygen at 2L/min. No gagging during procedure. Resp nonlabored. See VS record.
Patient Response
mmddyyyy 21:40 Judith Hiam
Breath sounds clearing
mmddyyyy 21:40 Judith Hiam
Reports breathing easier
mmddyyyy 21:40 Judith Hiam
Compliant with treatment regimen
Respiratory Treatments and Care
mmddyyyy 21:40 Judith Hiam
Humidified air per orders
mmddyyyy 21:40 Judith Hiam
Trach care per orders
mmddyyyy 21:40 Judith Hiam
Suction per orders and PRN
mmddyyyy 21:40 Judith Hiam
High Fowler's position
mmddyyyy 21:40 Judith Hiam
Teach rationale for nursing interventions

Skill 28.8 Performing Tracheostomy Care

Assessment Steps

1. Verify the health-care provider's order for tracheostomy care. Standard orders are to perform the care every 8 hours.
2. Assess the type of tracheostomy the patient has. If the inner cannula is disposable, you will need to obtain a new replacement cannula. If it is reusable, you will need to obtain a kit for cleaning the inner cannula.

Planning Step

1. Gather needed equipment and supplies: replacement cannula or tracheostomy care kit, hydrogen peroxide, sterile saline, sterile gloves, clean gloves, goggles and a mask, or a mask and face shield. You will need a tracheostomy holder if the patient does not use ties. You will also need a suction catheter and glove kit.

Intervention Steps

1. Follow the Initial Implementation Steps located on the inside front cover.
2. Suction the tracheostomy following the steps in Skill 28.7. ***This removes secretions and helps keep the tracheostomy patent during the cleaning of the inner cannula.***
3. Don clean gloves. ***This will allow you to touch the inner cannula to remove it without contaminating your sterile gloves or exposing yourself to blood or body fluids.***

Cannula Care

To Replace a Disposable Inner Cannula

4. Open the package containing the new inner cannula, keeping the cannula on the sterile inner surface of the package.
5. Remove the inner cannula by unlocking it, either by turning it slightly to the side or by pinching the connecting flanges ***so that it will easily slide out.*** Also remove the old tracheostomy dressing from beneath the faceplate.
6. Dispose of the inner cannula and used dressing in the biohazard trash.
7. Insert the new inner cannula by turning it so that the end you are holding is at about the 9 o'clock position. Then, as you insert it into the outer cannula, turn it gently to the 6 o'clock position. *Safety: Once the new inner cannula is inserted, ensure that it clicks into place or is tightened to stay in place.*
8. Go to Steps 15 to 19.

To Clean and Replace a Reusable Cannula

4. Open the tracheostomy care kit and set up your sterile field. Dump the contents of the kit onto the sterile field. ***This allows you to use the basin for your liquids.***
5. Open and pour hydrogen peroxide into the larger compartment in the basin to a depth of ½ inch. Add saline to a depth of another ½ inch to dilute the hydrogen peroxide. *Safety: Full-strength hydrogen peroxide can be irritating to the tissues. Follow facility policy regarding the use of hydrogen peroxide.*

(skill continues on page 604)

Skill 28.8 (continued)

6. Pour sterile saline in the other two compartments in the basin ***to be prepared to clean and rinse the inner cannula.***
7. Remove the inner cannula from the tracheostomy. Remember to unlock it by turning it slightly to the side or pinching the connecting flanges so that it will easily slide out.
8. Drop the inner cannula into the basin compartment containing the peroxide and saline ***to allow the cannula to soak.***
9. Remove the old tracheostomy dressing from beneath the faceplate and dispose of it in the biohazard trash.
10. Remove your clean gloves and sanitize your hands ***to prevent cross-contamination.***
11. Put on sterile gloves and arrange your supplies on your sterile field ***so that you can easily obtain what you need as you complete the procedure.***
12. Use the sterile small bottle brush to clean the inside and outside of the inner cannula with the peroxide/saline solution.
13. Place the inner cannula in a basin compartment containing only sterile saline and agitate it ***to rinse off the peroxide.***
14. Remove the inner cannula from the saline and use a sterile gauze 4×4 to dry the outside. Use both pipe cleaners together to dry the inside of the cannula by pulling them through it. *Safety: It is important to dry the inside and outside of the cannula to prevent introducing saline into the trachea and causing choking. Be alert to any threads from the gauze 4×4 that could cling to the cannula. It should be dry and debris free.*
15. Insert the cleaned inner cannula by turning it so that the end you are holding is at about the 9 o'clock position. Then, as you insert it into the outer cannula, turn it gently to the 6 o'clock position. *Safety: Once the cleaned inner cannula is inserted, ensure that it clicks into place or is tightened to stay in place.*

To Clean Faceplate

16. Dip a cotton-tipped applicator from your sterile field into the unused basin compartment containing sterile saline. Use the moistened applicator to clean around the stoma ***to loosen dried or crusted mucus.*** Get a new moistened swab for each swipe ***to prevent cross-contamination.***

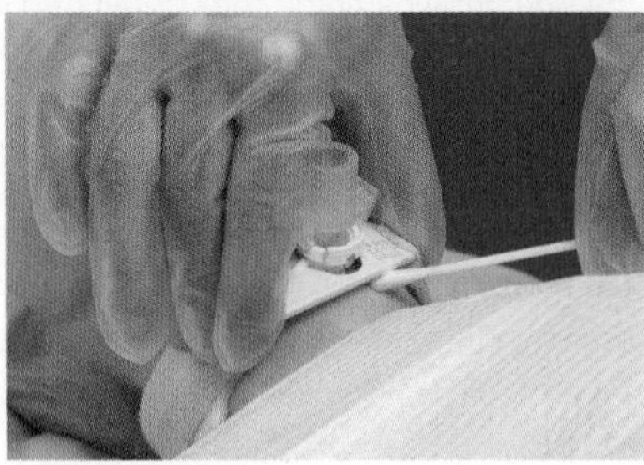

17. Dampen a sterile gauze 4×4 in the saline and clean the faceplate of the tracheostomy. Dry the faceplate with another gauze 4×4.

To Change the Tracheostomy Ties or Tracheostomy Holder

For Twill Ties

4. If you have an assistant, have him or her hold the tracheostomy faceplate in place while you insert one end of the tie into the slit at the side of the faceplate. *Safety: If you are working alone, do NOT remove the existing twill ties until the new ones are in place.*
5. Bring the other end behind the patient's neck and pull it through the slit on the other side of the faceplate.
6. Tie the two ends together at the side of the patient's neck ***so that he or she does not lay on a knot that could cause skin breakdown.*** *Safety: Ensure that you can fit one finger between the tie and the patient's skin to avoid making it too tight.*

For Velcro Holders

4. Insert the Velcro ends through the slits in the faceplate from back to front.
5. Ensure that the foam holder is laying smoothly behind the patient's neck.
6. Pull the Velcro through the slits and press it down against the foam, leaving about a one-finger space between the patient's neck and the holder. *Safety: Do NOT remove the old ties or holders until the new ties or holders are in place and secured. The patient will cough as you work with the tracheostomy and can cough it out if it is not secured.*

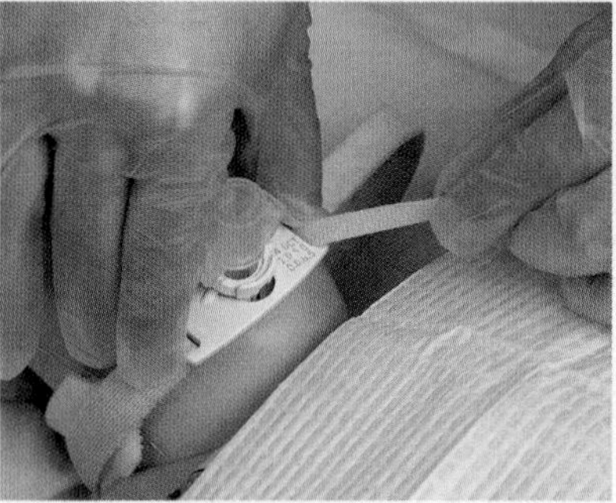

Completion of Tracheostomy Care

17. Replace the tracheostomy dressing with a clean tracheostomy one. This is placed so that the open ends point toward the patient's chin and are brought together above the tracheostomy. ***The dressing absorbs drainage and mucus from around the stoma.*** *Safety: If a split dressing is not available, avoid cutting a gauze 4×4 to make a tracheostomy dressing because the threads from the cut ends can enter the tracheostomy and cause infection and irritation. Instead, fold the gauze 4×4 in half and then each end at right angles to fit beneath the faceplate.*
18. Ensure that the tracheostomy collar is in place over the tracheostomy if ordered and that oxygen is being delivered per order.
19. Follow the Ending Implementation Steps located on the inside back cover.

Evaluation Steps

1. Determine the effectiveness of the procedure. Is the tracheostomy clean and patent?
2. Evaluate the patient's response to the procedure. Did he or she complain of pain, discomfort, fatigue, or shortness of breath?

Sample Documentation

10/11/22 2100 Trach care performed. Suctioned for mod amt of thick white mucus. Inner cannula partially obstructed with sm amt thick white mucus. Tolerated without c/o discomfort or fatigue. Writes "can breathe better" after procedure completed. ————
———— Nurse's signature and credentials

Skill 28.9 Maintaining Chest Tubes

Assessment Steps

1. Verify the physician's order for level of suction in the chest drainage system.
2. Assess for an emergency situation if chest tubes are being inserted at the bedside. Enlist the help of other staff members ***to help you gather and assemble all equipment as quickly as possible.***

Planning Steps

1. Gather needed equipment and supplies: chest tube with insertion tray, a drainage system, sterile water, connectors, petroleum jelly (Vaseline) gauze dressings, split drain sponges, an abdominal dressing pad, and padded Kelly clamps, as well as sterile gloves, masks, gowns, and goggles as needed.
2. Organize your equipment. Set up the suction and water seal per order ***to have the drainage system ready when the tube is attached.***

Intervention Steps

1. Follow the Initial Implementation Steps located on the inside front cover.
2. Assist the physician as required by opening packages, handing items, and pouring solutions. Reassure the patient during the procedure.
3. Once the tube is in place, attach it to the drainage system and remove the padded Kelly clamp.
4. Apply Vaseline gauze dressing or facility-recommended dressing around the chest tube site, sealing any area where an air leak could occur. Cover the gauze with drain sponges and abdominal dressing pads. Tape the dressing area completely ***to help prevent air from entering the chest cavity.***
5. Tape all connections thoroughly, taping away from the patient first and then back toward the patient. Attach the chest tube to the patient with a loop of tape ***to prevent tension on the insertion site as you tape the connections.***
6. Turn on suction as ordered until gentle bubbling is noted if it is a wet suction system.
7. Place drainage system securely on the floor and arrange the tubing so that there are no kinks or downward loops ***so that drainage can flow by gravity to the collection chamber.***
8. Maintain the drainage system in an upright position below the level of the chest at all times ***to prevent the water seal or suction fluids from being disturbed.***
9. Frequently assess the tubes for kinks or loops and the drainage in the tubing for clots, ***which could cause increased negative pressure in the chest cavity.*** *Safety: If clots are blocking the tubing, follow facility's policy and physician's orders. Do NOT milk or strip the tubes unless you are specifically ordered to do so.*
10. Ensure that Vaseline and gauze 4×4s are at the bedside in case of air leakage or other emergency. Follow facility's policy for appropriate action to take if the chest tube is dislodged.
11. Assess output in the collection chamber. Be aware of the color and amount draining each hour. *Safety: Notify the physician immediately if the drainage changes to a bright red color or is greater than 100 mL/hr.*
12. Assess for air leaks in the drainage system. Remember that wet suction will bubble gently in the suction chamber. If the patient has a pneumothorax, expect to see air in the water-seal chamber as well as tidaling in the chamber. As the pneumothorax resolves and the lung reinflates, the air in the water-seal chamber and the tidaling in the chamber will cease.
13. Mark output for your shift on the writable surface of the collection chamber. Mark the level of the output and then write the date, time, and your initials. Calculate drainage output for your shift by subtracting the amount in the drainage chamber when you started your shift from the amount in the chamber at the end of your shift.
14. Assist the patient to a comfortable position and reassure him or her regarding the chest tubes. Encourage the patient to change position, cough, and deep breathe every 2 hours ***to help reexpand the lung and remove drainage from the chest cavity.***
15. Follow the Ending Implementation Steps located on the inside back cover.

Evaluation Steps

1. Evaluate the effectiveness of the chest tubes. Is the patient breathing with less difficulty? Is the suction set correctly? Is the water seal at 2 cm of water? Are there signs of escaping pneumothorax? Are there any signs of additional air leaks?
2. Evaluate the patient's response to the procedure. Is the patient resting comfortably? Is pain medication needed for the incision site? Is the patient complaining of any other problems?
3. Evaluate the insertion site dressings. If there is a hemothorax, is the dressing dry and intact? Does it need to be reinforced or changed? Follow facility's policy for changing the dressing to the chest tube insertion site.

Sample Documentation

10/12/22 1825 Dr. Chapman inserted one chest tube for hemothorax. Attached to Pleuravac drainage system with wet suction at -20 cm. Water seal established with 2 cm water. Chest tube draining mod amt of dark red fluid, less than 100 mL/hr. All connections double-taped. Drsg at insertion site clean, dry, and intact. Resting quietly in bed in semi-Fowler's position eating ice chips. States he "can breathe better" after chest tube insertion. Requests pain med for incisional pain. ——————————

—————————— Nurse's signature and credentials

POST CONFERENCE

You were really worried when you walked into your patient's room the first morning and saw him with his tracheostomy, sounding all bubbly and coughing frequently. He pointed to the tracheostomy and mouthed the word "suction." Without much time to think, you grabbed a suction catheter and glove kit and set up quickly but without contaminating your sterile field or sterile supplies. You remembered as you suctioned to hold your own breath and not suction for longer than 10 seconds. It was obvious to you that the suctioning procedure tired your patient and made him a little short of breath. However, once you had suctioned his tracheostomy several times, he could breathe considerably better and mouthed "thank you." After that, you weren't afraid to suction him. His tracheostomy collar stayed in place pretty well, and you were able to replace his inner cannula the first day with your instructor's guidance. By the second day, you were feeling far more confident about all of his care. By the third day of clinicals, you were showing other students how to suction him.

Key Points

- Muscles, nerves, and chemicals all play a role in causing and controlling respirations.
- Impaired oxygenation may be due to hypoxia or hypoxemia caused by airway obstruction, secretions in the alveoli, chronic lung disease, and trauma.
- Respiratory assessment of the patient with impaired oxygenation must be very thorough to avoid missing subtle signs of hypoxia or hypoxemia.
- Crepitus indicates air under the skin, or subcutaneous emphysema, and the source of the leaking air must be found and treated.
- Diagnostic tests for which you will obtain specimens include sputum testing and throat cultures.
- Patients with impaired oxygen need to expand the lungs fully, which can be accomplished by turning, coughing, and deep breathing; use of an incentive spirometer; and nebulizer treatments with bronchodilators.
- CPT helps loosen and drain mucus from all the lobes of the lungs.
- Supplemental oxygen is available from different sources and with a variety of delivery devices. All require use of stringent safety precautions to prevent fire.
- The patient with chronic lung disease needs to conserve energy and preserve accessory muscles for breathing.
- Artificial airways vary from small plastic devices inserted in the mouth to tubes inserted through the nose, mouth, or an incision into the trachea.
- When caring for patients with artificial airways, you will suction to keep them patent. For tracheostomies, you will remove the inner cannula to clean or replace it.
- Chest tubes are inserted to re-establish intrathoracic pressure, remove air and drainage, and reinflate the lung.
- Chest tube drainage systems generally have three chambers: one for suction, one to create a water seal, and one to collect drainage.
- You are responsible for marking output for your shift, keeping the drainage unit upright and below the level of the chest, and keeping the tubing free from kinks and loops.
- You must know how to troubleshoot air leaks and what to do if the chest tube accidentally comes out or becomes disconnected from the closed drainage system.

Review Questions

Select the answer that is most appropriate for each of the following questions. Some questions may have more than one correct answer. Select all that apply.

1. Which is (are) true of chemical regulation of respirations?
   1. Chemoreceptors are located in the carotid and aorta and the brain.
   2. The cerebellum is responsible for brain control of respirations.
   3. The chemoreceptors in the brain cause an increase in the rate and depth of respirations in response to changes in blood pH.
   4. If the carbon dioxide level is higher than normal in the blood, the blood becomes more acidic and the pH falls below 7.35.
   5. If the oxygen level in the blood falls, this provides the stimulus to breathe in people who do not have chronic lung disease.
   6. Chemoreceptors in the carotid and aorta respond to decreased oxygen in the blood and send the message to the medulla.

2. A patient who has chronic lung disease is stimulated to breathe because the chemoreceptors detect:
   1. low oxygen in the blood.
   2. high oxygen in the blood.
   3. low carbon dioxide in the blood.
   4. high carbon dioxide in the blood.

3. You are caring for a patient who has lung disease. Yesterday, the patient was pleasant and cooperative. Today, the patient is irritable, restless, and a little confused. She is also complaining of a headache. What concerns you the most about this situation?
   1. The patient's complaint of headache. Along with her other symptoms, it could indicate an impending stroke.
   2. All of the symptoms concern you because they could all be signs of early hypoxia.
   3. The confusion concerns you the most because it could indicate the beginning of Alzheimer's disease.
   4. None of these symptoms concerns you greatly because the patient is probably just having a bad day.

4. You listen to the patient's lungs and hear adventitious breath sounds bilaterally. You note a frequent productive cough of thick yellow sputum. Which other assessments will you quickly make?
   1. Perform pulse oximetry to determine SaO_2
   2. Assess color of the lips, nailbeds, and mucous membranes
   3. Assess respiratory rate, character, and quality
   4. Palpate for crepitus
   5. Determine how much fluid intake the patient has had in the past 24 hours

5. Incentive spirometry is used to:
   1. deliver moisture and medication deep into the lungs.
   2. help prevent pneumonia and atelectasis.
   3. measure the rate and amount of air in a forceful exhalation.
   4. help the patient conserve energy when performing ADLs.

6. Your patient has a blood pH of 7.48 and is on oxygen at 8 L/min. Which oxygen delivery device is best for this patient?
   1. A simple face mask
   2. A Venturi mask
   3. A partial rebreathing mask
   4. A face tent

7. The health-care provider asks for a stat pulse oximetry reading on a patient wearing dark nail polish. What action will you take first?
   1. Ask the patient to remove her nail polish while you obtain a pulse oximeter
   2. Auscultate the patient's lungs for abnormal breath sounds
   3. Apply a pulse oximeter to the patient's finger to obtain the stat reading
   4. Obtain fingernail polish remover and remove the polish from one nail and then attach the pulse oximeter to that finger

8. When you look at the arterial blood gas results on your patient, you see that his pH is 7.32. What concern do you have for this patient?
   1. He is in alkalosis.
   2. He is in acidosis.
   3. He is in respiratory failure.
   4. He is hyperventilating.

ANSWERS 1. 1, 3, 4, 6; 2. 1; 3. 2; 4. 1, 2, 3; 5. 2; 6. 3; 7. 4; 8. 2

Critical Thinking Exercises

Answers available online.

1. Your patient had a chest tube inserted yesterday to drain a hemothorax and has been doing well. Suddenly the patient becomes restless and agitated, and respirations become more labored. When you take vital signs, you find the BP has dropped to 96/60, pulse is up to 110, and respirations are increased to 26 per minute. What will you do next?

2. Your patient with a tracheostomy is on a ventilator. His neck looks swollen this morning, and it has not been that way previously. What are your concerns?

Additional Resources

DAVIS edge. **Use the scratch off code on the inside front cover of your book to access online quizzes that will help you to improve your scores on course exams and prepare for the NCLEX-PN®.**

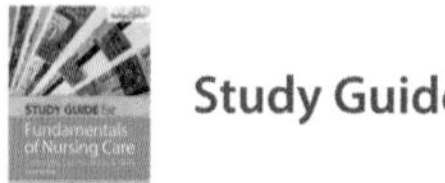

Study Guide

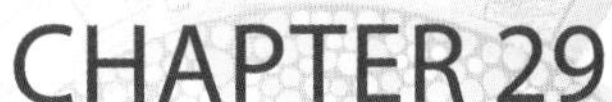

CHAPTER 29

Fluids, Electrolytes, and Introduction to Acid-Base Balance

KEY TERMS

Acidosis (ASS-ih-DOH-siss)
Aldosterone (al-DOS-ter-ohn)
Alkalosis (AL-kuh-LOH-siss)
Antidiuretic hormone (ADH) (AN-ti-DYE-yoo-RET-ik HOR-mohn)
Bicarbonate (bye-KAR-boh-nayt)
Buffer (BUFF-uhr)
Dehydration (DEE-hye-DRAY-shun)
Diffusion (dih-FYOO-zhun)
Electrolyte (e-LEK-truh-lyet)
Extracellular fluid (EKS-trah-SELL-yoo-lar FLOO-id)
Filtration (fil-TRAY-shun)
Fluid volume deficit (FLOO-id VOL-yoom DEF-ih-sit)
Intracellular fluid (IN-tra-SELL-yoo-lar FLOO-id)
Intravascular space (IN-tra-VAS-kyoo-lar SPAYS)
Osmosis (oz-MOH-siss)
pH

CHAPTER CONCEPTS

Acid-Base Balance
Fluid and Electrolyte Balance
Oxygenation
Nutrition
Patient-Centered Care

LEARNING OUTCOMES

1. Define various terms associated with fluids, electrolytes, and acid-base balance.
2. Describe the functions and movement of body fluids.
3. Identify body fluid compartments.
4. Explain how fluids are regulated in the body.
5. Describe fluid volume imbalances: fluid volume deficit and fluid volume excess.
6. Identify nursing actions to take for patients with fluid volume imbalances.
7. Explain the function of electrolytes in the body.
8. Identify normal ranges, functions, and dietary sources for selected electrolytes.
9. Discuss imbalances of electrolytes, including signs, symptoms, and causative factors.
10. Identify nursing actions to take for patients with electrolyte imbalances.
11. Describe the pH scale and where selected body fluids fall on it.
12. Briefly describe how the buffer system, respiratory system, and renal system regulate acid-base balance.
13. Identify four types of acid-base imbalances and nursing actions to take for them.
14. Discuss information found in the Connection features in this chapter.
15. Identify specific safety information.

CRITICAL THINKING CONNECTION

Clinical Assignment

You have been assigned the care of a patient admitted to the hospital with hyperkalemia. She has been in the intensive care unit with various treatments for hyperkalemia. You will be caring for her on the first day on the nursing unit after being moved out of intensive care. This seems a bit frightening to you because you are unsure what symptoms will indicate that she is having a problem with hyperkalemia again. In fact, you are not exactly sure what hyperkalemia is. You know that she has been seriously ill and is on telemetry, so you think it must have something to do with her heart.

Continued

CRITICAL THINKING CONNECTION—cont'd

Critical Thinking Questions:

1. What is hyperkalemia?
2. Which treatments are usually ordered for hyperkalemia?
3. What focused assessments will you need to make?
4. Which foods should the patient eat and which should she avoid?
5. Why is telemetry monitoring ordered for this patient?

While oxygen is the body's number one requirement to sustain life, water, food, and physical safety are almost as important. In this chapter, you will learn why water is the second most critical substance for sustaining life. You will also learn about the function of electrolytes and what happens when they are not in balance. In addition, you will be introduced to acid-base balance, acidosis, and alkalosis. Then you will learn about nursing actions to take for patients who have these types of imbalances.

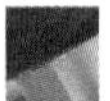

WATER

Water normally accounts for 50% to 70% of the body's total weight and serves as the liquid in which the body's solid components are dissolved. Age affects the percentage of water that comprises total body weight. For example, an adult male's body weight is made up of 60% to 65% water, while for an older adult this is only 50% to 55%. Infants and premature infants have the highest percentage of water in their body weight, with water making up 65% to 80% of their total weight.

Blood is composed of 80% to 83% water. ***Safety: Fluid loss interferes with homeostasis and impairs body functions so much that a person can only survive a few days without water intake.*** The volume of fluid in the body is directly affected by the amount of water ingested and absorbed from the gastrointestinal (GI) tract.

KNOWLEDGE CONNECTION

What percentage of body weight is made up of water in the following age groups: Infants? Adult males? Older adults? What is the most important to survival: water or food?

Distribution of Body Fluids

Body fluids are found in one of two water compartments: the intracellular space or the extracellular space. In healthy patients, approximately two-thirds of body fluids reside inside individual cells. Fluid within the cells is called **intracellular fluid** (ICF). The other one-third of the body's fluid is located outside the cells and is known as **extracellular fluid** (ECF). Box 29.1 shows the distribution of body fluids, with the contents of each water compartment.

Box 29.1

Distribution of Body Fluids

Intracellular Fluids

Two-thirds of the body fluids are found within the cells.

Extracellular Fluids

One-third of body fluids is found outside the cells, primarily in two areas:

- Interstitial space—the areas surrounding and between the cells. This fluid is also called *tissue fluid* or *interstitial fluid.*
- **Intravascular space**—includes the blood vessels and heart, which hold blood; the liquid portion of the blood which surrounds and holds the blood cells is called *plasma.*
- Very small amounts of additional fluids are found in certain body spaces, such as the cerebrospinal fluid around the brain and spinal cord, the fluids within the chambers of the eye, and synovial fluid in joints. These are not significant amounts, however, so they are not considered a part of fluid and electrolyte balance.

Fluid volumes are very closely related to the concentration of sodium chloride, also known as *table salt.* If individuals take in or retain too much sodium chloride, they will also retain excess water. Water will travel back and forth between ICF spaces and ECF spaces, depending on where there is more sodium chloride. One way to think of it is *where sodium goes, water follows.* That is why, after eating a large bag of buttered, salted popcorn, you find yourself thirsty and drinking lots of liquids.

The concentration of certain elements inside of cells is much higher than that outside of cells. The electrolyte potassium and protein molecules are found in much higher concentrations inside of cells than outside of cells, whereas sodium, chloride, and bicarbonate normally occur in higher concentrations outside.

KNOWLEDGE CONNECTION

Which water compartment contains approximately two-thirds of the body's water content? What are the two subdivisions within the extracellular compartment? What follows sodium?

Movement of Body Fluids

Fluids are continually moving across membranes to other compartments in an effort to maintain equilibrium between the compartments. This movement of fluid is controlled by several processes, including osmosis, diffusion, and filtration.

• WORD • BUILDING •

electrolyte: electro – electricity + lyte – untied
acidosis: acid – sour + osis – condition
alkalosis: alkal – alkaline + osis – condition

The tissues that form the blood vessel walls and the cellular membranes are described as *semipermeable.* This means that they allow passage of some substances, but not all substances, through the cell membrane or blood vessel walls.

A *solvent* is generally a liquid in which *solutes*, or solids, are dissolved to make a *solution*. The number of solutes present in the solvent determines the fluid's *osmolality* or concentration. When a difference in concentration exists in the fluid on two sides of a semipermeable membrane, the body attempts to balance those differences. Table 29.1 defines and describes the three types of movement of body fluids and gives examples of each.

KNOWLEDGE CONNECTION

Which does osmosis move: water or solute? Which does diffusion most commonly move: water or solutes? Compare the differences between osmosis and diffusion.

Movement of Absorbed Water From the Gastrointestinal Tract

When you drink a glass of water, the water you swallow passes through the esophagus and into the stomach. The bloodstream absorbs some of the water from the stomach and small intestine, but most of the water is not absorbed until it reaches the large intestine. Approximately 80% of the volume of water entering the first section of the large intestine, the *cecum,* is absorbed there. The water molecules must cross through the intestinal wall and capillary wall to enter the bloodstream.

Once the water has entered the bloodstream, it becomes part of the plasma and is circulated throughout the blood vessels until it reaches the capillary beds. This is where semipermeable capillary walls allow fluid, nutrients, and oxygen to move into the interstitial spaces. Carbon dioxide and other waste products are diffused from the interstitial fluid across the capillary wall into the bloodstream to be carried away and removed from the body. Waste products from the cells travel via the interstitial fluid into the bloodstream and on to the kidneys, where the waste products are filtered out into the urine.

The goal of all the fluid movement back and forth between water compartments is to maintain constant *relative* proportions of fluid and solutes.

Functions of Water in the Body

Water is required by the body for various functions, including the following:

- **Maintaining temperature:** Water helps to maintain body temperature, whether warm or cold. Because it takes longer for the temperature of liquid to change than it does for solid matter, the body's water protects from extreme changes. For example, when you step out of a warm house into a blizzard, your body fluids help to preserve heat. When the body is overheating, evaporation of fluid from sweat and from breathing will keep the body cool. However, water can only help the body to preserve heat for a certain length of time. When the body becomes dehydrated after large amounts of sweat are lost and not replenished, water is no longer available to decrease the body's temperature. ***Safety: When patients are dehydrated, they can lose the ability to regulate body temperature.***
- **Transporting electrolytes, minerals, vitamins, and waste products:** Water transports **electrolytes** such as sodium and potassium; an electrolyte is a salt that transmits electrical impulses when it is dissolved in water. Water also transports minerals such as zinc and copper and vitamins such as vitamin C and the B-complex vitamins to all the individual cells throughout the body. Water also transports waste products from the cells to the blood so that they can be eliminated in the urine.
- **Protecting the brain and spinal cord:** Water, as a component of spinal fluid, acts as a cushion for organs such as the brain and spinal cord, protecting these organs from damage from outside forces.
- **Lubricating the joints and digestive tract:** Water helps to lubricate joints such as the knees and elbows, reducing friction and allowing for smoother movement. It also provides for the smooth passage of food through the digestive tract, from the mouth through the large intestine.

KNOWLEDGE CONNECTION

Explain four functions of water in the body.

Regulation of Body Fluids

The most important factor determining water intake is thirst. The hypothalamus in the brain receives information from *osmoreceptors,* which detect when there is an elevated concentration of solutes in the blood. Increased concentration of the plasma (osmolality) results in low fluid levels in the blood. This stimulates thirst. However, if there is too much fluid or if there is a problem with the osmoreceptors, the hypothalamus in the brain does not cause you to be thirsty.

Water Intake

As you learned in Chapter 23, the average adult needs to consume somewhere between 1,440 and 1,920 mL of water per day, roughly between 1.5 to 2 liters each day. Some individuals may need more water intake, such as pregnant or nursing women, those individuals who work or exert in extremely hot environments, and athletes.

• WORD • BUILDING •

solvent: solvens – dissolving
solute: solutus – dissolved
osmoreceptor: osmo – impulse + receptor – receiver osmosis: osmo – impulse + osis – condition

Table 29.1
Movement of Body Fluids

Type of Movement and Definition	*Real-Life Example*	*How It Works in the Body*
Osmosis: when *water* moves through a semipermeable membrane to equalize concentration of solutes on each side of the membrane. 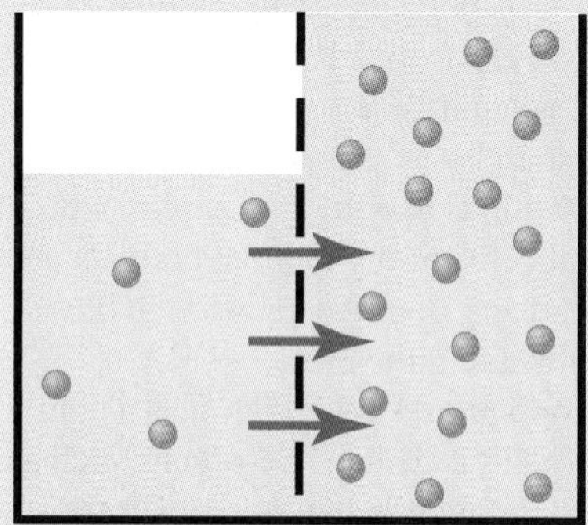 From Wilkinson JM, Treas LS. *Fundamentals of Nursing: Theory, Concepts & Applications.* Vol. 1. 3rd ed. Philadelphia, PA: FA Davis; 2016.	A raisin contains concentrated sugars and other solutes. When you soak it in a tablespoon of water, the raisin eventually plumps up as water crosses its skin (semi-permeable membrane) to equalize fluid in each side.	If a patient is given an IV solution that is more concentrated than plasma, some of the water in the red blood cells will leave the cells and cross the cell membrane to equalize the concentration in the fluid on the outside of the cell. This causes the red blood cell to shrivel, which is called *crenation*.
Diffusion: when *molecules* move from an area of higher concentration to an area of lower concentration to equalize the amount throughout the area or space. 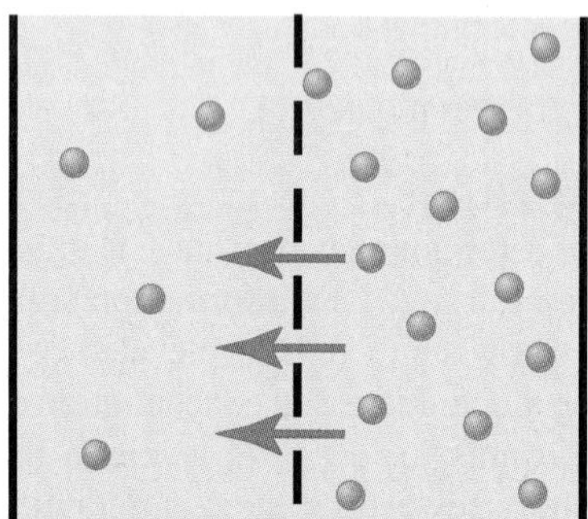 From Wilkinson JM, Treas LS. *Fundamentals of Nursing: Theory, Concepts & Applications.* Vol. 1. 3rd ed. Philadelphia, PA: FA Davis; 2016.	If you spray air freshener in one corner of a room, the molecules will *diffuse* from that area (higher concentration) to the rest of the room (lower concentration) until equalized; then it can be smelled throughout the room.	In the lungs, the blood in the capillaries around the air sacs contains higher levels of carbon dioxide and lower levels of oxygen than room air. When you inhale, room air that is higher in oxygen and lower in carbon dioxide is drawn into the air sacs. Oxygen molecules move into the capillaries (higher to lower concentration), and carbon dioxide molecules move out of the capillaries into the air sacs to be exhaled (higher to lower concentration).
Filtration: when solids are separated from liquids or gases by a barrier that only the liquids and very fine solutes can pass through.	A coffee filter holds ground-up coffee beans. Hot water passes through the beans and the filter. Tiny particles of the beans stay in the water, giving it flavor and color and turning it into coffee, but the grounds are separated out by the paper filter.	The liver filters blood to remove dissolved substances such as medications, over-the-counter drugs, alcohol, caffeine, and toxins from the blood.

Body Composition

Fatty tissue contains less water than muscular tissue, so body composition and size influence the volume of water in the body. Men, who typically are more muscular than women, tend to have a higher percentage of body weight due to water. Obese individuals and the elderly have a lower percentage of body fluid due to lack of muscle mass.

Hormonal Regulation

Several hormones help to maintain fluid levels in the body and to produce an appropriate volume of urine output. Antidiuretic hormone (ADH) and aldosterone both work on the kidneys to decrease urine production and increase body fluid level. Atrial natriuretic factor (ANF) causes the kidneys to excrete more urine to decrease the body fluid level. Box 29.2 explains how each of these hormones works to regulate fluids and electrolytes.

Normal Fluid Losses

The most obvious ways in which the body loses fluid is through elimination of urine and feces. Fluid lost through urine is controlled by ADH, aldosterone, and insensible fluid loss. *Insensible fluid loss* is that which cannot be directly measured, such as fluid lost during respiration and perspiration. Normal fluid loss for healthy patients varies from about 1 to 3 L per day, depending on fluid intake. Table 29.2 notes sources of fluid losses and gains.

Box 29.2

Hormones That Regulate Fluids and Electrolytes

Antidiuretic Hormone (Vasopressin)

When the blood becomes more concentrated, with less water than usual, the hypothalamus in the brain stimulates the release of **antidiuretic hormone.** This hormone acts on the kidneys, causing them to increase water reabsorption, which makes the urine more concentrated.

Aldosterone

When the blood volume becomes low, blood pressure falls. This is detected by the baroreceptors located in various blood vessels and the heart. These receptors send a message that causes the kidneys to release *renin.* Through a number of interactions (Fig. 29.1), aldosterone is then produced by the adrenal cortex. **Aldoseterone** regulates fluids and electrolytes by telling the kidneys to reabsorb more sodium and excrete more potassium. This causes more water to be reabsorbed by the kidneys and circulate in the blood. The principle of *water follows sodium* is at work here. When more water is reabsorbed, the blood volume increases and the blood pressure goes up.

Atrial Natriuretic Factor

When there is excessive blood volume, it causes the blood pressure to go up. The hormone atrial natriuretic factor is then produced. It causes the production of renin to be suppressed, which interferes with the production of aldosterone. Now the kidneys will excrete *more* sodium and therefore more water. This increases the urinary output and lowers blood pressure.

KNOWLEDGE CONNECTION

Which electrolyte does water follow? What are the effects of ADH on the body's fluid level? What effect does aldosterone have on the body's fluid level? How does ANF affect the production of urine? What will this do to the body's fluid level?

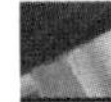

FLUID VOLUME IMBALANCES

Fluid volume imbalances involve not just gaining or losing fluid, but also losing electrolytes or having them become more concentrated. As a nurse, you will need to be very aware of your patients' fluid volume and electrolyte status throughout their care.

Fluid Volume Deficit

A true **fluid volume deficit** (hypovolemia) results when the patient loses both fluid and the electrolytes contained in that fluid. The most common cause for this is the loss of a large amount of blood through hemorrhage. When a patient loses only fluids, the remaining electrolytes become more concentrated. This is called **dehydration.** Hemorrhage and dehydration require different treatments.

Fluid volume deficit is caused by prolonged insufficient fluid intake or by loss of fluid. Patients with fluid loss may not always experience thirst, especially the elderly and patients with brain injuries. ***Safety: Young children should be offered fluids often. They can develop a fluid volume deficit if they are without fluids for a prolonged time.*** Extreme nausea, even though there is no vomiting, may prevent someone from drinking fluids for several days.

Another cause of fluid deficit is abnormal fluid losses. Losses can be due to bleeding, prolonged tachypnea, excessive sweating, fever, diarrhea, vomiting, or excessive urination due to diuresis. Severe depletion of fluid volume also occurs in hot climates or with extreme amounts of exertion or exercise. Fluid volume deficit can occur in varying degrees of seriousness, ranging from mild to life-threatening. (For signs and symptoms of fluid volume deficit, see Box 29.3.)

KNOWLEDGE CONNECTION

What is the difference between hypovolemia and dehydration? What causes fluid volume deficits?

• WORD • BUILDING •

dehydration: de – remove + hydr – water + ation – action

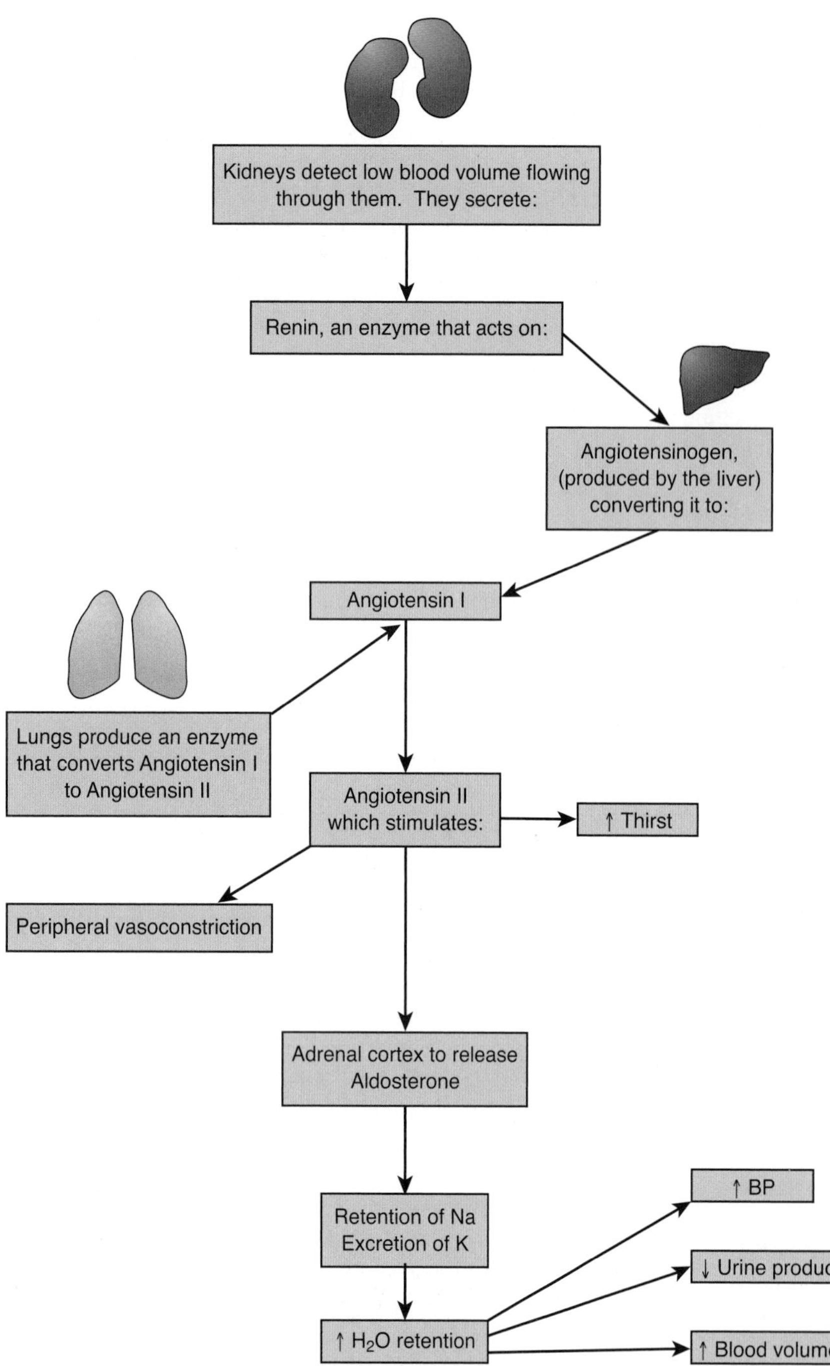

FIGURE 29.1 Renin-angiotensin-aldosterone system.

Elder Care Connection

Fluid Intake in Elders

Seniors, whether they live independently, with caregivers at home, or in a long-term care facility, are at high risk for dehydration. Many seniors experience a declining sense of thirst due to changes in the brain. When this occurs, either the senior or the caregiver will need to ensure that the senior is drinking water even when he or she does not feel thirsty. The recommended amount of fluid intake per day is about 1,800 mL, or 2 quarts. Alcohol and dietary supplements are less hydrating than water. Some liquids such as coffee and tea can also have a diuretic effect.

Elderly patients with cardiac or kidney disease, however, may be placed on a fluid restriction. These seniors will need to monitor how much fluid their physician or nurse practitioner has prescribed for them to take daily, monitor their daily weight, and watch for increased or decreased amounts of urine production.

Table 29.2

Estimates of Adult Fluid Loss and Gain Over 24 Hours

Loss or Gain	*Fluid Source*	*Volume*
Loss	Urine	1,200–2,100 mL
	Diuretics can cause loss up to:	*6,000 mL*
Loss	Insensible respirations	200–300 mL
Loss	Gastrointestinal tract	100–200 mL
	Vomiting can cause loss up to:	*6,000 mL*
Loss	Insensible perspiration	400–600 mL
	If environmental temperatures are high enough, can cause loss up to:	*1,000 mL/hr*
Gain	Water production through metabolism of ingested food	100–300 mL
Gain	Oral liquids	1,000–2,000 mL
Gain	Water in food	800–900 mL

Nursing Actions for Fluid Volume Deficit

When you care for patients with fluid volume deficit, whether due to hemorrhage or dehydration, you will take similar nursing actions. These include the following:

- Replace fluids orally and by IV as ordered by the health-care provider.
- Monitor electrolyte levels closely.
- Administer antiemetic medications ordered for nausea or vomiting, or antidiarrheal medication for loose stools.
- Monitor vital signs for low blood pressure, elevated pulse rate, and elevated temperature.
- Measure and monitor intake and output (I&O) for balance. Normally, the output total should be equal to or within 300 to 500 mL of the total intake. If a patient has a fluid volume deficit, urinary output *initially* will be less than the intake but should gradually increase as the patient becomes more hydrated. ***Safety: Persistent urinary output below 30 mL per hour may indicate renal failure.***
- Assess each patient to be sure that he or she has voided at least every 8 hours and notify the health-care provider if this does not occur.
- Administer IV fluids at the rate ordered. ***Safety: Even though a patient who has fluid volume deficit needs fluids, rapid infusion of IV fluids may cause fluid volume excess, or overload.***
- Assess the patient's oral mucous membranes for dryness and provide mouth care as needed.

Box 29.3

Signs and Symptoms of Fluid Volume Deficit

Be alert for signs and symptoms that may indicate the presence of or risk for developing fluid volume deficit. Be especially vigilant when monitoring infants, children, and older adults, who are at increased risk for fluid imbalances.

- Patient report of little or no fluid intake or urine output
- Patient report of frequent vomiting or diarrhea
- Flushed, pale, hot, dry skin with nonelastic turgor (nonelastic turgor is a very late sign)
- Complaints of thirst or nausea
- Dry, cracked tongue and lips
- Elevated heart rate
- Weak pulse
- Fever
- Low blood pressure
- In newborns, sunken or depressed fontanels
- Decreased level of consciousness (severe fluid volume deficit)
- Confusion (severe fluid volume deficit)

KNOWLEDGE CONNECTION

What assessments should be made for possible or actual fluid volume deficit? What nursing actions will you take for patients with fluid volume deficit? What is the danger of infusing IV fluids too rapidly?

Fluid Volume Excess

Most fluid volume excess (hypervolemia) is caused by retention of sodium and water in extracellular fluid. Causes of this include increased intake of dietary sodium; administration of IV fluids containing sodium; or retention of sodium or fluid as a result of medication or kidney, heart, or liver disease. Fluid volume excess causes decreased urinary output and excess fluid in the intravascular and interstitial spaces.

Infants, small children, frail elders, and patients with heart failure or renal failure are more susceptible to fluid overload than average adult patients. Even when fluids are ordered orally or intravenously, it can place the patient in fluid overload. (See Box 29.4 for the signs and symptoms of fluid overload.)

KNOWLEDGE CONNECTION

What is generally the cause of a fluid volume excess? What type of patients are considered more susceptible to fluid overload problems?

Box 29.4

Signs and Symptoms of Fluid Volume Excess

Signs and symptoms of fluid volume excess may appear suddenly. Assess the potential of each patient receiving IV fluids for risk of fluid volume excess.

- Increased respiratory rate, shortness of breath with exertion, or labored respirations
- Sudden onset of coughing
- Jugular vein distention
- Increased blood pressure or pulse pressure
- Full, bounding pulse
- Edema of extremities or dependent areas, such as feet, ankles, lower legs, and sacrum while in bed
- Auscultation of crackles or wheezes in the lungs and muffled or distant heart sounds
- Weight gain
- Increased urine production
- Pink or frothy sputum
- Decreased oxygen saturation level
- Anxiety or fear that is unexplainable by the patient

Nursing Actions for Fluid Volume Excess

When you care for patients with fluid volume excess, whether due to too much sodium, heart failure, or kidney failure, you will perform these nursing actions:

- Carefully monitor I&O for fluid volume excess (intake greater than output).
- Administer ordered diuretics and monitor for effectiveness.
- Assess daily weights at the same time of the day, preferably before breakfast, using the same scales and with the patient wearing the same type of garment.
- Monitor meal trays to ensure there are no extra salt packets or high-sodium foods because the patient will likely be on a low-sodium diet.
- If the patient is on a fluid restriction, determine the volume of fluid allowed on each shift and monitor it closely. Post the volume of fluids allowed for each shift above the patient's bed or on a marker board to serve as a reminder for patient, family, and staff. Collaborate with the dietary service to limit fluids sent on meal trays. Provide patient and family teaching to ensure their understanding and cooperation.
- Monitor vital signs for elevated blood pressure, increased pulse rate, bounding pulse, elevated temperature, and pulse oximetry every 4 hours.
- Auscultate breath sounds and heart sounds at least every 4 hours.
- Check dependent body sites for edema. Dependent sites are those that are hanging down or where blood can pool. When the patient is sitting in a chair, the lower legs, feet and ankles are in a dependent position. When the patient is lying on his or her back in bed, the sacral area is in a dependent position.
- Monitor urine output every 2 to 3 hours, or even every hour if inadequate urine excretion is suspected. Administer diuretics as ordered by the health-care provider. ***Safety: Some diuretics such as furosemide, a loop diuretic, are known to deplete the serum level of potassium, so check those levels often.***

KNOWLEDGE CONNECTION

What nursing actions would be appropriate for fluid volume excess?

Patient Teaching Connection

Diuretics and Potassium Levels

Many patients are prescribed diuretics to assist with elimination of excess fluids. Patients often call these drugs their "water pills." Some types of diuretics, such as loop diuretics, cause the patient to lose potassium and sodium. Furosemide (Lasix), a common loop diuretic, can also cause magnesium and calcium losses. Thiazide diuretics, such as hydrochlorothiazide, also cause potassium loss. Because hypokalemia is common with these types of diuretics, the health-care provider may also prescribe extra dietary potassium or potassium supplements. According to the Institute of Medicine, adequate intake of potassium for adults is 4,700 mg per day. Most patients will be prescribed a supplement dose of 20 *milliequivalents* (mEq), which equals about 1,500 mg per day. The patient must then obtain the rest of their potassium intake through their diet.

Teach your patients taking diuretics to follow up for their blood work as ordered. It is very important that electrolyte levels be checked regularly. Encourage patients to eat foods high in potassium, such as bananas, which provide about 500 mg of potassium each. Other foods high in potassium include yellow and orange fruits such as oranges and apricots, avocados, and sweet potatoes; other good sources include baked potatoes, yogurt, white beans, and halibut.

It is also very important to know if your patient is on a potassium-sparing diuretic, such as spironolactone. These types of diuretics do not cause potassium loss in the kidneys. Therefore, these patients should avoid excessive potassium in their diets and supplements containing potassium because of the risk of hyperkalemia.

• WORD • BUILDING •

hyperkalemia: hyper – excessive + kal – potassium + em – blood + ia – condition

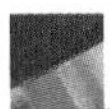

ELECTROLYTES

Electrolytes are chemical substances that, when dissolved in water, release either their positive or their negative electrically charged particles, called *ions*. These ions are capable of conducting electrical current. An *anion* is a negatively charged ion such as chloride (Cl^-). A *cation* is a positively charged ion such as sodium (Na^+) or potassium (K^+).

Electrolytes play various roles, including helping to transmit electrical impulses through nerve and muscle fibers and assisting to maintain balance between the ICF and ECF compartments. Table 29.3 provides the normal blood ranges, functions, and nutritional sources of the various electrolytes.

Table 29.3
Normal Blood Ranges, Functions, and Nutritional Sources of Electrolytes

Electrolyte, Cation, or Anion	*Normal Blood Range*	*Functions*	*Sources for Intake*
Sodium (Na^+) Cation	135–145 mEq/L Changes in direct proportion to Cl^-	Controls fluid osmolality and volume of blood Stimulates conduction of electrical impulses along nerves Works with calcium to regulate muscle contraction	Salt: Most individuals obtain 90%–94% from packaged, processed foods, including bacon, ham, canned vegetables, soy sauce, steak sauces, other sauces, salad dressings, processed cheeses, sandwich meats, salty snacks such as chips, jerky, pretzels, canned soups, broths Adding table salt to prepared foods
Chloride (Cl^-) Anion	97–107 mEq/L Changes in direct proportion to sodium Has inverse relationship with bicarbonate	Assists sodium in regulating fluid osmolality and volume Important for acid-base balance Production of gastric HCl	High-sodium–content foods listed above Lettuce, tomatoes, celery, olives, seaweed
Potassium (K^+) Cation	3.5–5.3 mEq/L	98% in ICF helps regulate fluid balance 2% in ECF is important for neuromuscular functions, *especially for the heart's contractility and rhythm*	Dried fruits, tomatoes, potatoes, spinach and other leafy greens, oranges, bananas, cantaloupe, red meat, chicken, fish, nuts, soy products
Magnesium (Mg^{2+}) Cation	1.6 –2.2 mg/dL	Assists neuromuscular function; dilation of arteries and arterioles; enzyme function; carbohydrate and protein metabolism	Leafy green vegetables, whole grains, beans, fish (halibut), almonds, soybeans
Calcium (Ca^{2+}) Cation	*Total Ca^{2+}*: 8.2–10.2 mg/dL *Ionized Ca^{2+}*: 4.64–5.28mg/dL	Strengthen skeletal bones and teeth *Ionized Ca^{2+}:* stimulates conduction of electrical impulses via nerves, which controls muscle contraction and relaxation, includes heart muscle Initiates enzyme action Cellular membrane permeability	Dairy products, green vegetables, shellfish, salmon, dried beans
Phosphorus (PO_4^{3-}) Anion	2.5–4.5 mg/dL May be higher in children	Vital for all tissues; muscle and red blood cell functions; metabolism of fat, protein, carbohydrates; manufacturing ATP energy source	Meats, fish, egg yolks, dairy products, nuts, beans, legumes, whole grains, soft drinks

Sodium

Sodium is the primary electrolyte involved in determining extracellular fluid volumes and controls fluid distribution throughout the body because *water follows sodium*. Sodium stimulates conduction of electrical impulses needed for skeletal and heart muscles to contract and relax.

In the blood, sodium is measured in milliequivalents; in food, it is measured in milligrams. ***Safety: The American Heart Association recommends that healthy adults consume no more than 2,300 mg per day.*** This is about 1 teaspoon of table salt. ***Safety: For people with hypertension, those over the age of 40, and African Americans, it is recommended that they consume no more than 1,500 mg per day because of their risk factors for cardiovascular disease.***

Most individuals think of sodium intake as "only that salt they have sprinkled on their food." However, a significant amount of sodium can be found in canned and processed foods. Even some prescription and over-the-counter medications contain sodium in the form of sodium bicarbonate. (See Table 29.3 for nutritional sources of sodium.)

Too much sodium or too little sodium can cause a variety of problems. See Table 29.4 for the signs and symptoms of both *hyponatremia* (too little sodium in the blood) and *hypernatremia* (too much sodium in the blood.)

Nursing Actions for Sodium Imbalance

Nursing actions for patients with hyponatremia include the following:

- Administering additional sodium, either orally, via nasogastric tube, or intravenously as ordered by the health-care provider. Examples of IV fluids are 0.9% sodium chloride (normal saline) and lactated Ringer's solution.
- Assessing vital signs for hypotension, increased pulse rate, or decreasing pulse volume.
- Monitoring I&O and evaluating balance.
- If hyponatremia is severe, assessing the patient for signs and symptoms of increased intracranial pressure (Box 29.5).

Table 29.4
Electrolyte Imbalances

Electrolyte Imbalance and Name	*Signs and Symptom*	*Causative Factors*
Sodium		
Deficit: hyponatremia	Anorexia, nausea, vomiting, headache, lethargy, muscle weakness or twitching, nonelastic skin turgor, tremors, seizures, swelling of optic nerve	GI suctioning, vomiting, diarrhea, ↑ blood sugar, congestive heart failure, renal disease, adrenal insufficiency, oxytocin, excessive infusion of D5W IV fluid, disease known as SIADH (syndrome of inappropriate antidiuretic hormone), administration of more than one tap-water enema, excessive diaphoresis
Excess: hypernatremia	Thirst, ↑ T, sticky mucous membranes, dry mouth, flushed skin, lethargy, restlessness, oliguria, ↑ irritability, hallucinations, seizures; pulmonary edema	Diabetes insipidus; heat stroke; watery diarrhea; ingestion of excessive corticosteroids, sodium chloride, or bicarbonate
Chloride		
Deficit: hypochloremia	Signs of hypokalemia and metabolic alkalosis: ↑ muscle excitability, tetany, ↓ R, shallow R, agitation, irritability, seizures, coma	↓ intake of Cl^- or Na^+ such as sodium-restricted diet; potassium deficiency, excessive diaphoresis, diarrhea, vomiting, diuretics, gastric suctioning, congestive heart failure, IV fluids without Cl^-, Addison's disease, metabolic alkalosis
Excess: hyperchloremia	Signs of metabolic acidosis, hyperkalemia, and hypernatremia: ↑ R rate and depth, dyspnea, ↑ P, ↓ cardiac output, arrhythmias, weakness, severe edema, ↓ LOC and coma	↑ Na^+ serum level, respiratory alkalosis, hyperparathyroidism, severe diarrhea, sodium retention caused by head trauma and ↑ intracranial pressure, renal failure, salicylate overdose, corticosteroid use, diuretic use, dehydration, metabolic acidosis

Table 29.4
Electrolyte Imbalances—cont'd

Electrolyte Imbalance and Name	*Signs and Symptom*	*Causative Factors*
Potassium ***Deficit:*** hypokalemia	Weak, rapid, or irregular P, ↓ BP, anorexia, nausea, vomiting, ↓ deep tendon reflexes, fatigue, muscular weakness and cramps, numbness, abdominal distention, ↓ peristalsis, ileus; may complain of seeing yellow haloes around objects if hypokalemia is caused by digoxin toxicity	Diarrhea; gastric suctioning; vomiting; bulimia; starvation; diuresis due to osmotic diuretics; digoxin toxicity; administration of carbenicillin, corticosteroids, and amphotericin B
Excess: hyperkalemia	Bradycardia and other arrhythmias, nausea, intestinal cramping, diarrhea, anxiety, muscle weakness, numbness or prickly sensations, flaccid paralysis	Renal failure, ketoacidosis, large burns, excessive use of K^+-sparing diuretics, too-rapid IV administration of K^+, severe dehydration ***Safety: Both severe deficit or excess can result in life-threatening arrhythmias.***
Magnesium ***Deficit:*** hypomagnesemia	Vomiting, anorexia, insomnia, arrhythmias, mood swings and hyperirritability, dizziness, ↑ neuromuscular irritability, muscle weakness and tremors, positive Chvostek's and Trousseau's signs	Starvation, malabsorption disorders, ketoacidosis, alcoholism and alcohol withdrawal, administration of gentamicin, hyperparathyroidism, vomiting
Excess: hypermagnesemia	↓ BP, ↑ P, ↓ R, hypoactive reflexes, muscle weakness and paralysis, drowsiness, lethargy, flushing, diaphoresis, cardiac arrest, death	Late renal failure, adrenal insufficiency, excessive administration of IV Mg^{2+} or oral antacids
Calcium ***Deficit:*** hypocalcemia	Muscle cramps and tremors; tetany; ↓ BP; tingling or numbness of fingers, toes, around the mouth; bronchospasm; carpopedal spasms; ↑ deep tendon reflexes; prolonged QT interval on EKG; positive Chvostek's and Trousseau's signs	Inadequate vitamin D consumption, malabsorption disorders, pancreatitis, peritonitis, alkalosis, hypothyroidism or hypoparathyroidism
Excess: hypercalcemia	Severe constipation, anorexia, nausea, vomiting, polydipsia, lethargy, fatigue, headache, polyuria, ↓ deep tendon reflexes, muscular weakness, bone fractures without trauma, confusion, slurred speech, psychosis, ileus development	Prolonged bedrest, excessive ingestion of calcium or vitamin D supplements, excessive serum level of digitalis, cancer, metabolic acidosis
Phosphorus ***Deficit:*** hypophosphatemia	Muscle weakness, bone pain, paresthesia of extremities and around the mouth, stuttering, chest pain, confusion, irregular P, ↑ susceptibility to infection, respiratory failure	↓ K^+ or ↓ Mg^{2+} serum level, vomiting, diarrhea, hyperventilation, burns, hyperparathyroidism, bone disease, diabetic ketoacidosis, alcoholism and alcohol withdrawal, bowel disorders, poor dietary intake
Excess: hyperphosphatemia	↑ P, tetany, anorexia, nausea, tingling of fingers and toes, irritability, carpopedal spasms, ↑ deep tendon reflexes, muscle twitching, tetany, seizures, ↓ cardiac output, coma	Renal failure, excessive intake of vitamin D or phosphorus, fluid volume depletion, conditions causing breakdown of large amounts of tissue

Box 29.5

Signs and Symptoms of Increased Intracranial Pressure

The earlier the signs and symptoms are detected, the better the patient's chance of escaping brain damage and permanent neurological deficits. Observe for even subtle changes in level of consciousness (LOC).

Early Sign

- Changes in LOC*

Late Signs

- Rising systolic blood pressure to hypertensive levels†
- Widening pulse pressure†
- Decreasing pulse rate to bradycardia†
- Pupillary changes
- Impaired body temperature control by the hypothalamus

* Decreases in LOC may be very subtle, such as decreased attentiveness or mild drowsiness, or obvious, such as profound unresponsiveness. Changes in LOC are also exhibited as excitement, ranging from subtle signs of increasing nervousness, anxiety, or agitation to strong unexplained anger or outbursts and erratic body movements.

†When seen together, these three signs are known as Cushing's triad.

Nursing actions for patients with hypernatremia include the following:

- Monitoring for elevated blood pressure and bounding pulse.
- Teaching patients to monitor their dietary sodium intake in an effort to prevent future problems. (See Table 29.3 for a list of foods high in sodium.)

Potassium

Potassium (K^+) is represented by the letter "K" because of its ancient name, Kalium. It is the most abundant cation in the intracellular fluid.

Although 3.5 to 5.3 mEq/L is considered to be the normal serum range for potassium, some health-care providers prefer to keep the serum potassium above 4.0 mEq/L in patients with heart problems to reduce risk of arrhythmias. The Institute of Medicine recommends a dietary intake of 4.7 g of potassium per day to help decrease long-term health problems (see Table 29.3).

Hypokalemia is a potassium level that is below the normal range, and *hyperkalemia* is an elevated level. ***Safety: Both too low and too high levels of potassium levels can affect the heart rhythm and cause life-threatening arrhythmias.*** (See Table 29.4 for further information regarding potassium imbalances.)

Nursing Actions for Potassium Imbalances

When caring for patients with real or potential potassium imbalances, it is critical for you to monitor them closely. When you care for patients with a potassium imbalance, you must be careful to prevent correcting the situation too much one way or the other.

Nursing actions for patients with hypokalemia include the following:

- Administering supplemental potassium chloride (KCl) as ordered in oral tablets, liquids, powders, or IV formulations. If the patient routinely takes certain diuretics, be certain to administer potassium as ordered by the health-care provider to prevent hypokalemia (see the Patient Teaching Connection feature).
- ***Safety: If the patient has less than 30 mL per hour of urinary output, hold all oral potassium supplements and check IV fluids for added potassium. Notify the health-care provider before administering potassium since doing so when urine output is very low could lead to kidney damage.***
- Monitoring the serum lab reports of all your patients, being especially mindful of the serum potassium levels if the patient
  - Is vomiting or having diarrhea,
  - Has a nasogastric tube to suction, or
  - Is taking loop diuretics.
- ***Safety: KCl is never administered by IV push or intramuscularly. Because of a high potential for death associated with IV potassium, most institutions require that it be mixed into a diluted IV solution by the pharmacy and then be double-checked by the nurse before it is administered to the patient.***
- Administering IVs containing KCL over several hours at the preferred rate of 10 to 20 mEq per hour. The infusion rate should never exceed 40 to 60 mEq per hour.
- ***Safety: When KCl is added to a 1,000-mL bag of solution, the KCl will concentrate at the bottom of the bag of IV solution. Agitate the solution well before infusing.***

Nursing actions for hyperkalemia include the following:

- Administering emergency medications for severe hyperkalemia, which may include sodium polystyrene sulfonate (Kayexelate) given via enema to bind with potassium, or the administration of IV insulin to push potassium back into the cells and lower serum levels.
- Restricting dietary intake of potassium-rich foods (see Table 29.3 for foods high in potassium).
- Monitoring the serum lab reports of all your patients, being especially mindful of the serum potassium levels if the patient is suffering from malnutrition or dehydration or has renal disease.

Real-World Connection

The Dangers of Potassium Chloride

Potassium chloride is a dangerous drug—so dangerous, in fact, that in some states it is given by injection to prisoners sentenced to die—which is why it is so very important to be careful when administering it to a patient. The following story illustrates just how careful you should be:

A student nurse on a medical-surgical clinical was administering medications. One of the patients was scheduled to receive a daily dose of potassium chloride (KCl) via the IV route. After the student read the order, she interpreted the order to mean IV push, which means to inject the drug directly into the IV line over a couple of minutes, rather than to dilute the KCl in a 1,000-mL bag of IV solution and infuse it over several hours. The student administered the KCl via direct IV push. The concentrated dose of KCl interrupted the electrical conduction in the patient's heart. The patient arrested and died.

This tragic but true event could have been prevented by using basic safety measures. Always make certain you are familiar with any medication you are going to administer no matter what it is—over-the-counter or prescription, narcotic or vitamin supplement, or electrolyte. If you are not familiar with the specific medication, always look it up in your drug reference book. ***Safety: When administering an electrolyte in less than 1,000 mL of fluid via the IV route, a second nurse should be asked to double-check and confirm the prepared medication, route, and rate before administration.***

Calcium

Calcium (Ca^{2+}) is the most common mineral in our bodies; 99% of it is combined with phosphorus and located in the bones and teeth, with the remaining 1% located outside the skeletal system in the blood. This 1%, known as the *total serum calcium level,* easily and rapidly exchanges back and forth between the blood and bone.

Ionized calcium, which is available for the body's use, stimulates the transmission of electrical impulses along nerve pathways, including the electrical conduction pathways of the heart that control contraction and relaxation of the heart. (See Table 29.3 for more information about calcium.)

Vitamin D is required for absorption of calcium from the GI tract. They are often combined in supplements for better absorption.

Hypocalcemia is defined as having lower-than-normal serum calcium. It is common with diseases that cause poor digestive absorption, such as anorexia or inflammatory bowel disease. Chronic low calcium levels can cause loss of bone and high blood pressure. (See Box 29.6 for information about osteoporosis, which is due to calcium moving from the bone to the blood.) *Hypercalcemia* is the term for too much calcium in the blood, which can cause a variety of conditions. (See Table 29.4 for more information about calcium imbalances.)

Nursing Actions for Calcium Imbalances

Nursing actions for hypocalcemia include the following:

- Administering oral calcium tablets or IV calcium along with vitamin D as ordered by the health-care provider for hypocalcemia. ***Safety: IV infusion of calcium can cause bradycardia and death if administered too rapidly. Use an infusion pump and assess the IV site and rate of infusion every 30 to 60 minutes.***

Box 29.6

Osteoporosis and Calcium Levels

A disease known as *osteoporosis* causes a higher level of calcium resorption than the level being deposited in the bones. *Resorption* is the process of removing calcium from the bones and absorbing it back into the bloodstream. The higher level of resorption leaves the bone structure weakened, with tiny holes or gaps within the bone, giving it a honeycomb appearance. Because of their weakened structure, the affected bones are easily fractured, sometimes without a trauma or fall.

For example, a patient may present for treatment reporting that he or she fell. Upon examination, a femur fracture is identified. Your first thought may be that the fall caused the fracture, which is normally the case. However, a patient with severe osteoporosis may experience a fracture without trauma, which then causes the individual to fall because the broken bone is no longer able to bear the person's weight. It is important to remember that even though a patient has a healthy serum calcium level, he or she may have a severe deficit of calcium in the bones. Bone density tests help detect this situation early.

- Monitoring the patient with hypocalcemia for muscle twitching, tetany (severe muscle spasms), and ECG changes.
- Assessing for spasms of the facial muscles and the arms and legs, as well as tingling around the mouth or tips of the fingers. The patient may become disoriented and confused.
- Being aware that patients suffering from hypocalcemia may also present with Trousseau's sign (Fig. 29.2) and Chvostek's sign (Fig. 29.3).

Nursing actions for hypercalcemia include the following:

- Encouraging fluids and monitoring IV infusions, as ordered, to help lower the calcium levels.
- Monitoring the patient for bradycardia, digestive complaints, and visual disturbances if also on digitalis (Lanoxin) because high calcium can cause digitalis toxicity.

Magnesium

Like calcium, magnesium (Mg^{2+}) is also part of the bone structure. About 50% to 60% of the body's magnesium is located within bone cells. It also assists with the work of the

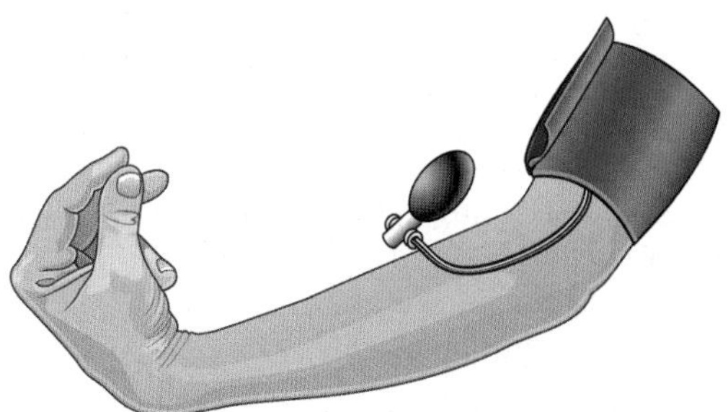

FIGURE 29.2 To check for Trousseau's sign, inflate a sphygmomanometer above systolic pressure. Flexion of the wrist and hand constitutes a positive sign (from Wilkinson JM, Treas LS. *Fundamentals of Nursing: Theory, Concepts & Applications*. Vol. 2. 3rd ed. Philadelphia, PA: FA Davis; 2016).

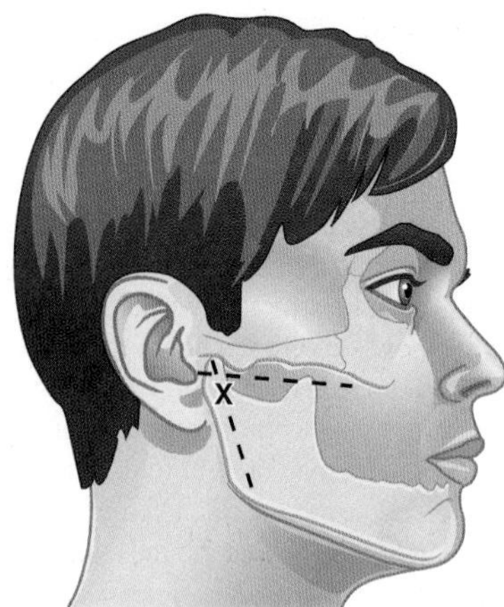

FIGURE 29.3 To check for Chvostek's sign, tap the face in front of the ear and below the zygomatic bone. Facial twitching constitutes a positive sign (from Wilkinson JM, Treas LS. *Fundamentals of Nursing: Theory, Concepts & Applications*. Vol. 2. 3rd ed. Philadelphia, PA: FA Davis; 2016).

heart, muscles, and nerve cells. Magnesium also helps to lower blood pressure by dilating the peripheral blood vessels. Research shows that magnesium can help protect the heart and support the immune system. Magnesium is sometimes used by patients who experience twitching and uncontrolled movements of their legs while trying to sleep. The magnesium works at the neuromuscular junctions, producing somewhat of a *sedative effect,* reducing the twitching of the muscles. (See Table 29.3 for more information about magnesium.)

Hypomagnesemia refers to a blood level of magnesium that is below the normal range. Decreased levels of magnesium can increase nervous system irritability and muscular contractility. Patients with alcoholism frequently develop hypomagnesemia along with other nutritional deficiencies.

A high level of magnesium, known as *hypermagnesemia,* will slow the nervous system responses, including the respiratory rate, and generally depress neuromuscular junctions. (See Table 29.4 for information about magnesium imbalances.)

Nursing Actions for Magnesium Imbalances

When caring for patients with magnesium imbalances, it is important to remember that both deficient and excessive levels of magnesium are closely linked to potassium and calcium imbalance.

Nursing actions for hypomagnesemia include the following:

- Assessing for imbalance in potassium and calcium as well as magnesium; restoring the magnesium level will also require restoring the balance of potassium and calcium
- Administering oral magnesium tablets as ordered for mildly low magnesium
- Monitoring I&O and assessing for fluid imbalances
- Teaching patients which foods are good sources of magnesium, such as nuts (cashews and almonds), seeds (sunflower, pumpkin, and flax), bananas, milk, oatmeal, and broccoli

Nursing actions for hypermagnesemia include the following:

- Monitoring IV calcium, if ordered
- Administering diuretic medications as ordered
- Assisting with scheduling the patient for dialysis if required to lower the magnesium level
- Asking about the patient's use of over-the-counter antacids and laxatives containing magnesium, which could contribute to elevated magnesium levels

Chloride

Chloride (Cl^-) accounts for approximately two-thirds of the body's anions and is commonly bound with sodium or potassium ions.

Chloride is found in interstitial fluid, lymph fluid, sweat, and gastric and pancreatic digestive juices, with lesser amounts in the blood. Chloride combines with hydrogen to form hydrochloric acid in the gastric juices of the stomach, which is used to break down foods. (See Table 29.3 for more information about chloride.)

Chloride is nearly always chemically bonded to another electrolyte in the body. As a result, chloride imbalances are most commonly seen in combination with other electrolyte imbalances. A below-normal serum level of chloride is known as *hypochloremia.*

When the chloride level is above normal levels it is called *hyperchloremia.* (See Table 29.4 for more information about chloride imbalance.)

Nursing Actions for Chloride Imbalances

When you care for patients with chloride imbalances, it will be important for you to follow these nursing actions:

- Encouraging foods high in sodium chloride for hypochloremia. These are listed in Table 29.3.
- Monitoring I&O carefully. If the patient routinely drinks water without electrolytes or drinks bottled water, the health-care provider may restrict the patient from drinking it.
- Measuring fluids lost through vomiting or diarrhea for appropriate replacement.
- Watching for signs of respiratory or neurological depression; high and low levels of chloride can change the acid-base balance of the body and cause serious neurological and respiratory changes.
- Monitoring the patient's I&O and laboratory results because hyperchloremia may be associated with metabolic acidosis.

Phosphorus

Phosphates are ions of the element *phosphorus,* but the two names are generally used interchangeably. Phosphate (PO_4^{3-}) is the primary intracellular anion and is essential to all body tissues, especially red blood cells and muscle cells. Phosphorus is used in energy exchange by cells. It also serves as part of the acid-base buffering system. Similar to magnesium, most of the body's phosphorus is stored in the bones and teeth.

Small amounts are found in nerve tissue and muscle cells. (See Table 29.3 for information about phosphorus.)

When there is a low magnesium level or a high calcium level, you will want to check for a low phosphorus level, known as *hypophosphatemia*. Phosphorus is abundant in the Western diet.

Hyperphosphatemia is the name for excessively high blood levels of phosphorus; few signs or symptoms accompany the elevation. (See Table 29.4 for information about phosphorus imbalances.)

Nursing Actions for Phosphorus Imbalances

When caring for patients with phosphorus imbalance, take the following nursing actions:

- Ask the patient about a history of malnutrition and laxative use.
- Administer oral medications, as ordered, that will bind phosphorus. Patients with chronic kidney disease may have high phosphorus levels.
- Encourage a low-phosphorus diet if ordered by the health-care provider.
- If the patient has hypophosphatemia, encourage dietary changes and administer supplements as ordered. If IV phosphorus is ordered, it must be infused no faster than 10 mEq per hour.

> **KNOWLEDGE CONNECTION**
> Which two electrolytes play a role in muscle contraction and relaxation? Which electrolyte can be depleted by diuretics?

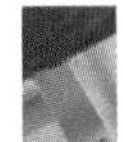

INTRODUCTION TO ACID-BASE BALANCE

Acid-base balance refers to the balance of the acids and alkaline bases of body fluids. A prolonged or extreme imbalance between the two will lead to death. ***Safety: An individual's blood pH must stay within a very narrow range that is slightly alkaline to ensure survival—between 7.35 and 7.45.*** Other body fluids each have a different pH (Fig. 29.4). Box 29.7 briefly explains the pH scale.

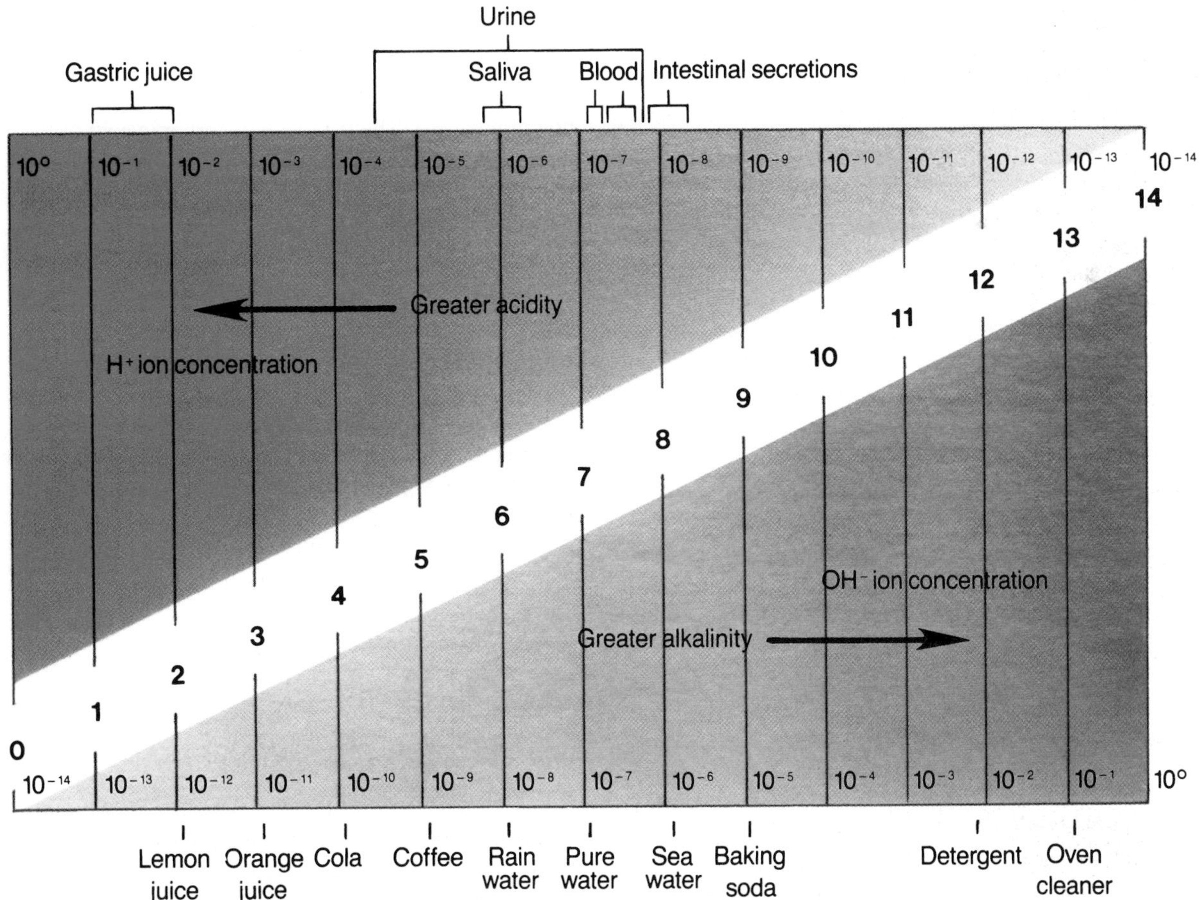

FIGURE 29.4 The pH scale. The neutral pH of 7 shows an equal concentration of H^+ ions and OH^- ions. Note the pH of various common household items indicated along the bottom edge. Then compare their pH to the pH of different body fluids indicated across the top edge (from Scanlon V, Sanders T. *Essentials of Anatomy and Physiology*. 7th ed. Philadelphia, PA: FA Davis; 2015).

KNOWLEDGE CONNECTION

What do the "p" and the "H" in pH stand for? What is the normal range of pH of human blood? Explain how the pH scale works.

Box 29.7

What is pH?

The **pH** scale is used to measure the acidity or alkalinity of a substance. The number on the pH scale corresponds to the "parts of hydrogen" (pH) in the substances. The scale ranges from 0 to 14. The number 7 on the scale is neutral, neither acidic nor alkaline. Pure water has a pH of 7. Substances with a higher concentration of hydrogen ions (H+) have a lower number on the pH scale and are more acid. Substances with a higher concentration of hydroxyl ions (OH^-) have a higher number on the pH scale and are more alkaline (see Fig. 29.4).

Regulation of Acid-Base Balance

Three systems work together in the body to regulate and maintain acid-base balance. Each system does its part to compensate for impairment in the other systems and correct any changes in pH. The following are the three systems:

1. Bicarbonate/carbonic acid buffer system
2. Respiratory system—the lungs control retention and elimination of carbon dioxide (CO_2), an acid
3. Renal system—the kidneys control retention and elimination of hydrogen (H), an acid, and sodium bicarbonate ($NaHCO_3$), a base

Note: Sodium bicarbonate ($NaHCO_3$) is commonly used interchangeably with bicarbonate (HCO_3^-) when discussing blood gases, as you will notice in this chapter.

Bicarbonate Buffer System

Bicarbonate ($HC03^-$) occurs naturally in the body as the main anion in the extracellular fluid. The normal range for bicarbonate is 22 to 26 mEq/L. It is an alkaline substance that helps decrease the acidity of the blood. Carbonic acid is formed when carbon dioxide combines with water. It is a weak acid that helps decrease the alkalinity of the blood.

A **buffer** is a substance that can bind with a strong acid or base to prevent major changes in the pH of body fluids. The bicarbonate buffer system consists of the following two chemicals:

1. **Sodium bicarbonate ($NaHCO_3$):** a weak base
2. **Carbonic acid (H_2CO_3):** a weak acid

To maintain acid-base balance, the following ratio must be met: 1 part carbonic acid to 20 parts sodium bicarbonate.

When sodium bicarbonate, which is a weak base, combines with a strong acid, such as hydrochloric acid, it forms two different substances: sodium chloride (salt), which is a base, and carbonic acid, which is a weak acid. When this occurs, the pH moves back into the normal range.

The kidneys help control the pH of the blood by releasing or reabsorbing sodium bicarbonate as needed. If carbonic acid, which is a weak acid, combines with a strong base, it helps decrease the strength of the base and move the pH back towards normal. The levels of carbonic acid are regulated by the lungs.

KNOWLEDGE CONNECTION

What is the ratio of carbonic acid to sodium bicarbonate that must be maintained to keep acid-base balance? How is carbonic acid formed? Which body system regulates sodium bicarbonate? Which body system regulates carbonic acid?

Role of the Respiratory System

In relation to acid-base balance, the lungs are responsible for one of two functions: either retaining more carbon dioxide (CO_2) to increase the acidity of the blood or removing excess carbon dioxide from the blood to decrease the acidity of the blood. To retain CO_2, the lungs slow the rate of respiration, allowing the formation of carbonic acid to help increase acidity. To remove excess CO_2, the lungs increase the rate of respiration so that they can exhale more CO_2 from the body into the atmosphere. The decrease in carbonic acid in the blood decreases the acidity. This relatively simple respiratory mechanism helps to maintain the pH within the normal range between 7.35 and 7.45. This action taken by the lungs can change the blood pH quickly, but the change does not last a long time.

KNOWLEDGE CONNECTION

How do the lungs help maintain normal pH? How quickly does this change the pH?

Role of the Kidneys

The kidneys have the ability to perform four basic functions as needed to maintain the proper blood pH:

1. Retain hydrogen (H^+)
2. Excrete H^+
3. Retain sodium bicarbonate ($NaHCO_3$)
4. Excrete $NaHCO_3$

When the blood becomes too acidic, the kidneys *remove* hydrogen ions from the blood and excrete them into the urine. Also, the kidneys reabsorb more bicarbonate back into the blood. Together these two actions will make the blood more alkaline, helping to return the pH back to normal. When the kidneys sense that the blood is too alkaline, they will retain more hydrogen ions in the blood and also will excrete more bicarbonate into the urine. Both of these actions make the blood more acidic, once again helping to return the pH back to normal.

This action of the kidneys works more slowly than the lungs, changing the pH balance over a period of days rather than hours. Once the pH changes are made, however, they are longer lasting than those made by the bicarbonate-carbonic acid buffer system or the respiratory system. Therefore, the kidneys could be described as the most effective of the three systems for balancing blood pH.

KNOWLEDGE CONNECTION

Which two body organs are involved in managing acid-base balance? What are the specific functions of each system that affect acid-base balance? Which system works most effectively to make pH adjustments?

Acid-Base Imbalance

An uncorrected acid-base imbalance will lead to either acidosis or alkalosis. **Acidosis** is an increase of acids in the blood and moves the pH to below 7.35. **Alkalosis** is an increase in blood alkalinity and moves the pH to above 7.45. Normally, there are minimal shifts back and forth in the blood pH between slightly acidotic and slightly alkalotic as conditions change. The buffer, respiratory, and renal systems are able to accommodate these shifts and bring the blood back to a normal pH, between 7.35 and 7.45.

The respiratory system responds quickly to minute changes in pH and works very rapidly, continuously adjusting as needed to help balance the pH. However, it is only capable of making small adjustments in the pH. When a larger pH adjustment is required, especially for a longer period of time, the kidneys will take action to return the pH to normal ranges.

Anatomy and Physiology Connection

The Brain and Acid-Base Balance

Chemoreceptors located in the aorta, carotid arteries, and medulla have the capability to sense or detect changes in blood levels of O_2 and CO_2, as well as disturbances in pH. When the pH lowers, the receptors send a message to the brain indicating that the blood's pH is too acidic. The medulla then signals the lungs to increase the rate of respiration, which will blow off more CO_2, helping to reduce the acidity of the blood. When pH increases, the receptors send a message to the brain indicating the blood's pH is too alkaline. The brain then signals the lungs to decrease the rate of respirations, which will allow retention of more CO_2, which combines with water and makes carbonic acid. This increases the acidity of the blood and moves the pH to normal.

Respiratory Alkalosis

When a patient is breathing rapidly and deeply, he or she will "blow off" more carbon dioxide than normal. Some mental states and illnesses that might cause this include fear and anxiety, fever, and overdose of aspirin. All of these cause *hyperventilation*. Remember that carbon dioxide combined with water makes carbonic acid, so when hyperventilation occurs, more carbonic acid is lost than with normal breathing. When acid is lost, the blood pH moves towards alkalosis. Because the lungs are unable to regulate pH normally, this is referred to as *respiratory alkalosis*.

Respiratory Acidosis

When a patient does not breathe as deeply and frequently as normal, he or she will retain more carbon dioxide than normal. Some conditions that could cause this include opioid pain medications, certain other types of medications, pneumonia, and chronic respiratory diseases such as emphysema and chronic bronchitis. All of these cause *hypoventilation,* which traps carbon dioxide in the lungs where it converts to carbonic acid. When acid is trapped, the blood pH moves towards acidosis. Because the lungs are unable to regulate pH normally, this is referred to as *respiratory acidosis*.

Metabolic Alkalosis

If a patient has a condition that causes either a marked loss of hydrogen ions or a marked increase of sodium bicarbonate, it will lead to *metabolic alkalosis*. Some conditions that cause this are severe vomiting and nasogastric suction. Both of these situations cause the patient to lose large amounts of hydrochloric acid from the stomach. Other possible causes of metabolic alkalosis include taking diuretic medications and overuse of antacids or taking sodium bicarbonate for heartburn. Diuretics can cause a loss of potassium in the urine, which stimulates the kidneys to excrete hydrogen ions to save potassium ions, leading to the pH increasing above 7.45. Antacids and sodium bicarbonate are alkaline, and excess amounts lead to alkalosis.

Metabolic Acidosis

If a patient has a condition that causes an increase in hydrogen ions or a very low level of bicarbonate ions, it will result in *metabolic acidosis*. Conditions that can cause this include prolonged diarrhea, intestinal disorders, and surgical removal of the colon. Because the intestinal tract contains large amounts of bicarbonate ions, damage to this area leads to loss of bicarbonate, causing the pH to lower. Two other conditions that also cause this situation are lactic acidosis, often the result of shock, and ketoacidosis, the result of uncontrolled diabetes mellitus. Both of these are types of metabolic acidosis. When patients are in kidney failure, their kidneys cannot respond to changes in pH, hydrogen ions are retained, and the pH falls below 7.35.

Nursing Actions for Acid-Base Imbalances

When you care for patients with acid-base imbalances, it is important to be aware of how both the lungs and the kidneys are functioning. In addition, take the following nursing actions:

- Monitor vital signs for tachypnea and bradypnea, tachycardia, and fever.
- Assess the patient's respirations for depth and pattern, dyspnea, length of inspiration versus expiration, and use of accessory respiratory muscles.
- Assess skin, mucous membranes, and nailbeds for cyanosis.
- Assess O_2 saturation and need for supplemental O_2.
- Monitor laboratory results of arterial blood gases (ABGs). Seriously ill patients may require endotracheal intubation and mechanical ventilation.

In Chapter 28, you were introduced to the laboratory diagnostic test called ABGs. (See Table 28.2 to review the normal ranges for ABGs and the significance of abnormal levels.)

KNOWLEDGE CONNECTION

Which two body systems are key in managing acid-base changes? What functions can each of these organs perform in efforts to maintain acid-base balance? Explain at least two causes of metabolic acidosis and two causes of metabolic alkalosis.

Nursing Care Plan for a Patient With a Fluid Imbalance

When you plan care for a patient with a fluid volume deficit or fluid volume excess, it is important to assess for signs and symptoms of electrolyte imbalance as well. To develop a thorough care plan, you will be thinking about many potential problems as well as those that you identify.

You have arrived at the hospital to work the day shift from 7:00 a.m. until 7:00 p.m., and you are assigned to provide nursing care for a 26-year-old female with Crohn's disease. She was admitted to the hospital around 4:00 a.m. with dehydration secondary to persistent diarrhea for 3 weeks. At home, she had gotten up to go to the bathroom and fainted, so her husband called an ambulance. You know that it will be important to be particularly alert to signs and symptoms of electrolyte imbalance as well as fluid imbalance.

Assessment

As you perform the beginning shift assessment on this patient, you find that her skin and mucous membranes are very dry. Her lips are cracked and chapped, her tongue shows deep furrows, and her eyes appear to be sunken in the orbital frame. Her pulse is 102 and is weak but regular. Her supine blood pressure is 96/52. When you check her skin turgor, it remains tented for longer than 3 seconds. She weighs 120 lbs (54.5 kg) and is 5 feet 2 inches (157.5 cm) tall. She informs you that her normal weight is 131 lbs (59.5 kg). She is oriented to all four spheres and is answering your questions appropriately. She tells you that she has not voided since before she went to bed at 11:00 p.m. Her laboratory work shows elevated sodium and low chloride in the blood. She tells you that in the past she had had short episodes of diarrhea due to her Crohn's disease but that she has never had it for this long and nothing she has taken stopped it for very long.

Nursing Diagnosis

You know that this patient is dehydrated, that she has had diarrhea for too long, and that it must be stopped to improve her dehydration. You are concerned about the appearance of her dry, cracked mouth, but more so regarding the fact that she has not voided in 9 hours. You know the minimum output indicating adequate kidney function is 30 mL per hour. The following nursing diagnoses are given for her:

- Fluid volume deficit
- Diarrhea
- Risk for impaired oral mucous membranes
- Knowledge deficit regarding management of her chronic disease

The first two nursing diagnoses are addressed in this care plan, but the other diagnoses are appropriate to be added as well.

Planning

Goals for this patient include adequate fluid volume, as evidenced by adequate intake of between 1,800 and 2,500 mL per day and output that is within 200 to 300 mL of the intake, moist oral mucous membranes, and elastic skin turgor by the time she is discharged from the hospital. Another desired outcome is that she will have four or fewer formed bowel movements per day before she leaves the hospital.

Interventions

Your nursing interventions are designed to help meet the needs identified in each nursing diagnosis. See the nursing care interventions and evaluations below.

Evaluation

As you evaluate your patient's responses to your interventions, you can decide if the action is effective, if it needs to be continued, or if it needs to be changed.

Nursing Care Plan for a Patient With a Fluid Imbalance—cont'd

Nursing Diagnosis: Deficient fluid volume related to prolonged diarrhea as evidenced by decreased BP, decreased skin turgor, and dry mucous membranes
Expected Outcomes: BP will stabilize with no signs of orthostatic hypotension, and I&O will be balanced prior to discharge.

Interventions	Evaluations
Monitor vital signs every 4 hours or more frequently, with blood pressure taken in lying, sitting, and standing positions, noting orthostatic hypotension; note elevated temperature, tachycardia, weak or thready pulse.	Day 1: 0800 – BP supine 98/62, sitting BP 90/58, standing BP 78/50. Requires assistance to sit on side of bed. Not able to ambulate due to dizziness accompanying BP drops. T – 100.4°F; P – 104 weak. Day 2: BP stability better by evening. 2015 – BP 108/78 supine, 104/66 sitting, 102/64 standing. T – 99.2°F; P – 82 reg & strong. No c/o dizziness. Able to be up to bathroom with assistance. Day 3: BP supine 128/76, sitting 126/78, standing 128/66; T – 98.8°F; P – 81 and regular. Alert and oriented. Able to be up unassisted. No dizziness.

Nursing Diagnosis: Deficient fluid volume related to prolonged diarrhea as evidenced by decreased BP, decreased skin turgor, and dry mucous membranes
Expected Outcomes: BP will stabilize with no signs of orthostatic hypotension, and I&O will be balanced prior to discharge.

Interventions	Evaluations
Maintain careful I&O record. Offer the patient 8 ounces of fluid every hour. She likes Sprite, hot tea, and water. Measure loose stools and include all IV fluids in intake.	Day 1: 24-hr intake – 3,350 mL. Output – 1,175 mL (700 mL was from 8 loose stools). IV @ 125 mL/hr. Drinking some fluid each hour when cued. Taking Sprite better than other fluids. Day 2: 24-hr intake – 3,420 mL. Output – 1,400 mL (250 mL was 5 loose stools). IV rate ↓ 80 mL/hr. Drinking fluids well. Day 3: Intake – 2,555 mL. Output – 2,400 mL (3 loose stools – 160 mL). IV has been discontinued.
Weigh the patient every morning.	Day 1: Wt. 125 lbs (56.8 kg) Day 2: Wt. down @ 124.5 lbs (56.6 kg) Day 3: Wt. up @ 126 lbs (57.2 kg)
Administer IV fluids and assess for signs and symptoms of fluid volume overload (shortness of breath, pedal or sacral edema, and increasing blood pressure or full bounding pulse).	Day 1: Tolerated IV NS 1000 mL w/ 20 mEq KCl at 125 mL/hr without s/sx of fluid volume excess. Site without erythema/edema. Day 2: IV ↓ 80 mL/hr; no signs of fluid volume excess. Site without erythema/edema. Day 3: IV discontinued.

Nursing Diagnosis: Diarrhea related to bowel inflammation as evidenced by many liquid stools per day
Expected Outcomes: Number of stools will decrease to less than three per day by discharge.

Interventions	Evaluations
Administer antidiarrheal medications as ordered and evaluate their effectiveness.	Day 2: Med helping; stools decreased to 8 in 24 hours; 5 loose BMs.
Auscultate bowel sounds every 4 hours and note any decrease in hyperactivity.	Day 2: Bowel sounds remain hyperactive. Day 3: Bowel sounds active; stools slowed to 3 in 24 hours, semiformed.

(nursing care plan continues on page 628)

Nursing Care Plan for a Patient With a Fluid Imbalance—cont'd

Interventions	Evaluations
Assure the patient that you will respond to her call light promptly or place a bedpan within her reach.	Day 2: No anxiety noted. Uses call light. No accidents. Day 3: Up to BR unassisted. Denies weakness/dizziness. Up to bathroom prn.
Place an incontinence pad beneath the patient to keep the bed clean.	No incontinence. Linens clean.
Demonstrate compassion and understanding regarding the patient's diarrhea.	No anxiety exhibited.

POST CONFERENCE

You learned how serious hyperkalemia can be. Your patient did well the first day you cared for her, but on the second day you noticed during your assessment that her heart rate was irregular, with a pattern of two beats and a skipped beat. You also noted that her urine output over the last 12 hours was less than 30 mL per hour. The monitor tech called and said your patient was having premature ventricular contractions. The patient told you that she felt weak and like her heart was "flip-flopping." You notified your instructor and the supervising nurse, who called the physician. Stat orders for a potassium level and basic metabolic profile (BMP) were received. Her blood work showed that her potassium level had risen from 4.8 to 5.6 mEq/L in 36 hours. Her BMP showed high levels of creatinine. The physician was again notified and ordered the patient transferred back to the ICU with acute renal insufficiency and hyperkalemia. You understood the need to act quickly and helped with the transfer. The ICU nurse told you that he would be administering IV insulin and glucose to the patient and that dialysis may be necessary. You felt really good, like a contributing part of the nursing team, because you had picked up on a key assessment indicating a potentially serious problem for this patient.

Key Points

- Body fluids are contained in two compartments: intracellular and extracellular fluids. The extracellular fluid compartment also includes the interstitial space and the intervascular space.
- Fluids move into and out of the fluid compartments through osmosis, diffusion, and filtration.
- Water has many functions in the body, including transporting, protecting, and lubricating.
- Regulation of body fluid is done by hormone regulation, normal losses, and water intake.
- Fluid volume deficit is the same as dehydration and is caused by prolonged insufficient fluid intake or prolonged loss of fluid. Young children and the elderly dehydrate more quickly than others.
- Fluid volume excess is the same as hypervolemia and is usually caused by excess sodium intake or compromised kidney, heart, or liver function.
- Nursing actions for fluid volume disturbances include careful recording of I&O, daily weights, administering or withholding fluids as ordered, and educating patients about ways to avoid similar problems in the future.
- Electrolytes are needed for fluids to move into and out of cells and for nerves and muscles (including the heart muscle) to work correctly. Some normal ranges are very narrow and must be monitored closely.
- The pH scale measures the acidity or alkalinity of a substance based on concentration of hydrogen or hydroxyl ions. Water is neutral and falls at 7 on the pH scale. Blood is slightly alkaline at 7.35 to 7.45.
- Acid-base balance in the body is regulated through three systems: the buffer system, the respiratory system, and the renal system.
- Acid-base imbalance results in one of four conditions: respiratory or metabolic acidosis and respiratory or metabolic alkalosis.
- Nursing care for acid-base imbalances includes careful monitoring of vital signs, respiratory status, oxygen saturation, and ABGs.

Review Questions

Select the answer that is most appropriate for each of the following questions. Some questions may have more than one correct answer. Select all that apply.

1. You will expect to find which of the following during the skin assessment of a patient with dehydration?
   1. Redness
   2. Dryness
   3. Dependent edema
   4. Blisters
   5. Prolonged skin tenting

2. The nurse is completing an I&O sheet for the patient. Which will the nurse include in the output?
   1. Sweat
   2. Peritoneal fluid
   3. Liquid stool
   4. Emesis
   5. Interstitial fluid
   6. Urine

3. The patient complains of shortness of breath and is expectorating pink frothy sputum. The nurse would assess for further signs and symptoms of:
   1. hyperkalemia.
   2. hypomagnesemia.
   3. fluid overload.
   4. fluid deficit.
   5. dehydration.

4. When teaching a patient about ways to avoid fluid overload, the nurse explains it is best to eat a diet that is low in:
   1. potassium.
   2. calcium.
   3. magnesium.
   4. sodium.
   5. phosphorus.

5. You know that your patient with chronic kidney disease will need more teaching if she says:
   1. "I will eat more oranges to prevent potassium buildup."
   2. "I will increase my milk intake to keep my calcium levels in the normal range."
   3. "I will avoid bananas so my potassium level will not get too high."
   4. "I can have scrambled eggs for breakfast as long as my calcium is not too high."

6. Your patient has a low potassium level, uncorrected by oral medications. The physician orders 30 mEq of KCl added to the IV of 1,000 mL of normal saline to infuse at 80 mL per hour. Which nursing intervention is of the most importance to perform today?
   1. Serve a diet with potassium-rich foods
   2. Restrict sodium in the diet
   3. Monitor blood levels of all electrolytes
   4. Make certain urine output is at least 30 mL per hour
   5. Monitor for fever and tachypnea

7. Your patient is admitted with alkalosis. Which laboratory finding would you expect?
   1. pH of 7.30
   2. pH of 7.48
   3. Decreased bicarbonate level
   4. Elevated carbon dioxide level

8. Which is true of respiratory acidosis?
   1. The patient is hyperventilating.
   2. The patient is hypoventilating.
   3. This causes the pH to elevate above 7.45.
   4. This causes the pH to drop below 7.35.

9. The patient for whom you are providing care has been receiving furosemide, a diuretic, in an effort to remove the excess water that has been retained as a result of heart failure. When you are preparing to assist the patient with a shower, she tells you that she is so tired today and that she just does not feel that her legs will hold her up long enough to take a shower. You know that she took a shower each of the past 3 days and wonder to what you might attribute this change. Which of the following laboratory results could explain her fatigue and muscle weakness?
   1. Hypokalemia
   2. Hyperchloremia
   3. Hypocalcemia
   4. Hypernatremia

10. If a patient's blood pH is 7.33, the patient is in:
    1. alkalosis.
    2. acidosis.
    3. hypovolemic shock.
    4. a state of dehydration.

ANSWERS 1. 2, 5. 2. 3, 4, 6. 3. 3. 4. 4. 5. 1. 6. 4. 7. 2. 8. 2, 4. 9. 1. 10. 2

Critical Thinking Exercises

Answers available online.

1. The patient is a 79-year-old male with chronic heart disease. His wife calls his physician's office to report that he is short of breath and not feeling well. She reports that he doesn't have a fever, and his heart rate and blood pressure readings on their home monitor were normal. You suspect heart failure, which can cause fluid retention. What assessment question should you ask that could best confirm your suspicion?

2. A patient with inflammation of the cecum is at risk for fluid volume deficit. Explain why this is so.

Additional Resources

DAVIS edge Use the scratch off code on the inside front cover of your book to access online quizzes that will help you to improve your scores on course exams and prepare for the NCLEX-PN®.

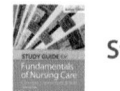

Study Guide

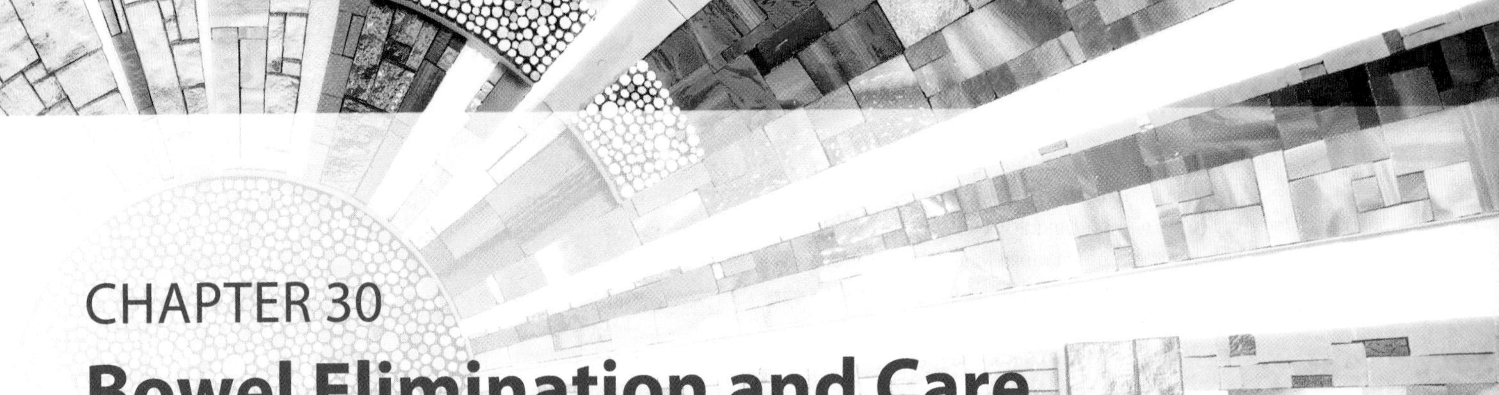

CHAPTER 30
Bowel Elimination and Care

Kathleen Hutchins-Otero

KEY TERMS

Colostomy (kol-OSS-tuh-mee)
Constipation (KON-stih-PAY-shun)
Defecation (def-uh-KAY-shun)
Diarrhea (DYE-ah-REE-ah)
Distention (dis-TEN-shun)
Fecal incontinence (FEE-kuhl in-KON-tih-nents)
Flatus (FLAY-tuss)
Guaiac test (GWYE-ac TEST)
Ileostomy (il-ee-OSS-tuh-mee)
Impaction (im-PAK-shun)
Kayexalate enema (kay-EKS-uh-layt EN-e-muh)
Melena (me-LEE-nah)
Occult blood (o-KULT BLUHD)
Siphon enema (SYE-fon EN-e-muh)
Steatorrhea (STEE-a-toh-REE-ah)
Stoma (STOH-mah)
Tenesmus (te-NEZ-muss)

CHAPTER CONCEPTS

Elimination
Patient-Centered Care
Safety

LEARNING OUTCOMES

1. Define various terms related to bowel elimination and care.
2. Describe normal bowel elimination patterns.
3. Identify normal and abnormal characteristics of feces.
4. Explain the significance of abnormal colors of feces.
5. Describe how to perform a thorough assessment of bowel function.
6. Discuss constipation and factors that contribute to it.
7. Describe nursing interventions to use for constipation.
8. Describe types of enemas, their purposes, mechanisms of action, and nursing considerations, as well as the contraindications and complications of enemas.
9. Discuss fecal impaction and nursing interventions for managing it.
10. Discuss diarrhea and factors that contribute to it.
11. Describe nursing interventions to use for diarrhea.
12. Discuss fecal incontinence and nursing interventions for managing it.
13. Explain the purposes of obtaining stool specimens.
14. Describe reasons for and types of alternative bowel elimination.
15. Discuss assessment and nursing care of ostomies.
16. Explain the purposes for colostomy irrigation.
17. Discuss information found in the Connection features in this chapter.
18. Identify specific safety information.
19. Answer questions about the skills in this chapter.

SKILLS

30.1 Administering a Cleansing Enema
30.2 Administering a Prepackaged Enema (Sodium Phosphate or Oil Retention)
30.3 Obtaining a Stool Specimen for Culture, and Ova and Parasites
30.4 Performing Guaiac Testing: Testing Stool Specimen for Occult Blood
30.5 Removing a Fecal Impaction
30.6 Changing an Ostomy Appliance
30.7 Irrigating a Colostomy

CRITICAL THINKING CONNECTION

Clinical Assignment

You are assigned to care for a 58-year-old male who had a total *colectomy* (removal of the colon) yesterday as a result of colon cancer. He has a permanent ileostomy as well as an abdominal incision with staples. You learn in shift report that his pain medication has been increased to better manage his discomfort.

Critical Thinking Questions:

1. How do you care for a new ileostomy?
2. How will you assess the stoma for evidence of adequate blood supply?
3. What type of output will you expect from the ileostomy?
4. What assessments will you make about his surgical incision?
5. How will you manage his pain to keep him comfortable?

Some nurses may view assisting with bowel elimination as nurse's aide work and low on the list of nursing priorities. However, understanding the importance of proper bowel elimination and the extent to which it can affect how a patient feels cannot be overstated. Problematic bowel elimination can cause mild to extreme discomfort as well as major health problems. In this chapter, you will learn the importance of proper bowel elimination, focused assessments related to bowel elimination, alternative methods of bowel elimination, abnormal patterns of elimination, and the appropriate nursing skills to promote proper bowel elimination.

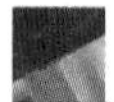

NORMAL BOWEL ELIMINATION

Bowel elimination occurs after nutrients are moved through the gastrointestinal (GI) tract, also known as the alimentary canal. This process begins in the *os,* or mouth, and ends as the waste products are eliminated as *feces,* or stool, via the anus. The process of bowel elimination is known as **defecation.**

Anatomy and Physiology Connection

Gastrointestinal Tract

The propulsion of a bolus of food through the GI tract is due to the rhythmic wavelike movements that begin in the esophagus and continue to the rectum, termed *peristalsis.* The mechanism of peristalsis is contraction of the circular and longitudinal muscles in the walls of the GI tract. As the muscles contract, the food bolus is pushed forward through the GI tract. In the stomach, enzymes break down the bolus of food, converting it into a semiliquid mass of partly digested food and digestive secretions known as *chyme.* Some absorption of water and alcohol occurs while food is in the stomach, but the stomach serves mostly as a reservoir, allowing chyme to slowly be emptied into the small intestine for further digestion and absorption. The chyme passes through the outlet of the stomach called the *pyloric sphincter* and into the small intestine, which is composed of the duodenum, jejunum, and ileum. It is here that most nutrients are absorbed into the blood via capillaries located in the villi and microvilli of the walls of the intestinal mucosa. The remaining chyme that is unable to be broken down for absorption passes through the ileocecal valve into the cecum portion of the colon, or large intestine. The ileocecal valve prevents backflow from the colon into the small intestine.

In the colon reside bacteria known as *normal flora,* whose purpose is to prevent infection and maintain health. The bacteria interact with the chyme, which produces a gas called **flatus.** As peristalsis moves the GI contents and flatus through the colon, it results in gurgles, clicks, and tinkling sounds, known as *bowel sounds.*

Most water absorption occurs in the colon, beginning in the cecum, followed by the ascending colon, transverse colon, descending colon, and finally the sigmoid colon, leaving a soft, formed mass of fecal material. As fecal material moves through the sigmoid colon into the rectum, the intestinal walls distend to accommodate the fecal mass. This **distention,** or stretching out of the intestinal walls and making them appear inflated, stimulates the walls' stretch receptors and sends impulses to the central nervous system, which in turn signals the muscular walls of the sigmoid colon and rectum to contract. This is known as the *defecation reflex* and is under voluntary control of the individual. The mass of waste will then pass through the internal and external anal sphincters, where it is expelled as feces.

Frequency of Elimination

Frequency of bowel elimination changes throughout the life span. Infants will normally have between three and six bowel movements daily. Children accomplish voluntary control of elimination between the ages of 2 and 3 years after their neuromuscular structures are developed. The frequency of bowel movements usually decreases to one or two bowel movements per day. This pattern usually is maintained throughout adulthood. However, peristalsis decreases as the individual ages, making elderly individuals more prone to **constipation,** or hard stools that are difficult to pass.

Some patients will normally have one bowel movement daily, while others may go several days between movements, and yet others may have several bowel movements each day.

• WORD • BUILDING •

defecation: de – remove + fec – dregs + ation – action
peristalsis: peri – around + stalsis – contraction
ileocecal: ileo – ileum + cecal – related to cecum

The goal of your elimination care is to maintain the patient's normal frequency pattern of bowel elimination, or as close to it as possible. At the very least, you must make certain the patient has a bowel movement at least every 3 days to prevent constipation.

KNOWLEDGE CONNECTION

Describe what happens during peristalsis. Explain the importance of normal flora in the GI tract. Explain the defecation reflex. What is the longest length of time a patient should be allowed to go without having a bowel movement?

Timing of Elimination

Because peristalsis begins with the introduction of food into the GI tract, the urge to defecate commonly occurs 30 minutes to 1 hour after eating. If the patient ignores the reflex and puts off going to the bathroom for a bowel movement until a later time, the stool remains in the intestines longer than necessary and can become dry and hard, contributing to the development of constipation. It is helpful to provide the patient time after each meal for toileting, offering assistance as needed.

Characteristics of Feces

Characteristics of stool include color, shape, consistency, odor, and frequency. A normal stool will vary depending on diet, amount of fiber and fluids, exercise, medications, and other habits. When a disease process is occurring in the GI tract, the changes in the characteristics of stool may provide clues as to the medical diagnosis, which is one of the reasons that assessment of bowel function is important. Table 30.1 presents a summary of normal and abnormal characteristics of stool.

Normal Characteristics

The typical stool is soft, formed, light yellowish-brown to dark brown, slightly odiferous, and falls into a slightly curved shape. Sometimes a normal stool may be a different color, such as red or green, simply due to variations in dietary intake. For example, eating green foods such as spinach may result in greenish-black streaks in the feces, while eating beets may result in red-tinted stools. Ingestion of iron supplements normally causes stools to be very dark brown or black.

Like frequency, the expected color and consistency of stool also are different across the life span. Normally newborns have black, shiny, sticky stools called *meconium.* Infants who are breastfed usually will have a bright yellow, pasty, seedy-appearing stool, while babies who receive formula or cow's milk will have a darker yellowish-brown or tan-colored stool that is much more firm and formed.

Abnormal Characteristics

If the patient has inadequate fluid intake or if transit time is prolonged, meaning stool is held in the body longer than usual, the stool may be a harder consistency and be passed in smaller balls or clumps, rather than a softer, longer, curved shape. If transit time is extremely short due to increased peristalsis, little or no water will be absorbed, and the stool will be liquid or semiliquid. Sometimes the rapid transit time does not allow bile to go through its typical chemical changes, giving feces a green color. Several liquid or watery stools per day are classified as **diarrhea.**

The stool consistency or shape may change due to variations in amount of fiber intake, an increase in amount of ingested fat, or changes in the structure of the intestine. Fiber

Table 30.1
Normal and Abnormal Characteristics of Stool

	Normal Characteristics	*Abnormal Characteristics*
Consistency	Soft, formed consistency	Liquid or semiliquid, watery, unformed, very hard and dry
Shape	Longer curved shape, cylindrical	Balls, clumps, or broken-off chunks; flat or ribbon-like; pencil-like
Color	Yellow in infants Light brown to dark brown in others	Bright red blood, black, coffee grounds appearance, pale, white, gray, or clay color
Presence of infection	Absence of pus, mucous, fat	Presence of pus, excessive mucus, foamy, or floating on water
Presence of parasites	Absence of parasites	Presence of worms or eggs
Odor	Slight odor	Foul odor, strongly odiferous, bloody or old-blood smell, metallic smell

intake will affect the bulk of the stool. It is very important to assess the appearance and color of the patient's feces and to take the appropriate actions if abnormalities are found. *Frank blood* is visible to the naked eye, and **occult blood** is hidden or not visible. To determine the presence of occult blood, a **guaiac test** must be performed on the stool sample. All abnormal appearance and color should be documented and reported. Refer to Box 30.1 for the significance of abnormal colors and appearance of feces.

KNOWLEDGE CONNECTION

Compare normal and abnormal characteristics of feces. Name at least two reasons that a stool may be pale or white. What is the term denoting excessive fat in the stool? What is the difference between frank and occult blood in a stool?

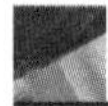

ASSESSMENT OF BOWEL ELIMINATION

A thorough assessment and data collection should be performed on admission to the hospital. Then assessment of bowel movements should be performed and documented every shift thereafter. Documentation should always include the following:

- Color
- Amount
- Consistency
- Unusual shape
- Unusual odor

Box 30.1

Significance of Abnormal Colors and Appearance of Feces

- Stool that appears fluffy, floats on water, and has a foul odor is due to an abnormally high content of undigested fat and is called **steatorrhea.** It may be due to disorders such as Crohn's disease.
- Stool that appears yellow and greasy and has a foul odor also may be due to pancreatitis and pancreatic cancer.
- Ribbon-shaped stool may indicate compression on the colon by a tumor, which may be colon cancer.
- Stool that contains blood, mucus, and pus generally indicates inflammation or infection of the intestinal mucosa.
- Stool may contain thread-like worms and granules that are parasite eggs.
- Stool that is pale or clay colored indicates a lack of bile in the intestines, which may be due to liver or gall bladder disease. Taking antacids or drinking barium for tests can also cause stool to be white.
- Small amounts of bright red blood in the stool may indicate hemorrhoids.
- Larger amounts of bright red blood will indicate bleeding or hemorrhage from the colon.
- Large amounts of maroon-colored blood indicates bleeding from the small intestines.
- Stool that is black and tarry with a foul odor indicates bleeding from the stomach; the blood has been partially digested, giving it the black, tarry appearance that is known as **melena**.

Data Collection

Data collection about the patient's normal bowel habits and any current problems the patient may be experiencing is part of assessing bowel function. Ask the patient the following questions:

- How often do your bowels normally move?
- Do you have any current problems, such as diarrhea or constipation, and how long has it been occurring?
- What is the normal number of stools you pass per day?
- What is the normal color of your stools?
- What is the normal consistency of your stools?
- Is your stool formed or unformed?
- Does abdominal cramping occur with or before a bowel movement?
- Do you experience any anal burning or itching?
- Is there pain with defecation?
- Do you feel urgency or pressure in the rectum (tenesmus)?
- Do you have any allergies?
- Do you take routine medications, and what medications have you taken for the elimination problem, both prescription and over the counter?
- Have you experienced recent changes in appetite?
- How much fiber do you eat?
- Do you have regular mealtimes?
- How much fluid do you drink in a day?
- What are your usual beverages?
- Are you experiencing nausea or vomiting?
- Do you have any food intolerances?
- Do you have any hemorrhoids?

Focused Assessment

Perform a focused assessment to determine the objective signs. First, assess the shape of the abdomen. The shape should be rounded or flat, but not distended or inflated. Distention related to the GI tract may be a sign of excessive gas, fluid, or stool.

Next, auscultate the bowel sounds using the diaphragm surface rather than the bell of your stethoscope to better hear the sounds. Listen in all four quadrants. Bowel sounds should be assessed at least once per shift and more often as indicated. As you listen to bowel sounds, you may hear different sounds signifying different situations for the patient.

If an impaction or intestinal blockage occurs, the peristalsis may increase or become hyperactive proximal to the blockage. The intestinal contents will churn and mix as the peristalsis pushes against the blockage. The intestine proximal to the

• WORD • BUILDING •

steatorrhea: steato – fat + rrhea – flow
tenesmus: teinesmos – stretching
impaction: impact – driven in + ion – action

Table 30.2
Bowel Sounds and Their Significance

Type	*Sound*	*Significance*
Normal	Soft gurgles, irregular clicks Between 5 and 30 per minute	Indicates normal bowel function
Hypoactive	Fewer than 5 per minute	May indicate constipation
Hyperactive	More than 30 per minute or continuous	May be heard when the patient has diarrhea
Borborygmi	Excessively loud gurgling May be high-pitched and tinkling in one quadrant and absent or decreased in the lower left quadrant	May indicate hunger or, if not hungry, can indicate bowel obstruction

blockage will distend while the intestine distal to the blockage may empty. The area distal to the blockage may have very distant or even absent bowel sounds. ***Safety: An absence of bowel sounds indicates a problem and should always be reported to the health-care provider.*** It is important to be aware that some individuals have very quiet and difficult-to-hear bowel sounds, necessitating that you listen carefully and for an adequate period of time. If you think that bowel sounds are absent, be certain to listen for at least 3 to 5 minutes in each of the four quadrants before declaring this. (See Table 30.2 for information about bowel sounds and their significance.)

Avoid palpating the abdomen until after you have assessed the bowel sounds because palpation may stimulate bowel sounds that were not there naturally. Normally, one's abdomen is soft when palpated, but it may become firm or hard with excessive gas, constipation, or obstruction of the bowel.

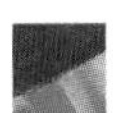

ALTERATIONS IN BOWEL ELIMINATION

The most commonly seen alterations in bowel elimination include constipation, fecal impaction, diarrhea, and fecal incontinence.

Constipation

Constipation is the term used for less frequent, hard, formed stools that are difficult to expel. Constipation may also include a bloated feeling. A patient with severe constipation may complain of loss of appetite, known as *anorexia,* as well as bloating, cramping, malaise, or not feeling well. Other patients may voice no complaints at all, making it important to identify the length of time since the last bowel movement. Elderly people who are not physically active are especially prone to constipation.

Factors Contributing to Constipation

A variety of factors can contribute to developing constipation. Many of these factors can easily be modified by the patient, which is why patient education is so important.

1. Decreased activity level: This occurs when a patient is ill or injured. Decreased activity results in slower peristalsis, leading to constipation.
2. Changes in food intake: Inadequate fiber intake decreases stool mass as well as decreasing peristalsis, leading to development of constipation. Too much fiber can result in excessive flatus, and too much fiber without adequate fluids can contribute to constipation. Eating at irregular times tends to lead to irregularity of bowel movements and constipation, while individuals who eat three meals daily at regular intervals tend to have more regular patterns of bowel elimination.
3. Decreased fluid intake: Too little fluid leads to harder stools as the body absorbs the majority of the fluid intake in an attempt to maintain fluid and electrolyte balance, leaving inadequate fluid in the colon to keep the stool soft. Some individuals find that hot or cold drinks help to stimulate peristalsis.
4. Medication side effects: Some over-the-counter medications containing aluminum (Amphojel) and calcium carbonate (Tums) can cause constipation. Iron supplements also cause constipation. Narcotic pain medications that contain opioids, such as codeine, hydrocodone, and oxycodone, cause severe slowing of peristalsis.
5. Surgery: Surgery, especially surgery on the GI tract, will decrease peristalsis and increase the risk for constipation. Anesthesia drugs can slow or completely halt peristalsis. Manipulation of the bowel changes the chemistry of the intestinal muscle cells, resulting in slowing of peristalsis. Postoperative pain can also suppress the urge to defecate. All postoperative patients should be assessed for adequate bowel elimination to prevent constipation.
6. Pregnancy: A decrease in stimulation of the muscles of the digestive tract and crowding of the sigmoid colon by the enlarging uterus both lend themselves to development of constipation.

• **WORD** • **BUILDING** •
incontinence: in – lack of + continence – ability to retain bodily discharge

7. Depression: Patients dealing with depression find that it can slow body processes, including peristalsis, affect appetite and activity level, and lead to constipation.
8. Aging: The natural aging process brings changes in bowel function that contribute to constipation, making it a greater risk for elders. Esophageal emptying and peristalsis slow as we age. The muscle tone of the smooth muscles of the GI tract decrease, contributing to constipation.
9. Laxative overuse or abuse: The patient may use laxatives so often that he or she is no longer able to have a bowel movement naturally. If the patient does not or cannot take laxatives as frequently as usual, he or she may become severely constipated or develop a fecal impaction.
10. Nerve damage or impairment: The nerves of the sigmoid colon, rectum, and both anal sphincters must be intact in order for the patient to sense the presence of the stool in the rectum and the need to defecate. If these nerves are damaged or communication between these nerves and the brain is interrupted, as with a severed spinal cord, the patient will be unable to identify when defecation is imminent and will not possess control over the sphincters to voluntarily retain or expel stool. This can result in constipation.

KNOWLEDGE CONNECTION

Describe at least eight factors that contribute to constipation. Explain specifically how opioid analgesics affect bowel elimination. What is meant by laxative abuse?

Nursing Interventions for Constipation

When you are caring for a patient with constipation, it is important to remember that the patient is often uncomfortable and may be uncomfortable discussing bowel issues with you. There are a number of interventions you can use to help the patient move his or her bowels and feel better. Box 30.2 contains independent nursing interventions to promote bowel elimination.

Increase Activity

Physical activity stimulates peristalsis. When a patient enters the hospital, his or her activity level probably will be decreased from the normal activities of home life. If allowed, the patient should be ambulated in the hallways at least three to four times daily and sat up in a chair for meals. When patients are ordered to remain on bedrest or to have limited ambulation, it is important that you do what you can to increase their physical activities within the restrictions of the physician's orders. Make certain that the patient on bedrest is turned, or repositioned, at least every 2 hours to help stimulate the normal peristalsis of the intestinal tract.

Box 30.2

Independent Nursing Interventions to Promote Bowel Elimination

There are various interventions that you may perform without a health-care provider's order. The following are examples of independent nursing interventions that are useful in promoting bowel elimination:

- Determine the patient's normal bowel movement frequency pattern.
- Carefully track and document frequency, amount, color, and consistency of bowel movements.
- Assess bowel sounds at least once a shift, noting hypoactive, hyperactive, or absent sounds.
- If patient is on bedrest: Reposition the patient at least every 2 hours and perform passive or active range-of-motion exercises at least twice a day (see Chapter 16).
- If patient is ambulatory: Increase activity by ambulating three to four times daily, getting up in chair for meals.
- Encourage fluids, including water and fruit juices, as allowed by health-care provider's orders.
- Encourage fiber intake as allowed by the patient's diet order, including whole grains, fruits, and vegetables.

Improve Fluid and Fiber Intake

When fluid intake is inadequate, the water that has been ingested is absorbed from the bowel into the bloodstream in an attempt to prevent dehydration. Without enough water to keep the stools soft, they become hard and difficult to expel. Unless contraindicated, fluid intake should be maintained between 1,500 and 2,500 mL per day in most adults. Teach your patient how much fluid intake he or she should have and why it is important.

If your patient is not drinking adequately, do not simply document the lack of fluid intake; find out what the patient likes to drink and then provide an adequate supply of those fluids. Water intake should be encouraged, but other fluids such as coffee, tea, carbonated drinks, juice, sports drinks, flavored drink mixes, milk, flavored bottled water, and broth are acceptable replacements. If the patient is debilitated, it will be your responsibility not only to encourage fluids but to provide the patient with whatever assistance is required to drink the fluids. Debilitated, elderly, or confused patients may not be able to drink more than a few sips at a time, thus making it necessary to provide a drink every 15 to 20 minutes in an attempt to provide adequate intake. This task may be delegated to the certified nursing assistant (CNA) or unlicensed assistive personnel (UAP).

It is important that the patient also has adequate fiber intake, generally 25 to 35 g per day. Encourage fiber intake as allowed by the patient's diet order, including whole grains, fruits, and vegetables. Again, you must educate your patient as to why fiber is needed and how much is required for normal bowel elimination. A patient is generally more compliant when he or she understands the purpose of an intervention. Box 30.3 lists foods high in fiber.

Provide Privacy

Be certain to provide patient privacy for elimination. As a nurse, you will become comfortable with and view elimination as a natural function and see no reason for embarrassment. However, that probably does not reflect how your patient will feel about it. It will be helpful for you to consider how you would feel if you had to expel a bowel movement in the presence of a stranger.

If the patient requires use of a bedpan or bedside commode (BSC), shut the room door, pull the privacy curtain, place the bedpan or assist the patient to the BSC, provide toilet tissue, and wait outside the curtain if at all possible. If the patient can be left unattended, leave the room and tell the patient you will return in a few minutes. Make certain the patient can reach the call light before you leave. If you must stay in the room, try to be as unobtrusive as you can.

If the patient is allowed bathroom privileges (BRP) and it is safe for him or her to sit unassisted in the bathroom, make certain the call light is within reach and the patient knows how to use it and close the bathroom door as well as the room door before leaving the patient's room. If you must remain present for standby assistance, make yourself busy straightening the room and making the bed. Provide whatever privacy can be safely afforded.

Privacy should also be provided when discussing elimination with the patient. Avoid asking a patient in the presence of visitors if he or she has had a bowel movement or to describe the characteristics of the stool.

Box 30.3

Food High in Fiber Content

Adequate fiber intake is important for healthy bowel elimination. Processed foods have little or no fiber. Some fruits and vegetables, especially raw, have high fiber content, as listed below:

- Apples, unpeeled
- Artichokes
- Beans
- Blueberries
- Broccoli
- Cabbage
- Carrots
- Cauliflower
- Cherries
- Corn
- Dried fruits
- Flaxseed
- Legumes
- Nuts
- Oatmeal
- Oranges
- Pears, unpeeled
- Plums
- Popcorn
- Prunes
- Raisins
- Raspberries
- Strawberries
- Sunflower seeds
- Whole-grain breads
- Whole-grain cereals
- Whole-grain flour

Assist With Positioning

The most comfortable and natural position for bowel elimination is the upright sitting position. If the patient is allowed to ambulate or have BRP, assist the patient to the bathroom. ***Safety: If the patient is unable to walk that far, use a BSC.*** When the patient is restricted to the bed, use a bedpan and place the patient in high or semi-Fowler's position. For details regarding placement of a bedpan, refer to Chapter 31.

Administer Medications

Medications for constipation may work by directly stimulating peristalsis, softening the stool, or adding bulk to the stool. Stool softeners and those that add bulk are safer than the laxatives that stimulate peristalsis. Patients may have already attempted to treat themselves with medications at home, so it is important to collect information regarding medications used at home from either the patient or family members.

Medications for constipation for hospitalized patients must be ordered by the health-care provider. Nurses can try a variety of independent interventions to relieve constipation before requesting medications to treat it (see Box 30.2).

KNOWLEDGE CONNECTION

Discuss how activity, fluids, and dietary fiber promote bowel elimination. What role does providing privacy play in bowel elimination?

Patient Teaching Connection

Preventing Recurrent Constipation

Patients need to be taught how to prevent the recurrence of constipation and its complications through the increase of fiber and fluid in their diets. Explain the importance of ensuring that the patient has a bowel movement at least every 3 days. Discuss the importance of eating at least three meals a day at regular intervals to stimulate regular peristalsis. Teach the patient to increase the fiber in his or her diet to a minimum of 25 to 30 g per day. Explain that fiber provides bulk, putting pressure on the walls of the intestines and stimulating the nerves of the small and large intestine. This stimulation increases peristalsis, which moves the waste products to the rectum for evacuation. The insoluble fiber found in fruits and vegetables will also hold fluids in the intestine, making the waste more moist and flexible.

If the patient is unable to ingest enough fresh fruits and vegetables, explain that fiber is available over the counter and by prescription in many forms, such as powders, capsules, tablets, and liquids. Explain that the amount of fiber should be increased slowly over 7 to 10 days and that taking too much too quickly will cause excessive flatus. The active bacteria in yogurt help to stimulate peristalsis, making it an excellent addition to the diet for prevention of constipation.

Teach that adequate fluids should be ingested to soften the stool. Water, fruit juice, flavored drinks, coffee, and tea provide fluid for the bowel. However, some fluids containing high levels of caffeine act as a diuretic and may actually lead to a drier stool. Too much caffeine may also increase peristalsis and cramping, as well as production of excessive flatus. It is recommended that caffeine intake be limited to 300 mg daily.

Administer Enemas

When medication does not relieve the problem of constipation, the health-care provider may order an *enema,* the instillation of a solution into the colon via the rectum, to relieve the problem. There are several types of enemas and each has a specific purpose. (See Table 30.3 for types of enemas, their purposes, mechanisms of action, and nursing considerations.) The water temperature of enemas should be between 105°F and 110°F to avoid burning the intestinal mucosa. Use a bath thermometer to check water temperature. If one is not available, pour a small amount of the solution on the inner side of your bare wrist. It should feel warm but never hot. Water that is too cold will cause abdominal cramping and may restrict the patient's ability to retain the water. Figure 30.1 shows examples of enema administration equipment and supplies.

Positioning the patient in the left Sims' or left lateral side-lying position allows gravity to help pull the solution into the intestine. The normal length to insert the tip of the tubing is 3 to 4 inches for administration of a cleansing enema to an adult. This generally allows instillation of enema solution into the rectum, sigmoid colon, and descending

Table 30.3
Types of Enemas

Type	*Volume for Adults*	*Purpose*	*Mechanism of Action*	*Nursing Considerations*
Tap water	500–1,000 mL	Cleansing	Hypotonic; allows fluid to move into interstitial fluid as well as be in the colon; distends colon and increases peristalsis	Hypotonic. ***Safety: Do NOT use for infants, children, or patients with congestive heart failure. Could result in fluid volume overload.*** Never give more than 3,000 mL total (i.e., three 1,000 mL enemas)
Normal saline (NS) (0.9%)	500–1,000 mL	Cleansing	Isotonic; adds fluid to the colon that does not move elsewhere; distends colon and increases peristalsis	Isotonic. Safe for use in children and congestive heart failure patients. Infants: use 50–150 mL Toddlers: use 150–350 mL School-age children: use 350–500 mL
Soapsuds (use castile soap only)	5 mL of castile soap added to 1,000 mL of tap water or normal saline	Cleansing	Works by distending the colon and by irritating the walls of the colon, which further increases peristalsis	***Safety: Mix castile soap in saline, not tap water, for infants, children, or patients with congestive heart failure.***
Hypertonic sodium phosphate	120 mL	Cleansing	Hypertonic; pulls fluid from interstitial spaces into the colon to soften the stool and increase peristalsis	Normally used only for adults.

Table 30.3
Types of Enemas—cont'd

Type	*Volume for Adults*	*Purpose*	*Mechanism of Action*	*Nursing Considerations*
Oil retention	120 mL	Softens hard stool (impaction)	Lubricates and softens hard stool mass, making it easier to remove	Normally used only for adults. Instill the enema 1 hour before removing an impaction.
Medicated enemas	As ordered	Exchange of substances and decreases inflammation	Steroid enemas decrease inflammation in the walls of the rectum and colon; **Kayexelate enema** pulls potassium from the body tissues and binds with it; excess potassium leaves the body when the enema is expelled	Must be retained for a specified period of time. May require a tube with a balloon to be inserted in the rectum to hold the medication in place.
Milk and molasses	As ordered	Cleansing	Hypertonic solution that pulls fluid into the colon and softens hard stool	Milk and molasses must be heated together to mix well, and then must be cooled to body temperature before administration; effective but messy.
Return flow (also called Harris flush and **siphon enema)**	500–1,000 mL	Remove flatus	Raising and lowering the enema container causes flatus to siphon back into the enema container	Prepare tap water or saline enema and administer 100–200 mL of solution and then lower the container below the level of the rectum for flatus to siphon out; repeat until no bubbles come back into the enema container.
High enema	500–1,000 mL	Cleanse higher up in the colon beyond the sigmoid	Distends the colon and moves up into the descending and transverse colon with position changes	Administer about half the fluid of a tap water or saline enema with patient in left Sim's position. Then turn patient to the back, then to the right side, and finish administering the fluid.

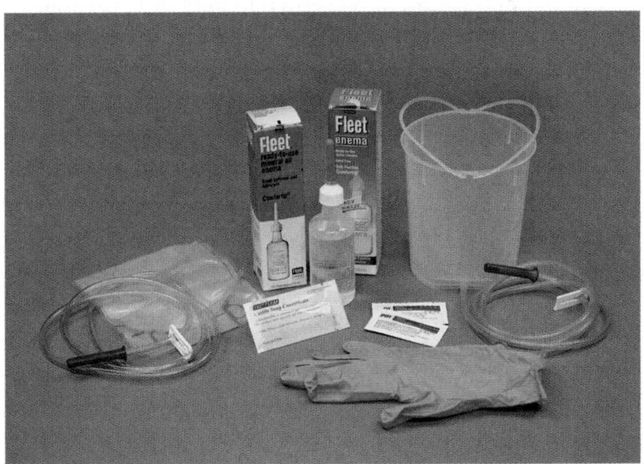

FIGURE 30.1 An enema bag, commercially prepared enemas, and an enema bucket with supplies for administration.

colon for lower bowel cleansing. ***Safety: Never attempt insertion of the tip of the tubing into the patient's rectum while the patient is in a sitting position, as on the toilet. The angle of the natural curve of the rectum and sigmoid colon changes when sitting. This can cause the tip of the tubing to scrape the intestinal wall, possibly damaging the mucosal lining, and increases risk of perforating the intestinal wall.***

Always preserve the patient's modesty and provide privacy for administration and elimination of an enema. Before beginning actual administration of the enema, position the patient in a Sims' or left lateral side-lying position (Fig. 30.2). Skill 30.1 (page 650) provides the steps for administering a cleansing enema. Skill 30.2 (page 652) explains how to administer a prepackaged enema, such as sodium phosphate (Fleets) and oil retention enemas.

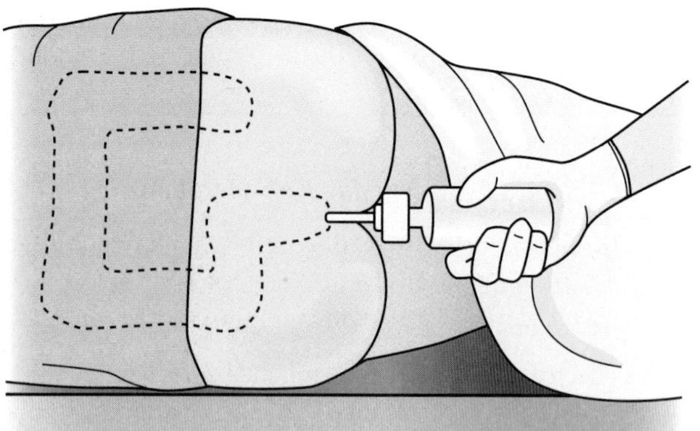

FIGURE 30.2 Patient positioned on left side in left lateral position for enema administration. Note the internal diagram of the colon.

Contraindications to Enemas

Numerous conditions may preclude you from administering an enema. It is your responsibility to assess for these conditions. Contraindications may include the following:

- Rectal surgery
- Severe bleeding hemorrhoids
- Ulcerative colitis or Crohn's disease
- Rectal fissure
- Rectal cancer
- Excessive bleeding potential due to disease or medication
- Certain heart conditions, such as myocardial infarction or unstable angina

Complications of Enemas

Enemas are normally viewed as simple procedures not requiring much knowledge or experience, but this is a myth. Administration of an enema can have serious consequences if the person administering it is not aware of the potential risks. Two serious complications are the vagal response and perforation of the intestinal wall, which can result in hemorrhage and infection.

- ***Vagal response:*** Any time you insert an enema tube into a patient's rectum, there is the possibility of stimulating the vagus nerve, which innervates not only the GI tract, but also the heart and bronchioles. ***Safety: When the vagus nerve is stimulated, it can drop the heart rate as low as 30 to 40 beats per minute (bpm) and cause constriction of the bronchioles of the lungs. As you know, a heart rate of 30 or 40 bpm is insufficient to support adequate blood pressure and circulation for longer than a few minutes, making it important to know the signs and symptoms to watch for*** (Box 30.4).

  If the patient complains of or exhibits any of these symptoms, you should immediately perform the following:
  - Stop the enema
  - Remove the tube from the rectum
  - Place the patient in the supine position
  - Assess pulse rate, skin color, and whether or not the patient is diaphoretic
  - Call for immediate assistance, but do not leave the patient
  - If the pulse rate is below 60 bpm, place the patient in the shock position, with the head lower than the feet
  - Assess blood pressure as soon as a cuff is available
  - Supply oxygen if needed

  The patient usually will recover quickly, increasing the heart rate back to the normal range and raising the blood pressure, but you must be prepared to react quickly and correctly if recovery is not immediate. When necessary, the drug of choice for raising the heart rate is atropine.
- ***Perforation of the colon:*** Always be gentle when inserting an enema tube; never force it or insert it farther than 4 to 6 inches. You should direct the tip of the tubing toward the umbilicus to follow the natural direction of the sigmoid colon. If you are not careful, it is possible to *perforate,* or go through, the intestinal wall. This can result in introduction of bacteria into the sterile peritoneal cavity, bleeding, and even hemorrhage. Again, never force the enema tubing if you meet resistance.

Box 30.4

Signs and Symptoms of Vagus Nerve Stimulation

During administration of enemas and impaction removal, you should constantly assess the patient for the following signs and symptoms of vagus nerve stimulation:

Symptoms

Complaints of:
- Chest pain
- Chest heaviness or pressure
- Shortness of breath or inability to breathe
- Dizziness
- Feeling like he or she is going to faint
- Nausea

Signs
- Pallor
- Clammy skin
- Pulse rate under 60 bpm

Please note that the patient does not have to exhibit all of the signs and symptoms; even one sign or symptom requires you to **stop administering the enema or removing the impaction** until it is established whether or not the patient can tolerate resumption of the enema.

KNOWLEDGE CONNECTION

Explain what to do if signs or symptoms of a vagal response are noted during enema administration. What can you do to reduce risk of intestinal perforation? Which enema solution is safe for administration to infants and patients with congestive heart failure? What is the normal enema volume for a cleansing enema for an adult? A 3-year-old child?

• WORD • BUILDING •

innervate: in – inside + nerv – nerve + ate – action

Supervision/Delegation Connection

Delegating Administration of an Enema

There will be times when you will need to delegate administration of an enema to a UAP or a CNA. Because you are held responsible for safe and competent administration of the enema, it is very important that you verify that the UAP or CNA has received specific training and is competent in performance of the skill. The training should be documented in writing for your best protection. It is your responsibility to assess the patient's condition and determine whether it is safe to have the UAP or CNA perform the skill. Make certain that the UAP or CNA clearly understands the vagal response, including the signs and symptoms and the actions to take if signs or symptoms are noted, and specifically to notify you immediately. It is also your responsibility to determine that the UAP or CNA understands appropriate steps to take to decrease the risk of perforating the intestinal wall.

Fecal Impaction

An **impaction** is a blockage of the movement of feces through the intestine by a mass of very hard stool. Fecal impaction may occur in the rectum, the sigmoid flexure, or any part of the large colon. It is more common in elders, patients on bedrest, and severely dehydrated patients. Any cause of constipation may lead also to impaction. One common cause, especially in elderly patients, is the abuse of laxatives. When laxatives are taken over a period of months and years, the bowel loses some of its natural contractibility, making bowel movements dependent on taking laxatives.

Sometimes small amounts of diarrhea are an indication of an impaction. In some situations, liquid stool from higher in the rectum or colon may seep around the solid impaction. When this happens, the patient may think he or she has diarrhea or may notice smears of liquid stool in the underwear or incontinence briefs. It is very important for the nurse to differentiate between diarrhea and the seepage of stool around an impaction. Remember that true diarrhea means that the patient is having several liquid stools per day. Small amounts of liquid stool seepage or just smears in the underwear are more indicative of fecal impaction, not diarrhea. If stool seepage is reported and treated as diarrhea, it will make the impaction worse. ***Safety: If an impaction is not relieved, obstruction or perforation of the bowel wall can occur.***

Nursing Interventions for Fecal Impaction

When your patient has a fecal impaction, it usually requires digital removal before administering a cleansing enema. This involves insertion of the gloved index finger into the anus to manually break the fecal mass into small pieces and remove them from the rectum. This procedure may be embarrassing as well as painful for the patient. To make the procedure less uncomfortable, it is helpful to instill an oil retention enema about 1 hour prior to digital removal. Some patients may even require mild pain medication to better tolerate the procedure. Skill 30.5 (page 655) presents the steps required to remove a fecal impaction.

There are several things you must consider before actually removing the impaction. First, review the facility's policy and procedures to determine which personnel are permitted to perform the procedure and whether or not a health-care provider's order is required. Most hospitals do not allow delegation of this procedure to a CNA or UAP. Next, review the patient's medical record for all of the patient's diagnoses. The same conditions that may contraindicate an enema may also contraindicate digital removal of impaction by the nurse. Once you have determined it is safe, you may proceed. Remember to monitor for signs of vagal nerve stimulation, just as you do with enema administration.

KNOWLEDGE CONNECTION

Explain how a patient with an impaction can exhibit signs of diarrhea.

Diarrhea

Loose or watery stools occurring three or more times a day are classified as diarrhea and may or may not be accompanied by cramping. **Tenesmus** is a persistent desire to empty the bowel when no feces is present, causing ineffective straining efforts. It may be due to inflammation in the rectum and may be experienced with bouts of diarrhea.

Elderly patients, infants, and small children dehydrate much quicker than do young or middle-aged adults, so it is important to assess these patients with diarrhea for dehydration often. Diarrhea that occurs frequently or lasts a long time can lead to fluid and electrolyte loss.

Some patients have conditions that cause intermittent diarrhea and constipation. Once the diarrhea leads to an empty bowel, peristalsis decreases and transit time is slowed. This allows more time for absorption of water, leading to formed and dryer stools, which may then result in constipation.

Factors Contributing to Diarrhea

Some of the factors that contribute to diarrhea can be controlled by the patient. Once again, teaching is very important when caring for patients with alterations in bowel elimination.

- ***Lactose intolerance:*** Some people are unable to digest lactose, a sugar found in milk and other dairy products. If they do ingest lactose-containing foods, it will usually cause them to have diarrhea. Some alternative dairy products are available with the lactose removed.
- ***Medication side effects:*** Antibiotics administered to treat infection can also kill some of the good bacteria that the body needs to stay healthy, specifically the normal flora found in the bowel. When the level of normal flora decreases, other microorganisms such as fungi are allowed to grow disproportionately, causing what is

called an *opportunistic infection.* Opportunistic infections grow in the bowel, causing diarrhea.

One of the more severe opportunistic infections is *Clostridium difficile,* otherwise known as *C. difficile.* If a *C. difficile* infection starts in a long-term care facility, it is difficult to keep it from spreading among the residents, who often have compromised immune systems.

- ***Anxiety and stress:*** High levels of stress or anxiety, as well as other emotional problems, can cause increased peristalsis and intestinal mucus production, which may result in diarrhea.
- ***Diverticulosis:*** This condition occurs when the muscular wall of the colon weakens and separates, allowing small pouches or pockets of the inner wall to protrude outward. These pouches easily trap fecal material and become inflamed. Such a pouch is called a *diverticulum.* When they become inflamed, the condition is referred to as *diverticulitis,* which can cause diarrhea and severe cramping sufficient to force a visit to a health-care provider. Diverticula have also been known to rupture, or *perforate,* allowing fecal material and bacteria to enter the sterile peritoneum and cause peritonitis, a life-threatening infection.
- ***Inflammatory processes:*** These conditions occur in response to autoimmune diseases such as Crohn's disease or by infectious microorganisms such as bacteria and viruses. The common name for bacterial or viral infections of the GI tract is *gastroenteritis.* Inflammation causes the mucosal lining and musculature of the intestinal tract to become edematous and increase mucus production. The edema and excessive mucus inhibit absorption and increase peristalsis. The result can be nausea, vomiting, cramping, or diarrhea. The transit time can be shortened dramatically, meaning that nutrients and water do not remain in the intestinal tract long enough to allow for absorption, resulting in dehydration and malnutrition.
- ***Food allergies:*** In response to food antigens, the body responds with an allergic reaction that can cause edema and inflammation of the intestinal walls with increased mucus production. The inflammation increases peristalsis, which decreases transit time, inhibits absorption, and results in diarrhea.

Laboratory and Diagnostic Connection

Diarrhea

It is important to differentiate between the possible causes of diarrhea because different causes require different types of treatment. Three laboratory tests are commonly performed to help identify the cause of diarrhea and other problems:

- *Guaiac test,* also known as an occult blood test, to test for the presence of blood in the stool
- *Culture and sensitivity* to identify microorganisms infecting the stool and the antibiotics that will kill the microorganisms
- *Ova and parasite test (O&P)* to test for presence of parasitic worms and their eggs

A stool specimen must be collected for these tests. The specimen should be placed in a specific container as indicated by facility policy and maintained at room temperature.

Nursing Interventions for Diarrhea

A variety of nursing interventions can help improve diarrhea. One important intervention is to modify food intake because the presence of food in the stomach can actually increase peristalsis. Your patient may be weak and is at risk for dehydration and electrolyte imbalance, so be very vigilant about encouraging fluids to replace what is lost.

MODIFY FOOD INTAKE AND INCREASE FLUIDS. Many health-care providers will order clear liquid diets during the first 24 hours of diarrhea caused by infection and inflammation. The clear liquids help to decrease the GI tract's digestive workload, allowing it time to rest and heal. Decaffeinated green or black teas, which contain tannin, and herbal teas such as chamomile may be used to soothe an inflamed colon and slow peristalsis. Sports drinks containing electrolytes, such as Gatorade, help to replace fluid and electrolytes lost with diarrhea. Pedialyte is an over-the-counter electrolyte replacement drink designed for infants and small children. (Refer to Chapter 29 for further details regarding fluid and electrolyte balance.) During the first 24 hours, avoid serving extremely hot or cold liquids, both of which can increase peristalsis. During this time, fluids are best tolerated if you serve them at room temperature or only slightly warmed or cooled.

If diarrhea lasts longer than 24 to 36 hours, full liquids along with any type of *cooked* fruits and vegetables, such as applesauce or carrots, may be given. Apple pectin is a common treatment for diarrhea. It is the primary ingredient found in over-the-counter antidiarrheal medications such as Kaopectate. ***Safety: Avoid serving apple juice because it will increase diarrhea.*** Aged cheeses and bananas are also considered therapeutic dietary additions for patients with diarrhea. Mashed bananas, applesauce, and cooked carrots are popular choices for infants with diarrhea. When diarrhea is due to loss of normal flora, yogurt containing active bacteria helps to replace normal flora and promote healing. It also can be used concurrently while taking prescribed antibiotics to prevent the loss of normal flora.

ADMINISTER MEDICATIONS. Various medications are available to treat diarrhea. Many are over the counter; others are only obtained by prescription. Medications to treat diarrhea may coat the mucous membranes of the bowel, inhibit peristalsis, or treat the disease or infectious process causing the diarrhea. Some medications stimulate absorption of intestinal fluids into the bloodstream and actually bind the toxins of the diarrhea-causing microorganisms so that they are removed during defecation. This not only helps to slow the diarrhea, but also helps in preventing dehydration.

Probiotics are microorganisms with health benefits, such as the microorganisms normally found in the intestines, which help digest food and produce vitamin K. They are useful in helping to prevent diarrhea caused by antibiotics and infections and help improve irritable bowel symptoms. *Lactobacillus acidophilus* is a probiotic supplement that comes in several forms. It can be used to replace normal flora or used concurrently with antibiotics to prevent loss of normal flora. It is also used as treatment for diarrhea caused by a virus known as *rotavirus.*

PROVIDE PERINEAL CARE. If the patient has diarrhea or is incontinent of stool, it is very important that you provide good perineal care to prevent the complications caused by feces on the skin. Feces are damaging to the skin and will result in irritation and excoriation if allowed to stay on the skin for extended periods of time. This destruction of skin results in loss of the body's first line of protection from infection.

Cleanse the skin around the perineum, rectum, and buttocks after each stool with a no-rinse bathing product, perineal wipe, or perineal cleaning product rather than soap and water. This is recommended because soap is alkaline and therefore irritating to the skin, and the mechanical friction of using a washcloth can cause skin damage. Rinse the skin well and pat dry. If stools are very frequent, it may be necessary to add the protection of a topical barrier cream to help prevent skin breakdown.

Fecal Incontinence

Continence, or rectal compliance, is the ability to voluntarily maintain the stool in the rectum until a convenient time for a bowel movement, as opposed to bowel or **fecal incontinence** where the voluntary control is lost. The degree or severity of incontinence may range from an occasional seepage of stool while passing flatus to continuous rectal seepage. If the nerves innervating the rectal sphincters have been damaged or severed, as in a spinal cord injury, the patient loses the ability to sense when the rectum is distended, necessitating expulsion of fecal material. Voluntary control of having a bowel movement is lost, resulting in fecal incontinence. Disoriented patients and those with arrested mental development may exhibit fecal incontinence.

Even though incontinence is beyond the patient's control, it can still be a source of guilt, serious embarrassment, and destruction of self-esteem. It can result in social isolation and perceived loss of intimacy.

Nursing Interventions for Fecal Incontinence

If the incontinence is caused by diarrhea, antidiarrheal medications may be ordered. If it is caused by seepage of stool around an impaction, the health-care provider may order removal of the impaction, enemas, and possibly stool softeners.

PROVIDE BOWEL TRAINING. When incontinence is chronic, bowel training may be initiated. The goal of bowel training is to establish regular bowel elimination. Assist the patient to the commode or onto bedpan at these times:

- When the patient arises each day
- After each meal
- Any time the patient says that his or her bowels have to move

Maintain a record of the patient's bowel activity. Once the time of day for the patient's normal bowel movement has been established, attempts are made to trigger defecation at that time. When a pattern of bowel elimination cannot be established, it is recommended to attempt to train the bowels to move within 1 hour after breakfast. This is an ideal time because the first meal of the day stimulates the strong peristalsis of the defecation reflex. Increasing fiber and fluids is also important when the patient is in a bowel training program.

PROMOTE SKIN INTEGRITY. Patients with fecal incontinence or uncontrolled diarrhea stools are at risk for skin breakdown. Topical barrier creams help to prevent excoriation, but if it is not possible to keep the patient clean and dry most of the time, a fecal incontinence pouch may be the best choice to protect skin integrity. Generally, the plastic baglike pouch has a peel-off backing around its opening. A moisture-proof barrier ring is generally used to attach the pouch to the patient's skin. The barrier ring also has a peel-off backing that must be removed before applying the ring to the skin around the anus. Apply carefully, ensuring that there are no leaks. Once the pouch is secured, fecal material drains into the pouch, which should be emptied before it is half full to prevent spills. Most systems are designed to be changed every 2 to 3 days unless a leak requires the pouch to be changed earlier.

PROVIDE EMOTIONAL SUPPORT. Whether or not the incontinence can be resolved, it is so important that you not only be professional and kind but that you also try to add an extra dose of compassion when you care for these patients. Teach nursing staff members and the patient's family members to avoid criticism or judgmental comments that may be hurtful. Be cautious in nonverbal communication as well, and avoid actions or body language that may imply that the patient is to blame or that cleaning the patient is offensive. That includes maintaining a neutral or even pleasant facial expression. Never refer to the pads used to protect the patient from fecal waste as *diapers* because this can be traumatizing to the adult patient. It is best to call them incontinence pads or briefs, or by a brand name such as Depends. Help to preserve your patient's dignity. Remember to consider: How would you feel if you were in the patient's situation?

KNOWLEDGE CONNECTION

Summarize the importance of promoting skin integrity. Describe a bowel training program. How can you help emotionally support a patient with fecal incontinence? List six possible causes of diarrhea. How can the nurse modify food and fluids to help the patient with diarrhea?

Elder Care Connection

Bowel Elimination and Aging

As healthy people age, it is common to find that their level of exercise and physical activity naturally declines. Those with health problems and debility may find their level of physical activity further hindered—and when an individual is less active, the need for the body's fuel, which is food, also decreases. When an individual eats less, he or she sometimes becomes more selective, leaning more toward favorite foods rather than focusing on maintaining a balanced and more nutritious diet.

Even issues such as improperly fitting dentures or *edentia,* the lack of teeth, decrease the ability to consume adequate levels of fiber. Any of these factors alone can result in decreased peristalsis and constipation, but when combined with the previously noted natural changes of aging, the increased risk for constipation in elders becomes obvious.

Diarrhea can result in fluid volume depletion in people of all ages but is more serious in infants and elders. A sudden water loss of as little as 5% of body weight requires treatment, while an 8% to 10% weight loss is considered to be a critical level of dehydration. If the water loss from diarrhea is not abated before the loss reaches 13% to 15% of body weight, death is likely. From 75% to 80% of an infant's weight is due to body water content, whereas an adult's is 65% to 70%, and the older adult's decreases to 55% to 60%. Elders also suffer a reduced sense of thirst. The combination of these two factors places the older adult at higher risk for dehydration as a result of diarrhea. Infants and small children will dehydrate from diarrhea the fastest of any age group because of their small size. Even though their percentage of body-water weight is higher than that of adults, their small size and weight cause even small losses of fluid to have a greater impact.

Obtaining a Stool Specimen

It will be your responsibility to collect a stool specimen when one is needed for testing. Skill 30.3 (page 653) shows the steps for collecting a stool specimen. Stool samples may be tested for the presence of parasites, parasitic eggs called ova, blood, and microorganisms. For an alert and oriented patient, you will need to explain the procedure in order to elicit his or her cooperation in the collection. It is important to use terminology that the patient understands when giving instructions about collecting the stool specimen. Include step-by-step instructions on how to collect the specimen, including washing of the hands. If the patient is an infant or is incontinent, collect the stool specimen directly from the diaper or incontinence brief.

Depending on facility policy, you may be the one to perform the test for hidden, or occult, blood while other tests will be performed by laboratory personnel. The test for blood may be referred to as a hemoccult test, a guaiac test, or simply an occult blood test and can be performed in the patient's bathroom. For further details, refer to Skill 30.4 (page 654).

Settings Connection: Medical Office

Patient Teaching for Stool Specimens

If you are instructing a nonhospitalized patient in how to obtain a stool specimen for occult blood testing, it is important to educate the patient regarding not only how to collect the specimen but dietary restrictions that should be followed for 2 to 3 days before specimen collection.

Specific food, medications, and supplements to avoid include the following:

- Anything containing red dye or food coloring
- Alcohol
- Antacids
- Antidiarrheals
- Gastric irritants such as nonsteroidal anti-inflammatory drugs (NSAIDs) or steroids
- Red Jell-O
- Red meats
- Red popsicles
- Vegetables and fruits high in peroxidase, an enzyme found in apples, bananas, grapes, and broccoli
- Vitamin C and iron supplements

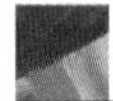

ALTERNATIVE BOWEL ELIMINATION

Certain disease processes and injuries can necessitate that a patient be provided with an alternative form of bowel elimination by surgically creating a bowel diversion. A bowel diversion is the redirection of the contents of the small or large intestine through an alternate exit site made through the abdominal wall. The fecal material, known as *effluent,* empties into an ostomy appliance, also called a bag or pouch. A need for a bowel diversion may be due to:

- Cancerous tumor
- Infarcted area in which the bowel walls have become ischemic and died
- Disease process such as Crohn's disease
- Ruptured diverticulum
- Ulcerative colitis
- Traumatic abdominal injury
- Bowel perforation

When the diversion is brought to the outside of the body through the abdominal wall, the new opening is called an

• WORD • BUILDING •

ostomy: ostium – little opening

ostomy, and the mouth of the ostomy is called a **stoma.** The name of the ostomy is determined by the area of the bowel that is brought out through the abdominal wall. If the ileum, a part of the small intestine, is used it is called an **ileostomy.** If a part of the large intestine, or colon, is used, it is called a **colostomy.** A colostomy is further identified based on the section of the large bowel utilized to form the stoma: the ascending, transverse, descending, or sigmoid colon (Fig. 30.3).

Colostomy

A colostomy stoma will have a single opening, termed a *single-barreled* or *end stoma,* if the distal colon is permanently removed, as with cancer of the descending or sigmoid colon. When a colostomy is performed due to severe inflammatory disease, such as Crohn's disease, the distal portion of the colon may not need to be removed, only allowed time to rest and heal the diseased portion. In this situation, the colon may be completely incised, or cut into two pieces. Both ends of the dissected colon are brought to the surface and two stomas are formed, a proximal and a distal stoma. This is known as a *double-barreled* colostomy stoma (see Fig. 30.3c). The stool will empty from the proximal stoma, and the distal stoma leads to the portion of the colon that is rested and allowed to heal. The only drainage from the distal stoma will be mucus produced by the mucosal lining of the intestine. The rectum and anus remain intact. After the distal portion of the colon heals, the loop is *anastomosed,* or surgically reconnected, and placed back into the abdominal cavity, and the abdominal wall closed. Normal elimination is then restored.

Another type of stoma seen in treatment of inflammatory disease is the *loop stoma.* A loop of bowel, usually the transverse colon, is brought to the surface of the abdomen. A plastic rod known as a *bridge* or *stay* is positioned under the loop of colon to keep it outside the body, and it is stitched to the abdominal wall. A slit is made in the loop and the colon is cuffed back on itself and also stitched to the abdominal wall. Stool will be expelled from the proximal opening. Occasionally the stool will seep from the proximal stoma into the distal stoma, and the patient will still have small amounts of stool coming from the rectum. This type of stoma can be difficult to fit a pouch over and is not used as often as a double-barrel colostomy.

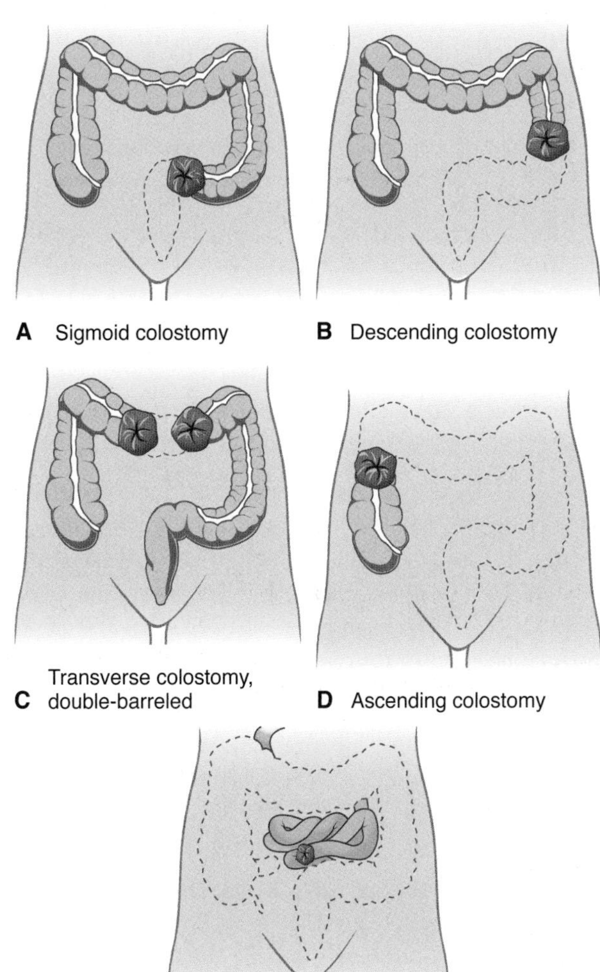

FIGURE 30.3 Locations of bowel diversion ostomies: (a) Sigmoid colostomy; (b) Descending colostomy; (c) Transverse colostomy, double-barreled; (d) Ascending colostomy; (e) Ileostomy (from Wilkinson JM, Treas LS. *Fundamentals of Nursing: Theory, Concepts & Applications.* Vol. 2. 3rd ed. Philadelphia, PA: FA Davis; 2016).

Stool Consistency Based on Location of the Colostomy

The stool consistency will depend on the section of the colon in which the stoma is located. If a colostomy is created in the ascending colon, effluent will be liquid to mushy with a foul odor. A right transverse stoma will expel mushy to semiformed effluent, while feces from a left transverse stoma will be semiformed to soft in consistency. A stoma created in the descending or sigmoid colon will produce soft to hard formed stools. This is because more water is absorbed from the feces as it has more contact with the colon.

Ileostomy

A diversion created in the ileum portion of the small intestine is known as an *ileostomy* (see Fig. 30.3e). This type of stoma is created at the end of the ileum due to the complete removal of the colon. Effluent from an ileostomy is liquid because the majority of the water is not absorbed until it reaches the colon. The effluent continually drains from the stoma, which requires that the patient constantly wear a pouch and empty it often. The effluent contains enzymes, making it very irritating to the skin surrounding the stoma. A loss of a large amount of ileostomy drainage can lead to symptoms of malnutrition and electrolyte imbalance.

Kock Pouch or Continent Ostomy

A *Kock pouch* is created for an ileostomy to help control the effluent. It is a diversion that uses the terminal portion of the

• **WORD • BUILDING •**

ileostomy: ileo – ileum + stomy – surgical opening

colostomy: colo – colon + stomy – surgical opening

ileum to form an internal pouch, or reservoir, to collect and store the effluent prior to evacuation from the body. A flap is formed that closes the reservoir, preventing leakage of the thin and watery effluent. Several times a day, the patient inserts a catheter to drain the reservoir. This type of stoma is also known as a *continent ostomy* because the patient has control over when the reservoir is drained. There are also several modified versions of the Kock pouch.

> **KNOWLEDGE CONNECTION**
> Contrast single-barreled, double-barreled, and loop stomas. Describe how an ileostomy is different from a colostomy located in the descending colon. Explain what a Kock pouch is.

Nursing Care of Patients With Ostomies

Many hospitals are now using nurses who have been specially trained to provide ostomy care. These enterostomal therapy nurses not only provide direct patient care and teaching, but also offer encouragement and emotional support, introduce the patient to ostomy support groups, serve as a resource person regarding different types of ostomy supplies, and serve as patient advocates. Their goal is to assist the patient to return to a normal life. However, even if enterostomal therapy nurses are available in your facility, it still is necessary for you to be able to assess and care for the patient with an ostomy. The enterostomal therapy nurse may not be available 24 hours a day, 7 days a week.

Assessment of the Ostomy

As with all nursing care, care of an ostomy begins with assessment or collection of data:

- What was the reason for the ostomy?
- When was the ostomy performed?
- What type of ostomy is it?
- What type of appliance, or ostomy bag, is in use?
- When was the appliance last emptied or changed?
- How much of the care is the patient able to perform, if any?

Now you will assess the patient and the stoma for objective data, noting the following:

- Contour and color of the abdomen, scars, and the surgical site; the presence of a dressing, sutures/clamps, and drains
- Appearance of the stoma, including size and edema, color, and moisture level
- Appearance of *peristomal skin,* the skin surrounding the stoma
- Characteristics of the effluent/fecal drainage
- Fit of the faceplate and fullness of the appliance bag

A new stoma should be pink to red, shiny, and moist (Fig. 30.4). Pallor, cyanosis, or a dusky color indicates impaired blood supply, while black depicts necrosis. Any impairment of blood supply should be reported to the physician and may require surgical intervention. Initially, there may be edema of the stoma, but the stoma should shrink to a small size over the first 2 to 3 weeks postsurgery. An established stoma will be smaller, pinkish-red, and drier in appearance. The peristomal skin should be free of irritation, excoriation, and erythema.

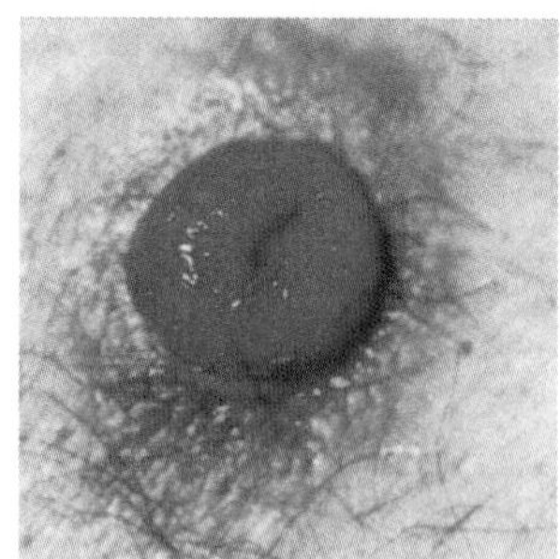

FIGURE 30.4 This healthy stoma is shiny, moist, and red (from Wilkinson JM, Treas LS. *Fundamentals of Nursing: Theory, Concepts & Applications.* Vol. 2. 3rd ed. Philadelphia, PA: FA Davis; 2016).

> **KNOWLEDGE CONNECTION**
> What assessments should be made for a new colostomy? What abnormal findings would require reporting to the physician?

Nursing Interventions

When you are caring for the patient with an ostomy, you may be the person who changes and cleans the appliance for the first few times. Eventually, you will need to teach the patient and a family member how to do this as well.

MEASURING A STOMA. Ostomy appliances come in different sizes. To determine the correct size flange and opening on the ostomy bag to use, the stoma must be measured. The stoma size is determined using a stoma measuring device made of card stock. The card has different sizes of holes cut out, each labeled with its corresponding size. The measuring device is placed over the stoma to determine the size of the opening on the ostomy bag that will best fit. The correct size will fit around the stoma and allow only a $\frac{1}{16}$ to $\frac{1}{8}$ inch of peristomal skin to show (Fig. 30.5). Once the correct size has been determined, it is used to select the corresponding size flange on the ostomy bag.

SELECTING AN OSTOMY APPLIANCE. Ostomy appliances also come in different types (Fig. 30.6). Some appliances are designed as a one-piece unit that has an attached adhesive disk that is applied directly to the patient's abdomen after the protective backing is peeled off the adhesive disk. Others are

• **WORD • BUILDING** •

enterostomal: entero – intestines + stom – surgical opening + al – related to

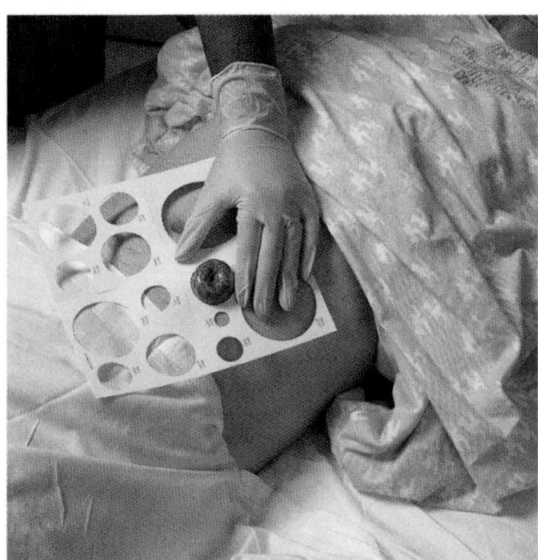

FIGURE 30.5 This nurse uses a device to measure the stoma size (from Wilkinson JM, Treas LS. *Fundamentals of Nursing: Theory, Concepts & Applications.* Vol. 2. 3rd ed. Philadelphia, PA: FA Davis; 2016).

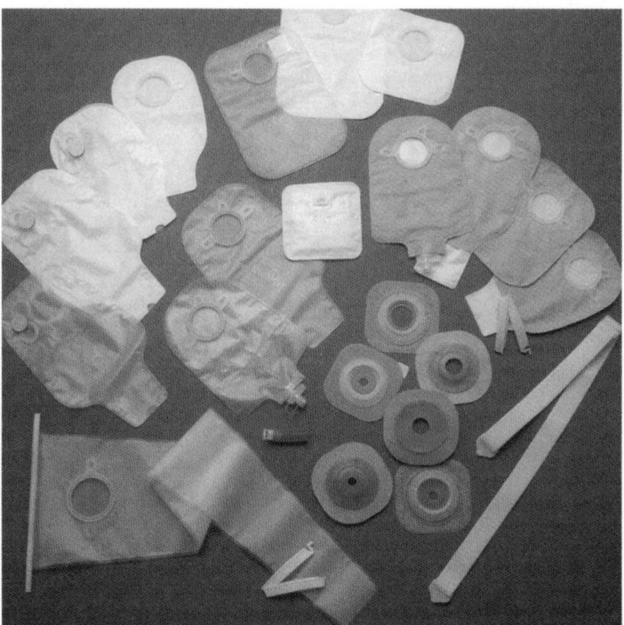

FIGURE 30.6 Ostomy supplies (from Wilkinson JM, Treas LS. *Fundamentals of Nursing: Theory, Concepts & Applications.* Vol. 2. 3rd ed. Philadelphia, PA: FA Davis; 2016).

designed as two-piece units; the bag attaches to an adhesive disk called a *wafer faceplate,* which adheres to the abdomen. The bag flange snaps onto the plastic flange on the wafer faceplate, somewhat like Tupperware lids attach. The faceplate is changed every 3 to 5 days or sooner if the adhesive backing begins to loosen from the skin. Once the adhesive on the faceplate begins to lose contact with the skin, it allows effluent to leak underneath the faceplate, which can cause severe excoriation of the skin. If leakage continues unheeded, infection and further ulceration of tissue can occur. Be sure to select the correct appliance based on what has been in use unless the enterostomal therapist indicates that a change should be made.

EMPTYING THE APPLIANCE. Empty the ostomy appliance bag when it is one-third to one-half full to prevent leaking and odor. Most bags have a drain located or open edge at the bottom that can be opened to empty it. Some patients prefer to remove the bag and apply a new one; others prefer to empty the bag, rinse it in cool water, dry it, and reapply. Ostomy supplies are generally expensive, making it difficult for some patients to afford them. This may limit how often the patient is willing to apply new bags. For further details regarding changing an ostomy appliance, refer to Skill 30.6 (page 656). For an example of electronic documentation of ostomy care, refer to Figure 30.7.

PROVIDING SKIN CARE. When applying or changing an appliance, assess the stoma and the skin around it to make certain there is no irritation, excoriation, or ulceration. Then use a soft washcloth, warm water, and mild soap to wash the stoma and skin, rinse thoroughly, and pat dry. Numerous products are available for use to help protect the skin around the stoma. An example is a protective barrier cream that may be used around the stoma to protect the small area of skin that shows after the appliance is in place.

PROVIDING EMOTIONAL SUPPORT. If the ostomy is new, assess the patient for how well he or she is dealing with the new stoma. Does the patient look at the new stoma or avert his or her eyes? Does the patient make eye contact with you? Ask questions regarding care of the stoma? Verbalize desire to learn about stoma care? This can be a blow to a patient's self-esteem, and the patient's attitude may largely depend on your reactions during provision of nursing care. Be careful to exhibit acceptance. Be matter of fact in your responses to the patient and in your demeanor as you provide ostomy care.

Irrigating a Colostomy

A colostomy irrigation is similar to an enema. Colostomies may be irrigated to evacuate stool due to constipation, or irrigation may be used postoperatively for stomas located in the descending or sigmoid colon. When irrigating a descending or sigmoid colostomy, the goal is to train the ostomy to evacuate at the same time each day. Because the stool is formed, it is possible to train the bowel to evacuate in the morning right after breakfast when peristalsis is naturally stimulated by eating breakfast. If the bowel is trained to move early in the day, some patients find that they can wear just a stoma cap rather than a bag for the rest of the day. This helps the patient have a greater sense of control. Skill 30.7 (page 658) provides more information on colostomy irrigation.

> **KNOWLEDGE CONNECTION**
>
> How do you determine which size of colostomy bag opening would best meet the patient's needs? How often should an appliance bag be emptied? How often should you change the faceplate and appliance bag? Explain two purposes for colostomy irrigation.

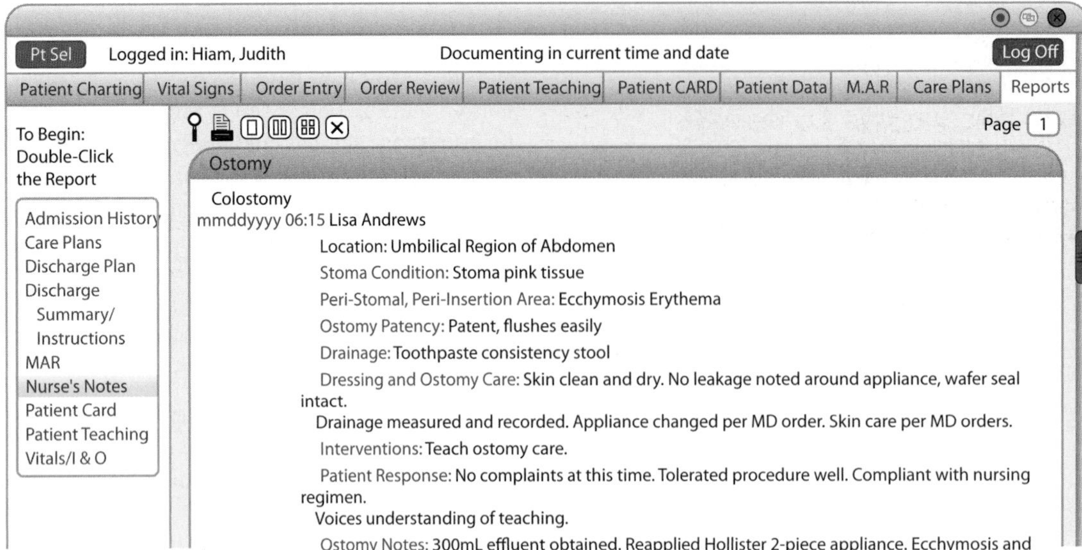

FIGURE 30.7 Sample electronic documentation of ostomy care.

Nursing Care Plan for a Patient With a New Colostomy of the Descending Colon

Your patient is a 39-year-old male who had severe ulcerative colitis that necessitated removal of the distal portion of his colon 1 day ago. He now has a permanent colostomy in the descending colon. He has refused to look at the stoma or drainage bag, but he has verbalized that he knows that he will have to learn how to take care of the colostomy. He has a very supportive wife and two teenage sons.

Assessment

Your first step in planning care for a patient with a colostomy is to gather all available data, including assessment of the colostomy stoma. Begin by seeking the answers to these questions:

- What patient teaching has already been done?
- Has referral to a support group been made?

The data you collect tell you that the patient's stoma is still edematous and a reddish color. It is moist and shiny, with a heavy coating of clear mucus. It is located on the left side of the abdomen. As you assess the stoma and effluent, you notice that the patient glances down at the stoma briefly a couple of times and then looks away. The rest of the time, he looks directly at you. The effluent is brown and semiformed with lots of mucus. The bag is about one-quarter full. A 1 ½-inch flanged colostomy bag with a drain in the bottom is currently in use. The peristomal skin is intact but slightly erythematous. There are no blisters or signs of bleeding. The patient acknowledges current incisional pain at a level of 7 on a scale of 1 to 10. He states that he has been trying to avoid asking for pain medication because he does not like to take it. No patient teaching or referral to an ostomy support group has been done. Toward the end of your focused assessment, he asks you if the "thing" will always look this gross, and how a person ever overcomes the feelings of disgust when caring for the colostomy.

Nursing Diagnoses

You are encouraged because the patient at least glanced at his stoma while you were performing the assessment. Having noted that he was looking at you most of the time, you were careful to make frequent eye contact with him so that he was able to observe your level of comfort and acceptance while looking at his stoma. You were careful to avoid making any type of facial expression that could be interpreted as unpleasant, unaccepting, or disgusted. He also asked you about overcoming feelings of disgust when caring for the colostomy, indicating that he is able to express at least some feelings about the stoma. This may indicate that he is ready to ask for help in adjusting to the change in body image.

The nursing diagnoses given for this patient include:

- Acute pain
- Impaired skin integrity
- Disturbed body image

Planning

Plan first to address his pain. When a person is in pain, it is difficult to deal with an altered body image. Reviewing his health-care provider's orders, you find that he does have pain medications ordered. You also review the medication administration record and find that he has not had anything for pain since late on the day of surgery. When you ask him about it, he tells you that he does not like to take pain medications, that "only wimps need drugs for pain." He also tells you that he has not been out of bed since surgery. You explain to him that pain impedes or slows the healing process, and that it is important to relieve his pain so that he can better deal with other aspects of his care as well as to speed the healing process so he can go home as soon as possible.

You know that he will need emotional support even after he is discharged, so you ask him if you may refer him to the local ostomy support group and schedule the first visit for the next day. While discussing the advantages of a support group, he tells you that his wife has voiced interest in learning how to care for his colostomy, and you encourage her participation.

Implementation

You are now at the stage of the nursing process to implement, or actually perform, the interventions that you have planned, as described in the care plan.

Nursing Care Plan for a Patient With a New Colostomy of the Descending Colon—cont'd

Evaluation
Once the interventions, or nursing actions, have been performed, you will want to evaluate whether or not they were effective (as described in the care plan). Did they accomplish what you intended? Did they help the patient's problem?

The patient is exhibiting more acceptance and says that it is not nearly as gross as he had feared it would be. He expresses gratitude to you for introducing him to the support group and for helping manage his pain better and adjust to his "new normal."

Nursing Diagnosis: Acute pain, related to surgical incision, as evidenced by c/o pain and reluctance to take pain medicines
Expected Outcomes: Analgesic will effectively reduce pain below 4 within 30 minutes of administration of injection. Patient will ambulate in hall a minimum of three times per day by tomorrow. Patient will demonstrate proper splinting of abdomen when coughing and ambulating by tomorrow.

Interventions	Evaluations
Use a pain scale of 1 to 10 to assess for pain and discomfort several times per shift, describing characteristics of pain.	Day 2: Initial c/o pain @ 7. Day 3: C/o pain @ 5. Day 5: C/o pain @ 4.
Encourage the patient to ask for pain medication before pain becomes severe enough to limit movement.	Day 2: Waited until pain was 7 before asking for meds, reminded to call earlier to try to keep pain below 4. Day 3: Called for med at level 5 pain.
Ambulate the patient in the hall at least 3–4 times/day, splinting his abdomen as needed.	Day 2: With assistance, ambulated 30 ft in hallway twice and 50 ft twice, tolerated with minimal increase in pain, states splinting helped; passed some flatus. Day 3: With standby assistance, ambulated 50 ft once and 100 ft three times. States he now feels much better after each ambulation.
Get the patient up in a chair for all meals and prn.	Day 2: Assisted to chair for all meals, tolerated w/o complaints. Ambulated w/assist in room. Day 3: To chair w/standby assistance. Tolerated w/o complaint. Then amb in hall twice w/o assistance. Day 5: Gets up for meals and walks ad lib without assistance or prompting.

Nursing Diagnosis: Impaired skin integrity, related to surgical procedure, as evidenced by irritated periostomal skin, stoma, and surgical incision
Expected Outcomes: Stoma will remain pink and moist until discharge. Edema will begin to decrease within 2 days.

Interventions	Evaluations
Assess the stoma for color, moisture, edema, and size daily on the 7/3 shift.	Day 2: Red, moist, lots of mucus, moderate edema, measures 1 ¼-in diameter. Day 3: Red, moist, lots of mucus, decreasing edema, 1 ¼-in diameter. Day 5: Healing, pinkish-red, moist, less mucus today, diameter is 1 1/16 in. Day 6: Pinkish red, moist, less mucus, 1-in diameter.
Assess peristomal skin for erythema, edema, and intactness of skin at least once per shift.	Day 2: Slight erythema, no edema, skin intact. Day 3: Slight erythema, no edema, skin intact. Day 5: No erythema or edema, skin intact.

(nursing care plan continues on page 650)

Nursing Care Plan for a Patient With a New Colostomy of the Descending Colon—cont'd

Interventions	Evaluations
Gently cleanse the stoma and peristomal skin each time the appliance bag is emptied and at least once per shift if the bag does not have to be emptied.	Day 2: Cleansed 3 times on 7/3. Day 3: Cleansed 4 times on 7/3. Day 5: Cleansed once on 7/3.
Empty the appliance bag when ⅓ to ½ full to prevent constant contact of stool on skin.	Day 2: Emptied 3 times on 7/3. Day 3: He emptied bag twice, emptied twice by nurse. Day 5: Emptied once on 7/3.

Nursing Diagnosis: Disturbed body image, related to new colostomy, as evidenced by avoidance of looking at stoma and comments about the stoma
Expected Outcomes: Patient will agree to visit with support group by day 4. Patient will observe stoma care by day 2. Patient will be able to explain various steps to prevent flatus and accidental spillage of effluent by discharge.

Interventions	Evaluations
Obtain the patient's permission to refer him to the local ostomy support group and make arrangements for visits to begin ASAP.	Day 2: Permission granted. Support group notified, will be here this afternoon.
Provide the patient with ample time to verbalize his concerns. Make time to sit with the patient 5–10 minutes a couple of times a day to encourage him to talk.	Day 2: Sat with him twice before support group came, he asked few questions; sat with him once after group, he asked more questions. Day 3: Sat with him; he verbalized concerns RE: odor control, other people "knowing" about ostomy. Discussion lasted 20–25 minutes. Day 5: Definitely more optimistic.
Make frequent eye contact during provision of colostomy care. Maintain a pleasant facial expression, smiling when appropriate.	Day 2: Makes eye contact only briefly. Day 3: Making much better eye contact. Smiled a couple of times during care and teaching.
Teach the patient that irrigating a colostomy located in the descending colon may allow him to regulate bowel movements and may even eliminate the need to wear an appliance during the day.	Day 3: Says this gives him "more hope." Day 5: As frequency of evacuation decreases, expresses more satisfaction.
Teach the patient to avoid foods that cause excess flatus.	Day 3: Verbally verifies understanding.
Teach the patient about products that he can use to reduce odors.	Day 3: Verbalizes understanding.
Encourage the patient and his wife to talk about their feelings regarding sexual activity.	Day 3: State they have already discussed with support group and understand, optimistic.

Skill 30.1 Administering a Cleansing Enema

Assessment Steps

1. Review the health-care provider's order and patient's age for type and volume to administer. ***This identifies what supplies are needed.*** If the health-care provider fails to indicate the volume of fluid to use, be certain to reference your facility's policy regarding volumes for the various age groups, such as small children. *Safety: Never administer an adult large volume of 1,000 mL to a small child. This could result in bowel rupture. Generally, the volume is 100 to 250 mL for small children and 250 to 500 mL for school-age children. Encourage the health-care provider to order the volume if there is any uncertainty.*
2. *Safety: Review the patient's medical record for conditions that might contraindicate administration of an enema, such as glaucoma, increased intracranial pressure, or recent rectal or prostate surgery. If such a condition is noted, notify the health-care provider for further clarification of the enema order. Also*

Skill 30.1 (continued)

assess for history of bowel disorders such as diverticulitis, ulcerative colitis, recent bowel surgery, abdominal pain or distention, and hemorrhoids. These may put the patient at risk for complications such as perforation.

3. Assess the patient's cognitive level and level of mobility and check orders for activity level. ***This determines whether a bedpan or bedside commode will be needed.***
4. Assess the patient's rectal sphincter control. ***This identifies the need to administer the enema solution while the patient is on the bedpan.***
5. Assess for last bowel movement, abdominal distention, and the presence of bowel sounds. ***This provides a baseline for evaluation of effectiveness.***

Planning Steps

1. Gather needed equipment and supplies: several pairs of clean examination gloves, a disposable protective gown, a waterproof pad, water-soluble lubricant, a "do not enter" sign to place on the room door, toilet tissue, washcloths and towel, a bath blanket, a bedpan with cover or bedside commode if needed, an enema administration set and solution for the type of enema ordered, and an IV pole.

Implementation Steps

1. Follow the Initial Implementation Steps located on the inside back cover.
2. Place the bedpan nearby or the commode near the bed ***for easy access after the enema is administered.*** *Safety: Arrange furniture and equipment to provide a clear pathway to the commode; if the patient is able to ambulate to the bathroom, open the bathroom door and clear the pathway. Position nonskid slippers and toilet tissue close by.*
3. Open and assemble the supplies. Close the clamp on the administration set tubing ***to prevent fluid from escaping before you begin the procedure.***
4. Prepare solution as needed and fill the container to the desired volume. *Safety: Water temperature should be between 105°F and 110°F (40.5°C to 43.3°C) to prevent burns and cold water cramping. Never heat water in a microwave oven.* If preparing an SS enema, add castile soap at a ratio of 5 mL per 1,000 mL normal saline or tap water. If the enema volume is 500 mL, then add only 2.5 mL of soap. *Safety: Add the castile soap only after you have all the water in the container. Otherwise you will have a great deal of soapsuds.*
5. Hang the container on the IV pole and prime the enema administration tubing: Open the clamp and allow solution to dispel all the air in the tubing. Then close the clamp. ***This prevents air from entering the colon, causing painful gas for your patient.***
6. Don clean procedure gloves ***to prevent the transmission of bacteria.***
7. Position the patient in the left lateral side-lying position or Sims' position, with a waterproof pad beneath the hips while you stand on the patient's right side. ***This allows gravity to assist with the retention of the solution by pulling the solution directly into the sigmoid and descending colon and allows you to visualize the anus.*** If the patient is short of breath, elevate the head of the bed very slightly.
8. Cover the patient with a bath blanket, exposing only the buttocks and rectum, ***to provide privacy and preserve modesty.***
9. If the patient does not have good sphincter control or cannot get out of bed, place the bedpan flat on the bed, directly beneath the rectum, up against the patient's buttocks ***to catch the enema fluid when it returns.***
10. Lubricate 4 to 6 inches of the distal end of the tubing with a water-soluble lubricant such as K-Y jelly ***to facilitate easy insertion into the rectum.***
11. If necessary, lift the superior buttock to expose the anus. Carefully and slowly insert the tip of the tubing 3 to 4 inches into the rectum, directing the tip toward the umbilicus ***so that it enters the rectum without causing trauma.*** Have the patient take slow, deep breaths ***to relax the sphincter.*** *Safety: If the tube does not pass easily into the rectum, allow a small amount of fluid to flow through the tubing for additional lubrication and try again. Do not force the entry.*
12. While holding the enema administration container at the patient's hip level, release the tubing clamp and begin instillation of the solution. Gradually raise the container to a height of 12 to 18 inches above the patient's hip level. Instill the solution slowly. ***Raising the height of the enema container too fast or too high increases the rate at which solution is instilled. The faster solution is instilled, the less the patient is able to receive and retain the solution. It also will result in more cramping and discomfort for the patient.***

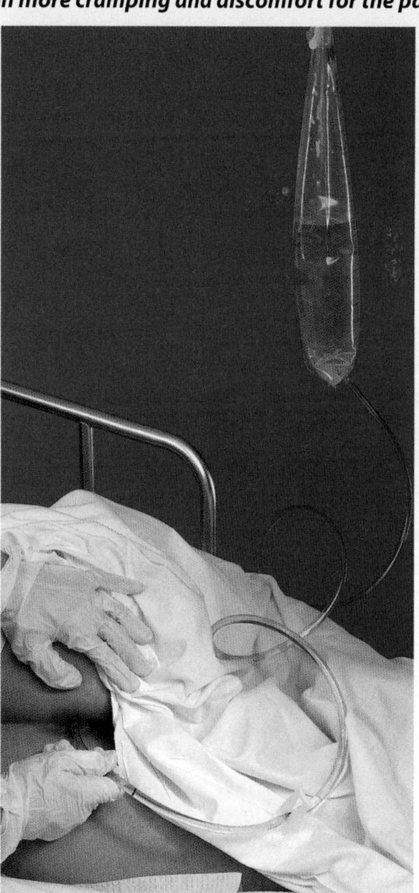

(skill continues on page 652)

Skill 30.1 (continued)

13. Continuously monitor the patient. If the patient complains of cramping, clamp the tubing for 15 to 30 seconds and instruct the patient to take slow, deep breaths through pursed lips or lower the container to decrease the flow. ***This will help the patient be more comfortable and be able to retain the solution longer.*** *Safety: Continually monitor the patient for signs and symptoms of vagal stimulation.*
14. Upon completion of instillation, clamp the tubing and carefully and slowly remove it from the patient's anus, covering the dirty tip with paper towels or toilet tissue. Clean the rectal area.
15. Cover the patient and instruct him or her to hold the enema solutions for approximately 5 to 15 minutes ***to improve the effectiveness of the enema.*** Place call light near.
16. Dispose of the enema supplies according to facility policy. Or if they are reusable, rinse with tap water and hang to dry in the bathroom.
17. Remove your gloves and perform hand hygiene.
18. When the patient is ready, apply clean examination gloves and assist the patient to the bathroom or bedside commode if allowed. Otherwise, place the patient on the bedpan and raise the head of the bed to 80 to 90 degrees, making certain that toilet tissue or disposable wipes and the call light are within the patient's reach. ***This puts the patient in a natural position for defecation.*** Provide privacy.
19. Remove gloves and protective gown. Wash hands.
20. After the patient has defecated, remove the bedpan or assist the patient back to bed. Then inspect the stool for color, consistency, and amount of return and document it.
21. After expulsion of the enema, apply clean examination gloves and assist the patient as needed to cleanse the anus and buttocks. Be certain to rinse and dry skin thoroughly ***to prevent chapping.***
22. Follow the Ending Implementation Steps located on the inside back cover.
23. Document the administration procedure, including the type and volume instilled, the patient's tolerance, and the return results, including the characteristics of the stool.

Evaluation Steps

1. Assess returned enema results, including the amount, color, and consistency.
2. Assess the patient's abdomen for distention and bowel sounds. Make certain the patient is comfortable and has no further needs before leaving the room.

Sample Documentation

12/29/22 0930 Bowel sounds hypoactive in all 4 quadrants. Abdomen slightly distended, but soft. States last BM was 3 days ago, and complains of a sense of "fullness and bloating" in abdomen. 1,000-mL NS enema administered rectally per health-care provider's orders. Received and retained full volume without difficulty or complaints of cramping. Assisted to bathroom. Expelled large volume of brown, soft, formed stool without difficulty. Perineal care performed. Bowel sounds active in all 4 quadrants. Abdomen now flat and soft. Expresses feelings of relief and improved comfort.
________________ Nurse's signature and credentials

Skill 30.2 Administering a Prepackaged Enema (Sodium Phosphate or Oil Retention)

Assessment Steps

1. Review the health-care provider's order and patient's age for type and volume to administer. ***This identifies what supplies are needed.*** If the health-care provider fails to indicate the volume of fluid to use, be certain to reference your facility's policy regarding volumes for the various age groups, such as small children.
2. *Safety: Review the patient's medical record for conditions that might contraindicate administration of an enema, such as glaucoma, increased intracranial pressure, or recent rectal or prostate surgery. If such a condition is noted, notify the health-care provider for further clarification of the enema order. Also assess for history of bowel disorders such as diverticulitis, ulcerative colitis, recent bowel surgery, abdominal pain or distention, and hemorrhoids. These may put the patient at risk for complications such as perforation.*
3. Assess the patient's cognitive level and level of mobility and check orders for activity level. ***This determines whether a bedpan or bedside commode will be needed.***
4. Assess the patient's rectal sphincter control. ***This identifies the need to administer the enema solution while the patient is on the bedpan.***
5. Assess for last bowel movement, abdominal distention, and the presence of bowel sounds. ***This provides a baseline for evaluation of effectiveness.***

Planning Steps

1. Gather needed equipment and supplies: several pairs of clean examination gloves, disposable protective gown, waterproof pad, water-soluble lubricant, "do not enter" sign to place on the room door, toilet tissue, washcloths and towel, bath blanket, bedpan with cover or bedside commode if needed, and prepackaged enema.

Implementation Steps

1. Follow the Initial Implementation Steps located on the inside back cover.
2. Place the bedpan nearby or the commode near the bed ***for easy access after the enema is administered.*** *Safety: Arrange furniture and equipment to provide a clear pathway to the commode. If the patient is able to ambulate to the bathroom, open the bathroom door and clear the pathway. Position nonskid slippers and toilet tissue close by.*

Skill 30.2 (continued)

3. Follow Steps 6–9 of Skill 30.1 regarding gloving, positioning, and draping.
4. Take the prepackaged enema out of the box and hold the bottle under warm running water. ***This helps to warm the solution in the bottle so that it does not cause cramping when instilled.***
5. Remove the plastic cap from the tip. Although the enema comes prelubricated, you may need to add more lubricant ***to make it easier to insert the tip into the rectum.***
6. Tilt the container slightly as you insert the tip 3 to 4 inches into the rectum. Slowly roll and squeeze the container until all of the solution is instilled ***to ensure that the container is completely emptied.***

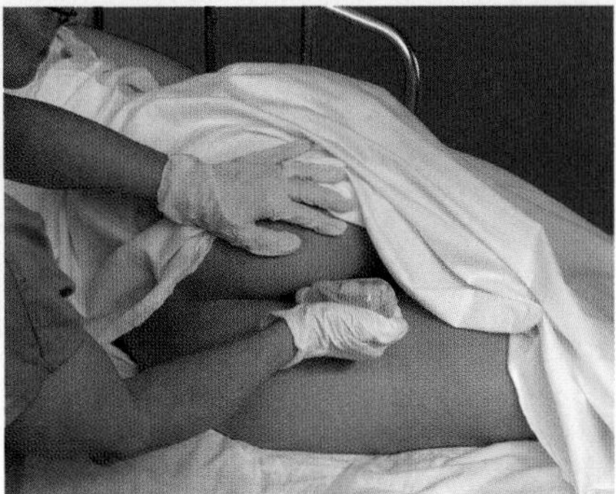

7. Withdraw the enema tip from the rectum and clean the area.
8. Cover the patient and encourage him or her to hold the enema solution for 5 to 10 minutes. **For an oil retention enema, the patient should be instructed to hold the oil for at least 30 minutes.**
9. Discard the empty container according to facility policy.
10. Follow Steps 18–24 of Skill 30.1.

Evaluation Steps

1. Assess returned enema results, including the amount, color, and consistency.
2. Assess the patient's abdomen for distention and bowel sounds. Make certain the patient is comfortable and has no further needs before leaving the room.

Sample Documentation

12/29/22 0930 Bowel sounds hypoactive in all 4 quadrants. Abdomen slightly distended, but soft. States last BM was 3 days ago, and complains of a sense of "fullness and bloating" in abdomen. Fleet enema administered rectally per health-care provider's orders. Received and retained without difficulty or complaints of cramping. Assisted to bathroom. Expelled large volume of brown, soft, formed stool without difficulty. Perineal care performed. Bowel sounds active in all 4 quadrants. Abdomen now flat and soft. Expresses feelings of relief and improved comfort ——————

—————————— Nurse's signature and credentials

Skill 30.3 Obtaining a Stool Specimen for Culture, and Ova and Parasites

Assessment Steps

1. Review the health-care provider's orders for type of test and stool specimen to obtain.
2. Review the patient's chart for activity restrictions, level of mobility, and cognition. ***This helps to determine if the patient can get up to the bedside commode or bathroom or requires use of a bedpan for collection of the specimen.***
3. Review facility policy and procedure ***to ensure that you are performing the procedure correctly.***

Planning Steps

1. Gather needed equipment and supplies: specimen container, tongue blade, bedpan if on bedrest or specimen pan for toilet or bedside commode if patient is able to get up, examination gloves, plastic bag in which to place the specimen container after specimen collection, and laboratory requisition.
2. Instruct the patient to notify you as soon as he or she has the urge to defecate ***so that you can obtain a stool specimen.***

Implementation Steps

1. Follow the Initial Implementation Steps located on the inside back cover.
2. Provide privacy during elimination.
3. If the patient is able to get up, place the specimen pan under the rim of the toilet or bedside commode at the back ***to catch the feces.***
4. Place the patient on the clean and dry bedpan or assist to the bedside commode or toilet.
5. Instruct the patient to empty the bladder if necessary before defecation ***to avoid contamination of stool specimen with urine.*** Tell the patient that toilet tissue should not be placed in the specimen pan or bedpan, whichever is used, ***to prevent contamination of the specimen.***
6. After the bowels have moved, remove the bedpan if one is in use; wear gloves to assist the patient to clean the perineal area as needed.
7. If the patient got up for the bowel movement, assist the patient back to bed and make him or her comfortable.
8. Wear gloves for collection of the stool specimen ***to prevent contact with blood or body fluids.***
9. Using a clean tongue blade, collect 1 to 2 inches of formed stool and place inside the appropriate specimen container for the ordered test. Take the stool specimen from at least two areas of the feces, collecting any abnormal specimen findings such as blood, mucus, or visible parasites or eggs. ***This allows the laboratory to test any abnormalities in the stool.*** If the stool is liquid, place 1 to 2 ounces of liquid stool in the specimen container. Close the container lid securely ***to prevent leakage.***

(skill continues on page 654)

Skill 30.3 (continued)

10. Complete and apply a label to the specimen container, including the patient's name, ID number, and room number; the health-care provider's name; the test to be run; and the date and time of specimen collection. Place the capped specimen container inside a plastic bag for delivery of the specimen to the laboratory. ***This protects you and anyone else handling the specimen from contact with blood or body fluids.***
11. Empty the bedpan or bedside commode of any remaining stool. Flush the toilet and clean the bedpan or bedside commode.
12. Follow the Ending Implementation Steps located on the inside back cover.
13. Deliver the specimen to the laboratory within 15 minutes of collection ***so that it can be tested while it is fresh, while any ova or parasites that may be present in the specimen are still alive.***
14. Document the type of stool specimen collected, including color and consistency of the fecal specimen, date and time of collection, and delivery time to the laboratory.

Evaluation Step

1. Assess the patient for comfort and needs before leaving room.

Sample Documentation

11/10/22 0915 Assisted to bathroom for defecation. Stool specimen collected for culture and sensitivity. Feces yellowish-brown, liquid consistency. Delivery to lab at 0925
———————— Nurse's signature and credentials

Skill 30.4 Performing Guaiac Testing: Testing Stool Specimen for Occult Blood

Assessment Steps

1. Review the health-care provider's order for type of test to be done.
2. Review the patient's chart to determine the patient's level of cognition and mobility. ***This helps to determine if the patient can get up to the bedside commode or bathroom or requires use of a bedpan for collection of the specimen.***
3. Review facility policy for this procedure. Read guaiac test card instructions.

Planning Step

1. Gather needed equipment and supplies: guaiac card with instructions for performing the test, tongue blade, bottle of developer, bedpan if on bedrest or specimen pan for toilet or bedside commode if the patient is able to get up, examination gloves, plastic bag in which to place specimen test card after specimen collection, and laboratory requisition.

Implementation Steps

1. Follow the Initial Implementation Steps located on the inside back cover, including explaining the purpose of the test.
2. Provide privacy during elimination.
3. Apply clean examination gloves.
4. If the patient is able to get up, place the specimen pan under the rim of the toilet or bedside commode ***to catch the feces.***
5. Place the patient on the clean and dry bedpan, or assist to the bedside commode or toilet.
6. Instruct the patient to empty the bladder if necessary before defecation ***to avoid contamination of stool specimen with urine.*** Tell the patient that toilet tissue should not be placed in the specimen pan or bedpan, whichever is used, ***to prevent contamination of the specimen.***
7. After the bowels have moved, remove the bedpan if one is in use; wear gloves to assist the patient to clean the perineal area as needed.
8. If the patient got up for the bowel movement, assist the patient back to bed and make him or her comfortable.
9. Use the wooden tongue blade for collection of the stool specimen. Select the specimen from two different areas of the stool, especially any part of stool that is red, maroon, black, or tarry in appearance. Use a separate tongue blade or wooden stick for each specimen. ***This allows for testing of the areas most likely to contain blood.***
10. Wrap the tongue blade in tissue and a paper towel, then dispose of it according to facility policy.
11. Read the specific kit instructions carefully before applying the stool sample and developer. Manufacturers may vary in which side of the card to apply the feces or how many drops of developer to use. According to test card instructions, apply a thin smear of feces to the two sample areas and close the flaps. Wait the instructed length of time before applying developer ***to ensure accurate results.***
12. According to specific kit instructions, apply the designated number of developer drops onto the opposite side of the card from the specimens, directly over each of the two feces smears. This allows the developer to penetrate the paper to the specimen. Also apply the designated number of drops directly onto the spot labeled "control."

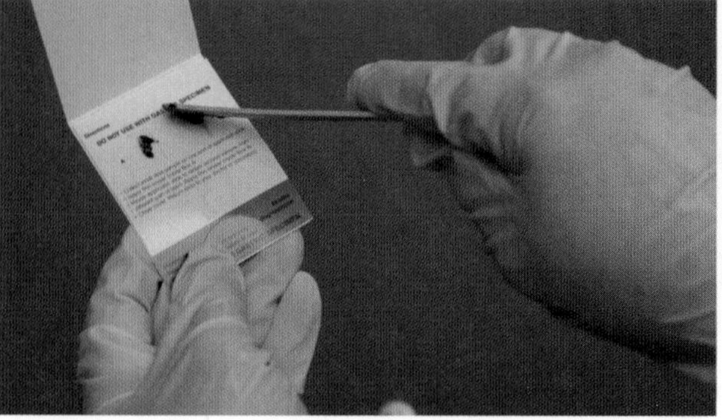

Skill 30.4 (continued)

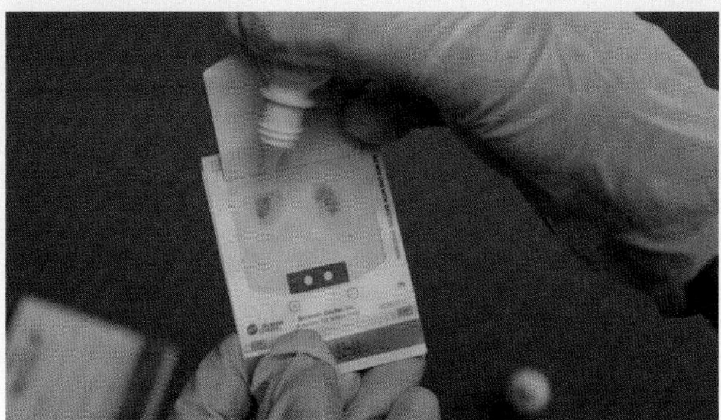

13. Wait for the designated length of time before reading the test results. If the color on the control site turns the paper a bluish color, ***this is indicative of a positive result.*** Compare the two feces sample sites to the control site. ***The test results are positive for the presence of blood if the feces smears turn a blue or bluish-purple color, similar to the control color. The test results are negative if the smears do not turn blue.***
14. Most facility policies require the guaiac test card to be placed in a plastic bag and delivered to the laboratory ***for verification of the test results.***
15. Follow the Ending Implementation Steps located on the inside back cover.
16. Document the characteristics of the bowel movement, including color, amount, and consistency of the feces and whether the results were negative or positive.

Evaluation Step

1. Notify the health-care provider according to facility policy regarding positive results for the presence of blood.

Sample Documentation

11/23/22 0835 Assisted to bedside commode for bowel movement. Specimen obtained and applied to guaiac test card. Feces were small amount of brown formed stool with small amount of bright red streaking throughout stool. Test results for presence of blood were positive. Specimen sent to lab for verification. Health-care provider telephoned about positive results.

Nurse's signature and credentials

Skill 30.5 Removing a Fecal Impaction

Assessment Steps

1. Review facility policy to determine who may perform this procedure and whether a health-care provider's order is required. If required, review the health-care provider's order.
2. Review the patient's medical record for conditions that might contraindicate digital removal of an impaction by a nurse.
3. Assess the patient's pulse rate and blood pressure to establish a baseline, as well as assessing for abdominal distention.

Planning Step

1. Gather needed equipment and supplies, such as several pairs of clean examination gloves, disposable protective gown, water-soluble lubricant such as K-Y jelly, waterproof pad, cover for bedpan (a disposable pad similar to the waterproof pad to be placed under the patient works well), toilet tissue, washcloths and towels, wash basin, and "do not enter" sign for room door.

Implementation Steps

1. Follow the Initial Implementation Steps located on the inside back cover.
2. Provide privacy and protect modesty as well as you can.
3. Position yourself on the right side of the bed. Position the patient in a left lateral side-lying or left Sims' position ***to facilitate access to the rectum and lower sigmoid colon.***
4. Cover the patient with a bath blanket, exposing only the rectum and buttocks, ***to provide warmth and privacy.***
5. Place a waterproof pad underneath the patient's hips ***to protect the linens.***
6. Position the bedpan on the bed close to the buttocks ***to help prevent unnecessary soiling of linens.*** Have toilet tissue within reach.
7. Generously lubricate your gloved index finger ***to reduce the discomfort of the procedure.***
8. Gently insert the finger into the anus and past both the outer and inner rectal sphincters until the fecal mass is located. Tell the patient to take slow, deep breaths during the procedure ***to help relax the sphincter.***
9. Slide the index finger between the outside of the fecal mass and the intestinal wall. Flex the finger toward the center of the fecal mass. ***This allows you to break up the mass so that it can be removed.*** *Safety: Never flex the finger toward the outside of the fecal mass, toward the intestinal wall. This increases risk of perforating the bowel wall.*
10. Using as little motion of the finger as possible, gently break up the fecal mass into small pieces and remove them from the rectum. ***This relieves the blockage caused by the impaction and causes the least discomfort to the patient.*** Place feces in the bedpan and repeat the process until the impaction is removed.
11. Continually monitor the patient for signs and symptoms of vagal stimulation. *Safety: If such symptoms are noted, stop the procedure immediately.*

(skill continues on page 656)

Skill 30.5 (continued)

12. After the impaction is removed, clean the anal area with toilet tissue or disposable wipes.

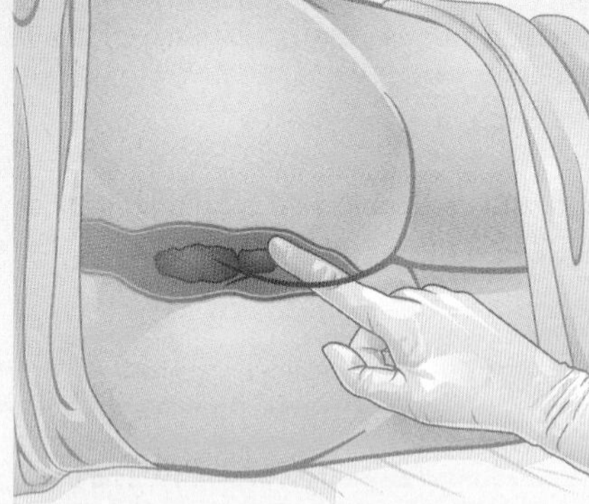

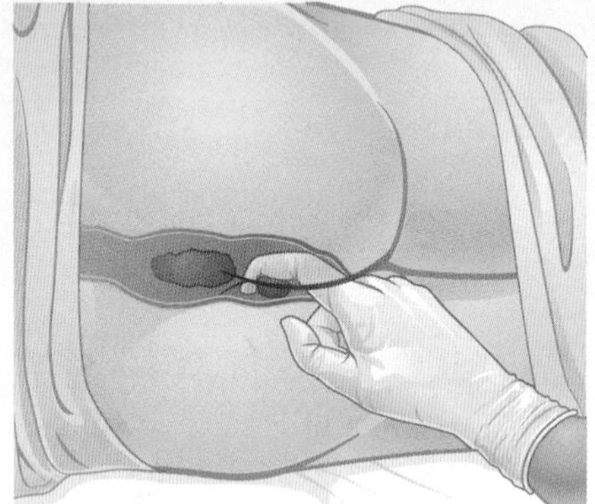

13. Remove contaminated gloves and dispose of in trash according to facility policy.
14. Apply clean examination gloves.
15. Cover the bedpan and place it in the bathroom while washing the patient.
16. Use warm soap and water to wash the anus area and buttocks ***to remove any fecal material and mucus.***
17. Remove the soiled pad from under the patient's hips and replace with a clean pad if needed.
18. Empty the contents of the bedpan into the toilet, noting characteristics of the feces before flushing.
19. Follow the Ending Implementation Steps located on the inside back cover.
20. Document the procedure; amount, color, and consistency of the feces; and the patient's tolerance of the procedure.

Evaluation Step

1. Assess the patient's comfort level and any further needs.

Sample Documentation

12/31/22 0830 States last BM was tiny and hard, 3 days ago and has been constipated ever since. Complains of rectal and abdominal pressure. Fecal impaction digitally removed per health-care provider's order without difficulty. Very large amount of brown, hard stool removed from impaction low in the rectal vault. Tolerated with only complaints of minor pressure in rectum. Perineal care performed. Bed returned to lowest position and call light within patient's reach. Instructed to notify nurse if further assistance or bowel elimination is required ———————— Nurse's signature and credentials

Skill 30.6 Changing an Ostomy Appliance

Assessment Steps

1. Review the patient's medical record and care plan for type of ostomy care to provide, date of and reason for ostomy construction, type of supplies to use, current patient condition, degree of self-care for ostomy, identified patient problems (including psychosocial issues and response to ostomy), and last time the appliance bag and faceplate were changed.
2. Assess the patient's bowel sounds, appliance bag and faceplate, and characteristics and amount of effluent/fecal drainage ***to verify type of supplies to use and determine whether the bag needs to be emptied before changing it.***

Planning Step

1. Gather needed equipment and supplies: stoma size measuring device; type of faceplate, bag, and supplies being used; clean examination gloves; wash basin and soap, washcloths, and towels; toilet tissue; bath blanket; two moisture-proof pads; and bedpan and cover or bedside commode as needed.

Implementation Steps

1. Follow the Initial Implementation Steps located on the inside back cover.
2. Provide privacy.
3. If patient condition allows, assist the patient to the bedside commode and arrange the supplies. Ostomy care is easier to provide on the commode. Plus, once at home, the patient probably will perform the procedure while sitting on the toilet. If the patient is unable to get out of bed, position him or her in the low semi-Fowler's position.
4. Cover the patient with a clean towel ***to reduce soiling of linens.*** If in bed, place a moisture-proof pad beside the patient and one across the patient's lap. If sitting on bedside commode, place one across the patient's lap. ***This will help protect the patient from contact with feces during the appliance change.***
5. Apply clean examination gloves ***to reduce contamination of hands.***
6. Unsnap the flange of the ostomy bag from the faceplate. Remove the bag and empty the contents into the bedpan if the bag is to be reused. Drain the contents if the bag is drainable. Place the entire bag in the bedpan and cover it until you have finished changing the appliance. ***This allows you to remove the feces using a bedpan.***
7. Gently clean drainage and feces and inspect the skin of the stoma and peristomal area. Gently wash with a cleansing agent with a pH of 5.5 and warm water.

Skill 30.6 (continued)

8. Gently remove the faceplate by pulling each edge toward the stoma ***to prevent tearing or stretching of the peristomal skin opening surrounding the stoma.*** Use adhesive remover if needed.

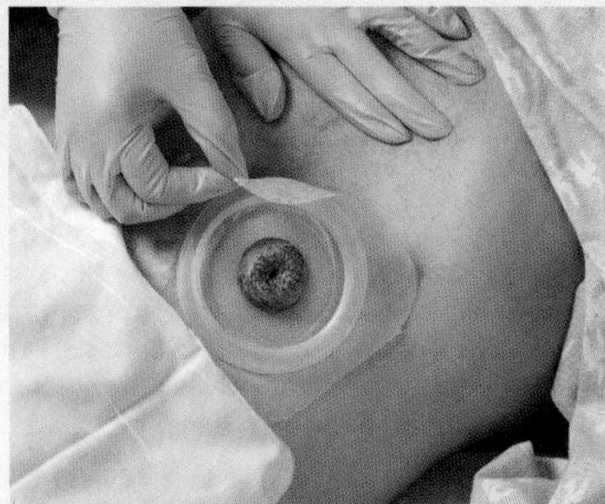

9. Gently clean, rinse, and dry the surrounding skin well ***to maintain the skin beneath the adhesive of the faceplate in good condition.***
10. Measure the size of the stoma, either by placing a standard stoma measuring guide over it, reusing a previously cut template, or measuring the stoma from side to side to approximate the circumference. It may be necessary to remeasure frequently during the postoperative period because the stoma will shrink as it heals.
11. Place a clean gauze 4×4 over the stoma ***to prevent contamination of the cleansed area until a new faceplate or bag is reapplied.***
12. Trace the size of the opening onto the paper on the back of the new wafer faceplate and cut the opening. The opening in the wafer should be approximately 1/16 to 1/8 inch larger than the circumference of the stoma ***to allow for skin movement with activity.***
13. Peel the backing off the wafer faceplate. You may wish to first hold the wafer between the palms of your hand to warm the adhesive ring.
14. Apply clean procedure gloves and apply any ostomy skin products that you are using, such as skin prep or skin barrier powder or karya paste.
15. Remove the gauze 4×4 covering the stoma and position the hole in the faceplate with the stoma centered in the middle of the opening ***to ensure that the faceplate is correctly positioned and will not cause pressure or allow leaking.***
16. Apply the adhesive side of the wafer faceplate by gently pressing it against the skin. Use care to make certain there are no wrinkles in the adhesive surface or in the skin under it. Gently rub the outer surface of the faceplate with your fingers ***to smooth and warm the adhesive disk to body temperature for better adhesion to the skin.***
17. If you are using a two-piece pouch, attach the bag to the faceplate by gently pressing the plastic flange onto the receiving flange on the faceplate. It works somewhat like a Tupperware lid seal. If the ostomy is new, avoid using excessive pressure on the newly traumatized area ***to reduce discomfort for the patient.***

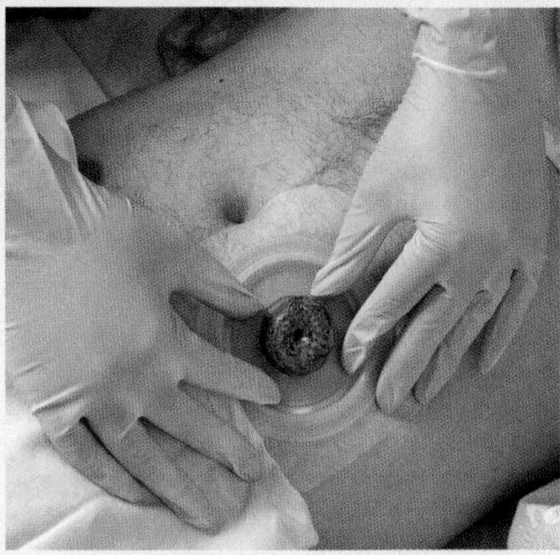

18. Remove contaminated gloves and wash hands.
19. Follow the Ending Implementation Steps located on the inside back cover.
20. Document the procedure, including assessment findings regarding the stoma and peristomal skin; amount, color, and consistency of effluent/fecal drainage; the patient's verbal and nonverbal responses; any abnormalities encountered or difficulties experienced; and patient teaching provided. Also document the effectiveness of teaching by noting the patient's response to the teaching. Make a note of the extent of patient participation in ostomy care.

Evaluation Step

1. Assess the patient for comfort and needs before leaving the room.

Sample Documentation

12/27/22 1000 New colostomy of left descending colon constructed 2 days ago. Stoma is red, edematous, moist and shiny. Peristomal skin is pink, intact, without edema or drainage. Bag 1/3 full of brown semiformed fecal drainage with clear mucus. Assisted patient to bedside commode for ostomy care. Stoma measured: 2-in. diameter. Bag emptied, rinsed with tap water, dried and reapplied. Patient observed procedure and asked questions regarding ostomy care, made good eye contact. Verbalized that she knew she could learn to take care of the new ostomy. Stated that she had originally thought the diagnosis of colon cancer meant an automatic death warrant and that she was glad to just be alive. Occasionally smiled during our interaction. Informed her that a representative from the local support group would be in to see her after lunch. Still up in chair with call light within reach. No complaints voiced. ————

———— *Nurse's signature and credentials*

Skill 30.7 Irrigating a Colostomy

Assessment Steps

1. Review the patient's medical record and care plan for type of ostomy care to provide, date of and reason for ostomy construction, usual bowel pattern, type of supplies to use, current patient condition, degree of self-care for ostomy, identified patient problems (including psychosocial issues and response to ostomy), last time the appliance bag and faceplate were changed, and date of last irrigation.
2. Assess the patient's bowel sounds, appliance bag and faceplate, and characteristics and amount of effluent/fecal drainage ***to verify type of supplies to use.***

Planning Step

1. Gather needed equipment and supplies: new faceplate, bag, and supplies being used; clean examination gloves; ostomy irrigation sleeve; irrigation administration set with cone-tipped tubing; irrigation solution; wash basin and soap, washcloths, and towels; toilet tissue; bath blanket; moisture-proof pad; IV pole; and bedpan and cover or bedside commode as needed.

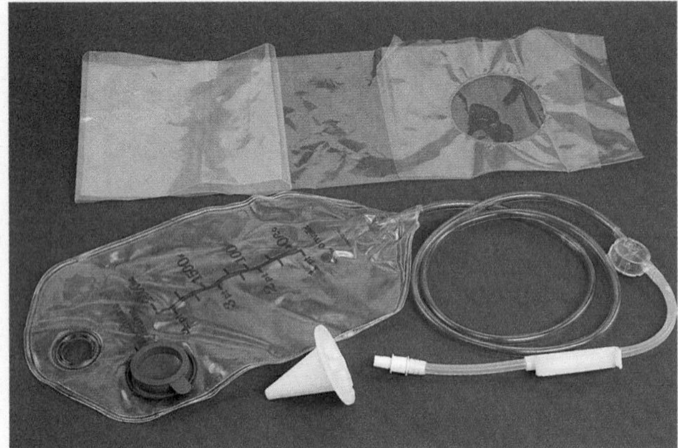

Implementation Steps

1. Follow the Initial Implementation Steps located on the inside back cover.
2. Provide privacy.
3. Prepare solution as needed and fill administration set container to the desired volume, usually between 500 and 1,000 mL. *Safety: Water temperature should be between 105°F and 110°F (40.5°C to 43.3°C) to prevent burns and cold water cramping. Never heat water in a microwave oven.*
4. Hang the filled irrigation administration container on the IV pole to a height level with the patient's shoulder once he or she is in a sitting position ***to provide for the least amount of pressure when beginning the irrigation.***
5. Assist the patient to sit on a chair facing the toilet (which he or she will most likely do at home) or to sit on the bedside commode. If the patient is unable to get out of bed, position the patient in a left lateral side-lying position ***to facilitate the best access to the colon.***
6. Place a moisture-proof pad across the patient's lap ***to reduce soiling of gown.*** If in bed, place a moisture-proof pad beside the patient underneath the stoma ***to protect the patient's abdomen from irrigation fluid.***
7. Apply clean examination gloves ***to prevent contamination of hands.***
8. Remove the old appliance and clean feces from the stoma and peristomal skin with toilet tissue and warm wet washcloth as needed.
9. Place the elastic belt around the patient's waist and clip the irrigation sleeve to the belt ***to more easily hold the sleeve in place.***
10. Place the open-ended tail of the irrigation sleeve in a bedpan if the patient is in bed, or between the patient's thighs into the bedside commode or into the toilet opposite the patient. ***This will ensure that the irrigation solution and return go into the bedpan, bedside commode, or toilet.*** Ensure that the end of the sleeve does not touch the toilet water.
11. Generously lubricate the tip of the insertion cone and your dominant gloved index finger ***to reduce patient discomfort upon insertion.***
12. Lift the top edge of the irrigation sleeve and place the cone in the stoma between the two sides of the sleeve. If the cone will not insert into the stoma, gently insert your lubricated index finger about 1 inch into the stoma opening. Give the stoma several seconds to relax and dilate. If the stoma opening is too tight for insertion of your index finger, use the smaller pinkie finger first. Then use the index finger to further dilate the opening. You will be able to feel the release of constriction around your finger. Once release is felt, remove the finger. ***Stomas will sometimes contract and require gentle dilation before insertion of the administration cone.***
13. While holding the cone in the stoma, release the tubing clamp, allowing solution to flow into the intestinal lumen.

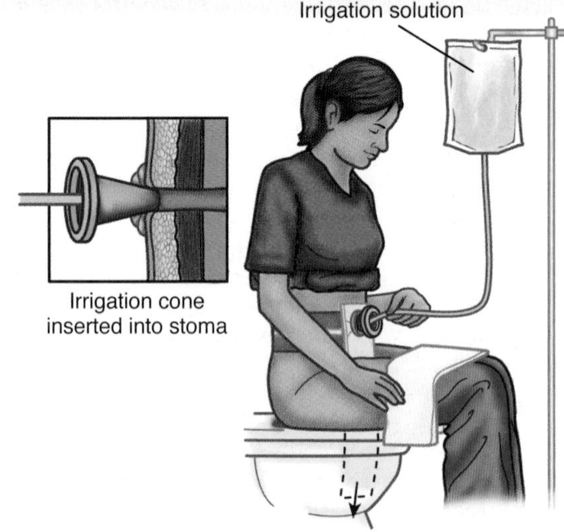

14. Stop or slow solution flow as needed ***to control retention and patient cramping.***
15. Once solution instillation is completed, remove the cone from the stoma and wrap the end of the cone in tissue or a paper towel ***until you can clean it properly.***
16. Close the top of the irrigation sleeve with a clamp ***to prevent any spilling of return solution.***

Skill 30.7 (continued)

17. Wait for evacuation to occur, which may be immediate or may take up to 30 minutes. Wash, rinse, and hang the irrigation administration equipment to dry in the patient's bathroom. ***The irrigation set can be reused by the same patient several times.***
18. Remove contaminated gloves, wash hands, and apply clean gloves.
19. After expulsion of irrigation is complete, remove the irrigation sleeve and elastic belt. Wash, rinse, and pat dry the stoma and peristomal skin, reassessing its condition as you do this ***to observe any changes that may have occurred during the irrigation.***
20. Apply a new faceplate and bag as needed.
21. Assess the characteristics of the returned contents before emptying into the toilet.
22. Assist the patient to return to bed or reposition as desired.
23. Follow the Ending Implementation Steps located on the inside back cover.
24. Document the procedure, including the type and volume of solution, difficulties encountered, and characteristics of the returned contents, including color, amount, and consistency of effluent/fecal drainage. Also document assessment findings regarding the stoma and peristomal skin, including color, edema, skin integrity, and moisture level of the stoma.

Evaluation Step

1. Assess for patient comfort and needs before leaving the room.

Sample Documentation

11/10/22 0800 Assisted to bedside commode. Colostomy irrigated with 500 mL of 0.9% normal saline without difficulty. Stoma was pinkish red, moist and shiny, no edema. Peristomal skin was intact, and without erythema or edema. Large amount of soft formed brown stool returned within 2 to 3 minutes of instillation. Patient unable to assist with procedure due to severe contractures of both hands. Conversed with nurse and made good eye contact throughout procedure. Faceplate clean and intact. Clean bag applied. Assisted to return to bed. No complaints voiced. ———
——— Nurse's signature and credentials

POST CONFERENCE

Your day turned out to be rather exciting in some ways. When you were assessing your patient, you noticed that his ileostomy was leaking under the faceplate, so you decided (with appropriate orders) to change the ostomy appliance. While you were doing so, you noticed that the stoma was a very pale pink. Remembering what you had learned, you pouched the ileostomy, then notified your instructor of your findings. He agreed with you that the stoma was too pale to be receiving good blood supply. The charge nurse was notified, who then called the physician. Because of your excellent assessment, the physician took the patient back to surgery to revise the stoma, ensuring that it would have good blood supply. The physician stated that had the stoma gone for 24 more hours in this condition, even more intestine would have had to be removed. You also learned the difficulties of keeping an ileostomy pouch emptied in a timely manner because it seemed to fill up quickly with liquid effluent.

Key Points

- Normal bowel elimination changes through the life span. Some adults may have one to two bowel movements daily, while others may go several days between movements. The urge to defecate commonly occurs 30 minutes to an hour after eating.
- Typical stools are soft, formed, light yellowish-brown to dark brown, slightly odiferous, and in a slightly curved shape. Abnormal characteristics include a variety of colors; foul odors; and a hard, dry consistency or a very loose to watery consistency.
- Various colors of bowel movement can be very significant. It may simply be due to foods the patient has eaten or can be indications of bleeding in various locations in the intestines.
- When performing a focused assessment of the bowels, ask about frequency, normal number of stools per day, normal color and consistency of stools, and if constipation or diarrhea is a current problem. Then auscultate bowel sounds and palpate the abdomen for firmness, distention, and pain.
- Constipation is the term for less frequent, hard, formed stools that are difficult to expel. Lack of fiber-rich foods and adequate fluids are often contributing factors, as well as a decrease in activity level, certain medicines and over-the-counter drugs, surgery, pregnancy, depression, aging, and nerve impairments.
- Nursing interventions for constipation include increasing activity, increasing fiber and fluid intake, providing privacy, and assisting with positioning to help facilitate a bowel movement. In addition, the health-care provider may order medications and enemas if necessary.
- Enemas are ordered to cleanse the bowel (tap water, normal saline, soapsuds, sodium phosphate, high enema, or

milk and molasses), soften feces (oil retention), deliver medications (steroids or Kayexelate), and relieve gas (Harris flush, return flow, or siphon).

- Enemas should not be given to patients with rectal conditions, excessive bleeding potential, and certain heart conditions. Complications of enemas include a vagal response, which causes a slowed heartbeat and other symptoms, and perforation of the colon.
- Fecal impaction occurs when a very hard mass of stool blocks movement of feces through the intestines. Nursing interventions for this include administering an oil retention enema to soften it and then digitally removing the hard mass.
- Diarrhea is defined as loose or water stools occurring three or more times in a day that may be accompanied by cramping. It may be due to lactose intolerance, intestinal infections, certain medications, anxiety, stress, diverticulosis, inflammation and infection of the intestines, and food allergies.
- Nursing interventions for diarrhea include modifying food and fluid intake, providing probiotics, and administering prescribed medications.
- Fecal incontinence is the inability to control the bowels. Nursing interventions for this include treating the underlying cause if due to diarrhea, administering medications as ordered, bowel training, providing skin care, and providing emotional support.
- Stool specimens may be ordered to test for infection, parasites and their eggs, and hidden blood. Patients bringing in a stool specimen to be tested for blood must avoid certain substances for 48 hours prior to the testing.
- Alternative bowel elimination is necessary as a result of tumors, cancer, damage to the intestines, and intestinal diseases such as Crohn's and ulcerative colitis.
- If part of the colon is used to create a stoma, it is called a colostomy. If the last portion of the small intestine is used, it is called an ileostomy. A continent ileostomy is called a Kock pouch.
- The normal healthy stoma is pink to red in color, shiny, and moist. The skin around it (peristomal skin) should be free of irritation, excoriation, and erythema.
- Nurses may be specially trained to care for ostomies (enterostomal therapists), but all nurses must know how to empty, clean, and change an ostomy appliance.
- Colostomy irrigation is done to relieve constipation and for bowel training when the stoma is in the descending or sigmoid colon. The colon may be trained to empty once per day with an irrigation so the patient doesn't have to wear a bag all day.

Review Questions

Select the answer that is most appropriate for each of the following questions. Some questions may have more than one correct answer. Select all that apply.

1. Which of the following would be the most accurate statement about digestion and elimination?
   1. All individuals have at least one bowel movement daily.
   2. An infant may have up to six bowel movements daily.
   3. GI peristalsis increases with age, making incontinence a normal finding.
   4. A stool is only considered normal if the color is a shade of brown.

2. Several medications have GI side effects and may lead to diarrhea or constipation. Indicate which of the following medications would be most likely to cause constipation in the patient.
   1. Amphojel
   2. Maalox
   3. Magnesium citrate
   4. Meperidine
   5. Amoxicillin
   6. Ferrous sulfate (iron)
   7. Imodium AD
   8. Milk of magnesia

3. A female patient is recovering from abdominal surgery 2 days ago. Her abdomen is distended and firm, and she complains of moderate to severe cramping and abdominal discomfort. As of yet, she has been unable to pass much flatus rectally. Which type of enema would be most helpful to this patient?
   1. Fleet Phospho-Soda enema
   2. Oil retention enema
   3. Harris flush enema
   4. Small-volume enema

4. Which of the following signs and symptoms may be an indication of vagal stimulation during the digital removal of an impaction?
   1. Complaint of rectal pressure
   2. Pulse rate of 42 beats per minute
   3. Complaint of difficulty breathing
   4. Moist skin
   5. Complaint of abdominal cramping
   6. Complaint of feeling faint

5. What of the following would be the best enema to administer to a patient before digital removal of an impaction?
   1. Siphon enema
   2. Oil retention enema
   3. Soapsuds enema
   4. Harris flush enema

6. Which of the following factors is most likely to result in diarrhea?
   1. Loss of intestinal normal flora
   2. Drinking excessive fluids
   3. Administration of opioid narcotics
   4. Manipulation of intestines during colon surgery
   5. Eating 10 to 15 g of fiber per day

7. The patient is to receive a cleansing enema for relief of constipation. Which of the following factors must be assessed prior to administration of the enema?
   1. Type of solution to administer
   2. Date of last bowel movement
   3. Type of diet the patient has been receiving
   4. Assessment of bowel sounds
   5. The patient's temperature

8. Which of the following assessment data might indicate the patient is having difficulty accepting his or her new colostomy?
   1. Asks questions about how to take care of the colostomy
   2. Observes as you irrigate the colostomy
   3. Looks at stoma and makes good eye contact with you during ostomy care
   4. Refuses to attempt care, and tells you to "just do it"

ANSWERS 1. 2. 2. 1, 4, 5, 7. 3. 3. 4. 2, 3, 4, 6. 5. 2. 6. 1. 7. 1, 2, 4. 8. 4

Critical Thinking Exercises

Answers available online.

1. You are caring for a 62-year-old female admitted to a hospital 45 miles from her hometown with a right midfemur fracture. Surgical repair was performed yesterday under general anesthetic. She has a history of arteriosclerosis and is very hard of hearing. Her dentures are at home, and no one can retrieve them for her until her daughter arrives in 3 days. She is an avid gardener and usually works in her gardens about an hour each morning before the temperature gets too hot. Each evening, she spends 30 minutes to an hour walking through the park admiring the trees, shrubs, and flowers. Her physician's orders include the following:
   - Bedrest
   - Assess circulation to right lower leg every 2 hours
   - Edentulous diet
   - Morphine sulfate 6 mg intramuscularly every 3 to 4 hours prn severe pain
   - Acetaminophen 250 to 500 mg orally every 4 to 6 hours prn lesser pain

   Which of the above factors puts this patient at risk for constipation?

2. Gerome Flygenhall has a new permanent colostomy located in the ascending colon. What teaching or services would be appropriate to provide for this patient? Be inclusive.

Additional Resources

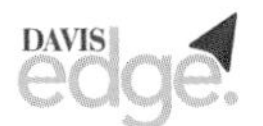

Use the scratch off code on the inside front cover of your book to access online quizzes that will help you to improve your scores on course exams and prepare for the NCLEX-PN®.

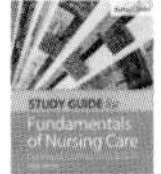

Study Guide

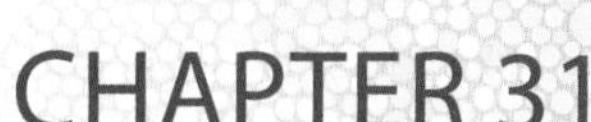

CHAPTER 31
Urinary Elimination and Care

KEY TERMS

Anuria (an-YOO-ree-ah)
Blood urea nitrogen (BLUHD yoo-REE-ah NYE-troh-jen)
Dialysis (dye-AL-ih-siss)
Dysuria (dis-YOO-ree-ah)
Hematuria (HEE-muh-TOO-ree-ah)
Incontinence (in-KON-tih-nents)
Indwelling catheter (IN-dwel-ing KATH-et-uhr)
Nocturia (nok-TOO-ree-ah)
Oliguria (AW-lig-YOO-ree-ah)
Polyuria (PAW-lee-YOO-ree-ah)
Renal calculi (REE-nuhl KAL-kyoo-lye)
Residual urine (ree-ZID-yoo-al YOOR-in)
Specific gravity (speh-SIF-ik GRA-vi-tee)
Straight catheter (STRAYT KATH-et-uhr)
Stress incontinence (STRESS in-KON-tih-nents)
Urge incontinence (ERJ in-KON-tih-nents)
Urinary diversion (YOOR-ih-NAIR-ee dih-VER-zhun)
Urinary retention (YOOR-ih-NAIR-ee rih-TEN-shun)
Urinary tract infection (UTI) (YOOR-ih-NAIR-ee TRAKT in-FEK-shun)
Void (VOYD)

CHAPTER CONCEPTS

Elimination
Infection
Patient-Centered Care
Safety

LEARNING OUTCOMES

1. Define various terms related to urinary elimination and care.
2. Describe normal contents and characteristics of urine and the significance of abnormal findings.
3. Identify normal voiding patterns.
4. Explain ways to assist patients with toileting.
5. Describe focused assessments to make about urine.
6. Discuss different types of urine specimens and urine tests.
7. List the steps for collecting a 24-hour urine sample.
8. Explain how to accurately measure intake and output.
9. Describe types of urinary incontinence.
10. Describe nursing interventions to help manage incontinence.
11. Identify steps in bladder training.
12. Identify purposes, types, and sizes of urinary catheters.
13. Explain guidelines for inserting catheters and draining urine from the bladder.
14. Discuss nursing care of patients with indwelling catheters.
15. Identify types of urinary diversions.
16. Describe the occurrence of, risk factors for, and prevention of urinary tract infections.
17. Plan care for a patient with a urinary tract infection.
18. Discuss information found in the Connection features of the chapter.
19. Identify safety issues related to urinary elimination and care.
20. Answer questions about skills in the chapter.

SKILLS

31.1 Assisting the Male Patient With a Urinal
31.2 Assisting With a Bedpan
31.3 Obtaining a Clean-Catch Midstream Urine Specimen
31.4 Performing a Bladder Scan
31.5 Inserting an Indwelling Urinary Catheter
31.6 Obtaining a Urine Specimen From an Indwelling Urinary Catheter
31.7 Inserting a Straight Catheter
31.8 Performing Continuous Bladder Irrigation
31.9 Applying a Condom Catheter
31.10 Irrigating a Closed Urinary Drainage System
31.11 Discontinuing an Indwelling Urinary Catheter

CRITICAL THINKING CONNECTION

Clinical Assignment

You are assigned to care for a 24-year-old male with a spinal cord injury due to a boating accident. He has an indwelling catheter. In report, you hear that there are physician's orders to irrigate the catheter every 8 hours prn for decreased output because he sometimes has mucus that blocks the catheter. The order is for a closed system irrigation. Also ordered is a 24-hour urine collection.

Critical Thinking Questions:

1. What is meant by a closed system irrigation?
2. How will you perform a 24-hour urine collection when the patient has an indwelling catheter?
3. How will you keep the urine cold for 24 hours?
4. What nursing care will you need to provide for this patient?

You may not have thought about the importance of normal urinary function until you entered nursing school. Now, however, you are learning how important it is for the body to rid itself of waste products. In this chapter, you will learn how to assist patients who are unable to urinate normally as well as those who need assistance with voiding. You will learn how to collect urine specimens in a variety of situations and how to insert and manage catheters.

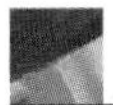

NORMAL URINARY ELIMINATION

You will hear various terms used in health care to refer to the elimination of urine. You may hear a nurse say that a patient has voided 300 mL of urine. **Void** is another word for urinate. An older term that you may also hear is *micturate,* which also means to void or to urinate.

Urinary elimination cleanses the blood of anything the body does not need. Urine is made up of approximately 95% water, with the remaining 5% being the solutes that are dissolved in the water, such as mineral salts and nitrogenous waste products. The kidneys eliminate these waste products before the blood levels rise high enough to be damaging, or toxic, to the body. The following are three waste products that must be removed:

1. *Urea,* which results from amino acid metabolism
2. *Uric acid,* which results from breakdown of ribonucleic acid (RNA) and deoxyribonucleic acid (DNA)
3. *Creatinine,* which is the waste product of muscle metabolism

The kidneys filter these waste products from the blood and eliminate them in the urine. In addition, they eliminate excess electrolytes, hydrogen ions as needed, and toxins.

Characteristics of Urine

The characteristics of urine include color, clarity, amount, and odor. With the use of testing materials, the pH and specific gravity of urine can also be determined.

Color and Clarity

Normal urine is straw-colored and clear without sediment. The color of urine is a primary indicator of whether or not the patient has had adequate fluid intake: the darker yellow the color, the lower the patient's hydration level. As dehydration worsens, the urine color may become dark yellow and then amber.

Urine can be cloudy, or have increased *turbidity,* due to the presence of fat globules, red or white blood cells, or bacteria, as well as due to sitting at room temperature for a long period. When blood is present in the urine—either visible or microscopic blood—it is referred to as **hematuria.** When the pH of urine is excessively alkaline, it can result in turbidity and the formation of certain types of crystals.

Sediment is any substance that settles to the bottom of a liquid. Components that may produce urine sediment include uric acid, bacteria, mucus, and phosphates.

Odor

Urine does have a very mild odor described as *slightly aromatic.* Other odors, such as a sweet or fruity smell, a strong ammonia-like smell, or a foul odor, are abnormal findings.

Amount

The amount of urine an adult produces in a day is the result of many metabolic occurrences in the body. The normal range of urine production is 1,000 to 3,000 mL in a 24-hour period. The acceptable *minimal* amount of urinary output per hour is 30 mL. For a person to have a balanced intake and output (I&O), there should be within a difference of approximately 300 to 500 mL in urine output compared to the total intake. As a nurse, you can make the decision to monitor a patient's I&O any time it is indicated. For example, if you are concerned that a patient is not making as much urine as you think he or she should, or you see beginning signs of fluid overload, you would want to begin strict monitoring of the I&O.

OLIGURIA. **Oliguria** is defined as urinary output of less than 30 mL per hour. It can be caused by decreased fluid intake, dehydration, illness, urinary obstruction, or renal failure. Oliguria also may be caused by hemorrhage or by severe loss of body fluids.

POLYURIA. Increased urinary output, or **polyuria,** is defined as output greater than 3,000 mL per day. It can be caused by

• **WORD • BUILDING •**

hematuria: hemat – blood + ur – urine + ia – condition
oliguria: olig – small + ur – urine + ia – condition
polyuria: poly – much + ur – urine + ia – condition

excessive fluid intake or by the consumption of alcohol, which affects the kidney's ability to reabsorb water. Certain medications, such as diuretics, or "water pills," increase urine production.

ANURIA. **Anuria** is the absence of urine production. It can be due to a temporary illness or urinary tract obstruction, or it can be a symptom of a serious underlying condition, such as kidney failure. If anuria is caused by a virus that causes vomiting and diarrhea, the kidneys will usually start producing urine on their own when hydration is restored. In more serious illnesses that shut down kidney function, the physician will order dialysis for the patient. **Dialysis** is the process of using a machine to filter waste products and salts and to remove excess fluid from the blood. This treatment may be temporary or long term depending on the cause of the anuria.

pH

The pH of urine is normally 4.5 to 8.0, depending largely on diet. A diet high in protein or cranberries will cause the pH to be lower, or more acidic; a diet high in citrus fruits, dairy products, or vegetables will cause the pH to be higher, or more alkaline. Determining the pH of the urine is helpful in the diagnosis and management of urinary tract infections (UTIs), which tend to make the urine more alkaline.

Specific Gravity

Specific gravity is the result of comparing the weight of a substance with the weight of an equal amount of water. The normal specific gravity for urine is 1.005 to 1.03. When the specific gravity is high, it means that the urine is more concentrated. When the specific gravity is low, the urine is more dilute. A low specific gravity may be caused by excessive fluid intake or impaired kidney function. A high specific gravity can be the result of dehydration, hemorrhage, or diabetes mellitus.

Anatomy and Physiology Connection

Urinary System

The urinary system is a multiorgan system consisting of the two kidneys containing millions of nephrons that filter the blood. The blood flows through the renal arteries into the kidney, into the nephron, and into the glomerulus, where filtration takes place. The blood pressure forces substances through the porous walls of the glomerulus to produce the filtrate. As the filtrate travels on through the proximal convoluted tubule, loop of Henle, distal tubule, and collecting tubule, most of the filtrate is reabsorbed, leaving only the waste products, toxins, excess electrolytes, and water to be excreted as urine.

Urine leaves the kidney by way of the ureter and travels by peristaltic action to the urinary bladder for storage. The ureters from both kidneys attach to the posterior base of the bladder, allowing urine to actually enter the bladder from the inferior or bottom side, not from the top or superior side of the bladder. Because of this, urine can *reflux,* or back up, into the kidneys if the valve at the cystoureteral junction does not close properly.

Urine is stored in the bladder, a sac made of smooth muscle, until the urge to void is felt when approximately 200 to 400 mL of urine has collected. The bladder can hold 1,000 mL or more of urine but usually is emptied long before it reaches that amount. The detrusor muscle in the walls of the bladder contracts, causing the bladder to empty. Urine leaves the bladder by way of the urethra and passes through two sphincters: the internal urinary sphincter at the neck of the bladder and the external urinary sphincter near the end of the urethra. In males, as the urine leaves the bladder, it passes through the prostatic urethra. The prostate gland surrounds this section of the urethra near the neck of the bladder; this explains how an enlarged prostate can inhibit or prevent urination. The urine then exits the body via the urinary meatus.

An important point to remember is that one continuous membrane lines the urinary system; it extends from the external urinary meatus all the way to the kidneys. This membrane allows bacteria to spread from outside the urinary meatus through the urethra into the bladder to ascend up the ureters and into the kidneys, where all the blood in the body is filtered. This direct pathway allows bacteria to spread to the blood, leading to a very serious systemic infection known as *urinary sepsis.* For this reason, proper perineal care and hygiene are very important to prevent UTIs.

KNOWLEDGE CONNECTION

How much urine do the kidneys normally make in a 24-hour period? When reviewing laboratory results for a patient, what would a specific gravity of 1.005 tell you about the patient's hydration status? A specific gravity of 1.033? What is the difference between anuria and oliguria?

Normal Voiding Patterns

The average individual urinates four to six times per day and does not routinely get up during the sleeping hours to void. Urinary frequency and volume of output are directly related to fluid intake. Because some individuals drink a large amount of fluid in a 24-hour period, you would expect them to urinate more frequently and have a larger output than those who have minimal fluid intake.

• WORD • BUILDING •

anuria: an – not + ur – urine + ia – condition
dialysis: dia – through + lysis – dissolving

Assisting With Toileting

When normally independent patients are in acute or long-term care settings, they often need assistance with personal hygiene and elimination. All members of the nursing team need to respond to patients' toileting needs in a timely manner to foster continued independence. When assisting patients with toileting, follow these guidelines:

- Offer the opportunity to use the bathroom or bedpan before and after meals and at bedtime.
- Male patients may use a urinal for voiding (Fig. 31.1). Some men find it difficult to void while sitting or lying in bed. If allowed, the male patient may stand at the bedside to void into the urinal. Skill 31.1 (page 683) describes how to assist a male patient with a urinal.
- Use a fracture pan, which is smaller and flatter, for patients who have had a hip or back surgery. The pan slips more easily under the buttocks and does not require that the patient be rolled from side to side. A fracture pan may also be used for patients who are very thin or if a regular bedpan causes back discomfort. In that situation, the patient may be rolled from side to side to place the fracture pan (see Fig. 31.1).
- Provide patients with privacy and avoid rushing them.
- Offer patients the opportunity to perform hand hygiene after toileting.

Patients who are unable to ambulate to the bathroom will use a bedside commode. A bedside commode is a portable chair with a toilet seat and collection bucket beneath it, which is removed for cleaning. The commode is placed near the patient's bed for easy access.

Patients with orders for bedrest are not allowed to be out of the bed to go to the bathroom or to use a bedside commode. These patients will need to use a bedpan for elimination (see Fig. 31.1). It may be embarrassing to them to ask for assistance, and they may delay as long as possible before asking for help. Always respond quickly to every patient's request for the bedpan to prevent incontinence or accidents. Skill 31.2 (page 683) shows the steps for assisting a patient with a bedpan.

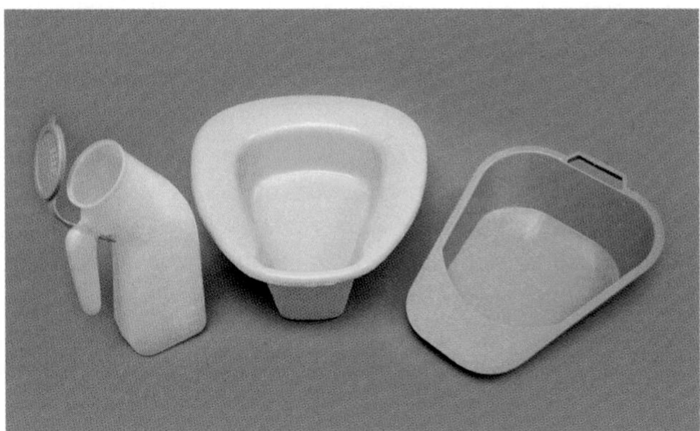

FIGURE 31.1 The urinal, bedpan, and fracture pan are all used to assist patients with urination.

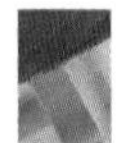

ASSESSING URINE AND URINARY OUTPUT

You will find that you are constantly assessing the function of the urinary tract, whether it is simply using your physical assessment skills, evaluating the results of diagnostic tests, or possibly even performing a test on the urine.

Focused Assessment

When you care for patients, you will learn to notice the color and characteristics of their urine on a frequent basis. Based on what you observe, you will be able to detect a great deal about their fluid status and the possible presence of infection. You will also learn to monitor for *edema,* or swelling, due to fluid retention. Edema due to kidney problems may be found in the hands, legs and feet, sacrum, and face. The quickest way to assess whether or not a patient is retaining water is to perform daily weights, at the same time each day, with the same scales, and with the patient wearing approximately the same amount of clothing. A weight gain of 2 pounds equals about a liter of fluid. Rapid weight gain, such as 2 or 3 pounds gained overnight, usually indicates fluid retention. Chapter 29 further discusses fluid volume excess.

The frequency of urination also is important. As mentioned earlier in the chapter, the average individual urinates four to six times per day and does not routinely get up during the sleeping hours to void. So if a patient makes extra trips to the bathroom during the night or voids more or less frequently than this, further assessment is needed. Patients who urinate with increased frequency may be exhibiting symptoms of a UTI, bladder inflammation, or diabetes mellitus.

Ask the patient if he or she is experiencing any burning or difficulty starting the stream of urine. Painful or difficult urination is called **dysuria.** Urination should not burn, and the patient should have voluntary control over the starting and stopping of the stream of urine. Burning during urination may be indicative of UTI or bladder or urethral inflammation.

Collecting Specimens and Testing Urine

In a hospital setting, you will be responsible for reviewing the laboratory reports for abnormalities and alerting the health-care provider. Therefore, you will need to know the significance of the tests and the possible results.

In some settings, you may assess specific gravity at the bedside or in the exam room rather than send a specimen to the laboratory. This can be tested with reagent strips. If you work in home health or a medical office, it will be common practice to perform some urine tests yourself. In the hospital setting, the specimens are generally sent to the lab for testing.

• WORD • BUILDING •

dysuria: dys – difficult + ur – urine + ia – condition

Clean-Catch Urine Specimen

A clean-catch, or clean-catch midstream, urine specimen (CCUA) is ordered to obtain uncontaminated urine for urinalysis (UA). It is important to give the patient adequate instructions on how to perform a CCUA. Instruct the patient to clean the urinary meatus with disposable antiseptic wipes prior to voiding. Instruct the patient to begin voiding and then to stop the stream and continue voiding into the specimen container. This removes contaminants from the skin and from the opening of the urethra that could enter the urine and become part of the specimen. It decreases the chance that the patient will be treated for a UTI due to a contaminated specimen. See Skill 31.3 (page 684).

Urinalysis

One of the most common diagnostic tests ordered in the health-care setting is a UA. Components of a UA are given in Table 31.1. This test is done to determine the presence of renal calculi, a UTI, a malignancy, and diseases affecting the kidneys. You will be responsible for obtaining urine specimens for UAs. ***Safety: When you obtain a specimen, transport it to the laboratory immediately or store it in a refrigerator. Urine that is left standing longer than 1 hour starts to break down, and the test becomes ineffective.***

Timed Urinary Collection

Another type of microscopic urine diagnostic test is a timed urinary collection; the most common timed urine specimen is a 24-hour urine collection. This type of specimen is helpful in evaluating kidney function by measuring the levels of various components in the urine, especially protein levels. The amount of protein the kidneys allow to pass into the urine can help diagnose kidney disease. It is very important that *all* the urine produced within the 24-hour collection time is added to the specimen jug. If urine from a single voiding is inadvertently flushed down the toilet, the 24-hour collection must be restarted. Follow these guidelines to correctly obtain the timed urine specimen:

- Ask the patient to void and discard the urine. This ensures that the 24-hour specimen begins with the patient having an empty bladder.
- Note the exact time that the urine is voided and discarded. This begins the 24-hour period.
- Post signs in the patient's room and on the door stating that the 24-hour urine collection is in progress. Include the date and time the collection started and the date and time it is to end.
- Collect every drop of urine that is voided during the next 24 hours, and pour it into the specified large-volume container. This container is kept on ice or refrigerated to prevent the urine from decomposing.
- If the patient has an indwelling urinary catheter, place the collection bag in a basin with ice. Empty the collection bag into the 24-hour urine container.
- If any urine is discarded during the 24-hour period, the entire specimen must be restarted.
- Exactly 24 hours after the collection began, ask the patient to void one last time and add the urine to the collection container. Then take the 24-hour specimen to the laboratory for testing. Remove the signs, and inform the patient that the collection is completed.

Reagent Testing

Sometimes urine is tested with reagent sticks, or dipsticks, to obtain immediate results (Fig. 31.2). When dipped into urine and the excess tapped off, each reagent pad changes color to indicate values of pH, specific gravity, protein, glucose, ketones, bilirubin, urobilinogen, blood leukocyte, and nitrite levels. This information can be used to screen for evidence of a UTI or the presence of abnormal substances in the urine. There are chemically impregnated pads on the stick that react to the urine. Each reagent pad must be read at specific times. The color changes on the pads are compared to a chart on the side of the dipstick bottle. If abnormal results are found, they should be confirmed by a UA. These dipsticks are often used to test urine quickly in medical offices and clinics. Box 31.1 lists the steps used in performing a urine dipstick test.

Straining Urine

Renal calculi, commonly referred to as *kidney stones,* can occur anywhere in the renal system from the kidneys to the urethra. When a stone passes out of the body, it is important to retain it and send it to the laboratory for analysis. The health-care provider may write an order to strain all urine. You will use a special urine strainer, shaped like a cone with a fine wire mesh at the narrow end (Fig. 31.3). Once the patient voids into a specimen pan placed in the toilet, pour the urine through the strainer. If a stone is collected, send it to the laboratory for analysis if ordered.

Measuring Intake and Output

It is very important for you to know whether or not the amount of urine produced by a patient is adequate. Remember that the minimum acceptable output is 30 mL per hour, or 240 mL in 8 hours. For knowledge of the urine output to be most useful, you will also want to measure the intake of fluid, otherwise known as measuring I&O. Not only will you measure the amount of fluid going in and fluid coming out, but you also will assess the balance between the intake and output, which means to compare fluid intake to urine output for each shift as well as the totals for each 24-hour period. When intake is greater than output, the patient is at risk for fluid overload. When output is greater than intake, the patient is at risk for fluid deficiency or dehydration. These fluid imbalances are discussed in Chapter 29.

To measure urine output of an ambulatory patient, place a specimen pan underneath the front rim of the toilet or bedside commode to catch the urine. The inside of the specimen

• **WORD • BUILDING •**

renal calculi: renal – related to the kidney + calculi – pebbles

Table 31.1
Urinalysis Results

Characteristic	*Normal Findings*	*Abnormal Findings*	*Possible Cause*
Color and appearance	Straw-colored to pale yellow	Lighter or totally clear	Increased fluid intake, diabetes insipidus
		Dark yellow	Concentrated from decreased fluid intake or dehydration Medications and diet can also affect the color of urine
	Clear	Cloudy or increased turbidity	Phosphate precipitation from setting, blood, epithelial cells, pus, fat droplets, bacteria, RBCs, WBCs
		Milky	Pus, fat globules
		Red or reddish-brown	Blood, sulfa drug
		Bright orangey-red	Pyridium (anesthetic drug for urinary burning)
		Yellowish- or greenish-brown	Bile in urine
		Green	*Pseudomonas* infection of urinary tract
pH	4.5–8.0	High pH (alkaline)	Vaginal discharge, diet high in citrate
		Low pH (acidotic)	Diet high in protein, cranberry juice
Specific gravity	1.005–1.03	Less than 1.005	Overhydration; dilute urine due to kidney impairment
		Greater than 1.03	Dehydration, hemorrhage, diabetes mellitus
Odor	Slightly aromatic	Strong fruity odor	Diabetes mellitus, starvation, and dehydration all cause formation of ketone bodies
		Fetid or foul odor	*Escherichia coli* infection
		Maple syrup odor	Maple syrup urine disease
		Fecal odor	Rectal fistula
Bacteria	Negative	+1 to +4 TNTC (too numerous to count)	UTI
Protein	Less than 20 mg/dL	Increased	Decreased renal function, some drugs, contamination with vaginal secretions
Leukocyte esterase	Negative	Present	Pyuria
Nitrites	Negative	Present	Infection
Glucose	Negative	Positive	Diabetes mellitus, Cushing's syndrome, liver and pancreatic disease
Ketones	Negative	Positive	Uncontrolled diabetes mellitus, pregnancy, carbohydrate-free diet, starvation

Continued

Table 31.1
Urinalysis Results—cont'd

Characteristic	*Normal Findings*	*Abnormal Findings*	*Possible Cause*
WBCs, leukocytes	Less than 5	Increased number	Urinary tract or vaginal infection
WBC casts	Negative	Present	Upper UTI
RBCs	Less than 5	Increased number	Damage to renal tubules, tumors, renal calculi, or infection
RBC casts	Negative	Positive	Upper UTIs
Crystals	Few/negative	Positive	Renal stones

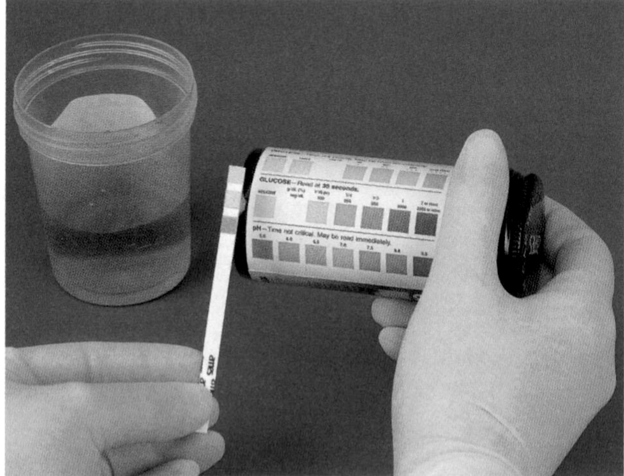

FIGURE 31.2 Urine dipsticks are used for quick testing at the bedside (from Wilkinson JM, Treas LS, Barnett KL, Smith MH. *Fundamentals of Nursing: Theory, Concepts & Applications.* Vol. 1. 3rd ed. Philadelphia, PA: FA Davis; 2016).

Box 31.1
Performing a Urine Dipstick

You may do a quick test of urine for abnormal findings using reagent strips, commonly referred to as urine dipsticks. To use these dipsticks correctly, follow these guidelines:

- Read the manufacturer's instructions before performing the test.
- Check the expiration date on the bottle of test strips.
- Put on clean gloves for the test.
- Remove one strip from the bottle and recap the bottle immediately to prevent contamination of other strips.
- Dip the test strip into the urine and begin timing. Tap against the side of the cup to remove excess urine.
- Hold the strip next to the bottle label, lining up the strip's small colored square pads to the corresponding ones on the bottle label.
- At each specified time, read the appropriate colored pad and note the results.

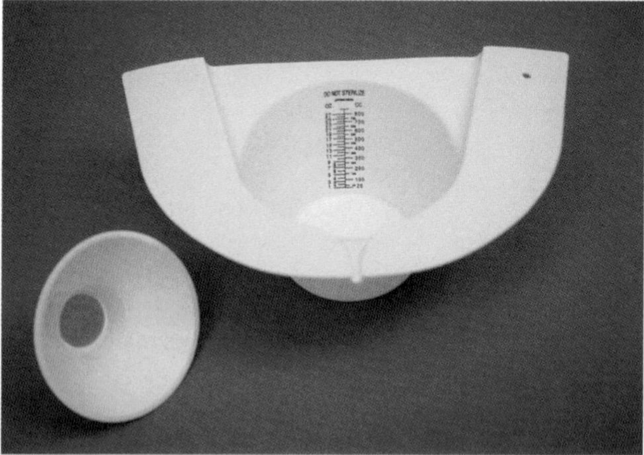

FIGURE 31.3 The urine strainer is used to detect the presence of stones. The specimen pan allows you to collect urine for testing or measurement.

pan is marked in milliliter increments (see Fig. 31.3). Males generally use the urinal to void; it is also marked in milliliter increments. If a bedridden patient voids in the bedpan, you will pour the urine into a graduated receptacle or a specimen pan to be measured before emptying it into the toilet.

Supervision/Delegation Connection

Monitoring Intake and Output

Monitoring I&O is a task that can be delegated to unlicensed personnel. As a nurse, if you are depending on someone else from the health-care team to aid you in assessing I&O, it is important to make sure he or she performs this assignment accurately and understands the importance of the task. Make sure you provide parameters to be reported to you during the shift if they occur. For example, you may need to know if the patient with a Foley catheter has less than 30 mL per hour of output for 2 consecutive hours or if the patient without a catheter does not void at least every 4 hours. If oliguria is overlooked and goes unreported for several hours, the patient may experience complications. Although the task of monitoring output can be delegated, licensed personnel are ultimately responsible. When working with unlicensed assistive personnel (UAP), provide clear instructions and expectations; never make the assumption that they know what needs to be reported to you. This is especially important when new members are added to your health-care team. Monitor I&O when a patient has an indwelling urinary catheter even if the health-care provider does not write an order for it.

Real-World Connection

Monitoring Urinary Output

Patients who have had abdominal surgery usually return to the medical-surgical floor with an indwelling urinary catheter in place. During morning report, the night shift nurse reported that Mrs. Jackson, who had a cesarean section the night before, had only 240 mL of urinary output for the previous 8 hours. Standard orders are to discontinue the urinary catheter the following morning, usually at 6:00 a.m. by the night shift nurse. Because the night nurse was concerned that the amount of urine was barely adequate, he made a clinical decision after emptying the drainage bag to leave the catheter in place until the health-care provider made rounds.

When the day shift nurse went into the room to assess the patient at 8:00 a.m., there was 60 mL of clear, dark amber urine in the drainage bag. When the patient's physician made rounds at 9:00 a.m., there was only 90 mL of urine in the bag. After reviewing the I&O record from the previous shift, the physician wrote the order to cancel the catheter removal that had been written the day before, as well as writing several new orders.

Nursing judgment constantly compels us to think critically about everything we encounter, especially before we take further action. Even though the patient had produced the minimum acceptable amount of urine, other factors were taken into consideration by the nurse before he made the correct decision regarding discontinuing the catheter. The physician appreciated and praised his clinical judgment. Eventually, the patient was taken back to the operating room and was found to have a large hematoma, or blood clot, in her abdomen that had to be removed.

KNOWLEDGE CONNECTION

You have asked a UAP to collect a final specimen from a patient who is in the process of collecting a 24-hour urine specimen. What instructions will you provide? When might reagent strips be used to test urine? What is the purpose of an order to strain all urine?

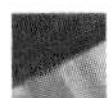

ALTERATIONS IN URINARY FUNCTION

Any single structure of the urinary system can malfunction, or a combination of structures can cause alterations in function of the system. The bladder may not empty completely, or it may not empty at all. The patient may be unable to control the urine as it leaves the bladder for various reasons. In addition, blockages may prevent the urine from traveling from the kidneys to the bladder to then be expelled, or the prostate gland in the male may be so enlarged that the patient is unable to empty his bladder.

Altered Bladder Function

When the bladder does not contract and empty, the patient may experience painful bladder spasms and distention. The nurse must take action to remove the urine from the bladder. When the patient cannot empty the bladder completely, the urine that remains in the bladder can become a good medium for bacteria growth, leading to infection. When the patient cannot control his or her urine output, it can be upsetting and embarrassing.

Urinary Retention

Urinary retention is the inability to empty the bladder at all or the inability to completely empty the bladder. It can be acute or chronic. With urinary retention, the kidneys are functioning normally and producing urine and the ureters are transporting the urine to the bladder to be stored, but for some reason the bladder is not emptying. An obstruction such as a kidney stone, an enlarged prostate gland, a tumor, a pregnant uterus, an infection, or scar tissue may cause retention. Other causes of urinary retention include UTIs, disorders or diseases of the nerves that regulate the bladder and urinary sphincters, postoperative complications due to anesthesia, inflammation, edema from surgery, and medications. An enlarged prostate is a frequent cause of urinary retention in older men. The prostate gland surrounds the urethra, and when the gland enlarges, it constricts the urethra and can prevent the bladder from emptying. After a period of time, the urine in the bladder can reflux into the kidneys, causing *hydronephrosis,* which is the stretching of the renal pelvis due to obstruction of the flow of urine from the bladder. If the obstruction is not relieved, hydronephrosis can lead to kidney atrophy and chronic renal failure.

Residual Urine

Residual urine is urine that remains in the bladder after the patient voids. It may be caused by bladder outlet obstruction or problems with the detrusor muscle's contractility. Normally, the maximum amount of urine left in the bladder after voiding is 100 mL. To determine if a patient has residual

• **WORD • BUILDING •**

hydronephrosis: hydro – water + nephr – kidney + osis – condition

urine, begin by palpating the bladder just above the symphysis pubis to evaluate if there is any bladder distention, because there might be with a large volume of residual. Then you may perform a bladder scan for an accurate estimation of the volume of urine that is present. A bladder scan is a noninvasive procedure that uses ultrasound to measure the amount of residual urine (Fig. 31.4). Skill 31.4 (page 685) lists the steps for performing a bladder scan.

Nocturia

When a person wakes often during the night to urinate, the condition is known as **nocturia.** Occasional nocturia may be caused by ingesting large amounts of fluid in the evening. If a patient has persistent nocturia, it may be due to an underlying disease process, such as heart failure, uncontrolled diabetes mellitus, a UTI, an enlarged prostate, or kidney disease. Nocturia should not be dismissed as a normal part of aging and should be evaluated by a health-care provider.

Urinary Incontinence

By 2 to 3 years of age, children have full control of their bladder. This control continues through adulthood for most people. However, there are situations in which this bladder control is lost during adulthood. This inability to control the passing of urine is urinary **incontinence.**

Incontinence is more common in women, although the incidence increases for both men and women as they age; however, this does not mean that it is a normal part of the aging process. When a patient experiences incontinence, he or she may be affected emotionally as well as physically. Patients may be forced to make lifestyle adjustments, giving up activities and social situations they once enjoyed because of loss of bladder control and the fear that people will be able to detect the smell of urine. Incontinence can cause hardships in the workplace as well. To make matters worse, because people often perceive incontinence as a normal part of the aging process, they may not seek treatment. Patients also may be too embarrassed to seek treatment.

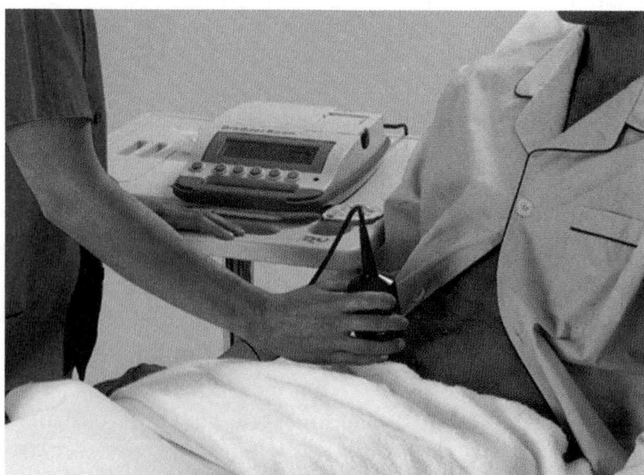

FIGURE 31.4 The bladder scan is used to detect the presence of residual urine in the bladder (from Williams LS, Hopper PD. *Understanding Medical-Surgical Nursing*. 5th ed. Philadelphia, PA: FA Davis; 2015).

TYPES OF INCONTINENCE. **Stress incontinence** occurs with increased abdominal pressure, which causes urine to leak out of the bladder. Stress incontinence is seen more in women than in men. Increased abdominal pressure can be caused by coughing, laughing, sneezing, vomiting, and heavy lifting or straining—anything that elicits a "bearing down" effect. Factors that may contribute to the development of stress incontinence include vaginal births, previous pelvic or vaginal surgery, genetics, hormone levels, and chronic medical conditions. When pelvic floor muscles become weak, they do not support the bladder and urethra, leading to urine leakage.

Urge incontinence, also known as *overactive bladder,* is the inability to keep urine in the bladder long enough to get to the restroom. Normally, most people void five to six times a day. When a patient experiences urge incontinence, he or she may urinate more frequently than normal in the daytime and experience nocturia two or three times per night. The patient may have urine leakage because of the inability to get to the bathroom quickly. This type of incontinence is caused by bladder spasms or contractions that lead to involuntary passing of urine. Triggers that may lead to urge incontinence include the sound of running water, drinking liquid, or placing your hands in warm water. Urge incontinence is often caused by a UTI, but many times the cause is not known. Muscle toning and strengthening exercises are sometimes successful treatments for urge incontinence. *Mixed incontinence* is diagnosed when a patient experiences both stress and urge incontinence.

Overflow incontinence occurs when the bladder is distended due to an obstruction, which prevents the bladder from emptying normally. Some urine may then leak past the blockage, causing overflow. In men, the most common cause of this obstruction is an enlarged prostate gland.

Other types of incontinence are less common. These include functional, total, and neuropathic incontinence. *Functional incontinence* occurs when the person is unable to reach a bathroom to urinate. This may be due to the unavailability of bathroom facilities or the person's inability to get on the toilet before urination occurs. *Total incontinence* is the loss of urine with no warning. In this situation, the person is unaware of the need to void and makes no effort to get to a bathroom. *Neuropathic incontinence* occurs when the nerves that control the bladder and surrounding structures are not getting the message to the brain that the bladder is full.

Nursing Interventions to Manage Incontinence

One treatment for stress incontinence involves teaching the patient to perform Kegel exercises, which will strengthen and tone the pelvic floor muscles. The exercises must be done regularly and indefinitely to be effective. Box 31.2

• WORD • BUILDING •

nocturia: noct – night + ur – urine + ia – condition

Box 31.2

Kegel Exercise Instructions

You may need to explain how to perform pelvic floor exercises to help prevent or control certain types of urinary incontinence. Instruct the patient using these guidelines:

- Have the patient lie supine.
- Have the patient place the hands on the lower abdomen to ensure that the abdominal muscles stay relaxed.
- Tell the patient to tighten the pelvic floor muscles (the muscles that stop the flow of urine or prevent you from passing gas) without tightening the abdominal or thigh muscles.
- Encourage the patient to hold the contraction for 5 to 10 seconds and then relax for 5 to 10 seconds. The patient should perform 40 to 60 exercises spread throughout the day.
- Advise the patient to not perform the exercises while urinating because it can cause urinary retention.

provides a description of how to teach a patient to perform Kegel exercises.

Encourage women to engage in a moderate exercise program on a regular basis to help decrease the incidence of incontinence. Studies have shown that women who engage in regular, moderately intensive physical activity have less urinary incontinence than women who lead sedentary lifestyles.

BLADDER TRAINING. Nurses can initiate a bladder training program without a physician's order to assist the patient in managing urinary incontinence. Bladder training involves assisting the patient to the bathroom at set times throughout the day, even if the urge to urinate is not recognized. For example, you would assist the patient to the bathroom after meals and every 2 hours during the day to increase awareness of the need to void. Follow these guidelines to increase the effectiveness of bladder training:

- Ensure that the patient is taking in adequate amounts of fluid, at least 64 ounces per day, to help maintain a healthy urinary tract and facilitate the elimination of waste.
- Teach patients to avoid caffeinated beverages and to drink more during the day and less in the evening to prevent nighttime incontinence.
- Offer fluids throughout the day, avoiding a large volume of fluid all at one time. Find out which fluids the patient prefers and offer an 8-ounce glass of fluid every 2 hours.
- Assist the patient to the bathroom or offer a bedpan every 2 hours and assess the patient frequently for incontinence. If the patient has been incontinent between toileting, decrease the length of time between offering the bedpan or assistance to the bathroom.
- Most people void in the morning, after meals, and before bed. Try to mimic the patient's normal voiding patterns.

In some circumstances, bladder training is not appropriate. If the patient is not able to understand the program or does not wish to participate, he or she is not a candidate for bladder training. In this situation, good skin care is very important to prevent skin breakdown. ***Safety: Clean the skin as soon as urinary incontinence is detected. When urine is left on the skin, the liquid portion evaporates and the chemicals left behind can cause skin irritation and skin breakdown.*** Change the patient's incontinence briefs and perform perineal care at least every 2 hours. In general, indwelling urinary catheters are not placed for long-term urinary incontinence because they can lead to UTIs, sepsis, urethral strictures, prostatitis, and the potential development of bladder cancer.

KNOWLEDGE CONNECTION

During data collection, you ask a male patient about problems with urination. He replies, "It seems to take me longer to pee than it used to." What is the patient experiencing? What are the differences in managing stress versus urge urinary incontinence?

Laboratory and Diagnostic Connection

Assessing Kidney Function and Failure

Blood urea nitrogen (BUN) results from the breakdown of protein by the body. The normal levels of BUN are 8 to 21 mg/dL in adults. Abnormal elevations in BUN may reflect infection or some degree of renal impairment. Creatinine is a waste product excreted by the kidneys. The normal level of creatinine in the blood is 0.6 to 1.21 mg/dL in an adult male and 0.5 to 1.11 mg/dL in an adult female. An increase in creatinine in the blood usually indicates decreased or impaired renal function. A health-care provider can use the serum creatinine level in a formula with age, gender, and race to determine the estimated glomerular filtration rate (eGFR). This helps to determine the stage of renal disease that a patient is in. A GFR less than 60 mL per minute when tested over 3 months indicates mild to moderate loss of kidney function. A GFR less than 15 mL per minute indicates renal failure. Physicians monitor serum creatinine and GFR over several months to determine the extent of chronic kidney disease and treat the patient to prevent further progression of the disease.

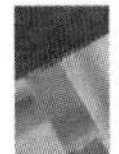

CARING FOR PATIENTS WITH ALTERED URINARY FUNCTION

Over your career, you probably will care for many patients with altered urinary function. The alteration may be related to the patient's original diagnosis and admission, or it may be due to an additional issue that developed after admission.

Urinary Catheters

One of the most common situations you will encounter is caring for patients who have an indwelling catheter in place or who need to have a straight catheter inserted to obtain residual urine or a sterile urine specimen. A *urinary catheter* is a tube usually made of rubber, plastic, latex, polyvinyl, or silicone that is inserted through the urethra into the bladder. It may be inserted and then quickly removed after the bladder is emptied, as in the case of a straight catheter, or it may remain in place when an attached balloon is inflated, anchoring it in the bladder.

Types of Catheters

There are many different types of catheters, including straight catheters, indwelling catheters, three-way catheters, and condom catheters. Box 31.3 describes different types of urinary catheters and their uses. Figure 31.5 shows cross-sections of different types of catheters.

INDWELLING CATHETERS. When you care for a patient with urinary retention, you will expect to receive orders to insert an **indwelling catheter,** also known as a *double-lumen catheter* or *Foley catheter,* to empty the bladder. The catheter will remain in the bladder, usually for a few days, and drain the urine on a continuous basis. Skill 31.5 (page 686) provides more information on inserting an indwelling urinary catheter. Skill 31.6 (page 689) provides information on obtaining a urine sample from an indwelling urinary catheter.

An indwelling catheter may be ordered for the following reasons:

- To relieve acute urinary retention or urinary obstruction
- To obtain accurate urine output measurements in severely ill patients
- To help prevent urine contact with an open wound in the sacral or perineal area
- To prevent complications during or after certain surgeries, such as urologic or abdominal surgeries
- To make the patient more comfortable at the end of life

It is your nursing responsibility to assess urinary output, including color, clarity, and amount, during your shift. Figure 31.6 shows indwelling catheters in both male and female patients.

In some circumstances, special catheters must be used. If an obstruction in the urethra or neck of the bladder is present, it may be difficult to pass the catheter into the bladder. If the obstruction is due to an enlarged prostate, a Coudé catheter may be the best choice (see Box 31.3).

If the catheter cannot be advanced into the bladder at all, a health-care provider may have to insert a suprapubic catheter (see Box 31.3). Once the suprapubic catheter is inserted, the catheter is advanced about an inch into the bladder, and the balloon is filled with 5 mL of sterile water to hold it in place. Figure 31.7 shows insertion of a suprapubic catheter.

STRAIGHT CATHETERS. If you are caring for a patient who is unable to fully empty his or her bladder and you have found residual urine in the bladder using a bladder scan, you could expect to receive orders to insert a **straight catheter,** also known as a *single-lumen catheter,* to empty the bladder. A straight catheter is a single tube with holes at the end. It may be made of red rubber, clear plastic, or silicone. The health-care provider may or may not also order a sterile specimen from the bladder for a UA or culture and sensitivity testing. This is also sometimes called an *in-and-out catheterization,* indicating that the catheter does not remain in the bladder. Straight catheters are also used by patients who must catheterize themselves on a regular basis to empty the bladder. An example of this would be the patient with a condition called *neurogenic bladder,* where the nerves to the bladder have been permanently damaged. The patient cannot control the nerves that cause the bladder to empty. The patient or a caregiver must insert a straight catheter to empty the patient's bladder several times per day, usually about every 4 hours.

In the hospital setting, you will use a sterile catheter insertion kit and a sterile straight catheter every time you insert a catheter. The hospital environment is full of pathogens, and you must take every precaution to prevent contamination of your sterile field or the sterile catheter, which would introduce harmful pathogens into the patient's bladder. (See Chapter 22 for a review of sterile technique.) Skill 31.7 (page 689) provides more information on inserting a straight catheter.

Elder Care Connection

Long-Term Care and Catheterizations

The Centers for Medicare & Medicaid Services of the U.S. Department of Health and Human Services states that only residents with appropriate justification should have indwelling urinary catheters. Appropriate use includes residents who have intractable urinary retention, stage 3 or stage 4 pressure injuries, terminal illness, or severe impairment such that positioning and clothing changes are uncomfortable or are associated with intractable pain.

Settings Connection: Home Health

Home Health Care and Catheterizations

In the home health-care setting, patients may need to perform self-catheterizations. Unlike the procedure in the acute care setting, self-catheterization at home is a clean rather than sterile procedure. Catheters are often washed and reused; patients wash their hands and put on nonsterile gloves when they perform the procedure. Those who may perform self-catheterization include patients with urinary retention, residual urine, or neurological conditions that prevent the bladder from emptying, or those who have a history of a spinal cord injury.

Box 31.3

Types of Catheters and Their Uses

Some catheters may be called by several different names. It is important to be familiar with the type of catheter, its function, and the various names it may be called.

- **Straight Catheter:** Also known as a *single-lumen catheter.* Used only for insertion into the urinary bladder to obtain a sterile urine specimen or a one-time drainage of urine from the bladder. It is aseptically inserted into the bladder through the urinary meatus, where either all the urine is drained or just enough urine for a specimen is obtained. Then the straight catheter is removed.
- **Indwelling Catheter:** Also known as a *double-lumen catheter* or a *Foley catheter.* Remains in the urinary bladder for a designated period of time. After insertion, one lumen is used to inflate a balloon near the tip of the catheter with 5 to 30 mL of sterile water; the amount of water is dependent on the size of the balloon. This inflated balloon sits at the junction of the bladder and the urethra, holding the catheter in place and helping to seal the exit from the bladder so that urine does not leak around the catheter (see Fig. 31.6). Urine continually drains out of the bladder through the lumen of the catheter into a drainage bag that hangs low on the side of the patient's bed. Indwelling catheters are inserted when the patient will need urine drainage for 1 or more days.
- **Three-Way Catheter:** Also known as a *triple-lumen catheter* or an *Alcock catheter.* Used in only one specific situation: After a male patient has had a transurethral resection of the prostate, the surgeon will insert a triple-lumen catheter with a 30- to 60-mL balloon to provide traction and help control bleeding. The third lumen in the catheter allows instillation of sterile fluid into the bladder during continuous bladder irrigation to help evacuate tissue and clots from the urinary bladder.
- **Coudé Catheter:** Used specifically to accommodate an enlarged prostate in male patients. It has a curved tip, allowing it to more easily pass through an enlarged prostate gland and enter the bladder.
- **Suprapubic Catheter:** Placed after trauma or surgery to the urethra or if an indwelling catheter cannot be inserted into the bladder. The physician makes a small incision above the pubic bone, passes an instrument through the abdominal wall and into the bladder, and then places the catheter. This procedure requires that the patient be given mild sedation or a local anesthetic.
- **Condom Catheter:** Also known as a *Texas catheter.* Used for males who are incontinent of urine to avoid the risk of infection related to insertion of an indwelling catheter. It is similar to a regular condom and is applied by rolling it onto the penis. It is a condom-like sheath with a 2-inch drainage tube connector on the tip that connects to a urinary drainage bag. The sheath collects the urine and allows it to drain through the drainage tube into the drainage bag, either a regular urinary drainage bag or a smaller bag that can be strapped to the thigh.

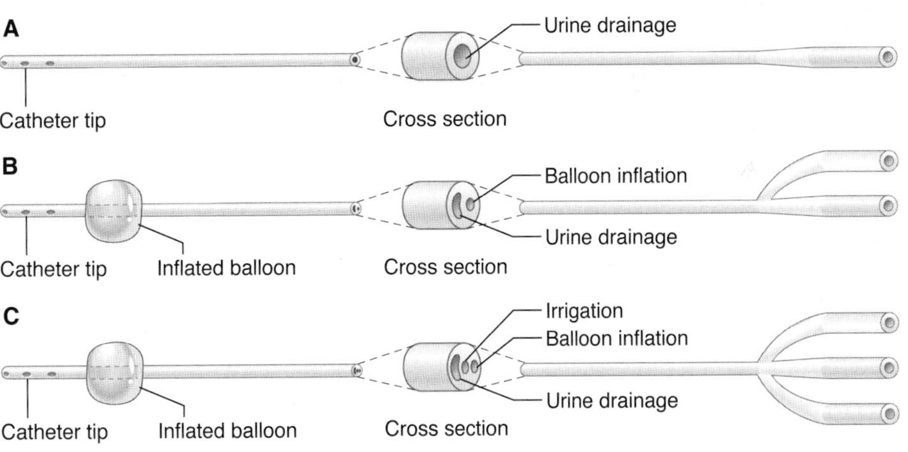

FIGURE 31.5 Types of catheters: (a) Straight catheter, also called a single-lumen catheter; (b) Indwelling catheter, also known as a double-lumen or Foley catheter; (c) Three-way catheter, also known as a triple-lumen catheter, used for continuous bladder irrigations (from Wilkinson JM, Treas LS, Barnett KL, Smith MH. *Fundamentals of Nursing: Theory, Concepts & Applications.* Vol. 1. 3rd ed. Philadelphia, PA: FA Davis; 2016).

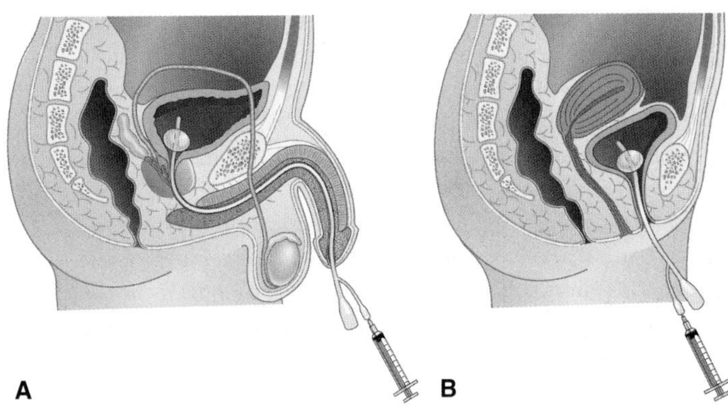

FIGURE 31.6 Placement of indwelling catheters: (a) Location of an indwelling catheter with the balloon inflated in a male; (b) Location of an indwelling catheter with the balloon inflated in a female (from Wilkinson JM, Treas LS, Barnett KL, Smith MH. *Fundamentals of Nursing: Theory, Concepts & Applications.* Vol. 2. 3rd ed. Philadelphia, PA: FA Davis; 2016).

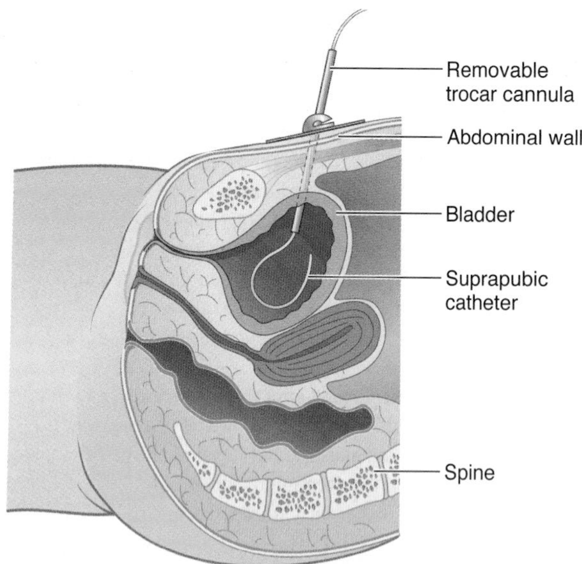

FIGURE 31.7 A suprapubic catheter is inserted through the abdominal wall directly into the bladder (from Wilkinson JM, Treas LS, Barnett KL, Smith MH. *Fundamentals of Nursing: Theory, Concepts & Applications.* Vol. 1. 3rd ed. Philadelphia, PA: FA Davis; 2016).

THREE-WAY CATHETERS. When the prostate gland enlarges in a male patient, it grows into the prostatic urethra and obstructs it, causing the opening through which urine can pass to narrow significantly. In this situation, the enlargement of the prostate is not due to cancer but is a benign condition called benign prostatic hypertrophy. A surgical procedure called transurethral resection of the prostate (TURP) is one option for treating this condition. In this procedure the physician removes the parts of the prostate that are blocking the urethra.

After this surgery, a *three-way catheter,* also known as a *triple-lumen catheter* or *Alcock catheter,* is inserted through the newly cleared urethra and into the bladder to allow for irrigation of the bladder. Because cutting has occurred, it is normal for blood and blood clots to pass through the three-way catheter and into the urinary drainage bag. The goal of nursing care after this procedure is to prevent any blood clots from obstructing the flow of the irrigation fluid into the bladder and back out again.

Continuous Bladder Irrigation

Irrigation fluid in large bags is hung from an IV pole, and the tubing is aseptically attached to the third lumen of the three-way catheter. The irrigation fluid runs continuously at a slow rate to wash out blood and prevent clots from forming (Fig. 31.8). If the urine in the collection bag becomes red or clots are evident in the tubing, increase the rate to flush them out. ***Safety: Assess for fluid return into the drainage bag frequently. It is possible for a blood clot to clog the urine drainage lumen, blocking urine and irrigation fluid from leaving the bladder. This is extremely important because irrigation fluid continues to flow into the bladder via the irrigation lumen, filling the bladder fuller and fuller. This can result in overdistention of the bladder and could potentially rupture the bladder if the urine lumen remains clogged.*** Skill 31.8 (page 691) presents information on how to perform a continuous bladder irrigation.

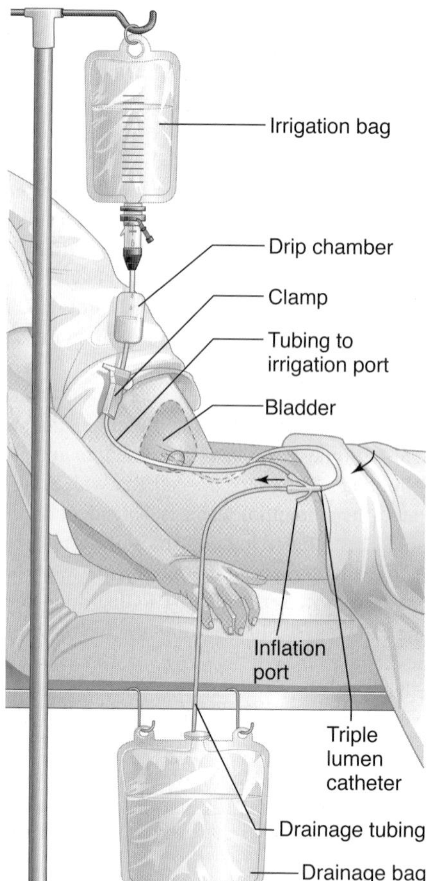

FIGURE 31.8 A continuous bladder irrigation consists of irrigation fluid from the large bag on the IV pole flowing through the triple-lumen catheter into the bladder and then out to the drainage bag on the side of the bed (adapted from Wilkinson JM, Treas LS, Barnett KL, Smith MH. *Fundamentals of Nursing: Theory, Concepts & Applications.* Vol. 2. 3rd ed. Philadelphia, PA: FA Davis; 2016).

To correctly calculate output with a continuous bladder irrigation, you must subtract the amount of irrigation solution instilled from the amount of fluid in the urinary drainage bag. For example, if 750 mL of saline was instilled during irrigation and a total of 1,000 mL of fluid has collected in the drainage bag, the amount of urine output would be 250 mL because you subtracted 750 from 1,000.

CONDOM CATHETERS. Condom catheters, also called external catheters, are not inserted into the bladder through the urethra, so they pose less of a risk for causing a UTI. Most condom catheters are held in place with a double-sided adhesive strip applied to the penis. It is important to apply the adhesive strip in a spiral. This prevents the strip from encircling the penis and potentially interfering with circulation. It also is important to keep the foreskin in place when applying a condom catheter to an uncircumcised male patient. Some types of condom catheters are held in place with wafers and skin adhesive. Skill 31.9 (page 691) shows the steps for applying a condom catheter using an adhesive strip.

> **KNOWLEDGE CONNECTION**
> List five reasons for inserting an indwelling catheter. What are four types of urinary catheters and why is each ordered? The UAP tells you that the output of a patient with a continuous bladder irrigation is 4,000 mL for an 8-hour shift. What additional information do you need to determine the amount of urine that was produced?

Catheter Size

Urinary catheters come in different sizes gauged by measuring the outer diameter of the catheter: the larger the number, the larger the catheter. The size is denoted with a number followed by *French (Fr),* which is the scale of measurement for urinary catheters. A child may need a size 8 French, while an adult may need a size 14 or size 16 French. When a patient in long-term care or home care has had an indwelling catheter for several years, it may be necessary to use even larger sizes, such as 20 or 22 French, because the urethra and cystourethral junction stretch over time. Catheters also come in different lengths according to their purpose. A 22-cm length would be appropriate for a female, while a 40-cm length would be appropriate for a male. However, in most health-care settings, a standard length of 40 cm is used. Catheters also come with different sizes of inflatable balloons, ranging from 5 to 30 mL.

Inserting Catheters

Insertion of any type of catheter requires a physician's order, which should be reviewed prior to the procedure. ***Safety: It is important to assess a patient for allergies to latex before inserting an indwelling urinary catheter. If the patient is allergic to latex, you will need to obtain a silicone catheter instead to prevent reactions.*** Always check for allergies to povidone-iodine (Betadine) as well because it is provided in most catheter insertion kits for cleansing the meatus and surrounding area prior to insertion. ***Safety: If the patient is allergic to Betadine, you will need to obtain a different cleaning agent according to your facility's policy.*** The type of catheter and the reason for catheterization will determine which supply kit you use. There are different kits for insertion of straight catheters and indwelling catheters. Figure 31.9 shows the contents of a straight catheter kit, and Figure 31.10 shows the contents of an indwelling catheter kit.

Insertion of a urinary catheter, in the hospital or another medical setting, requires stringent asepsis. Your sterile technique helps to prevent hospital-acquired UTIs. If you contaminate the catheter, your gloves, your sterile field, or sterile supplies, you must stop the procedure and start over with uncontaminated supplies. Failure to do so may cause your patient to experience infection, discomfort, added expense, and potentially death from sepsis. You may be the only person who knows if you have contaminated your sterile field or the sterile catheter during insertion. If that occurs, you must discard your supplies and begin again. ***Safety: Contamination of the catheter or sterile field can lead to a catheter-associated UTI (CAUTI).*** Refer back to Chapter 22 for review of sterile technique. Box 31.4 contains information regarding hospital costs associated with CAUTIs.

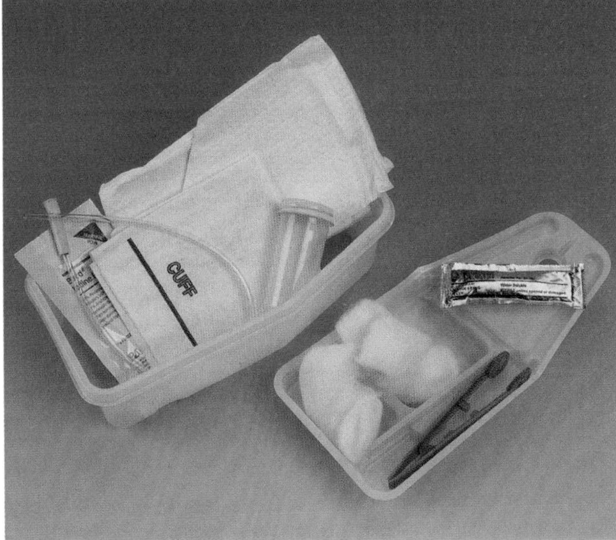

FIGURE 31.9 A prepackaged straight catheter kit (from Wilkinson JM, Treas LS, Barnett KL, Smith MH. *Fundamentals of Nursing: Theory, Concepts & Applications.* Vol. 2. 3rd ed. Philadelphia, PA: FA Davis; 2016).

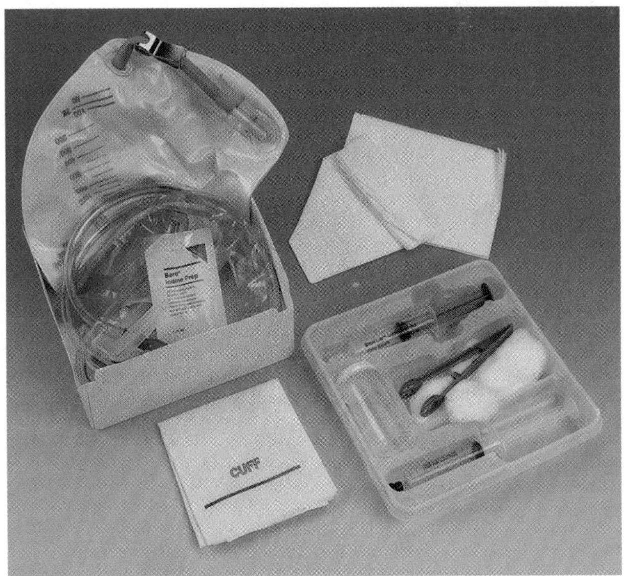

FIGURE 31.10 A prepackaged indwelling catheter kit (from Wilkinson JM, Treas LS. *Fundamentals of Nursing: Theory, Concepts & Applications.* Vol. 1. 2nd ed. Philadelphia, PA: FA Davis; 2011).

FEMALE PERINEAL ANATOMY. Before you begin the procedure of inserting a catheter, you will need to examine the patient's perineal anatomy. You may not see an obvious

• WORD • BUILDING •

cystourethral: cysto – urinary bladder + urethral – relating to the urethra

Box 31.4

Payment of Costs Related to Hospital-Acquired Urinary Tract Infections

The Centers for Medicare and Medicaid Services has determined that its insurance plans will no longer pay for any costs associated with catheter-related hospital-acquired infections. If a patient acquires a UTI after a urinary catheter is inserted in a hospital setting, the facility will not be paid for the costs of antibiotics, extra hospital days, or any other associated expenses. Your technique must be excellent when inserting urinary catheters and caring for patients with them.

urethral "opening" in the female patient unless she has had many urinary catheters in the past. The female urinary meatus often resembles a small dimpling of the tissue, almost like a tiny slit or crease, rather than the easily detectable opening that you will see in the manikin in the skills laboratory. In an elderly female, you may even find the urethral meatus in a slightly different location than indicated in textbook anatomy. The urinary meatus is generally located just below the clitoris, midway between the clitoris and the vaginal opening. In some elderly females, you may find the urinary meatus at the edge of or slightly inside the vaginal opening. A lack of hormones causes the tissue to *atrophy,* or shrink. This results in pulling the urinary meatus into the vaginal opening, making it more difficult to access with a catheter.

In certain circumstances, you may find that you are unable to separate the female patient's legs due to severe contractures or other conditions. In these instances, a possible alternative may be to insert the catheter while the patient is lying on her side. Turn the patient to the lateral position and view the urinary meatus from that angle before you prepare to insert the catheter. Patients who have long-term indwelling catheters may be easier to catheterize from this position.

MALE PERINEAL ANATOMY. Male patients may exhibit unusual urethral locations as well. The urethra of the male may open on the dorsum of the penis rather than at the tip of the penis, a condition known as *epispadias.* If the urethral meatus is located on the underside of the penis, the condition is termed *hypospadias.*

Some men have been circumcised, meaning that the foreskin that covers the glans penis has been surgically removed. This may be done due to cultural or religious preferences. For patients who have not been circumcised, you must retract the foreskin, or move it back from the glans, during catheterization. ***Safety: It is extremely important that you replace the foreskin to its original position after you have inserted the indwelling catheter. Failure to do so can cause constriction of blood flow to the glans penis, causing swelling and possible necrosis.***

If the patient has an enlarged prostate, you may meet resistance when you try to insert the catheter. If this occurs, twist the catheter slightly as you attempt to advance it. Sometimes this will be adequate to allow the catheter tip to enter the portion of the urethra that passes through the enlarged prostate. If that does not advance the tip beyond the prostate gland, the procedure may need to be attempted again using a Coudé catheter. This may need to be done by a physician, depending on facility policy.

Nursing Care of Patients With Indwelling Catheters

When you care for patients with indwelling urinary catheters, you will need to be aware of the position of the tubing and drainage bag and the flow of the urine into the bag and check for possible obstructions if output is low.

URINARY DRAINAGE BAGS. Urine drains from the catheter through tubing attached to a drainage bag, where it is stored until emptied. When caring for the patient with an indwelling catheter, monitor the drainage bag that collects the urine as it drains from the bladder several times during your shift. Empty the bag every 8 hours or more frequently if it becomes full. The numbers on the bag will provide you with only an approximate volume. Measure the exact volume of urine by emptying it into a graduated container. The task of emptying the catheter drainage bag can be assigned to a UAP, but monitoring urinary output during the shift is your responsibility. Unless otherwise ordered, output is normally recorded at the end of the shift. If the health-care provider has ordered hourly output readings or you are concerned about the amount of urine, use a urometer for the most accurate reading. A *urometer* is a small plastic measuring device attached to the urine drainage bag that accurately measures very small amounts of urine.

Follow these guidelines for care of the urinary drainage bag:

- Empty the catheter bag every 8 hours or when it is full and document the amount in the medical record.
- When emptying the bag, do not touch the drainage spout to any surfaces and wipe it with an alcohol swab before closing the spout.
- Always empty urine into a graduated container to obtain an accurate measurement. ***Safety: Each patient must have his or her own graduated container for measurement. Sharing these containers among patients can lead to cross-contamination and increase the incidence of CAUTIs.***
- Maintain the drainage bag below the level of the bladder at all times. If the bag is elevated, the tubing should be clamped first to prevent urine in the tubing from flowing back into the bladder, potentially causing a UTI.
- Keep the tubing free of kinks and coils.
- Hang the drainage bag on a moveable part of the bed; it should not lay on the floor. Avoid hanging it on the bed rails, however, because it could be raised above the level of the bladder when the rails are raised.

Evidence-Based Practice

Rapid Bladder Decompression

Clinical Question

Does rapid decompression of the urinary bladder cause more complications than gradual decompression?

Evidence

A literature review was done to quantify the risk of complications in relieving urinary retention due to obstruction. It was also done to determine if the risk of complications was higher with rapid versus gradual decompression of the bladder. Many nurses have been taught to clamp the catheter after 1,000 mL of urine has been drained from the bladder to prevent risk of complications such as hematuria and diuresis. The length of time that they were told to clamp the catheter varied. This research found that any complications were not clinically significant. There were no studies found comparing gradual versus rapid decompression.

Implications for Nursing Practice

This study and other research demonstrate that quick, complete emptying of the urinary bladder is safe and effective. However, it is always wise to assess the patient during the process and be ready to slow down decompression if needed. It is especially important to assess elderly patients with hypovolemia.

References

You can read more about this and similar studies at the following sites:

www.researchgate.net/publication/13849694_Management_of_Urinary_Retention_Rapid_Versus_Gradual_Decompression_and_Risk_of_Complications

www.ncbi.nlm.nih.gov/pubmed/23859894

http://journals.sagepub.com/doi/abs/10.1177/0049475512472432

TROUBLESHOOTING LOW OUTPUT. If no urine is collecting in the drainage bag, palpate the urinary bladder above the pubic bone to assess for a full bladder. Check for kinks in the catheter tubing. Ensure that the patient is not lying on the catheter or drainage bag tubing. Manipulate the drainage bag tubing so that the urine flows in a downward manner by gravity. If the tubing is looped downward, urine will pool and back up because it cannot run uphill. Have the patient change positions and see if the bladder will empty.

If the bladder feels distended (evidenced by palpating a firm area above the pubic bone), it is appropriate to perform a bladder scan. It is possible that the catheter is blocked by sediment or mucus. If none of the troubleshooting techniques improves output and the bladder definitely contains urine, notify the health-care provider to obtain orders to irrigate the catheter.

INTERMITTENT CATHETER IRRIGATION. A catheter can be irrigated, or flushed, with sterile saline to rinse out sediment or mucus that may be blocking the openings on the tube in the bladder. It is important to use good aseptic technique to prevent introducing pathogens into the closed urinary drainage system. This is accomplished by using a sterile syringe and noncoring blunt needle or other needleless access device (Fig. 31.11). The sterile saline is drawn up as ordered from a sterile container into a 20-mL syringe. The tube on the drainage bag contains an access port for this purpose. Clamp the drainage bag tubing below the port. This causes the saline to go into the bladder and not simply drain into the bag. Skill 31.10 (page 692) lists the steps for irrigating a closed urinary drainage system.

Catheter Care

You will provide perineal and catheter care together at least once a shift and any time the catheter becomes contaminated by a bowel movement to prevent UTIs. After cleansing the perineal area thoroughly, use clean water and a clean washcloth to perform catheter care. Hold the catheter in your gloved hand to prevent traction on the tubing as you clean the catheter. Using perineal wash or a disposable washcloth, clean the catheter with downward strokes from the insertion site toward the catheter bag. ***Safety: Always use downward strokes as upward strokes encourage the movement of microorganisms into the bladder.*** Rinse the catheter if appropriate. (See Chapter 15 for further information on perineal care.)

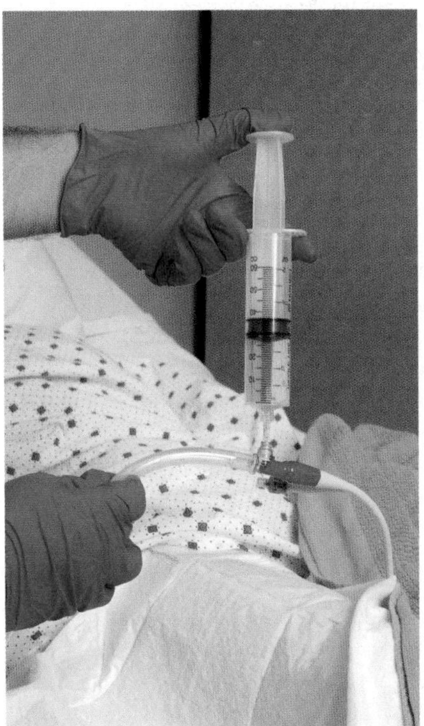

FIGURE 31.11 This nurse is irrigating a catheter using a noncoring blunt needle, maintaining the closed system (from Wilkinson JM, Treas LS. *Fundamentals of Nursing: Theory, Concepts & Applications.* Vol. 1. 2nd ed. Philadelphia, PA: FA Davis; 2011).

Discontinuing Catheters

Indwelling catheters inserted for surgical patients may remain in place for several days. You must have a health-care provider's order to discontinue an indwelling catheter. Skill 31.11 (page 693) shows the steps required to remove an indwelling urinary catheter. Upon removal of the catheter, it is important that you monitor for urinary retention, to determine if the patient has urinated within a maximum of 8 hours after the catheter was removed. Be certain to document when the patient voids and how much is voided. ***Safety: If a patient has not voided in the 8 hours after removing an indwelling catheter or has voided less than 240 mL, perform a bladder scan and notify the health-care provider.*** You may then receive an order to insert a straight catheter to empty the bladder or to reinsert an indwelling catheter if the bladder scan reveals an excessive amount of residual urine.

Caring for and Changing a Suprapubic Catheter

Suprapubic catheters may be required for long periods of time if the urethra cannot function normally. Dressings around the insertion site are changed using sterile technique to prevent the introduction of pathogens directly into the bladder. The tract from the bladder through the abdominal wall heals and forms a tunnel that the catheter is inserted through.

Suprapubic catheters that are in place for long periods usually are changed as needed. It is no longer recommended to change any catheters at routine times, such as every 30 days. Changing a suprapubic catheter is very similar to changing a Foley catheter. You will still use a sterile catheter kit, sterile gloves, and the correct size of sterile catheter. The patient is positioned on his or her back, and the drapes are applied to the lower abdomen. The differences involved in inserting a suprapubic catheter include the following:

- Only 3 to 5 mL of sterile water is placed in the balloon, so that amount will be withdrawn before an existing catheter is removed and replaced by a new one.
- Once the existing catheter is removed, clean around the suprapubic tract with the sterile swabs provided in the kit.
- Gently insert the lubricated catheter only 1 to 3 inches at a 10- to 30-degree angle to follow the suprapubic tract into the bladder.
- Insert 3 to 5 mL of sterile water into the balloon and tug very slightly to seat the catheter in the bladder opening.

KNOWLEDGE CONNECTION

What size catheter would you select for a male patient who has not had an indwelling catheter before? What can you do to help prevent CAUTIs when inserting an indwelling catheter? What are some anomalies of female perineal anatomy that you may see? What are male anomalies of perineal anatomy?

Urinary Diversions

In some situations, it is not possible to empty the bladder by draining it with a catheter because of an obstruction or interruption of the normal urine pathway. A **urinary diversion** means that the urine is eliminated by an alternative route rather than traveling through the bladder. These diversions may be established when there has been trauma to the bladder or the bladder has been removed as a result of bladder cancer. Occasionally, the ureters or bladder did not form correctly before birth, leading to a congenital condition requiring a urinary diversion.

One type of urinary diversion is the *ileal conduit.* The ureters are attached to a section of the small intestine that has been used to create a pouch and stoma. Urine drains continuously from the stoma. The patient wears an appliance over the stoma to collect the urine. Application of appliances to a stoma is discussed in Chapter 30. One of the greatest challenges with an incontinent urinary diversion is skin care. If the patient has a problem with irritation or skin breakdown, an enterostomal therapist or wound care nurse can recommend protective skin wipes or an ostomy powder to help protect the skin.

Additional types of urinary diversions include the *continent urostomy* and the newer *orthotopic bladder substitution.* For the continent urostomy, a pouch is created from the intestine, the ureters empty into the pouch, and a nipple valve is constructed (Fig. 31.12). The patient performs self-catheterization intermittently during the day to empty the pouch (Fig. 31.13). For the orthotopic bladder substitution, a part of the intestines is used to make a new bladder. The ureters drain into it, and the urethra drains the substitute bladder. The patient is able to void through the urethra but may experience incontinence and may have to perform self-catheterization intermittently (see Fig. 31.13).

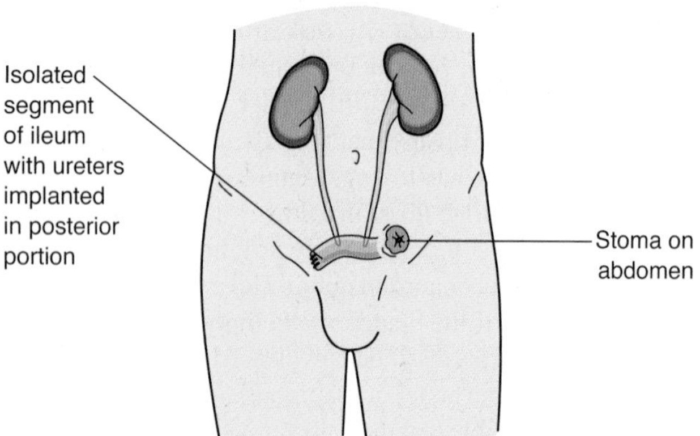

FIGURE 31.12 The continent urinary diversion. The pouch formed from intestine contains a valve that can be entered with a catheter to drain urine (from Wilkinson JM, Treas LS. *Fundamentals of Nursing: Theory, Concepts & Applications.* Vol. 1. 2nd ed. Philadelphia, PA: FA Davis; 2011).

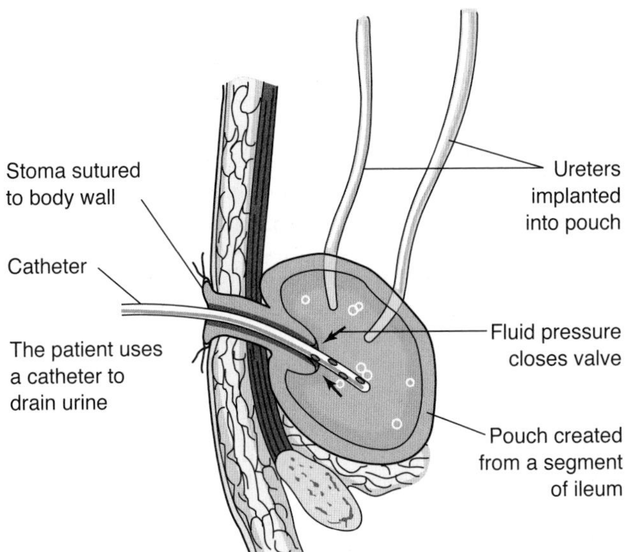

FIGURE 31.13 One type of urinary diversion, an ileal conduit. The ureters are implanted into a pouch made from a segment of the ileum that holds urine and opens to a stoma (from Wilkinson JM, Treas LS, Barnett KL, Smith MH. *Fundamentals of Nursing: Theory, Concepts & Applications*. Vol. 1. 3rd ed. Philadelphia, PA: FA Davis; 2016).

Urinary Tract Infections

A **urinary tract infection** (UTI) is caused by the presence of pathogens within the urinary tract. Any structure in the urinary tract may become infected, and the infection can spread from one structure to another. An infection in the urinary bladder is called *cystitis*. If the infection is left untreated, it can travel from the bladder up the ureters and into the kidneys. An infection in the kidney is called *pyelonephritis*, which can cause renal scarring and eventually lead to loss of kidney function. Approximately 80% of UTIs are caused by bacteria from the bowel, or *enterobacteria*. UTIs are more commonly seen in women than men because of the close proximity of the urethral opening to the anus, allowing bacteria to travel from the perianal area into the urinary tract.

The body's defense mechanisms help prevent UTIs. The pH of urine is acidic to help kill bacteria. Vaginal secretions also are acidic, which inhibits microorganisms from the rectum from migrating into the bladder. When a person voids, it flushes bacteria from the urinary tract. As women age, the changes to the reproductive tract increase the risk of acquiring a UTI. The pH of the vagina becomes more alkaline, which is less hostile to invading pathogens. Sexual intercourse, the use of diaphragms, and the use of spermicidal gels also can increase the incidence of UTIs. Encourage female patients who have recurrent UTIs to empty the bladder after intercourse and to use a method of birth control other than a diaphragm or spermicides.

In addition, if female patients have recurring UTIs, encourage them to avoid baths with the use of bath salts, perfumes, or bubble bath because these can irritate the urethra and cause infection that can migrate to the bladder. It also is important to empty the bladder frequently throughout the day to prevent pooling of urine in the bladder.

Symptoms of UTI include dysuria, urinary frequency, urgency, nocturia, low abdominal pain, and incontinence. If the patient has fever, chills, malaise, nausea, vomiting, and flank pain, the infection has most likely spread to the kidneys, causing pyelonephritis. In a physician's office, the diagnosis of UTI may be made using a urine dipstick test. The presence of nitrites and leukocyte esterase indicates a UTI. Nitrites can only be present if there are bacteria in the urine. A midstream clean-catch or straight catheter urine specimen may also be obtained for the purpose of performing a UA to diagnose a UTI.

The treatment of a UTI includes rest, increased fluid intake, antibiotics, and urinary analgesics. The treatment of pyelonephritis may include hospitalization for IV antibiotics. Patients are encouraged to drink cranberry juice or take cranberry extract tablets, which inhibit bacteria from adhering to the urinary tract. As a general rule, patients should consume 64 ounces of noncaffeinated fluid a day unless contraindicated.

KNOWLEDGE CONNECTION

List three types of urinary diversions. Explain how to prevent recurring UTIs in female patients. What are the symptoms of a UTI?

Settings Connection: Medical Office

Pediatric Considerations for Urinary Care

When you work in a health-care provider's office, you may see people of all ages with UTIs. It is important to recognize UTIs in children because their symptoms may be different than those seen in adults. UTI is second only to respiratory infections in children. Poor feeding, vomiting and diarrhea, and sleeplessness may occur. Children who once were toilet trained may have accidents. Children also may have personality changes. A child should be evaluated for a UTI if he or she presents with any of these symptoms.

UTIs occur more often in girls than boys. Girls should be taught from a young age to wipe from front to back. If a young girl does have recurrent UTIs, instruct her parents to have her shower rather than bathe and avoid bubble baths, which can lead to UTIs. To obtain a urine specimen from a child who is not yet toilet trained, you may use a sterile plastic urine collector bag with an adhesive patch placed over the genitals. Another type of device for collecting a urine specimen from a child may have the catheter extending from a test tube-like collection device.

Nursing Care Plan for a Patient With a Urinary Tract Infection

Your patient assignment is a 22-year-old female college student who was admitted with a severe UTI and possible pyelonephritis. She tells you that she is very busy with school, work, and a new boyfriend and that she does not have time to be sick. However, she states that she feels so awful with fever, chills, back pain, and painful urination that she knows she cannot keep up her schedule feeling this way. Figure 31.14 presents a concept map care plan for this patient.

Assessment

Her vital signs are outside of normal limits, with a temperature of 101.4°F (38.6°C), pulse rate of 106, respirations of 24, and BP of 116/70. She is also complaining of pain in her back. As you question her more closely, you learn that the pain is just below her rib cage on both sides, which you know is also referred to as *flank pain.* When you ask about her voiding patterns, she tells you that she is urinating "constantly" but only in small amounts and that she feels pain and burning when she urinates. She tells you that she got little sleep the past 2 nights because she was "up and down" all night long and because of the pain in her back, which she rates at an 8 on a 0-to-10 scale. Upon palpation, you find mild tenderness over her bladder area. Her skin turgor is adequate, and she has no signs of dehydration. She also tells you that she never wants to go through anything like this again, and she asks what she can do to prevent it from happening in the future.

As you review her history, you assess risk factors that would contribute to developing a UTI. She normally drinks diet cola only and rarely ever drinks water or juices. When she is well, she usually only voids two to three times per day because she has little time between classes for bathroom breaks. She denies nocturia until the current symptoms began.

When you review her laboratory and diagnostic test results, you learn that her white blood cell (WBC) count is elevated to 16,000/mm^3, indicating the presence of bacterial infection. Her UA shows cloudy yellow urine with a strong ammonia smell, with abnormal contents of casts, few WBCs, few red blood cells (RBCs), bacteria too numerous to count, and positive for nitrates.

Nursing Diagnoses

This patient has several indications of a UTI. In addition to this, her WBC is elevated to 16,000/mm^3 and she is complaining of

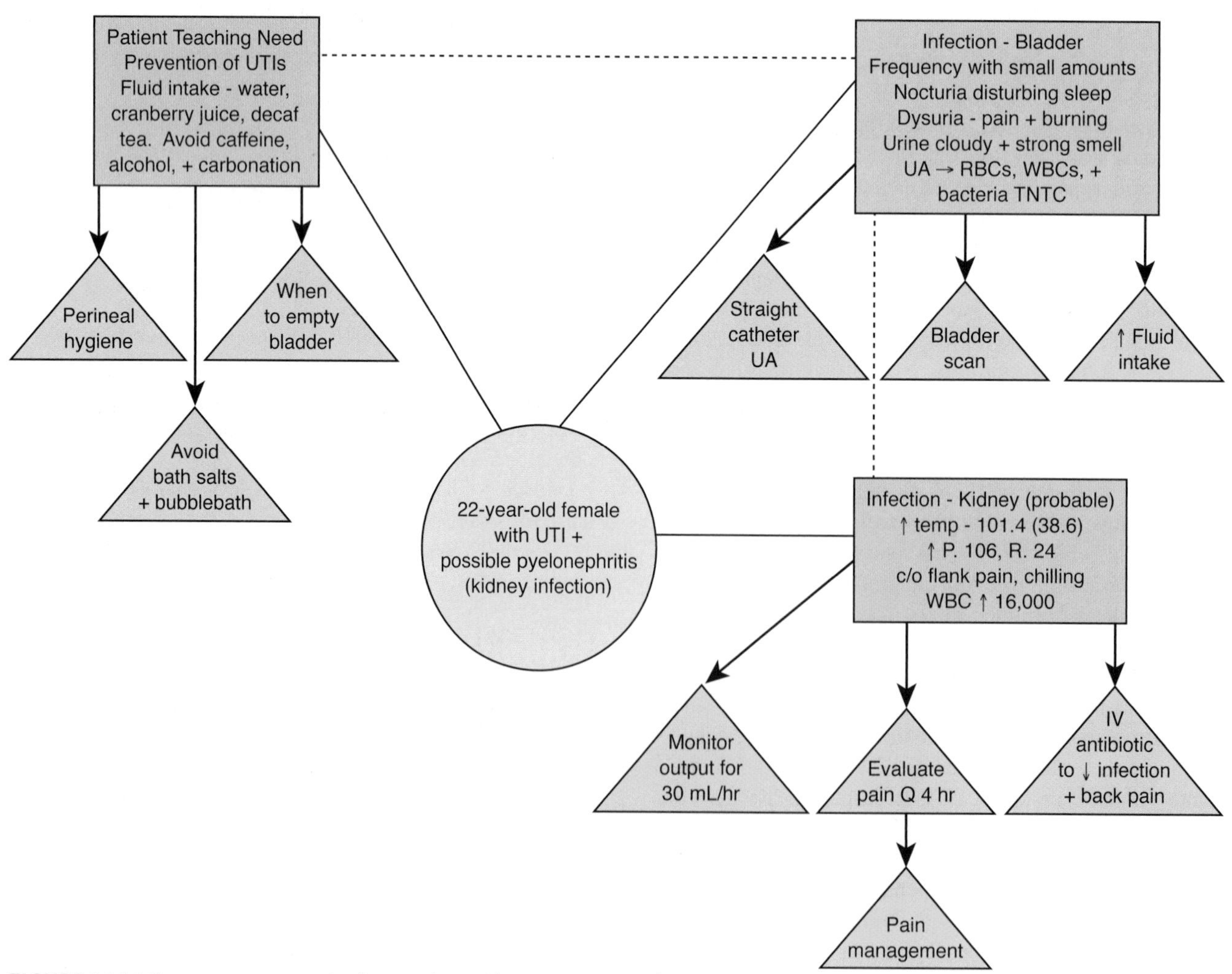

FIGURE 31.14 Concept map care plan for a patient with a urinary tract infection.

Nursing Care Plan for a Patient With a Urinary Tract Infection—cont'd

bilateral flank pain, which could indicate that the infection is spreading to the kidneys.

You also realize from her lifestyle that she is at risk for further recurrence of UTIs in the future.

The nursing diagnoses given for this patient are the following:

- Impaired urinary elimination related to UTI as evidenced by dysuria and urinary frequency
- Acute back pain related to probable kidney infection as evidenced by rating the pain at 8 and sleep disturbance
- Deficient knowledge of causes of UTI related to lack of exposure as evidenced by request for information

Planning

As you look at your options for interventions for this patient, you determine that improving her urinary functioning so that she can urinate without discomfort and with decreased frequency is a priority. You know that you need to take steps to help relieve her back pain so that she can rest, and that she must enhance her fluid intake to improve her urinary status. You also realize that you need to provide patient teaching about prevention and causes of UTI to help her from experiencing recurrent urinary problems.

Interventions

At this stage of the nursing process, you can now implement the interventions that you have planned.

Evaluation

The last step in the nursing process is to evaluate whether the interventions you have been implementing are helping the patient. The care plan below provides evaluations of those interventions. Continued follow-up should take place, but it looks like you are on the right track with your plan of care.

Nursing Diagnosis: Impaired urinary elimination related to UTI as evidenced by dysuria and urinary frequency

Expected Outcomes: The patient will exhibit normal elimination patterns of voiding clear yellow urine in amounts of 200 mL or more before discharge.

Interventions	Evaluations
Encourage intake of fluids that do not irritate the bladder, such as those without alcohol, caffeine, and carbonation. Encourage cranberry juice because it inhibits bacteria from adhering to the urinary tract. Determine the patient's fluid preferences and offer those that she likes.	Day 1: Unable to take fluids at first due to nausea. Later in day was able to take 120 mL of apple juice and 100 mL of grape juice. Day 3: Taking fluids better, as nausea resolves. Verbalizes understanding of importance of fluids and took 200 mL of cranberry juice even though she does not like it much.
Keep the call light within reach and ask the patient to call for assistance to the bathroom. Observe urinary output with each void for color, consistency, and amount. Evaluate discomfort with each void.	Day 1: Up to bathroom approximately every hour. Urinated 50–80 mL each void of strong-smelling, dark yellow, cloudy urine. Day 3: Urinating approximately every 2–3 hr, 150–200 mL at each void of light yellow urine. Cloudiness and odor have improved.
Administer antibiotics as ordered to treat the UTI. Assess for effectiveness by testing the urine with reagent strips at bedside, according to facility's policy.	Day 3: Antibiotics administered IV as ordered. Reagent strips show decrease in nitrates to normal levels.
Obtain straight catheterization urine specimen for culture and sensitivity (C&S) as ordered to determine infective organisms. Use meticulous sterile technique to prevent introduction of further infection.	Day 1: Straight cath performed using meticulous technique. Obtained 800 mL of cloudy, strong-smelling, dark yellow urine. Specimen for C&S sent to lab. Day 3: C&S shows presence of *Escherichia coli* and *Staphylococcus aureus* bacteria in urine; both are sensitive to prescribed antibiotic.
Perform a bladder scan to determine if the patient has residual urine in the bladder after emptying.	Day 2: Bladder scan done to check for residual urine. Less than 100 mL in bladder.

(nursing care plan continues on page 682)

Nursing Care Plan for a Patient With a Urinary Tract Infection—cont'd

Nursing Diagnosis: Acute back pain related to probable kidney infection as evidenced by rating pain at 8 and sleep disturbance
Expected Outcomes: Patient will rate back pain at 0 to 4 within 24 hours. Patient will report improving back pain as pyelonephritis responds to antibiotic therapy.

Interventions	Evaluations
Evaluate pain levels every 4 hours using a rating scale from 0–10. Be prompt in administering pain medication.	Day 1: Consistently rates back pain at a 7–8. Meperidine (Demerol) and odansetron (Zofran) administered as ordered at 4 p.m. and again at 8 p.m. Day 3: Rates pain at 3–5 and is taking hydrocodone/ acetaminophen (Lortab) every 6–8 hr.
Use distraction, gate theory techniques, or other methods to assist in pain relief.	Day 1: Watched TV for a brief period but slept most of the time. Day 3: Distracted by friends visiting, then watching movie with boyfriend. Did not ask for pain medication for 8 hr.
Administer IV antibiotics as ordered to treat kidney infection, which is causing the back pain. Assess the patient's response to antibiotics, including temperature, pulse, and respiration changes, as well as pain ratings.	Day 1: IV antibiotics administered as ordered through saline lock. Day 3: IV antibiotics discontinued and oral antibiotic started. Temp now 100.2°F (37.9°C), pulse 78, resp 18. Rates pain today at 3.
Monitor urinary output to ensure that the patient is producing amounts of at least 30 mL/hr to ensure adequate kidney functioning.	Day 1: Output total of 960 mL in 24 hr. Day 2: Output total of 1,600 mL in 24 hr. Day 3: Output total of 2,100 mL in 24 hr.

Nursing Diagnosis: Deficient knowledge of causes of UTI related to lack of exposure as evidenced by request for information
Expected Outcomes: Patient will verbalize understanding of causes of UTI and ways to prevent recurrence prior to discharge.

Interventions	Evaluations
Explain how a bladder infection can spread to the kidneys via the ureters. Emphasize the importance of early detection and treatment of a UTI to prevent spread to the upper urinary tract.	Day 3: Verbalized understanding when presented with a visual aid drawing of the urinary system.
Review perineal hygiene: Wipe front to back one time and dispose of toilet tissue. Wash front to back with a different area on the washcloth each time.	Day 3: Verbalized understanding of perineal hygiene and states that she always washes and wipes front to back.
Instruct the patient to avoid baths, especially with bath salts, perfumes, or bubble baths, which can irritate the urethra and lead to UTIs.	Day 3: Verbalized surprise that bath salts could irritate the urinary tract, stating she never thought about it before. States that she will stop using them to help prevent recurrence of UTI.
Instruct the patient to avoid excessive intake of alcohol and caffeinated and carbonated beverages and to increase intake of water, fruit juices (especially cranberry juice), decaffeinated teas or coffee, and flavored waters.	Day 3: Verbalized understanding of the value of cranberry juice and has learned that mixing it with lemon-lime–flavored water makes it easier for her to drink. States she will continue to drink it daily to prevent recurrences. Also verbalized the need to change her habits from drinking diet cola all day. States that the hospital stay has helped her stop that habit and she will drink flavored waters or juices from now on.

Nursing Care Plan for a Patient With a Urinary Tract Infection—cont'd

Interventions	Evaluations
Instruct the patient to empty the bladder every 3–4 hours throughout the day to prevent urine from pooling in the bladder.	Day 3: Verbalized surprise at this information and has decided when she can take bathroom breaks during her day to empty her bladder more frequently.
Instruct the patient to empty the bladder after intercourse and avoid the use of spermicides and diaphragm for birth control as these can lead to UTI in some people.	Day 3: Expressed gratitude for this information, stating she was completely unaware of the need to empty her bladder after intercourse to prevent recurrent UTIs.

Skill 31.1 Assisting the Male Patient With a Urinal

Assessment Steps

1. Check the physician's order for activity level so that you will know whether or not the patient can get out of bed.
2. Determine if the patient prefers standing or sitting to urinate.
3. Determine if the patient is able to stand independently or with assistance at the side of the bed.

Planning Step

1. Gather needed equipment and supplies: urinal, disposable wipes, and clean gloves.

Implementation Steps

1. Follow the Initial Implementation Steps located on the inside back cover.
2. Apply clean examination gloves.
3. If the activity order allows, position the patient for comfort either standing beside the bed or sitting on the side of the bed. If the patient is on bedrest, elevate the head of bed as much as the patient desires.
4. Place the urinal between his legs and place the penis inside the opening to the urinal.
5. When the patient is finished, provide disposable antibacterial wipes ***for patient hand hygiene.***
6. Measure the amount, color, clarity, and odor of the urine. In the older adult male patient, also note the size of the urine stream. Inquire if there was burning or difficulty starting the urine stream.
7. Empty the urinal, rinse it, and return it to the appropriate storage area.
8. Follow the Ending Implementation Steps located on the inside back cover.
9. If the patient is on I&O, record results on the I&O sheet at the bedside.

Evaluation Steps

1. Note the patient's ability to perform the activity and how much assistance was required.
2. Note any abnormalities in color, amount, odor, or consistency of the urine.

Sample Documentation

12/09/22 1910 Assisted to stand at bedside to use urinal. voided 450 mL cloudy, blood-tinged urine. Denies burning or difficulty starting and stopping urine stream. Assisted back to bed. Complains of general soreness throughout entire body. States he feels it is due to lying in bed. Denies a need for pain med. ———— Nurse's signature and credentials

Skill 31.2 Assisting With a Bedpan

Assessment Steps

1. Review the physician's order for elimination and activity level.
2. Determine what type of bedpan you will need. The patient's condition may determine whether or not a fracture pan is needed. ***If the patient is unable to roll from side to side, is very thin, or if a regular bedpan causes pain, a fracture pan must be used.***

Planning Step

1. Gather needed equipment and supplies: bedpan, clean gloves, toilet tissue, and premoistened cleansing wipes or warm wet washcloth.

Implementation Steps

1. Follow the Initial Implementation Steps located on the inside back cover.
2. Apply clean examination gloves.
3. Turn down the covers, exposing only as much of the patient as necessary.
4. Position the patient on the bedpan or fracture pan.
   - When using a regular bedpan, the patient should be assisted to roll to one side. Place the bedpan firmly against the buttocks and assist the patient to roll onto the back.
   - A fracture pan can be placed under the hips when the patient raises the hips, without turning from side to side.

(skill continues on page 684)

Skill 31.2 (continued)

If able, the patient can help by using a trapeze bar. The fracture pan can also be placed by turning the patient side to side, if the patient is able to do so.

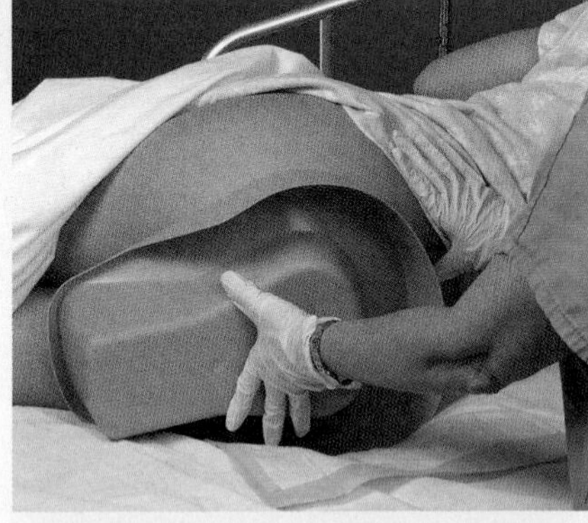

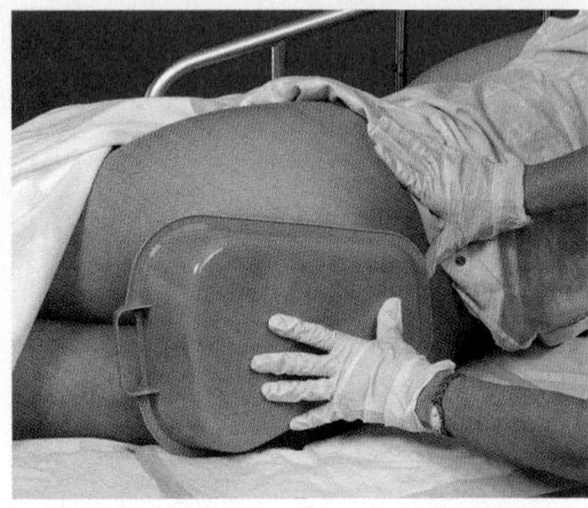

5. Raise the head of the bed unless contraindicated and replace the covers over the patient
6. Leave toilet paper or premoistened cleansing wipes and the call light within reach and pull the curtain ***to allow for privacy.*** Remove gloves and perform hand hygiene. If the patient is able to be left alone, step outside the room door ***to provide additional privacy.*** Inform the patient where you will be.
7. If you are monitoring I&O, ask the patient to dispose of the paper in the trash ***so that you can accurately measure output.*** Position the trash can close to the side of the bed.
8. Respond quickly when the patient signals that he or she is finished. Perform hand hygiene and don gloves if you have left the room previously. Move covers down.
9. If the patient was unable to wipe and cleanse his or her perineal area, perform this task for the patient.
10. Carefully support the bedpan ***to prevent spillage*** while assisting the patient to either lift the hips off the bedpan or turn to the side ***for removal of the pan.*** Replace covers.
11. Offer hand sanitizer or a washcloth with soap for the patient to wash his or her hands.
12. Provide perineal care as required (see Chapter 15).
13. Empty the bedpan into a graduated container if the patient is on I&O. Empty bedpan and graduated container into the toilet.
14. Clean the bedpan, and dry, cover, and store it in the bedside table or bathroom.
15. Follow the Ending Implementation Steps located on the inside back cover.
16. If the patient is on I&O, document appropriately on the I&O sheet at the bedside and on the flow sheet in the medical record.

Evaluation Steps

1. Note the amount, clarity, and color of the urine.
2. Evaluate the patient's response to being placed on the bedpan. Did he or she complain of pain or shortness of breath?

Sample Documentation

09/24/22 0725 Assisted onto fracture pan. Voided 325 mL clear yellow urine. Perineal care provided. No skin breakdown noted. Repositioned for comfort. ——————————— Nurse's signature and credentials

Skill 31.3 Obtaining a Clean-Catch Midstream Urine Specimen

Assessment Steps

1. Review the physician's order ***to determine type of specimen needed.***
2. Review the patient's chart ***to determine whether the patient can get out of bed for voiding.***

Planning Step

1. Gather needed equipment and supplies: sterile urine cup and cleansing wipes.

Implementation Steps

1. Follow the Initial Implementation Steps located on the inside back cover.
2. Assist the patient with these steps, or, if the patient is able to perform the procedure, instruct the patient regarding these steps:
   - Take the cap off of the specimen container and place the cap on a flat surface, open side up.
   - Avoid touching the inside of the specimen container or cap.

For female patients:

- Sit on the toilet. Spread the labia to expose the urinary meatus. Clean the meatus from front to back with a cleansing wipe. Use one wipe per pass. Wipe on each side and down the middle, disposing of each wipe after one pass. Do not allow the labia to close or contaminate the area being cleansed. ***Using each wipe only once prevents cross-contamination.***

Skill 31.3 (continued)

- Continue to hold the labia open and begin to urinate into the toilet. A couple of seconds after the urine stream has begun, place the specimen cup in the stream of urine, catching a sample of urine in the cup without stopping the urine stream. Obtain between 30 and 60 mL of urine for the sample.
- Remove the specimen cup and finish urinating into the toilet.
- Replace the lid on the cup without touching the inside of the lid.

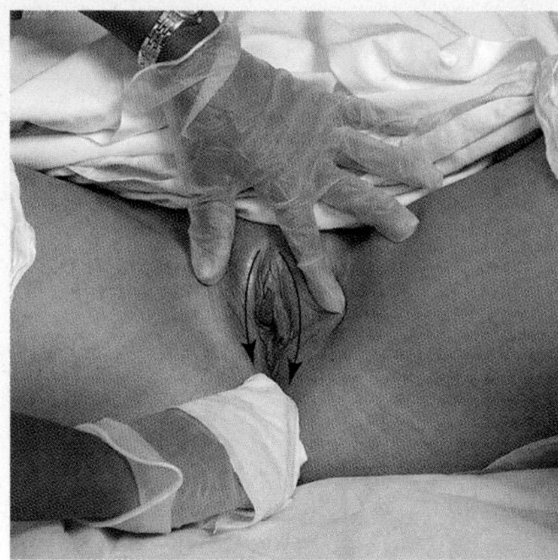

For male patients:

- Retract the foreskin if not circumcised. Clean the tip of the glans penis in a circular motion, moving from the meatus outward, and a few inches down the shaft of the penis. Dispose of the cleansing wipe. Use the second and third cleansing wipes and repeat the motion once with each wipe.
- Begin to urinate in the toilet. A couple of seconds after the urine stream has begun, hold the specimen cup in the urine stream to collect the specimen, without stopping the urine stream.
- Finish urinating into the toilet. *Safety: Replace the foreskin to its original position after you have completed the procedure.*
- Replace the lid on the cup without touching the inside of the lid.

3. Apply a computer-generated or barcoded label to the specimen cup.
4. *Safety: Place specimen cup in a biohazard specimen plastic bag and transport to the laboratory immediately. If the test is not performed immediately, store the specimen in the laboratory refrigerator to prevent components from breaking down.*
5. Follow the Ending Implementation Steps located on the inside back cover.

Evaluation Steps

1. Note the amount, color, clarity, and odor of the urine.
2. Note any difficulties with urination or with obtaining the clean-catch specimen.
3. Review test results when available and report abnormal findings to the physician.

Sample Documentation

10/23/22 0530 Midstream CCUA obtained for UA. 30 mL of dark amber, cloudy urine obtained. Labeled and sent to lab. ——————————
Nurse's signature and credentials

Skill 31.4 Performing a Bladder Scan

Assessment Step

1. Determine the need for performing a bladders scan: lack of adequate urine output although voiding, bladder distention, or a feeling of being unable to empty the bladder.
   Note: In most facilities, this is considered a nursing measure and no physician's order is required. Be sure to know and follow your facility's policy.

Planning Steps

1. Gather needed equipment and supplies: bladder scanner, conduction gel, and tissue or washcloth to remove the gel.
2. Ask the patient to void ***so that you are truly measuring residual urine.***

Implementation Steps

1. Assist patient to the supine position and drape so that only the lower abdomen is exposed ***to provide privacy for the patient.***
2. Follow the Initial Implementation Steps located on the inside back cover.
3. Clean the scanner head with antiseptic wipes ***to prevent transmission of microorganisms from one patient to another.***
4. Turn the machine on.
5. Select the patient's gender on the screen. ***Note: For some devices, if a female patient has had a hysterectomy you are to select male for the bladder scan. Follow the manufacturer's instructions for this.***
6. Palpate the symphysis pubis and apply approximately 2 tablespoons of conduction gel on the midline of the patient's lower abdomen, approximately 1 to 1 ½ inches above the symphysis pubis ***to ensure that the scanner can pick up the amount of residual urine in the bladder.***
7. Place the head on the gel and aim it towards the bladder, pointing slightly downward ***to ensure that the bladder reading is accurate.***
8. Press the scan button. Hold the scanner head steady until the scan is finished. Listen for the beep that will indicate the scan is completed. ***Releasing the button too soon will result in an inaccurate measurement of urine in the bladder.***
9. Read measurement of urine in the bladder ***to obtain the amount of residual urine in the bladder.***

(skill continues on page 686)

Skill 31.4 (continued)

10. Repeat the scan several times to ensure accuracy. Press DONE when finished and PRINT to obtain a printout of the results ***for accurate documentation in the patient record.***
11. Determine if you need to straight catheterize the patient or notify the physician based on the amount of residual urine found in the bladder.
12. Clean off the gel from the patient's lower abdomen.
13. Complete the Ending Implementation Steps found inside the back cover.
14. Document the procedure, amount of residual urine measured, and nursing actions taken.
15. Clean the scanner head and return the bladder scanner to correct location. Plug it in to charge, if appropriate.

Evaluation Step

1. Evaluate the amount of residual urine in the bladder. If there is more than 100 mL, follow your facility's policy regarding straight catheterization. *Safety: Be aware that for a patient who has had repeated straight catheterizations for residual urine, you may need to contact the health-care provider for an order to reinsert an indwelling catheter to prevent UTI risks with repeated straight catheterizations.*

Sample Documentation

06/14/22 1215 Bladder scan performed. 150 mL of residual urine measured. States she "feels like she needs to go but just cannot." ——— Nurse's signature and credentials

06/14/22 1245 Straight cathed and obtained 180 mL clear dark yellow urine. Dr. James notified. ——— Nurse's signature and credentials

Skill 31.5 Inserting an Indwelling Urinary Catheter

Assessment Step

1. Assess the patient for allergies to latex, povidone-iodine (Betadine), or tape.

Planning Step

1. Gather needed equipment and supplies: catheter tray, extra pair of sterile gloves, catheter leg strap, and bath blanket for draping the patient.

Implementation Steps

1. Follow the Initial Implementation Steps located on the inside back cover.
2. Put on clean gloves and drape the patient for privacy. Provide perineal care and examine the urinary meatus. ***This allows you to note any deviations from normal anatomy before you set up a sterile field.***
3. Position the patient before you set up the sterile field:
   - **For female patients:** Ask the patient to flex her knees and place her feet as far apart as possible.
   - **For male patients:** Position the male in the same manner or, if you prefer, have the patient lay flat with the legs close together. ***These positions allow you to set up the sterile field either between the patient's legs or on top of the legs.***
4. Remove the catheter kit from the outside plastic packaging. Turn the edges of the plastic bag to the outside without contaminating the inside of the bag. Place toward the end of the bed ***for use as a trash receptacle. The inside of the bag is still sterile, so if your gloves or forceps accidentally touch the inside as you discard items, they will not be contaminated.***
5. Position the catheterization tray:
   - **For female patients:** on the bed between the patient's legs.
   - **For male patients:** on the bed between the patient's legs or on the patient's lap on top of the thighs.
6. Open the distal flap of the tray first, then both side flaps, and then the flap closest to you last. *Safety: Touch only the 1-inch outer margin of the sterile wrapper with your bare hands to prevent contamination of your sterile field.*
7. Remove the sterile drape from the catheter kit without contaminating the contents of the tray.
   - **For female patients:** Place the sterile drape under the patient's buttocks, holding it by the 1-inch outer margin. ***This extends the sterile field from the perineum to the catheter tray. Avoid touching any of the drape surface.*** Remove the fenestrated drape (with a diamond-shaped opening in the middle) and lay it carefully over the perineum ***to provide a sterile field around the urethra and labia.***
   - **For male patients:** Place the sterile drape under the patient's buttocks or over the patient's lap or thighs; hold it by the 1-inch outer margin. ***This extends the sterile field from the perineum to the catheter tray.*** Remove the fenestrated drape (with a diamond-shaped opening in the middle) and place it carefully around the penis ***to provide a sterile field around the urethra and penis.***
8. Put on the sterile gloves provided in the catheter kit ***to prevent introducing pathogens into the urinary tract during catheter insertion.***
9. Lift out the plastic tray and place it on the sterile field, avoiding the 1-inch unsterile outer margin.
10. From the kit, pick up and open the lubricant and squeeze it onto a section of sterile plastic tray. ***Note: If the lubricant is in a syringe, you can squirt it onto a section of the sterile tray. Or, if you are catheterizing a male, you can later inject the lubricant directly into the urethra.***
11. Open the package of Betadine and empty the contents over the cotton balls. ***Note: Some kits may be packaged with Betadine swabs instead of cotton balls and liquid Betadine.*** *Safety: Use another type of antiseptic cleanser if the patient is allergic to Betadine.*
12. Lift out the sterile catheter, which will be encased in a clear plastic bag or sheath to provide extra security for maintaining sterility of the catheter.
13. Attach the syringe containing sterile water and screw the Luer-Lok tip to the colored port on the second lumen of the catheter. This second lumen is located at the Y-junction of the catheter. Do NOT inflate the balloon to test it. ***Note: Current***

Skill 31.5 (continued)

research indicates that this is not necessary and may cause problems with the balloon's function once the catheter is inserted.

14. Carefully remove the plastic cover from the catheter, maintaining strict asepsis of the catheter. Drop the plastic off to the side of your sterile field. *Safety: When you drop the plastic cover, you have less risk of contaminating your gloves than if you lay down the cover to the side of your sterile field.*
15. Now place the catheter with attached syringe into the sterile kit box within your sterile field. Use caution while you position the catheter. Place the first inch or two of the catheter in the lubricant you have squeezed onto the sterile field. This helps prevent the catheter from ***falling outside of the box and prepares it for insertion.***
16. Cleanse the urinary meatus.

For female patients:

- Use your nondominant hand to spread the labia to expose the urinary meatus. *Safety: This hand is now unsterile because you have touched the patient's skin.*
- While your nondominant hand continues to separate the labia, maintain exposure of the urinary meatus. With your dominant hand, pick up the Betadine swab or use the sterile forceps to pick up the Betadine-soaked cotton balls. Clean in the following order: Use one Betadine-soaked cotton ball or swab to clean the far labia minora from front to back. Drop the now-contaminated cotton ball or swab in the plastic bag you set up beyond your sterile field. *Safety: Do not remove your nondominant hand from the labia or let the labia close over the meatus. It will then be contaminated and must be cleansed again before proceeding with catheterization.*
- Use forceps to pick up a second cotton ball or swab. Cleanse the near labia minora from front to back. Drop the now-contaminated cotton ball or swab into the plastic bag.
- With the last cotton ball or swab, clean straight down from the clitoris over the urinary meatus and down past the vagina. Dispose of the cotton ball or swab as you have previously done.

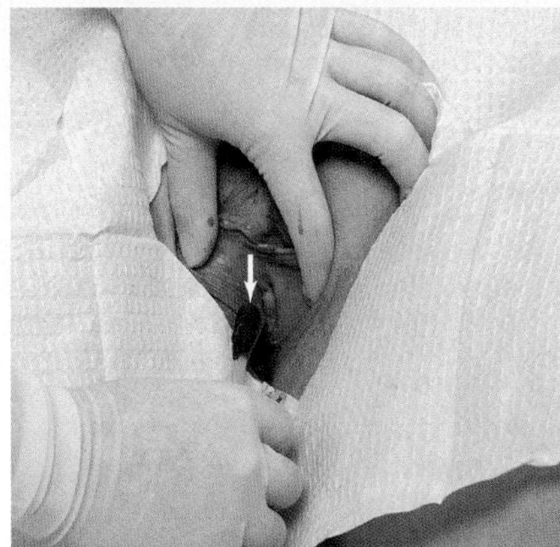

For male patients:

- Using your nondominant hand, grasp the penis shaft. Avoid using one or two fingers and the thumb; apply a full-handed grasp, retracting the foreskin if the man is uncircumcised. *Safety: This hand is now unsterile because you have touched the patient's skin.*
- Hold the penis at a 90-degree angle to the body while applying gentle traction. With your dominant hand, pick up the Betadine swab or use the sterile forceps to pick up the Betadine-soaked cotton ball. Begin cleansing at the urinary meatus, moving in concentric circles and covering the entire glans penis and a little ways down the shaft. Drop the now-contaminated cotton ball or swab in the plastic bag you set up beyond your sterile field. Use caution to avoid touching the sterile forceps or gloves to any potentially contaminated surface.
- Repeat the same cleansing motion three times with three separate cotton balls or swabs. *Safety: Remember to use each antiseptic wipe only once, moving in a concentric circle over the meatus, the glans, and a short distance down the shaft. Do not remove your nondominant hand from the penis after cleaning it to prevent contamination.*

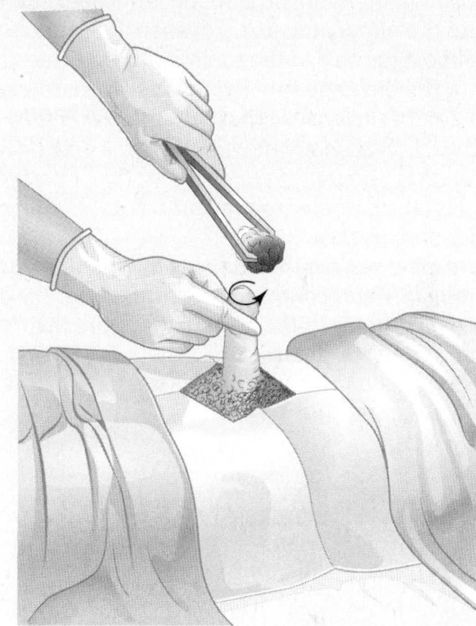

17. Pick up the sterile catheter with your dominant hand, dipping the tip in the lubricant you squirted on the plastic tray.

For female patients:

- Lubricate 1 to 2 inches of the catheter tip. Holding it about 1 inch from the tip of the catheter, insert it into the urinary meatus. Advance the catheter until you see urine flowing into the catheter tubing. At that time, advance the catheter another 1 to 2 inches ***to ensure that the catheter is fully in the bladder.*** *Safety: Do not let go of the catheter yet. Keep your dominant hand on the catheter to prevent it from sliding out of the bladder and urethra.*

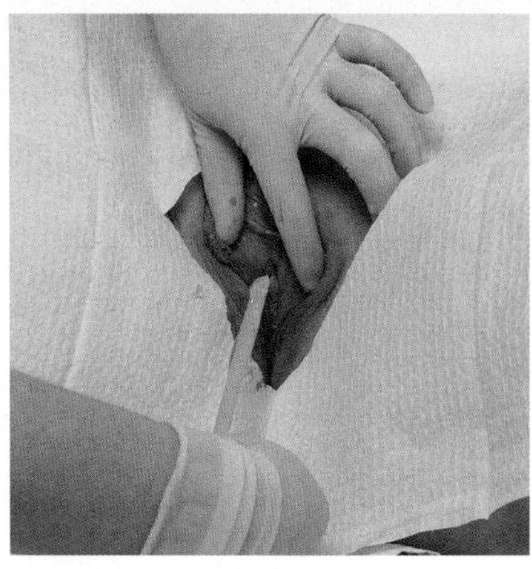

(skill continues on page 688)

Skill 31.5 (continued)

- Release the labia and, with your nondominant hand, pick up the syringe and inflate the balloon by depressing the plunger on the syringe completely. Pull ***gently*** on the catheter ***to seat the balloon at the cystourethral junction.***
- Twist the syringe off of the connection port and dispose of it in the plastic bag.

For male patients:

- Lubricate approximately 5 to 7 inches of the catheter ***to facilitate insertion and decrease discomfort to the patient.*** If the lubricant is in a syringe, the tip can be gently inserted into the urethra and the plunger depressed to fill the urethra with lubricant. Follow facility policy.
- With your dominant hand, pick up the lubricated catheter and insert it into the urinary meatus. Advance the catheter 7 to 9 inches, almost to the Y in the tubing, until you see urine flowing into the drainage tubing. Advance the catheter another 1 to 2 inches ***to ensure that the catheter is fully in the bladder.*** *Safety: If you inadvertently inflate the balloon while it is still in the urethra, you may damage the urethra.* Keep your dominant hand on the catheter ***to prevent it from sliding out of the bladder and urethra.***

  Note: If you meet resistance when inserting the catheter, the patient may have an enlarged prostate gland. Try gently twisting the catheter to the right to facilitate the tip of the catheter passing the prostate. *Safety: Do not force the catheter if you are unable to gently advance it.*

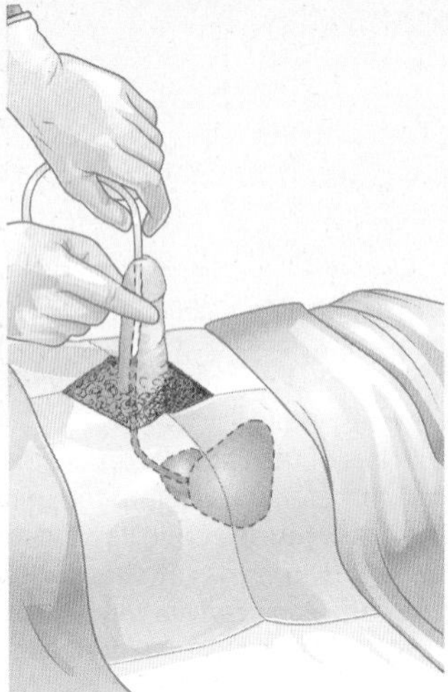

- Release the penis and, with your nondominant hand, inflate the balloon by depressing the plunger on the syringe completely. Pull gently on the catheter ***to seat the balloon at the cystourethral junction.***
- Twist the syringe off of the connection port and dispose of it in the plastic bag. Replace the foreskin if it was retracted. *Safety: If the foreskin is left in the retracted position, particularly with an indwelling catheter in place, it can cause a stricture-like effect, resulting in edema and possible necrosis of the head of the penis.*

18. Secure the indwelling catheter to the patient's thigh with a leg strap or tape. Some males may prefer to secure it to the lower abdomen. If you are not certain, simply ask the patient for his preference. To ensure adequate catheter length for patient movement, secure the catheter at the Y-junction. *Safety: This prevents tugging of the catheter, which in turn bangs the inflated balloon against the neck of the bladder where the urethra attaches. It also helps to prevent an ambulatory patient from stepping on the drainage tubing and accidentally pulling out the catheter.*
19. Cleanse all Betadine or other cleanser from the urinary meatus and surrounding area. ***If left on the skin, it may cause irritation.***
20. Depending on the structure of the bed, hang the catheter drainage bag from a part of the bed that moves with the patient when raised or lowered, or hang on a stationary piece of the frame that remains static directly below the patient's hips. Avoiding using the bed rails. *Safety: If the drainage bag is hung on the bed rails, it can be elevated above the level of the bladder when the rails are raised.* Hanging the drainage bag on the side of the bed nearest the door allows you to do a quick visual assessment of the amount and color of urine in the bag. *Safety: The drainage bag should not be elevated above the level of the patient's bladder unless it is first clamped close to the catheter connection to prevent urine from draining from the catheter tubing back into the bladder.*
21. Follow the Ending Implementation Steps located on the inside back cover.

Evaluation Steps

1. Evaluate how the patient tolerated the procedure. Did he or she complain of pain, burning, or other discomfort?
2. Evaluate the color, clarity, and amount of urine in the drainage bag after the procedure is completed. Avoid allowing more than 1,000 mL to drain at a time. Clamp the tubing in between drainings.

Sample Documentation

05/9/22 0800 #16 Fr Foley catheter inserted with sterile technique without resistance or complaints. Patent and draining via gravity to drainage bag. Immediately returned approximately 400 mL clear, pale yellow urine. Secured to leg with leg strap. Denies discomfort. ——————
—————— Nurse's signature and credentials

Skill 31.6 Obtaining a Urine Specimen From an Indwelling Urinary Catheter

Assessment Step

1. Check the physician's order ***to determine type of specimen to be obtained.***

Planning Steps

1. Gather needed equipment and supplies: sterile 10-mL syringe, sterile noncoring blunt needle or needleless access device, sterile specimen cup, alcohol wipes, and clean gloves.

Implementation Steps

1. Follow the Initial Implementation Steps located on the inside back cover.
2. Clamp the tubing below the level of the port for 15 to 30 minutes and allow urine to collect in the tubing above the clamp. ***This ensure that you will obtain a fresh sample.***
3. Put on clean gloves. Remove the cap from the specimen cup and place the lid on a flat surface with the open side up. Do not touch the inside of the sterile cup.
4. Clean the port on the tubing with alcohol and allow it to dry. ***This prevents the introduction of pathogens as the blunt needle penetrates the port.***
5. Using aseptic technique, insert the blunt needle into the port at a 45- to 90-degree angle and pull the plunger back slowly and steadily. Withdraw between 5 and 8 mL of urine for an adequate amount of urine for testing. *Safety: The indwelling urinary catheter is a closed drainage system that should not be interrupted. Do not disconnect the catheter from the drainage bag tubing to obtain a specimen because this will create a portal of entry for pathogens and increase the patient's risk of contracting an infection. Never obtain a urine specimen from the drainage bag.*

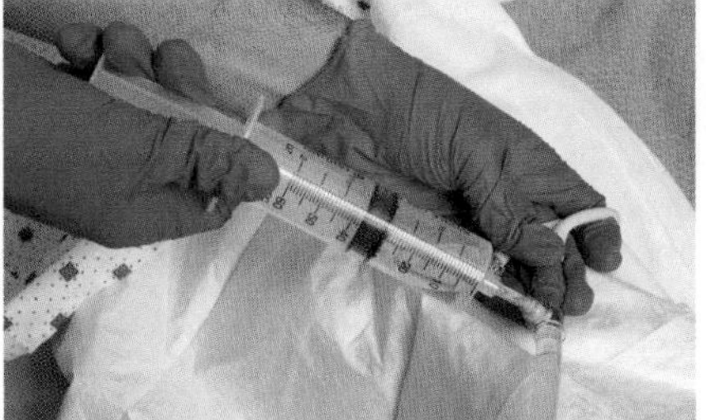

6. Hold the syringe over the specimen cup and carefully inject the urine into the cup using aseptic technique. Replace the lid on the specimen cup without touching the inside of the cup or lid.
7. Dispose of the blunt needle and syringe in the sharps container immediately.
8. Unclamp the catheter tubing, ***allowing free flow of urine.***
9. Apply a computer-generated or bar-coded label to the specimen cup.
10. Follow the Ending Implementation Steps located on the inside back cover.
11. Place the specimen cup inside the plastic biohazard specimen bag and transport it to the laboratory. It must be taken to the laboratory promptly or refrigerated.
12. Document the procedure in the medical record, including the characteristics of the urine.

Evaluation Steps

1. Evaluate the color, clarity, odor, and amount of urine. Ensure that you have obtained an adequate amount for testing.
2. Evaluate whether aseptic technique was maintained correctly.
3. Review testing results as soon as available and report any abnormal findings to the physician.

Sample Documentation

06/20/22 1300 Using aseptic technique, obtained 20 mL of clear yellow urine from port of indwelling catheter, placed in sterile specimen cup, labeled & hand-carried to lab for UA.
________________ Nurse's signature and credentials

Skill 31.7 Inserting a Straight Catheter

Assessment Steps

1. Check the physician's order ***to determine type of catheterization to be performed.***
2. Assess the patient for allergies to latex or povidone-iodine (Betadine).

Planning Step

1. Gather needed equipment and supplies: washcloth, towel, straight catheter tray with specimen cup, and extra pair of sterile gloves.

Implementation Steps

1. Follow the Initial Implementation Steps located on the inside back cover.
2. Put on clean gloves and drape the patient ***for privacy.*** Provide perineal care and examine the urinary meatus. ***This allows you to note any deviations from normal anatomy before you set up a sterile field.***
3. Position the patient as you did for an indwelling catheter (see Skill 31.5) before you set up the sterile field.

(skill continues on page 690)

Skill 31.7 (continued)

4. Position and open the sterile pack as you did for an indwelling catheter.
5. Set up your sterile field and place sterile drapes as you did for the indwelling catheter.
6. Apply your sterile gloves.
7. Open the lid of the specimen cup that came in the catheter kit and place the lid open side up on the sterile field. Leave the specimen container in the catheter kit basin ***to prevent it from tipping easily on the bed.***
8. Open the package of lubricant and squeeze it onto the bottom of the catheter kit basin.
9. Lubricate approximately 2 to 3 inches of the catheter tip for a female and 5 to 7 inches for a male ***to facilitate insertion and decrease discomfort to the patient.***
10. Open and prepare the package of Betadine cleanser as you did for the indwelling catheter. *Safety: Use another type of antiseptic cleanser if the patient is allergic to Betadine.*
11. Cleanse the urinary meatus (see Skill 31.5).

For female patients:

- Use your nondominant hand to spread the labia to expose the urinary meatus, just as you did for an indwelling catheter. *Safety: Remember this hand is now unsterile because you have touched the patient's skin.*
- Clean the far labia, near labia, and clitoris with antiseptic wipes as you did for an indwelling catheter. *Safety: Remember to use each antiseptic wipe only one time, cleansing from front to back. Do not remove your nondominant hand from the labia or let the labia close over the meatus because it will then be contaminated and must be cleansed again before proceeding with catheterization.*

For male patients:

- Hold the penis at a 90-degree angle to the body while applying gentle traction. *Safety: Once you grasp the penis with your nondominant hand and retract the foreskin if the man is uncircumcised, this hand is now unsterile because you have touched the patient's skin.*
- Clean the urinary meatus, the glans penis and a little ways down the shaft with antiseptic wipes as you did for an indwelling catheter. *Safety: Remember to use each antiseptic wipe only once, moving in a concentric circle over the meatus, the glans penis, and a little ways down the shaft. Do not remove your nondominant hand from the penis after cleaning it to prevent contamination.*

12. With your dominant hand, pick up the lubricated catheter and insert it into the urinary meatus. Advance the catheter until you see urine flowing from the end of the straight catheter into the catheter kit basin.
13. Once urine begins to flow, grasp the catheter close to the insertion site with your nondominant hand. Using same hand, pinch off the catheter to interrupt the urine flow while you use your dominant hand to place the end of the catheter into the specimen cup that is sitting inside the catheter kit basin. Allow urine to flow into the cup until it is one-half to three-quarters full.

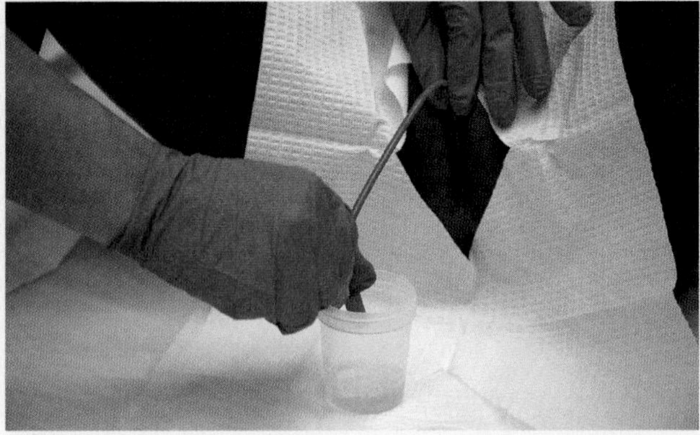

14. Pinch off the catheter again while you remove the end of the catheter from the specimen cup and lay it into the catheter kit basin. Still using your dominant hand, lightly screw the lid onto the specimen cup of urine. Then remove the cup from the catheter kit basin and set it nearby on the sterile field.
15. Allow urine to flow into the basin until the bladder is emptied.
16. Remove the catheter from the urethra by gently pulling it straight out.
17. Tighten the lid on the specimen cup, wipe off any urine on the outside of the cup, and set it aside.
18. Cleanse antiseptic solution from patient's genitals and pat the skin dry. *Safety: Replace the foreskin to its original position after you completed the procedure.*
19. Pour the urine from the catheter kit basin into a graduated container to obtain an accurate measurement. Record the volume of urine and then pour the urine down the toilet.
20. Apply a computer-generated or bar-coded label to the specimen cup.
21. Follow the Ending Implementation Steps located on the inside back cover.
22. Place the specimen cup inside the plastic biohazard specimen bag and transport it to the laboratory. It must be taken to the laboratory promptly or refrigerated.

Evaluation Steps

1. Evaluate how the patient tolerated the procedure. Did he or she complain of pain, burning, or other discomfort?
2. Evaluate the color, clarity, and amount of urine in the basin after the bladder has been completely drained.

Sample Documentation

05/9/22 0800 #14 Fr straight catheter inserted using sterile technique. 400 mL clear yellow urine obtained. 40 mL of urine obtained for sterile specimen and sent to lab. Denies discomfort. ———————— Nurse's signature and credentials

Skill 31.8 Performing Continuous Bladder Irrigation

Assessment Step

1. Check the health-care provider's order for continuous bladder irrigation.

Planning Steps

1. Gather needed equipment and supplies: IV pole, sterile continuous urinary irrigation setup (includes a sterile spike on one end of the tubing and a length of connecting tubing that will connect with the third lumen of the triple-lumen catheter), a 3,000-mL bag of sterile normal saline (NS) irrigation solution, and a sterile drape.
   Note: Normally a triple-lumen catheter is inserted in surgery by the surgeon after a TURP. The patient would normally not have a triple-lumen catheter inserted, unless the irrigation setup was connected to the third lumen. Then you would only have to hang bags of solution and maintain the irrigation. However, it is possible to receive a patient from surgery with the third lumen plugged by a sterile catheter plug. Or you may receive an order to insert the catheter and connect it to an irrigation setup. If so, you would require the supplies for inserting the triple-lumen urinary catheter.

Implementation Steps

1. Follow the Initial Implementation Steps located on the inside back cover.
2. Close the roller clamp on the irrigation setup tubing.
3. Uncap the sterile spike on the end of the irrigation setup tubing. Aseptically insert the spike into the port on the bag of NS irrigation solution. Keep the cap on the other sterile end of the irrigation setup tubing.
4. Hang the bag on the IV pole and unclamp the roller clamp. Remove the cap on the end of the tube and allow NS to flow through the tube to displace all the air in the tube, otherwise known as ***priming*** the tube. Then replace the cap, still using aseptic technique, and close the roller clamp to stop the flow of NS.
5. Cleanse the outside of the third lumen and the plug with two alcohol sponges. Remove the plug from the third lumen of the catheter using aseptic technique and insert the other end of the irrigation tubing into the lumen. *Safety: Keep the roller clamp closed until the tubing is attached.*
6. Open the roller clamp on the tubing, allowing irrigation solution to flow into the bladder until urine returns clear to light pink, without blood clots. *Safety: Make certain that the solution is also returning through the catheter drainage tubing into the drainage bag.*
7. Once the returning urine and solution remain light pink to clear, without clots, the flow rate of the irrigation solution is set. Regulate the rate as necessary so that it keeps the returning urine and irrigant at this color. If the urine becomes dark pink or red, or contains clots, increase the flow rate until the light pink color is again achieved.
8. Monitor flow and bladder distention for several minutes before leaving the room. Return within 15 to 30 minutes to reassess the amount of return and its color. If the urine color remains good, then you may monitor the return about every hour to assess the color of the urine in the drainage tubing and drainage bag. Repeat Steps 7 and 8 as needed.
9. Follow the Ending Implementation Steps located on the inside back cover.

Evaluation Steps

1. Evaluate the effectiveness of the irrigation by noting the color of the urine/irrigant return.
2. Evaluate output for the presence of clots.
3. Evaluate the patient's response to the continuous bladder irrigation. Does he complain of pain, bladder fullness, or cramping? Immediately respond to patient complaints. Assess for a distended bladder regularly.

Sample Documentation

06/20/22 1530 #20 Fr. triple-lumen catheter inserted without difficulty per physician's orders. Initiated continuous bladder irrigation with 3,000-mL bag of St. NS. Dark pink urine returned with dark red BB-size clots noted. Irrigant rate increased for 5 minutes until clots were no longer detected and urine was pale pink. Bladder palpated and nondistended. No complaints of cramping or discomfort.
———————— Nurse's signature and credentials

06/20/22 1545 Urine remains light pink without clots. No complaints of cramping or bladder spasms voiced. ————
———————— Nurse's signature and credentials

Skill 31.9 Applying a Condom Catheter

Assessment Steps

1. Assess the patient's genitals to determine size of catheter needed.
2. Assess for latex allergy.

Planning Step

1. Gather needed equipment and supplies: correct-size condom catheter, clean gloves, cleansing wipes, urine collection bag, skin prep, washcloth, towel, bath basin, soap, and scissors.

Implementation Steps

1. Follow the Initial Implementation Steps located on the inside back cover.
2. Place the patient in the supine position.
3. Position the sheet and towel so that there is no unnecessary exposure.
4. Provide perineal care ***to ensure that the area is clean and reduce the risk of introducing pathogens into the urethra.***

(skill continues on page 692)

Skill 31.9 (continued)

5. Apply skin prep around the shaft of the penis and allow drying according to package instructions ***to increase adhesion of the adhesive strip or condom catheter. Note: This may be all that is used to hold the condom catheter in place.***
6. If being used, apply the adhesive strip supplied by the manufacturer to the penis over the area of skin prep. Apply in a spiral pattern. Avoid wrapping a complete circle around the penis ***because it may have a tourniquet effect, cutting off circulation to the penis.***
7. Hold the penis in your nondominant hand. With your dominant hand, apply the catheter by slowly unrolling it over the glans penis and along the shaft of the penis. Leave 1 to 2 inches between the tip of the penis and the end of the condom catheter ***to allow urine to drain without leaking from the condom and to prevent pressure on the head of the penis.*** *Safety: Too much space left at the tip may allow the condom catheter to twist, causing urine to pool and loosen the adhesive. Constant urine contact with the skin can lead to maceration and skin breakdown.*

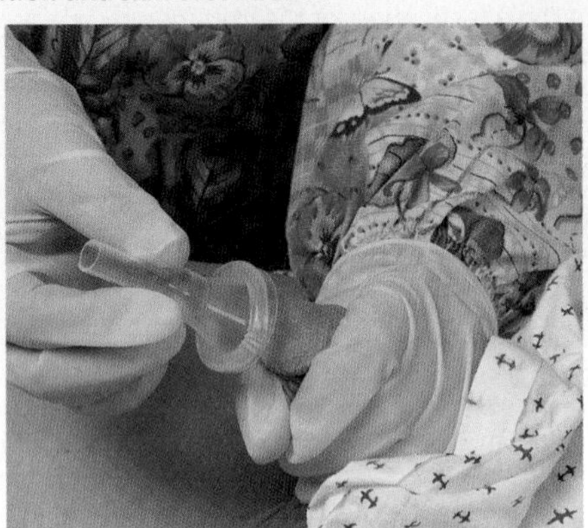

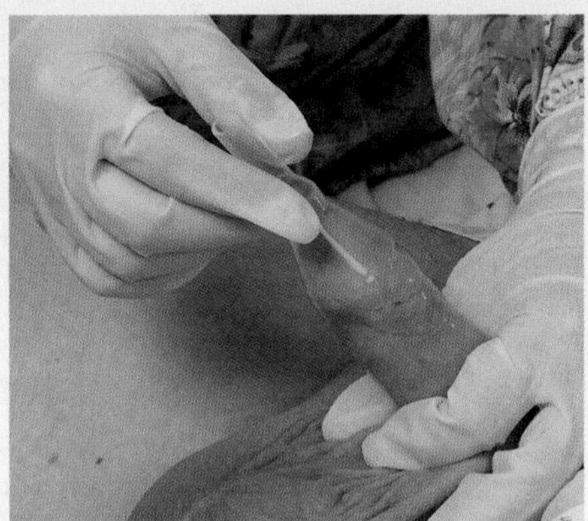

8. Attach the end of the condom catheter to the drainage bag and secure the tubing to the inside of the patient's thigh using a leg strap.
9. Follow the Ending Implementation Steps located on the inside back cover.

Evaluation Steps

1. Evaluate the catheter site within 30 to 60 minutes ***to make sure urine is flowing freely and there is no leaking.*** Also assess the penis for swelling and discoloration.
2. Assess the urine for color, amount, clarity, and odor. Make these assessments every shift.

Sample Documentation

04/1/22 1000 External condom catheter applied and attached to urine drainage bag. Skin intact. ——————
—————————— Nurse's signature and credentials

04/1/22 1045 Has drained 50 mL of clear dark yellow urine. No leakage. Penis without discoloration or edema. No C/O discomfort reported. ——————
—————————— Nurse's signature and credentials

Skill 31.10 Irrigating a Closed Urinary Drainage System

Assessment Steps

1. Check the physician's order for amount and type of irrigant.
2. Assess the patient's need for catheter irrigation. Note color and clarity of urinary output. Assess for bladder distention by palpating the bladder above the symphysis pubis.
3. Assess the patient's pain level and the need for any pain medication before the procedure.

Planning Steps

1. Gather needed equipment and supplies: bottle of sterile normal saline (NS) irrigation solution or other ordered solution, irrigation tray, 60-mL syringe with a tip that will accommodate a blunt needle, noncoring blunt needle, alcohol wipes, clean gloves, and waterproof drape.
2. Plan to keep the urinary drainage system closed during irrigation ***to help prevent introduction of pathogens and prevent UTI.*** Open irrigations are not recommended for this reason.

Implementation Steps

1. Follow the Initial Implementation Steps located on the inside back cover.
2. Apply clean gloves.
3. Empty the urine collection bag to allow for accurate output measurement.
4. Remove gloves, wash hands, and put on clean gloves.
5. Place the waterproof drape under the catheter port.

Skill 31.10 (continued)

6. Open the sterile irrigation tray without contaminating the inside of it.
7. Pour approximately 100 mL of sterile NS irrigation solution into the sterile irrigation container.
8. Attach the blunt needle to the syringe using aseptic technique.
9. Clamp the urinary drainage tubing below the level of the irrigation port.
10. Aseptically draw up between 30 and 60 mL of sterile NS into the syringe.
11. Cleanse the irrigation port on the Foley drainage tubing with an alcohol swab.
12. Insert the blunt needle into the irrigation port and slowly inject approximately 30 to 60 mL of the solution, holding the port slightly higher than the level of the bladder so gravity will assist the solution to run into the catheter and bladder. *Safety: If you meet resistance when irrigating the bladder, turn the patient slightly to the side and try irrigating again. Do not force the solution. If you continue to be unable to irrigate because of resistance, stop the procedure and notify the physician.*
13. After injecting the NS, remove the blunt needle from the port. If the health-care provider has ordered more than 60 mL, unclamp the drainage tube and allow irrigation solution to drain into the drainage bag. Then refill the syringe with 60 mL of NS and continue irrigation until the ordered amount has been used. Be certain to wipe the port with another alcohol sponge before piercing the port each time. ***Note: If the health-care provider has ordered a different solution and wants it to be left in the bladder as a bladder instillation, the solution will be instilled and then remain in the bladder for the length of time specified in the health-care provider's order (e.g., 30 minutes) with the tubing clamped. When the time has elapsed, return and unclamp the tubing.***
14. After completion of the irrigation, wipe the port one last time with a new alcohol sponge.
15. Remove all contaminated supplies and dispose of them in the appropriate biohazard container.
16. Empty the returned irrigant from the drainage bag, measure it, dispose of it in the toilet, and record.
17. Follow the Ending Implementation Steps located on the inside back cover.

Evaluation Steps

1. Evaluate the ease of performing the irrigation or any resistance met during the irrigation/instillation.
2. Note color, amount, and characteristics of the irrigant return. Evaluate for the presence of clots or mucus.
3. Evaluate the patient's reaction to the procedure. Did he or she complain of pain, pressure, or cramping?

Sample Documentation

10/29/22 1300 C/O full bladder, bladder palpated above the symphysis pubis. No urine noted in Foley drainage tubing at this time. Physician notified. Order for catheter irrigation received. —— Nurse's signature and credentials

10/29/22 1325 Foley catheter irrigated with 60 mL of sterile NS per physician's order. No resistance noted. Returned 225 mL of blood-tinged yellow solution immediately upon unclamping drainage tubing, followed by darker yellow urine containing small strings of mucus and small flecks of clotted blood. No complaints of pain or cramping. States the bladder feels so much better now. —— Nurse's signature and credentials

10/29/22 1400 Urinary drainage bag now holds approximately 350 mL of blood-tinged urine. —— Nurse's signature and credentials

Skill 31.11 Discontinuing an Indwelling Urinary Catheter

Assessment Step

1. Check the physician's order to ensure catheter is to be discontinued.

Planning Step

1. Gather needed equipment and supplies: clean examination gloves, 10-mL syringe with a Luer-Lok tip, and towel or disposable drape.

Implementation Steps

1. Follow the Initial Implementation Steps located on the inside back cover.
2. Apply clean examination gloves and provide perineal care for the patient if needed.
3. Empty and measure the urine in the drainage bag.
4. Place the patient in the supine position and place a towel or disposable blue pad between the patient's legs underneath the perineum.
5. Attach the syringe to the colored port used for balloon inflation.
6. Deflate the balloon by allowing the water in it to fill the syringe for 30 seconds. ***Note: Follow the manufacturer's instructions regarding balloon deflation. If directed, aspirate fluid by pulling back on the plunger. Some types of catheters may develop creases or ridges if this is done. Disconnect the syringe from the catheter.***
7. Ask the patient to take a deep breath. As the patient exhales, gently but quickly withdraw the catheter and allow it to rest on the towel or blue pad.
   - **For male patients:** Use your nondominant hand to grasp the penis shaft using a full-handed grasp. Use your dominant hand to steadily withdraw the catheter straight out of the urethra.

(skill continues on page 694)

Skill 31.11 (continued)

8. Remove the disposable blue pad with the catheter wrapped inside and dispose of it along with the empty drainage bag directly into the biohazard bag in the trash.
9. Provide perineal care as needed.
10. Explain to the patient that the catheter is now discontinued and that he or she should call for assistance when the urge to void is felt. Instruct the patient to void into a specimen pan so that you can measure urinary output. *Safety: Monitor the patient closely to ensure that he or she is voiding in adequate amounts after the catheter has been removed. If the patient has not voided in the 8 hours following the catheter removal, notify the physician.*
11. Follow the Ending Implementation Steps located on the inside back cover.
12. Document the procedure appropriately, noting the time the catheter was removed.

Evaluation Steps

1. Evaluate urinary output and perform a bladder scan according to facility policy to ensure that the bladder is emptying adequately.
2. Evaluate the need for recatheterization due to inadequate output.

Sample Documentation

06/14/22 1215 #18 Fr indwelling catheter discontinued per order without difficulty. Instructed to urinate into specimen pan the first time so it can be measured. ——
—— *Nurse's signature and credentials*

06/14/22 1500 Assisted to bathroom. Voided 350 mL of clear yellow urine. Bladder scan showed 25 mL of residual urine. ——
—— *Nurse's signature and credentials*

POST CONFERENCE

This has been one of your most interesting clinical experiences. Your patient was interesting and enjoyable. He seemed to enjoy having a student caring for him and said it gave him someone to talk with who was not so busy. The 24-hour urine specimen collection was a learning experience. You discovered that you had to keep the catheter drainage bag in a basin of ice during the collection period. You were rather relieved that he had a catheter because then you did not accidentally flush any urine during the collection period. After the collection period was over, you took the large container to the lab. The catheter irrigation was a new experience as well, but you were able to insert the blunt needle without contamination and flush the saline through the catheter.

Key Points

- Assessing the characteristics of urine includes color, clarity, amount, pH, and specific gravity.
- Assist patients with toileting before and after meals and at bedtime to mimic normal voiding patterns.
- Types of urine specimens and tests include CCUA, UA, timed collection, straining urine, and reagent testing.
- I&O monitoring can be an independent nursing action. It involves not only measuring the urine, but also evaluating the balance between I&O for fluid imbalances.
- Types of altered bladder function include urinary retention, residual urine, and nocturia and urinary incontinence.
- Urinary incontinence may be due to a variety of factors. These result in stress, urge, overflow, and functional incontinence.
- Nursing interventions for incontinence include bladder training, meticulous skin care, and teaching Kegel exercises.
- A variety of sizes and types of catheters exist. Catheters are sized by their diameter and measured in French units. Catheter types include straight, indwelling, and three-way catheters, each with a different purpose.
- After discontinuing an indwelling urinary catheter, it is important to monitor the patient for urinary retention. If the patient does not void within 8 hours after discontinuing the catheter, evaluate the need to recatheterize him or her. Call for health-care provider's orders if no standing orders exist.
- After a male patient has had a transurethral resection of the prostate, he will have a triple-lumen catheter in place, and continuous bladder irrigation will be used to prevent blood clots from clogging the catheter.
- Urinary diversions are created when the bladder is damaged or removed.
- Because one continuous membrane lines the urinary system, infection can travel from the urinary meatus to the bladder, up the ureters, and into the kidneys, where microorganisms are able to enter the bloodstream, causing sepsis.

Review Questions

Select the answer that is most appropriate for each of the following questions. Some questions may have more than one correct answer. Select all that apply.

1. Which of the following may decrease the incidence of UTI?
   1. Using a diaphragm
   2. Increasing fluid intake
   3. Voiding after intercourse
   4. Frequent voiding

2. Indicate the path of the flow of urine through the following structures by numbering them in order.
   1. Ureter
   2. Urethra
   3. Bladder
   4. Kidney
   5. Meatus

3. Your patient has been diagnosed with an enlarged prostate. He is at risk for which of the following?
   1. Urinary suppression
   2. Urinary retention
   3. Urinary incontinence
   4. Urinary diversion

4. When reviewing the UA results of a patient with the diagnosis of dehydration, which of the following would you expect to see?
   1. Specific gravity of 1.032
   2. pH of 7.0
   3. +Ketones
   4. +Nitrites

5. Which of the following statements made by a patient with incontinence would indicate a need for further teaching?
   1. "I can stop doing Kegel exercises when I no longer have a problem with leaking."
   2. "I can take medication that may help with my incontinence."
   3. "I may need surgery if other treatments don't work."
   4. "I should start a moderate exercise program."

6. You are initiating a 24-hour urine specimen collection for a patient as ordered by her health-care provider. Which of the following will you do first?
   1. Post signs in the room and on the door stating that a 24-hour urine collection is in progress.
   2. Place ice inside a 24-hour urine container.
   3. Ask the patient to void and then discard the urine.
   4. Ask the patient to void and then pour the urine into the 24-hour urine container.

7. You have removed an indwelling catheter from a postsurgical patient. Which of the following would need to be reported to the health-care provider?
   1. Eight hours after the catheter was removed, the patient has not voided.
   2. Bladder scan reveals 50 mL of residual urine.
   3. Voided urine is straw-colored without sediment.
   4. When assisted to the bedside commode, the patient complained of mild dizziness.

ANSWERS 1. 2, 3, 4 2. 4, 1, 3, 2, 5 3. 2 4. 1 5. 1 6. 3 7. 1

Critical Thinking Exercises

Answers available online.

1. You are caring for a patient who returned from the operating room several hours ago after having a transurethral resection of the prostate with continuous bladder irrigation. Thirty minutes ago you emptied the urine drainage bag, but now the amount of urine in the bag is decreased to 100 mL, and it is dark red. What should you do?

2. A 67-year-old female patient is complaining of dysuria, frequency, and urgency when she urinates. She is diagnosed with a UTI. She asks you how this infection occurred. How will you respond?

3. You are working at a walk-in clinic. A patient is being seen with signs of dehydration and a UTI. She states, "I don't understand how I can be dehydrated; I drink all day long." What questions would you need to ask?

Additional Resources

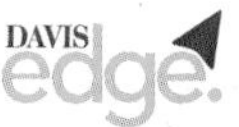

Use the scratch off code on the inside front cover of your book to access online quizzes that will help you to improve your scores on course exams and prepare for the NCLEX-PN®.

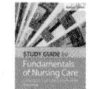

Study Guide

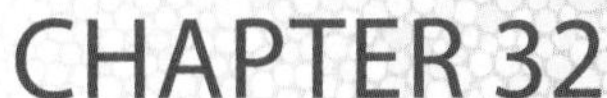

CHAPTER 32

Care of Elderly Patients

Alene Homan

KEY TERMS

Ageism (AYJ-izm)
Age-related macular degeneration (AYJ-rih-LAYT-ed MAK-yoo-lar dee-JEN-er-RAY-shun)
Alzheimer's disease (ALTS-HYE-merz di-ZEEZ)
Cataract (KAT-uh-rakt)
Cerebrovascular accident (ser-REE-broh-VAS-kyoo-lur AK-sih-dent)
Dementia (deh-MEN-cha)
Geri-chair (JAIR-ee CHAIR)
Glaucoma (glaw-KOH-mah)
Hallucination (huh-LOO-sih-NAY-shun)
Hemorrhagic stroke (HEM-o-RAJ-ik STROHK)
Illusion (ih-LOO-zhun)
Ischemic stroke (iss-KEE-mik STROHK)
Myocardial infarction (MY-oh-KAR-dee-uhl in-FARK-shun)
Resident (REZ-ih-dent)
Transient ischemic attack (TRAN-zee-ent iss-KEE-mik a-TAK)

CHAPTER CONCEPTS

Patient-Centered Care
Health Promotion
Cognition

LEARNING OUTCOMES

1. Define various terms associated with care of elderly patients.
2. Describe classifications of aging: young-old, middle-old, old-old, and elite-old.
3. Discuss the impact of the aging population on nursing.
4. Discuss common misconceptions about aging.
5. Describe changes that occur in the functions of each body system due to aging.
6. Explain recommended nursing actions to take for body system deficits.
7. Discuss the psychosocial problems of aging, including elder abuse.
8. Discuss nursing interventions to promote health and prevent illness and injury in the older adult.
9. Identify positive aspects of aging.
10. Describe ways to meet the needs of the resident in long-term care.
11. Compare the differences between acute care nursing routines and those in long-term care.
12. Discuss special considerations when assessing elderly patients.
13. Discuss the problem of polypharmacy in the older adult.
14. Discuss information found in the Connection features of the chapter.
15. Identify safety issues related to the care of elderly patients.

CRITICAL THINKING CONNECTION

Clinical Assignment

You are preparing for your clinical experience in an acute care hospital. You have been assigned to care for an 86-year-old female patient with a diagnosis of urinary tract infection (UTI), confusion, congestive heart failure (CHF), and diabetes. She was found lying on the floor in her kitchen unable to clearly explain what happened. In addition, she is dehydrated. She lives alone. Her daughter lives out of town and tries to visit monthly. In the shift report, the nurse says that there is some doubt that the patient has been purchasing and taking her medications for her CHF and diabetes. The daughter is coming today.

CRITICAL THINKING CONNECTION—cont'd

Critical Thinking Questions:

1. What are your feelings about caring for a confused patient?
2. What are the effects of a UTI on an elderly patient?
3. How might her CHF play a part in her current situation?
4. What do you expect to see and do when you enter the patient's room for the first time?
5. What are your major priorities when you plan care for this patient?
6. What will be needed for this patient to be able to return home alone?

This chapter contains information to help you relate to each of your older adult patients individually, not simply as "an old person." You will also learn about the physical and psychosocial changes of aging and how you can recognize and help prevent complications due to these changes.

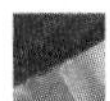

A DESCRIPTION OF AGING

Who are the elderly individuals in today's society? It is very easy for people to consider that anyone above a "certain age" is elderly. But how do we determine what that "certain age" is? Or is the term *elderly* to be associated with the ways in which one feels and behaves, as opposed to the actual chronological age that one is?

In the past, the age of 65 years has been associated with the time that a person becomes a senior citizen, or elderly. This is likely because 65 years was the magic age for retirement for many years. We now know that retirement can come at any age. Some people retire much earlier than 65, especially if they have the ability to support themselves. Others will work well past the age of 65, whether by necessity or by choice. Therefore, we no longer can identify an age as the marker for when someone becomes elderly. Many more criteria have to be assessed before that label can be assigned.

Classifications of Age Groups

For purposes of understanding how nurses care for the aging population, it is helpful to classify the different age groups of older adults. Each stage has its own nuances in terms of physiological and psychosocial changes that take place. Individuals will also experience changes related to developmental, sociocultural, and spiritual issues that occur within these stages of older adulthood. These will be described in more detail later in this chapter.

It is important to realize that, in today's world, people live longer than ever before, particularly in Western society. This is due in part to changes in the health-care system that make it better equipped to manage chronic disease conditions. With that in mind, it is not unusual that people do not see themselves as old because they continue to enjoy many of the same activities they enjoyed as a younger person even though they are now older.

Young-Old

The "young-old" are individuals aged 65 to 75 years. They also may be referred to as the young *elderly*. They have just started experiencing more of the physiological changes that are brought on by the aging process, although they may have experienced a somewhat gradual decline in physical health in the preceding decades. Common conditions seen in young-old individuals include elevations in blood pressure, higher cholesterol levels, and the onset of type 2 diabetes. Particularly in Western cultures, these conditions are prevalent due to sedentary lifestyles and the consumption of diets that are low in fiber and high in fat and animal proteins. Although the young-old may experience some changes in health, it is not uncommon to find them still working in the public or private sector, volunteering, and maintaining a social network of friends. It is within the next stage, middle-old, where physical and psychosocial changes begin to become more apparent.

Middle-Old

The "middle-old" are individuals aged 75 to 85 years. These are people who often have retired from working and who are experiencing the losses of spouses, family members, and friends to death. Physical changes are more apparent and often require that people refrain from doing things that formerly brought them pleasure, such as gardening, hobbies, and traveling. Although it is important to assess for depression in any patient, it is of particular importance to recognize that these individuals may be at higher risk for the development of a psychosocial disorder because of the implications of physical and social changes that affect their lives at this time.

Old-Old

The "old-old" are those who are 85 years and older. Often their health has significantly declined, leaving these people with the need for regular, and sometimes around-the-clock, assistance. According to the Congressional Budget Office, more than two-thirds of elderly persons 85 years and older report functional limitations. The manner in which these needs are met is often determined by the person's culture. In Eastern cultures, elderly citizens are valued and the old-old usually reside with family members. This family dynamic is carried forward as the younger generation in that home experiences this attitude toward caring for the elderly. In Western cultures, many times younger family members are working as well as raising their own children, so it is more common for the old-old to live in long-term care or assisted-living facilities. In Western civilization, when middle-aged individuals are caring for frail, elderly relatives and are also raising their dependent children, it is commonly referred to as "sandwiching," meaning that the middle-aged generation is sandwiched between raising a family and caring for aging relatives. By 2030, the National Institutes on Aging predicts that the oldest old will make up 7% of the world's 65 and older population.

Elite-Old

The "elite-old," also called *centenarians,* are 100 years of age or older. According to the 2010 U.S. Census, there are 53,364 Americans older than 100 years of age. This is up from 50,459 in 2000. Of those older than age 100 years, 80% are female. Again, this is testimony to better medical management of chronic conditions.

The Aging Population and Nursing

According to the National Institute on Aging, today 8.5% of people worldwide are age 65 and over. By 2050, this is expected to jump to nearly 17%. This means that there will be an increasing need for more nurses. Despite this, the Health Resources and Services Administration projects that the supply of nurses in the United States will fall by more than 1 million below the requirements needed to care for the population in the year 2020 unless extensive intervention is accomplished to recruit and retain more nurses.

> **KNOWLEDGE CONNECTION**
> What are the differences between the young-old, the middle-old, and the old-old? Are there similarities you can identify?

Misconceptions About Aging

It is not uncommon for others to categorize elderly people according to invalid assumptions. For example, some might stereotype elderly individuals as kind and nurturing, like doting grandparents. Other people, based on different experiences, might generalize that elderly people are confused, incompetent, or incapable of caring for themselves. Consider the many derogatory perceptions that people in today's society have of elders: Old people are hard of hearing, senile, confused, unhappy, depressed, in poor health, forgetful, cranky, and boring. Elderly people are often seen as afterthoughts who are incapable of having their own interests, desires, friendships, or activities. This practice of discrimination and prejudice against elders is referred to as **ageism.** The practice of ageism contributes to stereotyping, unequal treatment in the workforce, and denial of health care.

It is important to treat all patients as individuals, with unique characteristics and personalities, no matter the age of the patient. It is true that many of the patients you will care for will be elderly. Some may be confused and cranky, while others may be gentle and kind. In fact, your elderly patients will be quite similar to your younger patients, each one with different concerns and needs. It is never appropriate to practice ageism; rather, your purpose is to see your patients as individuals and to provide whole-person care.

Some individuals may resort to ageism because of a lack of knowledge about elders. Many traditional myths about elders are easily proven to be incorrect. When you care for elderly individuals, first assess their state of health, their psychological well-being, and their own perceptions of their abilities. The old adage, "You are only as old as you feel," is true. Numerous people who fall into categorization of young-old, middle-old, or old-old are younger in health, mind, and spirit than people of a much younger chronological age. Your nursing care should always be personalized based on the needs of the individual and not on your assumptions about a person based on his or her age.

> **KNOWLEDGE CONNECTION**
> If you are working with another nurse who states, "All old people are the same—cranky and needy," what appropriate response could you make to educate the nurse and to help dispel the myths about older adults?

PHYSICAL EFFECTS OF AGING

Throughout a patient's life span, each day brings physical changes that contribute to the health of the individual. In the early, formative years, these changes are centered on development and growth of physical structures within the body. During middle age, the physical changes revolve around maintaining homeostasis for optimal functioning. As a patient ages beyond 65 years, the physical changes begin to shift toward a decline in performance. The specific types of changes and the degree of change are often related to genetics, lifestyle choices, and the effects of chronic illness. For those reasons, some individuals will experience more health problems with aging than others. In the following section, specific information about physiological changes and associated nursing considerations will be explored.

> **Settings Connection: Medical Offices**
> **Older Adult Patients**
> If you work in a health-care provider's office or clinic, you will often see patients who are elderly. It is important to keep their special situations in mind. They may have several chronic conditions in addition to the reason they are being seen in the office that day. Avoid focusing on only the major complaint and take the whole patient into consideration.

Changes in Neurological Functioning

As people age, they are less able to process information supplied by both the neurological system and the sensory system. Reflexes slow because of sluggish nerve transmission and synapses. These slower reflexes are often the cause of injuries in elders because they may be unable to react quickly while walking, reaching, or driving. The decreased ability to feel cold and heat can lead to cold injuries and thermal burns.

Falls are the most common form of injury related to diminished neurological function.

A **transient ischemic attack** is a temporary decrease in the blood supply to the brain, causing sudden symptoms of dizziness, visual changes, weakness, numbness in one or more limbs, and difficulty swallowing. These attacks are sometimes referred to as "ministrokes," although the patient regains full use and feeling after the attack has passed. They may last a few minutes or a few hours.

A **cerebrovascular accident** (CVA), also known as *stroke* or *brain attack,* is also seen more often in the older adult. The cause of a CVA may be either a clot in a blood vessel or a bleeding blood vessel in the brain. When the cause of the CVA is a blood clot, it is referred to as an **ischemic stroke;** when the cause is a bleeding blood vessel, it is referred to as a **hemorrhagic stroke.** Either of these events interrupts normal blood flow to an area of the brain, resulting in death of brain tissue. Cerebrovascular accidents are often due to complications of conditions such as hypertension, atrial fibrillation, a diet high in saturated fats, elevated cholesterol levels, and diabetes. Depending on the portion of the brain affected by the stroke, the patient may be mildly to profoundly affected based on the degree of blockage and the length of time the brain has gone without the necessary oxygen. A left-brain CVA affects motor functioning on the right side of the body, may impair speech, and may cause memory loss. A right-brain CVA affects motor functioning on the left side of the body, can cause visual disturbances, and also may cause memory loss. The majority of CVAs occur in the right brain. Cerebrovascular accidents can cause a variety of communication issues, including aphasia, or the inability to speak, and dysphasia, which is difficulty speaking or understanding the spoken word. These debilitating effects from a CVA can be limited or, in some cases, can be prevented if the patient receives medical treatment within 3 to 4 hours.

Behavioral patterns can be affected without regard to the location of the CVA. Some behavioral changes exhibited after a CVA include depression, tearfulness, personality shifts, and apathy. Often these changes are permanent and can be quite distressing to the family. When you care for a patient who has had a CVA, focus on ways to promote and maintain safety, providing nonjudgmental, compassionate care, and support the family members as they adjust to changes in their loved one.

The most disturbing change that may occur after a CVA or other neurological disorder is a decrease in alertness, awareness, orientation, and the ability to communicate (dysphasia). Confusion, delirium, dementia, and depression are often found in elderly patients, especially after a CVA or with other types of neurological illnesses. *Delirium* refers to a state of mental confusion that usually is accompanied by illusions and hallucinations. A **hallucination** is a false perception having no relation to reality; the person may believe that he or she sees, hears, or smells something that is not really present. An **illusion** is a misinterpretation of sensory stimuli, such as seeing a coat rack but believing it is a human. The patient often is disoriented to time and place. **Dementia** is a decrease in intellectual functioning eventually resulting in the inability to care for oneself. It occurs gradually over months or years. Table 32.1 describes each of these conditions and the illnesses they often accompany.

Due to slowing of neurological processes, communication may be more difficult or take more time than with a younger adult. Speak slowly and be sure to face the patient when speaking to him or her. Allow plenty of time for the patient to respond. If you are in a hurry or feel busy, avoid seeming impatient because this may discourage the patient from attempting to communicate with you. Take the necessary time to engage in conversation with the patient; he or she just might have *something important to say.*

Table 32.2 provides information regarding the results of body system deficits, including neurological deficits, and the recommended nursing actions for these concerns.

Supervision/Delegation Connection

Caring for Confused Elderly Patients

In some states, the registered nurse (RN) or licensed practical/vocational nurse (LPN/LVN) can delegate certain tasks to unlicensed assistive personnel (UAP) when caring for confused elderly patients. These tasks may include performing hygiene routines, assisting with activities of daily living (ADLs), transferring between bed and chair, answering call lights promptly, providing adequate fluid intake and nutrition, and assisting the RN or LPN/LVN in maintaining environmental safety. If you choose to delegate when a patient is confused, be available to help the UAP because personal care may require two people under such circumstances.

Alzheimer's Disease

The most common type of dementia is seen in patients with **Alzheimer's disease,** which is strongly associated with aging. The diagnosis of Alzheimer's disease is based on symptoms because the only way this disease can be confirmed is by finding the characteristic neurofibrillary tangles in the brain on autopsy. It is seen most commonly in middle-old and old-old adults, but it has occurred in adults as young as 30 years.

Patients with Alzheimer's disease slowly withdraw from family and social interaction. They develop confusion that increases in severity until they reach a point where they do not recognize their own family members. They often wander at night and sleep during the day. Eventually they are unable to walk and speak, making sounds rather than words. Patients with advanced Alzheimer's disease require complete care and are totally dependent on others. When family members are the

• **WORD • BUILDING •**

cerebrovascular accident: cerebro – brain + vascular – relating to blood vessels; accident – event

ischemic stroke: isch – hold back + emic – blood; stroke – blow

hemorrhagic stroke: hemo – blood + rrhagic – bursting forth; stroke – blow

(Text continued on page 704)

Table 32.1
Changes in Orientation

Disorder	*Description*	*Reversible?*	*Associated Disorders and Conditions*
Confusion	Cannot think clearly; considered a cognitive impairment	Sometimes	Drug side effect Cerebrovascular accident Trauma Metabolic disorders Alzheimer's disease and other dementias Excessive stimuli from around-the-clock nursing care in critical care unit and lights always on Hypoxia
Delirium	State of heightened awareness; hallucinations and vivid dreams present; often has emotional outbursts	Yes	Drug side effect Drug intoxication Drug or alcohol withdrawal Febrile state Hypoxia
Dementia	Deterioration of cognitive functioning without a disturbance in consciousness	No	Alzheimer's disease Cerebrovascular accident Head injury
Depression	Alteration in emotional state marked by intense sadness or despondency, hopelessness, powerlessness	Yes	After a loss of loved one, relationship, home, independence, or financial security Coupled with certain medications Lifestyle changes

Table 32.2
Results of Body System Deficits and Recommended Nursing Action

Results of Body System Deficits	*Recommended Nursing Actions*
Neurological System Falls and broken bones	• Assess patient's safety. • Institute ways to improve safety.
Burns and other accidental injuries	• Check bath water temperature often. • Check on patient frequently. • Provide for sitters as needed and available. • Always explain what you are about to do before doing it. • Use a calming tone of voice when interacting. • Leave the light on at night if needed.
Self-inflicted injuries	• Assess risk for suicide or self-harm. • Refer to the health-care provider and appropriate mental health agencies.
Confusion	• Recommend Alzheimer's disease support groups. • Refer to home health services and Alzheimer's disease residential facilities as appropriate. • Encourage respite services for family members taking care of confused patients.

Table 32.2
Results of Body System Deficits and Recommended Nursing Action—cont'd

Results of Body System Deficits	*Recommended Nursing Actions*
Sensory System Decreased sensation	• Assess feet for injury, sores, or ingrown toenails and encourage follow-up with the health-care provider. • ***Safety: Monitor the temperature of the bath water to prevent burns.***
Poor vision	• Encourage patients to have regular eye examinations. • ***Safety: Provide adequate lighting for reading and moving about the room.*** • ***Safety: Provide a nightlight as needed.*** • ***Safety: Keep pathways clear of objects.*** • Provide magnifiers for reading.
Impaired hearing	• Encourage regular hearing evaluations. • Speak facing patient using lower tones. • Teach patients about availability of systems that can activate flashing lights for smoke detectors, ringing telephones, and doorbells. • Encourage use and maintenance of hearing aids.
Cardiovascular System Elevated cholesterol and blood pressure	• Encourage a heart-healthy diet. • Assess blood pressure every 8 hours or more frequently. • Encourage compliance of use of antihypertensive medications.

Decreased peripheral circulation	• Assess for:
	  • weak or absent peripheral pulses
	  • slow capillary refill
	  • decreased warmth of hands or feet
	  • pallor of extremities
	• Assess for environmental temperature comfort
	• Provide extra blankets as needed
	• Raise room temperature prior to bathing

Decreased cardiac output	• Assess lungs for adventitious breath sounds.
	• Auscultate heart for irregular rhythm or indistinct heart sounds every 8 hours.
	• Assess for:
	  • shortness of breath with exertion
	  • distended neck veins
	  • pallor
	  • bounding or thready radial pulse
	  • tachypnea
	  • pedal edema, weak or absent peripheral pulses
	  • cold or pale extremities
	  • confusion or restlessness
	  • decreased level of consciousness
	  • decreased urinary output
	• Monitor intake and output.
	• Encourage regular, moderate exercise.

Respiratory System Chronic respiratory conditions	• Assess lung sounds every 8 hours and prn. • Encourage patients to wash hands frequently and correctly with soap and water or use hand sanitizer.

Continued

Table 32.2
Results of Body System Deficits and Recommended Nursing Action—cont'd

Results of Body System Deficits	*Recommended Nursing Actions*
	• Instruct patients to stay 3 to 6 feet away from others who are ill with a respiratory illness. • Encourage compliance with respiratory medications and antibiotics. • Encourage patients to get flu and pneumonia vaccines. • Assure that bedridden patients are repositioned every 2 hours to prevent pneumonia. • Assess for fever, tachycardia, and tachypnea. Increase fluid intake unless contraindicated.
Inadequate O_2 supply to meet body demands during activity	• Plan nursing care to provide frequent rest periods. • Group nursing tasks together in short sessions to avoid constant interruption. • Observe for increases in respirations during activity. • Assess for pallor and cyanosis during activity. • Assess oxygen saturation level; apply and maintain supplemental oxygen as needed and ordered. • Elevate head of bed as tolerated by patient.
Gastrointestinal System Decreased peristalsis	• Encourage: • high-fiber foods and high fluid intake • activity • appropriate use of laxatives and stool softeners
Dryness of the mouth	• Perform mouth care every 8 hours or more often as needed.
Impaired sense of taste	• Encourage balanced, nutritional meals • Ensure meals are served at proper temperature.
Endocrine System Impaired blood sugar regulation	• Encourage balanced, nutritional meals and regular exercise. • Test blood sugar as ordered and administer ordered antidiabetic medications. • Monitor for hypoglycemia and hyperglycemia (see text on pages 836 and 837).
Reproductive System Decreased estrogen production in females	• Educate about lubrication products and locally applied estrogen creams to decrease vaginal dryness.
Decreased circulation to genitalia in males	• Encourage discussion of erectile dysfunction if it is a problem. • Discuss blood sugar and blood pressure control • Can help decrease development of erectile dysfunction
Genitourinary System Impaired emptying of bladder	• Encourage regular toileting schedule. • Scan the bladder to detect urinary retention. • Assess for signs and symptoms of UTI: burning during urination, urgency, frequency, cloudy urine, and a foul odor to urine. • Encourage fluid intake of liquids the patient likes to drink.
Decreased renal function	• Assess intake and output every 8 hours • Monitor for urine production minimum 30 mL/hr. • Assess renal function: blood urea nitrogen, creatinine, and glomerular filtration rate.

Table 32.2
Results of Body System Deficits and Recommended Nursing Action—cont'd

Results of Body System Deficits	*Recommended Nursing Actions*
Incontinence	• Implement bladder training when appropriate. • Assess for wet bed every hour; change wet linens as soon as detected. • Keep perineum and buttocks clean and dry. • Do not call adult waterproof underwear diapers. • Treat incontinent patients with respect. • Use barrier creams as indicated.
Musculoskeletal System	
Osteoporosis	• Encourage weight-bearing exercise. • Encourage increased calcium intake in foods and supplements. • Encourage compliance with other medications for bone strength. • Encourage the installation and use of handrails in tubs and around toilets in the patient's home. • Encourage the use of commercial "emergency help signal devices" that can be worn around the neck and activated when the patient falls or becomes seriously ill. • Encourage the use of assistive devices for stability.
Contractures	• Perform range-of-motion exercises at least once or twice per day if a patient is unable to ambulate. • Encourage neck, arm, and leg exercises that can be performed while sitting in a chair. • Use hand rolls to prevent contractures of hands. • Maintain proper body alignment both in bed and when sitting in a chair. • Encourage the patient to perform as much self-care as able. • Reposition at least every 2 hours.
Integumentary System	
Skin easily damaged	• Encourage protection of skin, such as wearing only closed-toed shoes. • Assess and cover all skin tears or open areas. • Apply creams and lotions to prevent cracking of skin. • Keep toenails trimmed straight across and consult a podiatrist for diabetics and as needed.
Increased capillary fragility	• Assess all injuries, even seemingly minor ones. • Be careful to avoid bumping or scraping the patient's arms and legs on bed rails, bed frames, wheelchairs, or chair legs. • Be extra gentle when handling the patient. Use tape sparingly. • Report bleeding gums. • Do not drag patient across sheets with repositioning.
Decreased circulation to skin and underlying tissue	• Turn immobile patients every 2 hours. • Encourage frequent position changes in patients who can turn themselves. • Place pillows between knees and ankles when in side-lying positions. • Change linens frequently and keep wrinkle free. • Position heels up off mattress (floating heels). • Use sheepskin elbow and heel protectors as needed. • Provide skin care several times per day if the patient is bedridden. • Assess pressure points for erythema at least every 4 hours, every 2 as needed. • Encourage adequate fluids and nutrition; provide protein supplements if needed.

primary caregivers, they may become overwhelmed; when this occurs, they, along with the patient, will need care and support.

It is difficult for family members to watch a loved one who has developed multiple medical problems "slip away" from them, particularly when one of the medical concerns is Alzheimer's disease or another form of dementia. Family members have to begin to say goodbye while watching their loved ones' awareness of them and the world slowly deteriorate. Family members often describe this process as taking care of someone they feel like they do not know because the cognitive changes seen in dementia seem to rob the patient of distinct personality features. While the nursing care for patients with dementia often focuses on maintenance of safety and assistance with ADLs, the care given to the caregiver is just as important and focuses on preventing burnout. Box 32.1 lists signs of caregiver burnout.

Real-World Connection

Alzheimer's Disease

A 75-year-old woman was caring for her elderly husband who had multiple illnesses as well as Alzheimer's disease. She was devoted to him and was his sole caregiver. Eventually, hospice was called in to provide additional in-home care. His wife struggled with watching his decline and accepting help with his care. She felt as though she was losing her husband and best friend as he became more and more withdrawn. The hospice nurse answered her questions honestly and allowed her to verbalize her sadness regarding the fact that he would not get better.

As her husband's physical and neurological function continued to decline, it was suggested that he be moved to a skilled nursing facility. This was extremely difficult for his wife to allow because she kept wondering if she could do more to be able to keep him home. Once again, the hospice nurse helped her see the reality of the situation. Using criteria recommended by the Alzheimer's Association (Box 32.1), the nurse assessed the wife's stress level and risk for burnout. The nurse also helped her understand that she was becoming overwhelmed, losing weight and sleep, and unable to keep her husband safe in the home setting. The nurse reassured the wife that he would be safe and attended to 24 hours a day, 7 days a week, at the skilled nursing facility.

Three weeks after his admission to the facility, he passed away peacefully, and his wife was grateful for the care he was given prior to his death. Although her husband did not survive, she was at peace with her decision and valued those last days with him because she could completely focus on being with him rather than trying to complete the innumerable tasks related to his care.

When you care for patients and family members in similar situations, it is important for you to help the family realize that it is not a sign of failure, but a sign of strength, to tap into the help available for both them and their loved one.

Changes in Sensory Functioning

Encompassing vision, hearing, taste, smell, and touch, the senses are also affected by slowing of the transmissions in the nervous system. Common visual disturbances in older adults include cataracts and glaucoma. **Cataracts** occur when the lens of the eye becomes cloudy, or opaque, causing visual blurring. **Glaucoma** is an eye disease characterized by increased intraocular pressure, which affects the optic nerve and can lead to blindness. **Age-related macular degeneration** is the destruction of the area in the retina where the optic nerve attaches, leading to the loss of central vision. In addition, many older adults complain of dry eyes due to less tearing and changes in visual acuity related to complications of untreated hypertension and diabetes.

As with neurological changes, decreases in the sensory abilities predispose patients to injuries. *Presbycusis,* or the normal decrease in hearing that accompanies the aging process, can increase the risk for injury if people cannot hear alarms and sirens. They often are unable to hear even the telephone unless they are present in the same room as the phone. When caring for a patient with decreased hearing, avoid shouting in an attempt to make them hear. It usually works best to lower the pitch of your voice, speak to the ear in which the patient hears the best, and slightly raise the volume of your voice. Another tactic that sometimes helps is to be on the same physical level as the patient and speak slowly, allowing him or her to read your lips. Inner ear disturbances can affect equilibrium, increasing the chance of falls. The number of olfactory nerves decreases, diminishing the sensation of smell, making it more difficult to detect things such as food spoilage

Box 32.1
Signs of Caregiver Burnout

When you are caring for a patient who has family members or friends involved in his or her care, it is important to pay attention for the signs of caregiver burnout. Even though caregivers are not necessarily sick, giving care to a loved one can be a very stressful experience. Ask these questions when assessing whether or not a caregiver is experiencing burnout:

- Does the caregiver feel that he or she must be the exclusive care provider?
- Does the caregiver feel that he or she is withdrawing from other friends, family, or activities because of the care he or she must provide for the loved one?
- Does the caregiver worry about the safety of the loved one?
- Is the caregiver anxious about finances and making health-care decisions for his or her loved one?
- Is the caregiver denying the impact of the disease and its effects on the family?
- Is the caregiver experiencing grief or sadness that the relationship with the loved one is deteriorating?
- Does the caregiver get frustrated or angry when the loved one does not listen?
- Is the caregiver experiencing personal health problems in addition to caring for the loved one?

or gas leaks. Touch sensation can be decreased as peripheral blood flow decreases. The taste buds become less sensitive, requiring stronger flavors to stimulate the patient's sense of taste. This is why many older adults tend to eat more sweet desserts than when younger, because they can better taste sweets than other tastes.

When patients do not taste and enjoy foods, they are less likely to consume the needed amount of nutrients to maintain their appropriate body weight. So, if an older patient wants to eat his or her dessert first at mealtime, this should be allowed. Avoid treating them as children, telling them they cannot have their dessert until after they have eaten the other things on their plate. Table 32.2 provides information regarding sensory deficits and the recommended nursing actions for these concerns.

Changes in Cardiovascular Functioning

As patients age, the heart muscle loses elasticity, the blood vessels narrow as arteries collect fatty deposits, and peripheral pulses are less palpable. Circulation is decreased, resulting in patient complaints of feeling cold, especially at bath time. These patients require a warmer room and warmer clothes than do younger people. These circulatory changes may occur without the patient's awareness, which puts the person at high risk for developing conditions such as coronary artery disease, hypertension, high cholesterol levels, **myocardial infarction** (also known as *heart attack*), or peripheral vascular disease. It is estimated that 10.6% of women and 21.1% of men between the ages of 60 and 79 have coronary artery disease. This increases to 18.6% of women and 34.6% of men at age 80 and older. Table 32.2 provides information regarding the cardiovascular changes that occur with aging and the recommended nursing actions for these concerns.

Changes in Respiratory Functioning

In an aging patient, lung elasticity is normally decreased. As with many body systems, the flexibility of the normally elastic lung tissue is reduced over time. The alveoli do not expand fully, which increases the risk for pneumonia, bronchitis, and complications of underlying chronic pulmonary disease.

Older adults are also more vulnerable to infections, particularly respiratory infection due to decreased immune function. Therefore, be sure to educate patients about ways in which to protect themselves from easily contracted infections. Table 32.2 provides information about ways to help patients protect themselves from respiratory illnesses.

Changes in Gastrointestinal Functioning

As peristalsis slows in the older adult, the cycle of food digestion slows, which can lead to poor appetite and decreased food intake. This may then result in malnutrition, weight loss, and an overall decrease in immune function. It is very important that you investigate the cause of a loss of more than a few pounds or kilograms in patients who are not trying to lose weight.

Constipation may result from numerous factors. Many medications list constipation as a side effect. As patients grow older, their lack of activity may slow down the entire gastrointestinal functioning, including evacuation. Aging can affect peristalsis, increasing the amount of time that feces remains in the large intestine, causing more water to be absorbed, leaving the stool dry and hard. Some older adults become very focused on the frequency of their bowel movements and become distressed easily if constipation occurs. Administer ordered medications such as stool softeners and laxatives to help prevent this problem. (See Chapter 30 for more information about constipation.)

Xerostomia is the medical term for an excessively dry mouth. This is a common complaint of older adults. There are several contributing factors. The sense of thirst is decreased, and the kidney's ability to conserve water diminishes. The cells in the salivary glands diminish in size and number, and dry mouth is a side effect of many medications. Table 32.2 provides information regarding deficits of gastrointestinal functioning and the recommended nursing actions for these concerns.

Changes in Endocrine and Genitourinary Functioning

As people age, the function of the pancreas decreases, which can lead to diabetes mellitus. Metabolism can slow, which means weight can increase. If patients are not able to exercise because of impaired mobility, the extra weight can affect their endurance and make controlling their diabetes more difficult.

As a complication of diabetes or other diseases, older adults may experience changes in renal function, leading to incomplete waste removal due to decreased efficiency of the filtering mechanism of the kidneys. This generally occurs gradually and eventually may lead to kidney failure. Figure 32.1 shows an elderly patient with renal changes.

With aging, the capacity of the bladder decreases because of loss of muscle tone. The bladder cannot hold as much urine as that of a younger adult, and older persons must go to the bathroom to empty the bladder more frequently. They often experience nocturia, which puts them at risk for falls and injuries when they are up at night. In addition, older adults are more at risk for developing UTIs due to more concentrated urine and decreased function of the immune response. (See Chapter 29 for more information about dehydration and the elderly.) Without proper attention, patients can develop urinary sepsis, a condition that warrants hospitalization and is often fatal. Table 32.2 provides information regarding endocrine and genitourinary system deficits and the recommended nursing actions for these concerns.

• WORD • BUILDING •

myocardial infarction: myo – muscle + cardial – heart; infarct – tissue death + ion – action

nocturia: noct – night + ur – urine + ia – condition

xerostomia: xero – dry + stom – mouth + ia – condition

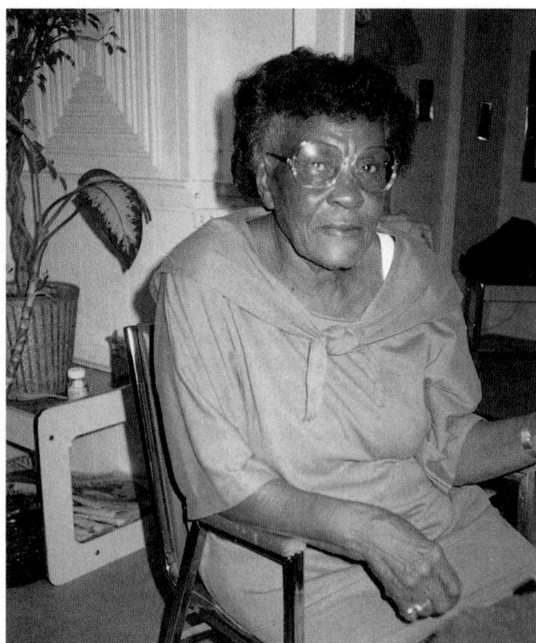

FIGURE 32.1 A patient with kidney failure does not necessarily look ill but experiences lack of energy, anemia, and elevated blood urea nitrogen and creatinine levels (from Polan E, Taylor D. *Journey Across the Life Span: Human Development and Health Promotion.* 5th ed. Philadelphia, PA: FA Davis; 2015).

Anatomy and Physiology Connection

Metabolization and Elimination of Medications

Most medications are metabolized and eliminated from the body via the hepatic and renal systems. After a medication is digested, it is absorbed into the bloodstream, where it can be transported through the portal vein to the liver, where most medications are metabolized, or broken down for use, leaving what is known as *by-products* or *end products.* The medication is then carried by the hepatic vein to the heart, where it is pumped out and circulated to the target organs. However, the drug is carried not only to the target organs but through the entire body and eventually back to the liver, where any remaining drug can be processed further.

The end products of medications are filtered and removed from the blood as it flows through the kidneys and then are excreted in the urine. If the liver or kidneys are not able to remove the toxins because of disease or impairment, they remain in the blood and circulate through the body. Essentially, this can lead to cumulative effects similar to a drug overdose. The by-products of metabolized medication are sometimes toxic to the liver. When the liver is exposed to excessively high levels or constant levels of a hepatotoxic drug, the liver can be seriously or even fatally damaged. An example of a drug that is toxic to the liver is acetaminophen, more commonly known as Tylenol. Many medications carry warnings that patients must have regular liver and kidney function testing while they are taking the drugs to detect damage to those organs that remove the medication from the body.

Changes in Reproductive Functioning

Older adults experience a normal decrease in hormone levels as they age. Men will experience a decline in testosterone, while women will experience a decline in estrogen. As this happens, men will still produce sperm, although they might not be as viable as sperm produced in younger years. Women will have gone through menopause during middle adulthood into early older age, which eliminates the possibility of childbearing.

This decrease in hormonal activity can change the older adult's sexual drive. Some older adults will gravitate toward less frequent sexual activity, while others will maintain an active sex life. Avoid stereotyping and assuming that seniors are uninterested in sexual relationships. Reassure patients about their own sexual needs and provide for privacy, caring for patients in a nonjudgmental fashion.

Erectile dysfunction (ED) is a condition in which men cannot achieve or maintain an erection. Medical disorders such as diabetes, kidney disease, chronic alcoholism, multiple sclerosis, atherosclerosis, vascular disease, and neurological disease can cause ED. Effective medications are available to treat ED.

It is most important for seniors to be educated about ways in which to protect themselves when they engage in sexual activity. The current generation of seniors did not grow up with the fear of sexually transmitted diseases, including HIV, AIDS, and hepatitis, so they may have questions about prevention. Table 32.2 provides information about reproductive system concerns and the recommended nursing actions for these concerns.

Changes in Musculoskeletal and Integumentary Functioning

As patients age, increased bone loss and muscle mass loss increase the risk for injury. As calcium is lost from the bones because of decreased absorption (and estrogen loss that takes place in women), osteoporosis can develop. Figure 32.2

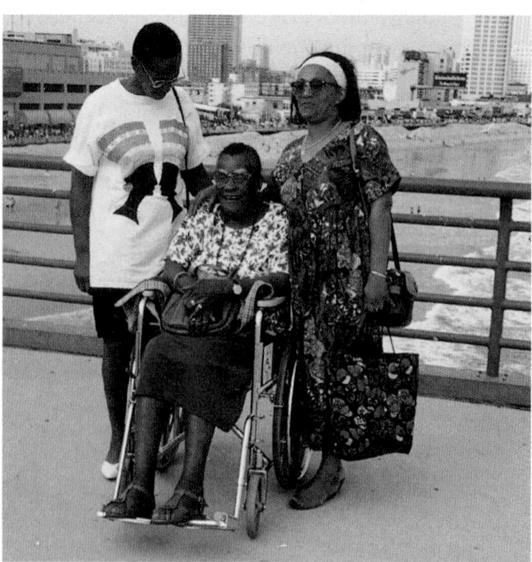

FIGURE 32.2 A patient with musculoskeletal disorders uses a wheelchair for mobility (from Polan E, Taylor D. *Journey Across the Life Span: Human Development and Health Promotion.* 5th ed. Philadelphia, PA: FA Davis; 2015).

shows a resident with a musculoskeletal condition that requires the use of a wheelchair. A decrease in muscle fibers and motor neurons causes a decrease in muscle mass and strength. Skin becomes less elastic and more prone to drying and breakdown. Nails thicken, and the skin bruises easily. Because of these changes and the changes related to diabetes, pay particular attention to the feet of patients with diabetes. They are less likely to be aware of dry, cracked skin on their heels, which can lead to an infection. They also may be unaware of a developing foot ulcer due to compromised blood flow that is often associated with diabetes.

The loss of subcutaneous fat and the decrease in sweat gland density over time change the older adult's ability to thermoregulate, meaning that they may chill more often than other individuals. Table 32.2 provides information regarding musculoskeletal and integumentary system deficits and the recommended nursing actions for these concerns.

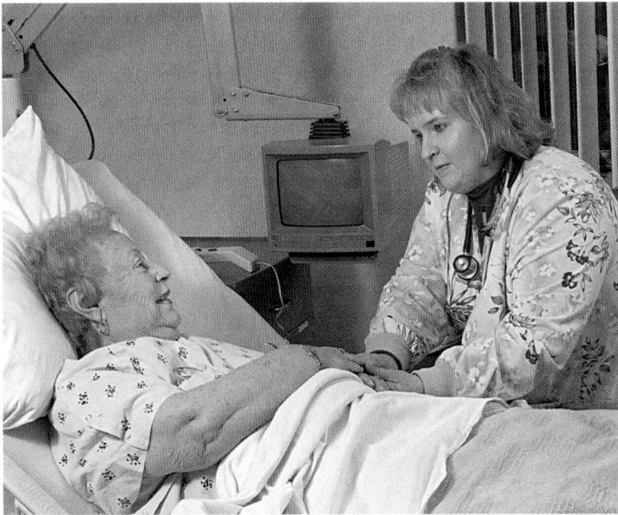

FIGURE 32.3 This patient is terminally ill and has been bathed, dressed, and made comfortable by the nursing staff (from Williams LS, Hopper PD. *Understanding Medical-Surgical Nursing*. 5th ed. Philadelphia, PA: FA Davis; 2015).

KNOWLEDGE CONNECTION

What might you teach an older adult about preventing UTIs? What would you teach an older adult about preventing osteoporosis?

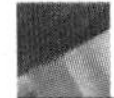

PSYCHOSOCIAL PROBLEMS OF AGING

When you perform an assessment on an older adult, keep in mind the numerous psychosocial concerns that he or she may have. Some of these were discussed earlier in this chapter, such as the loss of connection with loved ones that occurs in different types of dementia. Other concerns of older adults and their caregivers include the following:

- Fears about the dying process, as some people may struggle with spiritual beliefs
- Loss and grief as friends and family die or leave
- Safety concerns, including scams and crimes
- Elder abuse by caregivers
- Financial concerns regarding retirement and living arrangements
- Increased dependence on others

Loss, Grief, and Dying

It is a common misconception that because a person is older he or she is consumed with thoughts of death. Like most of us, thoughts of mortality do arise and are more prevalent if we receive a diagnosis of a terminal or untreatable disease. Figure 32.3 shows an elderly resident toward the end of her life. Older people also may feel their own mortality more strongly because of losing friends and family members to death with increasing frequency. For example, a middle-old couple moved to a retirement center and made many new friends, but in the first year of residency, approximately half of them died. While other people moved in and took their places, this change was difficult for the couple. Chapter 10 discusses the stages of grieving and therapeutic approaches you can use with your patients who are dealing with grief. Chapter 8 provides information regarding the spiritual aspect of your nursing care.

When you care for older patients who are dealing with loss and grief, you can include the following when planning and delivering nursing care:

- **Refer to support groups:** Most communities have numerous support groups that focus on different types of losses. They include those designed to support surviving spouses, those who have lost children, and those who have experienced any type of loss.
- **Educate about the importance of proper nutrition and exercise:** Older adults, especially those who live alone, may lose interest in food during an episode of loss and grief. Explain the importance of proper nutrition to keep the body strong and to help prevent new illnesses or worsening existing conditions. Exercise helps relieve stress and tension and can provide a time for focusing on something other than grief.
- **Encourage rest:** Because the grieving process can be exhausting, it is important for older adults to have the opportunity to rest when needed.
- **Help find comfort and meaning:** Sometimes this is as simple as sitting with the patient and allowing him or her to express feelings about the loss just experienced. There is no magic formula for helping the patient find comfort, but the presence of another human being who allows him or her to express feelings can prove to be quite comforting, particularly if the older adult has lost a close friend or spouse. Chapter 10 provides additional information about ways to help grieving patients.
- **Encourage spirituality, if the patient desires:** Older adults may find comfort in their spiritual beliefs during

times of loss. You may contact an appropriate person to assist the patient, such as a pastor, chaplain, priest, or shaman to assist them. Figure 32.4 shows an elderly person practicing his faith.

- **Allow the patient to grieve:** Provide privacy or sit in silence with the patient, as indicated, to allow the patient time to grieve. Recognize that each person may grieve differently, so be supportive and nonjudgmental during this time.

Safety From Scams and Crime

Older adults are considered easy prey because they are more trusting of individuals soliciting for money than younger individuals, making them frequent victims of those trying to defraud them of money.

It is not uncommon for such scams and crimes to take place over the telephone. The older adult does not know the caller, and sometimes it is easy for scammers to talk an elder into giving them credit card numbers or other identifying information, which they then use to defraud him or her. Because elderly people are often homebound and socially isolated, callers have an easy time gaining their trust, often because the callers are personable and sound official. ***Safety: Older adults should be cautioned about giving personal information over the telephone, via the mail, or over the Internet because so many of these schemes are indeed ways to pilfer money from unsuspecting people.***

Other scams involve people who come to an older adult's home and represent themselves as repairmen or utility workers. These people often are dressed for the part, and when they gain entry into the home they physically harm and rob the elderly person. Or they may give the false impression of having supplied the appropriate service when, in fact, they only completed small portions of the work or performed shoddy work. The elderly person then pays exorbitant amounts of money to these people, who leave false contact information and then disappear. ***Safety: Caution older adults not to allow anyone into their home whom they are not expecting and to always ask for identification before allowing an expected worker in.*** It is sometimes helpful if the elderly individual will consult a trusted family member or friend who might assist in determining the legitimacy of workers who are being considered for hire. However, many elderly individuals are struggling to maintain their sense of independence and are resistant to others helping them make their decisions.

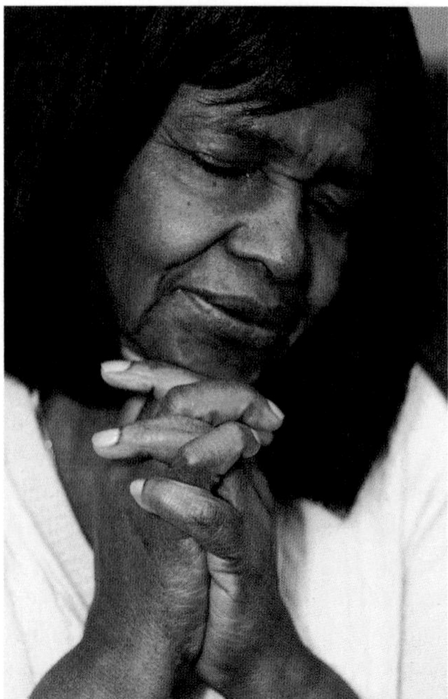

FIGURE 32.4 To meet the spiritual needs of elderly patients, provide opportunities for them to practice their faith.

Elder Abuse

It may come as a surprise to most to learn that according to the National Center on Elder Abuse, it is estimated that between 1 and 2 million seniors have been injured, exploited, or otherwise mistreated by a caregiver. This type of abuse can take place in many forms: *neglect,* which means that the caretaker has omitted providing basic necessary care, such as food or fluids, hygiene, or a safe environment; *psychological abuse,* which entails manipulation or mental cruelty; *physical abuse,* which involves any kind of physical harm done to the patient; *exploitation,* which involves using the older adult for personal gain, such as gaining access to the older adult's bank account and using it without his or her knowledge; and *sexual assault*, which involves any unwanted sexual contact.

Physical abuse is more recognized because of the outward signs that this type of abuse leaves behind. Be alert for these findings that could suggest abuse:

- **Excessive bruises in unexpected places:** This could be the caregiver's attempt to hide abuse by hurting the victim in places that would not normally be visible. Unexplained bruises on the genitalia and/or signs of sexually transmitted infection should also be assessed.
- **Bruises in multiple stages of healing:** This finding could potentially indicate that the older adult has been abused on an ongoing basis. When bruises are found in multiple stages of healing, it could be an indicator of infrequent abuse that occurs at different times or of frequent and varying kinds of abuse.
- **Bite marks:** Although less common than bruises and lacerations, bite marks may be found and be indicative of abuse.
- **Burns:** Burns in varying locations over the body often are indicators of abuse. The more frequent types of abusive burns come from cigarettes, which produce small round burns. When found, they are commonly seen on the palms of the hands, the soles of the feet, or on the abdomen.
- **Lacerations:** Like burns, the finding of multiple lacerations, particularly in various stages of healing, may indicate that the older adult is living in an unsafe environment where he or she is repeatedly brushing against objects that cut or that he or she is being purposely cut by a caregiver.

- **Fractures or dislocations:** Although there are no classic patterns of fractures that indicate elder abuse, keep in mind that repeated or multiple fractures or dislocations may be cause for concern.
- **Sedation:** Patients who are sedated may have been overdosed on medication. A caregiver may knowingly administer too much medication as a way to manage an elderly person, or a caregiver may accidentally be administering too much of a certain medication.
- **Dehydration or malnutrition:** These may be signs of poor dietary intake and may not indicate abuse. However, continued or repeated admissions for dehydration or malnutrition may indicate that the patient is not being provided with proper nutritional intake.
- **Excessively poor hygiene or unsuitable clothing:** This finding may indicate that the patient is not being cared for appropriately. Some elderly people are unable to see that their clothing is not clean and may show a lack of interest in personal hygiene. Therefore, be sure to investigate the situation before assuming that abuse is taking place. ***Safety: If elder abuse of any type is suspected, it should be reported immediately to the proper state authorities for investigation.*** (See Chapter 3 for more information on reporting abuse.)

Financial Concerns

While many people are ready to retire at age 62 or 65 years, others prefer to remain in the workforce until age 70 years or older. As they contemplate this change in work status, older people may express concerns about how they will provide for themselves and whether they will have enough money in the future when their income is fixed. Between the financial implications of older age and the physical changes that may take place, older adults may also have concerns about living arrangements. Many people wonder if they will have enough money to pay for a nursing home should they ever have to be admitted to one.

Although you cannot solve these problems, you can provide empathetic, therapeutic listening and refer the patient to appropriate resources for assistance. These resources may include social workers, social service agencies, the local Area Agency on Aging, and other senior assistive facilities.

POSITIVE ASPECTS OF AGING

In this chapter, we have discussed all the changes that aging brings, both physical and psychosocial. However, with those changes, aging also brings wisdom and insight. It is often within this stage of life that people have much knowledge to share with younger generations. Over the years, they have developed social skills, successfully raised families, excelled at a trade or business, learned from their own mistakes, experienced many things that others have yet to experience, and mastered concepts that younger adults have not yet grasped. They can utilize these rich pieces of knowledge as grandparents, civic leaders, volunteers, church workers, neighbors, and friends.

Be respectful of this special time in the life of an older adult and work to promote self-esteem as physical, psychosocial, and spiritual changes take place. If you avoid stereotypes and meet each patient where he or she is in the aging process, you can effectively care for the patient's needs personally and professionally while also promoting dignity. One way to accomplish this is by helping the elderly person be well groomed, as shown in Figure 32.5.

Settings Connection: Home Health

Caring for Older Adults

If you decide to work in home health care, chances are good that many of your patients will be older adults. This will require a good understanding of the physical, psychosocial, emotional, and spiritual needs of the aging adult.

In home health care, you will make visits to people who need assistance to remain in their homes rather than in a care facility. Many times these are elders who do not have family nearby to assist them but who are determined to remain at home if at all possible. With the assistance of home health nurses, nursing assistants, and therapists, many are able to do so.

KNOWLEDGE CONNECTION

List three things you can do to help an older adult patient who has recently lost his spouse. How might you help an elderly person avoid becoming a victim of a telephone scam?

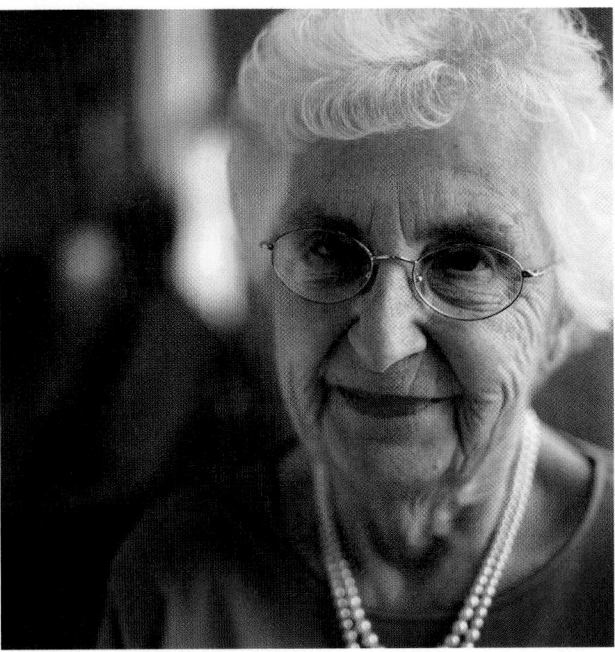

FIGURE 32.5 When you care for elderly patients, help promote dignity by assisting them to look their best (PunchStock).

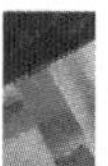

CARING FOR RESIDENTS IN LONG-TERM SETTINGS

While the aging process has the advantages of wisdom, more life experiences, and new and different opportunities, it also sometimes involves the loss of ability to live independently because of health problems, whether physical or mental. Many older adults may find it necessary to live in assisted living facilities, skilled nursing facilities, memory care facilities, or intermediate care facilities, all of which can be referred to as *long-term care* (LTC) facilities. You probably will have the opportunity to perform some of your clinical experiences in one of these types of facilities, and you will find that providing nursing care for these individuals is vastly different from the care you provide in an acute care setting. One difference is how you refer to those for whom you provide care.

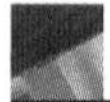

PATIENT OR RESIDENT?

You typically refer to the population within acute care facilities as *patients* or *clients*. Those individuals are in the facility temporarily because they require some type of diagnostics or treatment for health problems. Most individuals for whom you will provide care in LTC facilities are not there temporarily; they reside, or live, there. The facility is their actual home, their residence, and their place of refuge from society, although many of them would prefer to live somewhere else if they could. It is considered more appropriate to refer to these individuals as *residents* rather than *patients*.

Residents' Needs

Using the term *resident* may help you to maintain the focus of your role in providing nursing care. Even though an acute care patient and an LTC resident may have some of the same needs, you will have additional opportunities to meet more needs in the LTC setting. In acute care, you prioritize needs according to Maslow's hierarchy of needs, but it is performed within a much smaller time frame than in an LTC facility and may not require you to address needs from every level. When you care for patients in an LTC facility, your primary focus will be to provide ongoing life services for the residents—those things we all need and desire, which address all levels of Maslow's hierarchy of needs:

- Oxygen and fresh air, water and nutrition, healthy elimination
- Rest and sleep, comfort and pain relief
- Optimal health
- Safety and security
- Spiritual edification
- Freedom from anxiety and fear
- Love and affection, acceptance by others
- Self-respect and being respected
- Self-esteem and self-confidence
- Productivity and self-worth
- Simple enjoyment of and fulfillment in daily life

Helping to Meet These Needs

You will have ample chances to meet more of these needs than you will probably ever realize. When you enter an LTC facility, you have a unique opportunity to impact the lives of the residents and a chance to make their days brighter and more fulfilling. You have the opportunity to bring compassion, respect, comfort, and affection while you provide nursing care. One of the benefits for you is the opportunity to learn from a wealth of wisdom that the residents have to share. Many of them will have lived and experienced decades of life beyond that of the typical student. Encourage residents to reminisce and tell about events they have experienced. Listen attentively as you get to know the resident better, and you may gain knowledge or develop a better appreciation for the past.

The LTC setting is different from acute care in a variety of ways, including room contents, personal attire, personal care, nutrition and hydration, elimination and toileting, immobility and activity, medications, assessment, and documentation.

RESIDENT ROOMS. Even though LTC residents are living in a facility, it is still important to remember that their rooms are their personal residences and you should knock before entering. Residents may bring personal items, sometimes even pieces of furniture, to personalize their residences. Encourage residents to hang photographs and the artwork of grandchildren. Use personal blankets, pillows, and afghans when available. Provide whatever assistance is required to keep the room, floor, and bathroom clean, but allow the resident to arrange his or her possessions as desired. It may look cluttered to you, but it may be just the way he or she wants it. If the resident is immobile or has severe dementia, it will be your responsibility to maintain the room's appearance and organization so that safety is not sacrificed.

PERSONAL ATTIRE. The resident wears his or her own clothing and shoes unless the resident's condition is such that he or she requires continual medical and nursing intervention that is hindered by wearing personal clothing. Some residents will require that the LTC facility employees launder their clothing and sometimes their families will. If the facility launders the clothes, it is important for the resident's name to be written with a permanent marker on the label or inside the neck of all garments, even socks and underwear. ***Safety: Make certain that residents' shoes have nonskid soles to decrease the risk of falls. If the soles are somewhat slick, it is helpful to apply several strips of adhesive tape across the soles of the shoes. The cloth side of the tape helps prevent slipping on a tile floor.***

PERSONAL CARE. Some residents may be able to perform their daily hygiene without assistance, but many will need some help. For these residents, you will provide personal care but on a slightly different schedule than in acute care. For example, most residents will not take a complete bath every day. Aging skin becomes drier and more fragile, so many residents will prefer to take a complete tub bath or shower only two to three times per week. On nonbath days you will wash the resident's face, hands, feet, and perineal area daily and as needed. Most facilities have shower rooms or tub rooms, with several tubs and shower stalls that must be shared by all the residents. ***Safety: You will need to disinfect shower chairs, tubs, and mechanical lifts after each use. This is paramount to prevent cross-contamination.*** (See Chapter 14 for more information about disinfection.) Without stringent disinfection between residents, it is possible to spread diseases caused by highly contagious organisms such as *Clostridium difficile*. This bacterium causes severe diarrhea that has the potential to be fatal in elderly and immune-suppressed individuals, and it can spread quickly throughout a facility (see the Evidence-Based Practice feature).

Evidence-Based Practice

Infection Precaution and Control in Nursing Homes

Clinical Question

How do nursing homes meet goals for infection precautions and control?

Evidence

This study was done in 10 nursing homes across the country with 6 to 8 employees per home recruited to participate. Using in-depth interviews and open-ended guides, the researchers obtained data about when residents were placed on transmission-based precautions for contagious conditions and analyzed their findings. Infection control was considered a priority in all of the nursing homes in the study, and all of them had hand hygiene programs. The study found that isolation practices varied greatly among nursing homes. The decision to put a resident on transmission-based precautions seemed to be based on four things:

1. Perceived risk of transmission
2. Conflict with quality-of-life goals
3. Resource availability
4. Lack of understanding of infection prevention and control

Implications for Nursing Practice

This study highlights the need for clearer understanding of the transmission risk of multiple drug–resistant organisms (MDROs) in the nursing home setting as well as the need for more standardized infection control and prevention in LTC facilities.

Reference

You can read more about this study at https://www.ncbi.nlm.nih.gov/pmc/articles/PMC4575834/

Provide privacy for the residents by pulling the curtains between the bathing stations and ensure that the doors are kept closed while bathing facilities are in use. ***Safety: Immediately mop up all water that is splashed or dripped onto the floor to prevent falls.*** Whirlpool tubs are commonly used for bathing, providing the additional benefit of stimulating the circulation and débriding any wounds the resident may have. Safety is a real issue when bathing residents. It would be easy for residents with impaired mobility or dementia to drown in a whirlpool tub because of the depth of water. ***Safety: Never leave a resident unattended while he or she is bathing! Environmental temperature must be kept warm enough that the resident will not become chilled.***

Some residents are unable to stand or access the bathtub or whirlpool tub without the use of a mechanical lift. You learned about safe usage of this equipment in Chapter 16. ***Safety: Remember to obtain an adequate number of coworkers to provide safe handling while transferring residents via a mechanical lift.***

Provide hair care for residents on a daily basis and wash their hair at least once a week or more often if needed. Many LTC facilities have beauty and barber shops, allowing residents to schedule appointments with professional stylists. If the facility does not have these types of services available or if residents do not have someone who assists them in these matters, you will assist with styling their hair. It will help you to meet this need more easily if you think how you would feel if you were unable to perform these activities and no one else cared enough to assist you. Everyone wants to look their best to receive friends and loved ones when they come to visit; appearance is part of self-esteem.

Male residents may require assistance with shaving, some daily and others only two to three times per week. ***Safety: If a resident has supplemental oxygen being delivered, turn it off for at least 10 minutes before shaving with an electric razor to allow the higher oxygen levels in the room air to dissipate.*** If the resident cannot tolerate the removal of oxygen for that length of time, you will use a safety razor. ***Safety: Before using a safety razor, assess whether the resident is taking anticoagulants such as warfarin (Coumadin), which would put the resident at risk for excessive bleeding in the event you accidentally nick his skin.*** Follow the facility's policy regarding the use of electric and safety razors.

You will perform nail care more frequently in an LTC facility than in an acute care setting. Follow the facility's policy carefully regarding who may cut or trim nails, especially those of a resident with diabetes or peripheral vascular disease (refer to Chapter 15).

NUTRITION AND HYDRATION. Although you provide meals, snacks, and fluids to patients in acute care, the responsibility is more extensive in an LTC facility. It is your responsibility to make certain that each resident maintains adequate dietary intake by:

- Ensuring that dentures are inserted for meals
- Assessing whether the food needs to be finely chopped or pureed

- Feeding or assisting the resident to eat, as needed
- Monitoring and recording the percentage eaten at each meal
- Ensuring that adequate fluids are ingested, usually a minimum of 1,500 mL per day
- Providing supplemental protein and carbohydrate drinks as needed
- Monitoring for weight loss on a weekly or monthly basis

Most LTC facilities have a policy addressing interventions to implement when a resident eats 50% or less of the food served for a meal. The most common intervention is to provide a supplemental nutrition drink, such as Ensure, between meals. Accrediting agencies look for documentation that this has been done.

It is important that all residents who are able be taken to the dining room for each meal. Meals are a social event for most people, and this gathering allows residents to see, greet, and converse with their neighbors. Figure 32.6 shows residents socializing during a meal. For residents who are immobile, it is even more important to transfer them to the dining room for all three meals each day so that they have more opportunity to interact with others. You may transfer residents via a wheelchair or a special chair called a geri-chair. A **geri-chair** is a recliner with side arms, a lap belt, and wheels so that it can be navigated through the hallways. It is used for residents who are unable to sit unassisted.

The dining room in most facilities contains multiple tables with assigned seats for each resident. This allows the staff to deliver special diets to the correct residents. ***Safety: Always check the resident's meal card and diet before delivering the tray to the resident.***

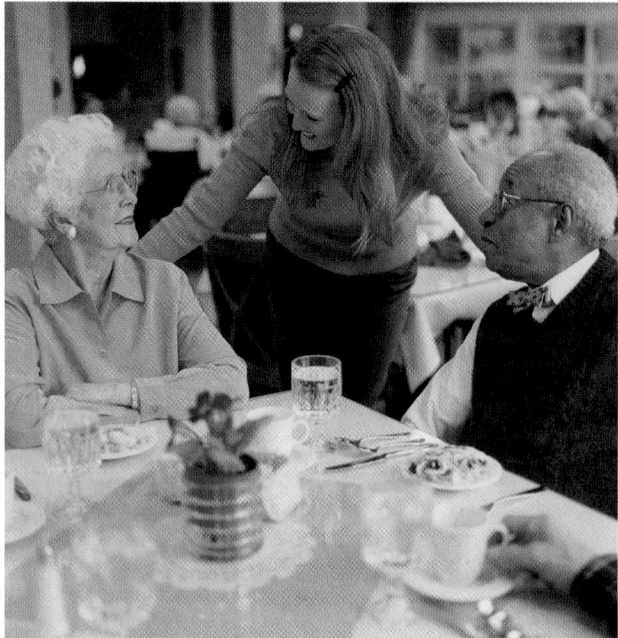

FIGURE 32.6 These residents are socializing during a meal (PunchStock).

When a resident is unable to feed himself or herself, you must assist him or her. It is important to sit in a chair next to the resident, rather than to stand. This puts you at eye level with the resident, which improves communication and allows the resident to see your face. It is important to make mealtimes as pleasant as possible. Converse with the residents and include them in conversations whether or not they are able to verbalize.

ELIMINATION AND TOILETING. Not all residents in an LTC facility are incontinent of bowel and bladder, but many are. Treat the resident with respect when you are changing the incontinence brief and washing the perineum after incontinence. (Also see the information about integumentary changes in Table 32.2.)

It is important to monitor and record whether or not each resident has a bowel movement on every shift. Residents with impaired mobility are particularly at risk for constipation. Most facilities have a policy requiring that each resident be provided with a stool softener or laxative if the resident does not have a bowel movement at least every 3 days. Careless tracking of daily bowel movements can result in fecal impaction, which is a very uncomfortable condition for the resident. (See Chapter 30 for more information about fecal impaction.)

IMMOBILITY. Residents can develop impaired mobility if you do not take action to prevent it. Encourage residents to get out of their rooms and to ambulate as much as possible. Encourage participation in exercise sessions and outdoor walks. Encourage those with gardening interests to help tend to the flower gardens if they are physically able. Lead groups of residents in chair exercises, which can help prevent loss of strength and preserve joint mobility.

Frequently reposition bedfast residents and those who are restricted to sitting in a chair and unable to walk. The longest any resident should remain in any one position is 2 hours. Repositioning, assessing pressure points for erythema, and applying lotion as needed are paramount to preventing pressure ulcers. (See Chapter 16 for more information about this.) Encourage residents, if they are able to do so, to sit in a chair for meals and to attend social events.

Also encourage the resident to do as much as he or she is able to do with regard to ADLs. For example, if a resident is only able to wash his or her face and hands and brush his or her teeth and hair, encourage the resident to do so. Avoid doing it all yourself in an effort to "just get it done" because you are busy. Participation in self-care helps to increase activity but also fosters confidence, independence, and self-esteem. (Also see the information about musculoskeletal changes in Table 32.2.)

ACTIVITY AND ENTERTAINMENT. Most LTC facilities schedule regular activities for the residents to participate in as they are able. Some examples include the following:

- Craft-making sessions
- Manicure sessions

- Domino tournaments
- Group singing and karaoke
- Movie time
- Current event discussion groups
- Daily reading aloud of the newspaper or Bible
- Paint-by-number pictures, watercolors, and finger painting
- Bingo
- Ice cream socials
- Book time, where a novel is read aloud each session until completed

Some LTC facilities may include music sessions in which residents are provided with instruments to play in accompaniment to someone playing the piano. Instruments may include triangles, cymbals, sticks, bells, tambourines, small hand drums, kazoos, or harmonicas. Encourage residents to participate in as many of these activities as possible. One of the best incentives is to include staff and family members who may be visiting at that time.

LTC facilities seek assistance from the local community to provide scheduled activities for residents, such as church services held in the facility chapel, vocal and instrumental talent sessions, monthly birthday celebrations, and holiday parties, as well as visits by children's groups, such as school classes, Sunday school classes, and Girl Scout and Boy Scout troops. Visits by children seem to be especially enjoyed and appreciated by the residents. Another good activity that has proved to be very therapeutic is pet therapy. Kittens, puppies, baby lambs, rabbits, or other small animals are scheduled to be brought in for petting and cuddling once or twice a month. Aquariums set up in the lobby or television area are another treat for residents and sometimes have a calming effect on residents experiencing an emotional event.

MEDICATIONS. As with acute care, most LTC residents will have ordered medications that you will administer and document. Remember that elders will often have stronger reactions to medications and are more at risk for toxicity because the kidneys and liver are unable to rid the body of the drug as quickly as younger adults do. ***Safety: Be vigilant in assessing for oversedation and toxicity in these residents.***

Vital Signs

Rather than assessing vital signs a minimum of three times per day as in acute care, vital signs are routinely assessed once a week or once a month according to the facility's policy. If the resident exhibits signs or symptoms of illness or suffers an injury, vital signs are assessed more frequently for a period of time as determined by the resident's condition and the facility's policy. ***Safety: When you administer medications to residents who require assessment of blood pressure or pulse, you will always check to be sure these vital signs fall within stated parameters before administering the medication.***

Documentation

Documentation for residents in LTC facilities is less frequent and detailed than that done in acute care. Routinely, the nurse makes one entry in each resident's record once per week or according to the facility's policy. Additional entries must be made for any change in condition, for signs or symptoms indicating possible problems, and when an accident occurs or injury is sustained. It will be your responsibility to know your employer's facility documentation policy. In addition, you will document medications according to the facility's policy.

Elder Care Connection

Working with the Elderly in Long-Term Care

In LTC, you will care for a variety of residents who are unable to care for themselves or are unable to be alone. Not all residents are elderly, but the majority are older than 60 years. It is important to create a homelike atmosphere for these residents because the facility is their home. See the following section for more on caring for elders in an LTC facility. Some specific types of LTC include intermediate and skilled care, memory care, and assisted living.

- ***Intermediate care*** is for health conditions that require daily nursing attention but not 24-hour nursing supervision. These patients are not acutely ill and may be disabled. They require mainly custodial care.
- ***Skilled care*** requires 24-hour nursing supervision and care and can include IV therapy, physical therapy, and wound care management. Facilities have a transfer agreement with local hospitals to care for patients with physical and psychological changes that require intervention beyond the capabilities of the LTC facility.
- ***Memory care*** is a specialized environment designed specifically for those suffering from dementia, especially Alzheimer's disease. Memory care is like assisted living with an increased level of support based on the severity of the cognitive impairment. The environment is created to provide the patients with objects and cues that may inspire a memory that can be comforting to the individual. Safety is of great concern in memory care. Often hallways are created in a circular pattern so that the patient can wander more safely. The atmosphere is quiet to decrease stimulation.
- ***Assisted living*** requires the least amount of care. These patients do not require around-the-clock attention but are unable to live totally independent. They may receive prepared meals, assistance with ADLs, housekeeping and laundry services, emergency services, and medication administration. Social activities may also be provided, and transportation for doctor appointments and shopping is often available as well.

PHYSICAL ASSESSMENT OF THE OLDER ADULT

Assessment Considerations for Hospitalized Elderly Adults

Although the physical assessment that you learned to do in Chapter 21 is identical to what you will perform for older adult patients, there still are elements that you need to focus on more intently to make this process as comfortable as possible. Box 32.2 provides tips for when you are performing a physical assessment on a hospitalized older adult.

In addition to the physical assessment, it is important to assess the patient for mental status and depression. A Mini Mental State Exam is often used to ask patients simple questions to determine their cognitive abilities. This may not be within the LPN/LVN's role, but you should be aware of this type of assessment.

Assessment Considerations for Residents in Long-Term Care

When you care for acutely ill patients in the hospital setting, you perform a head-to-toe physical assessment at the beginning of each shift on each patient and additionally as the patient's condition warrants further assessment. This is one of the biggest differences you will find in an LTC facility. A complete head-to-toe assessment is generally performed once a month unless the resident exhibits signs or symptoms of illness or suffers an injury, in which case assessment is performed based on the resident's condition and the frequency cited in the facility's policy. However, the assessments that are performed once a month include additional data beyond the traditional head-to-toe physical assessment. Some of the additional assessments that are made include the following:

- **General appearance:** characteristics such as emaciation, dry hair, or drooping on one side of the face
- **Adaptive equipment:** hearing aids, eyeglasses, dentures, and any prosthesis such as an eye or a limb
- **Ability to communicate:** includes verbal communication or nonverbal communication, with the method that is used if the resident is unable to speak
- **Level of cognition:** including degree of dementia if present
- **General eating habits:** how well the resident generally eats at mealtimes; dentition and ability to chew; type of diet, snacks, and supplements; level of hydration; swallowing or aspiration problems; required use of thickening agent in liquids
- **Special nutritional assistance:** nasogastric or percutaneous endoscopic gastrostomy feeding tubes, type and amount of nutritional supplement, frequency of instillation, tolerance of feedings, special body positioning required for feeding, and frequency of assessment of tube placement
- **Bowel and bladder elimination status and habits:** continent or incontinent, presence of Foley catheter or ostomy, and problems with diarrhea or constipation
- **Ambulatory status:** bedbound; whether one- or two-person assist, total assist, or mechanical lift is required for transfers; ambulates independently; able only to sit in a chair or lie in bed; requires use of cane walker, rolling walker, quad cane, single-prong cane, or gait belt to ambulate; or transferred with a wheelchair or geri-chair
- **Sleep habits:** how well the resident sleeps at night, whether or not the resident wanders, and whether the resident is routinely awakened by pain
- **Medical equipment:** such as oxygen, suction machine, splint, cast, and feeding pump
- **Activities:** include frequency of participation in activities, type of activities attended, and frequency of visitors

> **KNOWLEDGE CONNECTION**
>
> Discuss at least three safety issues about which you must be concerned when providing nursing care in an LTC facility. Explain why we refer to the LTC population as "residents" rather than "patients."

Box 32.2

Tips for Performing Physical Assessment on Hospitalized Older Adults

When you obtain a health history, be certain to consider the patient holistically. Beyond the physical presentation of the patient, there are often emotional, psychological, spiritual, or sociocultural needs that are pressing to an older adult. Before you perform the physical examination, consider which accommodations might make this process easier for the patient. These may include the following:

- **Extra attention to safety:** Because elderly patients may not be steady, consider how to make the physical assessment a safer experience. This may include assisting with transfers, helping the patient to move in the bed, and assisting the patient with disrobing and dressing as necessary.
- **Sessions:** Older adults may not be able to tolerate an entire physical assessment performed at once due to excessive fatigue. Plan your assessment to avoid tiring the patient. You may need to do part of the assessment and then allow the patient to rest a bit before you complete it.
- **Concentration and attention span:** Older adults may have difficulty answering a large number of questions about health history information, especially all at once. If possible, have a knowledgeable family member available to help answer health history questions with the older adult.
- **Extra time:** Avoid rushing the older adult during a physical assessment. Plan to spend extra time performing the assessment and to allow for questions to be answered. Patients will be more comfortable if they do not feel rushed.

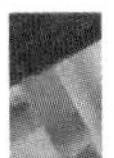

THE PROBLEM OF POLYPHARMACY IN ELDERS

When a patient is taking multiple medications, a potential concern exists for polypharmacy complications. The term *polypharmacy* refers to the ingestion of many medications. It is common for the older adult to have more than one health-care provider as he or she has developed various conditions over time. For example, the individual may have a primary care practitioner, a cardiologist for heart problems, a pulmonary specialist for respiratory disease, and an internal medicine health-care provider for diabetes, all of whom may also have physician assistants or nurse practitioners to assist them. All of these health-care providers may prescribe medications to treat separate conditions. Even though all of these medications are prescribed, their cumulative effects may cause adverse reactions or may result in drug-drug interactions because they are being taken together.

Ideally, each health-care provider should inquire regarding other medications the patient is already taking, but this does not always happen. Even when a health-care provider does ask a patient about medications he or she is currently taking, the health-care provider may still order a same-type drug but by a different name, thus putting the patient in jeopardy of overdose or drug toxicity.

Patients are often unaware of the reason for each of the different medications. They also may lack knowledge about the function of each medication and the possible interactions between drugs. Too often, health-care workers hear patients say, "I take a little white pill, a blue pill, and a pink pill," but they cannot identify the names of the medications or the reasons for taking them. ***Safety: It is paramount that you teach patients and family members to maintain a complete list of all medications and the dosages being taken. This list should accompany the patient any time he or she goes to the health-care provider's office or to the hospital. If at all possible, obtain all medications from the same pharmacy so they can be cross-referenced for interactions.***

Patient Teaching Connection

Teaching Patients About Medications for Multiple Conditions

When working with a patient who takes multiple medications, teach the patient the details of the drug regimen, including the following:

- Reasons for taking each medication
- Dosage for each medication; for example, one pill or two pills, the number of milligrams, etc.
  Note: The amount of milligrams/pill can change according to formulation.
- How often each medication is taken; for example, two or three times a day
  Note: Work with the patient to set times that work best for them and the particular medication.
- Whether the medication should be taken on an empty stomach or with food
- Safety precautions associated with each medication
- How to tell if the medication is effective
- Potential side effects of each medication
- Interacting substances; for example, if the medication would interact with alcoholic beverages

Also teach the patient how to store medications for maximum safety and how to devise an administration system because some patients do very well if they have a system for medication administration. Suggestions include a check-off calendar for each dose of each medication and a storage device that separates each dose for each day of the week.

Nursing Care Plan for an Elderly Patient

A 78-year-old female patient is admitted to the medical-surgical floor of an acute care hospital with the following medical diagnoses: bradycardia, nausea, CHF, mild dehydration, and hypokalemia. She lives alone but has family members who live in the same town. Figure 32.7 presents a concept map care plan for this patient.

Assessment

During your assessment, you discover that the patient has been taking the following medications at home: digoxin, Lasix, furosemide, Caduet, and potassium chloride (Klor-Con). She has seen several different health-care providers, and one prescribed the Lasix while another prescribed the furosemide. You know that these are two different names for the same medication, so in effect the patient is taking double the needed dose. She tells you that she ran out of the potassium chloride (Klor-Con) and has been without the medication for about a week. She also tells you that she has "no earthly idea" why she takes all these medicines, but she assumes that they "will make me better someday."

When you assess her vital signs, her temperature is 98.8°F (37.1°C), pulse 52 and irregular, respirations 20, and blood pressure 106/64. She is alert and oriented to time, place, and person. Her pupils are equal and reactive to light and accommodation. She is weak and unsteady on her feet when you assist her to the bathroom. She states she has been weak and has not felt well for the past few days.

When you review her lab work, you find that her potassium is low at 3.1 mEq/L (normal level: 3.5–5.3 mEq/L) and that her digoxin level is elevated at 2.2 (normal level: 0.5–2.0 ng/mL). Her urine specific gravity is slightly elevated as well, indicating dehydration.

(nursing care plan continues on page 716)

Nursing Care Plan for an Elderly Patient—cont'd

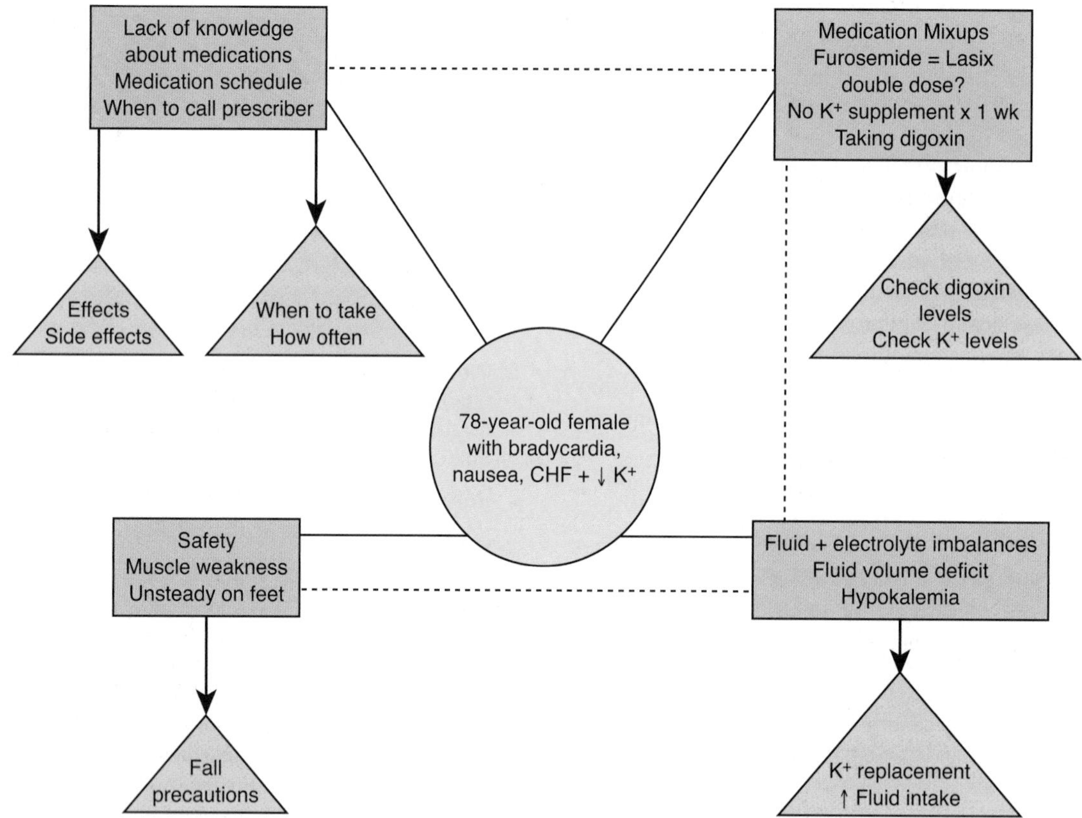

FIGURE 32.7 Concept map care plan for a 78-year-old female patient with bradycardia, nausea, congestive heart failure, and hypokalemia.

Nursing Diagnosis

When you review what you have learned about this particular patient, you understand that:

- She is taking two medications that are the same, prescribed by two different health-care providers, so she probably is getting too much diuretic.
- She has not taken her potassium supplement in a week, which is a further problem with the high dose of diuretic causing depletion of potassium.
- Her digoxin level is high and her heart rate is low, indicating digoxin toxicity.
- She is weak and unsteady on her feet, probably as a result of dehydration and hypokalemia.

You can identify that this patient has a significant risk associated with polypharmacy. This patient has been given the following nursing diagnoses:

- Risk for falls related to weakness as evidenced by unsteady ambulation, bradycardia, and hypokalemia
- Deficient knowledge related to medication purposes and schedules

Additional nursing diagnoses could also include deficient fluid volume and self-care deficit, toileting. For now, you will focus on the bulleted nursing diagnoses.

Planning

All patients are different, so only provide the interventions that will apply to this specific patient—and for this patient, you need to provide nursing care that will help her remain safe when ambulating and help her manage her medications appropriately to prevent further medication-related hospitalizations.

Consider that the patient is not aware that she is taking two medications that are the same, prescribed by two different health-care providers. Plan to teach about the medication regimen so that she has a working knowledge of why she takes these medications and what each should be doing for her. It also would be critical to teach her how often each medication should be taken and how much she should take at each dosing interval.

Consider that she is weak and unsteady on her feet due to her dehydration, digoxin toxicity, bradycardia, and hypokalemia. All these together place her at high risk for falls. It is very important that you protect her from injury while she is in the hospital, and you must take immediate steps to prevent potential falls.

Possible short-term goals for this patient would include the following:

- Patient will be steady during ambulation and have increased muscle strength by discharge.
- Patient will verbalize purposes and schedules for medications by discharge.

• WORD • BUILDING •

bradycardia: brady – slow + card – heart + ia – condition

hypokalemia: hypo – deficient + kal – potassium + em – blood + ia – condition

Nursing Care Plan for an Elderly Patient—cont'd

Implementation
At this stage of the nursing process, you can now implement the appropriate interventions for this patient. The care plan below provides nursing interventions for this nursing diagnosis.

Evaluation
The last step in the nursing process is to evaluate whether the interventions you have been implementing are helping the patient ambulate safely and master her medication regimen (see the evaluations in the care plan below).

Nursing Diagnosis: Risk for falls related to weakness as evidenced by unsteady ambulation, bradycardia, and hypokalemia

Expected Outcomes: Patient will ambulate 20 feet with standby assistance by discharge. Patient will experience heart rate of 60 or above consistently before discharge. Patient will have confirmed potassium levels within normal range (3.5–5.3 mEq/L) within 2 days.

Interventions	Evaluations
Evaluate the patient's fall risk using the Morse Fall Scale (see Chapter 13). Institute fall precautions. Post fall precautions on the door to the patient's room and in the patient's chart according to facility policy.	Day 1: Rated at a 35 on Morse Fall Scale and was identified as a medium fall risk. Placed on fall precautions immediately after admission and signs were posted on her door to indicate this. Day 3: She had experienced no falls or other injuries.
Instruct the patient not to get up unassisted. Check on the patient every 30 min to assist with any problems. Encourage the patient to use the call light; ensure that she knows where it is and how to use it. Keep needed items within her reach. Answer the patient's call light promptly so that she will not tire of waiting for help and attempt to get up alone. Respond to the bed/chair/leg monitor alarms immediately to prevent a fall. Assist the patient to ambulate to the chair or the bathroom when needed. Do not leave the patient alone while in the bathroom or on the bedside commode.	Day 1: Was on bedrest and used the bedpan. Nursing staff checked on her every 30 min, and she did not try to get up alone. Most of the time she would use the call light to ask for assistance, but occasionally she would call out to a staff member who walked by her room. Day 2: Able to get up to the bathroom with assistance. She was still weak but less unsteady on her feet and understood that she was not to get up alone. Day 3: She was able to go to the bathroom with standby assistance and was able to use her call light when she needed assistance.
Monitor vital signs every 4 hours. Assess heart rate and report pulse below 60. Hold Digoxin dose per protocol. Monitor telemetry readings once per shift and any time you are notified by the monitor technician. Assess blood pressure in three positions because heart rate is low and patient is at risk for falls.	Day 1: Heart rate remained below 60. The health-care provider was aware and felt it was due to digitalis toxicity. Blood pressure showed a significant drop (more than 30 mm Hg) when her position changed from sitting to standing. Day 3: Heart rate was 60. Telemetry readings remained in sinus rhythm throughout her hospital stay. Blood pressure was stable in all three positions.
Monitor potassium levels. Administer oral potassium as ordered. Administer IV potassium as ordered. Assess for signs and symptoms of hyper- or hypokalemia.	Day 1: Potassium was 2.9 mEq/L. The health-care provider ordered potassium added to her IV drip and started her on oral potassium. Tolerated both without difficulty. Day 3: Potassium level was back up to 3.5.
Teach the patient about her drug regimen, including brand names and generic names. Explain the importance of informing all health-care providers about all the medications she is taking. Review medications with the patient, explaining names, doses, and purposes of each.	Day 2: Able to verbalize the names of her medications when looking at a list. Able to identify the correct doses and times of day to take each medication. Verbalized understanding of the need to inform all health-care providers about each medication she is taking.
Ask the health-care provider for an order for home health care to follow the patient on discharge to ensure that she has a system for setting up and taking her medications correctly.	Day 3: The health-care provider ordered home health care follow-up for this patient. The home health nurse will visit after discharge from the hospital to ensure medication compliance.

POST CONFERENCE

During post conference, you share about caring for your patient. The first day, you simply felt overwhelmed by all her medications: 13 pills for her 9 a.m. meds. She was less confused that day because she had received IV fluids for dehydration and her UTI was responding well to antibiotics. She really looked happy when her daughter arrived. The second day was much better. Although you understood more about her medications, it was clear that your patient did not and that she had not been taking them correctly. You were able to begin teaching her about her medicines and how to take them. Her confusion was better by her second day in the hospital, and her daughter was also learning about the medications so that she could help her mother with them in the future. Your patient turned out to be an interesting and lively 86-year-old who offered to teach you how to knit. You confess that your ideas about her at the beginning were quite wrong and that you had unconsciously practiced ageism.

Key Points

- Older adults are classified as young-old, middle-old, old-old, and elite-old.
- The number of older adults in the United States will continue to increase substantially in the coming years.
- Physical changes take place in all of the major organ systems as patients age. Most of these involve a slow decrease of the organ system functioning.
- Older adults are at risk for elder abuse, scams, and crimes. The nurse should work with the patient and the caregivers to decrease the risks associated with these events.
- Positive aspects of aging include the development of wisdom and insight to share with younger generations. To help aging patients feel positive, meet them where they are in the aging process and ask about their lives.
- Meeting the needs of residents in LTC includes following Maslow's hierarchy of needs and providing opportunities for love and belonging, being respected, building self-esteem, and fulfillment in daily life. In LTC the rooms are homelike and residents wear regular clothing and shoes rather than gowns and slippers. The staff assists residents with ADLs, and the facility provides opportunities for activity and entertainment.
- In LTC, residents are not bathed as frequently due to skin changes, vital signs are taken weekly or monthly, and head-to-toe assessments are performed monthly. All of these are performed much more frequently in the acute care setting.
- Nurses should be active in dispelling the practice of ageism.
- Patients should be monitored for risks associated with polypharmacy.
- Nursing care of the older adult should always include a component for patient safety.

Review Questions

Select the answer that is most appropriate for each of the following questions. Some questions may have more than one correct answer. Select all that apply.

1. A nurse is caring for an elderly patient. Which physiological change is of the highest concern?
   1. Urinary retention
   2. Slowing of metabolism
   3. Impaired visual acuity
   4. Development of age spots on the skin

2. An elderly client with dementia is brought to the primary health-care provider's office. The client's daughter asks the nurse, "What is dementia?" Which nursing response is appropriate?
   1. "It is the deterioration of all cognitive functions."
   2. "It is the inability to think with usual clarity, speed, and coherence."
   3. "It is a feeling of intense sadness, helplessness, and hopelessness."
   4. "It is a perceptual disorder characterized by dreams and hallucinations."

3. An elderly clients states, "I can't afford to eat and buy all these medications." What nursing intervention would be most appropriate?
   1. Refer the client to chaplain's services
   2. Refer the client to available social services
   3. Help the client choose between food and medicine
   4. Give the client $100 of your money to help buy medicine

4. A nurse working in the hospital complains about his assignment, saying, "I don't have a single patient younger than 70 years old. I'll be babbling and confused by the end of my shift!" These comments reflect:
   1. humor in the workplace.
   2. the practice of ageism.
   3. an honest assessment of the assignment.
   4. caregiver burnout.

5. An elderly patient with diabetes is admitted with low blood sugar and a syncopal episode. He is confused and unable to give clear answers to most questions. He is noted to have multiple decubiti, poor hygiene, and several old and new lacerations with varying areas of ecchymosis. Which is of most concern to you, the nurse?
   1. The possibility that elder abuse is occurring
   2. Obtaining an accurate medical history
   3. The need for diabetic teaching
   4. The need for a tetanus shot because of his lacerations

6. The nurse is assessing an old-old client. Which assessment finding should the nurse consider as highest priority?
   1. Slowing of peristalsis
   2. Decreased sense of smell
   3. Loss of skin elasticity
   4. Temperature of 94°F

7. Which comment by the caregiver of an older adult patient with Alzheimer's disease would concern you the most?
   1. "I get tired, but my daughter comes to relieve me each day."
   2. "I can't sleep because I am afraid he will get out of the house."
   3. "This illness has affected the entire family, not just him."
   4. "The disease is progressing about the way we were told to expect that it would."

8. An 80-year-old patient is hospitalized with a UTI and peripheral vascular disease. In addition, he has glaucoma and diabetes. Which nursing actions would be appropriate for him?
   1. Assess finger stick blood sugar as ordered
   2. Assess peripheral pulses, capillary refill, warmth, and color of extremities
   3. Assess risk for suicide or self-harm
   4. Perform mouth care every 8 hours or more often as needed
   5. Protect from injury due to impaired vision
   6. Encourage weight-bearing exercise and increased calcium intake
   7. Scan the bladder to detect urinary retention
   8. Encourage fluid intake of liquids the patient likes to drink
   9. Administer antidiabetic medications as ordered
   10. Assess for improvement of signs and symptoms of UTI

ANSWERS 1. 3, 2. 1, 3. 2, 4. 2, 5. 1, 6. 4, 7. 2, 8. 1, 2, 5, 7, 8, 9, 10

Critical Thinking Exercises

Answers available online.

1. Describe how you might benefit from providing nursing care for residents in a long-term facility.

2. Describe how a young-old patient may differ from an old-old patient regarding physiological and psychosocial considerations. How would your approach in caring for both of these patients differ? How would your approach in caring for both of these patients be similar?

3. An elderly patient in an assisted living facility where you work tells you about a person he has recently met who is helping him invest his money. This person wants to be introduced to other residents for the same purpose. You have concerns that this could be a scam. What will you do?

Additional Resources

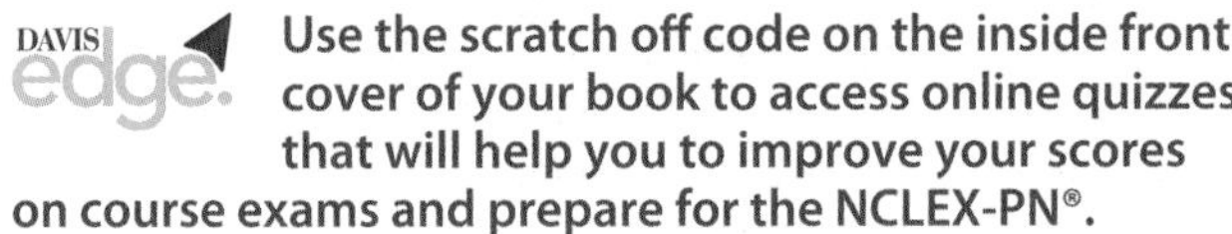

DAVIS
edge
Use the scratch off code on the inside front cover of your book to access online quizzes that will help you to improve your scores on course exams and prepare for the NCLEX-PN®.

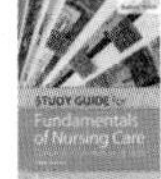

Study Guide

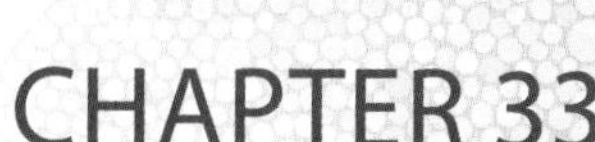

CHAPTER 33
Care of the Surgical Patient

Connie Hunt

KEY TERMS

Anesthesia (AN-es-THEE-zhah)
Antiembolism hose (AN-ti-EM-bo-lizm HOHZ)
Approximation (a-PROK-sih-MAY-shun)
Bier block (BEER BLOK)
Conscious sedation (KON-shuss sih-DAY-shun)
Corrective surgery (ko-REK-tiv SER-juh-ree)
Cosmetic surgery (koz-MET-ik SER-juh-ree)
Epidural anesthesia (EP-ih-DOO-ruhl AN-es-THEE-zhah)
Exploratory surgery (eks-PLO-ruh-tor-ee SER-juh-ree)
Extubation (EKS-too-BAY-shun)
General anesthesia (JEN-e-ruhl AN-es-THEE-zhah)
Intubation (IN-too-BAY-shun)
Laparoscopic surgery (LAP-a-ro-SKOP-ik SER-juh-ree)
Local anesthesia (LOH-kuhl AN-es-THEE-zhah)
Malignant hyperthermia (mah-LIG-nant HYE-per-THUR-mee-ah)
Palliative surgery (PAL-ee-AY-tiv SER-juh-ree)
Postanesthesia care unit (POHST-AN-es-THEE-zhah KARE YOO-nit)
Regional anesthesia (REE-jon-uhl AN-es-THEE-zhah)
Sequential compression device (sih-KWEN-shul kom-PRESH-uhn dih-vyess)

CHAPTER CONCEPTS

Safety
Patient-Centered Care
Comfort

LEARNING OUTCOMES

1. Define various terms associated with care of the surgical patient.
2. Differentiate among types of surgery by purpose and degree of urgency
3. Describe various surgical settings.
4. Discuss the components of the presurgical assessment.
5. Determine findings in a presurgical assessment that would be of concern.
6. Explain the various purposes of preoperative diagnostic testing.
7. Specify the important points to cover during preoperative teaching.
8. Explain the types and purposes of preoperative medications.
9. Describe the process and importance of obtaining informed consent.
10. Discuss the use of the preoperative checklist.
11. Compare the various roles and responsibilities of the surgical team members.
12. Identify types of anesthesia, with advantages and disadvantages of each.
13. Briefly discuss the intraoperative care of the surgical patient.
14. Discuss potential problems with nursing interventions for the patient in the postanesthesia care unit.
15. Identify patient care priorities when the surgical patient returns to the nursing unit.
16. Identify potential postsurgical complications, with emphasis on prevention and intervention.
17. Discuss information found in the Connection features in this chapter.
18. Identify specific safety features.
19. Answer questions about the skills in this chapter.

SKILLS

33.1 Applying Antiembolism Hose
33.2 Applying Sequential Compression Devices

CRITICAL THINKING CONNECTION

Clinical Assignment

You will be caring for a 67-year-old male patient who has been diagnosed with inflammatory bowel disease. He will be going to surgery today at 9:00 a.m. to have the diseased portion of the colon removed and the remaining intestines will be anastomosed, or reconnected surgically. This is called a segmental colectomy with anastomosis. Your instructor tells you that you will be responsible for completing most of the preoperative (preop) checklist and performing preop teaching. You will then care for this patient postoperatively (postop) after she returns to the nursing unit.

Critical Thinking Questions:

1. What portions of the colon could be removed in this procedure?
2. What special care might this patient need?
3. What will you include in preop teaching for this patient?
4. How will you ensure that the patient is ready to go to surgery?
5. How will you prepare to receive your patient back on the nursing unit after surgery?
6. How does caring for a patient immediately after return from surgery differ from caring for a patient 1 to 2 days after surgery?

This chapter will alleviate some of the mystery regarding what happens during surgery. You will learn how to provide nursing care in each phase of the surgical experience, including preop, intraoperative, and postop. You will learn how to assess and prepare your patients for surgery, the roles of the various operative personnel, and how to safely prioritize postop nursing care.

You have already learned that anxiety and fear are second priority *only* to basic physiological needs, such as oxygen, food, and water. This chapter will supply you with the knowledge necessary to alleviate much of your surgical patient's anxiety and fear, one of the easier yet more helpful interventions that you can perform for a perioperative patient.

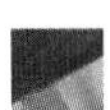

PURPOSES OF SURGERY

Surgery is performed for a number of reasons, including treatment of a disease or injury, such as removal of the gallbladder to treat inflammation and gallstones, termed a *cholecystectomy.* Surgical procedures that treat or cure disease are classified as *curative surgeries.* Other purposes for surgery include the following:

- **Correction: Corrective surgery** is done to repair an anatomical or congenital defect. An example is to repair a cleft palate so that a child can nurse or eat normally.
- **Cosmetic: Cosmetic surgery** may be performed to change or improve one's physical appearance. Examples of this type of procedure include a face lift or breast augmentation.
- **Exploration: Exploratory surgery** is done to provide further data and determine a diagnosis for a problem. For example, abdominal pain sometimes requires exploratory surgery to determine the cause.
- **Palliation: Palliative surgery** alleviates symptoms and provides comfort but does not necessarily cure the disease or heal the injury. An example of palliative surgery is removing as much of a tumor as possible, known as *debulking* a tumor. This type of surgery can decrease pain and relieve pressure, but it will not cure the cancer.

KNOWLEDGE CONNECTION

Compare curative surgery to palliative. Explain how cosmetic surgery is different from curative, corrective, and palliative. Which one do you think would be least likely to be covered by health insurance? What does exploratory surgery mean?

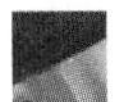

DEGREES OF URGENCY

Correlating with the various reasons to perform surgery are degrees of urgency, meaning how quickly the surgery must be scheduled. The degrees of urgency include the following:

- **Elective surgery:** Any surgery that is voluntary and scheduled a week or more in advance. Elective surgery includes those surgeries intended to improve a patient's quality of life, either physically or psychologically. The surgery may be medically necessary, such as a cataract removal. Alternatively, it may be patient desired, such as breast augmentation.
- **Urgent surgery:** Surgery required within 24 hours of diagnosis to prevent complications that may occur with waiting. An example of urgent surgery is a hip pinning following fracture to prevent complications associated with immobility and emboli formation.
- **Emergency surgery:** Surgery that cannot be delayed and usually is scheduled within 2 hours to prevent serious complication or death. Examples include a stable gastrointestinal bleed or subdural hematoma evacuation.
- **Salvage surgery:** Surgery required when cardiopulmonary resuscitation is in progress on the way to the

• WORD • BUILDING •

perioperative: peri – around + operative – related to an operation

cholecystectomy: chole – bile + cyst – bladder + ectomy – surgical removal

operating room (OR) or the patient's life or limb is threatened. Examples of this type of surgery include surgery for such things as a gunshot wound or a ruptured aneurysm.

KNOWLEDGE CONNECTION

Classify the following surgeries for purpose and degree of urgency:

- Repair of hand after exploding fireworks almost blew the thumb off
- Liposuction of abdomen
- Appendectomy because of acute severe right-sided, lower abdominal pain
- Tonsillectomy for history of repeated strep infections of the throat and tonsils
- Open reduction of fractured femur with excessive bleeding into thigh
- Removal of cancerous tumor wrapped around the spinal cord in a patient with advanced metastatic cancer of the brain and bone who suddenly lost all function and sensation below the waist

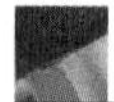

VARIOUS SURGICAL SETTINGS

In the past, surgery was performed only in hospitals. However, improved technology has allowed health-care professionals to safely perform certain surgeries in a number of different settings. This allows for reduced expenses and decreased time away from home for the patient. It also reduces hospitals' demands for nursing personnel to provide postop patient care, decreasing their costs.

Outpatient Surgery

Outpatient surgery is performed on a patient who is not admitted to the hospital as an inpatient. The patient arrives at the site prior to surgery, has the procedure, spends certain hours in the recovery room, and returns home the same day. The perfect candidate for outpatient surgery is a patient with few to no pre-existing medical conditions. Surgeries performed on an outpatient basis include only minor surgical procedures with minimal postop risk of complications. They may be performed in a stand-alone surgery center or in a medical office. They may also be performed in a hospital outpatient surgery department where the patient is not admitted as an inpatient and generally does not stay overnight.

Stand-Alone Surgery Center

A stand-alone surgery center is a facility designed to only provide perioperative care for minor surgical procedures during the day. It is generally open for a specified length of time each day, such as from 7:00 a.m. to 7:00 p.m. All types of anesthesia can be administered as needed and postop. Recovery room services are provided until the patient is awake and stable enough to be discharged to home. An example of a surgery well suited for a surgery center is a knee arthroscopy on a young adult. The patient is scheduled to arrive at the surgery center 1 to 2 hours prior to surgery, undergoes the procedure, and after several hours in recovery is released to go home. Procedures in this setting may be described as *day surgery.*

Medical Office

Certain procedures that are considered very minor and do not require anesthesia other than an injection of a *local anesthetic,* an agent that will numb the site, may be performed in the medical office. An example of a surgery well suited for a medical office is a *vasectomy.*

Hospital Outpatient Surgery Department

Many hospitals now offer surgery on an outpatient basis as well as on an inpatient basis. The patient comes to the facility for the surgical procedure but is not admitted as an inpatient and generally does not spend the night there. Compared to a freestanding surgery center or medical office, a hospital-based outpatient surgery department allows for more extensive surgery on higher-risk patients who may have to be given general anesthesia that puts the patient to sleep. The difference is that the hospital has readily accessible personnel and laboratory facilities. A hospital also allows for overnight stay should the patient develop complications. An example of surgery well suited for hospital-based outpatient surgery is a tonsillectomy on an 8-year-old, in whom the risk of bleeding is highest between 6 and 8 hours after surgery.

Inpatient Surgery

Inpatient, hospital-based surgery is performed on patients who have been admitted to the hospital. Patients are sent to surgery from an inpatient bed, emergency room, or intensive care unit. These patients may require hospitalization before surgery to stabilize a pre-existing or acute condition that requires surgical intervention. An example of this type of surgery is a patient admitted for abdominal pain who required insertion of a nasogastric (NG) tube and IV therapy. Once the NG tube was inserted, the patient was diagnosed as having a gastrointestinal bleed, which required surgical intervention to prevent hemorrhage.

KNOWLEDGE CONNECTION

What would you consider to be advantages of inpatient hospital-based surgery? What do you feel would be an advantage of surgery performed in a daytime surgery center? What types of surgeries might be inappropriate to perform in a daytime surgery center?

• WORD • BUILDING •

anesthetic: an – without + esthe – sensation + tic – producing

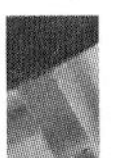

PREOPERATIVE CARE OF THE SURGICAL PATIENT

When most new nursing students think of caring for the surgical patient, they may think of just caring for the patient during surgery or postsurgery. However, it is important to realize that there is a tremendous amount of care to be provided preop as well. In fact, the more thorough the preop teaching, the better the patient generally does postop because of a reduction of fear/anxiety and increased compliance with postop care. Patients presenting for surgery should bring with them a personal history of medical problems and prior surgeries, family histories of disease or illness, and personal indications for surgery. Your job is to help optimally prepare the patient and, where appropriate, the patient's family for the surgery and anesthesia.

Presurgical Assessment

Presurgical assessment includes a preliminary process of assessment and preop testing to ensure that the patient is healthy enough to undergo surgery and **anesthesia,** which is the loss of sensation, with or without loss of consciousness, accomplished by the administration of inhaled or injected medications. Presurgical assessment also helps the surgeon determine if the patient should or can be scheduled for surgery at a freestanding surgical center or medical office or if the patient would be better cared for in a hospital setting.

After assessment and testing, a patient judged to be a safe candidate for surgery is said to have received *presurgical clearance.* Patients may have their presurgical clearance done in the surgeon's office, a freestanding laboratory facility, or the hospital's laboratory. This process helps to identify pre-existing medical conditions. Examples include hypertension and diabetes, which need to be optimized before adding the threat of surgery and anesthesia. A physician may decide to delay portions of the presurgical assessment until the patient arrives at the surgical site.

Safety: The primary goal of the presurgical assessment is patient safety.

Patient History

You will want to begin your preop assessment with the goal of obtaining a detailed patient history. The history is one of the best measures of patient status, so it is important that your questioning be targeted, specific, and complete. Taking the patient's history has eight steps:

1. **Exploring the patient's understanding of the need for surgery to be performed:** This will help you to make sure the patient knows what procedure is being performed and why. Be certain the patient understands his or her options as well as the expected results of the surgery. The patient should be able to explain in his or her own words why surgery is required and what will be done.
2. **Asking about any previous surgeries and anesthetics:** This will help you find out about any problems that may have occurred with previous surgeries. An example includes severe nausea or an allergic reaction.
3. **Asking about the patient's family health history:** This includes asking about any family history of anesthetic problems.
4. **Asking about current medication use, including prescription medications, over-the-counter medications, and herbal medications:** This may provide clues to pre-existing medical problems as well as identify potential drug interactions that may occur with anesthetic exposure. This is a particularly important assessment because some medications and herbs must be stopped for a specific length of time prior to surgery to prevent complications, such as extended bleeding time.
5. **Asking about medication allergies and intolerances:** This is necessary to prevent exposures to known harmful medications. Asking should remind you to see that the patient has an allergy band applied and the chart is correctly labeled for allergies.
6. **Asking about alcohol and illegal drug use, abuse, and addiction:** This will help you anticipate potential drug interactions and problems with pain management after surgery. It can also alert you to observe for withdrawal signs and symptoms related to abuse of and addiction to illegal drugs.
7. **Asking about tobacco use:** Tobacco use can contribute to intraoperative and postop problems with oxygenation and ventilation. This information directs care toward the prevention of postop hypoventilation and pneumonia.
8. **Asking females about the possibility of pregnancy, specifically to determine the date of the patient's last menstrual period:** Unless it is an emergency, surgery during pregnancy should be avoided.

> **KNOWLEDGE CONNECTION**
>
> Identify eight types of data that should be collected as part of the patient's medical history. What is the primary goal of performing a presurgical assessment and medical history prior to scheduling a surgical procedure? Why should you ask about previous surgeries the patient has had? What role does asking about family health history play?

Review of Systems

The review of systems is designed to identify the presence or absence of pre-existing diseases that may affect either the surgical procedure or the administration of anesthesia. Pre-existing disease may also be the cause for surgery. An example is a case of severe arthritis and the need for a joint replacement, or it may be a factor that increases perioperative risks. It is especially important to assess organ systems that can be affected by the anesthetics, such as the central nervous and cardiovascular systems. It is also important to assess organ systems that affect the actions of anesthetics, such as the pulmonary and renal systems, and the accessory gastrointestinal organs, such as the liver.

CARDIOVASCULAR SYSTEM. Ask about pre-existing *arrhythmias,* which are heart rhythm irregularities, chest pain, and myocardial infarction, the medical name for a heart attack. This is important because of the risk for reinfarction during surgery. Ask about hypertension and, if present, ask about medications used and compliance; also assess the degree of control of the blood pressure. A patient with poorly controlled hypertension may have begun to develop end-stage renal damage, meaning the kidney function has deteriorated to minimal functioning. This would clue you to the need for preop testing of renal function. If the patient has a history of heart failure, you would be clued to assess for edema in the extremities; auscultation of heart sounds, noting muffled S_1 and S_2; and auscultation of breath sounds, noting crackles or rhonchi. If there are signs and symptoms of heart failure, surgery probably will be cancelled until the patient's symptoms abate.

RESPIRATORY SYSTEM. Ask the patient about dyspnea, both exertional and at rest. This can provide clues about pulmonary and cardiac disease. If the patient has a history of asthma or other chronic obstructive pulmonary disease (COPD), inquire about inhaler and oxygen use. These patients will be at a higher risk for airway irritation intraoperatively and postop. It also would be pertinent to inquire if the patient takes corticosteroids because they tend to inhibit wound healing.

CENTRAL NERVOUS SYSTEM. As you are asking questions of your patient, assess if your patient is able to follow commands and understand your teaching. If the patient does not follow simple requests or answer your questions, make certain that the lack of response is not because of a language barrier. Evaluate any neurological deficit so that you have a clear understanding of adjustments that need to be made in delivering care. For example, a patient with dementia might benefit from having a family member remain at the bedside in the preop holding area and immediately after surgery in the **postanesthesia care unit** (PACU). Normally this might not be allowed, but for a patient with severe dementia it might make the difference in reducing stress, confusion, or lack of cooperation.

RENAL SYSTEM. Many anesthetic agents and medications are eliminated through the kidneys, so it is important to assess for pre-existing renal disease because failure to eliminate medications can result in toxicity. In addition, the patient with renal dysfunction almost always is anemic, which has the potential to compromise oxygenation. Coagulation deficits also may be present in patients who are on dialysis. Tests that will help determine the health status of the kidneys are the *creatinine* and *estimated glomerular filtration rate* (eGFR). Creatinine, which is an end waste product of metabolism, is removed from the blood by the kidneys. Therefore, an elevated serum level of creatinine points toward kidney problems. The creatinine levels are also used to calculate the eGFR, which provides data about kidney function. However, the eGFR is applicable only to nonpregnant patients between 18 and 70 years of age who are not obese and who do not have severe nutritional deficiencies.

MUSCULOSKELETAL SYSTEM. Arthritis is the most common musculoskeletal disease found in older surgical patients. Arthritis can compromise positioning. In addition, medications taken for arthritis, such as aspirin and nonsteroidal anti-inflammatory drugs (NSAIDs), such as ibuprofen and naproxen, affect platelet function, which increases the risk of bleeding.

GASTROINTESTINAL SYSTEM. Malnutrition and anemia can compromise wound healing, while obesity increases the risk of pulmonary and cardiac compromise. Malnutrition is characterized by several laboratory tests, including low serum *prealbumin, albumin, transferrin, hematocrit* (Hct), and *hemoglobin* (Hgb) levels. Prealbumin, a protein produced primarily by the liver, is good evidence of the patient's protein status and serves as one of the best indicators of malnutrition. Albumin, a protein produced in the liver, is a good indicator not only of nutritional status but also of liver function itself. Transferrin is a glycoprotein produced by the liver that carries over half of the body's iron. When the serum level of transferrin remains low, it can interfere with production of Hgb, which can lead to anemia. Together, low Hgb and Hct results serve as the primary determinant of anemia. Obesity is a risk factor for hypertension, coronary artery disease, stroke, reflux and aspiration, and airway difficulties.

The liver is the primary organ for drug metabolism, so any pre-existing hepatic disease, such as hepatitis, cirrhosis, or alcoholism, has the potential to decrease the rate and efficacy of drug clearance. In addition, the liver is responsible for the production of clotting factors to assist with clotting of blood and bile for digestion. It regulates carbohydrate, amino acid, and lipid metabolism. It stores the fat-soluble vitamins A, D, E, and K; the water-soluble vitamins A and D; and iron and copper. Therefore, liver disease increases the risk of bleeding and malnutrition as well as poor wound healing. The tests that provide clotting information are the *prothrombin time* (PT) and the *international normalized ratio* (INR); these tests are ordered together. When the clotting sequence is prolonged, it provides information regarding the status of the liver as well as an elevated risk for bleeding. Another test called the *activated partial thromboplastin time* (APTT) provides further data that indicates whether or not the patient has an increased risk for bleeding.

ENDOCRINE SYSTEM. Most patients with pre-existing endocrine disease will have the disease well controlled before surgery. However, the patient with diabetes is at the greatest risk for sudden increases and decreases in blood sugar levels due to NPO status, emotional stress preop, and the physical stress of surgery itself. The presence of diabetes will require frequent monitoring of the blood glucose levels postop as well as possible administration of sliding scale insulin.

HEMATOLOGICAL SYSTEM. The patient with a low *red blood cell* (RBC) count or Hgb level is at risk for problems with oxygenation because the RBCs carry the Hgb that is responsible for carrying oxygen to cells throughout the body. Patients with low platelet counts are at risk for excessive bleeding and hemorrhage. Even when the platelet count is normal, if the PT, INR, and APTT are excessively long, the patient still may be at risk for bleeding during surgery. Patients with low *white blood cell* (WBC) counts have decreased immunity. These patients are at greater risk for infection than are individuals with normal WBC levels.

Physical Examination

A complete physical examination may or may not have been done in advance of the day of surgery by the surgeon or medical provider. If it was not performed prior to admission, the admitting physician and/or surgeon should perform the examination to ascertain patient stability. The anesthesia provider also may perform an assessment to determine whether the patient is a good candidate for anesthesia.

KNOWLEDGE CONNECTION

Which body systems are important with regard to the metabolism of anesthesia agents? Which laboratory test results provide you with data regarding the patient's nutritional status? Which tests are significant for a patient who has chronic respiratory problems and requires surgery? What significance would a low WBC count have for a patient about to have surgery? How might having severe arthritis affect a patient who undergoes surgery? Which laboratory tests provide you information regarding the patient who is at risk for bleeding/hemorrhage problems?

Preoperative Diagnostic Testing

The ordering of preop laboratory tests should be based on the patient's individual history and physical examination, with consideration of the specific surgery to be performed. Also, most facilities have standing orders requiring that certain laboratory tests be performed on all surgical patients.

Laboratory and Diagnostic Connection

Standard Preoperative Laboratory Tests

Most facilities require the following basic tests as the minimum for all preop patients:

- ***Complete blood cell count*** (CBC): Done to detect low Hgb and Hct indicating anemia, which could place the patient at risk for hypoxia if heavy blood loss occurs. It is also important to ensure that the WBC count does not indicate a current infection and that the platelet count is within normal range. A low platelet count would put the patient at risk for coagulation problems. ***Safety: A patient with a normal platelet count is not ensured to be free of coagulation problems because there are various other components that also affect the clotting process.***
- ***Urinalysis*** (UA): Done to rule out urinary tract infection (UTI) and to look for protein, which could indicate impaired renal function. An elevated specific gravity also could indicate that the patient is dehydrated, which would require infusion of IV fluids prior to surgery.
- ***Electrocardiogram*** (EKG): Done to detect cardiac arrhythmias or signs of ischemia, which is lack of oxygen delivery to the heart muscle via the coronary arteries.

Some facilities have a standing policy to perform a preop pregnancy test, known as the *human chorionic gonadotropin (hCG) test,* on all females of childbearing age. It is imperative to know whether or not a woman is pregnant prior to performing surgery on her. This is especially important in the first trimester, when anesthesia medications as well as postop medications may interfere with fetal development.

Laboratory tests should be ordered in correlation to the history and physical examination findings to evaluate the extent and control of disease progression. Lab tests can detect imbalances that require preop correction, such as a low serum potassium (K^+) level. They also provide an assessment of perioperative risk.

Before going into surgery, the anesthesia provider and often the surgeon or internist will evaluate preop laboratory test results and the preop EKG for any abnormality that requires correction before surgery. Sometimes, scheduled surgery must be cancelled. For example, if the patient has been taking warfarin to prevent blood clots, clotting times will be assessed before surgery. The patient would have stopped taking the warfarin in advance to prevent surgical bleeding. But the clotting values may not have returned to normal values yet, which might require postponement of the surgery. If a new abnormal finding is seen on EKG, surgery may be postponed for a cardiologist evaluation.

KNOWLEDGE CONNECTION

What three diagnostic tests are generally performed on every preop patient? How might routine medications that a patient has been taking be a problem for the surgical patient? Which test is sometimes performed preop, but only on women?

Preoperative Patient Teaching

Research has shown that a patient who receives good preop teaching tends to do better postop and to have a smoother, shorter recovery period. Preop teaching provides the patient and family with information, skills, and instructions that will support optimal healing, be conducive to the shortest recovery period, and serve to prevent or reduce postop complications.

It is common and expected that the patient and the patient's family will feel anxiety in relation to a scheduled surgery. Keep in mind that the average layperson does not have even the *basic* knowledge related to nursing and medical care that you now have and may take for granted. By assisting the patient and family to understand what will happen and what the patient will and may experience, you can relieve some of these "fears of the unknown." There also may be legitimate fear related to the results of the surgery, including possible disfigurement or death. This fear is a preop issue that can impair communication, alter one's cognitive ability to process information, and immobilize one's ability to function. In order to limit the patient's anxiety prior to surgery, provide the following:

- Information regarding preop preparations, including diagnostic tests, NPO status, skin shave or scrub, intestinal preparation, insertion of tubes or IVs, and administration of preop medications (see the Evidence-Based Practice feature)
- What the patient can expect in the OR, including equipment, bright lights, cold temperatures, and masked staff members wearing caps and gowns that make it difficult to identify each one
- A description of the general roles of the various OR team members who will be responsible for the patient's care
- What the patient will and may experience postop once in the PACU, also known as the *recovery room*
- Actions the patient can take to help prevent complications, decrease discomfort, shorten recovery time, and optimize healing

Sometimes a little knowledge allows the patient or family members to feel they have a little bit of control over the situation. Your skill in anticipating and assessing their knowledge needs and providing the appropriate teaching to meet those needs will help to allay their fears and reduce their anxiety. It will also help to increase their active participation in and compliance with medical advice and recommendations. (Refer back to Chapter 12 for further details regarding patient teaching.)

Evidence-Based Practice

Preoperative Bathing or Showering With Skin Antiseptics to Prevent Surgical Site Infections

Clinical Question

Is preop bathing or showering with skin antiseptic necessary to prevent surgical site infections?

Evidence

It has been common practice to have patients bathe or shower using an antiseptic skin wash to decrease the presence of skin bacteria prior to surgery. This was believed to decrease hospital-acquired surgical site infections. Such infections usually cause higher hospital costs and require the patient to stay in the hospital longer.

A review was done of seven trials involving 10,157 patients who bathed using either chlorhexidine (an antibacterial skin wash), soap and water, or no special preop washing. This review did not find any clear evidence that bathing or showering with chlorhexidine prior to surgery was any more effective than soap or other wash products in preventing surgical site infections.

Implications for Nursing Practice

While having patients bathe or shower before surgery is important, it is not necessary for them to use chlorhexidine or other antibacterial skin washes to prevent surgical site infections. One factor not included in this study was the use of antibiotics before and during surgeries to help prevent surgical site infections.

Reference

You can read more about this study at http://onlinelibrary.wiley.com/doi/10.1002/14651858.CD004985.pub5/pdf

KNOWLEDGE CONNECTION

What are the benefits of performing preop teaching? List the types of things that should be taught preop.

Patient Teaching Connection

Preoperative Teaching for Outpatient Laparoscopic Cholecystectomy

A patient is scheduled for an outpatient laparoscopic cholecystectomy, a type of **laparoscopic surgery** in which the gallbladder is removed using a specialized scope and instruments. Rather than opening the abdominal cavity with a standard 4- to 6-inch (10.16- to 15.24-cm) incision, the scope is inserted into the abdominal cavity via three or four tiny incisions between ½ and ¾ inch (1.27 to 1.85 cm) in length. This laparoscopic approach reduces the risk of infection, decreases postop pain, and shortens recovery time. Initial teaching should be done in the physician's office during the same visit at which the decision was made to schedule the surgery. The following is the information that the patient needs to know prior to his or her arrival at the outpatient surgery center on the day of surgery:

1. Do not eat or drink anything for a specified period of time (according to the physician's protocol, generally 6 to 12 hours) before surgery.
2. Avoid smoking 24 hours preop. Advise to ask health-care provider for nicotine patches if desired.

• **WORD • BUILDING** •

laparoscopic: laparo – flank + scop – look + ic – related to

3. Arrange for a driver to take the patient home afterward.
4. Shower with antibacterial soap the night before surgery.
5. Bring the completed registration/admission packet supplied preop as well as any advance directives the patient may have.
6. Confirm the date and time of the surgery and the physical location and phone number of the surgery center.
7. Leave jewelry and valuables at home.
8. Discuss any medications or herbal supplements that must be held preop.

Along with these instructions, an explanation of what will occur on the day of surgery should be included (Box 33.1). Additional specific preop teaching topics will be taught the morning of surgery before the patient goes to the OR. These topics include the following:

- Turn, cough, and deep-breathing exercises, which are addressed below
- The specific device the patient's surgeon uses to stimulate venous return from the lower extremities, such as antiembolism hose, ankle and leg exercises, or a sequential compression device, which are discussed in the following section of this chapter
- The approximate length of time the patient will be in the OR and recovery
- The importance of asking for pain medication before the pain becomes severe
- The importance of informing staff of nausea as soon as it is detected in an attempt to prevent vomiting
- Showing the family where they can wait for the physician's report

Turn, Cough, and Deep-Breathing Exercises

One important risk reduction strategy is promotion of optimal ventilation to prevent pneumonia and *atelectasis,* collapse of one or more lobes of the lung. The most common things you will teach to help prevent these respiratory complications is how to effectively cough and deep breathe and why it is important to turn from side to side every 1 to 2 hours. Turning from side to side prevents secretions from pooling in one area of the lungs, known as *stasis.* Pooled secretions provide the perfect medium for bacterial growth, which leads to hypostatic pneumonia. Turning also stimulates deeper inhalation, which, along with coughing and deep breathing, helps with the elimination of anesthetic gases. Deep breathing helps to expand the lungs more fully and works to prevent atelectasis.

Explaining the rationale behind the repeated instruction to "take a deep breath" will help the patient understand that this intervention is designed to aid in the elimination of anesthetic gases and to promote gas exchange. The deep breathing and coughing should be initiated as soon as the surgical procedure is completed and anesthesia is discontinued. (See Chapter 28 for more information about respiratory care.)

Incentive Spirometry

Incentive spirometry may also be instituted to promote deep breathing. It can increase lung volume and encourage coughing to clear mucus from the airway. This skill should also be taught and practiced before surgery and reinforced after surgery. (See Chapter 28 for more on incentive spirometry.)

Stimulation of Lower Extremity Circulation

One of the most common and serious complications of surgery is formation of a *thrombus,* or blood clot. Normally, contractions of the leg muscles help to compress leg veins and stimulate venous return of blood to the heart. When a patient is less active or is restricted to bedrest, the result is less contraction of the leg muscles. This allows venous blood flow to slow and blood to pool in the veins and eventually coagulate and form clots.

The condition of forming these clots is commonly referred to as *deep venous thrombosis*. Research shows that even traveling on long air flights allows sufficient slowing of venous return to increase an individual's risk of blood clots in the legs.

A clot impairs circulation in the legs and causes inflammation of the vein at the site of the attached clot. A clot can break loose from the vein wall and be carried into the circulation that is returning blood back to the heart and pulmonary circulation to be reoxygenated. Once the clot is carried to the lungs, it becomes known as a *pulmonary embolism* (PE), which causes severe respiratory distress and has the potential to be fatal. Therefore, prevention of thrombus formation is key.

Prevention involves stimulation of the venous return of blood to the heart so that the blood does not begin to pool. The patient should be instructed regarding three ways to stimulate lower extremity circulation: leg exercises, antiembolism hose, and sequential compression devices.

LEG EXERCISES. You will want to teach leg exercises to your patient as a method of preventing clot formation. The exercises are designed to flex and extend the leg muscles so that as the muscles contract, they compress the leg veins, assisting them to return blood back to the heart. The exercises are the easiest and most natural way to stimulate peripheral circulation. They prevent venous stasis and deep venous thrombosis or clots. Teach your patients to perform the following exercises:

- Ankle circles with the toes extended, 10 times in each direction, both clockwise and counterclockwise
- Ankle pumps, alternating ankle flexion and extension for a total of 10 times each

• WORD • BUILDING •

antiembolism: anti – against + embol – stopper + ism – condition

thrombosis: thromb – blood clot + osis – condition

Box 33.1

Example of Outpatient Surgery Teaching

The following dialogue is an example of preop teaching you might provide for a patient scheduled for an outpatient surgery:

"Feel free to stop me at any point during this teaching session and ask any questions that come to mind. Otherwise, you may forget them by the time I am through speaking. Okay? Your surgery is scheduled on Tuesday, March 9, 2015, at 7:30 a.m. Be certain you do not eat or drink any type of fluid, including water, after 10 p.m. on Monday night, the night before your surgery. Bring all your completed paperwork and preoperative lab results with you and arrive at the surgery center by 6 a.m. Give the paperwork to the receptionist. She will take you to the holding area, where we will prepare you for surgery.

You will change into a hospital gown and be asked a lot of questions, and your IV will be started. Your chart will be reviewed, and consent for surgery will be explained and signed. Bring a written list of any questions that you may have so that you do not forget any of them. We will do some preoperative teaching, show you how to deep breathe and cough to prevent pneumonia, and discuss postoperative pain and nausea medications. You will meet the anesthesiologist, Dr. Nancy Blehm, and talk with her and your surgeon before being taken into surgery. You will be given medication in your IV to decrease the likelihood of nausea postoperatively as well as medication to relax you and probably make you drowsy. You may have up to two family members accompany you while in the holding area, where you typically will be for 30 to 60 minutes.

We will then take you from holding to the OR, where you will again be asked more questions; some will be the same ones you have already answered, such as 'Are you allergic to any medications?' This is part of a protocol we do for your safety. The room will probably feel cold, but we will provide you with as many blankets as you need. Everyone in the OR will be dressed in scrubs and will be wearing masks. The anesthesiologist will place electrodes on your chest so that she can monitor your heart and a blood pressure cuff on your arm to monitor your blood pressure. She will then administer sedative medication into your IV line to make you drowsy. Dr. Blehm will monitor your breathing, oxygen levels, heart rhythm, and all your vital statistics that are necessary to keep you safe and well. You will have your own personal circulating nurse whose primary responsibility will be to act as your advocate and see that everything runs smoothly for you. You will be asleep in no time, and when you begin to wake up you will probably be in the recovery room.

This type of surgery typically lasts between 30 and 60 minutes, and combined with the recovery time, you will probably be ready to go home within 3 to 4 hours. We will direct your family to the waiting room, where the surgeon will come to find them after surgery. We will keep your family informed of your condition and notify them if there are delays. If you wish, you may have one family member at the bedside while in recovery. If you are not nauseated after waking up, you will be allowed ice chips first; if you tolerate them, you will be allowed to sip dark cola or lemon-lime sodas and munch on saltine crackers. Once you are fully awake, able to take fluids without nausea, and have urinated, you will be discharged to go home. A prescription for pain medication will be provided prior to discharge. Do you have any questions I might answer for you?"

- Leg flexion and extension: Bend the knees and place the feet flat on the bed. Keeping the plantar surface of the foot on the bed, bring one foot at a time as close to the buttock as possible. Then slide the same foot toward the foot of the bed until the leg is fully extended. Repeat this using the other leg. This should be done 10 times for each leg.

ANTIEMBOLISM HOSE. **Antiembolism hose** or stockings are often called AE hose or TED hose. *TED* stands for *thromboembolic disorder,* the primary diagnosis for use of the hose. They are a pair of strong support hose that are applied to compress the leg veins. This compression assists leg veins to return blood back to the right side of the heart where it can be sent through the pulmonary artery to the lungs to be reoxygenated. This helps to prevent blood from pooling in the leg veins because of inactivity and bedrest. Instruct the patient preop regarding the purpose and importance of the hose. The hose are sometimes applied preop, dependent on physician's orders and according to facility policy.

It is pertinent that the TED hose fit the patient's legs properly. Make sure to measure the appropriate leg dimensions before selecting the size to apply. For thigh-high hose, measure the length of the leg from the gluteal fold to the bottom of the heel. Then measure the circumference of the calf and the thigh at their largest diameters. Cross-reference these measurements on the TED chart to determine which size of hose to select.

It is important to prevent the hose fabric from bunching together, especially at the ankle and knee joints (Fig. 33.1). Also, the tops of thigh-high TEDs tend to roll down. If the fabric bunches together or the tops roll down, those areas will work like a tourniquet and restrict venous blood return, exacerbating pooling of blood. Monitor the TEDs every couple of hours to ensure that they are kept smooth and are not restricting circulation. Assess pedal pulses each shift to ensure arterial blood flow to the feet.

Remove the hose at least twice per day to prevent excessive pressure or tension on any one spot. Good times to remove the TED hose are during the morning bath and during delivery of bedtime care. This allows you the opportunity to assess the skin of the legs and feet for areas of erythema, breaks in the skin, and edema. Wash and dry the legs and feet well before reapplying the hose. Performing this again before bedtime

• WORD • BUILDING •

thromboembolic: thrombo – blood clot + embol – stopper + ic – related to

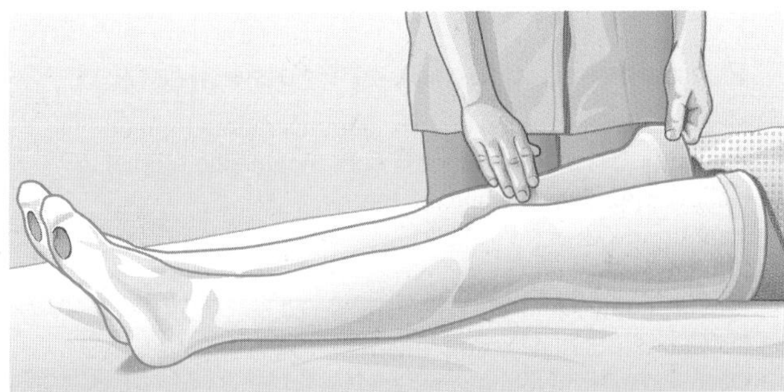

FIGURE 33.1 Antiembolism hose should be worn pulled all the way up and kept smooth, without wrinkles, bunching, or the top edge rolling down (from Wilkinson JM, Treas LS. *Fundamentals of Nursing: Theory, Concepts & Applications.* Vol. 1. 3rd ed. Philadelphia, PA: FA Davis; 2015).

helps to make the patient comfortable for sleep. Skill 33.1 (page 749) provides more information on application of TED hose. Figure 33.2 gives an example of electronic documentation of TED hose.

SEQUENTIAL COMPRESSION DEVICES. **Sequential compression devices** (SCDs) may also be known by brand names, such as Pneumatic Air Stockings. They consist of compression sleeve pads capable of having air pumped into and out of them. They are designed to wrap around the legs and come in thigh-high or knee-high lengths. The sleeve pads connect via tubing to a compression pump, which intermittently pumps air into the sleeves until they are filled and then empties the air, deflating the sleeves around the legs (Fig. 33.3). This process results in intermittent compression of the legs, aiding venous return of blood to the heart. You will want to teach the patient the purpose and significance of their use in order to gain compliance and cooperation in reapplying them after ambulation or toileting. Skill 33.2 (page 751) provides more information on application of SCDs.

KNOWLEDGE CONNECTION

What are the purposes for turning, coughing, deep breathing, and using an incentive spirometer? Why do we use sequential compression devices? What must be done prior to applying a pair of TED hose? Which body system do TED hose help? Explain what a PE is and why it is dangerous. Which body system will leg exercises stimulate?

Postoperative Pain and Discomfort Control

Teach your patient that medication will be ordered for pain, nausea, and vomiting, and various other discomforts that may be anticipated postop. Explain to the patient that it is always best to keep pain under control by asking for medication before the pain gets too severe. Tell the patient that research shows that the body recovers and heals faster when pain is properly controlled. Explain the pain scale that you will be using to assess the patient's level of discomfort. Look and listen for verification of understanding. Never assume that what you taught is understood just because you said it. If the patient voices concerns regarding addiction to pain medications, carefully explain the need to manage pain so that the patient will be able to turn, cough, deep breathe, and ambulate, which help to prevent other complications. Also explain that the patient will be given strong pain medicines only as long as necessary and then will be transitioned to milder medications. If the patient is still concerned, inform your supervisor.

KNOWLEDGE CONNECTION

Once you have *taught* something to a patient, what must you do to determine its effectiveness? What phase of the nursing process would this be? What phase of the nursing process would taking a medical history be? And patient teaching?

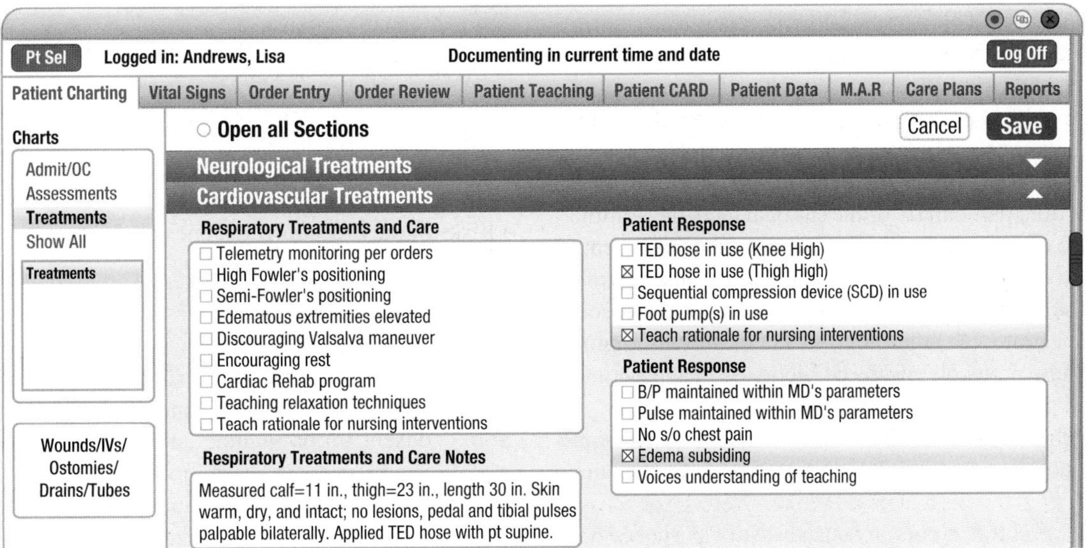

FIGURE 33.2 An example of electronic documentation of TED hose.

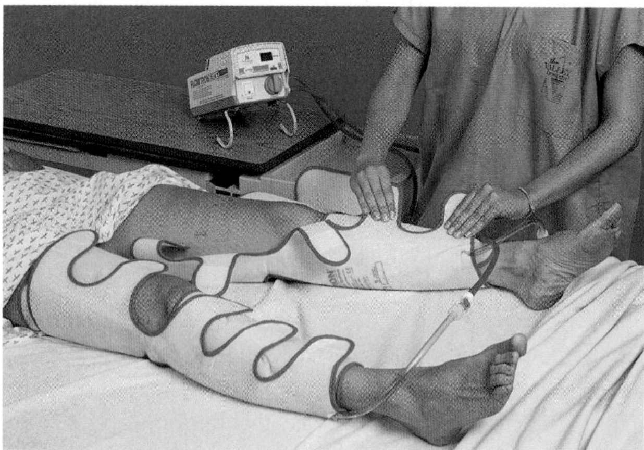

FIGURE 33.3 Sequential compression devices are applied by wrapping the compression sleeve pads around the legs and then connecting them to the pump unit via connecting tubes (from Wilkinson JM, Treas LS. *Fundamentals of Nursing: Theory, Concepts & Applications*. Vol. 1. 3rd ed. Philadelphia, PA: FA Davis; 2015).

Box 33.2

Purposes and Goals of Premedication

There are various reasons for the administration of preop medications. The most common ones include the following:

- Relieve apprehension and anxiety
- Provide sedation
- Provide analgesia
- Provide amnesia
- Decrease anesthetic requirements
- Decrease gastric volume and acidity
- Prevent nausea and vomiting
- Dry secretions and prevent aspiration
- Prevent bradycardia
- Facilitate induction
- Decrease allergic reaction
- Decrease stress of parental separation
- Prevent infection
- Prevent clot formation

Preoperative Medications

The administration of preop medications is designed to address a specific patient need. It is based on the patient's history, examination, laboratory tests, or surgery. The purpose and goal of premedication will dictate the specific medication choice. One purpose for administering preop medications is a safety issue: the prevention of aspiration during anesthesia and recovery. Anticholinergics such as atropine, scopolamine, and glycopyrrolate may be given preop to dry secretions. They thereby decrease the risk of aspiration and increased airway irritability. These drugs are indicated for patients who have pre-existing problems with secretions, have previously had a stroke, or have Parkinson's disease, as well as for toddlers, small children, and patients whose surgery will result in the stimulation of oral mucous membranes because stimulation of the oral mucosa can increase salivation 10-fold, potentially placing the airway at risk.

Other indications for premedication include the desire to decrease intraoperative anesthesia requirements and the need to induce analgesia. This is especially important when preop patient preparation may prove uncomfortable, as may be the case with placement of IV lines or the injections associated with regional blockade. These medications generally reduce anxiety and have sedating effects.

Antibiotics may be given prior to surgery to decrease the risk of infection, particularly of the surgical incision. Antibiotics are also used to prevent bacterial endocarditis in patients with a history of congenital or rheumatic heart disease and valve disease with regurgitation. Many hospitals have developed written protocols regarding the use of antibiotic prophylaxis. These protocols ensure antibiotic use in appropriate patients and prevent inappropriate use when unnecessary.

An antiemetic such as ondansetron or metoclopramide is sometimes administered preop to reduce postop nausea and vomiting.

Box 33.2 presents a comprehensive list of purposes for which preop medications may be administered. Most will be administered intravenously when the patient arrives in the holding area before surgery.

KNOWLEDGE CONNECTION

What determines which preop medication will be ordered?

Informed Consent

As you learned in Chapter 3, an informed consent must be completed and signed by the patient prior to surgery being performed. This means that the patient must be informed and understand the procedure for which he or she is about to give consent. The consent form should list the correct surgical procedure that is to be done. Most will include a partial list of possible risks or complications, some of which are life-threatening. No abbreviations are used when completing the consent form. The physician is responsible for providing the following explanations:

- The procedure to be performed
- The expected or desired outcome of the procedure
- Alternatives that are available in place of the procedure
- The expected outcomes of the alternatives or of simply not having the procedure at all
- Risks of the procedure and anesthesia

Once the physician has explained all these things, the patient must be allowed to ask questions and register any concerns. Once all of the patient's questions and concerns have been addressed, it is required that the patient acknowledges verbally that he or she understands the procedure and risks. Some consent forms include an area in which the patient writes, using layperson's terminology, what he or she understands the surgery to be. For example, the patient who is having a cholecystectomy might write "take out my gallbladder." Figure 33.4 presents an example of a surgical consent form.

REQUEST AND CONSENT FOR SURGICAL, MEDICAL OR DIAGNOSTIC PROCEDURES
AND ACKNOWLEDGMENT OF RECEIPT OF INFORMATION

Patient: *Emma May*

Patient NO: *#48476006110* DATE: *MM/DD/YYYY* TIME: *1645*

The hospital and your physician are required by law to obtain your consent to perform the surgical, medical or diagnostic procedure(s) listed below. Signing this form will acknowledge that you request and consent to your physician performing the recommended procedure(s). Your signature also confirms that your physician has explained to you the procedure(s), the risks of the procedure(s), the alternatives, if any, and risks of the alternatives and the risks or consequences of foregoing all treatment. **Please READ THIS ENTIRE FORM CAREFULLY** and then before signing it, ask your physician any additional questions you may have. Your request and consent is valid until you withdraw it.

1. I hereby request and authorize *Dr. Brad Monett* with hospital personnel and/or other trained persons of his/her choice and/or Medical/Physician Assistant/Nursing Student ______ to perform upon (patient) *me, Emma May* the following surgical, medical or diagnostic procedure(s) *Left total knee replacement* ______ to include any necessary or advisable anesthesia and disposal of tissue removed during surgery. I further request and authorize my physician and his assistant(s) to perform any other procedure that in his or their judgment is advisable for my well-being. This additional request and authority is extended as I recognize that during the above listed procedure(s), unforeseen conditions may require different or additional procedures.

2. I hereby request and consent to the administration of such anesthetics as are necessary. I further request that the choice of anesthetic to be used shall be made by professional anesthesia personnel.

3. I acknowledge that some of the risks known to be associated with surgery and anesthesia and which may be applicable to the proposed procedure(s) are:

INFECTION	**LOSS OF AN ARM OR LEG**
SEVERE BLOOD LOSS	**LOSS OF BLADDER FUNCTION**
IMPOTENCE	**LOSS OF BOWEL FUNCTION**
DISFIGURING SCARS	**PARALYSIS BELOW THE WAIST**
LOSS OF FUNCTION OF AN ORGAN	**PARALYSIS BELOW THE NECK**
LOSS OF FUNCTION OF AN ARM OR LEG	**BRAIN DAMAGE**
LOSS OF AN ORGAN	**DEATH**

4. I am aware that the practice of medicine and surgery is not an exact science and acknowledge that no guarantees or warranties have been made to me concerning the results of the procedure(s). I acknowledge that even though my physician has advised me of all known risks, up to and including the rare but possible severe risks as revealed in item 3 of this form, that additional unforeseeable and unpreventable situations could arise in the course of my care which might result in injury.

5. I HEREBY STATE THAT I HAVE READ AND UNDERSTAND THIS REQUEST AND CONSENT AND THAT ALL MY QUESTIONS ABOUT THE PROCEDURE(S), ALTERNATIVE PROCEDURE(S), AND RISKS OF EACH HAVE BEEN ANSWERED IN LANGUAGE THAT I UNDERSTOOD AND THAT ALL BLANKS WERE FILLED IN PRIOR TO MY SIGNATURE.

Signed: *Emma. L May*
Patient or person authorized
to request procedures for patient: ______

Relationship or Capacity: ______

Witness to signature: *K. Gann, LPN*

I have explained the procedure(s), alternative(s) and risks to the person or persons whose signature or signatures are affixed above.

Dr. Brad Monett
Signature of Physician

FIGURE 33.4 Surgical consent form. (Courtesy of King Kingfisher Regional Hospital, Kingfisher, OK. Used with permission.)

The patient or authorized person then signs the form granting permission for the surgery. The nurse generally signs it only as a witness to the fact that it was the patient or authorized person's signature (Fig. 33.5). When nurses sign consent forms as a witness, they must sign with their full names, not initials, and then follow with their credentials (e.g., LPN or LVN).The physician also must sign the consent form acknowledging that it was he or she who explained everything to the patient.

Safety: As part of this informed consent process, for procedures involving either a left or right designation for the surgery (such as left leg or right ear), you should mark the correct side and site of the planned surgical procedure with an indelible ink marker. Mark it right onto the patient's body to reduce the risk of error. For example, if the left breast is to be removed, a large "X" and something similar to "this side only" or "yes" is written on the left breast. Some health-care providers and nurses even write "Not this side!" or "no" on the nonoperative side in a further attempt to prevent removal of the wrong body part.

KNOWLEDGE CONNECTION

What are your responsibilities as a nurse regarding obtaining consent for surgery? What should health-care providers do to reduce the risk of performing surgery on the wrong side of the patient's body when a left or right designation is required for the site procedure?

Preoperative Checklist

As a nurse, one of your final preop responsibilities to the patient is to confirm that all preop tasks have been completed and that the patient is ready to go into surgery. Using a preop checklist can facilitate a last-minute confirmation as well as provide documentation. An example of a preop checklist may be seen in Figure 33.6.

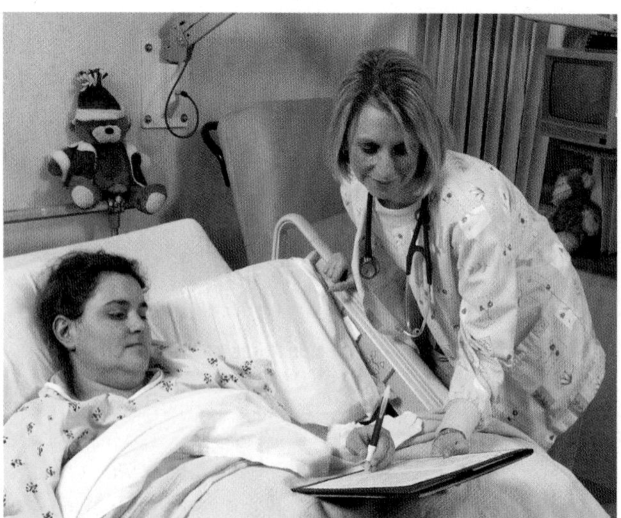

FIGURE 33.5 This nurse is witnessing the patient sign a surgical consent form (from Williams LS, Hopper PD. *Understanding Medical-Surgical Nursing*. 5th ed. Philadelphia, PA: FA Davis; 2015).

The Holding Area

The patient will be transported from his or her room via a gurney or a wheelchair to the holding area. The patient will remain in the holding area until he or she is taken into the surgery suite (Fig. 33.7). If the facility's policy permits, allow the family to accompany the patient to the holding area and provide them a few minutes to hug or kiss each other goodbye. Depending on the facility's policy, if the patient is a child, the parents may be allowed to accompany the child into the holding area. Direct the family to the appropriate waiting area where the physician will come to talk with them after surgery.

Once the patient is in the holding area, any remaining preop orders will be carried out. An IV may be initiated while the patient is in the holding area. The circulating nurse will confirm the identity of the patient, making sure that allergy and identification bands are in place. The nurse will confirm completion of preop orders and preparation. The nurse will also check for the presence of the signed consent form and ordered laboratory tests. Only when this has been completed will the patient be brought into the surgery suite.

KNOWLEDGE CONNECTION

What types of things are on the surgery checklist? What are the circulating nurse's responsibilities in the holding area?

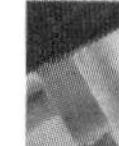

INTRAOPERATIVE CARE OF THE SURGICAL PATIENT

The OR is a specialized environment, created with one primary goal in mind: patient safety. To safely perform a surgical procedure requires numerous personnel and specialized equipment and instruments (Fig. 33.8). Each surgical team member has specific responsibilities that must revolve around that which is *in the patient's best interest.* The nurses working in the OR play a specialized role in patient care, advocating for the patient, who is unable to advocate for himself or herself because of the administration of anesthesia.

Surgical Team Members

Patient care is the responsibility of the entire surgical team, which at the minimum consists of the following:

- Anesthesia provider
- Surgeon
- First surgical assistant
- Circulating nurse
- Scrub nurse

Pre-op Surgical Checklist **Client Name**

_____ I.D. BAND ON _______________
_____ NPO AS ORDERED
_____ PRE-OP TEACHING COMPLETED
_____ INFORMED CONSENT SIGNED
_____ HISTORY AND PHYSICAL ON CHART
_____ ALLERGIES
_____ LAB RESULTS
_____ CBC: HGB _____ HCT _____ WBC _____ PLATELETS _____
_____ POTASSIUM _____
_____ URINALYSIS _____
_____ PREGNANCY TEST SERUM _____ URINE _____
_____ PT _____ PTT _____ BLEEDING TIME _____
_____ TYPE AND SCREEN _____ CROSSMATCH _____-___ UNITS
_____ ECG ON CHART
_____ CHEST X-RAY REPORT ON CHART
_____ SHOWERED/BATHED
_____ HOSPITAL GOWN ON
_____ PREPS COMPLETED AS ORDERED
_____ ANTIEMBOLISM STOCKINGS
_____ JEWELRY TAPED/REMOVED: DISPOSITION _____
_____ VALUABLES: DISPOSITION _____
_____ DENTURES, PROSTHESIS REMOVED
_____ HAIR PINS, WIGS, MAKEUP, NAIL POLISH, ONE ACRYLIC NAIL REMOVED
_____ CONTACT LENSES REMOVED
_____ VOIDED
_____ VITAL SIGNS: T _____ P _____ R _____ BP _____
_____ PRE-OP MEDICATIONS GIVEN _____ SIDE RAILS UP _____
_____ IV STARTED _____
_____ EYE GLASSES AND HEARING AID(S) TO OR
_____ OLD CHART TO OR
_____ X-RAYS TO OR
_____ FAMILY LOCATION _____
_____ NEXT OF KIN _____
CLIENT READY FOR SURGERY _____
TIME _____ (NURSE SIGNATURE)
COMMENTS:

FIGURE 33.6 Sample preoperative checklist (from Williams LS, Hopper PD. *Understanding Medical-Surgical Nursing.* 5th ed. Philadelphia, PA: FA Davis; 2015).

Anesthesia Provider

The anesthesia provider has the responsibility for sustaining the patient's life and ensuring that the patient remains comfortable. The provider may be a physician or a registered nurse (RN) with specific anesthesia training. A *medical doctor anesthesiologist* (MDA) is a physician who has education, experience, licensing, and credentialing in administration of anesthesia. A *certified registered nurse anesthetist* (CRNA) is an RN who has gone through extensive education and training to deliver anesthesia care. This training is most common through completion of a master's degree in nursing. The CRNA administers anesthetics under the supervision of a physician, who may be an MDA or may be the surgeon performing the procedure. An *anesthesiologist assistant* (AA) is an allied health professional who works under the direction of a licensed anesthesiologist to develop and implement anesthesia care plans. All AAs possess a premedical background and a baccalaureate degree.

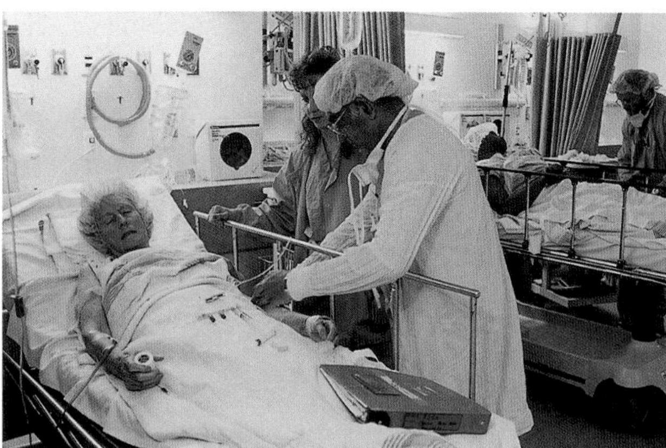

FIGURE 33.7 Surgical holding area (from Williams LS, Hopper PD. *Understanding Medical-Surgical Nursing*. 5th ed. Philadelphia, PA: FA Davis; 2015).

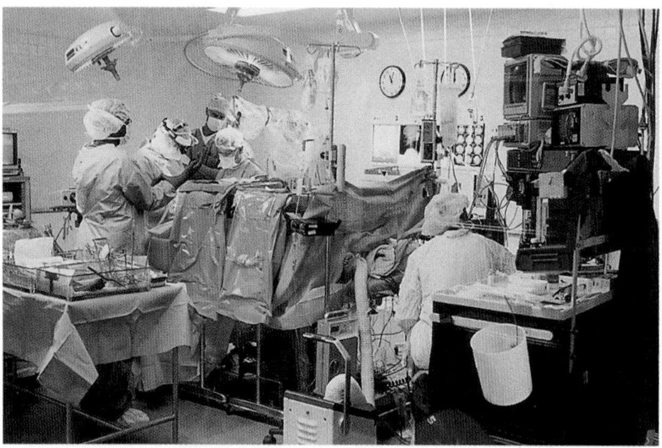

FIGURE 33.8 An operating room in use; anesthesia is on the right (from Williams LS, Hopper PD. *Understanding Medical-Surgical Nursing*. 5th ed. Philadelphia, PA: FA Davis; 2015).

AAs also complete a comprehensive didactic and clinical program at the graduate school level.

Surgeon

The surgeon is a physician who has been granted surgical privileges to perform a surgical procedure in a facility based on education, experience, licensing, and credentialing. The surgeon may perform the procedure independently. Alternately, the surgeon may have a first surgical assistant, which is common in more complex and lengthy surgeries.

First Surgical Assistant

The first surgical assistant may be another physician, a physician assistant, or a registered nurse. The *registered nurse first assistant* (RNFA) is a registered nurse who has received additional education and extensive training in the field of surgery. The RNFA directly assists the surgeon throughout the procedure. The RFNA's duties may include controlling hemostasis, assisting with instrumentation, manipulating and incising tissue, and suturing or stapling and closing the incision. The RNFA also may be directly involved with patient care preop and during recovery.

Circulating Nurse

The circulating nurse is a registered nurse; this role cannot be delegated to a licensed practical/vocational nurse (LPN/LVN). The circulating nurse is responsible for management of the care of the patient throughout the surgical procedure. The circulator is the primary patient advocate and is responsible for ensuring that everything that is done in the OR is in the best interest of the patient, who can no longer speak for himself or herself once the anesthesia has been administered. The circulating nurse ensures that the correct procedure is performed. The circulating nurse also maintains the patient's rights, provides appropriate privacy and preservation of modesty, and preserves the patient's dignity. The circulating nurse, who is not scrubbed, can leave the room if needed. She or he can also obtain supplies from cabinets within the room, opening them directly onto the sterile field.

The circulating nurse is responsible for coordination of the surgical team and any additional personnel who might be required for successful completion of the procedure. It is this nurse's job to maintain the safest environment possible for the patient while carefully observing the patient's condition from his or her arrival in the OR until the patient has been transferred to the PACU. This involves specifics such as calling a time-out before surgery (which will be addressed a little later). It also includes taking sponge and needle counts to ensure that these items are not left inside the operative site.

Scrub Nurse

The scrub nurse can be an RN, an LPN/LVN, or a certified scrub technician. It is the scrub nurse's job to set up the sterile field with all the appropriate sterile instruments and supplies immediately prior to actually beginning the procedure. It is also the scrub nurse's responsibility to then ensure that the sterility of the field is maintained while actively assisting the surgeons working within the sterile field during surgery. This includes passing sterile instruments, surgical sponges, suture and needles, staple guns, suction tips, or other equipment to the surgeons.

> **KNOWLEDGE CONNECTION**
> Explain the various roles and responsibilities of the surgical staff.

Preparation of Surgical Suite

Before any surgical procedure begins, the OR nursing staff are responsible for preparing the surgical environment. This will first involve preparing the room by making sure that the room has been disinfected and is ready to accept the patient. All equipment needed for the procedure will be brought into the room and set up as much as the room will allow prior to the introduction of both the patient and personnel. This is important because once room setup begins it will be the responsibility of the OR nursing staff to make sure that the equipment remains sterile. Frequently, the OR nursing staff will work from both experience and prepared "cheat sheets." These sheets contain information about equipment needed for a particular type of surgery, as well as individual surgeon preferences for equipment and glove sizes. To set up the room, the scrub nurse must first scrub so that he or she is in a position to begin working with and setting up sterile supplies. The surgical scrub is designed with the primary goal of preventing infection through the most cost-effective, simplest method known to reduce wound infection: handwashing.

Safety: As another step in patient protection, a time-out is called when a patient enters the OR. Initiated by the circulating nurse, a time-out is designed to prevent the risk of the wrong patient, wrong site, and wrong surgery. During the time-out, the RN will verify and document verification of the:

- Patient's identity and date of birth
- Presence of signed consent in the chart
- Correct site of surgery: If the surgery has a left or right distinction or involves multiple structures, such as fingers, or multiple levels, such as in spinal surgery, the surgical sites should be marked with a permanent marker.
- Correct procedure
- Presence of correct x-ray or other films
- Presence of needed special equipment

> **KNOWLEDGE CONNECTION**
> Who calls the time-out? What is its purpose?

Types of Anesthesia

Anesthetic agents are administered to decrease or completely block sensory perception. Some agents either partially or completely decrease the level of consciousness. The different types of anesthesia include:

- **General anesthesia:** The patient is totally unconscious.
- **Conscious sedation:** The patient is asleep but not totally unconscious; this is commonly used for diagnostic procedures.
- **Regional anesthesia:** Specific nerves and the region innervated by the nerves, such as a finger, an arm, or the lower half of the body, are blocked from sensory perception by injection of a local anesthetic numbing agent such as lidocaine.
- **Local anesthesia:** A very small area of tissue is blocked from sensory perception by injection of a local anesthetic numbing agent such as lidocaine; common uses are dental work, suturing lacerations, and biopsies.

The decision regarding the type of anesthesia is based on the type of surgery to be performed, the patient's preexisting medical conditions, and the preference of the surgeon and anesthesia provider. A patient having open heart surgery requires a general anesthetic. A patient having a knee arthroscopy may be a candidate for general or regional anesthesia. Depending on the site, a biopsy can sometimes be done under local anesthesia. Conscious sedation is commonly used for diagnostic procedures such as a colonoscopy or an esophagogastroduodenoscopy. It can also be used for closed reduction of fractures and in medical and dental offices for certain anxiety-producing procedures.

General Anesthesia

General anesthesia has five objectives:

1. Loss of consciousness
2. Amnesia regarding the procedure
3. Pain relief
4. Skeletal muscle relaxation
5. Blocking reflexes such as coughing and gagging, as well as endocrine and autonomic responses

Because no one medication is capable of meeting all of these objectives, general anesthesia requires the administration of multiple agents. Narcotics are used for pain relief. Benzodiazepines are used to reduce anxiety and to provide amnesia and sedation. Muscle relaxants are used for skeletal muscle relaxation. They also facilitate placement of the endotracheal tube or laryngeal mask airway to control ventilation. IV anesthetics are used for sedation and to induce and maintain anesthesia. Inhalation agents are used to induce and maintain loss of consciousness.

An advantage of general anesthesia is that it can be used for procedures that take longer to complete. They also decrease patient anxiety, reduce memory of the procedure, and provide complete comfort for the patient throughout the surgical procedure. Disadvantages include risk of aspiration due to vomiting, respiratory or cardiac arrest, brain damage, stroke, and death.

Conscious Sedation

Twilight sleep is a state of hypoconsciousness, or partial anesthesia, in which medications have reduced the patient's sensation so that less pain is experienced. **Conscious sedation** provides a controlled minimal level of sedation that allows the patient to be relaxed and in twilight sleep. However, the patient is still able to maintain his or her own airway and respond purposefully. Various medications may be used to attain this state of decreased consciousness, such as opioids, hypnotics, and sedatives. The use of conscious sedation depends on the procedure to be done, the patient's health, and both the patient and physician's preferences. The advantages include patient comfort, less risk, and the ability to easily waken the patient. The one disadvantage of conscious sedation is that it can only be used for certain short procedures.

> **KNOWLEDGE CONNECTION**
> Contrast general anesthesia and conscious sedation. Which is the more risky of the two?

Regional Anesthesia

Regional anesthetic techniques are used to isolate the administration of a local anesthetic, such as lidocaine, to a specific nerve or region to prevent transmission of sensory information to and from that section of the body. This results in numbness or loss of feeling as well as loss of ability to voluntarily move the area. Common types of **regional anesthesia** are spinal anesthesia, epidural anesthesia, peripheral nerve block, and local anesthesia.

SPINAL ANESTHESIA. Spinal anesthesia, sometimes called a *spinal block,* involves injection of the anesthetic into the cerebrospinal fluid in the subarachnoid space (Fig. 33.9A). The nerves below the site of injection are blocked from central nervous system transmissions. It is commonly used for delivery of a baby, perirectal surgery, and abdominal or lower extremity surgery.

A primary advantage of spinal anesthesia includes no loss of consciousness and more rapid recovery. It also allows for reduction of aspiration due to vomiting, and potential for decreased need for pain medications in the immediate postop period. A disadvantage is that the type of surgical procedure may limit this as an option. In addition, the patient may require additional IV agents to be administered for anxiety because the patient potentially will be awake with this type of anesthesia.

Side Effects. Possible side effects include urinary retention, hypotension, and headache. If the patient is unable to empty the bladder, it may be necessary to perform a catheterization to drain the bladder or place an indwelling catheter that will be left in until sensation returns to the lower half of the body.

The patient should be monitored for hypotension due to vasodilation of the peripheral blood vessels, which allows blood pressure to drop excessively. The vasodilation occurs because of blocking of the sympathetic vasomotor nerves.

Some patients develop a post–spinal anesthesia headache due to leakage of spinal fluid during the spinal anesthetic. The anesthesia provider may participate in treatment of a spinal headache if necessary. These patients should be monitored closely.

Sometimes spinal anesthesia affects a higher level of the spinal cord than intended because the anesthetic seeps above the injection site and does not limit sensation blockage to below the site. The danger with this side effect is that it may paralyze the respiratory muscles and decrease the heart rate. Monitor the vital signs closely and position the patient in a high Fowler's position if this becomes a problem. It is rare but possible that the patient's ventilation may require support until the anesthetic wears off.

EPIDURAL ANESTHESIA. **Epidural anesthesia** differs from spinal anesthesia in that a small catheter is inserted into the epidural space of the spinal column to provide continual administration of a stronger anesthetic agent. Some physicians utilize epidurals for postop pain control as well as during surgery. The second difference is the area of instillation of the anesthetic. Because the anesthetic agent is instilled into the epidural space, it does not come in contact with the spinal cord as it does with spinal anesthesia, thus making it safer for the patient (Fig. 33.9B). The advantages and disadvantages are similar to those of spinal anesthesia.

Side Effects. If the anesthesia provider inadvertently injects the anesthetic agent too deeply into the subarachnoid space,

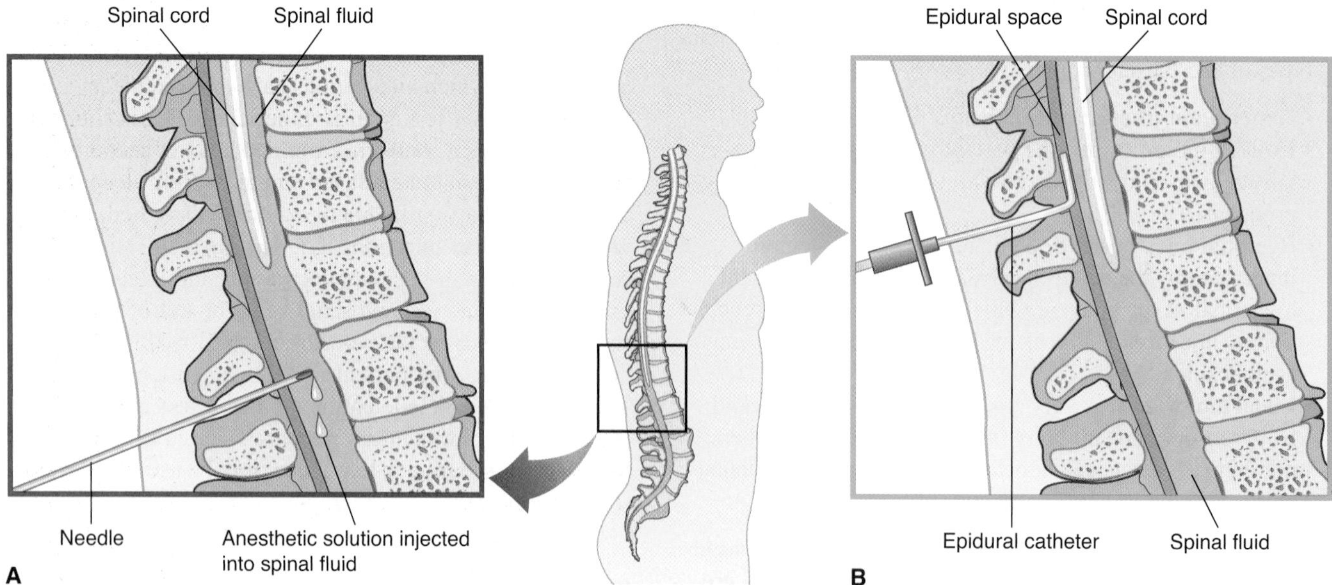

FIGURE 33.9 (a) Spinal anesthesia is the injection of a local anesthetic agent into the subarachnoid space. It blocks sensation and movement below the injection site. (b) Continuous epidural anesthesia can be used to provide postoperative analgesia (from Wilkinson JM, Treas LS. *Fundamentals of Nursing: Theory, Concepts & Applications*. Vol. 1. 3rd ed. Philadelphia, PA: FA Davis; 2015).

this too can result in respiratory depression and paralysis. This requires support of respirations until the respiratory nerves and muscles regain their ability to function.

PERIPHERAL NERVE BLOCK. If anesthesia is desired for an area such as an arm or leg, a peripheral nerve block may be the anesthesia of choice. The anesthetic is injected into a nerve or group of nerves to depress transmission of signals to and from the site. The advantages include no loss of consciousness and a lower risk of side effects. A common type of peripheral nerve block is the **Bier block**. A tourniquet is placed around an extremity to decrease venous return while continuing to allow full arterial delivery of oxygenated blood to the site. The anesthetic agent is injected intravenously in the extremity or portion of the extremity that is distal to the tourniquet. The anesthetic causes loss of sensation in the area as long as the tourniquet remains in place. The disadvantage of the Bier block is that the tourniquet cannot be left in place longer than 2 hours. Using it therefore limits the length of time that anesthesia may be effective.

The continuous peripheral nerve block is a type of extended anesthesia in the operative area that uses an elastomeric reservoir ball; an example is the On-Q pain relief system, which lasts about 72 hours after surgery. This decreases the need for as much opioid medication postop. The reservoir balls may have an automatic flow rate or a variable flow rate, which continually delivers anesthetic medication. It may also have an on-demand button for the patient to push for breakthrough pain. In most cases, the patient can remove the thin catheter that goes through the incision site by gently pulling on the reservoir ball after the 72-hour period. The ball loses its shape as the anesthesia leaves the reservoir and resembles an empty balloon after 3 days.

Local Anesthesia

Local anesthesia is supplied through the use of agents such as lidocaine. These agents may be administered by injection or applied topically to mucous membranes for loss of sensation of a very small area, such as the nose and throat or for a skin or soft tissue biopsy. The advantages are that the patient remains awake and alert, fewer risks are involved, and the anesthetic takes less time to wear off. The only disadvantage is that it can only be used for small areas.

> **KNOWLEDGE CONNECTION**
> What type of surgery might be performed using a spinal block? Conscious sedation? Bier block?

Intraoperative Interventions

Numerous interventions must be performed in the OR besides the actual surgical procedure performed by the surgeon. Many of these interventions are related to safety of the patient.

Miscellaneous Interventions and Equipment

Sometimes the patient's IV is not started until the patient is in the OR. Many of the supplies and equipment that are used, as well as the interventions performed, provide safety for the patient. Cardiac monitor electrodes are applied to the patient's chest for monitoring cardiac rate and rhythm. Grounding pads are applied to allow safe usage of electrical equipment. ***Safety: Safety straps are used to secure the patient to the operating table.***

Automated vital sign machines and pulse oximeters are applied to monitor the patient's blood pressure, pulse, and oxygen saturation levels. The anesthesia provider also monitors the patient's temperature throughout the surgery. This is done to ensure that the patient does not become hypothermic or develop **malignant hyperthermia,** which is a rapid and severe rise in body temperature that occurs while under a general anesthesia because of an inherited genetic trait. The anesthesiologist or nurse anesthetist administers the appropriate anesthesia. For a general anesthesia, he or she will administer appropriate medications to sedate the patient. He or she will also perform **intubation,** which is the insertion of an endotracheal tube into the patient's trachea to maintain an open airway and administer inhalant anesthesia and oxygen (Fig. 33.10). In addition, the anesthesiologist or nurse anesthetist attaches the ventilator for use once the patient is sufficiently sedated to paralyze the respiratory muscles.

Specific interventions may be performed, such as insertion of a Foley catheter or a NG tube. Suction is kept readily available for use by the anesthesia provider to maintain a clear airway and for use by the operating team to maintain visibility within the operative site. The suction is used to remove blood and other body fluids that pool within the operative site.

In an effort to protect the patient from microorganisms and infection, special ventilation systems have been installed to prevent air from the rest of the facility from entering the OR. Room temperature and humidity are controlled within tight ranges to decrease bacterial growth. Surgical hand scrubs are performed by the OR team members, who may not wear artificial nails or jewelry. Sterile instruments, equipment, overhead light handle covers, supplies, gowns, and gloves are also used to protect the patient, as are clean face masks and hair coverings. The gowns, gloves, masks, and hair coverings are accompanied by face shields or goggles as well as shoe covers. These items protect the OR team members from any blood-borne pathogens that may be carried in the patient's body fluids.

Positioning the Patient

Once the anesthesia has been initiated, an important task of the OR team is to provide appropriate and safe positioning of the patient. The team may use straps, wedges, pillows, and surgical table attachments to maintain positioning. Special surgical tables or extension pieces may be required for morbidly obese

• WORD • BUILDING •

hyperthermia: hyper – excessive + therm – heat + ia – condition
intubation: in – inside + tub – tube + ation – action

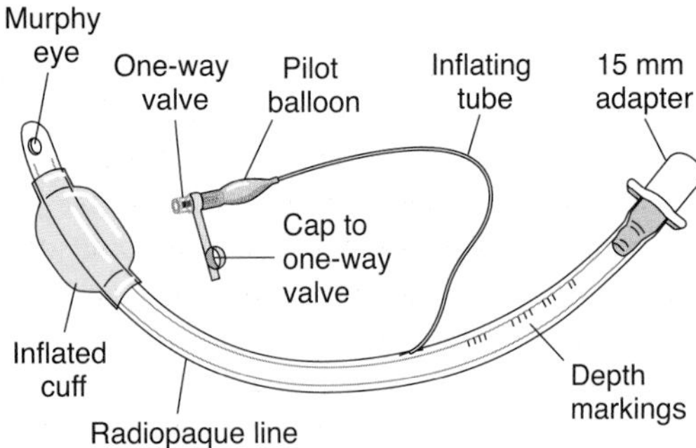

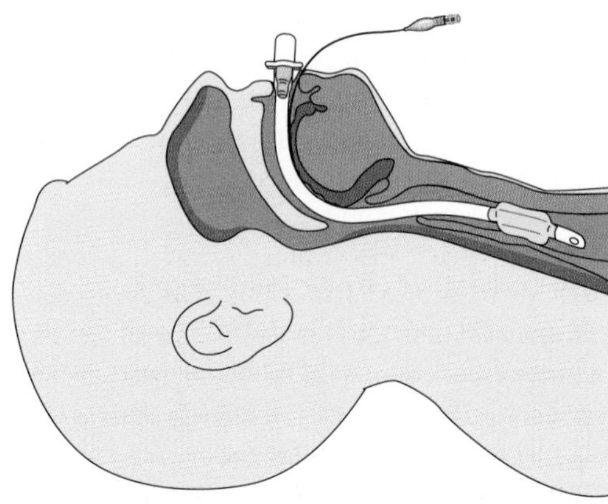

Placement of tube in airway

FIGURE 33.10 Endotracheal tube (from Williams LS, Hopper PD. *Understanding Medical-Surgical Nursing*. 5th ed. Philadelphia, PA: FA Davis; 2015; modified from Barnes TA. *Respiratory Care Principles*. Philadelphia, PA: FA Davis; 1991).

and extremely tall patients. Variables to be considered in positioning the patient include the need for:

- Access to the surgical site
- Access to the patient's airway
- Monitoring of vital signs
- Maintaining patient body alignment
- Patient safety
- Patient comfort

Skin Preparation

Shaving hair from the operative site is no longer routinely done. Research has shown that it increases the risk of infection by allowing microbes easier access through the patient's first line of defense, via microscopic nicks to the skin. Therefore, the hair on the operative site is generally just clipped very short unless it is necessary to remove all hair. If the hair is to be clipped, this may be done by the nurses caring for the patient preop. The scrub nurse is generally responsible for shaving the operative site if it is required.

Surgical Scrub

Once the patient has been positioned for the surgery, the operative site skin will be vigorously scrubbed with an antimicrobial wash and paint. The combination of an antiseptic agent and the friction of application helps to further reduce the microbial count. The antiseptic solution will be applied using a sponge or sterile instrument, working in concentric circles from the center of the surgical site to the periphery. A combination alcohol-iodine solution (DuraPrep) is the most commonly used agent. Alcohol is used for a rapid microbial kill with fast drying, while the iodine provides for a water-insoluble persistent film. Skin preparation should be documented by the circulating nurse on the intraoperative record.

Draping the Patient

After the skin is cleansed and dried with a sterile towel, surgical draping can begin. The drape allows for isolation of the surgical site and localizes the sterile field to the surgical site. Draping will also maintain patient privacy. Drapes should be applied in such a way as to allow for the full possibility of surgical incisions and for any potential additional incisions. They should also be applied in a way that allows the placement of surgical drains that might be placed at the end of surgery.

The Surgical Procedure

More and more surgeries are being performed using endoscopic techniques. While more technically difficult, endoscopic techniques minimize surgical trauma, speed recovery and discharge, and reduce postop complications. However, there are many types of surgery that require an incision of several or more inches for introduction of instruments and performance of required maneuvers.

Although a detailed description of every surgical procedure is not possible in this text, it is possible to identify descriptors that help to explain the procedure. For example, some common descriptors are:

- **–ectomy:** to remove, as in tonsillectomy (removal of tonsils) or lobectomy (removal of lobe of the lung)
- **–otomy:** to cut or separate, as in craniotomy (cutting of bones of the cranium or skull)
- **–ostomy:** to create an opening, as in colostomy (opening into the colon for elimination of wastes)
- **Transplant:** to uproot and replant, as in kidney transplant (removal of kidney from donor to recipient)
- **Ablation:** to remove from, as in surgical ablation of heart tissue for atrial fibrillation

Tissue Specimens

Tissue samples may be obtained for biopsy or other testing, or cultures may be obtained for laboratory analysis. If needed, the scrub nurse will assist in placing the sampled tissue into collection medium and will make the transfer of collected specimens to the circulating nurse, who prepares patient labels for the containers and completes appropriate requisitions. The circulating nurse is responsible for the transfer of tissue specimens to the appropriate laboratory.

Needle, Sponge, and Instrument Counts

Safety: An additional intervention to promote patient safety is the counting and recording of the numbers of sponges, needles and

other sharps, and instruments used during a procedure to prevent the unintentional retention of foreign items in the surgical wound. The count is performed and documented between the scrub nurse and the circulating nurse at the following points:

- As the room is set up before the procedure is started
- When additional supplies are opened and added to the sterile field
- When the scrub nurse is replaced by a second scrub nurse at any point during the procedure
- Before closure of each surgical cavity
- At the end of the case prior to closure of the surgical incision
- After skin closure

Final Intraoperative Interventions

At the end of the surgery, the anesthesia provider will lighten the anesthetic to the point that the endotracheal tube can be removed, called **extubation,** prior to transport, if possible. The circulating nurse completes documentation. She or he then assists the anesthesia provider in the safe transfer of the patient to the PACU or to an intensive care specialty unit. Upon arrival to the PACU or intensive care specialty floor, the anesthesia provider or circulating nurse provides a verbal report to the nurse who will be providing postanesthesia nursing care. He or she also provides the postanesthesia nurse with either the written anesthesia record or a computerized record that contains information about the patient's preop status, need for surgery, and intraoperative summary of the surgery and anesthetic course. Any complications will be identified, as will any special needs. The report information will be documented in the PACU record.

While the circulating nurse transports the patient from the OR, the scrub nurse breaks down the room and takes instruments to central sterile (the area of the hospital the primary function of which is to sterilize supplies and equipment) for cleaning, disinfection, and resterilization. There, instruments are cleaned and disinfected with an automatic instrument washer, similar to a dishwasher. Disinfection does not sterilize; it only reduces the microbial count. The cleaned instruments are sorted and grouped into specific surgery instrument packs. They are then sterilized to render them free of all microorganisms in an *autoclave,* a machine that uses heat and steam pressure for a specified length of time to ensure that no microorganisms survive.

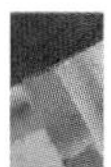

POSTOPERATIVE CARE OF THE SURGICAL PATIENT

Admission to the PACU begins the transition from the OR to postop care. In the PACU, the RN will maintain close observation and assessment of the patient, usually observing no more than two patients at a time. This close patient observation and assessment continues until the patient is ready to transfer back to his or her room, where other nurses provide further postop care.

Postanesthesia Assessment and Care

Patients are monitored continuously by the PACU nurse, with documentation of the assessments done on admission, every 15 minutes, and again upon discharge to the patient's room. Assessments and documentation may be more frequent, as often as every 5 minutes, if the patient is still intubated, deterioration occurs, or an intervention is initiated because of a change in condition.

In the PACU, the immediate priority is to maintain a patent airway and verify respiratory and cardiac function. This requires immediate application and observation of a pulse oximeter, EKG monitor, blood pressure monitor, and supplemental oxygen. It also requires assessment of respiratory rate, depth, and characteristics. Anesthesia may compromise both cardiac and pulmonary function, and, depending on type, the surgery itself may compromise both as well. ***Safety: Suction must be readily available for use in maintaining an open airway.***

After the admission assessment is completed and the patient is deemed stable, the PACU nurse will develop a plan of care directed toward anesthetic and surgical recovery.

Potential Patient Problems and Nursing Care

Postop problems and side effects are limitless because the patient is more vulnerable in the unconscious state. Respiratory problems, cardiovascular problems, gastrointestinal problems, hypothermia, and pain and discomfort are possible following general anesthesia. (See Table 33.1 for examples of these potential concerns and nursing care to help prevent further complications.)

Real-World Connection

Postoperative Complications

The student nurse was caring for a postop patient who had just returned from having a laparoscopic cholecystectomy (removal of the gallbladder). The student had performed an initial assessment and assessed vital signs upon the patient's return to the nursing unit; all findings were within normal limits except for incisional pain at a 7. The patient was drowsy but responded to voice and followed simple commands to take deep breaths and splint the incision while coughing. Pain control was provided by a patient-controlled analgesia pump with morphine. The pump was programmed for continual infusion of a low dose of morphine as well as intermittent doses to be delivered according to the preset parameters and frequency of patient use.

The instructor entered the room about 90 minutes later to check the patient's status while the student was gone to lunch. Upon entering the room, the instructor observed

• WORD • BUILDING •

extubation: ex – out of + tub – tube + ation – action

the patient with circumoral cyanosis, cyanotic nailbeds, and erratic, shallow respirations at 5 per minute. The apical pulse was very irregular, beating at a rate in the 60s and 70s and then within seconds speeding up to rates over 130 per minute.

Supplemental O_2 was applied at 4 L per minute via nasal cannula. Telemetry was applied for monitoring cardiac rate and rhythm. The physician was notified and the morphine discontinued. The patient required stimulation and was encouraged to turn, cough, and deep breathe every few minutes over the next hour to maintain the respiratory rate above 10.

Within 60 minutes, the patient's vital signs had stabilized and again were within normal limits, except for a tachycardia of 110. The patient had awakened enough to get up to the bathroom with assistance to void. The final outcome was positive, but these events serve to demonstrate how quickly a postop patient can deteriorate. This deterioration can occur even after anesthesia has been discontinued, the patient has been extubated and has returned to the nursing unit from the PACU, and assessment findings and vital signs have indicated the patient was stable. A postop patient's condition can turn in the blink of an eye.

The PACU nurse must also note and carry out any postop physician's orders that are to be performed while in recovery. These may include obtaining x-rays, administering antibiotics, or applying ice packs.

The patient can be discharged for transfer to his or her room or to go home *only* after meeting all the criteria for discharge. These criteria include both recovery from anesthesia and the absence of any anesthetic or surgical complications. Prior to discharge, the nurse will make and document a final assessment and complete the PACU record documentation. The transfer report provides information about the patient's current status; pre-existing medical history; and a summary of the surgery, anesthetic, and PACU course. Complications will be identified, as will special needs. Then the PACU nurse will notify the receiving nurse on the floor of the impending transfer and report any special patient needs. This gives the receiving nurse time to gather and prepare any additional supplies or equipment so that they are ready for use when the patient arrives.

Return to the Patient's Room

If the surgical patient is an inpatient before going to surgery and is thought to be returning to the same room, it is best to prepare the room to receive the patient postop as soon as the patient is transported to the OR. This prevents the patient

Table 33.1
Potential Patient Problems in the PACU With Nursing Interventions

Potential Problems	*Nursing Care*
Respiratory Concerns • Obstructed airway (may be due to laryngospasm or laryngeal edema after extubation, excessive secretions, or the tongue over the airway • Respiratory depression due to anesthesia and narcotics • Pre-existing conditions such as COPD	• Prepare suction equipment and suction the patient as needed. • Monitor the respiratory rate, depth, and pattern at least every 15 minutes, or more often if necessary, until the patient is stable and more awake. • Apply supplemental oxygen at the appropriate liter flow and with the appropriate delivery device. • Monitor breath sounds and oxygen saturation level. Elevate the head of the gurney if necessary. Encourage the patient to take deep breaths as he or she becomes more awake ***Safety: Most patients will have an oral or nasal airway placed once the endotracheal tube is removed to help maintain a patent airway until the patient is sufficiently awake to handle his or her own secretions.*** (See Chapter 28 for more information about artificial airways.)
Cardiovascular Concerns • Abnormal rate (bradycardia, tachycardia) • Rhythm disturbances • Hypotension • Hypertension	• Each patient will be placed on a monitor so heart, respiratory, and oxygen saturation patterns can be observed. • Auscultate heart sounds, noting muffled or distant S_1 or S_2. • Monitor blood pressure closely, noting even small decreases. • Administer IV fluids adjusted according to patient condition. • Assess the patient's skin color and temperature and whether the skin is moist or dry. • Assess the strength of the apical, radial, and pedal pulses and capillary refill in all four extremities. • Monitor for excessive bleeding from the surgical site and drains. Excessive blood loss may be visible or internal. Because bleeding can be unseen, assess the size of the operative site and surrounding area for edema or, if the abdomen, distention.

Table 33.1
Potential Patient Problems in the PACU With Nursing Interventions—cont'd

Potential Problems	*Nursing Care*
	• Always be alert to falling blood pressure and tachycardia that occurs suddenly, persists, or rapidly reoccurs even with fluid administration.
Gastrointestinal Concerns • Very slowed or completely stopped peristaltic action due to anesthesia • Nausea • Vomiting	• Administer antiemetic medications ordered for prn use. • Use suction as needed. • Keep an emesis basin, washcloth, and towel within reach. A cool wet cloth on the forehead or neck may feel good to the patient experiencing nausea. • Auscultate for bowel sounds at least every 4 hours. *Additional interventions if vomiting does occur:* • If the patient is still sedated, position the patient on his or her side to prevent aspiration. Someone should stay with the patient to provide suction as needed until vomiting ceases. • Assess the emesis for color, consistency, and amount. • Provide mouth care after vomiting. • Record on intake and output sheet. • Administer antiemetic medications as ordered. If they are ineffective, notify the surgeon for new antiemetic orders. • Patients are generally kept NPO or restricted to ice chips (or clear liquids if ordered and bowel sounds are present).
Thermoregulation Concerns • Hypothermia due to cold environment in OR, exposure, and length of time under anesthesia	• Monitor temperature and complaints of being cold, including teeth chattering, chilling tremors or shakes, and mottling of skin. • Apply additional warmed blankets as needed. If cloth blankets are not adequate, use warm air flow blankets to raise the patient's body temperature. • Assess patient temperature to differentiate between hypothermia and the tremors and shaking caused by general anesthesia as consciousness is regained, which the patient may interpret as being cold.
Postop Pain and Discomfort • Incisional pain as anesthesia wears off	• Administer pain medication as ordered, generally via the IV route • Treat pain according to the patient's evaluation of its severity

from being brought back to a room that is not ready to receive a postop patient. If the postop patient is to be transferred to a new floor and room, the recovery room nurse should notify the floor where the patient will be sent after surgery that a postop patient will be transferred to the floor. If this is done as soon as the patient is received in the PACU, then the receiving nurse has time to prepare the room and make it ready for the postop patient.

Room Preparation

Room preparation includes obtaining needed supplies and preparing a surgical bed with a lifting or draw sheet and disposable waterproof pads if needed. (Refer to Chapter 15, Skill 15.10, for steps in making a surgical bed.) In addition, the furniture should be arranged so that the gurney can be positioned parallel to the bed and the heads of the gurney and bed are aligned with each other. This better positions the patient so that after transferring from the PACU gurney into his or her bed, the patient is properly positioned at the head of the bed (Fig. 33.11). It also prevents the staff from having to lift the patient a second time to move him or her toward the head of the bed.

The room should be arranged to provide easy access with the gurney. Move chairs, the over-bed table, and the bedside table out of the way so that nothing impedes a direct path from the door to the side of the bed. Remove unnecessary clutter from both tables to accommodate the supplies you will be using immediately upon return of the patient. Store patient belongings in the closet and drawers until needed. Box 33.3 lists the equipment and supplies that should be ready for use at the bedside. Postop patients may return with numerous pieces of equipment that require space and reorganization of furniture to accommodate them. Failure to adequately prepare the room, supplies, and equipment can result in decreased efficiency of care. It can also create unsafe conditions should the patient suddenly develop problems.

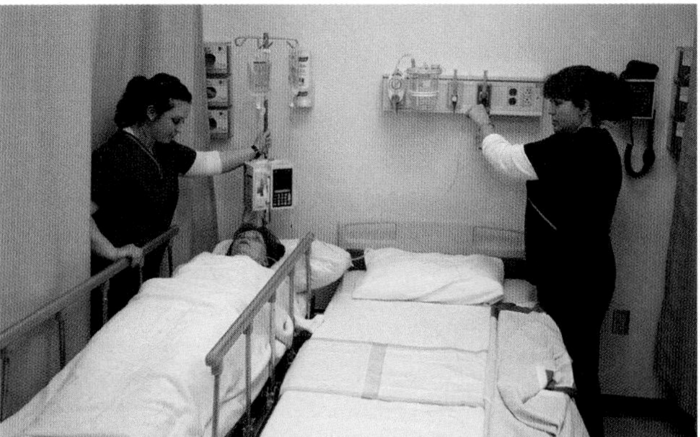

FIGURE 33.11 When transferring a postoperative patient from a gurney to a nursing unit bed, align the head of the gurney with the head of the bed before transferring the patient.

Box 33.3

Equipment and Supplies Needed for Postoperative Patient Care

There are many supplies and pieces of equipment that are required for proper postop care. Certain things will be needed as soon as the patient is transferred from the gurney to the bed, such as vital sign equipment. Some are safety related, allowing you to be prepared for an emergency situation that could develop, such as the suction equipment. Others are needed simply to meet the patient's needs after surgery. Having all your supplies will also save you the footwork and time of making multiple trips to gather supplies one or two at a time as you need each one. Additionally, the postop patient should not be left alone for at least the first 15 to 30 minutes after returning to the room. Equipment and supplies to gather include the following:

- Vital sign equipment, including a pulse oximeter
- Penlight
- IV pole with infusion pump
- Suction equipment
- Oxygen setup with delivery device
- Emesis basin
- Washcloths and towels
- Clean patient gown
- Box of tissues
- Mouth care supplies with lip lubricant
- Several extra pillows for positioning
- Extra blankets
- Pen and paper to record vital signs
- TED hose and/or sequential compression device according to health-care provider's orders
- Small pillow for splinting (for abdominal surgeries)
- Small cup of ice chips if health-care provider's orders allow
- Specimen pan to measure urinary output
- Ice pack if ordered

Initial Postoperative Patient Assessment

Transfer the patient from the gurney to the bed using as much assistance as needed for safety. If the patient is able to help, allow him or her to do so. This is a good time to multitask. While transferring the patient to the bed, assess the patient's skin color and temperature and whether it is dry or moist, the color of urine in the Foley drainage bag, and whether the IV site is intact.

FIRST PRIORITY. Once the patient is in the bed, your immediate priority is to complete an initial assessment with vital signs to determine the patient's condition and establish a baseline for subsequent comparisons. The assessment should begin with the number one priority: airway and gas exchange. Is the airway patent? Is there an oral or a nasal airway in place? Or is one needed? Assess respiration rate, depth, and pattern. Assess color of the skin, noting pallor or cyanosis. Assess oxygen saturation, noting if it is below 95%. Apply supplemental oxygen if ordered or if the patient's respiratory status indicates a need.

SECOND PRIORITY. Determine the patient's level of responsiveness and ability to follow instructions by instructing the patient to take several deep breaths while you are applying the pulse oximeter, blood pressure cuff, and cardiac monitor if ordered or according to facility policy. Begin assessing for cardiac stability by obtaining a pulse rate and blood pressure. Note a weak or thready pulse, tachycardia, bradycardia, or other arrhythmias, as well as hypotension or hypertension. Auscultate heart sounds, breath sounds, and bowel sounds. Note muffled or distant S_1 or S_2; absent, decreased, or adventitious breath sounds; and hypoactive or absent bowel sounds (Fig. 33.12). Assess peripheral circulation by assessing peripheral pulses and temperature of all four extremities, noting weak or absent pulses and cool or cold hands or feet. Check pupils for equality of size and response to light stimulus.

SURGICAL SITE. Assess the surgical site and dressing for bleeding and drainage. Using an ink pen, draw a circle around any area of drainage on the dressing, along with notation of the current date and time. This allows you to later gauge additional amounts of bleeding or drainage. Any drains should be assessed and attached, if ordered, to the appropriate suction. If Hemovac or Jackson-Pratt drainage devices are in use, ensure that they are activated. (Refer to Chapter 26 to review

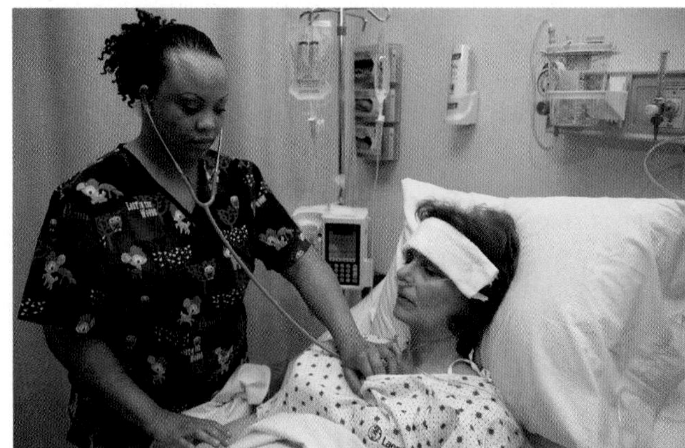

FIGURE 33.12 Once a patient is returned to the nursing unit from the PACU, a complete assessment should be performed to determine the patient's condition.

care of drains.) ***Safety: Make sure you wear gloves when working with drains and dressings.*** If the dressing is saturated with blood, reinforce the dressing with sterile gauze 4×4s or larger abdominal combined dressings, also known as *ABD pads*, and notify the surgeon. You should not remove the initial surgical dressing without a direct health-care provider's order. Assess for abdominal distention and rigidity, which may be indicative of internal hemorrhage.

FLUIDS AND RELATED EQUIPMENT. Assess the type of IV fluid hanging, IV patency, and rate of infusion. Assess the IV site for erythema, edema, and intactness of site dressing. If the patient has a Foley catheter connected to gravity drainage, assess its intactness, patency, color, clarity, and volume of urine output. ***Safety: Make certain the tubing is properly secured to the leg or, if a male prefers, the abdomen.*** This reduces trauma to the neck of the bladder and the internal sphincter, where the inflated balloon constantly tugs against them if it is allowed to dangle unsecured from the urinary meatus. This can cause discomfort, such as a burning or pulling sensation, and increase the feeling that the patient needs to void.

Real-World Connection

Importance of Securing Foley Catheter Tubing

On an evening clinical, a student nurse was assigned to care for a confused elderly male patient who had a Foley catheter. Upon completing his initial shift assessment, the student reported to his instructor that the Foley catheter tubing was not secured to the patient's leg as the student had been taught to do. The instructor agreed with the student that he should immediately secure the tubing to prevent urethral irritation and discomfort. The student correctly secured the catheter tubing immediately. Shortly thereafter, the hospital staff nurse intercepted the student and informed him that she had removed the securing device from the catheter tubing because hospital policy had been changed and they no longer followed this "outdated" procedure. The student reported this interaction to his instructor, who promptly went in search of the staff nurse to discuss and view this new policy. The staff nurse reiterated what she had told the student but could not produce a policy in writing for the instructor. Before further action could be taken, the student rushed to inform the instructor and staff nurse that the patient was found bleeding from the penis and the catheter, with the still-inflated 30-mL balloon laying on the floor. The patient had accidentally stepped on the tubing when he got up from the chair and pulled out the catheter with the bulb still inflated, tearing the penis open with a 2-inch laceration, exposing the damaged urethra inside. This patient suffered needlessly because the catheter was not secured properly.

PAIN AND DISCOMFORT. Thoroughly assess the patient's pain level using the facility's preferred pain scale. (See Chapter 19 for further information regarding use of pain scales.) Be certain not only to assess the site and the intensity of the pain but also to include characteristics of the pain. For example, is the pain sharp or stabbing? Dull, aching, or cramping? Is it limited to the surgical incision site? Or is it, for example, in the shoulder from which the arm was extended during surgery? Determine what medications were administered during surgery and in the PACU to reduce the risk of overmedicating the patient. Once you have completed the assessment, administer analgesics according to the health-care provider's orders, evaluating the medication's effectiveness. Remember, the pain is as bad as the patient says it is, not as bad as you think it should be.

SAFETY INTERVENTIONS. ***Safety: Make sure that the call bell is within reach of the patient, the side rails are raised for safety, and the bed is lowered to its lowest position.*** The head of the bed is generally raised for patient comfort unless contraindicated by the type of surgery. The bedside table with needed supplies, including water or ice chips if allowed, should be brought within the patient's reach.

DOCUMENTATION. Document your assessment, including the six vital signs, as soon as possible. Begin an intake and output record.

Supervision/Delegation Connection

Postoperative Assessment

Delegation of postop assessment and vital signs to unlicensed assistive personnel (UAP) is not appropriate until the patient's condition is determined to be stable. You are responsible for observing the postop patient and assessing him or her according to the patient's individual responses to surgery and anesthesia. Even though vital sign assessment may be safely delegated to UAPs in certain other situations, this is not one of them.

Continued Assessments

You should remain at the bedside until you are certain that the patient is stable. After your initial assessment is complete, continue to monitor the patient's level of consciousness and respiratory and cardiac status—including vital signs—at 15-minute intervals for the first hour.

After the first hour of monitoring vital signs every 15 minutes, if the patient is stable, assessments can be lengthened to every 30 to 60 minutes according to facility policy. (See Box 33.4 for an example of a frequency schedule.) The assessments are performed at progressively lengthening intervals over the first 24 hours postop. Most hospital units have a standardized postsurgical care plan in place that details postsurgical care routines regardless of the type of surgery. If your patient shows any signs of instability, call for assistance without leaving the bedside.

Box 33.4

Example of Postoperative Vital Sign Frequency

After a general anesthetic, it is necessary to monitor the patient's postop vital signs frequently to detect developing problems as early as possible. Each facility will have its own policy delineating vital sign frequency, but the following is a commonly used schedule:

- Every 15 minutes × 4
- Every 30 minutes × 4
- Every 1 hour × 4
- Every 2 hours × 4
- Every 4 hours × 4
- Then every 8 hours

PAIN CONTROL. Pain assessment remains a major priority throughout the entire postop period. It is important to remember that simply because the patient has fallen asleep after complaining of pain, this does not mean that you should withhold pain medication that may be administered. Anesthesia can make a patient groggy, but the patient may still experience discomfort. The postsurgical orders will specify available interventions. These may include use of a patient-controlled analgesia (PCA) pump, IV administration, or administration of oral medications. Remember, you have a number of nonpharmacologic interventions available to assist with pain control as well, including repositioning, use of warm blankets, music, and touch. However, these alternatives do not replace pain medication when the patient needs medication unless he or she has cultural or personal beliefs that prohibit use of analgesic pain medications.

FLUID AND ELECTROLYTE BALANCE. The patient's fluid and electrolyte balance should be monitored closely. ***Safety: If the patient does not have an indwelling Foley catheter, you should make certain the patient voids within 8 hours.*** If the patient cannot void within the specified length of time, it may be necessary to obtain a health-care provider's order to either perform a straight catheterization or insert an indwelling urinary catheter. Be certain to measure all urine output as well as emesis and other drainage. The patient may still be NPO and dependent on IV fluids for hydration. Keep the mouth and lips moist to reduce dryness, cracking, and discomfort due to dry mucous membranes. ***Safety: Monitor the IV fluid and rate of infusion and perform an IV site assessment at least every 2 hours.*** Make certain the intake and output are balanced to prevent fluid overload or dehydration.

POSTOPERATIVE ORDERS. Postop orders may also include additional specific assessments to be made. These may include hourly urine output or neurological examinations and specific actions to be taken, including turning the patient every 2 hours and when to get the patient out of bed. Postop orders may also include assessing specific patterns that, if present, require notification of the surgeon, including parameters for blood pressure, pulse, temperature, and oxygen saturation. ***Safety: All preop orders are discontinued when a patient goes to surgery. New ones must be written when the patient returns to the nursing unit.*** (Box 33.5 provides further discussion on preop versus postop orders.)

Postsurgical Complications

Some postsurgical complications may occur that are specific to the type of surgery that was performed. There are also some complications that may occur independently of the type of procedure. It is your role to help prevent these complications with accurate and pertinent assessments and delivery of appropriate nursing actions or interventions and to intervene promptly if signs of these complications are noted.

Fever

It is somewhat common for the postop patient to run a low-grade temperature, within the range of 99°F to 99.8°F (37.1°C to 37.6°C), after surgery, but more elevated temperatures of 101°F (38.3°C) or higher may be a sign of infection. The more commonly seen infections include pneumonia, wound infection, and UTI, particularly if an indwelling catheter is present.

NURSING CARE. A fever of 101°F requires notification of the surgeon. The surgeon will frequently order blood, urine, sputum, and wound cultures to determine the source of infection before ordering antibiotics to treat the infection. The surgeon also may order acetaminophen, a medication that reduces fever and is classified as an *antipyretic* medication. High fevers (greater than 102°F) may require application of cool wet cloths to the forehead, neck, axilla, and groin.

Atelectasis

Atelectasis can cause postop hypoxemia, most commonly due to excessive secretions or decreased lung volumes. Low blood pressure can also contribute to atelectasis. Nonspecific

Box 33.5

Preoperative Orders Versus Postoperative Orders

The standard of care is that all preop orders are automatically discontinued when a patient goes to surgery. This standard requires that new orders be written for any care that is to be delivered postop. The following pointers will help to keep you a safe and accurate practitioner.

- All preop orders are canceled when the patient goes to surgery.
- The physician must write new postop orders, including orders for any medications taken preop that are to be administered postop.
- If the physician writes "resume preoperative meds," you must clarify with her or him which specific medications are to be resumed. Never assume that it really means all of the medications that were taken before surgery.
- After clarifying with the physician, list the specific medications individually in the computer.

signs of hypoxemia range from agitation to excessive sleepiness, tachycardia to bradycardia, and hypertension to hypotension. Patients will present with diminished to absent lung sounds. Patients who meet any of the following criteria should be considered at risk for atelectasis:

- Has received general anesthesia, particularly if a smoker
- Has abdominal surgery pain
- Is on bedrest or restricted activity
- Has chronic respiratory disease

NURSING CARE. Once again, prevention is key. Implementation of treatment strategies early, before the patient becomes symptomatic, will help to prevent the development of atelectasis. Treatment includes coughing and deep breathing exercises, incentive spirometry, repositioning, and promotion of increased mobility with early ambulation. Humidified oxygen is administered as indicated.

Pulmonary Embolism

PE occurs as the result of a venous clot that is released into the circulation, lodges in a vessel in the lungs, and obstructs blood flow and gas exchange. It is a leading cause of perioperative morbidity, with deaths generally occurring within 30 minutes of an acute event (Fig. 33.13). The patient will complain of acute shortness of breath and will immediately develop tachycardia, increased respiratory rate, and hypoxemia, even if already on oxygen. If severe, the patient may go into cardiac arrest.

Patients at risk for PE include those who have venous stasis or blood pooling; *hypercoagulability,* which is increased risk of clotting; or abnormalities of the blood vessel walls. These risk factors are increased in elderly patients and obese patients; in those with varicose veins, immobility, malignancy, and congestive heart failure; and in patients who have had pelvic or long-bone surgery.

NURSING CARE. Because a PE can be life-threatening, prevention is important. TED hose and sequential compression devices may have been applied before or after surgery. Maintain both until the patient is able to get out of bed and ambulate to promote blood flow. See that the patient performs postop leg exercises to stimulate venous circulation and prevent stasis. An anticoagulant may be ordered for subcutaneous administration for patients who must remain on bedrest or who had surgery on the skeletal system, such as repair of a hip fracture or knee replacement.

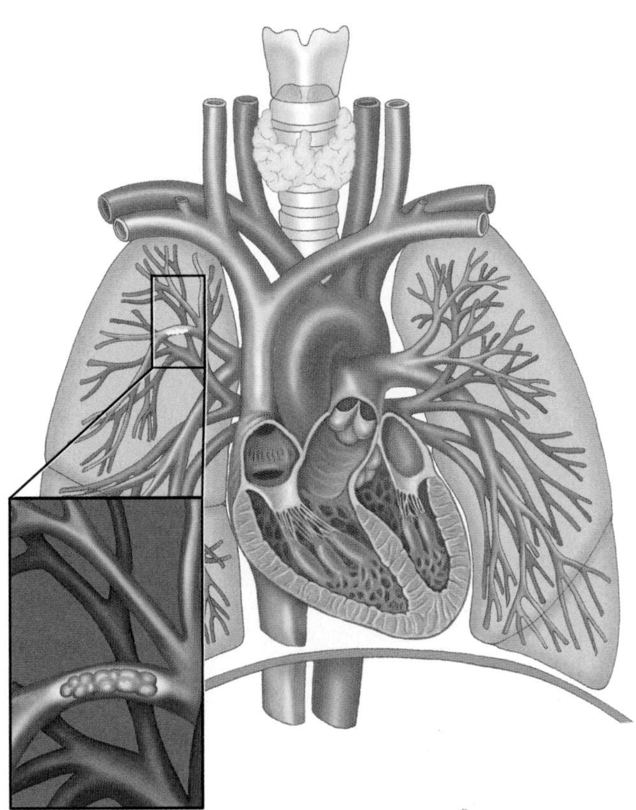

FIGURE 33.13 Pulmonary embolism (from Williams LS, Hopper PD. *Understanding Medical-Surgical Nursing*. 5th ed. Philadelphia, PA: FA Davis; 2015; modified from Barnes TA. *Respiratory Care Principles*. Philadelphia, PA: FA Davis; 1991).

Nausea and Vomiting

Nausea and vomiting, while not life-threatening, is distressing for patients. It may be caused by the agents used in the OR, NPO status, pain medications used after surgery, or an NG tube that is not functioning appropriately.

NURSING CARE. Assess for nausea and treat as soon as possible to prevent vomiting. Surgeons commonly order an antiemetic to be available on an as-needed basis for patient comfort. For surgeries associated with nausea and vomiting, the anesthesia provider or PACU nurse may have given a dose of the antiemetic already, so check the OR and PACU records first before administering the first dose.

Urinary Retention

Urinary retention after surgery may occur due to use of a regional anesthetic such as a spinal or narcotics administered for pain after surgery.

NURSING CARE. Monitor intake and output carefully. If the patient is unable to void, assess the bladder for distention. If distention is present, try to assist the patient to void by helping him or her to the bathroom unless contraindicated; if the patient is male, you may help him stand to void. Running water also may be helpful. If the patient remains unable to void, the surgeon may order bladder catheterization. However, to decrease the risk of infection, the catheter usually is not left in place. A catheter is placed in the OR for surgeries after which voiding is known to be difficult or output monitoring is critical.

Wound Infection

The edges of the surgical incision should meet and be aligned with one another, known as **approximation.** Wound *dehiscence* refers to a separation of the wound edges. Occurring most commonly 7 to 10 days postop, it is seen in approximately 2%

of all midline abdominal incisions. It is associated with 15% to 40% mortality, with infection being the most common underlying cause.

Patients at risk for alterations in wound healing include those with diabetes, malnutrition, suppressed immune function, advanced age, and infection. A patient taking corticosteroids for a chronic condition such as rheumatoid arthritis or obstructive pulmonary disease should be considered to be immunosuppressed because of the medication's action in reducing the body's normal anti-inflammatory response.

NURSING CARE. While dressing changes are routinely the responsibility of the nurse, sometimes a surgeon will prefer to remove the initial surgical dressing on the first postop day. Unless the health-care provider orders otherwise, you should assess the wound daily, noting possible signs of infection such as poor approximation of incision edges, dehiscence, erythema, edema, color, amount, and odor of drainage. ***Safety: Perform proper handwashing prior to wound assessment or dressing change, and use clean or sterile gloves as appropriate.*** If a surgical drain is present, look for erythema, edema, and drainage around the insertion site. Also assess the color, amount, and odor of drainage from the drain itself. Accurate assessment allows for early detection of and intervention for infection. Document your assessment, noting changes from previous assessments. In addition to monitoring the wound, assess temperature for fever and monitor the WBC count for elevation related to infection. If dehiscence occurs, cover the wound with a large sterile dressing or sterile surgical towel moistened with sterile normal saline. Notify the surgeon immediately (Chapter 26 details wound assessment and management).

Nursing Care Plan for a Patient Who Is Postoperative Following Colectomy

You are assigned to care for Jeremy Lackey, a 67-year-old male admitted the previous evening with the diagnosis of inflammatory bowel disease. He has just returned from surgery where he underwent a segmental colectomy with anastomosis. This means the surgeon removed the diseased segment of his colon and rejoined the ends of the remaining portions. Now you need to get started developing Mr. Lackey's care plan. Figure 33.14 presents a concept map care plan for this patient.

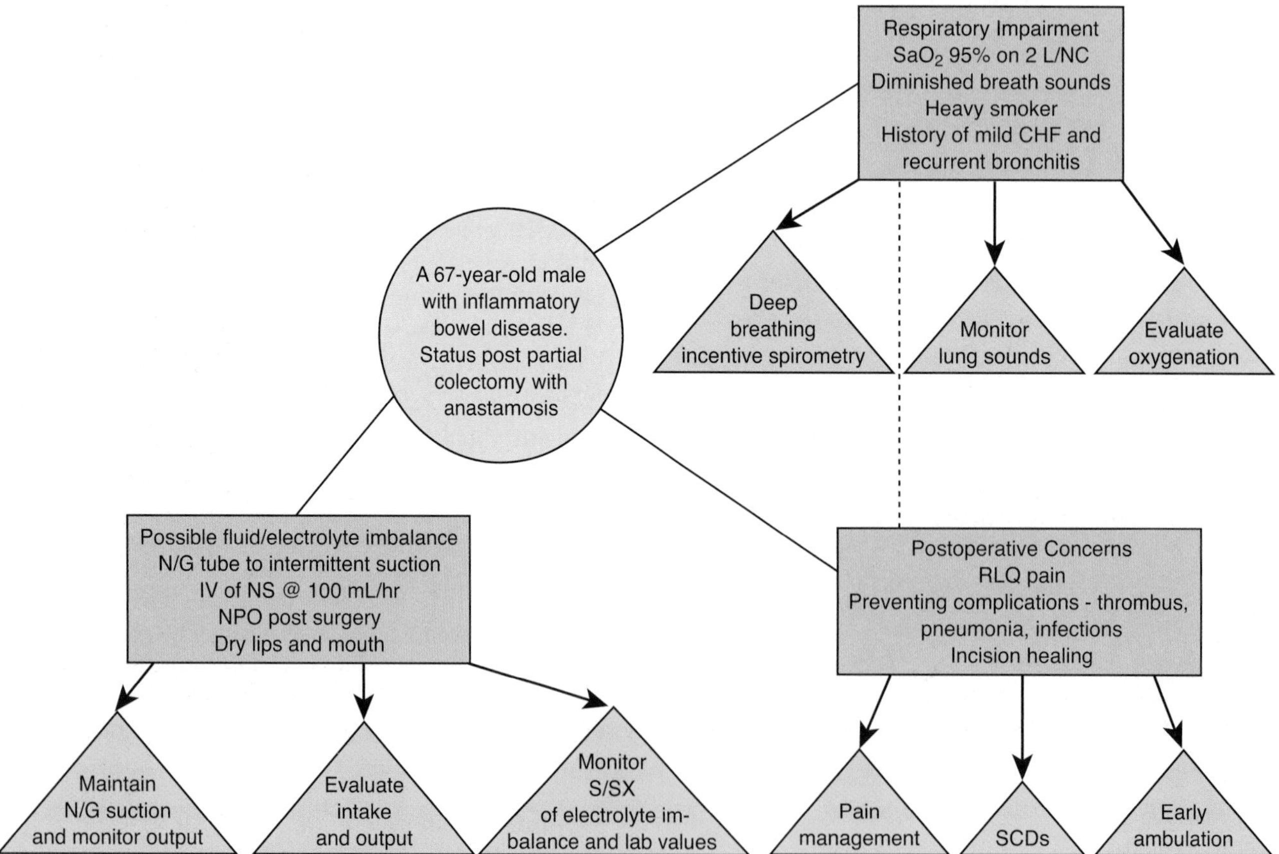

FIGURE 33.14 Concept map care plan for a patient having abdominal surgery.

Nursing Care Plan for a Patient Who Is Postoperative Following Colectomy—cont'd

Assessment

Development of a care plan begins by first gathering all the available data. You will need to determine postop problems you can anticipate for this patient. But you know that a physical assessment is your priority at this time.

- What is his LOC?
- Are his vital signs stable?
- What is the status of his respiratory system?
- What is the status of his cardiovascular system?
- What is the status of his neurological system?
- Is the patient comfortable or experiencing pain? Nauseated?
- What equipment is in use? IV pump? PCA? SCDs?
- What are the patient's postop needs?
- Have postop orders been carried out yet?
- Did the patient receive preop teaching?

You have just documented the assessment. A synopsis of the assessment findings includes the following information:

Still groggy but responsive to voice and follows simple commands; oriented to 4 spheres. Pupils equal and responsive to light bilaterally. BP – 118/66, T – 98.2°F, AP – 96 regular and distinct, R – 19/minute shallow and even, SpO_2 – 95% with O_2 on @ 2 L/min per nasal cannula. Breath sounds diminished in all 5 lobes but improve when cued to take deep breath; no adventitious breath sounds. C/O dry lips and mouth. Requesting ice chips. Right lower quadrant abdominal pain @ 4, down from 9 before analgesic. NG tube to low suction patent, draining dark green contents. Denies nausea. Abdominal dressing dry and intact. Abdomen flat and soft. No bowel sounds auscultated. IV of 1,000 mL 0.45% NS infusing in left forearm @ 100 mL/hr via infusion pump. Site without erythema or edema. Has not voided since returning from OR. Bladder not palpable. SCDs on both legs with capillary refill time less than 3 seconds and strong pedal pulses bilaterally.

The chart reflects that preop teaching was done with the patient and family, and understanding of teaching was evidenced. You note that he is a heavy smoker and has had several bouts of bronchitis over the last 5 years. He has a history of mild congestive heart failure for which he takes a diuretic to prevent water retention. Postop orders are now noted. There is no additional care to deliver at this time.

Nursing Diagnosis

The first priorities as you review his data are that he smokes, has a medical history of bronchitis, and has diminished breath sounds—plus he had a general anesthetic and is currently experiencing decreased physical activity. He has supplemental O_2. The congestive heart failure could potentially cause some respiratory issues and will have to be watched

The nursing diagnoses for this patient are:

- Impaired gas exchange
- Acute pain
- Risk for electrolyte imbalance

Planning

Now you need to plan what nursing interventions should be performed to prevent the possible problems and actual problems that you know to expect. You want to individualize the plan of care, making certain the interventions meet Mr. Lackey's specific needs. You plan for ways to improve his respiratory status and gas exchange, to manage his pain effectively, and to keep his fluid and electrolytes in balance.

Implementation

Now you can begin to carry out the interventions that you have planned. The following Care Plan lists nursing interventions for these nursing diagnoses.

Evaluation

The last phase of the nursing process is to evaluate whether the interventions you have been implementing are helping Mr. Lackey's respiratory efforts and preventing pneumonia. You will also want to evaluate whether or not the medications are keeping the patient comfortable and with a pain level less than 3 to 4 the majority of the time. What is the total intake and output (I&O)? Is he adequately hydrated? Are his electrolytes balanced? The following Care Plan provides evaluations of the nursing interventions.

Nursing Diagnosis: Impaired gas exchange, related to smoking, history of bronchitis, abdominal incision pain, and general anesthesia, as evidenced by diminished breath sounds and shallow respirations

Expected Outcomes: O_2 saturation will remain above 95%. Breath sounds will be clear to auscultation and will not be diminished by second postop day. Temperature will remain below 100.4°F. No evidence of pneumonia, supported by clear chest x-ray at discharge.

Interventions	Evaluations
Assess vital signs, noting increased respiratory rate, decreased depth, irregular pattern, decreased SpO_2, increased pulse rate, dropping blood pressure, and increased temperature. Use facility postop frequency schedule.	Day 1: Within normal limits all day. 10 p.m.: 122/74, 98.2°F orally, 88 reg & strong, 18 shallow & even. SpO_2 has remained above 95% since noon.
Encourage the patient to turn, cough, and deep breathe 5 times every 2 hours.	Day 1: Good resp effort, cough productive of small amount clear sputum.

(nursing care plan continues on page 748)

Nursing Care Plan for a Patient Who Is Postoperative Following Colectomy—cont'd

Interventions	Evaluations
Auscultate breath sounds every 4 hours, noting decreased, absent, or adventitious sounds.	Day 1: Diminished in 5 lobes; few fine crackles in RLL @ 10 p.m.
Assist the patient to use an incentive spirometer every 1 hour for 8 hours, then every 2 hours. Initial goal is volume of 700 mL; increase by 100 mL as patient meets each goal.	Day 1: Met 700-mL goal 2nd hr. Met 900-mL goal 5th hr. Met 1,250-mL goal 12th hr. Still @ 1350 mL @ 10 p.m.
Maintain supplemental O_2 @ 2 L/min per nasal cannula.	Day 1: O_2 con't @ 2 L/min per nasal cannula. No dyspnea. Skin remains pink.
Elevate the head of the bed 30–60 degrees prn.	Day 1: Only needed head of bed up once for brushing teeth.
May use bedside commode.	Day 1: Only used urinal today.
Assist the patient to dangle for 5–10 minutes 2 times on day of surgery—ambulate in room tomorrow a.m.	Day 1: Dangled 5 min @ 3:00 p.m. & tolerated it without dyspnea, stated pain increased only while getting up to sitting position, felt good once upright.
Ambulate 4 times/day in halls—to begin 1 day postop.	
Have suction setup ready in room.	Day 1: Handling own secretions.

Nursing Diagnosis: Acute pain, related to surgical manipulation of abdominal contents as evidenced by abdominal incision
Expected Outcomes: Pain level will be below 5 within 60 minutes after analgesic administration; patient will be able to maintain pain below 3 with oral analgesics at discharge.

Interventions	Evaluations
Use 0–10 scale to assess pain at each contact with the patient.	Day 1: Highest pain rating was immediately after return from PACU @ 10. Maintained less than 5 remainder of day with analgesics.
Turn the patient every 2 hours, maintain proper body alignment, position, and support with pillows for comfort.	Day 1: Erythema on sacrum resolves 5–10 min after repositioning. No other erythema noted. Skin remains intact over pressure points. Body alignment maintained with pillows. Does not like to lay on left side.
Encourage the patient to splint the incision when coughing or moving.	Day 1: Had to be reminded to splint while coughing but said it does help a little.
Provide back or foot massage 1–2 times per shift.	Day 1: Reported that massages of back felt great and seemed to help him relax.
Administer morphine 4–6 mg IV every 2 hours prn pain. Evaluate effectiveness within 20–30 minutes.	Day 1: 4 mg only controlled pain for 45–60 min. 6 mg kept pain less than 5 most of day.
Administer promethazine 50 mg IM every 4–6 hours prn nausea/vomiting or to potentiate morphine per order. Evaluate effectiveness within 30–60 minutes.	Day 1: Only required once for potentiation of first dose of morphine 4 mg. Decreased pain from 5 to 3.

Nursing Care Plan for a Patient Who Is Postoperative Following Colectomy—cont'd

Nursing Diagnosis: Risk for electrolyte imbalance, related to nasogastric suction
Expected Outcomes: Electrolytes will remain within normal limits each day. Urine output will remain within 300 mL of IV intake.

Interventions	Evaluations
Monitor I&O every shift. Note if output is *less* than total intake by more than 300 mL.	Day 1: NPO. IV In – 3,000 mL; Out – 2,875 mL.
Make certain the patient voids at least every 8 hours. Assess characteristics.	Day 1: Voiding without difficulty; urine clear, yellow.
Provide mouth care and lip moisturizer every 4 hours.	Day 1: Applies lip moisturizer himself. Lips more moist than immediately postop.
Keep NG tube connected to low, intermittent suction. Secure the tube to the patient's nose, avoiding pressure on naris. Pin the tube to the patient's gown.	Day 1: No erythema noted on naris.
Continue IV infusion of 1,000 mL 0.45% NS with 30 mEq KCl @ 125 mL/hr per order.	Day 1: IV still @ 125 mL/hr. Site Rt. forearm, 18-gauge intracath, no edema/erythema, site dressing dry/intact.
Monitor laboratory results for elevated or decreased potassium, sodium, and chloride.	Day 1: Postop potassium 3.3 mEq; obtained order to increase IV potassium.
Assess drainage characteristics every 2 hours. Measure and empty at end of shift.	Day 1: NG tube patent, drainage thick, dark green. 24-hr Out – 525 mL.
Assess for peripheral edema every 4 hours.	Day 1: None.

Skill 33.1 Applying Antiembolism Hose

Assessment Steps

1. Review the health-care provider's order to determine the type of hose ordered. ***They come in knee-high and thigh-high lengths.***
2. Measure the patient's legs according to type ordered.
   - **For thigh-high:** Measure the length of the posterior aspect of the leg with the patient in the supine position, measuring from the gluteal fold to the plantar surface of the heel. Then measure the circumference of the largest part of the calf and the largest part of the thigh.
   - **For knee-high:** Measure the length from the posterior knee to the plantar surface of the heel. Then measure the circumference of the largest part of the calf.

   Cross-reference the measurements on the manufacturer's chart to determine the correct size. ***This ensures proper fit.***
3. Assess skin integrity of both legs and feet. ***This establishes a baseline against which you can measure future skin integrity and makes you aware of problems with the skin.***

Planning Steps

1. Gather needed supplies: antiembolism hose and powder. ***Being prepared saves time and footwork.***
2. Plan to have your patient lie supine for a minimum of 15 minutes prior to application of hose. ***This aids venous return of blood to the heart and reduces the risk of trapping pooled venous blood in the lower legs.***

Implementation Steps

1. Follow the Initial Implementation Steps located on the inside back cover.
2. Make certain that the patient's legs are clean and dry. ***This reduces microorganisms and prevents maceration from applying the hose over moist skin.***

(skill continues on page 750)

Skill 33.1 (continued)

3. Grasp the top edge of the hose and slide your nondominant hand into the hose and down to the heel of the hose, where you grasp the fabric of the heel with your hand.

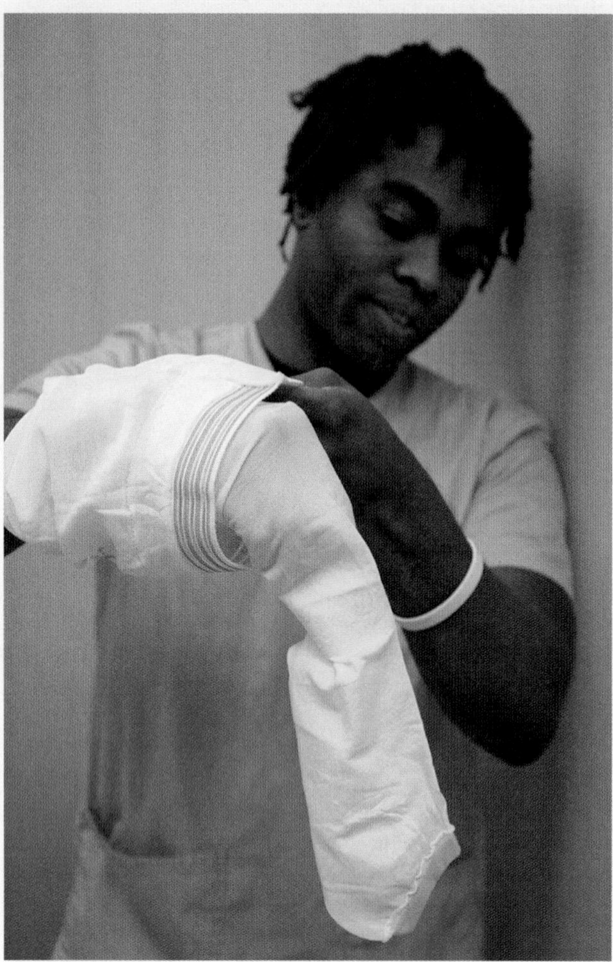

4. Use your dominant hand to slowly pull the hose inside out, turning it down to the heel. ***This enables you to slide the tight hose over the foot and calf more easily.***
5. With the patient's toes pointed down, grasp the turned foot of the hose and center it over the toes. Then ease the hose over the heel, making certain the heel is also centered in the hose before proceeding to slide it over the calf. ***This helps to ensure more even compression over the foot and leg.***

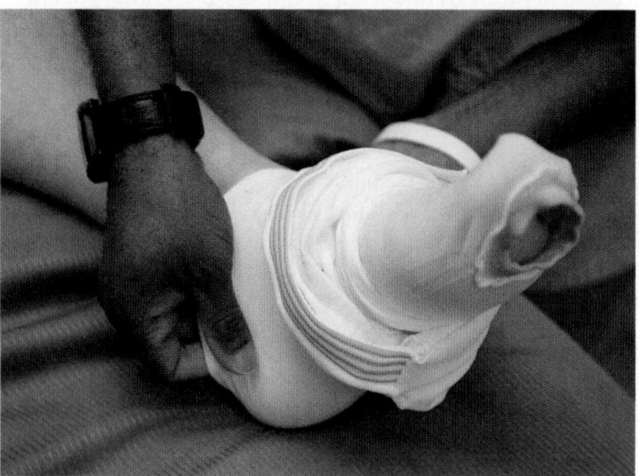

6. Smooth all wrinkles from the hose and pull the hose up to its full length. Avoid allowing the hose to bunch, wrinkle, or fold over at its top. ***This prevents constriction of venous circulation and pressure ulcers.***
7. If the hose style has closed toes rather than open toes, gently pull the hose at the end of the toes to provide more room for the toes and nails. ***This helps to prevent capillary compression in the toes and sore toenails due to pressure at the corners of nail.***
8. Repeat the process for the other leg.
9. Follow the Ending Implementation Steps located on the inside back cover.
10. Remove hose at least twice per day: during bath and p.m. care. Wash and dry the legs; assess for pressure areas or impairment of skin integrity before reapplying hose. ***This allows the skin to be exposed to air and stimulates circulation. It adds to the comfort of the patient and helps him or her to rest afterward.***
11. Assess pedal pulses each shift. ***This ensures adequate arterial circulation to the feet.***
    Note: Hose should be hand-washed daily and allowed to air dry to prevent soiled hose from smelling and irritating the skin. Therefore, the patient will require two pairs: one pair to wear while the other pair is drying.

Evaluation Steps

1. Do the stockings fit smoothly without wrinkles? Do they come up to the correct height on the legs? ***This ensures proper fit.***
2. Are you still able to palpate the pedal pulses? ***This ensures that the stockings are not so tight that they block arterial blood flow to the feet.***

Sample Documentation

10/5/22 1930 Legs measured for thigh-high TED hose. Thigh = 29 in. Calf = 16 in. Length = 29 in. Skin of legs and feet intact and without erythema or edema. TED hose applied. Pedal pulses strong bilaterally. Purpose of TEDs explained. Verbalized understanding of purpose. States had worn them before. ————————

———————— Nurse's signature and credentials

Skill 33.2 Applying Sequential Compression Devices

Assessment Steps

1. Verify the health-care provider's order for the length of the device. Measure the length of the legs, if needed. ***These devices come in different lengths.***
2. Measure the circumference of the thigh if the thigh-high length is ordered. ***This ensures the proper amount of compression.***
3. Read the manufacturer's instructions for application and use of sequential compression devices. ***Each brand-name SCD will work slightly differently.***

Planning Step

1. Gather needed equipment and supplies: compression sleeves, compression pump or motor, and connecting tubing. ***Being prepared saves you time and footwork.***

Implementation Steps

1. Follow the Initial Implementation Steps located on the inside back cover.
2. Assist the patient to the supine position ***to prevent venous pooling and to make access to the legs easier.***
3. Cleanse the lower extremities if necessary and apply antiembolism hose if they have also been ordered. ***SCDs should be applied over clean skin and are often ordered in addition to antiembolism stockings.***
4. Attach the pump unit to the foot of the bed according to the manufacturer's instructions. ***Following the manufacturer's instructions ensures proper use and increases safety.***
5. Apply compression sleeves to the patient's legs according to the manufacturer's instructions. ***Following the manufacturer's instructions ensures proper fit and use while increasing safety.*** *Safety: Ensure that the cord does not cause a fall risk.*
6. Connect the tubings to the compression sleeves and the pump according to the manufacturer's instructions. ***This allows air for compression to enter the compression sleeves from the pump.***
7. Assess to make certain there is room for you to insert two fingers between the compression sleeves and the patient's legs. ***This prevents excessive compression.***
8. Turn on the pump.
9. Assess pedal pulses, skin color and temperature, sensation and movement of toes, presence of edema, and capillary refill of toes every 8 hours. ***This ensures adequate circulation and nerve function.***
10. Instruct the patient to call for assistance to remove the SCDs if he or she is allowed to ambulate. ***This helps to prevent falls.***
11. Follow the Ending Implementation Steps located on the inside back cover.

Evaluation Steps

1. Assess several cycles of inflation and deflation of the devices. Make certain the tubings are not kinked and preventing correct inflation. ***This ensures proper function.***
2. Assess patient comfort ***to validate correct placement and pressure of devices.***
3. Remove sleeves at intervals ***to assess the skin beneath them and for signs/symptoms of deep vein thrombosis.***

Sample Documentation

9/7/22 1115 Skin of legs and feet pink, warm, dry, intact. Pedal pulses strong and equal. Cap refill brisk bilaterally. Calf-high SCDs applied to legs. States they "feel good." ——— Nurse's signature and credentials

POST CONFERENCE

You cared for the same patient, Mr. Lackey, for all 3 days of your clinical experience. It was quite a time of learning for you. You listened as the staff nurse told the patient about the surgery. You taught the patient about turning, coughing, and deep breathing after surgery. You had to move very quickly to get everything done on the preop checklist before the OR transport came to take him to surgery. In fact, you had barely finished administering the ordered preop medications when the transport arrived. The nurse signed off with you on the checklist, though, and you felt good about getting it all done correctly.

You were not really prepared for how sick the patient was when he returned to the nursing unit after the surgery. He had a NG tube, an IV, and a catheter in place, and he was moaning in pain. For just a moment or two, you nearly panicked. However, with your instructor's assistance, you calmed down quickly and went about caring for this gentleman. You focused on meeting his needs, assessing his status, monitoring his vital signs, and reassuring his family. Each postop day he was more improved, and you were able to remove the NG tube and the catheter.

Key Points

- Surgeries are classified by purpose and degree of urgency. Purposes of surgery include correction, cosmetic, exploratory, and palliative. Degrees of urgency include elective, urgent, emergency, and salvage.
- Surgery may be performed in freestanding surgery centers, medical clinics, or hospitals.
- Factors that increase risk of surgery and anesthesia include previous reaction to anesthesia, smoking, obesity, pre-existing medical conditions, malnutrition, immunosuppression, and impairment of the hepatic, renal, or pulmonary systems.
- Presurgical assessment components include the patient history, review of systems, and physical examination.
- Findings in a presurgical assessment that would be cause for concern include pregnancy, signs and symptoms of heart failure, low Hgb and Hct count, increased bleeding time tests, and a low or high WBC count.
- Preop diagnostic testing is ordered to correlate with the patient's history and type of surgery, as well as standard preop testing required by the facility. These are done to be sure that the patient is healthy enough to tolerate the surgery and to prevent complications during and after surgery.
- Preop teaching should include what the patient can expect before, during, and after the surgery; practicing any postoperative exercises to be done; explaining how pain will be managed; and making the patient aware of the presence of any tubes or drains after surgery.
- Consent forms for surgical procedures must include the patient's or guardian's signature. Signature also implies informed consent, meaning the patient understood what was going to be done, what the alternatives were, risks and possible complications, and expected outcomes.
- Completing the preop checklist is the responsibility of the nursing unit nurse and the circulating nurse.
- The surgical team consists of the anesthesia provider, surgeon, first surgical assistant, circulating nurse, and scrub nurse. Each have unique responsibilities and work together to provide the safest and most effective surgical environment for the patient.
- There are several types of anesthesia: general; conscious sedation; regional, which includes spinal and Bier block; and local.
- Patent airway and gas exchange are the top priority in the PACU and after return to the nursing unit. You should thoroughly assess each postop patient upon return from the PACU to the nursing unit.
- Prevention of postsurgical complications is the responsibility of the nursing staff. Such complications include fever greater than 101°F, atelectasis, pulmonary emboli, nausea and vomiting, urinary retention, and wound infection. Specific nursing interventions are necessary to help prevent each of these complications.

Review Questions

Select the answer that is most appropriate for each of the following questions. Some questions may have more than one correct answer. Select all that apply.

1. Which of the following patients is scheduled for palliative surgery?
   1. A patient scheduled for tonsillectomy due to repeated throat infections
   2. A patient scheduled for repair of a gastric ulcer due to lack of healing with medication
   3. A patient scheduled for removal of an untreatable cancerous brain tumor due to its impingement on the optic nerve
   4. A patient scheduled for breast enlargement so that her body shape will be better balanced
   5. A patient scheduled for a hysterectomy (removal of female reproductive organs) due to severe endometriosis

2. For which of the following patients would it be appropriate to schedule his or her surgery in a surgery center as opposed to a hospital setting?
   1. A patient with severe chronic respiratory disease who needs an appendectomy
   2. A patient with an above-the-knee amputation who needs a breast biopsy
   3. An elderly patient with hypertension and diabetes who needs a resection of the colon
   4. A patient with hemophilia who needs a tonsillectomy

3. Which of the following pieces of medical history would be pertinent regarding a patient being assessed to undergo a major abdominal surgery?
   1. Recent seizures
   2. History of rubella
   3. Has had multiple lacerations sutured
   4. Takes medication for cardiac problems
   5. Is allergic to milk

4. A male patient about to be scheduled for a major surgery tells the physician that he has been diagnosed with some kind of serious problem of his liver but can't remember the name of the disorder. About which of the following might the physician be concerned as a direct result of the patient's statement?
   1. The patient's ability to tolerate IV fluids
   2. The patient's ability to urinate after surgery
   3. The ability of the patient's blood to clot
   4. The patient's ability to maintain adequate body temperature during anesthesia

5. Which of the following tests are performed on most surgical patients preop?
   1. Electrocardiogram, complete blood count, and urinalysis
   2. Magnetic resonance imaging, serum sodium level, and esophagogastroduodenoscopy
   3. Lumbar puncture, urine culture and sensitivity, and blood type
   4. Chest x-ray, finger stick blood sugar, and electrolytes

6. Which of the following types of information should you teach preop patients?
   1. Preop prep
   2. What to expect in the OR
   3. Roles of the surgical team members
   4. Actions to prevent complications
   5. Name of each surgical team member

7. What interventions can you perform to stimulate a postop patient's circulation?
   1. Antiembolism hose
   2. Immediate ambulation on return from PACU
   3. Sequential compression devices
   4. Leg exercises

8. What are the purposes for administering preop medication?
   1. Decrease risk of infection
   2. Prevent aspiration during anesthesia
   3. Decrease intraoperative anesthesia
   4. Convenience to surgical staff

9. What are the primary responsibilities of the circulating nurse in surgery?
   1. Serving as the primary patient advocate
   2. Keeping notes of the surgical procedure
   3. Calling time outs
   4. Maintaining patient rights

ANSWERS 1. 3, 2. 2, 3. 1, 4, 5, 4. 3, 5. 1, 6. 1, 2, 5, 7. 1, 3, 4, 8. 1, 2, 9. 1, 3, 4

Critical Thinking Exercise

Answers available online.

1. Identify assessment findings you might detect in a new postop patient that would cause you concern.

Additional Resources

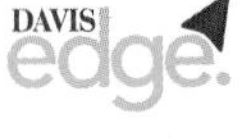

Use the scratch off code on the inside front cover of your book to access online quizzes that will help you to improve your scores on course exams and prepare for the NCLEX-PN®.

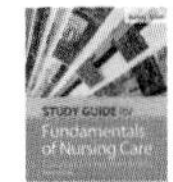

Study Guide

CHAPTER 34

Phlebotomy and Blood Specimens

KEY TERMS

Aerobic (air-OH-bik)
Anaerobic (AN-air-OH-bik)
Anastomoses (uh-NAS-tuh-MOH-seez)
Blood culture (BLUHD KUL-chur)
Evacuated tube (ih-VAK-yoo-AYT-ed TOOB)
Hematoma (HEE-muh-TOH-mah)
Hemoconcentration (HEE-moh-KON-sen-TRAY-shun)
Hemolysis (hee-MAH-lih-siss)
Lymphostasis (LIM-foh-STAY-siss)
Petechiae (pee-TEE-kee-ee)
Phlebotomy (fleh-BOT-uh-mee)
Sclerosed (skle-ROHZD)
Septicemia (sep-tih-SEE-mee-ah)
Tortuous (TOR-choo-uss)
Tourniquet (TOOR-ni-ket)

CHAPTER CONCEPTS

Safety

LEARNING OUTCOMES

1. Define various terms associated with phlebotomy and blood specimens.
2. Identify veins commonly used for venipuncture as well as sites to avoid.
3. Explain how to find and access a vein, including tips for accessing veins in difficult situations.
4. Identify types of equipment used to perform venipuncture.
5. Describe the correct technique for cleansing a venipuncture site.
6. Identify the order of draw for collection tubes when performing venipuncture.
7. Describe the process of venipuncture using the evacuated tube method, syringe method, and butterfly infusion set.
8. Describe how to properly label specimens.
9. Describe complications that can occur as a result of venipuncture and ways to prevent them.
10. Explain when and how to perform a dermal puncture.
11. Discuss information found in the Connection features in this chapter.
12. Identify specific safety information.
13. Answer questions about the skills in this chapter.

SKILLS

34.1 Applying a Tourniquet
34.2 Performing Venipuncture
34.3 Collecting a Blood Culture Specimen
34.4 Performing Dermal Puncture for a Finger Stick Blood Sugar

CRITICAL THINKING CONNECTION

Clinical Assignment

You have been assigned to clinical experience in a medical office, where you will draw blood from several different patients throughout the day. The physician is a family practice physician, so the patients may be of different ages. You are concerned about being able to perform successful venipunctures on all of the patients, especially the elderly patients and the younger children. In addition, you have concerns about how to obtain specimens from patients

CRITICAL THINKING CONNECTION—cont'd

whose veins tend to roll. One of your big concerns is the possibility of a patient fainting when you draw his or her blood.

Critical Thinking Questions:

1. What actions will you take when drawing blood from elderly patients?
2. What actions will you take when drawing blood from young children?
3. How will deal with a patient who feels faint?
4. How can you minimize rolling veins?

Phlebotomy is the puncturing of a vein to withdraw blood. Although most hospitals and clinics hire specially trained individuals, known as *phlebotomists,* for this purpose, it is common for the nurse to draw blood samples as well. In this chapter, you will learn which veins are best to use and tips to make vein access easier. You will learn how to perform *venipuncture*, which means entering the vein with a needle for the purpose of drawing blood. You will also learn the correct labeling procedure for specimens and how to perform dermal punctures.

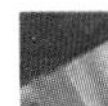

PHLEBOTOMY

As you have already learned, protection from body fluids is always required when caring for patients. It is of particular importance when performing venipuncture because of the potential for exposure to blood and blood-borne pathogens. ***Safety: Always follow personal protective equipment guidelines when performing venipuncture.***

Purposes of Phlebotomy

Blood contains white blood cells (WBCs), red blood cells (RBCs), platelets, oxygen, carbon dioxide, electrolytes, water, vitamins, minerals, proteins, hemoglobin, enzymes, hormones, antibodies, and waste products. The blood acts as the primary source of transportation for all of the substances required by body cells. The blood carries the waste products to the lungs and kidneys, where they can be eliminated from the body. Because blood has so many functions vital to life, blood samples are necessary to help identify problems with organ functions and enable us to diagnose disease and measure its progression.

Preparation of the Patient

A physician's order is required for each laboratory test to be done. Be certain to review the order prior to performing a blood draw and follow facility policy for each order.

As with all interventions, identify your patient using two different methods, which is mandated by The Joint Commission. Usually this is done by asking the patient to tell you his or her first and last name and birthdate. Verify that the computer-generated label matches the information. A third identification check for blood samples includes comparing the label with the patient's identification bracelet. If you are in a medical office, you may request that the patient confirm that the name on the label reads correctly. Positive patient identification can also be made using barcode technology. Scan the bar code on the patient's identification band that is matched against the blood collection order in the handheld computer or other mobile device.

Explain the procedure to the patient in terms that the patient will understand. This helps to reduce anxiety and fear and allows the patient to cooperate with you as you draw the blood sample. Assure the patient that you will be as careful and gentle as possible, but do not give false assurance that the venipuncture will *not* hurt.

Patients should be positioned in the supine or semi-Fowler's or high Fowler's position if they are in bed for this procedure. If you are performing this procedure in a medical office setting, the patient should be seated in a chair. ***Safety: If the patient has problems with hypotension or syncope (fainting), or if the patient voices or exhibits signs of anxiety regarding needles, assist the patient in the supine position before attempting to draw blood. Never attempt phlebotomy while a patient is standing.***

KNOWLEDGE CONNECTION

Why is it important to explain what you are about to do before every procedure? What will you do to protect yourself from contact with body fluids during phlebotomy?

Selecting an Appropriate Vein for Venipuncture

The most commonly used site for venipuncture is the antecubital fossa, which is the shallow depressed area laying anterior to the elbow. However, other sites also may be used. Your selection will vary with each patient. Figure 34.1 shows the superficial veins of the inner aspects of the arm.

The median cubital is generally the vein of choice, followed by the cephalic vein and the basilic vein.

• WORD • BUILDING •

phlebotomy: phlebo – vein + tomy – cutting

venipuncture: veni – vein + puncture

Anatomy and Physiology Connection

Veins and Arteries

There are some differences in veins and arteries. Veins carry deoxygenated blood and waste products from the capillaries back toward the heart, while arteries carry oxygenated blood and nutrients from the heart to the capillaries to be delivered to the body's tissues. The blood pressure (BP) is higher in arteries than in veins, thus necessitating that the artery walls be thicker than those of veins. Both arteries and veins have many **anastomoses,** or junctions where veins join other veins and arteries join other arteries, providing alternate routes for blood flow if one pathway should become obstructed.

Another difference is that veins have valves and arteries do not. The blood in veins must fight against gravity to return to the heart. These valves help to prevent backflow of blood, making it important to avoid damaging the valves when you access the vein for phlebotomy.

Veins on the dorsal side of the hand can also be used to draw blood if the antecubital areas are unavailable, but because they are not secured by as much tissue as the antecubital veins, they tend to roll more than arm veins. They also produce more discomfort with venipuncture than do veins in the antecubital area (Fig. 34.2). If the hand veins do not produce an appropriate site, the wrist veins may be used.

When a blood sample is required in newborns and infants younger than 2 years, dermal puncture is used if at all possible. If a venipuncture is necessary, one of the veins on the dorsal side of the hand is preferred. For newborns, the scalp veins may be accessed but you must be specially trained to perform venipuncture of a scalp vein.

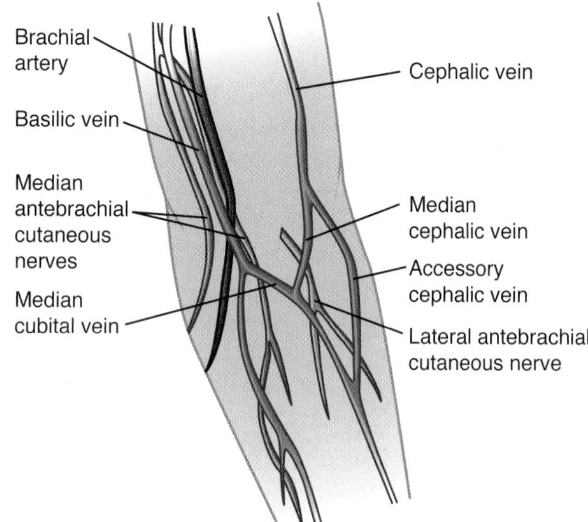

FIGURE 34.1 Superficial veins of the forearm (from DiLorenzo M, Strasinger S. *Blood Collection, A Short Course.* 3rd ed. Philadelphia, PA: FA Davis; 2010).

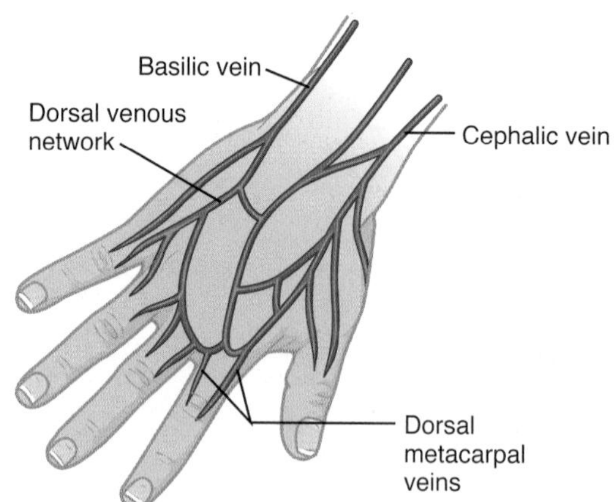

FIGURE 34.2 Superficial veins of the hand (from DiLorenzo M, Strasinger S. *Blood Collection, A Short Course.* 3rd ed. Philadelphia, PA: FA Davis; 2010).

Sites to Avoid

Some veins should not be used for venipuncture because of certain conditions that can alter the quality of the blood specimen. For example, venipuncture should not be performed in an arm with IV access devices because the fluids and medications may dilute or alter the specimen. Use the other arm.

If a patient has had a mastectomy on one side, avoid drawing blood from that arm. Once lymph tissue has been surgically removed, the lymph fluid does not move and remains static, a condition known as **lymphostasis.** To decrease risk of infection, use the opposite arm for venipuncture.

An arm with edema due to other causes should be avoided because the fluid causing the edema may alter test results. Also, if the patient is on dialysis, avoid using the arm where the shunt or fistula is placed. Use the opposite arm instead.

Avoid any sites with altered skin integrity, including the following:

- Rashes
- Incisions or sutures
- Open areas
- Burns
- Severely macerated or softened, weeping skin
- New tattoos
- Abrasions
- Edema
- Contusions

Inserting a needle in these areas could increase the risk of infection. Drawing from an edematous area can result in dilution of the blood sample with serous tissue fluid. Do not perform venipuncture on scarred tissue, even though it is technically "intact." This includes scars from burns, trauma, surgery, and drug abuse.

Avoid using veins that are **tortuous,** or have many twists and turns, and veins that are **sclerosed,** which means that they feel hard and ropey. These conditions may cause decreased blood flow through the area, which could alter the test results. Also avoid sections of veins where valves can be palpated to prevent damaging the valves.

KNOWLEDGE CONNECTION

What is the first vein of choice to use for phlebotomy? The second choice? What veins or sites should be avoided?

Finding a Vein

When inspecting an arm or hand for venipuncture, what you can *see* is not as important as what you can *feel.* Select a vein based on how the vein feels, not on how it looks. Before palpating for a vein, apply a tourniquet around the upper arm several inches above the antecubital area. A **tourniquet** is a flat latex strip that can be snugly wrapped around the arm to occlude the venous return of blood toward the heart. This causes the vein to distend so that it may be better visualized and palpated.

Wearing clean exam gloves, use your index or middle finger to palpate the skin over the areas of the arms or hands where you know the veins are located. Avoid using your thumb to palpate because it is less sensitive. A good vein will be elastic and feel bouncy when palpated. The vein should feel soft, not hard. Feel for the shape and direction of the vein. The size of the vein, of course, is important—the larger the better. Box 34.1 provides a description of how you can learn to locate veins with your eyes closed.

Locating and Accessing Veins in Difficult Situations

Sometimes it is difficult to locate a suitable vein for phlebotomy or to access it once a vein is selected. Some of the situations in which this may occur include the following:

- Obesity
- Dehydration
- Tiny, fragile veins
- Rolling or collapsing veins

Here are a few tips to try in these situations:

- Let gravity assist in filling the veins. Position the patient in such a way that the proposed arm is able to hang dependent, below the level of the heart, for several minutes.
- Apply warm packs. As you learned in Chapter 18, heat dilates veins, allowing more blood to fill them. A warm, wet towel can be applied to the arm and covered with plastic wrap to help hold the heat. Leave in place for 3 to 5 minutes.
- Use an alcohol swab and apply rubbing friction to the area in an attempt to stimulate the vein to distend.
- Massage the arm upward from the wrist to the elbow to help distend the veins.

If the patient is obese, it may be very difficult to palpate a suitable vein through all the tissue. To exert adequate pressure to occlude the veins deep in the tissue will require rather tight application of a tourniquet. If the tourniquet must be applied tighter than usual or the patient's skin is fragile, apply the tourniquet over the gown or shirt sleeve to reduce skin tears and discomfort.

The best vein to feel for venipuncture is the median cubital vein, which normally is the most prominent, followed by the basilic and the cephalic veins. If you are unable to locate a vein in the antecubital area, try the hands and wrists. Most of all, be patient. Allow time for the heat, gravity, tapping, and friction to do their work. Be certain to remove the tourniquet frequently to prevent damage to tissue and veins.

Box 34.1

Finding a Vein With Your Eyes Closed

While learning what a vein "feels like," a good exercise to improve your sensitivity to the feel is to practice with your eyes closed.

- Hold the hand and forearm of a classmate and close your eyes. The classmate will serve as your eyes while you get used to the feel of a vein versus the feel of an area without a palpable vein.
- Lightly bounce your index or middle finger up and down repeatedly on the skin surface, moving across the dorsal side of the hand, where the veins usually are the most easily detected. As you detect the difference in the elasticity and bounce indicating a vein, your partner can verify whether or not you are over a vein.
- After feeling the veins of the hand, move up the arm toward the wrist, then the forearm, and finally to the antecubital areas where the veins usually are not as prominent as they are on the hands.
- Then trade positions with the classmate and allow the classmate to feel while you serve as the eyes.

This exercise will also be useful when you learn to initiate IV access for infusion of fluids and PRN locks in Chapter 38.

KNOWLEDGE CONNECTION

Which sense is most important in locating a suitable vein for phlebotomy—sight or sensation? List several tips that you can use when having trouble locating a vein.

Cleansing the Site

You have learned sterile technique in previous chapters and will be required to put it to use again when performing phlebotomy. You will cleanse the selected site with 70% isopropyl alcohol or chlorhexidine or another bacteriostatic solution according to facility policy. ***Safety: When drawing a specimen for blood alcohol level, alcohol should not be used to cleanse the site because it can contaminate the specimen.*** Clean the site starting at the point where you intend to pierce the skin with the sterile needle and moving outward in concentric circles until an area of 2 to 3 inches has been cleansed. ***Safety: Once you wipe the skin of the next larger concentric circle, do not go back over the previously cleansed center with the same antiseptic wipe because this will bring contamination from the outer edges back to the center of the "cleansed" area.*** Make concentric circles small and tight so that you do not leave dry, contaminated areas between the circles where you cleansed. Allow the site to dry before making the initial puncture. If the alcohol has not dried, it will cause a stinging sensation to the patient and may cause the sample to be hemolyzed. Keep the needle sterile at all times throughout the phlebotomy process.

When drawing blood cultures and arterial blood gases, use povidone-iodine (Betadine) or chlorhexidine gluconate for cleansing the site. If you have excess povidone-iodine on the site, you may wipe if off using *only* a *sterile* gauze pad, such as a 2×2-inch gauze pad.

Equipment and Supplies

A variety of access devices can be used for phlebotomy; each has its own advantages. The three types we will discuss are the evacuated tube system, syringe and needle, and butterfly or winged infusion set. There are also different types of tubes that you must use. Box 34.2 presents a list of equipment used in venipuncture.

Evacuated Tube System

To use the evacuated tube system, you will need a double-pointed needle, an evacuated tube, and a plastic barrel-shaped holder, which are diagrammed in Figure 34.3. The **evacuated tube** is a plastic or glass tube closed with a colored rubber stopper or a rubber stopper surrounded by a colored plastic top, from which a certain amount of air has been evacuated. Evacuation of the air leaves a vacuum inside the tube that will cause blood to flow into the tube once the tube is activated. The volume of blood that enters the tube equals the specific volume of air that was evacuated. The tube is activated by pushing the rubber stopper onto the sheathed pointed end of the needle that has been screwed into the plastic holder.

The rubber stoppers are color coded according to the type of additive the tube contains. Each laboratory test has a designated tube-top color and additive that must be used when drawing the blood sample (Fig. 34.4).

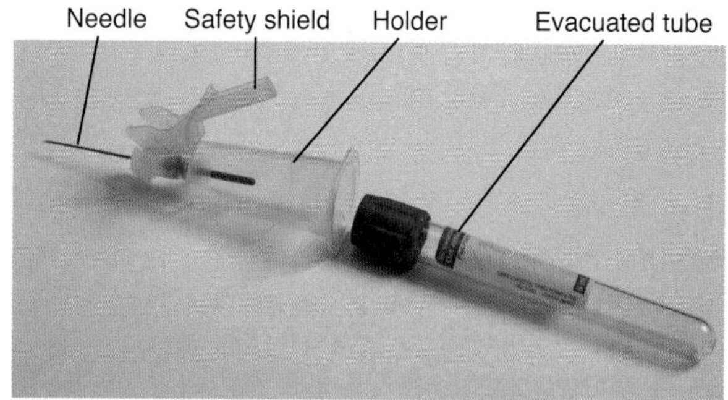

FIGURE 34.3 An evacuated tube system (from DiLorenzo M, Strasinger S. *Blood Collection, A Short Course.* 3rd ed. Philadelphia, PA: FA Davis; 2010).

Box 34.2

Venipuncture Equipment

It saves an extraordinary amount of time and energy to gather all needed supplies and equipment prior to initiating work at the patient's bedside. Make it a habit to be prepared before beginning venipuncture. The common items you will need to perform venipuncture include the following:

- Requisition for specific laboratory tests
- Labels for collection tubes
- Examination gloves
- Alcohol or chlorhexidine gluconate povidone-iodine wipes
- Tourniquet or BP cuff
- Either a (1) double-pointed needle and a plastic tube holder or a (2) 1-inch, 21- or 23-gauge needle or a butterfly infusion set and a syringe
- Specific collection tubes for ordered tests
- 2×2-inch gauze pad
- 1-inch tape or bandage
- Plastic zippered or sealable bags for transportation of blood samples to laboratory

NEEDLES. Needles come in different lengths from ½ inch to 2 inches. The common lengths used for phlebotomy vary from ½ inch for a newborn to 1 ½ inches for an obese adult. The diameter of the needle is known as the gauge of the needle, and they range from 16 to 30 gauge. Remember that the larger the number, the smaller the size. Most phlebotomy is performed using between 20-gauge and 23-gauge needles. Preserve the sterility of the needle throughout the phlebotomy process. ***Safety: Needles are used only once! Never restick a patient using the same needle.***

To use the evacuated tubes, you will need a special double-pointed needle designed solely for the evacuated tube system. One end of the needle is covered with a rubber sheath that screws into the needle end of the plastic tube holder. The other end of the needle is the portion that will be inserted into the patient's vein.

PLASTIC TUBE HOLDER. You will also need a plastic tube holder, a round barrel that has a small opening on one end into which the needle is screwed, and is open on the other end, which allows insertion of the evacuated tube (refer to Fig. 34.3). The tube is loosely inserted into the holder while the actual venipuncture is made. Once the needle tip is inside the patient's vein, the evacuated tube is activated by carefully pushing the rubber stopper of the tube onto the sheathed end of the needle. This movement forces the rubber sheath to scrunch up against the hub of the needle. Pushing the tube onto the needle activates the vacuum in the tube so that it will pull blood from the vein into the tube. The tube holder with needle still in place is disposed of in the sharps container after use.

The advantage of this system is its ease of use and the reduced risk of needle-stick injuries, especially when drawing blood for multiple tests. The contaminated needle is left uncapped, with the safety device engaged, and disposed of in a sharps container, which is made of hard plastic that is impervious to puncture by needles (Fig. 34.5). ***Safety: Always use safety needles. Never recap a contaminated needle. Activate the safety device as soon as you withdraw the needle from the patient's arm (Fig. 34.6).***

BD Vacutainer® Venous Blood Collection Tube Guide

Tubes with BD Hemogard™ Closure	Tubes with Conventional Stopper	Additive	Inversions at Blood Collection*	Laboratory Use
Gold	Red/Black	• Clot activator and gel for serum separation	5	For serum determinations in chemistry. May be used for routine blood donor screening and diagnostic testing of serum for infectious disease.** Tube inversions ensure mixing of clot activator with blood. Blood clotting time: 30 minutes.
Light Green	Green/Gray	• Lithium heparin and gel for plasma separation	8	BD Vacutainer® PST™ Tube for plasma determinations in chemistry. Tube inversions prevent clotting.
Red		• None (glass) • Clot activator (plastic)	0 5	For serum determinations in chemistry. May be used for routine blood donor screening and diagnostic testing of serum for infectious disease.** Tube inversions ensure mixing of clot activator with blood. Blood clotting time: 60 minutes.
Orange	Gray/Yellow	• Thrombin	8	For stat serum determinations in chemistry. Tube inversions ensure complete clotting, which usually occurs in less than 5 minutes.
Royal Blue		• Clot activator (plastic serum) • K_2EDTA (plastic)	8 8 0 5 8	For trace-element, toxicology, and nutritional chemistry determinations. Special stopper formulation provides low levels of trace elements (see package insert).
Green		• Sodium heparin • Lithium heparin	8 8	For plasma determinations in chemistry. Tube inversions prevent clotting.
Gray		• Potassium oxalate/sodium fluoride • Sodium fluoride/Na_2 EDTA • Sodium fluoride (serum tube)	8 8 8	For glucose determinations. Oxalate and EDTA anticoagulants will give plasma samples. Sodium fluoride is the antiglycolytic agent. Tube inversions ensure proper mixing of additive and blood.
Tan		• K_2EDTA (plastic)	8 8	For lead determinations. This tube is certified to contain less than .01 μg/mL (ppm) lead. Tube inversions prevent clotting.
	Yellow	• Sodium polyanethol sulfonate (SPS) • Acid citrate dextrose additives (ACD): Solution A - 22.0 g/L trisodium citrate, 8.0 g/L citric acid, 24.5 g/L dextrose Solution B - 13.2 g/L trisodium citrate, 4.8 g/L citric acid, 14.7 g/L dextrose	8 8 8	SPS for blood culture specimen collections in microbiology. Tube inversions prevent clotting. ACD for use in blood bank studies, HLA phenotyping, and DNA and paternity testing.
Lavender		• Liquid K_3EDTA (glass) • Spray-coated K_2EDTA (plastic)	8 8	K_2EDTA and K_3EDTA for whole blood hematology determinations. K_2EDTA may be used for routine immunohematology testing and blood donor screening.*** Tube inversions prevent clotting.
White		• K_2EDTA with gel	8	For use in molecular diagnostic test methods (such as but not limited to polymerase chain reaction [PCR] and/or branched DNA [bDNA] amplification techniques).
Pink		• Spray-coated K_2EDTA	8	For whole blood hematology determinations. May be used for routine immunohematology testing and blood donor screening.*** Designed with special cross-match label for patient information required by the AABB. Tube inversions prevent clotting.
Light Blue	Clear	• Buffered sodium citrate 0.105 M (≈3.2%) glass 0.109 M (≈3.2%) plastic • Citrate, theophylline, adenosine, dipyridamole (CTAD)	3-4 3-4	For coagulation determinations. CTAD for platelet function assays and routine coagulation determination. Tube inversions prevent clotting.
Clear	Red/Gray	• None (plastic)	0	For use as a discard tube or secondary specimen collection tube.
Partial-draw Tubes (2 ml and 3 mL: 13 x 75 mm)		**Additive**	**Inversions at Blood Collection***	**Laboratory Use**
Red		• None	0	For serum determinations in chemistry. May be used for routine blood donor screening, immunohematology testing,*** and diagnostic testing of serum for infectious disease.** Tube inversions ensure mixing of clot activator with blood. Blood clotting time: 60 minutes.
Green		• Sodium heparin • Lithium heparin	8 8	For plasma determinations in chemistry. Tube inversions prevent clotting.
Lavender		• Spray-coated K_2EDTA (plastic)	8 8	For whole blood hematology determinations. May be used for routine immunohematology testing and blood donor screening.*** Tube inversions prevent clotting.
Small-volume Pediatric Tubes (2 mL: 10.25 x 47 mm, 3 mL: 10.25 x 64 mm)		**Additive**	**Inversions at Blood Collection***	**Laboratory Use**
Light Blue		• 0.105 M sodium citrate (≈3.2%)	3-4	For coagulation determinations. Tube inversions prevent clotting.

* Invert gently, do not shake

** The performance characteristics of these tubes have not been established for infectious disease testing in general; therefore, users must validate the use of these tubes for their specific assay-instrument/reagent system combinations and specimen storage conditions.

*** The performance characteristics of these tubes have not been established for immunohematology testing in general; therefore, users must validate the use of these tubes for their specific assay-instrument/reagent system combinations and specimen storage conditions.

BD Tube Guide. Courtesy and © 2008 Becton, Dickinson and Company.

FIGURE 34.4 BD Vacutainer tube guide (from the *BD Vacutainer® Venous Blood Collection Tube Guide*. Franklin Lakes, NJ: Becton, Dickinson and Company; 2010).

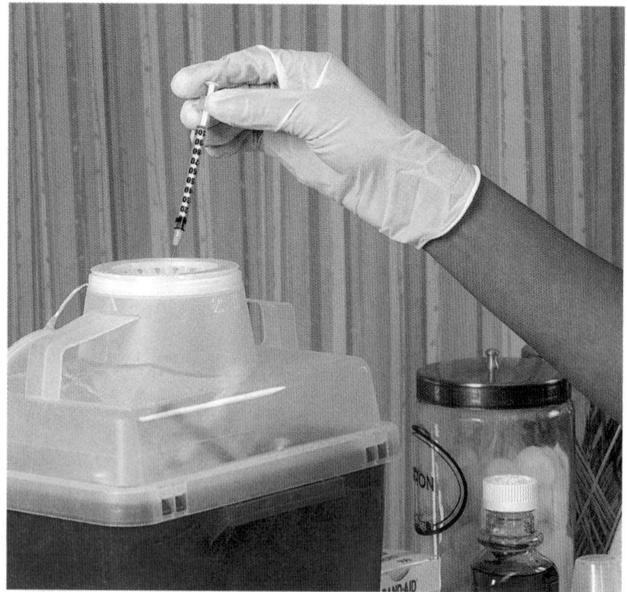

FIGURE 34.5 Always dispose of needles, glass, and other "sharps" in clearly labeled sharps containers. These containers must be puncture proof and clearly marked, and typically are red so they are easily identified (from Wilkinson JM, Treas LS. *Fundamentals of Nursing: Theory, Concepts & Applications*. Vol. 1. 2nd ed. Philadelphia, PA: FA Davis; 2011).

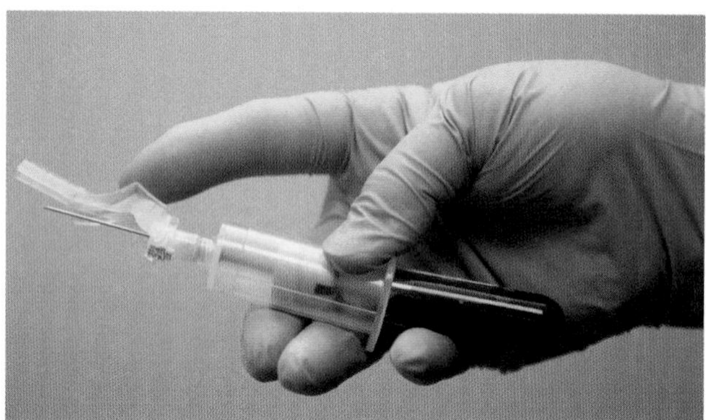

FIGURE 34.6 Activate the safety device immediately to reduce the risk of contaminated needle-stick injuries.

Needle-and-Syringe Method

The vacuum in the evacuated tube system may be too strong and cause vein collapse of the smaller and more fragile veins in the elderly and children. For these veins, it may work better to use a needle and a syringe for venipuncture (Fig. 34.7). The syringe will allow you to control the rate at which the blood is pulled from the vein. The slower the extraction of the blood, the less chance there is of vein collapse. A small needle, such as a 1-inch-length, 22- or 23-gauge needle, can be used for this method. Anything smaller can destroy the RBCs, which release the hemoglobin and cellular contents into the plasma. This destruction of RBCs is known as **hemolysis.**

Blood drawn with a syringe is immediately transferred to the correct evacuated tube to prevent blood clots from forming. To do this, a device is used that allows for the blood transfer without using the syringe needle or removing the rubber stopper in the tube. After the blood is collected, the safety needle is activated and removed, and then the syringe tip is inserted into the hub of the transfer device. Then the evacuated tubes are filled by pushing them onto the rubber-sheeted needle in the transfer device (Fig. 34.8).

Butterfly or Winged Infusion Sets

The butterfly or winged infusion set is especially useful for small or fragile veins (Fig. 34.9). The needle size may vary from 21 to 23 gauge and from ½ to ⅝ inch in length. The needle has two rubber wings at the base that fold upward to allow for easy holding. Tiny tubing extends from the needle for 6 to 8 inches and attaches to either a plastic holder or a Luer-Lok syringe. The advantage is that having the syringe farther from the needle allows for easier maneuvering. The winged needle also allows for stabilization of the needle with a piece of tape, making it ideal for use with children or elderly adults. The winged infusion sets also come with safety devices attached to the needle, which should be activated immediately after withdrawing the needle from the patient's skin.

> **KNOWLEDGE CONNECTION**
>
> How do you activate an evacuated tube? What is hemolysis? What equipment is needed for each of the three methods of performing venipuncture?

Tubes With Color-Coded Tops

As mentioned previously, the tops of phlebotomy tubes are color coded to designate the combination of additives that are within the tube. These additives are specific to certain laboratory tests so that the different colored tops indicate different laboratory tests. Each manufacturer uses slightly different colors and additives. At the facility where you work, you will need to memorize the colors and the tests for which they are used. Table 34.1 lists tube-top colors and some of their designated tests.

In addition to using aseptic technique, using the correct *the order of draw* is a very important aspect of phlebotomy. Additives from tubes that are drawn first can contaminate the subsequently drawn blood samples, requiring that certain tubes be drawn in a designated sequence. Table 34.1 includes the tube-top colors, their additives, the order in which to draw the tubes, and common tests.

Different types of anticoagulants are added to different tubes for different tests. All tubes that have anticoagulants in them have to be mixed immediately after they are filled. This is done by gently inverting the tube three to eight times, depending on the type of tube. Follow your facility's lab guidelines for the number of times to invert each tube. ***Safety: Avoid shaking a tube containing blood and an anticoagulant because it can cause hemolysis. Gently invert all anticoagulated tubes the specified number of times.***

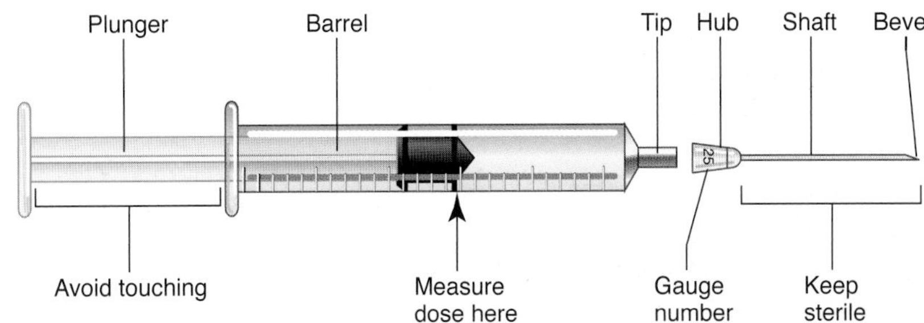

FIGURE 34.7 Parts of a syringe and needle (from Wilkinson JM, Treas LS. *Fundamentals of Nursing: Theory, Concepts & Applications*. Vol. 1. 2nd ed. Philadelphia, PA: FA Davis; 2011).

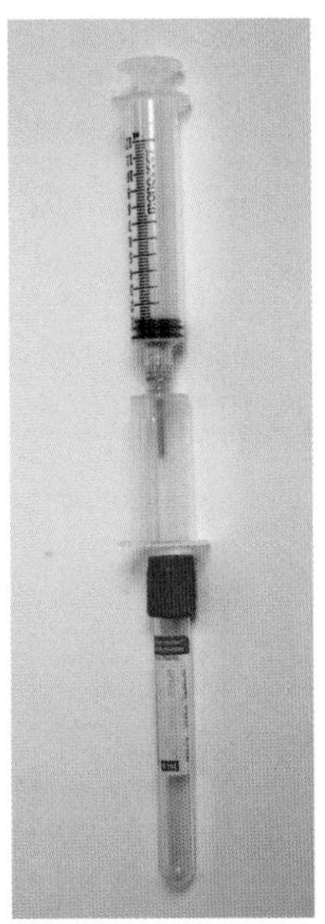

FIGURE 34.8 Using a transfer device to transfer blood from a syringe to an evacuated tube (from DiLorenzo M, Strasinger S. *Blood Collection, A Short Course*. 3rd ed. Philadelphia, PA: FA Davis; 2010).

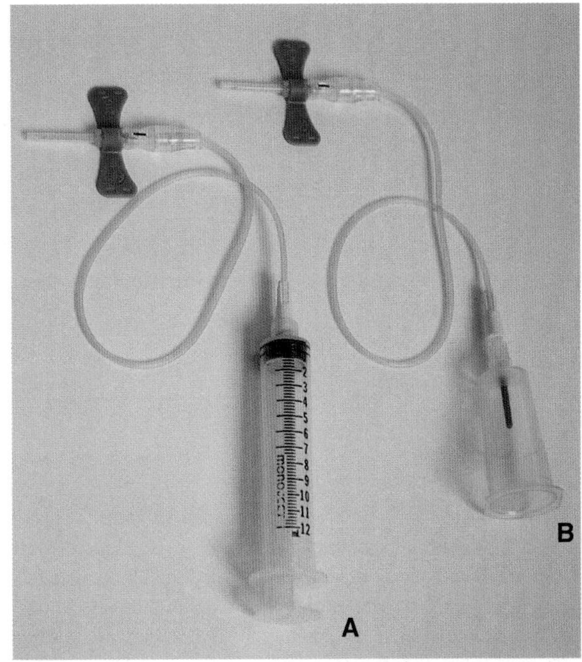

FIGURE 34.9 Butterfly collection sets: (a) Butterfly needle attached to a syringe; (b) Butterfly needle attached to an evacuated tube holder (from DiLorenzo M, Strasinger S. *Blood Collection, A Short Course*. 3rd ed. Philadelphia, PA: FA Davis; 2010).

LABELS. All specimens must be labeled before they are sent to the laboratory. Most facilities use computer-generated labels. Always apply the labels after the specimen is drawn and always attach the label before you leave the room. ***Safety: Attach the label to the collection tube in the patient's room or exam room after the blood specimen is drawn.*** Labeling the collection tubes before actually obtaining the specimen allows for two errors to occur:

1. The labeled collection tube may be used for drawing blood from the wrong patient.
2. Completing the label ahead of time may lead to inaccuracy regarding time of draw.

Box 34.3 presents the required data for labeling specimens.

Tourniquet

Tourniquets are most commonly flat, nonlatex strips about 1-inch wide and 16- to 18-inches long. All tourniquets are one-time use only and then are disposed of. The tourniquet is placed around the arm 3 to 4 inches above the site for venipuncture. The tourniquet is applied tight enough to occlude the superficial veins that you will be using but should allow blood to flow in the deeper arteries. If you are using the antecubital site for drawing blood, the tourniquet should be placed about 3 to 4 inches above the antecubital area, and there should be a palpable radial pulse. ***Safety: The tourniquet should never be left in place for longer than 1 minute.*** Leaving the tourniquet on longer can cause hemolysis or **hemoconcentration,** a concentration of RBCs in the blood sample due to a decrease in the volume of plasma allowed to flow. If the tourniquet is applied too tightly, it can result in pinpoint areas of hemorrhage, known as **petechiae,** or cause bruises, called **hematomas.**

In patients whose veins are difficult to locate or are fragile, as is common in elderly patients, a sphygmomanometer or BP cuff can be used in place of a tourniquet. It allows for a more even distribution of the pressure applied to the arm to occlude the venous return. This prevents the *rupture* or *"blowing"* of tiny and fragile veins. It also allows for better

• WORD • BUILDING •

hemoconcentration: hemo – blood + con – together + centr – center + ation – action

Table 34.1
Evacuated Tube-Top Colors, Draw Sequence, and Designated Tests

Draw Sequence	*Tube-Top Color*	*Tests*	*Additive*
First	Yellow or blood culture bottles	Blood culture	Sterile media bottles
Second	Light blue	Coagulation tests such as partial thromboplastin time, prothrombin time	Sodium citrate
Third	Red, red and gray, or gold	Chemistry tests, serology, blood bank	None or clot activator or gel separator
Fourth	Green	Ammonia, stat electrolytes, arterial blood gases	Heparin, may have gel separator
Fifth	Lavender or pink	Complete blood count, crossmatch, sedimentation rate	Ethylenediaminetetraacetic acid (EDTA)
Sixth	Gray	Glucose, lactic acid, blood alcohol level	Potassium oxylate or sodium fluoride
Seventh	Yellow	Blood bank studies, DNA and paternity testing	Sodium polyanetholsulfonate (SPS) and acid citrate dextrose (ACD)

Box 34.3
Required Data for Labeling Specimens

Avoid labeling blood specimen tubes prior to the blood draw to reduce the inaccuracy of recording the time the blood specimen was drawn and inadvertently mismatching the labels to another patient's blood specimen tubes. There may be more than one patient with the same name, so be careful to include all needed identifying data. The label should include the following information:

- Patient's first and last name
- Hospital identification number (inpatient) or date of birth (outpatient)
- Health-care provider's name
- Type of test ordered
- Date and time specimen was collected
- Your initials

distention of the distal veins. The cuff is pumped to 40 mm Hg to allow blood to flow into but not out of the veins.

Gloves

Nonlatex exam gloves without powder are always worn when palpating for a vein and when performing phlebotomy due to the risk of contact with blood. The Occupational Safety and Health Administration mandates that gloves must be worn and changed after every patient. The gloves should fit tightly enough to aid with vein detection using your fingertips. Other personal protective equipment, such as goggles, may be worn due to the risk of splashing. ***Safety: Always wash your hands before application and after removal of gloves. Change gloves between patients to avoid cross-contamination.***

KNOWLEDGE CONNECTION

When should tubes of blood be labeled? What data should be on the label? How long can you safely leave a tourniquet on a patient's arm?

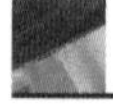

PERFORMING VENIPUNCTURE

Once you have located a vein using the tourniquet, remove the tourniquet while you cleanse the site and make certain all supplies are positioned within easy reach. Using either alcohol or an antiseptic designated by facility policy, cleanse the site starting in the center and making concentric circles outward until a 2-inch area has been prepared. Allow the site to dry for 30 to 60 seconds. Do not fan the site with your hand or blow on it to speed drying. Make certain the site is not touched while it is drying and during reapplication of the tourniquet. If the site is accidentally contaminated before the dermal puncture is made, the site must be cleansed again.

Reapply the tourniquet 3 to 4 inches above the proposed site, tucking the tourniquet from the top so that the ends will not flop onto the cleansed area (see Skill 34.1, page 766). Aseptically uncap the needle. Hold the plastic tube holder or syringe in your dominant hand, with the needle bevel facing upward, your thumb on top, and your fingers underneath the holder to allow you to press fingers against the patient's arm for stabilization while changing tubes.

Position the needle at an angle of 15 to 30 degrees. If the vein is shallow, use 15 degrees, and if the vein is deeper, increase the angle as needed up to 30 degrees. When making the dermal puncture, use a swift, smooth motion to decrease discomfort. As the needle enters the vein, you may feel a lessening of resistance against the needle. If the vein is not successfully accessed with the initial puncture, *do not probe blindly*. Use the index finger of your nondominant hand to carefully palpate the vein proximal to the tip of the inserted needle to determine where the needle tip is in relationship to the vein. If the needle is not in the vein, it must be in one of four positions: either it is above the vein, to the right of the vein, below the vein, or to the left of the vein. While palpating, take care not to contaminate the needle or the needle insertion site. Once you have determined the relative position of the vein and needle, redirect the needle to enter the vein. ***Safety: Only move the needle forward or backward to prevent tissue damage. Do not move the needle side to side.***

Once the needle enters the vein, gently push the evacuated tube onto the needle. Keep the needle stable and be careful not to push the needle through the vein. The evacuated tube will stop filling at a predesignated volume. If using a syringe, use your nondominant hand to slowly pull back on the plunger, allowing the syringe to fill to the required amount. If you pull the plunger back too quickly, it can cause the vein to collapse or hemolysis of RBCs to occur

When more than one tube is required, keep in mind the correct order of draw. As each tube is filled, continue to keep your dominant hand braced against the patient's arm. Avoid moving the needle while removing or advancing the tube onto the needle. Once the last tube is pushed onto the needle, remove the tourniquet. *Remember that the tourniquet should stay on the arm no longer than 1 minute.*

Once the last tube has filled completely, remove it from the holder, and withdraw the needle from the patient's arm. Immediately apply a 2×2-inch gauze pad to hold pressure on the puncture site. Activate the needle safety device promptly.

Hold pressure on the site for a full 1 to 2 minutes until the bleeding stops, or longer if needed. If you withdrew multiple tubes of blood or the patient is known to have a tendency to bleed longer, it may be helpful to have the patient elevate the arm above the heart level while holding direct pressure on the puncture site. ***Safety: Do not allow the patient to flex the elbow to hold the pressure on the site, as it tends to increase hematoma formation.*** The bleeding should always stop within a maximum of 3 to 5 minutes unless the patient is on anticoagulants, which may require you to hold pressure on the site for 10 minutes or longer. After the bleeding has stopped, secure the gauze pad to the site with a piece of tape or a self-adhering wrap. Instruct the patient that the tape or wrap should be removed after 15 minutes and to avoid carrying anything heavy with that arm for 1 hour.

Complete and inspect the labels for accuracy of information. Then attach the labels to each tube before leaving the patient's side to avoid accidental mismatching of specimens and patient labels. In some facilities, you will ask the patient to verify that their name is correct on the label and spelled correctly. Place the specimens inside a designated container such as a plastic bag for transport to the laboratory. Dispose of contaminated items in the appropriate sharps container. Remove gloves and wash your hands. The specimens should be immediately transported to the laboratory. Document the procedure.

Skill 34.2 (page 767) details the steps in performing venipuncture.

KNOWLEDGE CONNECTION

Describe the process of drawing a blood specimen. Where are contaminated items disposed of?

Laboratory and Diagnostic Connection

Drawing Blood Culture Specimens

Normally the blood is sterile within the vascular system. But when the patient is suspected of having an infection in his or her blood, otherwise known as **septicemia,** blood specimens may be drawn to determine if organisms are present in the blood, and, if so, which specific organism is the culprit. This test is known as a **blood culture.** Blood culture specimens are normally drawn during temperature spikes to better detect if organisms are present in the blood. When blood cultures are ordered, special care must be taken when drawing the blood specimen to ensure that no contamination of the specimen occurs.

Blood culture specimens usually are drawn in two separate long-necked bottles that fit into the plastic tube holder and advance onto the sheathed end of the needle. The first one that is drawn is used to determine if **anaerobic** organisms are present. Anaerobes are organisms that can live and replicate without oxygen. The second specimen drawn is for **aerobic** organisms, or those that grow and replicate in the presence of oxygen. When drawing blood culture specimens, it is critical to maintain asepsis and to draw the correct volume of blood. Always check the facility policy for volume of blood to be drawn for the specific type of specimen bottles used. Skill 34.3 (page 769) details the steps in collecting a blood culture specimen.

COMPLICATIONS OF PHLEBOTOMY

Several complications may occur during phlebotomy. There are several actions you can take to try to prevent these complications.

- Hematoma—bruising that occurs when blood leaks out of the vein into the tissue:
  - Remove the tourniquet prior to removing the needle from the vein.

• WORD • BUILDING •

hematoma: hemat – blood + oma – tumor
anaerobic: an – without + aero – air + bic – related to life
aerobic: aero – air + bic – related to life

- Hold pressure over the puncture site for at least 1 to 2 minutes. Hold longer—3 to 5 minutes—if the patient is on anticoagulants.
- If a hematoma does form, apply a cold cloth or small ice pack.
- Infection due to nonintact skin after a venipuncture:
  - Use strict aseptic technique for venipuncture.
  - Cleanse the site thoroughly and correctly.
- Patient complains of feeling faint, light-headed, or nauseated:
  - Offer a cold cloth or compress applied to the forehead and neck.
  - Assist the patient to a supine position or to lower the patient's head to between the knees.
  - If the patient experiences syncope during the blood draw, immediately remove the tourniquet and needle, and hold pressure on the site.
- Failure to obtain blood can be the result of several problems, which can be fixed as follows:
  - **The needle is not in the vein:** Palpate the vein proximal to the needle and redirect the needle.
  - **The needle is against a valve or wall of the vein:** Pull back on or rotate the needle slightly.
  - **The evacuated tube has lost its vacuum:** Insert another tube.
  - **The vein has collapsed because an evacuated tube that was too large was used or the plunger of the syringe was pulled back too quickly:** Remove the evacuated tube or cease pulling back on the syringe plunger. Remove the tourniquet to allow additional blood flow to the arm. Reapply the tourniquet and use a smaller tube or draw back on the syringe plunger more slowly.
  - **The vein rolls:** Use the index finger and thumb of your nondominant hand to anchor the vein both above and below the intended insertion site while making the puncture.
  - **The veins are tiny or fragile:** Use a winged infusion set with a syringe rather than an evacuated tube system in which the vacuum may be too strong for a fragile vein. Once access has been gained, pull back on the syringe plunger very gently and slowly to decrease the risk of rupturing or collapsing the vein.

If these attempts to fix the problem fail, remove the needle and perform venipuncture in the other arm using a fresh sterile needle.

KNOWLEDGE CONNECTION

What are possible complications of phlebotomy? What nursing actions should you take to reduce the risk of these complications? If they do occur, what should you do?

Settings Connection: Home Health

Drawing Blood in the Home Setting

If you work as a home health nurse, you may be required to draw blood specimens from homebound patients who are unable to make the trip to a lab or medical office. These patients may need close monitoring of certain blood levels to manage diseases and illnesses or manage medications. You will take all the equipment and supplies needed with you. You will be very careful to use aseptic technique at all times in the home. After you perform the venipuncture and obtain the specimen(s), you will also be responsible for transporting the tubes to the nearest laboratory used by the ordering health-care provider.

Evidence-Based Practice

Blood Tests and Hospital-Acquired Anemia

Clinical Question

Can drawing blood for tests cause hospital-acquired anemia?

Evidence

A retrospective study was done at a hospital in Providence, RI, using a chart review of electronic health records. A total of 479 patients who were not anemic on admission to the hospital were included in the study. Between admission and discharge, 65% were found to have a hemoglobin lowered by 1.0 g/dl or more and 49% of the patients developed anemia. It was determined in the study that using smaller tubes helped decrease the patient's anemia risk.

Implications for Nursing Practice

Those with a lower body mass index and longer hospital stays had a higher risk for developing hospital-acquired anemia, which turns out to be quite common. Decreasing the frequency of blood draws and using smaller volume tubes for blood testing can help decrease the incidence of hospital-acquired anemia.

Reference

You can read more about this study at www.hindawi.com/journals/anemia/2014/634582/.

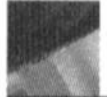

DERMAL PUNCTURES

Dermal punctures are a simpler way to obtain blood specimens for some tests. They are used when veins are inaccessible and are the preferred method of obtaining blood specimens from children younger than 2 years. The site for puncture in children older than 2 years and in adults is the fleshy portion just to the side of the center of the fingertip. Avoid the tip end of the finger as well as the sides, where there is less flesh between the skin and the bone (Figs. 34.10

and 34.11). ***Safety: Do not puncture the index finger because of its high number of nerve endings, which makes puncturing it more painful.*** The pinkie finger has less flesh and is rarely used except on patients with severely calloused hands, which do not bleed easily with a dermal puncture. In this situation, the pinkie finger may be pierced because it is less calloused and will generally bleed better.

In children younger than 2 years, the heel is used rather than a fingertip. The puncture should be made on the medial and lateral aspects of the fleshy portion of the plantar surface of the heel. Avoid piercing the posterior edge or sides of the heel where the skin is closer to the calcaneus bone.

The skin is punctured using a spring-loaded lancet that is self-limiting regarding the depth and width of the puncture. The blood is collected in a micro-collection tube or a capillary tube, or it is applied directly to a testing strip for a test such as a finger stick blood sugar (FSBS). Figure 34.12 shows one type of FSBS testing monitor, and Figure 34.13 shows lancets, a micro-collection tube, a capillary tube, and one type of FSBS strip.

Settings Connection: Medical Office

Dermal Puncture Sites

In newborns and infants up to 2 years of age, the heel is used for skin punctures. The fingers cannot be used in part because of inadequate blood flow produced by the tiny fingers, but most importantly to avoid damaging the nerves and bone that are closer to the surface than in an adult. Make the puncture along the medial or lateral aspect of the *heel pad* but avoid moving too far to either side and extending beyond the plantar surface so that you actually puncture the side of the heel and foot (Fig. 34.10). In older children and adults, the preferred site for dermal puncture is the fingertip. Make the puncture on the palmar surface of the most distal phalanx of one of the fingers (Fig. 34.11). Avoid puncturing the very tip of the finger or along the sides of the finger where the tissue is thinner.

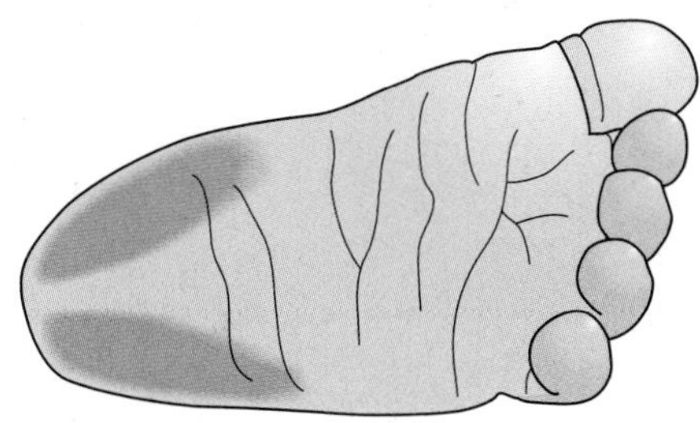
For infants: Perform skin puncture on the lateral aspects of the plantar surface of the heel
FIGURE 34.10 For infants, perform skin puncture on the lateral aspects of the plantar surface of the heel.

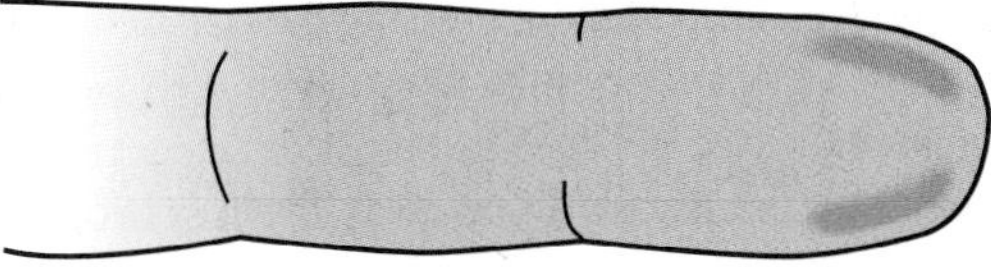
For older children and adults: Perform skin puncture on the lateral aspects of the palmar side of the distal phalanx (fingertip)
FIGURE 34.11 For older children and adults, perform skin puncture on the lateral aspects of the palmar side of the distal phalanx (fingertip).

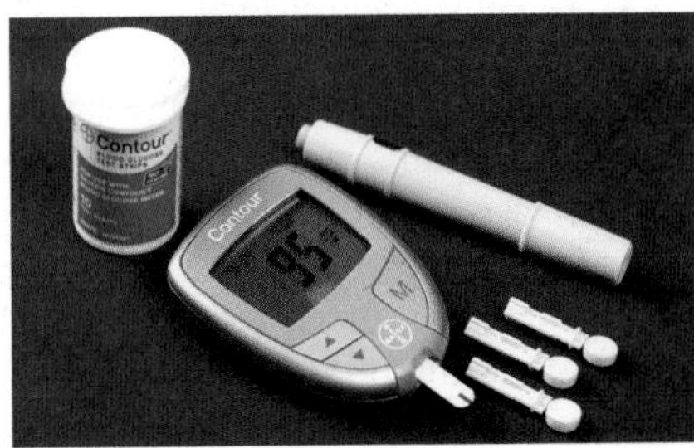
Contour
FIGURE 34.12 Finger stick blood sugar monitor, bottle of strips, and lancet holder (from Wilkinson JM, Treas LS, Barnett KL, Smith MH. *Fundamentals of Nursing: Theory, Concepts & Applications*. Vol. 2. 3rd ed. Philadelphia, PA: FA Davis; 2016).

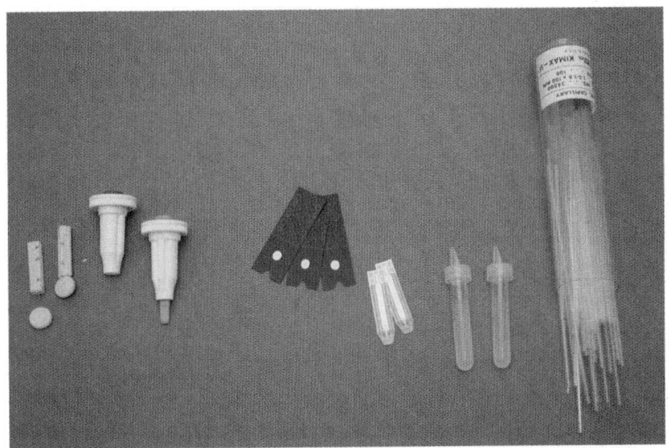
FIGURE 34.13 From left to right: Two styles of lancets to make skin puncture; two types of finger stick blood sugar strips upon which the drop of blood is placed; microcollection tubes and capillary tubes in which the blood sample is placed.

Performing Dermal Puncture

Before dermal puncture, warm the patient's hand if it is cold by placing it in warm water for a few minutes. The heat will dilate the vessels, providing better blood flow when the skin is pierced.

Begin by cleansing the site with alcohol and allowing it to dry. Wearing gloves, hold the patient's hand lower than the heart to allow for better capillary filling. Keep the fingertip lower than the palm of the patient's hand, holding it between your thumb and index finger. If you are using a spring-loaded lancet, place the device firmly against the sides of the fleshy aspect of the fingertip without pressing the device hard enough to indent the skin. Do not stick the sides or the tips of the fingers where the tissue is thin. Then press the lancet release button to activate the lancet. Wipe away the first drop of blood with sterile gauze to avoid alteration of the specimen by the dried alcohol on the skin or tissue fluid from the puncture site.

Now firmly squeeze the fingertip, alternately squeezing and releasing the pressure to express the blood sample. Avoid strenuously massaging or milking the puncture site to produce blood flow because this can cause hemolysis and dilution of the sample with tissue fluids. If a capillary tube is being used to collect the specimen, hold the tube horizontally and touch the tip of the tube *lightly* to the drop of blood, but do not allow the tube to touch the puncture site itself. If the tube is not held horizontally, air bubbles will be introduced into the sample. When done correctly, capillary action will draw the blood into the tube. Avoid scraping the capillary tube against the skin in an attempt to collect the blood because this can cause hemolysis. Once the tube is filled, tap the end of the capillary tube into the sealant clay to seal it.

If a microcollection tube is used, hold the tip of the collection scoop beneath the puncture site so it touches the underside of the blood drop and then allow the blood to run through the scoop and down the inside of the tube. Avoid touching the collection device to the puncture site or scraping it over the skin. When the tube is filled, apply the color-coded top and invert it 5 to 10 times.

If an FSBS is to be performed, use the designated strip for the specific monitor that will read the blood sample. Lightly touch the strip to the drop of blood and allow capillary action to pull the blood onto the strip so that the monitor can read the glucose level. Skill 34.4 (page 770) provides more information on performing a dermal puncture for an FSBS.

After the blood sample is collected, hold a 2×2-inch gauze pad over the puncture site with gentle but firm pressure to stop the bleeding. Dispose of contaminated items in the sharps container. Remove gloves and wash your hands. Document the procedure.

KNOWLEDGE CONNECTION

What sites are used for dermal punctures in adults? In infants?

Supervision/Delegation Connection

Phlebotomy

Phlebotomy should not be delegated to unlicensed personnel. Only certified phlebotomists, laboratory technicians, or licensed nurses should draw blood specimens. Dermal punctures for FSBS can be safely delegated to certified nursing assistants and unlicensed assistive personnel who have been specifically trained in how to perform the procedure.

Skill 34.1 Applying a Tourniquet

Assessment Steps

1. Assess the fragility of the patient's skin ***to determine if the tourniquet should be placed over the sleeve of the patient's gown.***
2. Assess the antecubital areas of both arms ***to evaluate the quality of the veins.***

Planning Steps

1. Select the vein that feels most suitable.

Implementation Steps

1. Follow the Initial Implementation Steps located on the inside back cover.
2. Place the rubber tourniquet under the upper arm, midway between the shoulder and the antecubital areas.
3. Bring the two ends around the arm and cross them over the upper arm (for right-handed individuals), with the left end crossing below the right end or, for left-handed individuals, with the right end crossing below the left end.

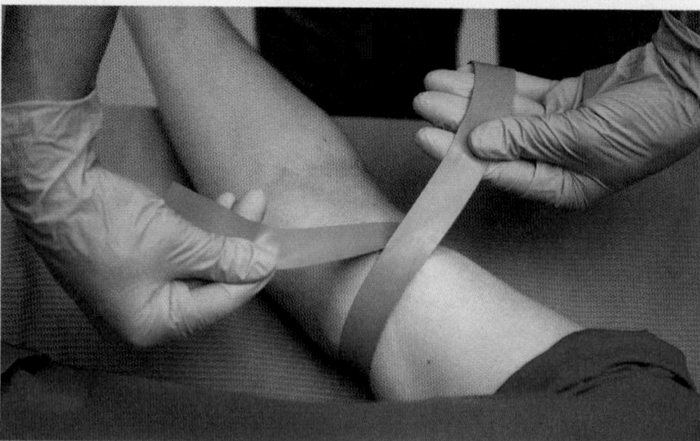

Skill 34.1 (continued)

4. With your nondominant hand, grasp the tourniquet where it crosses over itself and grasp the lower tubing end with your dominant hand.

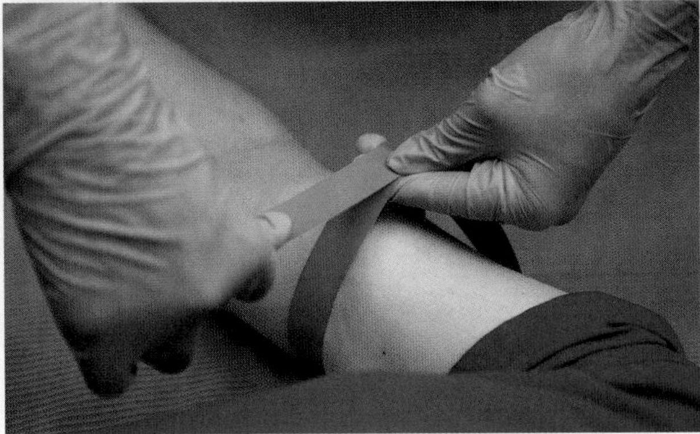

5. Pull the end in your dominant hand until it is taut, and use your nondominant hand to maintain the tension where the two ends cross.
6. Using your dominant hand, tuck the end of the tourniquet into the top side of the band that is now wrapped around the arm and held in place by your nondominant hand.

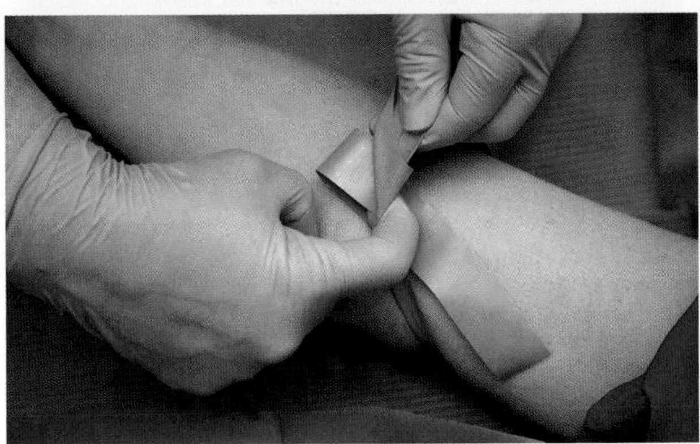

7. Gently release your nondominant hand's grasp and allow the tourniquet to tighten against the patient's arm. Both tails of the tourniquet should arise from the top of the band now surrounding the arm ***to prevent contamination of the site after cleansing.***

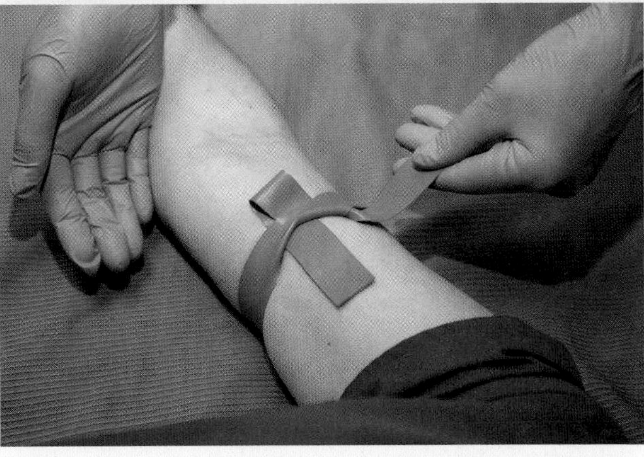

Evaluation Step

1. Evaluate if there is adequate distention of the intended vein. If so, proceed with venipuncture.

Skill 34.2 Performing Venipuncture

Assessment Steps

1. Review the health-care provider's order ***to determine the type of test for which blood is to be drawn.***
2. Obtain the computer-generated label and compare it to the health-care provider's order.

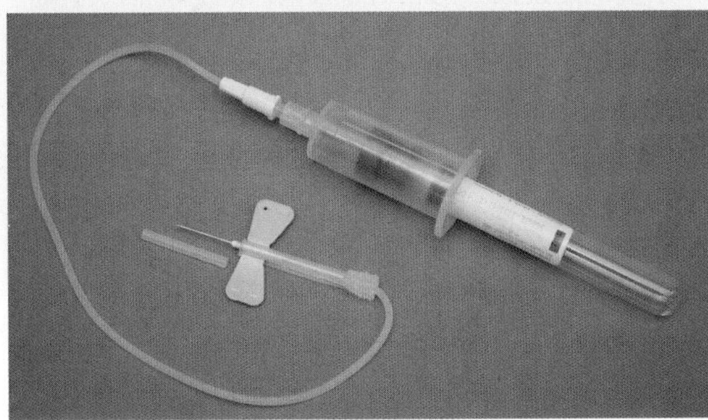

3. Determine whether special conditions such as fasting or specific times are required.
4. Assess the patient's veins ***to determine which type of phlebotomy equipment will be best to use.***

Planning Steps

1. Gather needed equipment and supplies: tourniquet; clean gloves; alcohol sponges, chlorhexidine, or facility-specified antiseptic; laboratory requisition; correct colored-top tubes for ordered tests; labels; sterile 2×2-inch gauze pad; and tape. ***Gathering all needed supplies saves you time and effort.***
    - **Evacuated tube system:** plastic tube holder and double-pointed needle or winged infusion set
    - **Syringe and needle system:** 5- or 10-mL syringe depending on the amount of blood needed for the test(s) and whether you are using a needle or winged infusion set
2. Screw the needle or winged infusion set onto the plastic tube holder or syringe ***so that it is ready to use.***

(skill continues on page 768)

Skill 34.2 (continued)

3. If more than one test is ordered, determine the order in which the tubes should be drawn.

Implementation Steps

1. Follow the Initial Implementation Steps located on the inside back cover.
2. *Safety: Wash your hands to prevent cross-contamination. This is particularly important because of the invasive nature of this skill.*
3. *Safety: Verify patient identity by checking the ID band and use a second method of identifying that this is the correct patient.*
4. Arrange supplies within arm's reach, positioned so that you do not have to turn around or lean over to pick up the tubes once the needle is positioned in the vein.
5. Apply gloves.
6. Apply the tourniquet 3 to 4 inches above the intended puncture site, with the tails of the tourniquet extending from the top side ***so that they will not contaminate the site after cleansing it.***
7. Palpate the intended vein ***to ensure that you have selected a good vein and that it is adequately distended.***
8. Cleanse the site with 70% alcohol or chlorhexidine or as designated by facility policy. *Safety: If povidone-iodine is to be used, make certain the patient is not allergic to iodine or shellfish.*
9. Allow the site to dry for 30 seconds while you perform the following step:
   - **Evacuated tube system:** Place the first tube loosely into the plastic tube holder. *Safety: Do not advance the rubber stopper onto the sheathed needle. This will result in loss of vacuum from the tube.*
   - **Needle and syringe system:** Pull back and forth on the syringe plunger two or three times ***to make certain it is not stuck.***
10. Uncap the needle. Position the needle so that the bevel is up.
11. ***If you are using a winged infusion set known as a butterfly on either the plastic tube holder or syringe,*** fold the two wings just proximal to the needle upward. Hold the two wings together between your index finger and thumb.

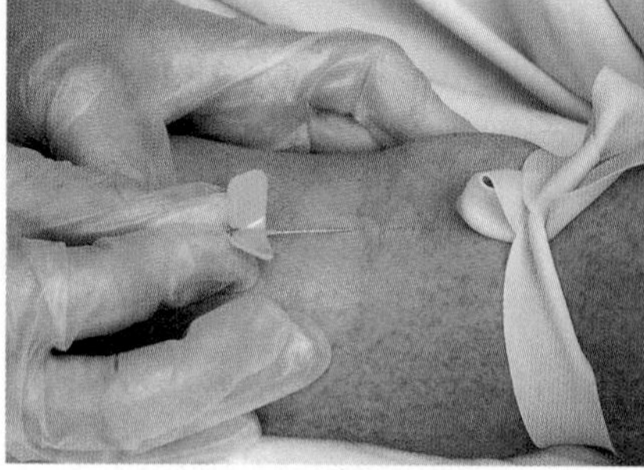

If Using an Evacuated Tube System

12. Hold the plastic tube holder so that it rests on your fingertips and your thumb is on top of the holder, letting the tube lay loosely in the holder. If this does not feel comfortable, you may delay the insertion of the tube into the holder until you have gained access to the vein.

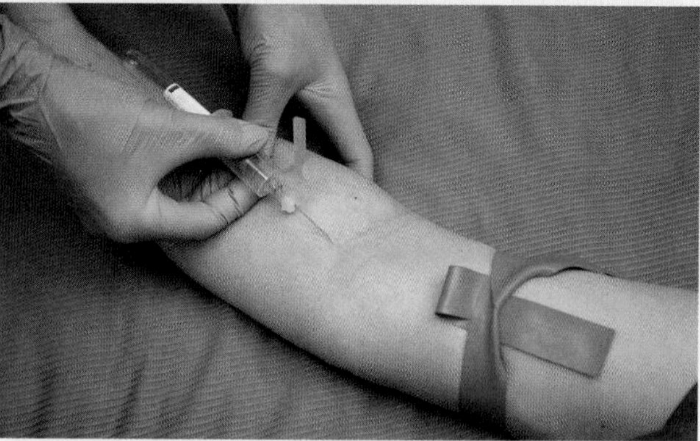

13. Using an angle between 15 and 30 degrees, pierce the skin in a swift, continuous motion.
14. Monitor for a slight "popping" sensation or release of resistance against the needle point, which you will feel when you enter the vein.
15. Once in the vein, brace your hand that is holding the phlebotomy device firmly against the patient's arm.
16. Using your nondominant hand, gently push the rubber stopper of the tube onto the sheathed end of the needle, using a slight pushing and twisting motion, making certain to maintain the stability of the needle ***so that it will not be pushed through the vein.*** Blood should begin to enter the tube.
17. When the tube stops filling, gently remove the tube from the holder with your nondominant hand, using a twisting motion as you pull the tube off the needle. Again, make certain to brace your dominant hand that is holding the plastic tube holder against the patient's arm ***to stabilize the needle and prevent pulling it out of the vein.***
18. Gently invert the tube of blood two to three times and lay it aside. Pick up the next tube to be filled. Carefully repeat the process. Once the last tube is advanced onto the needle, using your nondominant hand, release the tourniquet while the tube fills.
19. When tube stops filling, remove it from holder as described above. Using your nondominant hand, place a 2×2-inch gauze pad over the needle insertion site while removing the needle from the patient's arm, applying firm pressure to the site immediately after the needle is withdrawn. *Safety: Immediately activate the needle safety device to prevent the risk of needle stick.*
20. Place a piece of tape over the gauze pad to maintain pressure on the puncture site. You may want the patient to elevate the arm above the heart in an outstretched position, without bending the elbow, ***to decrease bleeding.***

If Using a Needle and Syringe System

12. Hold the syringe so that it rests on your fingertips and your thumb is on top of the syringe.
13. Using an angle between 15 and 30 degrees, pierce the skin in a swift, continuous motion.
14. Monitor for a slight "popping" sensation or release of resistance against the needle point, which you will feel when you enter the vein.

Skill 34.2 (continued)

15. Once in the vein, brace your hand that is holding the syringe firmly against the patient's arm.
16. Pull the plunger back slowly and gently begin drawing blood into the syringe. Avoid pulling the plunger back too quickly ***because this can collapse fragile veins.*** Fill the syringe to the required volume.
17. Release the tourniquet using your nondominant hand.
18. Place the 2×2-inch gauze pad over the needle insertion site while quickly removing the needle from the patient's arm, applying firm pressure immediately after the needle is withdrawn. *Safety: Immediately activate the needle safety device to prevent the risk of needle stick.*
19. Once bleeding has stopped, place a piece of tape over the gauze pad ***to hold pressure on the site.*** You may want the patient to elevate the arm above the heart in an outstretched position, without bending the elbow, ***to decrease bleeding.***
20. Remove the safety needle from the syringe and place it in the sharps container.
21. Hold the syringe and attach it to the blood transfer device so that the device is at the bottom. Then advance an evacuated tube onto the internal needle of the blood transfer device. Keep the tube vertical, and it will fill from the bottom. Do not push on the plunger of the syringe. Follow the correct order of draw.

For Either System

22. Invert tubes the number of times required by lab guidelines to mix the blood with the anticoagulant.
23. Dispose of the contaminated needle, syringe, and disposable plastic tube holder in the sharps container.
24. Label each tube of blood according to facility policy before leaving the patient's bedside. ***This helps to ensure that the correct tests will be performed on the correct patient.***
25. Place specimens in a plastic bag or specified container.
26. Follow the Ending Implementation Steps located on the inside back cover.
27. Deliver the specimens to the laboratory per facility policy.

Evaluation Steps

1. Reassess the puncture site to ensure that bleeding has stopped before leaving the room.
2. Remind the patient to remove the gauze pad and bandage in 1 to 2 hours.

Sample Documentation

09/19/22 1530 Blood drawn for CBC from right antecubital and sent to the lab. Pressure dressing applied. No bleeding from site. ——— Nurse's signature and credentials

Skill 34.3 Collecting a Blood Culture Specimen

Assessment Steps

1. Review the health-care provider's order ***to verify the test to be performed and to determine whether the culture specimen can be drawn at any time or only during a temperature spike.***
2. Determine if blood for other laboratory tests is to be drawn at the same time as the blood culture specimen. ***This may save the patient from an additional needle stick.***
3. Review facility policy regarding the correct volume of blood that is to be drawn for the blood specimens.
4. Obtain the computer-generated label and compare it to the health-care provider's order ***to ensure correctness of order.***
5. Assess the patient's veins ***to determine which type of phlebotomy equipment will be best to use.***
6. Assess whether or not the patient is allergic to povidone-iodine or shellfish. ***This prevents unwarranted allergic reactions.***

Planning Steps

1. If multiple tests are ordered, plan to draw the blood culture specimen first.
2. Gather needed equipment and supplies: gloves, alcohol wipes, povidone-iodine swabs, tourniquet, double-pointed needle or winged infusion set, two evacuated tube system culture bottles, plastic holder, one clean 2×2-inch gauze pad, two sterile 2×2-inch gauze pads, labels, requisition, and other tubes if further tests are to be performed. ***Gathering all needed supplies saves you time and effort.***
3. Plan the sequence in which blood will be drawn. An anaerobic culture specimen is always drawn first, then an aerobic culture specimen, and then blood is drawn in the correct sequence for additional laboratory tests.
4. Screw the needle or winged infusion set onto the plastic holder ***so that it is ready to use.***
5. Prepare two culture bottles. Remove the caps from each bottle. Cleanse each bottle top with at least two povidone-iodine swabs and allow to dry. Lay a ***sterile*** 2×2-inch gauze pad over each of the bottle tops.

Implementation Steps

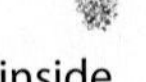

1. Follow the Initial Implementation Steps located on the inside back cover.
2. Apply gloves ***to protect yourself from blood-borne pathogens.***
3. *Safety: Verify patient identity by checking the ID band and use a second method of identifying that this is the correct patient.*

(skill continues on page 770)

Skill 34.3 (continued)

4. Apply the tourniquet and select the vein to be used.
5. Remove the tourniquet. *Safety: Avoid leaving the tourniquet in place for longer than 1 minute.*
6. Cleanse the site vigorously with alcohol wipes, using at least two separate wipes and cleansing at least a 2-inch circle. ***This helps remove body oils from the skin's surface.***
7. Cleanse the site again using two povidone-iodine swabs if the patient is not allergic to iodine. (If allergic, cleanse the site again with a fresh alcohol wipe.)

   Begin at the center and move outward in concentric circles. Allow the site to dry for 1 minute, allowing the iodine to dry. ***This is necessary for the iodine to have adequate time to kill any bacteria on the skin's surface.***
8. Reapply the tourniquet, avoiding contamination of the site.
9. Wipe the tops of the bottles with the sterile 2×2-inch gauze pads ***to wipe away any iodine residue.***
10. Uncap the needle. Holding the needle with the bevel up and, using a 15- to 30-degree angle, swiftly and smoothly insert the needle into the vein. Remember to inform the patient just prior to piercing the skin.
11. Once the needle is in the vein, use your nondominant hand to place the ***anaerobic*** culture bottle into the holder and push it onto the sheathed needle. Be certain to brace your dominant hand, which is holding the needle, against the patient's arm ***to provide stability and prevent the needle from going through the vein.***
12. After the first bottle is filled, remove the bottle from the plastic holder and set it aside.
13. Insert the ***aerobic*** culture bottle into the holder and gently push it onto the sheathed needle.
14. Remove the tourniquet while the second bottle is filling.
15. When the second bottle is filled, remove it from the holder.
16. Cover the puncture site with the clean 2×2-inch gauze pad and remove the needle from the patient's arm, applying firm pressure to the site as soon as the needle is withdrawn. ***This prevents hematoma formation.***
17. Immediately activate the needle safety device and place the contaminated needle in the sharps container. ***This helps to reduce the risk of contaminated needle-stick injuries.***
18. When bleeding is stopped, apply a piece of tape over the gauze pad ***to hold pressure on the puncture site.*** Have the patient elevate the arm above the level of the heart ***to reduce the risk of hematoma formation,*** but do not allow the patient to bend the arm at the elbow. ***This is known to increase bleeding into the subcutaneous tissues.***
19. Complete and apply labels to both the anaerobic and aerobic specimen bottles before leaving the patient's bedside.
20. Follow the Ending Implementation Steps located on the inside back cover.
21. Transport the specimens to the laboratory per facility policy.

Evaluation Steps

1. Assess the site to make certain bleeding has stopped.
2. Remind the patient to remove the gauze pad and bandage in 1 to 2 hours.

Sample Documentation

03/05/22 2100 Blood cultures drawn from left antecubital without difficulty. Specimens taken to lab. —————— Nurse's signature and credentials

Skill 34.4 Performing Dermal Puncture for a Finger Stick Blood Sugar

Assessment Steps

1. Review the health-care provider's order ***to determine the type of test that is to be performed.***
2. Review the instructions for the correct use of the finger stick blood sugar monitor.

Planning Step

1. Gather needed equipment and supplies: gloves, alcohol wipes, dry cotton balls, lancet, finger stick blood sugar monitor with correct strips, bandage, and pen and paper.

Implementation Steps

1. Follow the Initial Implementation Steps located on the inside back cover.
2. Apply gloves ***to protect you from blood-borne pathogens.***
3. Inquire if the patient has a preference as to which finger is pricked. ***This is a simple choice that will allow the patient to feel that he or she has some control over the care received.***
4. Have the patient dangle the hand off the side of the bed or chair ***to allow gravity to help fill the capillaries.*** If the hand is cold, have the patient wash hands with warm water and soap ***to increase blood flow to the hand.***
5. Cleanse the fingertip site with alcohol and let dry.
6. Hold the spring-loaded lancet against the fleshy fingertip pad, just slightly off center, avoiding the very tip or the sides of the fingertip. Press the release button, which causes the lancet to pierce the skin.

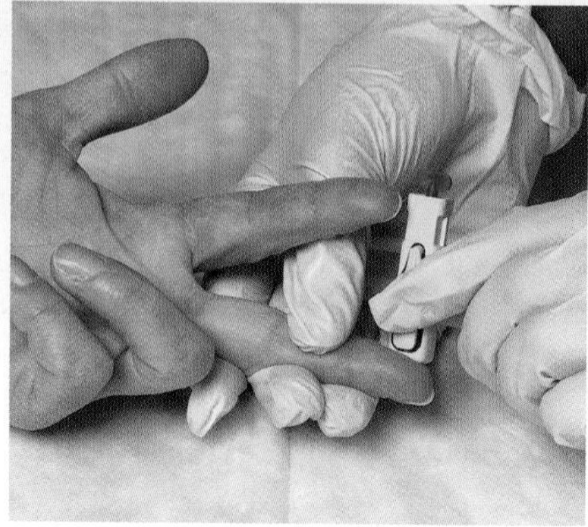

Skill 34.4 (continued)

7. Apply gentle pressure to elicit a drop of blood, wiping away the first drop with a dry cotton ball. ***This prevents the alcohol residue and tissue fluids from diluting the blood sample.***

   Note: For some glucometers, it is not necessary to wipe away the first drop of blood. Follow the manufacturer's instructions.

8. Squeeze the next drop and touch the end of the monitor strip to the edge of the drop, allowing the strip to draw the blood into itself. Avoid scraping or touching the strip against the skin.

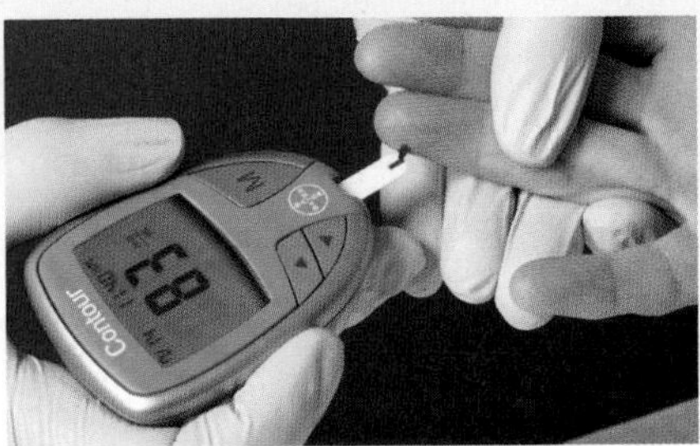

9. Use a cotton ball to hold firm pressure on the puncture site while waiting for the monitor to process the blood glucose level. Apply a bandage if the patient desires.
10. Dispose of the lancet in the sharps container and the strip in the biohazard trash.
11. Follow the Ending Implementation Steps located on the inside back cover.

Evaluation Steps

1. When the monitor produces the glucose level, write it down on paper. Do not rely on your memory.
2. Evaluate if the glucose level requires further action, such as notification of the health-care provider or administration of insulin.

Sample Documentation

07/18/22 1630 FSBS - 213 mg/dL. Regular insulin 3 units given subcutaneously in left abdomen. ——— Nurse's signature and credentials

POST CONFERENCE

When you meet with your instructor and fellow students, you are pleased to report that you were able to obtain all the blood specimens ordered in the medical office. For one elderly patient, you had to try every tip you learned in this chapter, but you were finally able to get the specimen. No one fainted or even yelled, and you left feeling confident that you would be able to perform venipunctures in the future. The clinical medical assistant was very helpful and reminded you of tips to make the venipunctures and blood specimen collections easier to accomplish.

Key Points

- The Joint Commission requires use of two methods to identify patients prior to procedures.
- The most common vein choice for phlebotomy is the median cubital.
- Sites where phlebotomy should be avoided include an arm with an IV, an arm on the side of a mastectomy, skin with altered integrity, scarred or edematous tissue, and tortuous or sclerosed veins.
- It is more important to be able to feel a vein than to see it.
- Use your index or middle finger to palpate for a vein.
- Tips to aid in accessing veins include the application of warm moist compresses, hanging the arm dependently, applying friction using an alcohol wipe, using your finger for gentle tapping over the vein site, using a BP cuff instead of a tourniquet, and anchoring the vein above and below the intended puncture site.
- The order of draw is yellow or culture bottles, red, light blue, red tiger-top, green, lavender, gray, and orange or yellow/gray.
- Always use safety needles. Never recap contaminated needles. Dispose of contaminated needles in the sharps container.
- Use between a 20-gauge and 23-gauge needle for phlebotomy.
- Wear gloves and maintain asepsis during phlebotomy.
- Label specimens after they are drawn while you are still in the patient's room.
- Never leave a tourniquet on for longer than 1 minute.
- Dermal punctures in older children and adults should be performed on the lateral aspects of the palmar side of the fingertip.
- Dermal punctures in infants are performed on the lateral aspects of the plantar surface of the heel.

Review Questions

Select the answer that is most appropriate for each of the following questions. Some questions may have more than one correct answer. Select all that apply.

1. When selecting a vein for phlebotomy, which of the following are true?
   1. Use the vein that looks the largest, no matter what its condition.
   2. Avoid areas where the vein is crooked or feels hard and ropelike.
   3. The site of choice is the dorsal side of the hand.
   4. Use the right arm of a patient who has had a left mastectomy.
   5. Use the right arm of a patient who has an IV in the right arm.

2. Which of the following needle sizes would be an appropriate choice to use for phlebotomy in a 45-year-old patient?
   1. 16 gauge
   2. 19 gauge
   3. 21 gauge
   4. 23 gauge
   5. 30 gauge

3. The tourniquet should be applied where in relation to the intended puncture site?
   1. 6 inches distal to the site
   2. 3 inches distal to the site
   3. 6 inches proximal to the site
   4. 3 inches proximal to the site

4. A "good" vein for phlebotomy should meet which of the following criteria?
   1. It should feel bouncy.
   2. It should feel rigid.
   3. It should feel knobby.
   4. It should feel elastic.

5. When performing phlebotomy using a needle and syringe, drawing back on the plunger can result in which of the following complications?
   1. Collapse of vein
   2. Hematoma
   3. Infection of site
   4. Rolling the vein
   5. Blowing the vein

6. Activation of the needle safety device should occur when?
   1. Before the initial stick
   2. During the draw of blood
   3. Immediately after the tourniquet is released
   4. As soon as the needle is withdrawn
   5. After placing tape over the puncture site

7. A patient who has had venipuncture performed will need more teaching if she says:
   1. "I shouldn't lift anything heavy with this arm for an hour."
   2. "I will take the wrap off of my arm tomorrow morning."
   3. "I will hear from my doctor about my test results."
   4. "Yes, the name on the label is my name correctly spelled."

8. A patient has several blood tests ordered. You have gathered the correct tubes, which include a red top, green top, and light blue top. In which order will you draw them?
   1. Green, red, light blue
   2. Light blue, green, red
   3. Red, light blue, green
   4. Light blue, red, green

9. Which of these will always be drawn first if multiple tests are ordered?
   1. Blood cultures
   2. Light blue top
   3. Red top
   4. Lavender top

10. When performing a dermal puncture for blood sugar on an adult patient, where should the puncture be made?
    1. On the lateral aspect of the heel
    2. On the lateral aspect of the finger tip
    3. On the end of the fingertip
    4. On the left earlobe

ANSWERS 1. 2, 4, 2. 2, 3, 3. 4, 4. 1, 4, 5. 1, 5, 6. 4, 7. 2, 8. 4, 9. 1, 10. 2

Critical Thinking Exercise

Answers available online.

1. Explain steps you should take to avoid hemolysis.

Additional Resources

DAVIS edge. **Use the scratch off code on the inside front cover of your book to access online quizzes that will help you to improve your scores on course exams and prepare for the NCLEX-PN®.**

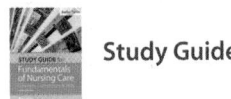

Study Guide

CHAPTER 35 Researching and Preparing Medications

David W. Smith

KEY TERMS

Adverse effect (AD-vers e-FEKT)
Allergic reaction (ah-LER-jik ree-AK-shun)
Brand name (BRAND NAYM)
Chemical name (KEM-i-kuhl NAYM)
Desired effect (dee-ZYE-urd e-FEKT)
Generic name (je-NER-ik NAYM)
Medication administration record (med-i-KAY-shun ad-MIN-iss-TRAY-shun REK-ord)
Mucosal route (mew-KOH-suhl ROOT)
Nursing drug guide
Oral route (OR-uhl ROOT)
Over-the-counter medication (OH-ver-the-KOWN-ter med-i-KAY-shun)
Parenteral route (pah-REN-tur-uhl ROOT)
Physician's Desk Reference
Prescription medication (pre-SKRIP-shun med-i-KAY-shun)
Side effect (SIDE e-FEKT)
Therapeutic level (thair-uh-PYOO-tik LEV-el)
Topical route (TAH-pik-uhl ROOT)
Toxicity (tahk-SI-si-tee)

CHAPTER CONCEPTS

Safety
Patient-Centered Care

LEARNING OUTCOMES

1. Define various terms associated with researching and preparing medications.
2. Differentiate between the chemical, generic, and brand name of medications.
3. Explain when generic prescriptions might be used.
4. Discuss two general categories of medications.
5. Summarize the routes of medication administration.
6. Describe the schedule for controlled drugs, with an example of a drug in each schedule.
7. Contrast desired effects, side effects, and adverse effects of medications.
8. Describe allergic reactions, including anaphylaxis.
9. Identify resources to use when researching medications.
10. Discuss types of medication interactions that may occur.
11. Identify common classifications of medications and safety assessments to make prior to administering them.
12. Explain information and abbreviations found in prescriber's orders.
13. Calculate drug dosages using a formula.
14. Explain how to obtain medications for administration.
15. Determine the seven rights, patient rights, and safety checks to perform to prevent medication errors.
16. Describe guidelines to use when preparing medications.
17. Explain ways to prevent medication errors.
18. Discuss how to handle medication errors.
19. Discuss information found in the Connection features of the chapter.
20. Identify safety issues related to researching and preparing medications.

CRITICAL THINKING CONNECTION

Clinical Assignment

You will be caring for a patient who is taking many medications, and you will administer her medications for the first time in clinical tomorrow morning. She takes eight oral medications as well as a nitroglycerin patch and an insulin injection. You have no idea what most of the oral medications are for, and you cannot imagine how

CRITICAL THINKING CONNECTION—cont'd

to say their names. You are a bit familiar with the nitroglycerin patch because your grandfather wears one. You are extremely nervous about administering the insulin injection because you can only think about all the things that can go wrong. You are fearful that you might make an error and harm your patient.

Critical Thinking Questions:

1. What is the classification, therapeutic effects, and major side effects of the nitroglycerin patch?
2. What are the seven rights of medication administration?
3. How would you prepare for medication administration?
4. How would you teach the patient about each medication?

In this chapter, you will learn how to look up information about medications before you administer them. You also will learn general information about the classifications and effects of medications, as well as important assessment keys prior to administration of certain groups of drugs. In addition, you will learn the steps for preparing medications safely and in a way that helps prevent medication errors.

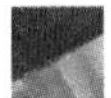

FUNDAMENTALS OF MEDICATIONS

A great deal of information about medications is available to you. There are thousands of medications that you could be administering, and new ones are continuously being developed. All that information is overwhelming to the average person. Even television commercials to promote medications extol their virtues and then quickly follow with a list of side effects and cautions. It is important to know about every medication before you take it or administer it to a patient. You will need to know about the names, categories, classifications, therapeutic effects, side effects, adverse effects, and interactions of medications, as well as the legal regulation of drugs and how to research a medication before you administer it.

Names, Categories, and Routes of Medications

A single medication actually may be called by three different names: its chemical name, generic name, and brand name. It is important to be aware of the overlap in the types of names of medications as well as the differences in those names.

Names of Medications

The **chemical name** is the name of the exact ingredients of the medication. It reads like a chemical formula. For example, the chemical name for a common anti-inflammatory is *(±)-2-(p-isobutylphenyl) propionic acid.* The chemical name is not used in prescribing or administering medications. Instead, the other two names are used.

The **generic name** is assigned by the U.S. Adopted Name Council. It usually is based, at least in part, on the chemical name but is more of a shorthand version. In our example in the previous paragraph, the generic name of the common anti-inflammatory is *ibuprofen.* Generic names are not capitalized and are not owned by the pharmaceutical company that developed the drug, so they are also sometimes referred to as the *nonproprietary name.* All medications have a generic name even if they are not available for purchase in generic form.

The **brand name,** also called the *trade name,* of a drug is usually shorter and easier to remember. This name is owned by the pharmaceutical company, so it is sometimes referred to as the *proprietary name.* One drug might have many brand names because it is made and sold by a variety of companies. In our example, the anti-inflammatory ibuprofen is sold under a variety of brand names, such as *Motrin, Advil, Medipren,* and *PediaProfen,* as well as *Amersol* in Canada. Brand names are capitalized and often are registered, requiring the ® symbol to be used in print.

GENERIC PRESCRIPTIONS. When a drug is first developed in the United States, it is patented by the pharmaceutical company that does the research and development. That company then sells the drug for a period of time with no competition from other manufacturers because it owns the patent; the price is designed to help offset the costs of the research and development. Approximately 20 years after the company begins selling the drug, the patent expires, which allows the drug to be sold as a generic medication and manufactured by other pharmaceutical companies under a different brand name. At this point, the generic medication will be less expensive than the brand-name medication because it is no longer the exclusive property of the pharmaceutical company that developed it; therefore, the generic medication can be manufactured and offered at less expense even though it is exactly the same medication as the brand-name medication.

Categories of Medications

Two general categories of medications exist: prescription and over the counter. **Prescription medications** are available with a written direction from a health-care provider with prescriptive authority. This includes physicians; nurse practitioners; and, in some situations, physician assistants (PAs), depending on state laws. The prescription includes the patient's and health-care provider's identifying information, the medication name and dose, instructions to the pharmacist, any special instructions, and directions to the patient.

Over-the-counter (OTC) medications are available without a prescription; they are also referred to as *nonprescription medications.* They may be purchased by the consumer for use at recommended dosages. Before a medication is offered OTC, it must be determined safe at the dose available. The medication also may be available in a stronger dose that requires a prescription. Our earlier example of ibuprofen is available OTC in 200-mg tablets, but it also is available by prescription in a stronger dose of 800-mg tablets. Follow the manufacturer's guidelines for safe dosage on OTC medications.

Routes of Medication Administration

Medications can be delivered by several routes. It is always important to know which route is ordered because some medications can be given by more than one route. These routes will be discussed in more detail in the remaining chapters of this book.

- **Oral route:** Taken through the mouth, either by swallowing or buccal (between cheek and gums) placement
- **Sublingual route:** Absorbed under the tongue, such as ondansetron ODT. ODT stands for *orally disintegrating tablet,* which is placed under the tongue
- **Mucosal route:** Absorbed through the mucosa, such as medications applied through the rectum, vagina, eye, or ear, and inhaled into the lungs and bronchi
- **Topical route:** Applied to the skin; includes creams, ointments, lotions, and transdermal patches
- **Parenteral route:** Given beneath the skin; includes all injections, such as *intradermal* (between the layers of the skin), *subcutaneous* (beneath the skin), *intramuscular* (within muscle layers), and *intravenous* (into the vein)

KNOWLEDGE CONNECTION

What is the difference between the generic name of a drug and a generic prescription? How might a drug be available both by prescription and OTC? By which route would the pneumonia vaccine be delivered?

Legal Regulation of Medications

Over time, many laws have been enacted regarding the regulation of drugs. Several are designed to control the sales and use of narcotics, which are highly addictive. Some laws have been enacted to protect the public by regulating the manufacture and sale of all medications by the U.S. Food and Drug Administration (FDA). Box 35.1 gives a brief synopsis of the impact of several of these laws.

The Comprehensive Drug Abuse and Control Act categorized drugs according to their abuse potential using a schedule from I to V. All drugs in these schedules are considered controlled drugs and must be handled using specific guidelines. Box 35.2 provides a definition of each level and examples of the drugs in each. Schedule II drugs are kept under double lock and must be counted at the end of every shift. When medications are kept in a computerized cabinet, access already is limited, and the count is automatically done by the computer and/or two nurses. Other drugs may be included in the count as well depending on facility policy. All of these medications given during the shift must be accounted for and signed out for administration to a patient.

Real-World Connection

Drug Abuse in Nursing

While no research shows that nurses abuse drugs at a higher rate than the general population, nurses certainly deal with high work-related stress and easy access to drugs. The American Nurses Association suggests that up to 10% of the nursing workforce may be dependent on drugs or alcohol.

One nurse began taking medications that were prescribed for her patients, known as *diverting drugs,* as a way to deal with the emotional pain of watching her sister die of cancer. The nurse could not relieve her sister's pain, but she could relieve her own. Over time, she diverted more and stronger medications until she was taking a tourniquet and a syringe filled with hydromorphone (Dilaudid) to the bathroom in the pocket of her scrubs. She would apply the tourniquet and inject the hydromorphone directly into her vein and then return to work in an impaired state.

One night, she apparently overdosed and was found unconscious in the bathroom, snoring loudly. Once she came to, the police escorted her off of the nursing unit in handcuffs. She faced a variety of criminal charges, including falsifying records, forging prescriptions, and possession of a controlled substance without a prescription.

This nurse's story ends well, though. She entered a drug treatment program and then continued in the Peer Assistance Program available through her state's board of nursing. As part of her recovery, she bravely told her story to nursing students to help them understand how easy it can be to abuse drugs. She also told the students about how difficult recovery can be but that it is worth all the effort it takes. By complying with all the requirements of the Peer Assistance Program, she was able to get her nursing license back again and work in a setting without dispensing medications.

Effects and Interactions of Medications

Medications are prescribed to achieve a specific effect, such as pain relief. At the same time, other effects may occur that are not intended. Medications can interact with one another and cause a more intense effect or a decrease in effectiveness. Medications also can interact with food and supplements such as vitamins and herbs, causing a response that either is greater or less than desired.

Medication Effects

The **desired effect** is the reason a medication is prescribed or the purpose for which it is given. For example, if the patient has high blood pressure, the health-care professional prescribes a medication to lower the blood pressure, which is the desired effect.

• WORD • BUILDING •

mucosal route: mucosal – related to mucus; route – road
parenteral route: par – beside + enteral – intestinal; route – road

Box 35.1

Laws Regulating Medications

Many laws have been passed regarding medication quality and safety. The following four laws impact the way drugs are developed, marketed, stored, and named today.

- **Food, Drug, and Cosmetic Act of 1938:** Established a government agency to approve all new drugs and determine that the drug was safe for humans. This agency became the U.S. FDA.
- **Durham-Humphrey Amendment of 1952:** Specified the criteria for prescription medications and OTC medications.
- **Kefauver-Harris Amendment of 1962:** Established the FDA as responsible for giving drugs official (generic) names and specified criteria for deeming a drug safe and effective before it is offered for sale.
- **Comprehensive Drug Abuse and Control Act of 1970:** Established Schedules I through V, categorizing drugs according to their potential for abuse; set guidelines for the manufacture, distribution, and sale of controlled substances; addressed the need for treatment for drug abuse and dependence; and made it illegal to possess a controlled substance without a legal prescription for it.

Box 35.2

Schedule (Controlled) Drugs With Examples

The Comprehensive Drug Abuse and Control Act of 1970 set up a classification of drugs by their abuse potential and medical usefulness and set guidelines for the manufacture, distribution, and sale of controlled substances. Often referred to as the "drug schedule," this law sets the requirements for storing and handling controlled drugs.

- **Schedule I:** These drugs are highly addictive and have no medical purpose; therefore, they are sometimes referred to as "street drugs." Examples: heroin, LSD, peyote, and mescaline.
- **Schedule II:** These drugs have high potential for abuse and do have accepted medical use. Examples: morphine, codeine, fentanyl, oxycodone, methadone, meperidine, amphetamines, and short-acting barbiturates.
- **Schedule III:** These drugs, while having potential for abuse, are at less risk to be abused than those in Schedules I and II. Examples: lower doses of barbiturates, acetaminophen with codeine, paregoric, and anabolic steroids.
- **Schedule IV:** These drugs have a lower potential for abuse than Schedule I, II, and III medications. Examples: central nervous system depressants such as chloral hydrate, diazepam, lorazepam, meprobamate, and phenobarbital.
- **Schedule V:** These drugs have the lowest potential for abuse. Examples: medications with very small amounts of codeine and atropine, such as cough medications with codeine, and antidiarrheals, such as diphenoxylate with atropine (Lomotil). A prescription may not be required, but the consumer will sign for the medication and provide identification when purchasing it.

A **side effect** occurs when an unintended outcome takes place. This outcome may not necessarily be unexpected. For example, a patient taking a medication for hypertension may feel dizzy upon standing for a few seconds. When the patient stands, the effect of the blood pressure medication prevents the body from adjusting as quickly to a change in position, resulting in a momentary decrease in blood to the brain, which causes dizziness. This type of side effect is minor, and the patient may adjust to it. However, if the medication lowers the blood pressure too much, the patient may feel dizzy most of the time or may even faint. The prescriber may need to adjust the dose or change the medication because of more severe side effects.

Adverse effects also are unintended but are more severe or harmful than side effects. Often these effects are unexpected at the normal medication dose. They may be due to the patient's inability to tolerate the normal dose or to his or her specific reaction to the drug. The following are some reasons that adverse reactions might occur:

- Chronic illness that affects the body's ability to metabolize and excrete the drug
- Drug allergies
- Liver or renal impairment or failure
- History of previous drug reactions

Severe adverse effects are those that are life-threatening; require medical intervention to prevent permanent damage or death; and could lead to hospitalization, disability, or congenital damage to an infant.

Allergic reactions occur when the patient's body reacts to the medication as a foreign invader to be destroyed. Generally, the first time the patient takes the offending medication, no reaction occurs. At this point, the body recognizes it as a foreign substance and forms antibodies against it. Then the next time the patient takes the medication, the body reacts with an allergic response. Sometimes the allergic response occurs much later, after the patient has taken the drug several times.

A typical mild allergic reaction causes a rash, hives, and itching. It usually resolves when the medication is discontinued. Sometimes the prescriber may have the patient take diphenhydramine (Benadryl) or another antihistamine concurrently with the drug and continue to take the drug as prescribed. The antihistamine helps prevent the mild allergic response.

ANAPHYLAXIS. A more severe reaction, referred to as an *anaphylactic reaction,* is life-threatening. It causes swelling of the airways, shortness of breath, respiratory arrest, decreased blood pressure, and eventually circulatory collapse. This type of reaction occurs as soon as the medication reaches the bloodstream, so if you are administering the medication through an IV line, the reaction will occur immediately. ***Safety: If you suspect an anaphylactic reaction, stop the medication at once and follow facility procedure for responding to anaphylaxis.*** The patient may have to be intubated and given ventilator support. Expect to administer IV fluids to increase blood volume and bring up the blood

• WORD • BUILDING •

anaphylactic reaction: ana – against + phylactic – protective; reaction – adverse effect from contact with a substance

pressure. You may also be ordered to give additional IV medications such as epinephrine to stimulate the heart. ***Safety: Always check the chart for allergies before administering any medication.***

Sometimes patients describe themselves as allergic to a medication, but when asked about the reaction, it is more typical of unpleasant side effects. For example, a patient may say, "Dilaudid makes me really sick. I vomit if I take it." This most likely is a description of the side effects of nausea and vomiting, which are common with hydromorphone (Dilaudid). Make sure the prescriber is aware, but he or she still may prescribe the medication along with another medication to relieve the side effects. ***Safety: If the patient says he or she is allergic to a medication, you must record it as an allergy, along with documenting the patient's description of the reaction when the medication is taken.***

Classifications of medications that often cause allergic reactions include the following:

- Antibiotics, especially penicillin and sulfa drugs
- Iodine and dyes injected for certain procedures
- Vaccines
- Anticonvulsants, also known as seizure medications

TOXICITY. When medications are administered as ordered, the goal is for the patient to have therapeutic levels of the drug in the bloodstream. A **therapeutic level** is the amount of medication in the blood needed to achieve the desired effects on the target organ or organs. In many cases, the amount of medication required for the desired effect is far below the amount of medication that could cause harmful toxic effects. Most medications are not likely to cause a toxic effect unless they are taken in amounts greater than prescribed.

However, it is possible for patients to experience toxic effects of a medication. Certain medications can accumulate in the body rather than being completely excreted. As this happens, the patient will exhibit symptoms of **toxicity,** or too much of the medication in the body. If the patient continues to take the medication, severe toxic effects such as multiple organ failure and even death can occur.

Laboratory and Diagnostic Connection

Determining Digoxin Toxicity

One medication that can cause toxicity is digoxin, a cardiac glycoside that can accumulate in the body. Blood levels are drawn periodically to determine the amount of drug in the blood and whether the levels are elevated above therapeutic ranges. If the levels are elevated, the patient may develop symptoms of digoxin toxicity, which include nausea, vomiting, halos of light around objects, blurred vision, objects appearing to have a yellow cast, irregular heartbeat, and bradycardia. Blood levels greater than 2.0 ng/mL indicate toxic levels of digoxin in the blood. While the laboratory may notify the health-care provider of toxic levels, nurses should be certain that the health-care provider is aware of the laboratory results.

If the blood levels are elevated, the prescriber usually discontinues the medication for a few days to allow the medication to be removed from the bloodstream and then restarts it at a lower dose. ***Safety: It is your responsibility to check the most recent blood levels of medications in the patient's chart and to hold any questionable dose until you speak with the prescriber.*** For example, a patient is taking digoxin; you check his chart for the level drawn yesterday morning, and find that it was 2.1 ng/mL. You will not give another dose of digoxin until you notify the health-care provider of the 2.1-ng/mL level and receive new orders. If you do not take the time to check this and just give the medication as ordered, you will make the patient even more toxic by administering another dose. The following are some common medications that may cause toxicity:

- Digoxin
- Gentamicin
- Imipramine
- Vancomycin
- Warfarin
- Phenobarbital
- Procainamide
- Valproic acid

Drug Interactions

Medications can interact with one another, causing increases or decreases in the desired effects. For example, the patient may be taking warfarin (Coumadin), an anticoagulant that prevents blood clotting. If the patient also takes a medication containing aspirin or ibuprofen, which also has anticoagulant properties, it will delay the ability of the blood to clot for longer than desired by the prescriber. This can lead to excessive bruising and spontaneous bleeding from the nose, gums, eyes, vagina, kidneys, and intestines. It also can lead to life-threatening hemorrhage if it is not reversed. Pharmacists keep close watch on prescribed medications to detect dangers of drug interactions, but patients must be educated to prevent interactions between prescription drugs and OTC preparations.

Medications can interact with certain foods. Patients are advised to avoid such foods while taking the particular drug, or they are advised to avoid taking the drug with specific foods or beverages. For example, the antibiotic tetracycline should not be taken with dairy products because proteins in these foods cause decreased absorption of the drug. Grapefruit juice should not be consumed with certain medications taken to lower cholesterol because the juice interferes with the enzymes that break down the drugs, causing the blood levels of the medication to become too high.

• WORD • BUILDING •

toxicity: toxic – poison + ity – condition
anticoagulant: anti – against + coagulant – congealing
antibiotic: anti – against + biotic – living thing

Vitamins and herbal supplements can interact with medications and interfere with their effectiveness. St. John's wort, a popular herbal supplement taken to relieve mild to moderate depression, can interact with many medications. It can interact with birth control pills by increasing the breakdown of estrogen, which decreases the effectiveness of the medication. St. John's wort also can interact with narcotics because it decreases the rate of excretion of these drugs from the body, leading to increased effects and side effects of some narcotics. ***Safety: You are responsible for looking up medications before you give them and for being aware of any potential drug-drug, drug-food, or drug-supplement interactions.***

> **KNOWLEDGE CONNECTION**
>
> Why might nurses be at risk for drug abuse? What would happen if you gave a patient a medication when his or her blood levels were already above therapeutic levels? List three types of drug interactions.

Researching Medications

No one can know or remember everything about all medications. A wealth of information is available about each individual medication, plus an overwhelming number of medications exist, with new ones being developed frequently. You must always look up medications to determine facts about them that you do not know or about which you are unsure. It is important to know how to obtain information about a medication when you need it. A variety of books and Web sites are available, as well as nursing drug guide apps for phones and tablets. Pharmacists are also an excellent resource when you have a question about a medication or potential drug interaction.

Some of the more common books that you may use for medication research include nursing drug handbooks, the *Physician's Desk Reference,* and pharmacology textbooks.

Nursing Drug Guides

While the *Physician's Desk Reference* is designed to be a comprehensive guide for health-care providers and prescribers, other references are more specific for nurses. **Nursing drug guides** include generic drugs listed in alphabetical order with information about their classification and brand names; absorption, distribution, metabolism, and excretion; indications for use; dosages; contraindications, cautions, and interactions; nursing interventions; and patient teaching. Drugs that are a combination of two different medications must be looked up separately. For example, Zestoretic is a combination of lisinopril and hydrochlorothiazide. To obtain information about this drug, you would need to look up each component separately.

Nursing drug guides are smaller books than the PDR and can easily be kept on the medication cart or in the medication room for quick reference. The information is less detailed than that in the PDR and is more geared for nurse's needs. Figure 35.1 shows a nurse looking up a medication in a nursing drug guide.

Physician's Desk Reference

The ***Physician's Desk Reference*** (PDR) is a comprehensive book containing detailed information about a large number of medications. It contains the same information as that contained in drug package inserts provided by pharmaceutical companies. It also contains photographs of many oral medications if you need to identify a tablet or capsule. This book is found at some nurses' station in hospitals and is used by health-care providers to prescribe medications, as well as by nurses to research medications.

Pharmacology Textbooks

You probably will use some type of pharmacology textbook in your nursing course. Most of these include classifications of drugs with explanations of the effects and uses for each class. As a nurse, you will often perform the same type of nursing interventions for all of the drugs in a particular classification. For example, all antihypertensive medications lower blood pressure. Therefore, you will always want to check the blood pressure before administering an antihypertensive to ensure that the blood pressure is not already so low that the medication will drop it too low.

Internet Resources

Many sites provide drug information. Be sure to use a reliable site, such as www.pdrhealth.com or www.medlineplus.com. Often, the drug information online is written for the patient, not for the nurse or other health-care provider. These sites may be easier to read but may omit important assessment and evaluation data.

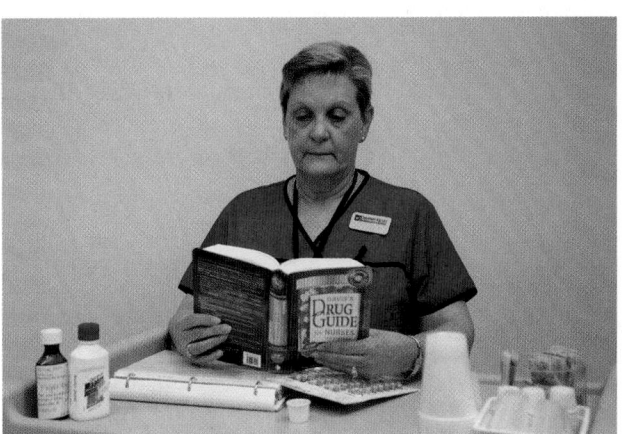

FIGURE 35.1 This nurse is looking up a medication in a nursing drug guide prior to preparing the medication for administration.

Classifications and Effects of Medications

Because it is impossible to learn about every medication, you will find it helpful to learn information about groups of drugs that work in a similar manner and have similar effects and side effects. Table 35.1 includes some of the major classifications and their purposes.

KNOWLEDGE CONNECTION

List four resources you can use to look up information about medications you will administer. Why is it important to check the patient's vital signs before administering an antiarrhythmic medication? What laboratory value will you check before administering a thiazide or a loop diuretic?

Table 35.1
Classifications and Purposes of Medications

Classification	*Purpose*	*Nursing Concerns*
Cardiovascular Medications		
Antianginals	Increase blood flow and oxygen supplied to the heart muscle by causing the coronary arteries to dilate.	Because they dilate arteries, they also lower blood pressure. ***Safety: Check blood pressure and pulse before administering them.***
Antiarrhythmics	Regulate an irregular heartbeat; act on the nerve impulses in the heart; often slow the heartbeat and decrease blood pressure.	***Safety: Check vital signs before giving these medications. Hold if blood pressure or pulse is low and check with prescriber before administering.***
Anticoagulants	Delay blood clotting; sometimes called *blood thinners;* prescribed to treat or prevent heart attack, stroke, and blood clot formation.	Because they delay blood clotting, side effects include internal or external bleeding. Blood tests such as prothrombin time, international normalized ratio (INR), and partial thromboplastin time are ordered to monitor anticoagulation. ***Safety: Assess for tarry stools, bleeding gums, bleeding from the rectum or vagina, and nosebleeds.***
Antiplatelet agents	Also prevent blood clotting but work by making platelets less sticky so they are less likely to form clots.	Antiplatelet agents do not affect clotting time or INR. ***Safety: Check for platelet count and check for signs and symptoms of bleeding.***
Antihyperlipidemics	Prescribed to treat high cholesterol and triglycerides in the blood, which contribute to plaque formation inside the arteries, causing narrowing and restriction of blood flow. This can contribute to heart attack, stroke, high blood pressure, and other conditions.	Check liver function tests; assess for muscle pain and weakness, which could indicate myopathy.
Antihypertensives	Prescribed to lower blood pressure; often more than one drug is prescribed because they work in different ways.	***Safety: Check lab values and blood pressure before administering to prevent hypotension.***
Cardiac glycosides	Prescribed to slow and strengthen the heartbeat; include all drugs that contain or are derived from digitalis. Used to treat congestive heart failure and atrial arrhythmias, such as atrial fibrillation.	Check digoxin blood levels before administering to prevent toxicity. ***Safety: Because these medications cause the heart to slow, assess the apical pulse before administering them. If the rate is below 60, do not administer and notify prescriber.***

Table 35.1
Classifications and Purposes of Medications—cont'd

Classification	*Purpose*	*Nursing Concerns*
Diuretics	Prescribed to decrease edema and fluid retention; rid the body of excess fluid through the urine. Cause kidneys to increase salt and water output, which decreases excess fluid in the blood and lowers blood pressure.	Patients taking potassium-sparing diuretics should not eat foods high in potassium or take potassium supplements. ***Safety: Check potassium levels before administering thiazide or loop diuretics.***
Vasodilators	Prescribed to widen blood vessels, lower blood pressure, and increase circulation.	Side effects include headache, nausea, and hypotension. ***Safety: Assess blood pressure before giving vasodilators to avoid causing hypotension.***
Gastrointestinal Medications		
Antacids	Used to neutralize stomach acid. Products contain aluminum, magnesium, calcium, or a combination of them.	Most common side effects are either constipation or diarrhea. ***Safety: Antacids interact with some medications. Ensure that you do not give them at the same time.***
Anticholinergics	Ordered to block the action of the parasympathetic nervous system; slow peristalsis and reduce stomach acid production; sometimes called *antispasmodics*; prescribed for irritable bowel syndrome, ulcers, Parkinson's disease, and asthma.	Can reduce gastric motility, causing constipation, and can cause urinary retention; assess frequently for distended bladder and abdomen.
Antiemetics	Ordered to relieve nausea and vomiting.	May be given via injection or suppository, if patient is vomiting and unable to keep an oral medication down. Phenergan gel is applied to inner wrists to be absorbed through the skin.
Gastroesophageal reflux disease medications	Given to reduce or block amount of acid produced by the stomach.	Check liver and kidney function tests for abnormal results.
Laxatives and stool softeners	Given to relieve constipation; stool softeners keep water in the feces of the large intestine; some laxatives increase peristalsis to move the feces through the bowel quickly, and other laxatives, such as milk of magnesia, pull water into the intestine to prevent dry, hard feces.	Do not continue to give regularly ordered stool softeners if the patient is having liquid stools. If the patient has not had a bowel movement for 2 days, it is appropriate to give an ordered prn laxative on the third day. This will prevent prolonged constipation or fecal impaction. ***Safety: Assess the need before giving stool softeners or laxatives.***
Endocrine Medications		
Antidiabetics	Oral hypoglycemics stimulate the pancreas to produce more insulin when it is not making enough to meet the body's needs; insulin itself can be given only by injection because it would be destroyed	***Safety: Always check the patient's finger stick blood sugar prior to administering an antidiabetic medication.***

Continued

Table 35.1
Classifications and Purposes of Medications—cont'd

Classification	*Purpose*	*Nursing Concerns*
	by gastric acid, and insulin injections are prescribed when the pancreas no longer makes enough insulin, even in response to oral hypoglycemics; in some cases, both oral hypoglycemic and insulin injections are ordered.	
Steroids	Ordered to relieve inflammation and to treat diseases such as asthma and bronchitis; may be ordered as skin cream, such as hydrocortisone, to treat local inflammations, and as injections directly into inflamed joints or into muscle to decrease systemic inflammation.	Watch for signs of infection because steroids mask infections. Check fasting blood sugar levels because steroids increase blood sugar. This type of medication should not be stopped abruptly. Patients should be tapered off steroids. ***Safety: Assess blood pressure before administering oral or injectable steroids because they cause hypertension.***
Reproductive hormones	Estrogen is ordered to minimize symptoms of menopause and decrease osteoporosis; counteracts the effects of testosterone, so may be used to treat prostate cancer. Testosterone is ordered to increase strength and virility in males and block estrogens in females with certain types of cancers.	Estrogen may cause blood clots. Assess for edema, swelling, depression, and hepatic dysfunction. Testosterone can affect blood glucose, and topical applications can cause virilization in female sex partner if exposed to drug on patient's skin.
Thyroid replacement hormone	Ordered to replace thyroid hormone that is not being produced in sufficient amounts by the body.	***Safety: Assess patient for excitability, tachycardia, irritability, and anxiety, which can indicate an excessive dose.***
Immune System Medications		
Antibiotics	Used to treat infections caused by bacteria by interfering with the way bacteria live and reproduce, allowing the immune system to more easily eliminate the infection; to be effective, antibiotics must be taken regularly for the prescribed amount of time, and bacteria must be completely killed or the infection can recur.	Administer with food when appropriate to prevent stomach irritation, nausea, and vomiting. Tetracycline antibiotics should be given on an empty stomach and never administered with milk or dairy products. ***Safety: Check the patient's allergies before administering antibiotics. Assess for rash, itching, or hives.***
Antifungals	Used to treat fungal infections such as athlete's foot, yeast infections, and systemic fungal infections.	Often in the form of topical creams or ointments, but some are given IV for severe systemic infections.
Anti-inflammatories, including steroids	Prescribed to decrease the symptoms of inflammation and to relieve pain from muscle strain/sprain and arthritis; there are two types: steroids (see Endocrine Medications) and nonsteroidal anti-inflammatory drugs (NSAIDs).	Often cause gastrointestinal side effects such as heartburn, nausea, vomiting, and ulcers. ***Safety: Assess for signs of bleeding ulcers such as tarry stools, especially in the elderly.***

Table 35.1
Classifications and Purposes of Medications—cont'd

Classification	*Purpose*	*Nursing Concerns*
Antivirals	Prescribed to treat viral infections.	These medications do not cure the diseases but help minimize some symptoms.
Nervous System Medications		
Analgesics	Prescribed to relieve pain, often called *pain medicines;* include narcotics and nonnarcotics. Narcotic analgesics act on the brain to relieve pain and are addictive; nonnarcotic analgesics include NSAIDs and acetaminophen.	Side effects of narcotics include nausea, constipation, vomiting, and slowing of respirations. ***Safety: Assess patient for effectiveness of medication in relieving pain.***
Antianxiety medications	Antianxiety medications are prescribed to relieve anxiety and promote calm, rest, and sleep.	***Safety: Antianxiety medications are prone to addiction.***
Anticonvulsants	Ordered to decrease seizure activity due to epilepsy or other causes.	***Safety: Check blood levels of seizure medications before administering them to prevent toxicity.***
Antidepressants	Prescribed to relieve depression and to treat certain types of pain, such as migraine headaches; selective serotonin re-uptake inhibitors increase the function of neurotransmitters in the brain; older drugs, particularly monoamine oxidase inhibitors (MAOIs), are prescribed for depression and to treat Parkinson's disease but can interact with certain foods to cause severe hypertension.	***Safety: Teach patients taking MAOIs to avoid foods high in tyramine, including smoked, aged, or pickled meat or fish; aged cheeses and sausages; and red wines. Ingesting these foods can lead to hypertensive crisis. The patient should be monitored for suicidal tendencies.***
Sedative and hypnotic medications	Sedatives act on the brain to promote calm and sleep; hypnotics induce sleep and fall into two classes: benzodiazepines and nonbenzodiazepines. Benzodiazepines carry a higher risk for dependency, toxicity, and abuse.	***Safety: Caution patients not to get up alone after taking sedative or hypnotic medications.***
Respiratory Medications		
Antihistamines	Prescribed to block the action of histamine, which decreases allergy symptoms, including mild respiratory allergies such as hay fever and sinus conditions; also used to prevent or treat motion sickness symptoms.	These medications may cause drowsiness; patient should not drive or engage in potentially hazardous activities until the response to the drug is known.
Antitussives	Used to control coughing; nonprescription cough medicines usually contain	***Safety: If the cough is productive, an expectorant should be used rather than a cough suppressant.***

Continued

Table 35.1
Classifications and Purposes of Medications—cont'd

Classification	*Purpose*	*Nursing Concerns*
	dextromethorphan to suppress coughs or guaifenesin as an expectorant; prescription-strength cough medicine may contain codeine, a narcotic, which also suppresses coughing.	
Bronchodilators	Prescribed to open airways to ease shortness of breath associated with asthma and emphysema. May be administered IV, orally, and as an inhalant.	Bronchodilators have side effects of agitation, insomnia, tremors, anxiety, and nausea. ***Safety: Monitor theophylline blood levels because these drugs may cause toxicity.***
Expectorants	Used to thin mucus so that it can be coughed out, which helps prevent lung congestion leading to pneumonia.	Instruct patient to increase fluid intake to help loosen and thin mucus; he or she should drink at least eight glasses of fluid daily.

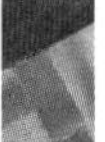

PREPARING TO ADMINISTER MEDICATIONS

Anyone can remove a medication from the packaging and hand it to a patient to swallow. This is not medication administration. Preparing medications is not a task you can perform mindlessly. You must stay focused and think critically throughout the entire process.

Reading Medication Orders

Medication orders are written by health-care providers with prescriptive authority, such as physicians, nurse practitioners, and PAs. All medication orders must include the:

- Date and time of the order
- Name of the medication, either generic or brand
- Dosage of medication
- Frequency for taking the medication (e.g., twice per day)
- Route of administration, such as oral, intramuscular, or IV
- Patient's name (in the hospital setting, the order will be written on a health-care provider's order page that is stamped with the patient's name)
- Specific reason for administrating the medication
- Signature of the prescriber

Figure 35.2 shows an example of a prescription.

Because medication names can be similar, it is very important to verify any order that seems unclear. ***Safety: If the dose, route, or frequency is not appropriate for the medication, notify the prescriber and verify the order.***

The frequency ordered for a medication may vary greatly. It may be ordered several times per day, it may be ordered only as needed (prn), or it may be ordered to be given one time only. Read orders carefully to ensure that the frequency is appropriate and then follow the order. Box 35.3 provides details regarding specific ordered frequencies.

Computerized Health-Care Provider Order Entry

As the changeover is being made to electronic health records, health-care providers' prescriptions for medications have also become computerized as medication administration records. This change is positive for a number of reasons. It decreases errors in reading prescriber's handwriting and therefore decreases errors in medication administration. Allergy and adverse drug reaction warnings immediately appear on the computer screen if the ordered medication is inappropriate for the patient. In addition, drug-drug, drug-food, and drug-lab interaction warnings appear. The computer software ensures that only appropriate dosage forms, routes, and schedules are selectable. All of these features help make computerized health-care provider order entry a safer method of prescribing medications. When an electronic method of transcribing is not in use, the medication order is transcribed from the health-care provider's order sheet in the chart to the **medication administration record** (MAR), which usually is kept in a notebook on the medicine cart or computerized cabinet. The MAR lists the medications and the times they are to be given. The nurse initials in the correct box under the date and across from the time to indicate that a medication has been administered. The MAR may be designed in such a way that the nurse writes the time the medication is to be administered beneath the date and then writes his or her initials next to the time as the medication is given. Medications given on a prn basis are documented in the nurses' notes, as are medications that are withheld for some reason. An explanation is provided in the documentation. In long-term care facilities, the back side of the MAR contains an area for documenting prn medications and medications

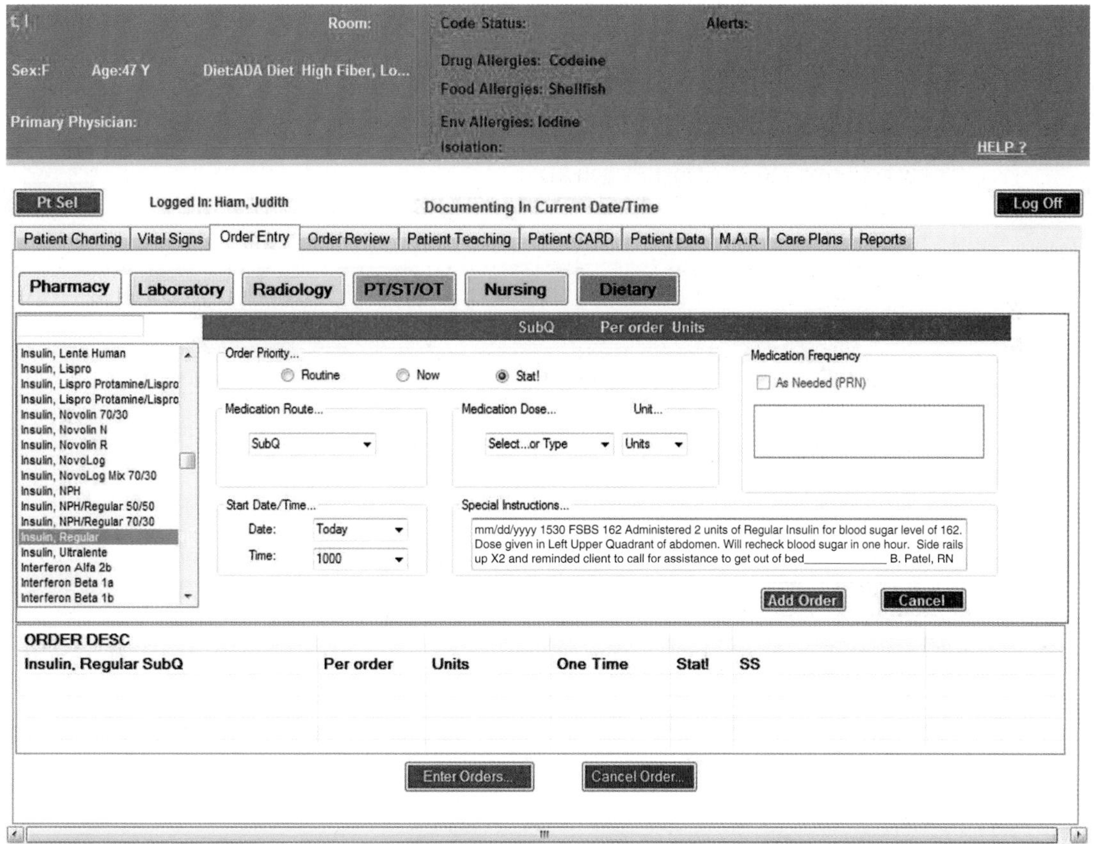

FIGURE 35.2 An example of a computerized physician order entry medication prescription (from Wilkinson JM, Treas LS. *Fundamentals of Nursing: Thinking, Doing, and Caring*. Vol. 2. 3rd ed. Philadelphia, PA: FA Davis; 2016).

Box 35.3

Specific Ordered Frequencies

Medications are ordered at specific frequencies that are scheduled at routine times in the health-care facility. Below are the usually ordered frequencies for most medications. Pay close attention to the frequencies written in medication orders and do not confuse them.

- **Daily:** One time per day, may be morning or evening
- **Twice per day:** Every 12 hours, or morning and evening
- **Three times per day:** Every 8 hours or with meals
- **Four times per day:** Every 4 hours; usually at 9 a.m., 1 p.m., 5 p.m., and 9 p.m.; for antibiotics, may be every 6 hours, usually 12 a.m., 6 a.m., 12 p.m., and 6 p.m.
- **As needed (prn):** As needed within specified time limits. Example: Lortab 7.5 mg every 4 hours prn pain. Patient can take it no closer together than every 4 hours.
- **Stat:** Immediately, no more than 15 minutes. Example: Nitrostat spray sublingual stat.
- **One time:** Give medication one time only and do not continue to administer it. Example: Miconazole 100 mg 1 vaginal suppository to be given one time only.

that were not given. It is possible for errors to be made when orders are transcribed. When computerized ordering systems are used, there is less risk of human error, but mistakes still can occur (Fig. 35.3). ***Safety: Always compare the order on the MAR with the prescriber's original order to detect any possible errors before you prepare and administer medications.***

Abbreviations Used in Medication Orders

Standard abbreviations are often used to save time when prescribers write medication orders. Over the years, however, errors were made due to misinterpretations of some abbreviations. Therefore, The Joint Commission (formerly JCAHO) has determined that some medication abbreviations can no longer be used to prevent confusion and errors. In addition to that list, the Institute for Safe Medication Practices (ISMP) has compiled a list of error-prone abbreviations, symbols, and dose designations. Box 35.4 includes acceptable abbreviations commonly used in medication orders, along with their meanings.

Calculating Drug Dosages

Ideally, the dose of medication available to you will be the exact dose that the prescriber orders, but that does not always occur. If the available medication is in a different dose than what is

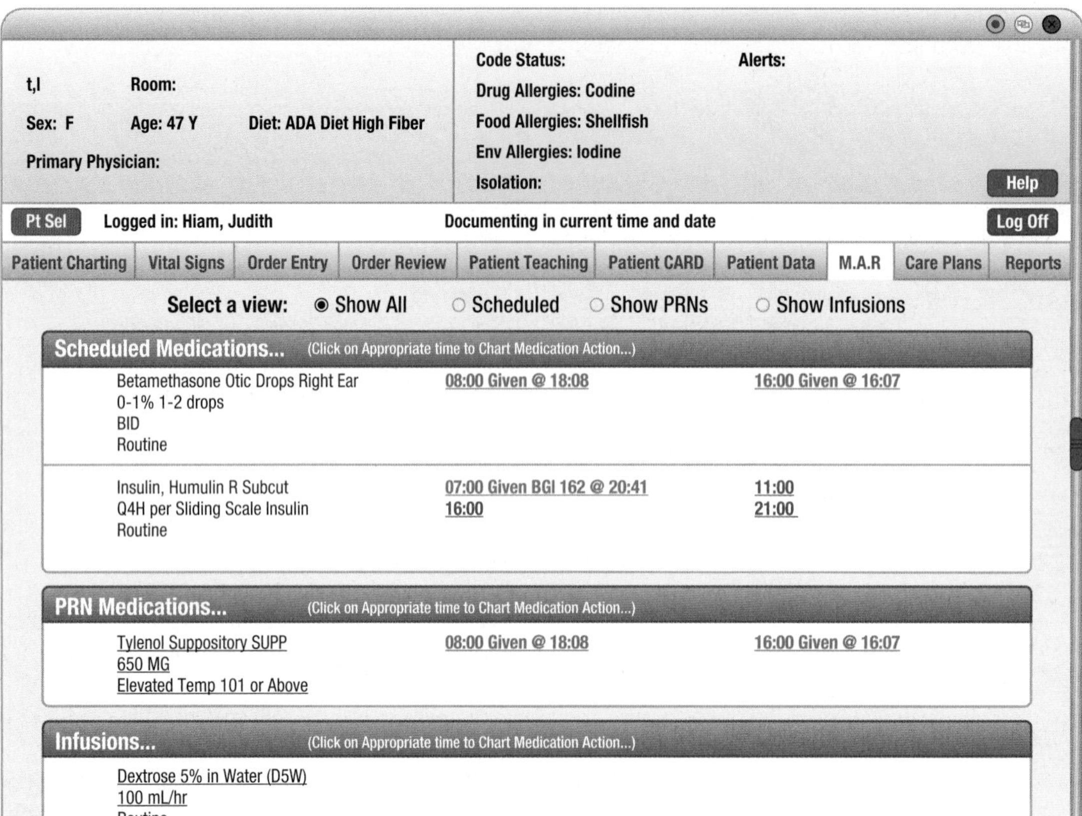

FIGURE 35.3 An example of an electronic medication administration record.

Box 35.4

Medical Abbreviations Commonly Used in Medication Orders

As you interpret medication orders, you will find medical abbreviations that are commonly used. Some abbreviations are officially not to be used and appear in a list in Chapter 5. Others are not encouraged by the ISMP because they can be confused with other abbreviations and contribute to medication errors.

g	grams
gr	grains
h	hour
IM	intramuscularly
IV	intravenously
kg	kilograms
mg	milligrams
mL	milliliters
PO	*per os* in Latin, which means by mouth
q	every

ordered, you must calculate how much of the available medication to administer to your patient. For example, the prescriber may order 1,000 mg of an antibiotic. However, the pharmacy may stock the medication only in 500-mg capsules. It will be your job to determine how many capsules to give the patient.

The same is true of liquid medications. When at home, you might take a teaspoon of a liquid, but in the hospital it may be ordered by milligrams or the amount of the drug dissolved in liquid, expressed as milligrams per milliliter (mg/mL). You will then be required to calculate how many milliliters of liquid to administer to give the desired milligrams of medication. For example, the health-care provider may order amoxicillin liquid 250 mg per feeding tube every 6 hours. The bottle of amoxicillin might be labeled 250 mg/5 mL. That means that every 5 mL of liquid you pour out contains 250 mg of dissolved antibiotic.

If that is confusing, think of it this way: You add 4 teaspoons of sugar to 4 ounces of water and mix it well. When you measure out 1 ounce of water, it will contain 1 teaspoon of dissolved sugar, or 1 teaspoon/ounce. The same is true of medications dissolved in liquid, but the measurements are in the metric system rather than the household system, so the measurement is in milligrams/milliliter.

Systems of Measurement

Medication measurements are mostly made using the metric system. For example, most medications are ordered in milliliters, milligrams, or micrograms. Occasionally an older system of measurement called the *apothecary system* is used when medications are ordered that have existed for a very

• **WORD • BUILDING •**

apothecary system: apothecary – shopkeeper; system – set of principles and procedures

long time. For example, aspirin was originally measured in grains (gr), as was morphine. Grains are a measurement in the apothecary system (Table 35.2). The Joint Commission does not recommend use of the apothecary system because of the confusion it may cause.

The metric system is more accurate and standardized, so it has gradually replaced the apothecary system. The household system is the measurement system used with cooking: teaspoons, ounces, and pints. When a patient is discharged with medication orders, they are written in household measurements (for liquids) so that the patient will be able to measure the medication at home.

Sometimes it may be necessary to convert between systems. This is not common, but in case you need to do so, Table 35.2 provides equivalents between systems that will help you if you need to make such a conversion. Sometimes it is necessary to convert between different units of the metric system. Table 35.3 provides conversions between micrograms, milligrams, and grams.

Calculations

Calculations are not required often, but when they are, you need to have confidence that you can correctly perform them. It is recommended that you have your calculations checked by your instructor while you are a student and have a more experienced nurse check them when you first enter practice.

Many ways exist to arrive at the correct dose. There are several different formulas that you can use to calculate the correct amount of medication to administer. However, if you have math anxiety or get confused when using formulas, it may be easiest to learn one formula that can be used in the most common situations. This book utilizes one formula with several applications.

To correctly use a formula, you must know where to insert each number and then carry out the mathematical operations correctly. In this formula, the problem is set up as a fractional equation, and then cross multiplication must be performed to solve for the correct amount to administer, or x. The *H* stands for the dose you have on hand, or the dose available. The *D* stands for the dose that is ordered by the prescriber. The *V* stands for the vehicle, which is either a tablet or liquid. To set up the problem, arrange the information in this manner:

$$\frac{H}{V} = \frac{D}{x}$$

The next step is to cross multiply:

$$Hx = VD$$

Now you will solve for x:

$$x = \frac{VD}{H}$$

This is more easily understood by using numbers in place of the letters. For example, if an order is for amoxicillin liquid 500 mg per feeding tube every 6 hours and you have on hand amoxicillin 250 mg/5 mL, you will need to determine how many milliliters of liquid medication to administer (x). In this problem, $H = 250$, $D = 500$, and $V = 5$. When you plug those numbers into the formula, it should look like this:

$$\frac{250}{5} = \frac{500}{x}$$

Now, when you cross multiply, it should look like this:

$$250x = 2{,}500$$

To get rid of the x, you must divide what is in front of it into both sides of the equation. In this case, you must divide 250 into 2,500 to find $1x$.

$$1x = \frac{2{,}500}{250}$$

Table 35.2
Measurement Systems Equivalents

Apothecary	*Metric*	*Household*
Weight Measures 1 grain (gr)	60 or 65 milligrams (mg)	
½ gr	30 mg	
¼ gr	15 mg	
	1 kilogram (kg)	2.2 pounds (lbs)
Volume Measures 1 fluid dram	5 milliliters (mL)	1 teaspoon
3–4 fluid drams	15 mL	1 tablespoon
1 fluid ounce	30 mL	2 tablespoons

Table 35.3
Converting Between Units of Measurement in the Metric System

Micrograms	*Milligrams*	*Grams*
1,000,000	1,000	1
100,000	100	0.1
1000	1	0.001

*To change between units of measurement in the metric system, move the decimal three places to the **right** to convert to a smaller unit. Move the decimal three places to the **left** to convert to a larger unit.

When you do the math, the answer becomes:

$$1x = 10 \text{ mL}$$

Therefore, you will administer 10 mL of amoxicillin to the patient to equal 500 mg of dissolved drug.

CONVERTING BETWEEN SYSTEMS USING THE FORMULA. You can also use this formula to convert between systems of measurement. For example, if your order is for 5 grains of aspirin and the aspirin label on hand in the patient's medication drawer indicates that it contains 300 mg in 1 tablet, you can determine how much aspirin to administer. Because the aspirin that you have for use is labeled in milligrams, you need to know how many milligrams is equal to the ordered dose of 5 grains. In this situation, H = 300 mg, D = 5 gr, and V = 1 tablet. By looking at Table 35.2, you can see that 60 mg is equivalent to 1 gr. Set up the formula with numbers in place:

$$\frac{60 \text{ mg}}{1 \text{ gr}} = \frac{300 \text{ mg}}{x \text{ gr}}$$

When you cross multiply, you get $60x = 300$. When you divide both sides of the equation by 60 to solve for x, you get $x = 5$ gr. This tells you that the health-care provider's order for 5 gr is equal to 300 mg, meaning that what you have available is equivalent to the amount the health-care provider ordered. So you will give 1 tablet of aspirin to your patient.

To practice this skill, refer to the Study Guide for more problems.

CALCULATING MILLIGRAMS PER KILOGRAM OF BODY WEIGHT. Medications may be ordered in a different way to be more exact about the amount needed for the patient's body weight. You may see this ordered for pediatric patients to prevent overdose of medications in different-sized patients, especially newborns. For example, the prescriber might order 50 mg/kg of ampicillin daily for a child who weighs 22 lbs. If the patient's weight is in pounds, you will need to convert it to kilograms using the formula above (2.2 lbs equals 1 kg; see Table 35.2):

$$\frac{2.2 \text{ lbs}}{1 \text{ kg}} = \frac{22 \text{ lbs}}{x \text{ kg}}$$

Now cross multiply: $2.2x = 22$

Divide each side by 2.2: $x = 10$

You are solving for the number of kilograms the 22-lb child weighs, so you know that the child weighs 10 kg.

Once you have the patient's weight in kilograms, you can determine how much medication to give. It is the health-care provider's intent that the patient will receive 50 mg of medication for every kilogram of body weight. The patient weights 10 kg, so you must multiply that by 50 mg to determine the dose the patient will receive:

$$10 \text{ kg} \times 50 \text{ mg} = 500 \text{ mg total daily dose}$$

You will learn another formula for calculating IV flow rates in Chapter 38.

> **KNOWLEDGE CONNECTION**
>
> List three systems of measurement used in preparing medications. Why were some abbreviations put on a "do not use" list? If the health-care provider orders digoxin 0.25 mg to be given PO daily and the Lanoxin tablets in the drawer are labeled 0.125 mg, how many tablets will you administer to your patient?

Obtaining Medications

In hospital settings, medications may be found in a variety of storage systems. These include computerized cabinets, carts, and locked bins in the patient rooms.

Computerized Cabinets

To provide inventory control as well as safe medication storage, many acute care facilities use a computerized cabinet. One type is called Pyxis®. You must have a password to enter the system, which records your identity as the person who removed the medication. You then type in the patient's name, and a list of ordered medications for that patient appears on the screen. When you choose a medication, the drawer containing it opens, allowing you to remove the medication. When you close the drawer, the medication is automatically charged to the patient. Narcotics are kept in this system as well. When removing narcotics from the system, it is important to count the medication and make sure the count is correct. When the drawer containing the narcotic opens, two nurses will count the narcotic each time and then enter the amount they are removing. Figure 35.4 shows this type of computerized cabinet.

Medication Cart

A medication cart may be used in some acute and long-term care facilities. It is restocked by pharmacy staff every 24 hours in the hospital setting. In long-term care, the medications are packaged in 30-day punch cards and kept in the resident's section of the drawer. There is a separate locking drawer for narcotics storage, and the entire cart locks as well. ***Safety: Always lock the medication cart when you are not obtaining medications from it.***

Locked Bins in Patient Rooms

In some settings, the patient's medications are kept in a locked bin built into the closet in the patient rooms. The bin can be unlocked and stocked from the hallway, and it can be unlocked and accessed in the patient's room. This prevents nurses from having to run back and forth to medicine rooms or carts to obtain medications. However, narcotics are kept in the medication room under two locks.

Rights Involving Medications

Prior to administering any medication, you must ensure that everything is correct and that the patient is willing and able to take the medication. Seven rights of administration help

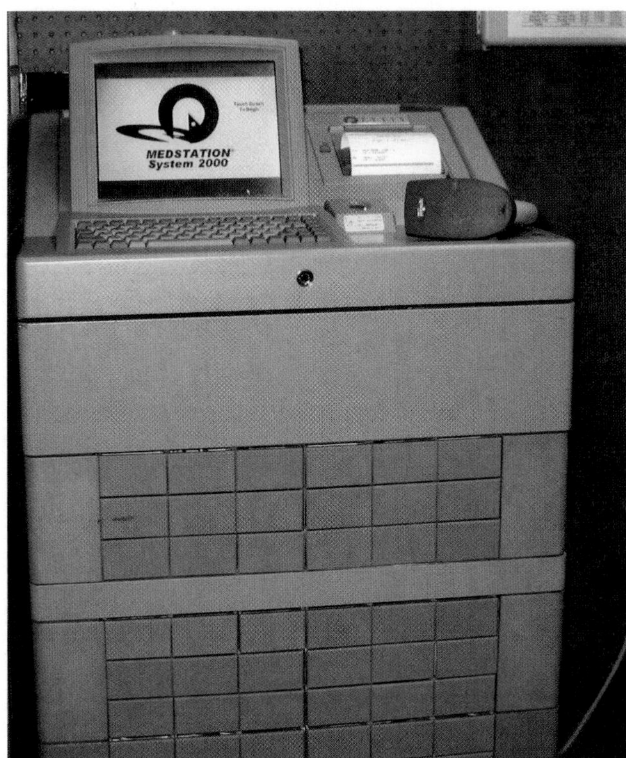

FIGURE 35.4 This is a type of computerized medication cabinet (from Wilkinson JM, Treas LS. *Fundamentals of Nursing*. Vol. 1. 3rd ed. Philadelphia, PA: FA Davis; 2016).

prevent you from making any errors. Patients' rights are established to protect them from being forced to take medications that they do not wish to take.

Rights of Medication Administration

To prevent medication errors, you need to check the seven rights of administration prior to giving any medication to a patient. Ensure that you have the:

- **Right Medication:** Remember that orders may have changed since the last time you administered medications to this patient. Check for new medication orders and orders to discontinue previous medications. ***Safety: Always verify that you have the correct medication by reading the label and comparing it with the MAR. Do not identify medications by their size, shape, or color because many drugs have very similar appearances.***
- **Right Dose:** You must carefully read the ordered dose and ensure that it is within the appropriate range for the patient. Check the original prescriber's order to be certain about a dose. ***Safety: Pay close attention to the placement of decimals, because this can cause overdosing or underdosing if you misread it.***
- **Right Route:** Ensure that you know the route by which you are to administer the medication. Some medications, such as hydrocortisone, may be given orally, topically, and as an injection. ***Safety: Pay close attention to the ordered route. If you administer a medication by the wrong route, it is considered a medication error.***
- **Right Patient:** ***Safety: Use two methods of identifying your patient.*** Ask the patient to confirm his or her name and check the patient's armband or other identifying information and compare it to the MAR. If a patient is confused or hard of hearing and you say, "Mr. Smith?," he may answer with "Yes" even though he is not Mr. Smith. When two patients share a room, it is very important to identify each patient for each medication and procedure. Do not rely on "Bed A" and "Bed B" distinctions.
- **Right Indication:** Ensure that you know why the patient is getting the medication. Some medications, such as a beta blocker, lower blood pressure and heart rate. ***Safety: Pay close attention to the order indication, vital signs, and lab values.***
- **Right Date and Time:** Some instructors break this apart and have seven rights of medication administration. Orders may be written for a medication to be given every other day, so it is important to note the date and to administer the medication as ordered. Some drugs are given for a period of time, such as 10 days, and then automatically discontinued unless reordered. If you give a medication on a day it is not ordered to be given, it is considered a medication error. Based on the facility, to give a medication at the right time, it must be administered within ½ hour before or ½ hour after the scheduled time. For example, if a medication is ordered at 9:00 a.m., you can give it between 8:30 a.m. and 9:30 a.m. ***Safety: Be aware of when medications are due and administer them within the 1-hour window of time.***
- **Right Documentation:** You must document correctly and completely to meet this right. You will document on the MAR with your initials under the correct date and time. If the medication is a narcotic, you also must document the medication, amount, route, and the patient's name in the narcotic record. If the medication is to be administered prn, you will write the date, time, medication, and reason for administering it on the back of the MAR or in the nurses' notes, depending on facility policy. You also must document the patient's response to it after a period of time has elapsed, usually an hour for oral medications. If you do not give a medication for some reason, such as a patient refusing a medication or feeling nauseated, you must initial, circle the time on the MAR, and explain why the medication was not given on the back. ***Safety: Document all medications, given or not given, according to facility policy.***

When you check these rights and confirm that they are correct, you decrease the chances of making a medication error.

Patient Rights

Patients also have rights regarding medication administration. They have the right to know what the medication is for and how it will affect them. They have the right to refuse a medication. The patient can choose not to take a medication and should not be judged negatively for his or her choice. For example, a patient on chemotherapy for cancer may choose to stop taking the medication because of the side effects. While you might not make that same choice, you need to respect the patient's choice.

Patients also have the right to question their medications. They are now encouraged to question a medicine if it does not look like what they take at home, or it is not being administered at the frequency they normally take. Some patients know their own medications and routine far better than the nurse in the hospital does. ***Safety: If the patient questions a medication, research it thoroughly before administering it. This is an important safety check regarding the correct administration of medications.***

Safety Checks

When you prepare medications for administration, it is very important for you to stay focused on the task at hand. Ensure that you have no distractions, such as idle conversations or interruptions. When you prepare medications, you will obtain all the medications ordered for a patient at the time they are to be given. It is best not to prepare medications for two patients at one time because it is too easy to get confused. To prevent errors as you prepare medications, perform these three safety checks:

1. Verify the medication, dose, route, patient, indication, date, and time as you remove the medication from the cart, bin, or Pyxis® machine.
2. Verify the medication, dose, and route against the MAR prior to placing it in the medication cup and returning the container to the drawer, if applicable.
3. Verify the patient, medication, indication, dose, and route at the bedside prior to opening it and administering it to the patient.

If you are administering a number of medications to a patient at one time, it is a good idea to count the number of ordered medicines on the MAR and count the number of medicines in the cup to ensure that you are giving the correct amount. For example, if a patient has eight oral medications ordered at 9:00 a.m., you would count the number of medicines in the cup to be sure you have eight ready to administer.

Some facilities use bar codes for inventory control, charges, and patient identification when administering medications. After preparing the medications, you take them to the bedside still in their bar-coded packaging. You use a bar code scanner to scan the code on the patient's identification bracelet and then scan in the bar code on the medications. If a medication is not ordered for that patient, the scanner will beep to let you know that there is a problem. This is yet another way to ensure that the right medications are being given to the right patient. However, it does not take the place of the nurse making all the correct checks when preparing medications.

Supervision/Delegation Connection

Medication Administration

You must always administer the medications that you prepare. Do not delegate that task to anyone. For example, you cannot prepare medications and then leave them at the bedside for the certified nursing assistant (CNA) or unlicensed assistive personnel (UAP) to administer later, such as after the patient's bath. In hospitals, preparation and administration of medications is strictly a function of a licensed nurse and cannot be delegated to a CNA or UAP. In some states, specially trained medication aides are allowed to administer medications to the residents in a long-term facility. In that situation, it is your responsibility to oversee the medication administration if it is performed by a medication aide.

Guidelines for Preparing Medications

Before you administer any medication, whether oral, topical, inhaled, injectable, or IV, follow these guidelines:

- Check the orders on the MAR and compare them with the original health-care provider's order. Check for any discrepancies and validate that the order is correct.
- Look up any medication with which you are unfamiliar. If you are unsure about the purpose or effect of a medication, look it up. As you review the orders, determine if you need to check the patient's chart for any laboratory values prior to administering the medications and then obtain the information required.
- Wash or sanitize your hands according to facility policy.
- Obtain the ordered medications from the computerized cabinet, medicine cart, or patient bin. As you do so:
  - Verify the seven rights of medication administration.
  - Check medication allergies and compare them with the ordered medication.
  - Perform the first two safety checks.
- Determine if all medications are provided in the same dose and unit of measurement as ordered. If not, perform drug calculations to ensure that you have the correct number of tablets or capsules and that you have the correct amount of liquid medication.
- Place the unopened medications in a medicine cup.
- Close and lock the medication cart or patient medication bin. If you are using a computerized cabinet, clear your password.
- Immediately take the medication to the patient's bedside. If the patient is unavailable, store prepared medications according to facility policy. Label the medicine cup(s) with the patient's name and room number prior to storing them.
- Perform the third safety check at the bedside with two patient identifiers prior to opening the individually packaged medications.
- If using a bar-code system, scan the patient's identification bracelet with the bar-code scanner, and then scan each medication before you open it.

- Assess any required vital signs, labs, or any other essential patient conditions before administering the medications, such as blood pressure or pulse if the medication will decrease or increase those readings. Ascertain that it is safe to give the medication to the patient.
- Administer the medications to the patient. Stay with the patient to ensure that all medications are swallowed and no problems occur (see Chapter 36).
- ***Safety: Do not leave medications at the patient's bedside or ask another person to administer them for you. Administer only what you prepare.***

KNOWLEDGE CONNECTION

List the seven rights of medication administration. What are the three safety checks to make when preparing a medication and when do you perform them? How can you be sure that you have the correct number of medications for patients who take large amounts at one time?

Evidence-Based Practice

Medication Administration Errors in Hospitals, Long-Term Care Facilities, and Home Health Settings

Clinical Question

Do medication administration errors (MAEs) decrease with the use of automated dispensing cabinets, bar coding, and electronic prescribing orders?

Evidence

This study analyzed six randomized controlled trials (RCTs) and seven controlled trials (CTs) that were conducted in hospitals and other institutions and focused on adult patients, pediatrics, and other age groups. The study assessed automated dispensing cabinets, bar coding, and electronic prescribing orders and found that there was a reduction in MAEs in five of the six RCTs using these medication administration tools.

Implications for Nursing Practice

This study highlights the need for using automated dispensing cabinets, bar coding, and electronic prescribing in order to decrease MAEs. It is important to be diligent when pulling medications and checking the patient identifiers, route, time, date, and indication for each medication.

Reference

You can read more about this study at

Keers R, Williams S, Cooke J, et al. Impact of Interventions Designed to Reduce Medication Administration Errors in Hospitals: A Systematic Review. *Drug Safety*. 2014;37, 317-332. https://www.researchgate.net/profile/Tanya_Walsh/publication/261839601_Impact_of_Interventions_Designed_to_Reduce_Medication_Administration_Errors_in_Hospitals_A_Systematic_Review/links/57642e3908aedbc345ecbf32.pdf. Accessed September 12, 2018.

MEDICATION ERRORS

The best way to prevent medication errors is to be extremely careful during preparation, question anything that does not seem correct about the order, and know what you are giving, including the expected effects of the medication and the potential side effects. Check the vital signs or blood levels of a patient prior to administering medications to prevent toxicity or adverse effects. Calculate drug dosages carefully and have them checked by another nurse before preparing the medication. Box 35.5 gives tips for preventing medication errors.

Safe Medication Practices

The ISMP exists to improve medication safety by educating the health-care community and consumers about safe medication practices. They have developed guidelines for various issues identified as likely to cause errors in medications. In cooperation with the FDA, they have also developed a strategy to prevent confusion between medications with similar names by using "tall man letters." Box 35.6 lists FDA-approved generic drug names using tall man letters. Additional drug names using tall man letters can be found on the ISMP Web site, as well as a list of error-prone abbreviations, symbols, and dose designations. You can report medication errors to the

Box 35.5

Tips for Preventing Medication Errors

It is easy to confuse some medication names and doses. You must be very careful to read names and doses exactly to prevent errors. You also must focus completely on the task at hand when preparing medications for administration.

- **Read drug names carefully.** Many drug names are similar and can be confusing. Examples include Zantac and Xanax, baclofen and Bactroban, Plavix, and Pradaxa, Zostrix, and Zestril.
- **Read doses carefully, especially those with decimals.** Look for a 0 in front of the decimal to call attention to its presence so that it will not be overlooked. Example: 0.125 mg and 0.25 mg are both doses of digoxin. Also, doses in different units of the metric system can be the cause of an error. Example: Thyroid hormone is provided in micrograms (mcg) but may be ordered in milligrams (mg); 0.1 milligram is equal to 100 micrograms.
- **Never administer a medication you are unknowledgeable about.** If you do not know what the medication is for or what the expected effects are, you must look it up. Even if it is inconvenient and time-consuming, you must know what you are administering and if the dose is within the appropriate range.
- **Focus on medication preparation without distractions.** Prepare medications for one patient at a time.
- **Ask for clarification.** If an order is unclear, outside of usual dosage parameters, or seems inappropriate for the patient, clarify the order with the prescriber.

Box 35.6

FDA-Approved List of Generic Drug Names With Tall Man Letters

Drug Name With Tall Man Letters	Confused With
acetaZOLAMIDE	acetoHEXAMIDE
acetoHEXAMIDE	acetaZOLAMIDE
buPROPion	busPIRone
busPIRone	buPROPion
chlorproMAZINE	chlorproPAMIDE
chlorproPAMIDE	chlorproMAZINE
clomiPHENE	clomiPRAMINE
clomiPRAMINE	clomiPHENE
cycloSERINE	cycloSPORINE
cycloSPORINE	cycloSERINE
DAUNOrubicin	DOXOrubicin
dimenhyDRINATE	diphenhydrAMINE
diphenhydrAMINE	dimenhyDRINATE
DOBUTamine	DOPamine
DOPamine	DOBUTamine
DOXOrubicin	DAUNOrubicin
glipiZIDE	glyBURIDE
glyBURIDE	glipiZIDE
hydrALAZINE	hydrOXYzine
hydroMORPhone	MORPhine
hydrOXYzine	hydrALAZINE
medroxyprogesterone – methylPREDNISolone – methylTESTOSTERone	
methylprednisolone – medroxyPROGESTERone – methylTESTOSTERone	
methylTESTOSTERone – medroxyPROGESTERone – methylPREDNISolone	
mitoXANTRONE	MORphine
niCARdipine	NIFEdipine
NIFEdipine	niCARdipine
prednisoLONE	predniSONE
predniSONE	prednisoLONE
risperiDONE	rOPINRole
sulfADIAZINE	sulfiSOXAZOLE
sulfiSOXAZOLE	sulfadiazine
TOLAZamide	TOLBUTamide
TOLBUTamide	TOLAZamide
vinBLAStine	vinCRIStine
vinCRIStine	vinBLAStine

Source: FDA. Name Differentiation Project. Fda.gov. www.fda.gov/Drugs/DrugSafety/ MedicationErrors/ucm164587.htm.

ISMP Web site to help them identify and develop strategies for preventing such errors in the future. The Web site is www.ismp.org/tools/tallmanletters.pdf.

Handling a Medication Error

Although all staff make every effort to avoid a medication error, sometimes an error does occur. It may be that you discover the error or that you make an error. ***Safety: The most important thing is that you are honest about the mistake so that the patient can be protected from harm.***

If you find an error made by another nurse, follow the facility policy for reporting it. In most situations, you will report it to the unit nurse manager or his or her assistant. Because you found the error, you will fill out the incident report (see Chapter 3). Avoid making judgmental statements about anyone who makes a medication error because it can happen to very good nurses at times. All it takes is distraction from the task at hand, lack of focus, or not being thorough in knowledge about the medication.

If you make an error, be honest and report it yourself following facility policy. Complete the incident report and notify the health-care provider. This is a humbling experience, but you must put the patient's well-being above your own pride. Most hospitals have a nonpunitive approach to error reporting to prevent staff from failing to report incidents that could bring harm to a patient.

An example to illustrate this occurred to a nursing student on a leadership rotation toward the end of her practical nursing program. The student was administering medications to all the residents on one hall in a long-term care facility. She checked the MAR, prepared the medications for a male resident, and then administered them. She then prepared the medications for the resident's roommate and administered them. When she returned to the MAR, she realized that she had made two errors: She had given each resident his roommate's medications. The student was extremely distressed and went to her instructor with the error. They notified the health-care providers for each resident and completed incident reports. The student monitored vital signs every hour and finger stick blood sugars every hour as ordered for 4 hours. Neither resident suffered any ill effects, but the situation could have been life-threatening.

Real-World Connection

Pediatric Medication Administration

A nurse made a potentially fatal error when drawing up heparin for an infant's IV line because of failing to pay close attention to the ordered strength of the medication. This nurse drew up heparin 10,000 units/mL to flush the infant's line instead of the ordered 1,000 units/mL.

When you prepare medications for children, you must be constantly focused on the correct dose for the weight of the child. You will give only a portion of an adult dose, and it is critical that your dosage calculations be correct. Have them checked by another licensed health-care professional to verify that you are administering the correct dosage. In addition, always be certain that you have the correct strength of the medication.

Elder Care Connection

Age-Related Concerns of Medication Administration

When you prepare medications for elderly patients, keep in mind that they are more at risk for toxicity because of decreased liver and kidney function, which causes the medication to build up in the blood. It is very important to check blood levels of medications and signs and symptoms of toxicity prior to administering medications to the elderly.

POST CONFERENCE

Although you were nervous, you managed to prepare all of your patient's medications after looking them up in your nursing drug guide. When your instructor asked about each medication, you were ready with the answers. You even calculated a dose correctly. You checked the patient's fasting blood sugar and finger stick blood sugar levels before administering the insulin. The patient's potassium level was 3.3, so you and your instructor talked with the PA prior to administering the ordered furosemide (Lasix). The PA told you to give the Lasix and wrote an order to increase the potassium supplement to 20 mEq bid. Your instructor had to remind you, once you got to the bedside, to assess the blood pressure before administering Lasix and another antihypertensive. You learned a great deal about your patient's medications and will know them well next time.

Key Points

- Medications have three names based on chemical ingredients, generic assigned names, and brand names.
- Medications fall into two categories: prescription and OTC. Sometimes a medication can be in both categories due to different strengths.
- Controlled drugs fall into one of five schedules based on their potential for abuse. Schedule II drugs must be kept under double lock and counted at the end of each shift.
- Medications are prescribed for desired effects, but they also may cause side effects, which usually are mild and expected, as well as adverse effects, which are more severe and harmful.
- Allergic reactions to drugs may range from mild, causing itching, rash, and hives, to anaphylaxis, which causes swelling of the airways and shortness of breath and can possibly lead to shock and death.
- Some medications can accumulate in the bloodstream and cause toxicity. Nurses are responsible for checking the most recent medication blood levels prior to administering medications known to cause toxicity. Hold any ordered dose if blood levels are elevated and notify the prescriber.
- Drugs can interact with other drugs, with foods, and with supplements. Nurses are responsible for researching medications prior to administration to be aware of any potential interactions.
- Read prescriber orders closely and carefully, paying close attention to decimals and abbreviations. If the dose, route, or frequency is not appropriate for the medication or the patient, notify the prescriber and verify the order.
- The seven rights of medication administration help prevent you from making medication errors while preparing medications.
- The three safety checks occur when you remove the medication from the storage area, before you return the container or remaining medication to the storage area, and at the bedside before you open and administer the medication.
- You must admit to any medication error you make for the sake of the patient's well-being.
- In hospital settings, medication may be found in computerized cabinets, medication carts, and locked bins in patient rooms.
- Before you administer any medication, whether oral, topical, inhaled, injectable, or IV, follow the guidelines for preparing medications.

Review Questions

Select the answer that is most appropriate for each of the following questions. Some questions may have more than one correct answer. Select all that apply.

1. The drug name that is assigned and is not owned by the pharmaceutical company that develops the drug is the:
   1. chemical name.
   2. proprietary name.
   3. brand name.
   4. generic name.

2. You are preparing to administer a Schedule II drug. What special considerations are necessary?
   1. It is kept under double lock or with limited access in a computerized medication cabinet.
   2. It has a lower potential for abuse than Schedule III drugs.
   3. The remaining medications must be counted.
   4. The count must match the total in the record book.
   5. If kept in a computerized medication cabinet, the count is totaled by the nurse and the computer.

3. When you administer an antihypertensive medication at a dose within normal ranges, the patient's blood pressure drops to 84/60. This is a/an:
   1. side effect.
   2. adverse effect.
   3. allergic reaction.
   4. anaphylactic reaction.

4. A patient tells you that he is allergic to a muscle relaxer because it makes him sleep all day. You know that this is a common side effect of this medication. What action will you take?
   1. Record it as an allergy in the chart only
   2. Explain to the patient that he is not really allergic to the medication
   3. Record it as an allergy in the chart with an explanation of the reaction
   4. Notify the health-care provider immediately of the allergy and check for blood levels of the drug in the chart

5. A patient is taking a medication to lower cholesterol. You know that the patient needs more teaching about the medication when he says:
   1. "I will take my medicine each morning with grapefruit."
   2. "This medicine is to help lower my blood pressure."
   3. "If I experience any adverse effects or problems, I will contact my doctor."
   4. "I need to eat a low-fat diet and exercise as well as take this medication."

6. A patient on birth control pills tells you that she is also taking St. John's wort as an herbal supplement for mild depression. Which response will you make?
   1. "You need to be on a prescription drug for depression, not treat yourself."
   2. "St. John's wort increases estrogen breakdown, so it can decrease the effectiveness of your birth control pills."
   3. "St. John's wort decreases the rate of excretion of estrogen, so it can increase the side effects of birth control pills."
   4. "Have you looked up the medications you are taking to see if it interacts with any of them?"

7. You are using the PDR to look up a medication to determine its effects and side effects. The best way to obtain information is to first look up the medication in the:
   1. Brand and Generic Name Index and then read about it in the Product Information Section.
   2. Product Identification Section and then read about it in the Product Information Section.
   3. Manufacturer's Index and then locate it in the Product Identification Section.
   4. Product Category Index and then the Manufacturer's Index.

8. The nurse knows the seven rights of medication administration are which of the following?
   1. Right patient
   2. Right route
   3. Right indication
   4. Right dosage
   5. Right documentation
   6. Right medication
   7. Right date and time

9. Which of the following is(are) commonly used medical abbreviations?
   1. IM
   2. SQ
   3. kg
   4. mL
   5. TID
   6. QID
   7. mg

ANSWERS 1. 4, 2. 1, 3, 4, 5, 3. 2, 4. 3, 5. 1, 2, 6. 2, 7. 1, 8. 1, 2, 3, 4, 5, 6, 7, 9. 1, 3, 4, 7

Critical Thinking Exercise

Answers available online.

1. You have prepared oral medications for your patient and have taken them into his room. The patient is in the bathroom taking a shower. His wife says, "Just leave the medicine on the bedside table. I will see that he takes it." What will you do and why?

Additional Resources

DAVIS edge. **Use the scratch off code on the inside front cover of your book to access online quizzes that will help you to improve your scores on course exams and prepare for the NCLEX-PN®.**

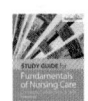

Study Guide

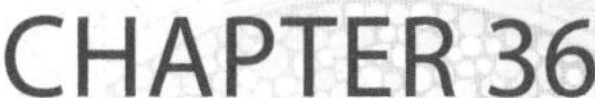

CHAPTER 36 Administering Oral, Topical, and Mucosal Medications

KEY TERMS

Buccal route (BUK-uhl ROOT)
Capsule (KAP-suhl)
Dry-powder inhaler (DRYE-POW-duhr in-HAY-luhr)
Elixir (ih-LIK-ser)
Enteric-coated (en-TER-ik-KOH-ted)
Metered-dose inhaler (MEET-uhrd DOHSS in-HAY-luhr)
Narcotic (nar-KOT-ik)
Rectal route (REK-tuhl ROOT)
Respiratory route (res-PIH-ra-tor-ee ROOT)
Solution (so-LOO-shun)
Sublingual route (sub-LING-gwuhl ROOT)
Suspension (sus-PEN-shun)
Sustained-release (sus-TAYND-rih-LEESS)
Syrup (SIH-ruhp)
Tablet (TAB-let)
Transdermal route (tranz-DER-mahl ROOT)
Vaginal route (va-JYE-nuhl ROOT)

CHAPTER CONCEPTS

Safety
Patient-Centered Care

LEARNING OUTCOMES

1. Define various terms associated with oral, topical, and mucosal medications.
2. Differentiate between the use of oral, sublingual, and buccal routes of administration.
3. Describe the variety of oral, topical, and mucosal forms of drugs.
4. Explain how to prepare liquid medications.
5. Describe special considerations for administration of narcotic medications.
6. Describe special precautions needed when administering medications to patients on tube feedings.
7. Discuss principles to use when administering medicines through an enteral tube.
8. Explain the differences in administering medications to children, adults, and older adults.
9. Discuss guidelines for administering medications via the topical and transdermal routes.
10. Describe guidelines to follow when administering eye, ear, and nasal medications.
11. Discuss vaginal medications and how they are administered.
12. Identify purposes of rectal medications and contraindications for this route.
13. Differentiate between the use of a metered-dose inhaler and a dry-powder inhaler.
14. Identify nursing responsibilities when administering oral, topical, and mucosal medications.
15. Explain how to document medication administration on paper and in electronic medication administration records.
16. Discuss ways to prevent errors in medication administration and documentation.
17. Explain what to do if a medication error occurs.
18. Discuss information found in the Connection features of this chapter.
19. Identify safety issues related to the administration of oral, topical, and mucosal medications.
20. Answer questions about the skills in this chapter.

SKILLS

36.1 Administering Oral Medications
36.2 Administering Medications Through an Enteral Tube

SKILLS—cont'd

36.3 Administering Topical and Transdermal Medications
36.4 Administering Eye and Ear Medications
36.5 Irrigating the Eye and Ear
36.6 Administering Vaginal Medications
36.7 Administering Rectal Suppositories
36.8 Administering Inhaled Medications

CRITICAL THINKING CONNECTION

Clinical Assignment

You are assigned to care for a 22-year-old female with developmental disabilities and a seizure disorder. She suffered brain damage at birth and is unable to chew and swallow. She lives in a long-term care facility and was transferred from that facility to the hospital for management of her seizure disorder, as well as treatment of eczema, constipation, and a vaginal yeast infection. She has a percutaneous endoscopic gastrostomy (PEG) tube, and you will be administering her feedings and medications through it. You have never administered a tube feeding before, much less medications through a PEG.

Critical Thinking Questions:

1. How would you administer a PEG tube feeding?
2. How would you give liquid and tablet medications through a PEG tube?
3. How would you administer medications that are not compatible?

Administration of medications following the seven rights is a huge responsibility. You must know not only the medication, dose, indication and route ordered, but also how to correctly administer medications via every route. In this chapter, we will focus on administration of drugs via the oral, topical, mucosal, and inhaled routes. Injected and IV routes are discussed in Chapters 37 and 38, respectively.

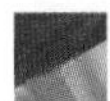

ROUTES OF ADMINISTRATION

Many drugs are available in multiple forms that can be administered by several routes. It is important to know the purposes, uses, and variations of each route. For example, variations of the oral route include the **sublingual route** (under the tongue) and the **buccal route** (between the cheek and gum). In addition to understanding how to administer the medications via all the routes, you also will need to learn which types of preparations are suitable for each route.

Oral Route

The *oral route* of administration is the method by which medications are taken through the mouth or oral mucous membrane. When you think of administering medications by the oral route, you most often think of medications that are swallowed. This route is commonly referred to as "by mouth" or PO (*per os* in Latin); it includes drugs that enter the bloodstream directly through the oral mucosa. Medications enter the bloodstream through the oral mucosa when the sublingual and buccal routes are used. Sublingual medications are placed beneath the tongue to be absorbed, and buccal medications are placed between the cheek and gum to be absorbed. Oral medications are available in various forms, including tablets, capsules, and liquid medications.

Tablets and Caplets

A **tablet** is made of powdered ingredients compressed into various sizes and shapes. Tablets are the most common form of oral medication, and the majority are designed to be swallowed. They are broken down by the digestive system and absorbed into the bloodstream. Caplets are similar to tablets but are oblong in shape, making them easier for some people to swallow. Tablets that are not swallowed whole may be in forms that can be chewed, or they may melt on contact with saliva. An example of the latter form is hyoscyamine sulfate (Levsin).

Chewable tablets, such as chewable low-dose aspirin, are an alternative for patients who have difficulty swallowing large capsules or tablets. Chewing also breaks down the medication for increased activity in the stomach, such as in chewable antacids.

Enteric-coated tablets contain an outer coating that does not dissolve until the medication reaches the intestines. This coating protects the stomach from ingredients in the medication that may be irritating, thus preventing nausea, vomiting, and ulcer formation. Some medications are destroyed by stomach acids, and the enteric coating prevents the acids from inactivating the drug before it reaches the intestines.

Another type of coated tablet is a film-coated tablet. This coating prevents contact with the active ingredient during normal handling, which could cause damage to the medication.

Sustained-release tablets, also called *controlled-release, delayed-release, extended-release,* or *modified-release* tablets, are designed to slow the absorption of the drug. These medications are absorbed slowly over time for a continuous effect. ***Safety: Do not crush or break sustained-release or enteric-coated tablets.*** Crushing a sustained-release tablet will cause the patient to receive all of the drug at one time, leading to severe adverse effects and possible overdose. Crushing an enteric-coated medication will cause the medication to be absorbed in the stomach rather than the intestine, leading to gastric irritation or possible destruction of the medication.

Buccal tablets are designed to dissolve between the cheek and gum. As it dissolves, the tablet is absorbed through the

• WORD • BUILDING •

sublingual route: sub – under + lingu – tongue + al – related to
buccal route: bucc – mouth or cheek + al – related to; route – road

walls of the numerous blood vessels in the inner cheek. Similarly, sublingual tablets dissolve under the tongue and are absorbed by the blood vessels there. These medications do not have to be digested to enter the bloodstream.

Capsules

A **capsule** is a gelatin shell containing a powder or pellets of medication. It may be preferred over tablets because it is swallowed more easily. Capsules may contain sustained-release pellets that dissolve over time for lasting medication effect.

If the patient is unable to swallow the capsule, it can be opened and the contents mixed with 1 to 2 teaspoons of soft food, such as applesauce or ice cream. ***Safety: Never put crushed tablets or opened capsules in a full serving of ice cream or applesauce. The patient may refuse to eat the entire serving, and you will not know how much medication has been ingested.*** Not all capsules can be opened and safely administered in this way. Check your nursing drug guide or discuss with a pharmacist before opening capsules. Medications that should not be crushed are listed in Box 36.1. Skill 36.1 (page 811) provides more information regarding administration of oral medications.

Liquid Medications

Liquid oral dosage forms include syrups, elixirs, solutions, and suspensions. Health-care providers often prescribe liquid medications to patients who cannot swallow solid dosage forms and for those with nasogastric or PEG tubes. Definitions for each type of liquid oral form are found in Box 36.2. ***Safety: Always shake a suspension prior to administering it to mix the drug with the liquid. Failure to do so could cause ineffective medication action when doses are poured from the top of the bottle and an overdose of medication when doses are poured from the bottom of the bottle.***

Box 36.1

Medications That Should Not Be Crushed

Some medications should not be crushed because crushing can cause them to be absorbed too quickly or because they are designed to dissolve in the intestines rather than the stomach. In addition, some medications can irritate mucous membranes in the esophagus and stomach if they are crushed. Medications that should not be crushed include the following:

- Buccal or sublingual tablets
- Effervescent tablets
- Enteric-coated tablets
- Liquid-filled gel caps
- Medications that may taste too bitter to swallow
- Mucous membrane irritants
- Neoplastic agents (chemotherapy for cancer treatment)
- Orally disintegrating medications
- Sustained-release tablets

For a complete list of that should not be crushed, go to the Institute for Safe Medication Practices Web site at www.ismp.org.

Box 36.2

Forms of Liquid Medication

Liquid medications come in a variety of forms to make them easier to swallow. Some should be used with caution in certain circumstances.

- An **elixir** may contain sweeteners or flavorings. It also may contain water and alcohol. It is generally clear in appearance, although some may contain colorings. Patients with a history of alcohol abuse or who are receiving disulfiram (Antabuse) should avoid elixirs because of the alcohol content.
- A **solution** is a liquid that contains a dissolved substance.
- A **suspension** contains fine particles of medication mixed with, but not dissolved in, a liquid. When the mixture sits, the particles drift to the bottom of the liquid.
- A **syrup** is a concentrated aqueous preparation of sugars, with or without flavoring agents, and medicinal substances.

When administering a liquid medication, shake the preparation if it is a suspension or if settling may have occurred. When you are pouring a dose from a bottle, you usually will use a plastic medicine cup. For infants and young children, you may use calibrated droppers or syringes. While pouring the liquid medication, hold the measuring device at eye level (Fig. 36.1A). You will notice that the top of the liquid is not

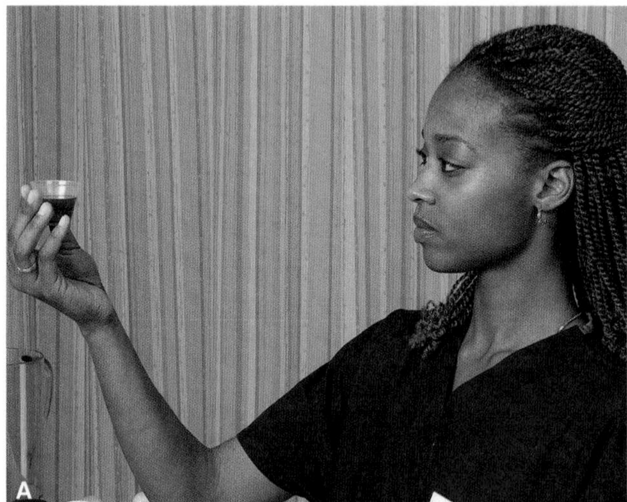

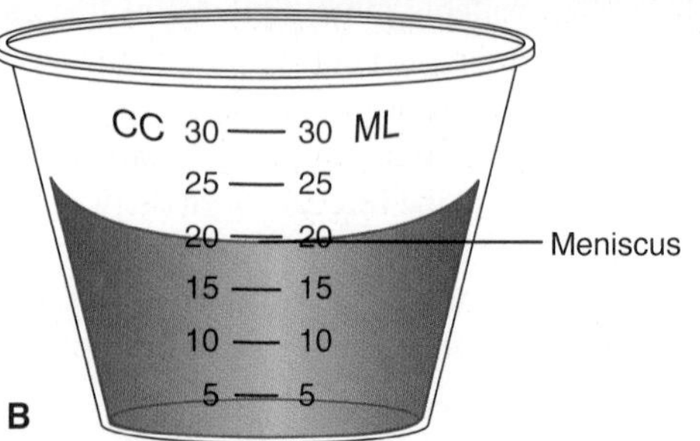

FIGURE 36.1 This nurse is measuring liquid medication at eye level (Part A from Wilkinson JM, Treas LS. *Fundamentals of Nursing: Theory, Concepts & Applications*. Vol. 1. 3rd ed. Philadelphia, PA: FA Davis; 2016).

level but instead curves up on the sides and is slightly lower in the middle. This is called the *meniscus* (Fig. 36.1B). ***Safety: When reading the amount of liquid in a medicine cup, read it at the lowest level of the meniscus.***

If you are pouring a liquid medication from a multiple-dose bottle, hold the label in the palm of your hand as you pour. In this way, no medication can accidentally be poured over the label and obscure the information on it.

In clinical settings, most liquid medications are packaged in single doses, also referred to as the *unit dose system.* It may not be necessary to pour out and measure liquid medications.

Some liquid medications, such as oral iron preparations, can stain the teeth. ***Safety: Administer liquid medications that can stain teeth by having the patient drink it out of the medicine cup using a straw.*** Have the patient drink a full glass of water afterward to prevent any of the medication from staying in contact with tooth enamel.

Holding Oral Medications

It is important to know when to withhold medications as well as when to administer them. ***Safety: If the patient is NPO, do not administer routine medications unless ordered to do so.*** For example, in some situations the prescriber may write an order to give the medicines with a sip of water. If the patient is complaining of nausea or is vomiting, withhold the medication and notify the prescriber. If you give the medication, the patient may vomit all or part of it.

> **KNOWLEDGE CONNECTION**
> Which types of tablets cannot be crushed? How would you administer the contents of a capsule to a patient unable to swallow it? Explain how to pour liquid medications.

Administration of Oral Narcotic Medications

Narcotic medications are made with opium and opium derivatives that control and relieve pain. Narcotics are controlled substances that may be formulated for oral, topical, injectable, and IV administration.

In the hospital setting, you may frequently administer oral narcotics to your patients. As you learned in Chapter 35, narcotics have a high potential for abuse and are regulated by law according to schedules. However, when narcotics are ordered by the prescriber for pain, it is appropriate to administer them. Often, the prescriber will order a strong narcotic for moderate to severe pain and a less potent drug for mild to moderate pain. In those situations, you will use your nursing judgment as you assess the patient's pain level and how he or she rates the pain. Refer to Chapter 19 for information on assessing and managing pain.

Historically, nurses have undermedicated patients for pain rather than overmedicating them. It is important to assess vital signs, especially respiratory status, prior to administering narcotics because they depress respirations and lower blood pressure. In addition to specific pain and vital sign assessments, obtaining narcotics for administration requires more steps than preparing other medications. (See Chapter 35 for information on obtaining and preparing narcotics.) ***Safety: Remain with the patient until narcotic medications are swallowed to ensure that he or she does not "cheek" the medication. In rare situations, a patient might save up a number of narcotic medications to attempt suicide later by taking them all at once.***

COUNTING NARCOTIC MEDICATIONS. Nurses must count narcotics and other controlled substances at specific times, most commonly at shift changes. The oncoming nurse counts the narcotics with the off-going nurse. Any discrepancies must be accounted for and the narcotics record amended. If the count on the narcotics record does not match the number of narcotics in the drawer, report it immediately following facility policy, as federal law requires strict inventory and records with controlled substances compared to other prescription drugs. In some facilities, it is a policy that the off-going nurse cannot leave until the discrepancy is resolved. If it cannot be resolved, it may be policy for the nurses to participate in a urine drug screen to determine if diversion is occurring.

If you do not use a full dose of a narcotic, discard the unused narcotics and record the waste according to facility policies. For example, if you have an order for 50 mg of meperidine (Demerol) to be administered PO and the meperidine in the drawer is in 100-mg tablets, you would administer only half of a tablet. The remaining half must be discarded according to facility policy. In most cases, you will dispose of it in a chemical waste container with another licensed nurse as a witness. Then you will record the narcotic drug wastage on the narcotic record and have the witness cosign with you. ***Safety: In most situations, you will not dispose of wasted narcotic medications by flushing them down the toilet because this contributes to drugs in the environment.***

> **KNOWLEDGE CONNECTION**
> What are narcotic drugs? How should you handle and administer narcotics? Describe the procedures for properly disposing of unused narcotics.

Enteral Tube Route

Patients who are unable to swallow food and medications may have a nasogastric or gastrostomy (PEG) tube placed. When that is the case, you will prepare oral medications and administer them through the enteral tube. (For a review of feeding tubes and formulas, see Chapter 24.)

• WORD • BUILDING •
narcotic: narkotikos – benumbing

Medication Considerations

Medications in tablet form will need to be crushed to a fine powder and mixed with 20 mL of water to be administered through the feeding tube. A mortar and pestle or a pill crusher may be used. When possible, the prescriber will order liquid medications, but if that is not possible, tablets will be crushed. Some medications, however, cannot be crushed because doing so will affect their absorption or desired effects (refer to Box 36.1).

Most capsules can be opened and mixed with water to be administered through the feeding tube. However, the contents of certain capsules must be mixed with juice rather than water and administered through a large-bore tube. ***Safety: Always mix omeprazole (Prilosec) and lansoprazole (Prevacid) with apple or orange juice rather than water and flush the tube with juice.*** This helps preserve the enteric coating on the granules and helps prevent clumping of the granules, which can then clog the tube. It is important to consult with the pharmacist before opening capsules and administering the contents through a feeding tube, especially with antireflux medications. Some sustained-release capsules may be opened and mixed with 20 mL of water and then instilled via the tube. However, there are some sustained-release medication capsules that cannot be opened for tube instillation. Sustained-release medications that are crushed or capsules that are opened against the manufacturer's recommendations may result not only in a quicker onset of action, but also in a more intense or stronger effect as well as severe adverse reactions.

Some medications should be taken on an empty stomach. Other medications can interact with the ingredients in tube-feeding formulas and cause decreased effectiveness. Box 36.3 gives details about certain medications and their interactions with tube-feeding formulas. Because such interactions are known to occur, it may be necessary to turn off a continuous tube feeding for a period of time before and

Box 36.3

Common Medication and Enteral Formula Interactions

Always check for incompatibilities prior to administering medications through an enteral tube. The following medications are known to interact with tube-feeding formulas. Recommendations of how to overcome those interactions are discussed below.

Phenytoin (Dilantin) Suspension

If this antiseizure medication is given through an enteral tube and mixes with the formula in the patient's stomach, its absorption may be decreased by nearly 70%. When administering phenytoin, follow facility policy regarding stopping the continuous tube feeding. It is recommended that you stop the feeding for 1 to 2 hours prior to administering the phenytoin and then flush the tube with 60 mL of water after administering it to prevent the medication from adhering to the tube. Dilute phenytoin with 20 to 60 mL of water to improve its absorption before administering it through an enteral tube.

Carbamazepine (Tegretol) Suspension

This is another antiseizure medication that is not well absorbed when administered via an enteral tube. This drug may adhere to the feeding tube itself. It is recommended that you dilute this medication with an equal volume of water or normal saline before administering it through an enteral tube to help prevent adherence to the tube. In addition, always flush the tube with at least 30 mL of water before and after administering any medication.

Warfarin (Coumadin)

This is an anticoagulant medication that is crushed and administered through an enteral tube. It can bind to the proteins in the tube feeding formula, decreasing its absorption and effectiveness. It is recommended that a continuous tube feeding be stopped for at least 1 hour before and 1 hour after warfarin administration to help prevent this interaction. If the medication is still less effective than required, it may be necessary for the health-care provider to change the order to low-molecular-weight heparin (Lovenox), which is injectable only.

Fluoroquinolones

This is a class of antibiotics whose absorption is decreased by interactions with minerals in the feeding formula, such as calcium, magnesium, aluminum, and iron. It is recommended that you stop the tube feeding for at least 1 hour before and 2 hours after administering these types of antibiotics. It is also important to thoroughly crush the tablets and dilute them in 20 to 60 mL of water. *Safety: Do not administer ciprofloxacin (Cipro) suspension through a feeding tube because it may adhere to the tube and cause occlusion.*

Proton Pump Inhibitors

These medications help prevent symptoms of gastroesophageal reflux disease by decreasing the amount of acid produced by the stomach. Because of their action, these medications are inactivated by gastric acid and are designed to dissolve in the duodenum. As discussed in the chapter text, omeprazole (Prilosec) and lansoprazole (Prevacid) may be opened and the granules mixed with apple or orange juice for administration down a large-bore enteral tube. Then the tube should be flushed with more juice rather than with water.

If these medications must be administered through a small-bore enteral tube, you must dissolve the intact enteric-coated granules in a sodium bicarbonate 8.4% solution to prevent the drug from being destroyed by the stomach acid. Consult the pharmacist for assistance in this situation.

Another proton pump inhibitor, pantoprazole (Protonix), is available in a delayed-release suspension that contains enteric-coated granules. It is recommended that the suspension be drawn up in an oral syringe and mixed with apple juice for administration through an enteral tube.

However, another type of proton pump inhibitor, esomeprazole (Nexium), which is available as delayed-release capsules and a delayed-release oral suspension, should be mixed with water before administering through an enteral tube.

after administering the medications. ***Safety: Consult drug book references and the facility pharmacist to determine which medications may or may not be opened, crushed, mixed with formula, or administered via an enteral tube.***

Certain medications are known to cause clumping with tube-feeding formula when given through an enteral tube. Small-bore feeding tubes can easily become obstructed if such clumping occurs. Even though some of the medications that cause clumping are liquids, they should not be administered through an enteral feeding tube. Box 36.4 lists the medications that are known to cause clumping when administered with tube-feeding formula.

Administration of Medication Through the Feeding Tube

When you administer medication through a feeding tube, it is important to keep several principles in mind. ***Safety: Always flush the feeding tube with 30 to 60 mL of water before and 20 to 30 ml after administration of medications to prevent interactions with formula in the tube, adherence of the drug to the tube, and clogging of the tube.***

It is ultimately your responsibility to know and follow the correct method of administration for each medication you give. Most medications will dissolve best in water that is room temperature or slightly warm as opposed to cold water. There are conflicting theories regarding whether mixing medications together prior to administration will result in physical reactions that can alter or destroy their desired effects, so it is recommended that you administer each medication separately, never mixing the crushed pills or liquids together. This also makes it possible for you to identify each drug during administration; this is pertinent in case an interruption occurs during the administration process. For example, if you were administering medications through an enteral tube and accidentally spilled one medication, you could identify which medication the patient did not receive. Another situation might be that while you are at the bedside preparing to administer the medications, the health-care provider walks in and discontinues one of the medications that you have already crushed. In this example, you would be able to identify which medication to stop. If the medications were all mixed together in one cup, you would be unable to remove the discontinued medication.

When administering multiple medications, you must also flush the tube between medications with 20 to 30 mL of water to clear the medicine out of the tube before instilling the next medicine. This further reduces the risk of an adverse reaction occurring due to mixing two or more drugs together in a small amount of water. ***Safety: Avoid mixing crushed pills or liquids together in the same cup to be as accurate as possible while administering medications.*** Skill 36.2 (page 812) provides more information on administering medications through an enteral tube.

If you are administering medications through a nasogastric tube that is connected to suction for gastric decompression, it is very important that you discontinue the suction and clamp the nasogastric tube for 30 minutes after you administer the medications. Otherwise the medication will be immediately suctioned out of the stomach through the tube. ***Safety: Be sure to resume the suction in 30 minutes to prevent distention, nausea, and vomiting from occurring because the tube is clamped too long.***

Box 36.4

Medications That Cause Clumping When Administered With Enteral Feeding Formulas

The following medications should not be administered with tube feeding formulas:

- Brompheniramine (Dimetapp)
- Ferrous sulfate (Feosol elixir)
- Guaifenesin (Robitussin)
- Lithium citrate (Cibalith-S)
- Monobasic sodium phosphate (Fleet Phospho-Soda)
- Potassium chloride liquid
- Pseudoephedrine hydrochloride (Sudafed syrup)

Supervision/Delegation Connection

Unlicensed Personnel and Medication Administration

If you are working in a setting where you supervise unlicensed personnel who administer medications, be very sure that they are knowledgeable about all aspects of medication administration in their scope of practice. Take time to observe each staff member when they prepare and administer medications. Ensure that the medicines are being administered correctly. Because you are the licensed person, you are responsible for the medications administered by those you supervise. Avoid assuming that your unlicensed staff members always know what to do.

KNOWLEDGE CONNECTION

How much water should be used to flush an enteric tube before and after administration of medications? In how much water should a crushed medication be dissolved? How will you know if it is safe to crush a medication or open a capsule or administer a medication with a particular formula?

Administering Medications to Special Populations

Administration of medications to elders and to children can pose certain challenges. The elderly patient is more at risk for side effects and medication interactions, while children may be more resistant to swallowing medications. (See Boxes 36.5 and 36.6 for tips on administering medications to these special populations.)

Elder Care Connection

Medication Organizers and Punch Card Systems

Medication Organizers

Many elderly patients in home health care use medication organizers, which contain separate storage compartments for the medications to be taken at breakfast, lunch, dinner, and bedtime. These containers can be prepared for an entire week at a time. They offer the added benefit of allowing the client and the nurse to see if the medications have been taken.

Punch Card Systems

Most long-term care facilities use a punch card system for administering medications. Each card contains a 30-day supply of medication, which is numbered in descending order. Punch out the medication in order and you will be able to tell exactly how many tablets or capsules remain. Reorder a resident's medications when a 7-day supply remains to avoid interruption in medication availability.

Box 36.5

Administering Medicines to Older Adults

Older adults may have problems taking medications because of difficulty swallowing. In addition, their reactions to and metabolism of medications may be different from those of younger adults because of the effects of aging on different body systems.

It is important to keep the following considerations in mind when you are administering medications to the elderly:

- **Difficulty swallowing:** You may need to crush medications and mix them in 1 to 2 teaspoons of applesauce or ice cream for the older person to swallow. If medications cannot be crushed, you may need to obtain an order for a liquid medication.
- **Metabolism of medications:** Because aging causes patients to be more sensitive to medication effects and side effects, it is important to assess frequently for toxicity and undesired effects. Aging also affects the ability of the body to prevent medications from affecting the central nervous system, so assess for increased side effects of confusion or disorientation.
- **Multiple medications:** Many elderly people are taking a large number of medications for a variety of chronic conditions. Be alert to possible interactions of these medications with each other and with OTC medications, including supplements and herbal remedies.
- **Adverse drug reactions:** It is important to monitor laboratory results to determine if medications should be held and the prescriber consulted. Monitor liver and kidney function tests for toxic effects of certain medications. When elderly patients are taking multiple medicines, consider any new sign or symptom to be drug related until determined differently.

Box 36.6

Administering Medicines to Infants and Children

One major focus of administering medications to infants and children is getting them to take the medicine. Some devices and ideas to improve this include:

- **Administration devices:** Infants may spit out liquid medications. Use of an oral syringe is recommended because it offers more accurate dosing and is easy to use. Teach parents to remove the cap from the end of the syringe and to keep it out of the infant or child's reach to prevent choking. Place the syringe toward the back of the mouth in the cheek pouch and depress the plunger to administer the medication.
- **Small doses:** The amount of medication ordered for children is generally a fraction of an adult dose. Double-check the appropriate pediatric dosage for the patient's weight, usually ordered in milligrams per kilogram of body weight. Overdoses can easily occur. Some facilities require two nurses to check a pediatric medication dose before it is administered.
- **Objectionable taste:** If a child refuses a medication because of its taste, speak with the pharmacist about adding a flavoring syrup to it. If the taste cannot be masked, you can offer a frozen juice bar to the child first because it will help numb the taste buds. Praise the child when he or she takes the medication.

Topical Route

The *topical route* of administration involves applying a drug to the skin or mucous membranes. Topical drugs typically are used for their action at one specific site. In addition to the skin, other topical routes may include the vagina, anus, eyes, and ears; however, these are sometimes distinguished from topical drugs applied to the skin.

Topical drugs usually act locally, but they also may have systemic effects. There are several different classes of topical preparations, each with unique characteristics (Box 36.7).

Box 36.7

Types of Topical Medication Preparations

The following is a list of the most common types of topical medications:

- **Creams** typically are *viscous* (thick) emulsions, with some *emollient* (moisturizing) ability. Creams are commonly used for topical steroids and in medications to relieve itching.
- **Gels** are not as thick as creams. They usually are clear but may contain coloring. Phenergan gel is applied to the inner wrists to help relieve nausea.
- **Lotions,** like creams, are emulsions, but are less viscous and moisturizing. Some may be drying, such as calamine lotion for poison ivy.
- **Ointments,** like creams, are highly viscous and have an emollient base. They often are dispensed in tubes. Ointments are used for antibiotic and steroid topical medications.

When you administer topical medications such as creams and ointments, you will generally apply a thin coat of the medication to the affected area. Certain topical medications are ordered to be applied "liberally," or with a thick coat of medication. It is important that you know the appropriate application amount by researching the medication in a nursing drug guide. Use a cotton-tipped swab or a tongue depressor to apply the medicine. Avoid touching the opening of the tube or dispenser to the patient's skin to prevent contamination. Wear gloves when you administer topical medications to decrease the chance of contact with blood, body fluids, and medication.

Some topical medications should not be covered with an occlusive dressing because it can alter the absorption of the drug. If you are uncertain about covering a topical medication, check with the pharmacist before applying an occlusive dressing. Skill 36.3 (page 813) provides more information about administering topical medications.

Transdermal Route

The **transdermal route** is a method of applying a drug to the skin using a patch. The drug is absorbed through the skin into the bloodstream for a systemic effect (Fig. 36.2). The transdermal route delivers a slow, constant dose of medication. Transdermal patches are drugs bonded to an adhesive bandage and applied to the skin. Several drugs are now prepared in patch form, including nitroglycerin, nicotine, and oral contraceptives.

Safety: Before applying the patch, write the date, time of application, and your initials on the patch. When applying transdermal patches, avoid touching the medicated portion with your fingers. Wear gloves during the application, and apply each patch to a different place than the previous patch. Be sure to remove the previous patch first to avoid giving the patient an overdose of medication. Try to choose a site that has the least amount of hair, such as the upper arm or lower abdomen. It may be necessary to shave an area on the upper chest or arm so that the patch will adhere. Do not cut patches to fit smaller areas. Skill 36.3 provides more information on applying a transdermal patch.

> **KNOWLEDGE CONNECTION**
> Describe the different types of topical preparations. Why are certain drugs administered topically or transdermally?

Mucosal Route

Drugs may be absorbed through the mucous membranes in the eyes, nose, rectum, and vagina. This route is sometimes preferred because the drugs enter directly into the bloodstream, resulting in faster onset of action. For example, if a patient has nausea and vomiting, you may administer medication via a rectal suppository to relieve the nausea and vomiting. The drug is absorbed into the bloodstream for a rapid effect that could not be obtained by administering it orally.

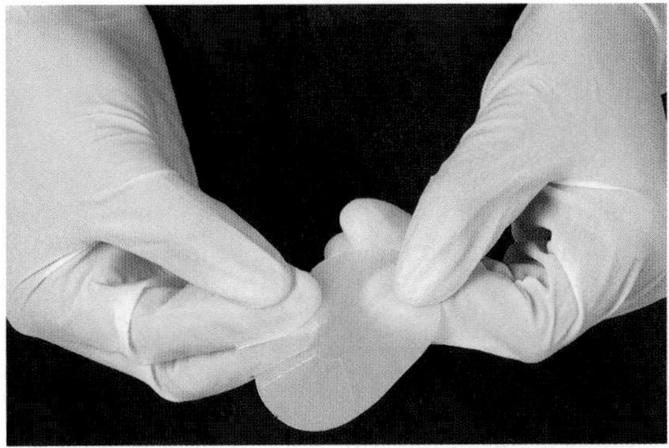

FIGURE 36.2 A transdermal patch is used for delivery of systemic medications (from Wilkinson JM, Treas LS. *Fundamentals of Nursing: Theory, Concepts & Applications.* Vol. 2. 3rd ed. Philadelphia, PA: FA Davis; 2016).

Some mucosal medications are administered for local effects, such as a vaginal medication to treat a yeast infection or an eye medication to treat glaucoma.

Eye Medications

Drugs administered to the eye take the form of drops or ointments and usually are applied in the lower conjunctival sac. Eye medications may be ordered to lubricate the eye, to prevent or treat conditions such as glaucoma or infection, or for diagnostic purposes. Examples of eye medications include timolol (Timoptic) for glaucoma, gentamicin (Garamycin) for bacterial infections such as conjunctivitis or "pink eye," and prednisolone (Inflamase) for inflammation.

When you administer eyedrops, you will place them into the middle part of the lower conjunctival sac. Have the patient tilt his or her head back and look upward. Gently pull the lower lid down to expose the sac. Gently brace your hand against the patient's forehead or cheek to prevent injury to the eye if the patient moves his or her head. Administer the drop of eye medication into the conjunctival sac.

To apply eye ointment, gently squeeze a line of ointment into the conjunctival sac. Instruct the patient to close his or her eyelids and move the eyes around while keeping the eyelids closed. ***Safety: Avoid applying pressure to the eyeball at all times. Also, avoid touching the tip of the tube or dropper to the patient's eye or skin to prevent contamination by pathogens.*** A tissue may be used to wipe from the inner to outer part of the eye along the eyelash. Advise patients not to rub their eyes after applying eyedrops or ointments.

In some situations, the drug that is administered for a local effect may be absorbed into the bloodstream and cause unwanted systemic effects. To prevent this, after you administer the eyedrops, press your gloved fingertip gently against the lacrimal ducts on either side of the nose for a few seconds.

• WORD • BUILDING •

transdermal route: trans – across + dermal – related to the skin; route – road

lacrimal: lacrim – tears + al – related to

Skill 36.4 (page 815) provides further information about administering eye medications.

Ear Medications

Drugs administered in the ear are in the form of drops. These drugs may be used to soften cerumen, relieve pain, treat infection or inflammation, or facilitate removal of a foreign body, such as an insect or a small object. Examples of eardrops include ciprofloxacin/hydrocortisone (Cipro HC) for infection and carbamide peroxide (Debrox) to soften earwax for removal.

To instill eardrops, position the patient lying on his or her side with the affected ear up. For adults and children older than 3 years of age, gently pull the pinna up and back. For children younger than 3 years of age, pull the pinna down and back. This helps straighten the ear canal, which allows the drops to penetrate to the middle ear. Aim the dropper so that the medication drop rolls down the wall of the canal and does not drop directly onto the tympanic membrane, which would cause pain. ***Safety: Avoid touching the dropper to the surface of the ear to prevent the introduction of pathogens into the bottle of ear medication. Ask the patient to remain with his or her head positioned with the affected ear up for at least 2 minutes. A cotton ball can be placed loosely in the ear to absorb excess medication. Safety: Do not administer eardrops to patients with damage to the tympanic membrane.*** If in doubt, ensure that the tympanic membrane has been examined with an otoscope by a health-care professional prior to administering the medication. Skill 36.4 provides more information about administering eardrops.

Eye and Ear Irrigations

You may have orders to irrigate a patient's eyes or ears with saline to flush away debris and contaminants. Sometimes you will be irrigating to remove a foreign body from the eye or ear, such as an insect in the ear or piece of sawdust in the eye. Occasionally, a small child will place a foreign body in a body orifice, including the ear. It is important to know that irrigation is contraindicated for the removal of a foreign body that could absorb fluid and enlarge. For example, a dry bean will absorb irrigation fluid and become even more securely wedged in the ear. Skill 36.5 (page 816) provides more information on eye and ear irrigation.

Nasal Medications

Nasal medications are administered to reduce inflammation, facilitate drainage, or treat infections in the nasal cavity. Drugs administered via the nasal mucosa are rapidly absorbed into the bloodstream. Some medications are administered for local effects on the nasal mucosa. Mucinex nasal spray (guaifenesin), for example, is used to promote sinus and nasal drainage by reducing swollen nasal membranes. Other drugs administered via the nasal route are given for systemic effects and are simply absorbed through the nasal mucosa. These medications include nicotine (Nicotrol Inhaler), calcitonin (Miacalcin), and sumatriptan (Imitrex).

Nasal decongestant sprays can be counterproductive if used for long periods of time. While they relieve congestion with administration, they also can cause a rebound effect with long-term use. This causes swelling of the nasal mucosa, leading to congestion, which causes the need for more nasal spray. If long-term use continues, the arteries in the nasal passage will shrink and scar, causing lesions and nosebleeds. Generally, it is not recommended to use nasal decongestant sprays for more than 3 days. Steroid nasal sprays, such as budesonide (Rhinocort), generally do not cause these rebound effects.

To administer nasal sprays, it is very important to position the patient with the head flexed forward so that the spray enters the sinuses and does not go down the throat.

Vaginal Medications

Medications administered via the **vaginal route** come in the form of suppositories, creams, aerosol foams, or tablets that are inserted into the vagina and dissolve there. Some preparations come with a disposable tubular applicator with a plunger to insert the medication. Other medications come with a prefilled applicator that can simply be inserted and the plunger depressed. This route typically is used to treat local infections such as yeast infections, but they also may be used for treatment of vaginitis, for endometrial atrophy, and for contraception with spermicidal agents.

When you administer creams using an applicator, you will attach the applicator to the end of the tube containing the cream. As you squeeze the tube, the cream will fill the applicator, pushing the plunger backward. When the applicator is filled with cream, you will detach it from the tube of medication and insert it into the patient's vagina. Gently insert the applicator into the vagina along the posterior vaginal wall for approximately 3 inches (8 cm) and depress the plunger to disperse the cream. Always wear gloves when administering vaginal medications to prevent contact with blood and body fluids. Gently depress the plunger until all of the cream is inserted. Instruct the patient to remain lying down for between 5 and 15 minutes so that the medication can be absorbed. Some medications are ordered to be given at bedtime to prevent loss of the cream when the patient stands upright.

When you administer a vaginal suppository, you will first lubricate the tip of the suppository with a water-soluble lubricant. Insert the suppository with the index finger. Vaginal tablets are diamond shaped and fit into the end of an applicator with a plunger. After placing the tablet in the applicator, you may apply water-soluble lubricant to it. Gently insert the applicator into the vagina along the posterior vaginal wall for approximately 3 inches (8 cm) and depress the plunger. This will push the tablet deep into the vagina, where it will dissolve and the medication will be absorbed. The patient may wish to wear a perineal pad to protect clothes from drainage due to the cream, foam, or suppository. Skill 36.6 (page 817) provides more information about administering vaginal medications.

Rectal Medications

Rectal medications typically are available in suppository or enema form, but ointments and creams also may be administered. Medications given via the **rectal route** are inserted directly into the rectum and may be ordered when nausea or vomiting is present or when the patient cannot take anything by mouth. While it is a safe and convenient route, many people object to its use. Small children can be especially distressed by rectal administration of medications.

Rectal administration of medications may be used to directly treat local pain and inflammation. Hydrocortisone (Anucort-HC), for example, is a rectal suppository used for swelling and inflammation due to hemorrhoids. Sometimes seizure medications may be administered via the rectal route. Diazepam rectal gel (Diastat) is a medication approved for epilepsy. The rectal route may also be used for laxative purposes. Rectal suppositories are often administered to stimulate a bowel movement. One example is bisacodyl (Dulcolax) suppositories.

Medications may also be administered by enema. An example of this is a sodium polystyrene sulfonate (Kayexalate) enema, which is given to help decrease dangerously high potassium levels in the blood. (See Chapter 30 for a more thorough discussion on enemas.)

If a patient has cardiac dysrhythmia or had a recent myocardial infarction, avoid using the rectal route for medication administration because insertion may stimulate the vagus nerve and trigger a dysrhythmia. Evaluate the appropriateness of administering medications via the rectal route to patients with undiagnosed abdominal pain or who have recently undergone surgery of the bowel, rectum, or prostate because insertion of the medication could cause trauma or injury.

Rectal suppositories are bullet shaped, with a rounded tip and a blunt end. When you administer a rectal suppository, you will first lubricate the tip with a water-soluble lubricant. Wear gloves to avoid possible contact with blood or body fluids. Insert the suppository rounded tip first and, with your index finger on the blunt end, push it past the internal anal sphincter so that it will be retained in the rectum. Because rectal suppositories are made using a wax base, they are generally kept in the refrigerator to prevent melting. Skill 36.7 (page 818) provides more information about administering rectal suppositories.

Respiratory Medications

Medications administered by the **respiratory route** are dispersed in fine droplets and inhaled into the lungs and bronchial airways, usually through the use of inhalers or nebulizers (Fig. 36.3). The respiratory route of medication administration is often used to treat pulmonary conditions such as asthma and chronic obstructive pulmonary disease.

The onset of action following pulmonary administration is rapid. Nebulizers use compressed air forced through liquid medication, resulting in a fine mist that is inhaled into the bronchi and bronchioles to dilate them. Bronchodilators are given to open constricted airways and include albuterol

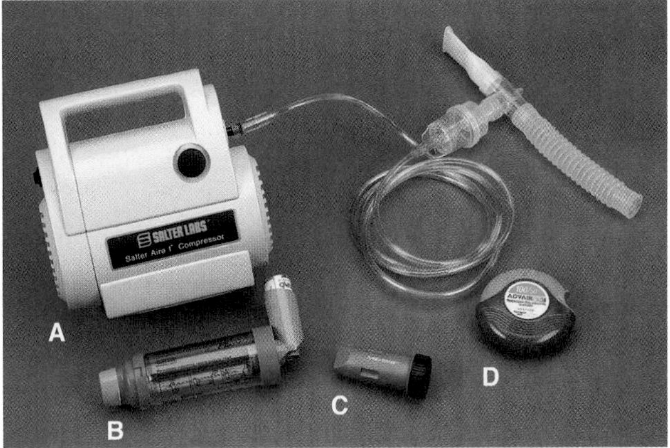

FIGURE 36.3 Different types of inhalers: (a) Ultrasonic nebulizer delivers medication and humidity as a fine mist; (b) Metered-dose inhaler delivers measured doses (this one has a spacer); (c) Dry-powder inhaler (Turbuhaler); (d) Diskhaler (from Wilkinson JM, Treas LS. *Fundamentals of Nursing: Theory, Concepts & Applications*. Vol. 1. 2nd ed. Philadelphia, PA: FA Davis; 2011).

(Ventolin, Proventil) and ipratropium bromide (Atrovent). Certain mucolytic drugs such as acetylcysteine (Mucomyst) also may be administered using a nebulizer. For more information on administering a nebulizer treatment, please refer to Chapter 28. Other methods of administering respiratory medications are metered-dose inhalers and dry-powder inhalers.

METERED-DOSE INHALERS. **Metered-dose inhalers** (MDIs) are pressurized medication dispensers that spray a premeasured amount of drug into the lungs. They are the most efficient way to get medications into the airways. Medications such as short-acting bronchodilators are delivered quickly to treat an acute asthma attack. MDIs are also used to deliver anti-inflammatory agents and bronchodilators for long-term management of asthma. ***Safety: Instruct patients to avoid leaving MDIs in the car because heat may cause them to explode or rupture.***

Some patients have difficulty using an MDI correctly, so it is important to teach the proper technique for administration. Skill 36.8 (page 819) provides more information on administering medication via an MDI.

MDI Maintenance. Wipe the mouthpiece of the MDI after use to remove excess medication. If a spacer is being used, rinse it daily in warm water and then allow it to air dry. It can be difficult for patients to tell how much medication is left in an MDI. Newer metered-dose inhalers have a counter on the back showing the number of doses remaining in the inhaler (Fig. 36.4). This helps the patient know when the inhaler is nearing empty so that a new one can be ordered. As with other medications, discard expired inhalers and replace with new ones.

• WORD • BUILDING •

dysrhythmia: dys – abnormal + rhythm – measured motion + ia – condition

Patient Teaching Connection

Using a Metered-Dose Inhaler

Instruct the patient to first shake the inhaler to mix the contents before delivery. Have the patient remove the mouthpiece cover and hold the inhaler 1 to 2 inches away from the mouth. This prevents large droplets of medication from landing on the tongue and being rapidly absorbed, leading to increased severity of side effects such as nervousness, tremors, and tachycardia. Patients may be accustomed to placing the mouthpiece directly into the mouth, but newer research indicates that the 1- to 2-inch distance is preferred.

Instruct the patient to inhale deeply as he or she depresses the canister, then hold the breath for 10 seconds. Teach the patient to then breathe out slowly through pursed lips. Frequently the order for MDI administration is to take two puffs. If that is the case, the patient should wait 1 full minute before taking the second puff to allow the medication to be completely absorbed.

In some situations, especially when the patients are elders or children, it may be difficult for them to coordinate depressing the canister with deep inhalation. In that case, a spacer may be used. This is a chamber that attaches to the inhaler mouthpiece and holds the medication after the canister is depressed. The patient can then inhale the medicine in several more shallow breaths.

Instruct patients to rinse their mouths with water and spit it out after using steroid inhalers. Steroids in the oral cavity can lead to a yeast infection called *thrush,* so rinsing out the mouth after use prevents the steroid from remaining in the oral cavity. If patients are using two types of inhalers, such as a bronchodilator and a steroid, instruct them to wait 5 minutes between the use of each inhaler. Instruct the patient to use the steroid inhaler last and then to rinse the mouth immediately after use.

DRY-POWDER INHALERS. Unlike MDIs, **dry-powder inhalers** (DPIs) do not contain a pressurized canister and do not spray out medication; rather, they rely on the force of the patient's own inhalation to dispense a dose of dry-powder medication. Common DPIs include the Rotahaler, Spinhaler, Diskus, and Handihaler.

Diskus inhalers are a frequently prescribed type of DPI. These are flat disks containing a number of small chambers, each loaded with an individual dose of dry medication. When you slide the thumb grip away from you, it reveals the mouthpiece and a lever. When the lever is pushed, it opens the door to the chamber. The patient must place the mouthpiece of the diskus directly into his or her mouth and close the lips around it. When the patient inhales deeply, the dry powder is breathed into the lungs. ***Safety: Ensure that patient does not exhale directly into the DPI because the exhalation will disperse the powder.*** Patients with severe asthma may not be able to produce enough air flow to successfully use these inhalers. Skill 36.8 gives more information on how to administer medication via a DPI.

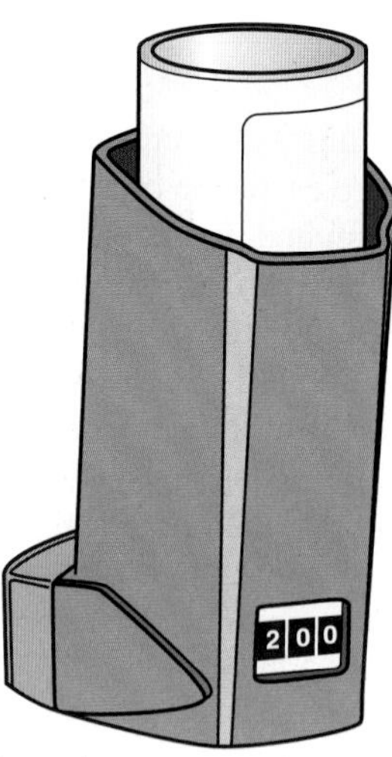

FIGURE 36.4 Inhaler with counter on the back that shows the remaining doses.

KNOWLEDGE CONNECTION

List four types of topical preparations. Under what circumstances might you question administering a medication rectally? Explain the differences between an MDI and a DPI.

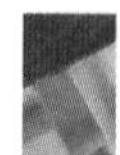

NURSING RESPONSIBILITIES FOR ADMINISTERING ORAL, TOPICAL, AND MUCOSAL MEDICATIONS

As discussed in Chapter 35, you are responsible for assessing the patient, monitoring laboratory results, and evaluating the information before you administer any medications.

- Assess the patient for the appropriateness of medication administration. For example, you have an order from a prescriber for a daily stool softener for a patient. When you question the patient about his or her bowel movements, you learn that the patient is having three or four soft stools each day, described as "almost diarrhea." In that case, it would not be appropriate to administer the stool softener without discussing it with the prescriber first.
- Check all laboratory results to determine if it is safe and appropriate to administer an ordered medication, because some medications can reach toxic levels or exceed the therapeutic effect. For example, if the patient is taking warfarin (Coumadin), it is important to check the prothrombin levels (pro time) or international normalized ratio (INR) in the laboratory results first. This medication is an anticoagulant, and it is possible that the blood will

not clot adequately if too much of the drug is in the bloodstream. The patient may bleed from the vagina, rectum, nose, or gums. If the pro time or INR is above the therapeutic range, you need to hold the medication and notify the prescriber.

- Always check drug allergies prior to administering any medication. It also is important to check the ingredients of combination medications for patients who are allergic to determine if a sensitivity exists. An example is if you have an order to apply triple antibiotic ointment to an open area on a patient's arm. You will need to determine the names of the three antibiotics in the ointment and compare them to any allergies the patient might have. If the patient is allergic to neomycin, for example, he or she could react to the ointment as well as the systemic medication.
- Check the timing prior to administering medications and ensure that you are dispensing them appropriately. ***Safety: For prn medications, you must check to see the last time the medication was given to ensure that the timing is within the ordered parameters.*** If a medication is ordered every 4 hours prn, check the documentation to determine the last time it was given. Be sure that you administer the drug at least 4 hours from the last dose.

Laboratory and Diagnostic Connection

Coordinating Medication Administration With Blood Specimens

It is very important that you administer medications on time, especially when laboratory values are to be drawn. The laboratory staff plans to obtain blood specimens based on the expected time that medications are to be given. For example, a digoxin level is ordered to be drawn 8 hours after the medication is administered. If the patient is taken to another department for a diagnostic procedure and the medication is not given on time, alert the laboratory staff right away. Otherwise, the digoxin level may be drawn only 4 hours after administration, leading to an artificially elevated blood level and possible inappropriate changes in the medication dose.

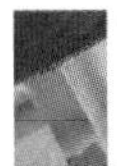

DOCUMENTATION OF MEDICATION ADMINISTRATION

Medication administration may be documented in one of two ways: on paper or electronically. More acute care hospitals are moving to the electronic version of medication administration records (MARs) because these systems help prevent medication errors due to built-in safeguards. However, the electronic system is expensive and may be cost prohibitive for smaller facilities and long-term care facilities.

Documentation on a Paper MAR

MARs provide documentation of the date and time a medication is administered, as well as the person who dispensed it. As discussed in Chapter 35, the record contains a grid with the date and time marked.

After you administer a medication in a hospital setting, you will immediately document it on the MAR. On most paper MARs, the ordered medications are listed on the left side with the times of administration. Across the top of the page, the dates are listed. You will initial in the appropriate section, across from the medication and time, and beneath the correct date, or write in the time followed by your initials. Some facilities have a policy that you write in the time you administered the medication, followed by your initials. Then you draw a single line through the time to indicate the medication has been administered.

If a medication is not given for some reason, follow facility policy for documenting the omission. Often, the procedure is to initial in the section or box across from the medication and then circle your initials. This signals that an explanation documenting why the medication was not given will be found in the nurses' notes or on the reverse side of the MAR.

Paper MARs contain an area to correlate the nurse's initials with his or her full name and credentials. Figure 36.5 shows the area at the bottom of the MAR where the nurse writes his or her name to identify his or her initials.

Medications are transcribed from the prescriber's order sheet to the MAR. ***Safety: There is potential for errors to occur during transcription of medication orders.*** This is why it is always necessary for you to check the original prescriber's order to be certain that you are administering the medications as intended in that order.

Paper MARs also contain identifying information, including the patient's name, room number, and identification number; the health-care provider's name; and the patient's allergies, which are listed in red ink. The medication listing includes the name of the medication (generic is preferred) and the dose, route, and frequency of administration.

On a paper MAR, when a medication is discontinued the entire section is highlighted in yellow all the way across the MAR and the word "discontinued" is written next to the medication on the list. Sometimes the abbreviation "disc" is used. The older abbreviation "d/c" is no longer acceptable because it could be mistaken for other words. ***Safety: Always read the MAR carefully before administering medications.*** Occasionally a medication may be marked as discontinued, but the section has not been highlighted in yellow, causing the potential for error.

Documentation of Special Situations

When a medication is ordered to be administered prn, or "as necessary," you will document it on the MAR in the section for prn medications. On some MARs, the prn medications are listed at the bottom of the MAR as they are given. Because these medications are not given at scheduled times, you must write in the time you administered the medication. In

HOSPITAL MEDICATION ADMINISTRATION RECORD

Codes For Injection Sites

A - Left Anterior Thigh
B - Left Deltoid
C - Left Gluteus Medius
D - Left Lateral Thigh
E - Left Ventral Gluteus
F - Left Lower Quadrant
G - Left Upper Quadrant
H - Right Anterior Thigh
I - Right Deltoid
J - Right Gluteus Medius
K - Right Lateral Thigh
L - Right Ventral Gluteus
M - Right Lower Quadrant
N - Right Upper Quadrant

Mary Smith 086432
age 46 John Miller, M.D.

ALLERGIES: PCN, Sulfa

DATE ORDERED	DATE REORD.	DRUG - DOSE - ROUTE - FREQUENCY	ADMIN. TIME	DATE MM/DD/YYYY	DATE MM/DD/YYYY	DATE MM/DD/YYYY
MM/DD/YYYY		Lanoxin 0.25mg po Q D	0900	09 JW		
MM/DD/YYYY		Rocephin i gm IV Q D	1200	1200 JW		
MM/DD/YYYY		Zinacef i gm IV Q 8 hr	0800	08 JW		
			1600			
			2400			
SIGNATURE / SHIFT INDICATES			7-3	JW		
NURSE ADMINISTERING MEDICATIONS			3-11			
J Wilson, RN			11-7			

FIGURE 36.5 Documentation on an MAR.

addition, you must document the reason you gave the medication in the nurses' notes or other appropriate location, following facility policy.

It is very important to check back with the patient in 30 minutes to 1 hour to see if the medication relieved the problem. This is the evaluation phase of the nursing process. Document the patient's response to the medication. If the medication does not relieve the problem, you will then contact the prescriber and document that you have done so. Document any new orders received.

Narcotic medications are often given on a prn basis. In addition to the special documentation needed for prn medications, you also must sign out narcotic drugs in the narcotic record or narcotic book. As discussed in Chapter 35, it is extremely important to sign out these types of medications and ensure that the count is correct. In facilities that use electronic MARs, it is not necessary to sign out the narcotic medication separately because the computerized system counts the drug for you. Skill 36.1 provides an example of documenting a prn narcotic medication.

Documentation on an Electronic MAR

Electronic MARs, or eMARs, are part of an electronic system designed to reduce administration errors. This system uses bar-code reading technology to monitor the administration of medications. The eMARs record patient health information into a computer database, including medication, allergies, past or present illnesses/injuries and hospital visits, and family history. Figure 36.6 shows an example of documentation of a rectal suppository on an eMAR.

The principles of electronic documentation are the same as for paper records. The health-care provider orders the medication, and the pharmacist dispenses it with a bar-code attached and then delivers the medication to the computerized medication cabinet or medication cart. This offers a method of inventory control as well. The patient's identification band contains a special medication bar code. You can access your patient's ordered medications via a computer or handheld device. The screen will show the medications due at a particular time for a particular patient. When you scan the bar code of each medication with the scanner, similar to checking out at a grocery store, the computer screen shows any warning messages, interactions, or considerations before administering the medication. You will then determine if further action is needed before you administer the medication.

When you go to the patient's room, you will still use two methods of identification for the patient and then scan the medication bar code on the patient's identification band. The administration of the medication is automatically recorded in the eMAR, and the medication is automatically charged to the patient. If you are using a handheld device, it may be necessary to download your administration of medications into a main computer. Follow facility policy because different software programs may require different pathways for documentation.

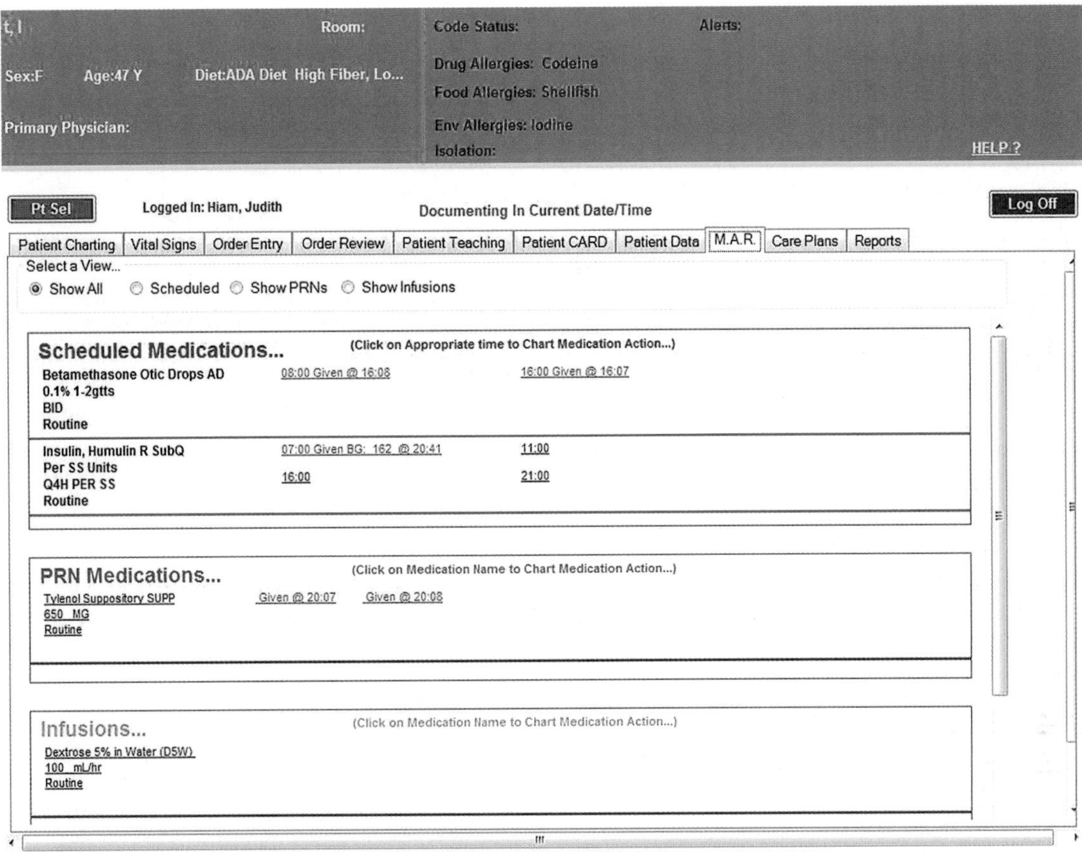

FIGURE 36.6 Electronic MAR documentation sample (from Wilkinson JM, Treas LS. *Fundamentals of Nursing: Theory, Concepts & Applications.* Vol. 2. 3rd ed. Philadelphia, PA: FA Davis; 2016).

Documentation on MARs in Long-Term Care

In many long-term care facilities, documentation of medications is done prior to taking the medication to the resident. This is known as the "PIG" method of administration, which stands for "Punch, Initial, Give." If for some reason the medication is not administered to the resident, you will circle your initials and document the reasons and results in the nurses' notes or on the MAR. Accurate and thorough documentation is vital for regulations, reimbursement, and quality of care.

Some long-term care facilities use MARs as well. In that situation, the eMAR is available on a laptop computer found on the medication cart. Pictures and room numbers of the residents appear on the screen once you have logged in. You then touch the resident's picture to access the resident's medication record. When you administer the medication, you enter your initials at the appropriate time. When no more medications are due for that resident for the rest of the day, the resident's picture changes from color to black and white. In this way, you can tell at a glance which residents still have medications due.

Documenting Withheld or Refused Medications

Under certain circumstances, a drug may be withheld or refused. If a patient refuses a medication, take the time to ask the reason behind the action. If it is due to unpleasant side effects, you may be able to take some actions to minimize those side effects. If the patient believes the medication is not effective, document this and discuss it with the prescriber. Encourage patients and residents to take prescribed medications by explaining the desired effect of the drug. If the patient or resident continues to refuse, do not force the issue. Notify the prescriber and document in the nurses' notes the date, time, and reason for withholding a drug. Then document the name of the prescriber notified and the prescriber's response. All actions must be documented to safeguard the patient.

> **KNOWLEDGE CONNECTION**
>
> How do a paper MAR and an eMAR differ? What must be included in the documentation of a prn medication? How will others know which nurse is represented by the initials on the MAR? How will you document a medication that was not given?

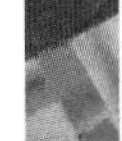

PREVENTING ADMINISTRATION AND DOCUMENTATION ERRORS

It is your responsibility to do everything possible to prevent an error in administering and documenting the medications that you give to patients. It is extremely important to check and double-check each step of the medication administration process. To help you prevent administration and documentation errors, follow these guidelines:

- Always check the original prescriber's order against the order on the MAR. Investigate any discrepancies before administering any medications.
- Check frequently for new or changed medication orders. Avoid working solely from a computer printout pulled at the beginning of the shift because medication orders often change throughout the shift.
- Read medication orders very carefully, being aware of drugs with similar names and distinguishing between abbreviations.
- Look up any unfamiliar medication to ensure that you are administering the appropriate dose and that you can assess for the intended effects and any side effects.
- Be certain that it is appropriate to administer the medication: check laboratory results, vital signs, or other parameters prior to administration.
- Always perform the three safety checks before administering a medication.
- Ensure that you follow the seven rights of medication administration every time you prepare and give a medicine.
- Question any orders that require more than one to two tablets or capsules or that exceed the recommended dose.
- Document medications as soon as you have administered them to prevent another nurse from coming behind you and administering them again.
- Check carefully for discontinued orders to avoid administering an incorrect medication.
- Ensure that you carefully supervise any unlicensed person whose job description includes administration of oral, topical, or mucosal medications.

Real-World Connection

Consequences of Medications Not Administered

The unlicensed staff members working in a group home for adults with developmental disabilities were responsible for administering oral, topical, and mucosal medications. A few residents had PEG tubes in place with medications ordered to be crushed and administered through the tube. One resident, a 19-year-old female, had a severe seizure disorder. She went into a seizure that could not be stopped, and eventually she died.

When a family member was packing up her belongings, he noticed some of her medications had been dropped into the grill that covered the top of the heating and cooling unit next to her bed. When the grill was removed, many of the resident's pills were found there, including her antiseizure medications. Apparently one unlicensed staff member lacked the knowledge or the desire to crush the medicines and administer them through the PEG tube. All the medications were signed out as administered on the MAR for the past several months. While the family never knew who was responsible, they were still left to wonder if their loved one would not have died if she had received all of her medications correctly.

Remember that you are responsible for supervising unlicensed staff and ensuring that they are correctly performing medication administration.

If a Medication Error Occurs

Even when you are very careful, sometimes you make a medication error because you are human. The important thing is that you admit the error and take steps to protect your patient from injury or harm. Sometimes you may find an error made by another nurse. It is equally important to report that as well to protect the patient. Avoid being punitive or hypercritical of others if they make an error. Be supportive of other staff because it could be you making an error the next time. One very seasoned nurse explains that she worries more about new nurses who never make mistakes because they probably do but are not admitting to them.

If you make a medication error, follow these steps:

- Put the patient first. Check for adverse effects from the medication. Take a set of vital signs and determine any abnormalities.
- Notify the prescriber and explain what happened.
- Carry out additional orders for assessing and monitoring the patient's response to the incorrect medication administration.
- Complete an incident report, following facility policy regarding further documentation or notification.
- Avoid being too hard on yourself or other nurses if an error occurs. It is very upsetting to make an error and cause possible harm to a patient. It is so important for nurses to be supportive of one another and to help solve the problems that might lead to future errors.

KNOWLEDGE CONNECTION

List three ways to prevent making an error related to the order on the MAR. Give an example of a medication order that you would question. Explain what documentation is required if a medication error occurs.

Skill 36.1 Administering Oral Medications

Assessment Steps

1. Check the original prescriber's order, ensuring that it matches the order in the MAR, ***to prevent oversight of a transcription error.***
2. Assess the need for measuring vital signs or finger stick blood sugar before administering the medication. ***This prevents administering medications that are outside the parameters ordered.***
3. Assess laboratory results to determine the appropriateness of medication administration ***to determine if the patient has toxic levels of any medication or laboratory contraindications to administering the medication.***
4. For oral medications, assess whether the patient is able to swallow whole tablets or capsules ***to determine whether to crush the medications or to open the capsules prior to administration, if appropriate.***
5. For sublingual and buccal medications, assess the mouth for lesions, gum disease, and color of mucous membranes ***to prevent administering medications that will not be well absorbed.***

Planning Step

1. Plan to crush medications if patient is unable to swallow them whole. *Safety: Do not crush enteric-coated tablets because these drugs are irritating to the esophagus and stomach lining, and breaking their enteric coatings may lead to gastric irritation. Do not crush or break sustained-release drugs because doing so may lead to rapid absorption of large amounts of drug.*

Implementation Steps

Prepare the Medication

1. Wash hands and follow standard precautions.
2. Obtain the medication from the patient's drawer or from the computerized cabinet.
3. Follow the steps for preparing medications for administration, found in Chapter 35.
4. Verify the seven rights of medication administration ***to ensure that you have the right patient, right medication, right dose, right route, right date, right indication, and right time.***
5. Perform two safety checks ***to ensure that you are obtaining the right medication for the correct patient.***
6. For liquid medications:
   - Shake suspensions ***to evenly distribute the medication in the liquid base.***
   - Hold the bottle so that the label is in the palm of your hand ***to prevent drips from obscuring the label.***
   - Hold the medicine cup at eye level and pour the liquid to the desired amount ***to ensure accurate measurement.*** Read the level at the center, or lowest point, of the meniscus.

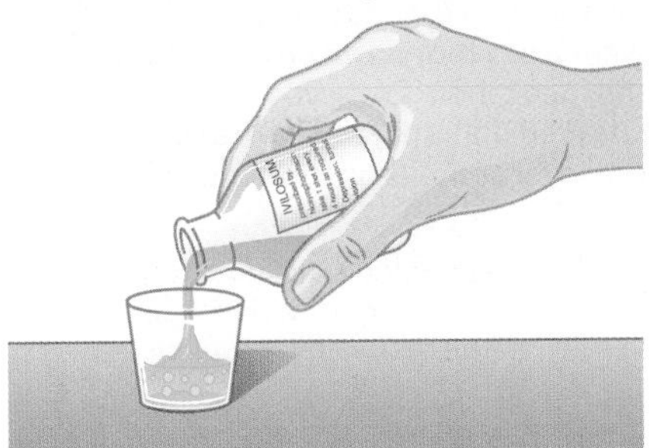

For scored tablet medications:
   - Place the tablet in the tablet cutter.
   - Select the designated dose as ordered by the provider.
   - Split the tablet with the tablet cutter and place in a medicine cup.

Administer the Medication

7. Follow the Initial Implementation Steps located on the inside back cover.
8. Perform a third safety check ***to ensure that you are administering the right medication to the correct patient.***
9. Tell the patient the name of the medication, explain its action, and explain how to take the medication ***to ensure the patient's cooperation.***
10. Pour water into a cup for the patient, if needed.
11. Assist the patient to a sitting position ***to prevent choking or aspiration while he or she is taking the medication.***
12. Open the unit dose packaging and drop the medication into the medicine cup without touching it with your fingers. ***This prevents opening medications that will not be used and helps you identify each medication as you are about to administer it.***
13. Hand the medication to the patient. Hand water to the patient and offer more if needed, unless the patient is on a fluid restriction.
14. If the patient cannot hold the medication, don gloves, place the medication in a medication cup, and tip the cup into the patient's mouth.
15. Remain with the patient until the medication is swallowed ***to ensure that the patient does not choke or "cheek" the medication.***

For Sublingual and Buccal Drugs

- *For* ***buccal administration,*** instruct the patient to place the medication in the mouth against the cheek until it dissolves completely.

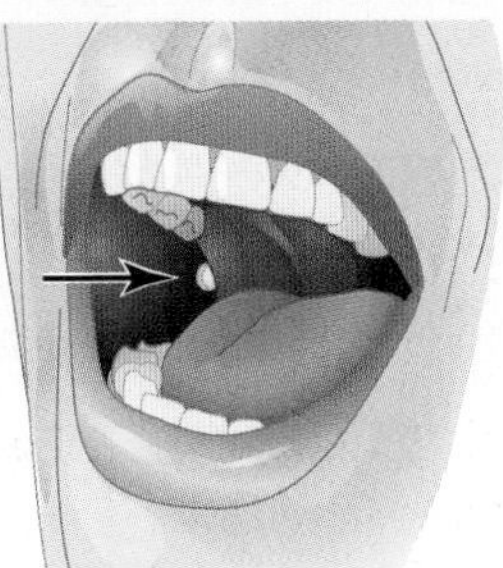

- *For* ***sublingual administration,*** tell the patient to open the mouth and lift the tongue. Place the medication under the tongue and instruct the patient to keep the medication there until it dissolves completely.

(skill continues on page 812)

Skill 36.1 (continued)

- Administer buccal or sublingual tablets whole. Instruct the patient not to chew, swallow, or spit out these tablets before they dissolve completely.

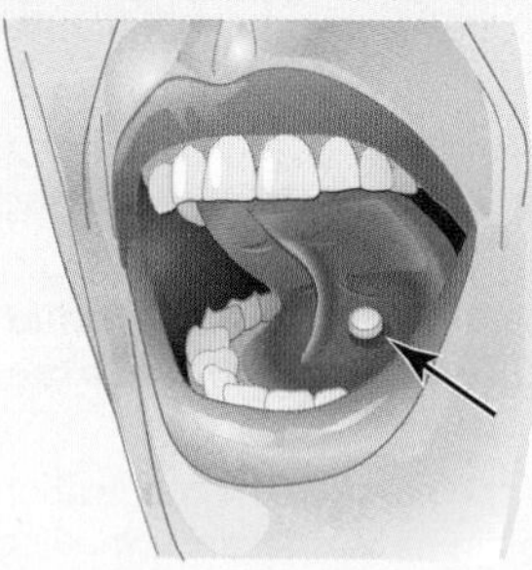

16. Follow the Ending Implementation Steps located on the inside back cover.
17. Document the medication administration on the MAR and in the nurses' notes for prn medications. Document any medication that is withheld or refused in the nurses' notes.

Evaluation Steps

1. Assess the patient receiving medications via the buccal or sublingual route within 5 to 10 minutes ***because the medication is rapidly absorbed via these routes.*** Determine if the medication has been effective and follow orders for repeating.
2. Assess patients taking oral medications in 30 minutes after the medications are given. Assess for desired effects and adverse effects of the medications.
3. If the patient is experiencing adverse effects such as nausea or vomiting, notify the prescriber if no orders for an antiemetic are available.

Sample Documentation

07/09/22 1400 C/o right shoulder pain. States the pain is at a 7 on a 0–10 scale and is sharp at times, throbbing at other times. Lortab 5 mg given PO for c/o right shoulder pain ———————————— Nurse's signature and credentials

07/09/22 1440 States pain is better after medication. Rates it at a 3 now. ———————————— Nurse's signature and credentials

Skill 36.2 Administering Medications Through an Enteral Tube

Assessment Steps

1. Check the original prescriber's order, ensuring that it matches the order in the MAR ***to prevent oversight of a transcription error.***
2. Assess for any contraindications to medication administration. Check laboratory results, check vital signs for results outside parameters, and check bowel sounds ***to ensure that the medication will be digested and absorbed.***
3. Assess for the need for any prn medications ***so that you can prepare all medications at the same time.***
4. Assess the PEG tube insertion site for redness, edema, or purulent drainage, ***which could indicate infection.***
5. Check placement of the nasogastric or PEG tube by aspirating stomach contents, checking the pH of stomach contents, and measuring the length of the tube as described in Chapter 24.
6. Check the amount of residual tube feeding in the patient's stomach. If you obtain 100 mL or more, delay administering the medication according to facility policy.

Planning Steps

1. Determine whether all nonliquid medications may be crushed or opened for administration through the tube. Consult with the pharmacist if you are unsure. *Safety: Do not crush enteric-coated tablets because these drugs are irritating to the esophagus and stomach lining, and breaking their enteric coatings may lead to gastric irritation. Do not crush or break sustained-release drugs because doing so may lead to rapid absorption of large amounts of drug.*
2. Determine the need to turn off the feeding pump before or after medication administration (refer to Box 36.3).

Implementation Steps

Prepare the Medication

1. Wash hands and follow standard precautions.
2. Obtain the medication from the patient's drawer or from the computerized cabinet.
3. Follow the steps for preparing medications for administration, found in Chapter 35.
4. Verify the seven rights of medication administration ***to ensure that you have the right patient, right medication, right dose, right route, right date, right indication, and right time.***
5. Perform two safety checks ***to ensure that you are obtaining the right medication for the correct patient.***
6. Crush tablets that are safe to be crushed by placing them in a mortar and crushing with a pestle or by using a pill-crushing device. Ensure that you get all the powder out of the mortar or the pill crusher. Mix the medication with 20 mL of water.
7. For liquid medications:
   - Shake suspensions ***to evenly distribute the medication in the liquid base.***
   - Hold the bottle so that the label is in the palm of your hand ***to prevent drips that could obscure the label.***
   - Hold the medicine cup at eye level and pour the liquid to the desired amount ***to ensure accurate measurement.*** Read the level at the center, or lowest point, of the meniscus.
8. Place liquid medicines and crushed or opened medicines mixed with a small amount of water in separate medication cups. Do not mix the medications. *Safety: Mixing can cause medication interactions.*

Skill 36.2 (continued)

Administer the Medication

9. Follow the Initial Implementation Steps located on the inside back cover.
10. Perform a third safety check ***to ensure that you are administering the right medication to the correct patient.***
11. Tell the patient the name of the medication and explain the procedure ***to ensure the patient's cooperation.***
12. Ensure that tube placement and residual feeding have been checked (see Assessment Steps).
13. Clear the tube with 30 to 60 mL of water first. Follow the procedure in Chapter 24 for administering fluid through a nasogastric or PEG tube. ***Clearing the tube removes formula that might adhere to the tube walls and interact with medications, as well as ensuring that the tube is patent before medications are administered through it.***
14. Administer the first medication through the tube and follow it with 20 to 30 mL of water. This may be done using a syringe with gentle pressure or by allowing it to flow in via gravity.
15. Administer the second medication through the tube and follow it with 15 mL of water.
16. Repeat Step 15 until all the medications have been given.
17. Clear the tube with 20 to 30 mL of water to ensure that all the medication is out of the tube and is not adhering to the sides.

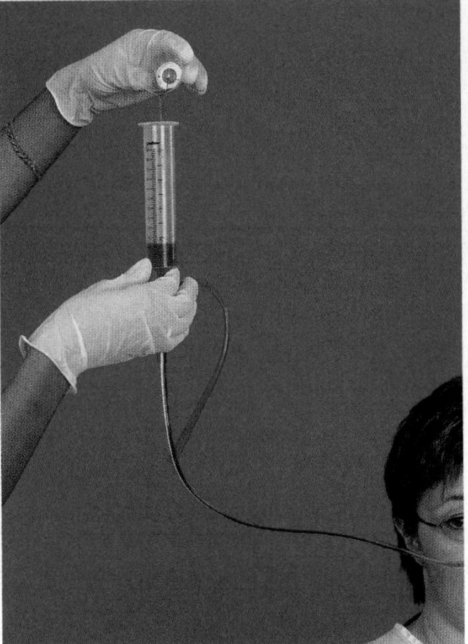

18. Restart the continuous tube feeding or hold the tube feeding for 1 to 2 hours depending on the medications you have administered.
19. Keep patient in a sitting position for 30 minutes. ***This helps to minimize aspiration.***
20. Follow the Ending Implementation Steps located on the inside back cover.
21. Document the medication administration on the MAR.
22. Document fluid given via tube on the intake portion of the intake and output record. Include liquid medications and all water.

Evaluation Step

1. Assess the patient 30 to 45 minutes after the medications are given. Assess for desired effects and adverse effects of the medications.

Sample Documentation

07/10/22 0900 Lansoprazole (Prevacid) 15 mg administered via PEG tube. Medication capsule opened and mixed with 15 mL of apple juice per pharmacist's instructions. Tube cleared with 30 mL of water before and after med admin. ——————————

—————————— Nurse's signature and credentials

Skill 36.3 Administering Topical and Transdermal Medications

Assessment Steps

1. Check the original prescriber's order, ensuring that it matches the order in the MAR, ***to prevent oversight of a transcription error.***
2. Assess the need for measuring vital signs or finger stick blood sugar before administering the medication. ***This prevents administering medications that are outside the parameters ordered.***
3. Assess laboratory results to determine the appropriateness of medication administration ***to determine if the patient has toxic levels of any medication or laboratory contraindications to administering the medication.***

Planning Steps

1. For topical medications, determine if the area should be covered after application.

(skill continues on page 814)

Skill 36.3 (continued)

2. Gather needed supplies: gauze and tape or an adhesive bandage ***if topical medication is to be covered;* tongue blade or cotton-tipped swab *for application of a topical cream or ointment.***

Implementation Steps

Prepare the Medication

1. Wash hands and follow standard precautions.
2. Obtain the medication from the patient's drawer or from the computerized cabinet.
3. Follow the steps for preparing medications for administration, found in Chapter 35.
4. Verify the seven rights of medication administration ***to ensure that you have the right patient, right medication, right dose, right route, right date, right indication, and right time.***
5. Perform two safety checks ***to ensure that you are obtaining the right medication for the correct patient.***

Administer the Medication

6. Follow the Initial Implementation Steps located on the inside back cover.
7. Perform a third safety check ***to ensure that you are administering the right medication to the correct patient.***
8. Tell the patient the name of the medication and explain the procedure ***to ensure the patient's cooperation.***

For Topical Medications

9. Remove the existing dressing if one is in place.
10. Cleanse the area with sterile gauze and normal saline or follow orders for cleansing with another solution. Pat dry. ***Cleansing removes the previous layer of ointment or cream, and patting dry prevents irritation or abrasion to the injured area.***
11. Assess the appearance of the wound or lesion. Note redness, swelling, size, and drainage ***to assess for infection and healing.***
12. Apply a small amount of topical ointment or cream to a cotton-tipped applicator or tongue blade ***to prevent touching the tube of cream or ointment to the wound.*** In some facilities, it may be required that you put a small amount of ointment or cream in a medicine cup and then take it to bedside.
13. Spread a thin coat of medication onto the affected area. ***This allows the medication to penetrate the area and does not waste medicine.***
14. If the lesion is to be covered, apply sterile gauze without touching the area that will cover the wound ***to prevent contamination.***
15. Write the date, time, and your initials on one piece of tape and apply it to the dressing as you tape it in place. ***This identifies the last time the dressing was changed and by whom.***
16. Follow the Ending Implementation Steps located on the inside back cover.
17. Document the appearance of the wound or lesion and the type of dressing applied if one was used.

For Transdermal Medications

9. Locate and remove the existing patch.
10. Cleanse the area with an alcohol swab and wash with normal saline or follow orders for cleaning with another solution ***to remove any remaining medication so that it will no longer be absorbed.***
11. Select a new location for the patch you will apply. Choose an area with minimal body hair on the trunk or upper arms. Clip hair if necessary for the patch to stick.
12. If the area is oily or sweaty, cleanse it with an alcohol pad or soap and water.
13. Write the date, time, and your initials on the patch.
14. Remove the adhesive backing and apply the patch in the selected location.
15. Follow the Ending Implementation Steps located on the inside back cover.
16. Document the time, date, and site of application of the patch on the MAR according to facility policy.

Evaluation Steps

1. Assess the patient for any complaints of increasing discomfort 30 minutes after application of topical medication, ***which could indicate a reaction to the medication.***
2. Notify the prescriber if no improvement is visible over several days. ***The medication may need to be changed.***
3. Assess the patient for adverse effects of transdermal medications ***because they have systemic effects.***

Sample Documentation

07/12/22 1600 Neosporin ointment applied to skin tear on left forearm. 2 cm × 3 cm open area; oozing serous fluid. Covered with sterile gauze and two strips of tape. ——— Nurse's signature and credentials

07/12/22 1645 No complaints of pain or burning at wound site. ——— Nurse's signature and credentials

Skill 36.4 Administering Eye and Ear Medications

Assessment Steps

1. Check the original prescriber's order, ensuring that it matches the order in the MAR ***to prevent oversight of a transcription error.***
2. Assess the eye or ear. If discharge or crusting is present around the eye, clean with warm water and a washcloth before administering the medication. If wax or discharge is noted from the ear, gently wipe using a cotton ball.
3. Ensure that the tympanic membrane is intact prior to administration of ear medications. Check the health-care provider's notes, or check the patient's ear with an otoscope if documentation is not available. ***Medications should not be put into the ear of a patient with a nonintact eardrum because this allows the medications to enter the middle ear.***
4. Determine the patient's age ***for correct administration of eardrops.***

Planning Step

1. Gather needed supplies: tissues and cotton balls.

Implementation Steps

Prepare the Medication

1. Wash hands and follow standard precautions.
2. Obtain the medication from the patient's drawer or from the computerized cabinet.
3. Follow the steps for preparing medications for administration, found in Chapter 35.
4. Verify the seven rights of medication administration ***to ensure that you have the right patient, right medication, right dose, right route, right date, right indication, and right time.***
5. Perform two safety checks ***to ensure that you are obtaining the right medication for the correct patient.*** *Safety: Ensure that you are applying the medication to the correct eye or ear. Abbreviations for right, left, or both eyes and ears are no longer recommended for use because of medication errors related to their use.*
6. Warm eardrops to room temperature by holding the bottle between the palms of your hands. ***Administering cold eardrops can cause nausea.***

Administer the Medication

7. Follow the Initial Implementation Steps located on the inside back cover.
8. Perform a third safety check ***to ensure that you are administering the right medication to the correct eye or ear of the correct patient.***
9. Tell the patient the name of the medication and explain the procedure ***to ensure the patient's cooperation.***

Administering Eyedrops

10. Assist the patient to a sitting position and ask him or her to tilt the head back slightly.
11. Gently pull the lower lid down to form a pouch, exposing the conjunctival sac.
12. Position the eyedropper ½ to ¾ inch above the eye.
13. Instill the prescribed number of drops and have the patient close his or her eyes for 1 to 2 minutes. Wipe off any excess medication with a tissue.

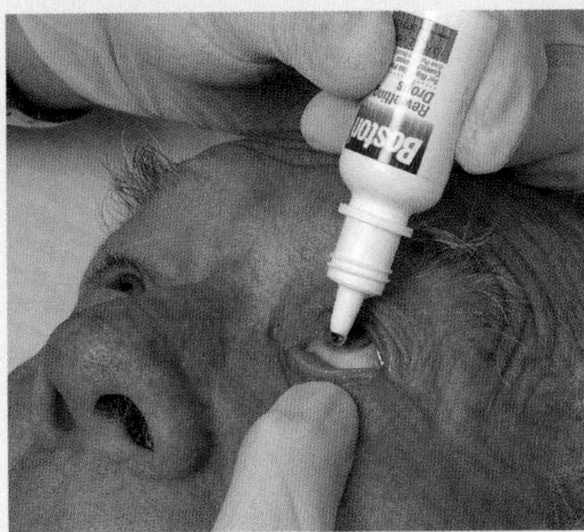

14. Follow the Ending Implementation Steps located on the inside back cover.
15. Document administration of the eyedrops on the MAR.

Administering Eye Ointments

10. For eye ointments, assist the patient to a sitting position and ask him or her to tilt the head back slightly.
11. Gently pull the lower lid down to form a pouch, exposing the conjunctival sac.
12. Squeeze a ribbon of ointment into the pouch from the inner canthus to the outer canthus approximately 1 inch.

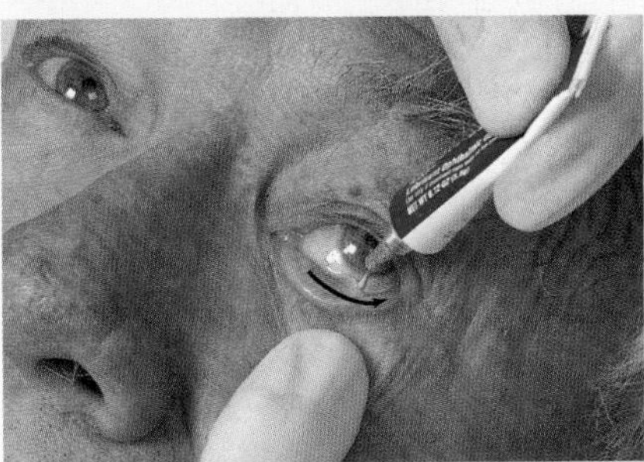

13. Instruct the patient to close the eyelids for 2 to 3 minutes and gently move the eyes around under the lids to distribute the ointment. Wipe away any excess medication with a tissue. *Safety: Avoid touching the tip of the bottle or tube to the eye because this can cause pathogens to enter the medication.*
14. Follow the Ending Implementation Steps located on the inside back cover.
15. Document administration of eye ointment on the MAR.

Administering Ear Medications

10. Assist the patient to a lateral position with the affected ear up.

(skill continues on page 816)

Skill 36.4 (continued)

11. For adults and children older than 3 years, gently pull the outer part of the ear (pinna) up and back. ***This straightens the ear canal, which allows the medication to penetrate farther into the ear.***

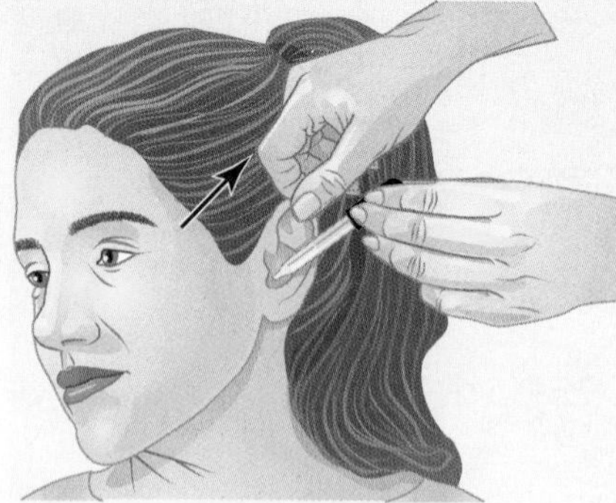

12. For children younger than 3 years, pull the pinna down and back. ***This straightens the ear canal, which allows the medication to penetrate farther into the ear.***

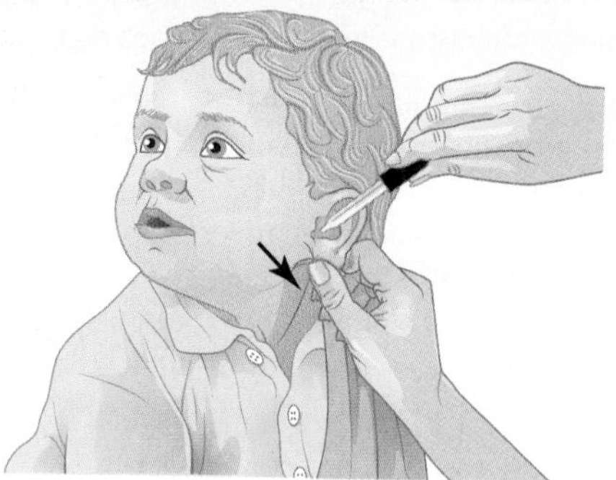

13. Instill the prescribed number of drops, making sure the drops fall against the side of the ear canal and not on the tympanic membrane, ***to prevent pain.***
14. Keep the patient's head turned for 5 to 10 minutes to ensure the medication enters the ear properly.
15. Place a cotton ball loosely in the ear for 15 minutes, if desired, and then remove. *Safety: Do not leave the cotton ball in the ear because it provides a warm, dark, moist environment for pathogen growth.*
16. Follow the Ending Implementation Steps located on the inside back cover.
17. Document the administration of eardrops on the MAR.

Evaluation Steps

1. Assess the patient for effects of the medication in 30 to 45 minutes.
2. Evaluate improvement in eye or ear discomfort. If the medication is not effective over a few days, notify the prescriber ***as a different medication may be needed.***

Sample Documentation

07/14/22 1105 Timoptic 0.5% one drop administered to both eyes per order after return from surgery. No c/o pain or discomfort. Resting quietly, respirations even and unlabored at 18 per minute. ——————

—————— Nurse's signature and credentials

Skill 36.5 Irrigating the Eye and Ear

Assessment Steps

1. Check the original prescriber's order, ensuring that it matches the order in the MAR, ***to prevent oversight of a transcription error.***
2. Assess the purpose of the irrigation: removal of a foreign body, washing out excessive cerumen from the ears, or removal of chemicals in the eyes.
3. Ensure that the tympanic membrane is intact prior to ear irrigation ***to prevent damage to the middle ear.***
4. Assess the need for cleansing of the eye or ear prior to irrigation. If exudate is present, plan to cleanse the area with moistened cotton swabs.

Planning Step

1. Gather needed supplies: irrigation solution (generally normal saline or tap water), basin for pouring irrigant, 35- to 60-mL syringe, basin for catching irrigant, clean gloves, and waterproof pad.

Implementation Steps

1. Follow the Initial Implementation Steps located on the inside back cover.
2. Explain the procedure to the patient ***to ensure the patient's cooperation.***

For Eye Irrigation

3. Assist the patient to lie on the side of the affected eye or to lie on the back with his or her head turned to the side of the affected eye, ***allowing best access from the inner to the outer canthus.***
4. Place a basin along the side of the patient's head ***to catch irrigant as it flows from the eye.***
5. Draw up 30 mL of solution into the syringe, keeping the tip of the syringe sterile at all times ***to prevent introduction of pathogens into the eye.***
6. Use your nondominant hand to hold the patient's eye open and ask the patient to look up.
7. Gently depress the plunger of the syringe 1 inch, aiming a stream of irrigant toward the conjunctival sac flowing from the inner canthus to the outer canthus. ***This prevents damage to the cornea.***
8. Repeat the irrigation process until the irrigation solution returns clear or the ordered amount of solution has been used.
9. Dry the outside of the eyelids with swabs or tissue.

Skill 36.5 (continued)

10. Follow the Ending Implementation Steps located on the inside back cover.

For Ear Irrigation

3. Warm the solution to body temperature by holding the bottle of irrigant under warm running water. *Safety: Instilling cold solution into the ear can cause nausea and dizziness.*
4. Assist the patient to sit up and tilt his or her head toward the unaffected ear. Ask the patient to hold the basin under the affected ear.
5. Draw up 30 mL of solution into the syringe.
6. Straighten the ear canal by pulling the pinna up and back or, if the patient is under the age of 3, by pulling the pinna down and back.
7. Aim at the top wall of the ear canal and gently depress the plunger of the syringe. *Safety: Aiming the irrigation syringe directly into the canal can cause damage to the tympanic membrane.*
8. Repeat the irrigation process until no more debris returns in the irrigation fluid or until the ordered amount of fluid has been used.
9. Dry the outside of the ear with cotton swabs or tissue.
10. Follow the Ending Implementation Steps located on the inside back cover.
11. Document the type and amount of fluid used, the type and amount of debris obtained, and how the patient tolerated the procedure.

Evaluation Steps

1. Evaluate the patient's tolerance of the procedure. Determine if the procedure caused pain, discomfort, or nausea.
2. Evaluate the effectiveness of the irrigation; determine if the eye or ear is clear of debris or foreign body.

Sample Documentation

07/23/22 1325 Left ear irrigated with 60 mL warmed normal saline to remove cerumen buildup. Moderate amount of dark brown wax removed, then irrigation return clear. C/o mild pain during procedure, relieved after procedure completed. ———————— Nurse's signature and credentials

Skill 36.6 Administering Vaginal Medications

Assessment Steps

1. Check the original prescriber's order, ensuring that it matches the order in the MAR ***to prevent oversight of a transcription error.***
2. Assess the patient for complaints of itching, burning, or pain in the vaginal area.
3. Inspect the vaginal area for discharge and inflammation.

Planning Step

1. Gather needed supplies: applicator for cream or tablet, a washcloth and towel to cleanse the area if discharge is present, and a water-based lubricant if inserting a tablet.

Implementation Steps

Prepare the Medication

1. Wash hands and follow standard precautions.
2. Obtain the medication from the patient's drawer or from the computerized cabinet.
3. Follow the steps for preparing medications for administration, found in Chapter 35.
4. Verify the seven rights of medication administration ***to ensure that you have the right patient, right medication, right dose, right route, right date, right indication, and right time.***
5. Perform two safety checks ***to ensure that you are obtaining the right medication for the correct patient.***
6. Attach the applicator to the tube of vaginal cream and squeeze until the applicator is filled and the plunger is pushed out, or insert the diamond-shaped tablet into the end of the appropriate applicator. Apply water-based lubricant to the tablet.

Administer the Medication

7. Follow the Initial Implementation Steps located on the inside back cover.
8. Perform a third safety check ***to ensure that you are administering the right medication to the correct patient.***
9. Tell the patient the name of the medication and explain the procedure, ***to ensure the patient's cooperation.***
10. Assist patient into the dorsal recumbent or Sims' position.
11. Gently retract the folds of the labia ***to expose the vaginal orifice.***
12. Cleanse the area with a washcloth and warm water if discharge is present.
13. Lubricate the tip of the applicator or vaginal suppository with a water-soluble lubricant ***to make insertion more comfortable for the patient.***
14. Insert the applicator gently into the vagina. Depress the plunger completely ***to distribute the medication.***

(skill continues on page 818)

Skill 36.6 (continued)

15. Withdraw the applicator and wipe residual medication from the vaginal area.

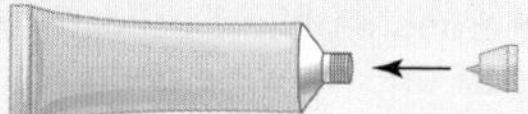

Invert cap and pierce end of medication tube

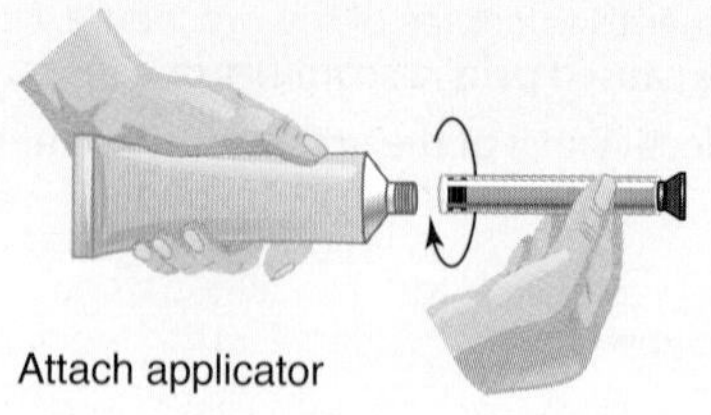

Attach applicator

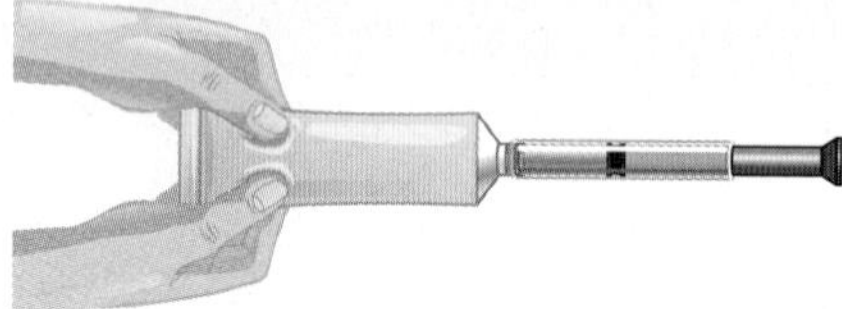

Squeeze medication into applicator

16. Encourage the patient to remain in the recumbent position for 20 to 30 minutes after administration ***to allow for absorption of the medication.***
17. Apply a perineal pad ***to prevent discharge of medication onto undergarments when the patient is upright.***
18. Wash applicator with soap and water, rinse, and dry. Store for future use.
19. Follow the Ending Implementation Steps located on the inside back cover.
20. Document the drug administered on the MAR.

Evaluation Steps

1. Evaluate the patient's response to the medication. Ask about relief of itching, burning, pain, and discomfort.

Sample Documentation

07/12/22 2010 Nystatin 100,000 units vaginal tablet inserted with applicator. Instructed to remain in dorsal recumbent position for 20 minutes. Peri pad given to protect underwear. ——————————

—————————— Nurse's signature and credentials

Skill 36.7 Administering Rectal Suppositories

Assessment Steps

1. Check the original prescriber's order, ensuring that it matches the order in the MAR, ***to prevent oversight of a transcription error.***
2. Assess the need for the medication as this route can be used for a laxative, hemorrhoid treatment, or delivery of a systemic medication. If it is a systemic medication, assess for the need to continue using the rectal route, such as for vomiting.
3. Assess bowel status. Do not administer if the patient has diarrhea without consulting the prescriber ***because the medication likely will not be absorbed.***

Planning Step

1. Obtain the suppository from the refrigerator. Usually it will be stored there ***to prevent melting of the wax base.*** Obtain water-soluble lubricant.

Implementation Steps

Prepare the Medication

1. Wash hands and follow standard precautions.
2. Obtain the medication from the patient's drawer or from the computerized cabinet.
3. Follow the steps for preparing medications for administration, found in Chapter 35.
4. Verify the seven rights of medication administration ***to ensure that you have the right patient, right medication, right dose, right route, right date, right indication and right time.***
5. Perform two safety checks ***to ensure that you are obtaining the right medication for the correct patient.***

Administer the Medication

6. Follow the Initial Implementation Steps located on the inside back cover.
7. Perform a third safety check ***to ensure that you are administering the right medication to the correct patient.***
8. Tell the patient the name of the medication and explain the procedure ***to ensure the patient's cooperation.***
9. Assist the patient to the left Sims' position. ***This position allows best access to the rectum and sigmoid colon.***
10. Lubricate the tip of the suppository with a water-soluble lubricant ***to make insertion more comfortable for the patient.***
11. Instruct the patient to take a deep breath to help relax the anal sphincters.
12. As the patient exhales, insert the suppository 1 to 3 inches with the index finger, ensuring that it is past the internal anal sphincter ***to facilitate retention.***

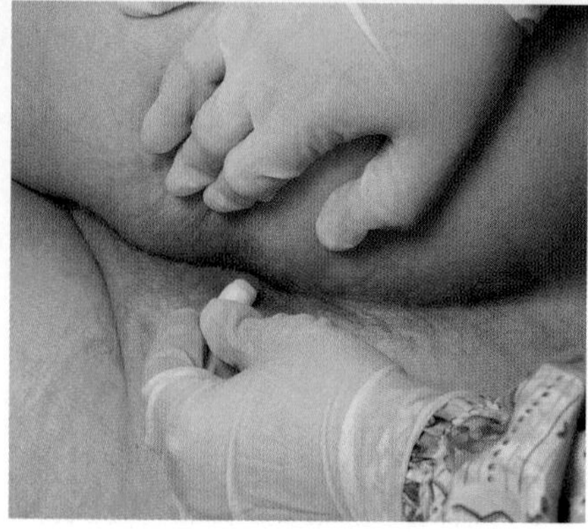

Skill 36.7 (continued)

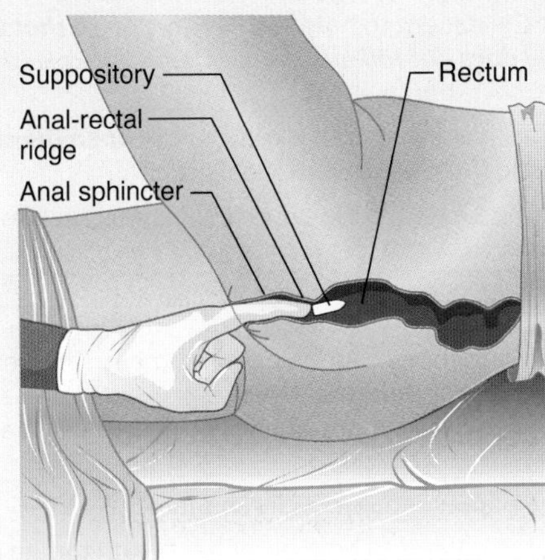

13. Clean and dry the rectum after insertion.
14. Remove gloves and wash hands.
15. Instruct the patient to hold the suppository in the rectum as long as possible ***to allow it to melt and the medication to be absorbed.***
16. Ask the patient to remain in the left Sims' or left lateral position for 5 to 10 minutes ***to help him or her retain the suppository.***
17. Assist the patient to the bathroom, if needed, when the urge to expel the suppository is strong.
18. Follow the Ending Implementation Steps located on the inside back cover.
19. Document medication administration on the MAR. If it is a prn medication, document in nurses' notes the reason for the medication and the response.

Evaluation Steps

1. Evaluate the patient's response to the medication. If it is given as a laxative, note the color, amount, and consistency of the bowel movement and document it.
2. If the suppository is given for other purposes, evaluate the systemic response in 30 to 45 minutes and report any adverse effects.

Sample Documentation

07/13/22 2115 Dulcolax suppository administered via rectum for c/o constipation. States no B.M. in 2 days "but it feels like it is right there." Remains in left Sims' position to retain med. ——— Nurse's signature and credentials

07/13/22 2200 Up to bathroom with assist. Expelled moderate amount dark brown stool. States feels "much better now." ——— Nurse's signature and credentials

Skill 36.8 Administering Inhaled Medications

Assessment Steps

1. Check the original prescriber's order, ensuring that it matches the order in the MAR ***to prevent oversight of a transcription error.***
2. Assess lung sounds ***to determine respiratory status.***
3. Assess the need for measuring vital signs prior to administering inhaled medications.

Planning Step

1. Obtain a glass of water and emesis basin for the patient to use when rinsing his or her mouth after administration of inhaled medications.

Implementation Steps

Prepare the Medication

1. Wash hands and follow standard precautions.
2. Obtain the medication from the patient's drawer or from the computerized cabinet.
3. Follow the steps for preparing medications for administration, found in Chapter 35.
4. Verify the seven rights of medication administration ***to ensure that you have the right patient, right medication, right dose, right route, right date, right indication, and right time.***
5. Perform two safety checks ***to ensure that you are obtaining the correct medication for the patient.***

Administer the Medication

6. Follow the Initial Implementation Steps located on the inside back cover.
7. Perform a third safety check ***to ensure that you are administering the right medication to the correct patient.***
8. Tell the patient the name of the medication and explain the procedure ***to ensure the patient's cooperation.***

For MDI

9. Assist the patient into the upright position ***to help expand the lungs fully when he or she is taking a deep breath.***
10. Prior to administering the medication, tell the patient to rinse out his or her mouth.
11. Remove the mouthpiece cap.
12. Shake the inhaler ***to mix the medication and prepare it to spray.*** If a spacer is to be used, attach it to the mouthpiece of the MDI.
13. Instruct the patient to tilt the head back slightly and breathe out completely.
14. Have the patient open his or her mouth while you hold the inhaler 1 to 2 inches away. ***This allows the spray that enters the mouth to be a fine mist rather than large droplets that may be absorbed by the oral mucosa and cause excessive side effects.*** If a spacer is used, have the patient close the lips around the mouthpiece of the spacer.

(skill continues on page 820)

Skill 36.8 (continued)

15. Press down on the inhaler to release one puff of medication as he or she takes a deep, slow breath in.

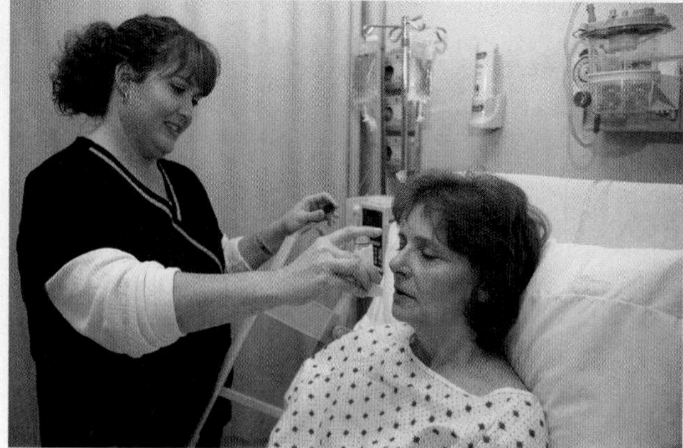

16. Once the medication is inhaled, instruct the patient to hold his or her breath for 10 seconds ***to allow the medication to go into the lungs.***
17. If two puffs of medication are ordered, have the patient wait 1 minute before taking the second puff. ***This allows the first puff to be absorbed before the second puff is taken.***
18. Have the patient rinse out the mouth after the last puff of medicine. Make sure the patient spits out the water and does not swallow. ***This is especially important if the medication is a steroid because leaving it in the mouth can lead to thrush.***
19. Encourage the patient not to drink, eat, or brush the teeth immediately after using the MDI ***because this can affect absorption of the medication.***
20. Follow the Ending Implementation Steps located on the inside back cover.
21. Document the administration of the MDI on the MAR and any other form according to facility policy.

For DPI

9. Assist the patient into the upright position ***to help expand the lungs fully when he or she is taking a deep breath.***
10. For diskus-style DPIs, move the thumb grip away from you, ***which will open the diskus and reveal the mouthpiece.***
11. Instruct the patient to hold the DPI upright ***so that the powder drug does not fall out.*** *Safety: Do not shake DPIs because they are in powder form.*
12. Move the lever away from the patient ***to open the chamber containing the next dose of medication.***
13. Instruct the patient to exhale in a direction that is away from the DPI device. *Safety: If the patient exhales into the DPI, the dose of powder will be dispersed so that it is not available to be inhaled.*
14. Place the mouthpiece in the patient's mouth and tell him or her to seal the lips around it. A spacer is not necessary with a DPI; the medication is automatically inhaled when a breath is taken.
15. Have the patient inhale deeply and forcefully.
16. Instruct the patient to hold his or her breath for the count of 10.
17. Have the patient rinse out the mouth after the last puff of medicine. Make sure the patient spits the water out and does not swallow it.
18. Follow the Ending Implementation Steps located on the inside back cover.
19. Document the administration of the DPI on the MAR and any other form according to facility policy.

Evaluation Steps

1. Assess lung sounds 30 to 45 minutes after the inhaler is administered to determine improvement.
2. Evaluate the patient for side effects of inhaled medications, especially nervousness, insomnia, restlessness, and nausea.

Sample Documentation

07/15/22 0915 Assisted with MDI. Required reminders not to put MDI mouthpiece in the mouth but to hold it 1 to 2 inches away. Also had difficulty coordinating spraying the MDI and inhaling at the same time. Able to perform correctly on the second inhalation with fewer cues. ——— Nurse's signature and credentials

POST CONFERENCE

You learned a great deal about the administration of medications in this clinical experience. You applied topical medication to the patient's eczema on her arms and legs. After contacting the pharmacist, you learned that you were not supposed to cover this type of medication. You gave a rectal suppository for constipation and a vaginal cream to treat her yeast infection. The patient was taking Tegretol suspension for her seizures. You knew that you had to dilute it with an equal volume of water and flush the tube carefully afterward to prevent it from adhering to the tube. The patient also had Prilosec ordered for acid reflux. You learned to open the capsule, and then you mixed it with apple juice rather than water and flushed the tube afterward with the apple juice. In your research, you learned that the potassium chloride liquid she was taking could cause clumping of the tube-feeding formula. In the facility, the patient had had problems with her tube becoming obstructed easily. You informed the nurse, who talked with the doctor. The patient was discharged to the facility with new orders to discontinue the potassium chloride and to give the Prilosec with 8 ounces of orange juice daily to supply potassium.

Key Points

- Drugs are available in a variety of forms, including tablets, capsules, liquids, eyedrops and eardrops, nasal drops, rectal and vaginal suppositories, and inhalers.
- When you administer oral narcotic medications, you must be sure that the patient's vital signs are stable. You also are responsible for keeping an accurate count of narcotics and for disposing of any unused medications correctly with a witness and signatures.
- Several classifications of medications require special administration techniques when given via an enteral tube due to interactions with the tube feeding formula. You are responsible for knowing how to correctly administer these medications via the enteral tube.
- When preparing medications to administer through an enteral tube, prepare each separately in individual medication cups. When administering them, separate each medicine with 20 to 30 mL of water to prevent interactions between the medications or interactions with the formula and to prevent drugs from adhering to the tube.
- Topical medications are often administered for local effects, while transdermal medications are given for systemic effects. You must evaluate the desired effects and side effects of both routes of medications.
- Eye medications are placed in the lower conjunctival sac to prevent damage to the cornea during administration.
- Ear medications should only be given to patients whose tympanic membrane is intact. Administer eardrops carefully, aiming the dropper so that the medication rolls down the wall of the ear canal and does not drop directly onto the tympanic membrane, which causes pain.
- Nasal medications are often given to reduce congestion, but some nasal sprays can cause a rebound effect with long-term use. This causes swelling of the nasal mucosa, leading to more congestion and the need for more nasal spray.
- Rectal medications are administered for local or systemic effects. This route is contraindicated in patients with certain cardiac conditions or in those with bowel or rectal disorders.
- Metered-dose inhalers contain liquid medication delivered as a mist and inhaled into the airways. To avoid intense side effects, it is recommended that patients hold the mouthpiece 1 to 2 inches away from the mouth during administration, which will prevent large drops of the drug from landing on the tongue and being rapidly absorbed.
- Dry-powder inhalers provide longer-acting effects. These inhalers contain a dry powder that the patient inhales deep into the airways. Do not allow the patient to breathe into the DPI because that will disperse the powder and waste the dose.
- Document medications on the paper MAR according to facility policy. Include the medication, dose, route, frequency, date, time, and your initials. When an eMAR is used, the bar-code technology documents and charges the medications as they are prepared and administered.
- Always check the seven rights of medication administration and perform the three safety checks when preparing medications to help prevent making a medication error.
- If a medication error is discovered, you must document it on an incident report or according to facility policy whether or not you made the error. Put the patient first and always admit to any medication error that occurs.

Review Questions

Select the answer that is most appropriate for each of the following questions. Some questions may have more than one correct answer. Select all that apply.

1. Your patient has been prescribed timolol maleate (Timoptic) eyedrops. Where should you instill the eyedrops?
   1. The cornea
   2. The pupil
   3. The eyelid
   4. The lower conjunctival sac

2. Which of the following techniques is(are) correct when inserting a rectal suppository?
   1. Position the patient on his or her right side with the left leg flexed.
   2. During insertion, tell the patient to hold his or her breath.
   3. Lubricate the tip of the suppository.
   4. Gently insert the suppository, directing it with the index finger.

3. A patient has been prescribed an MDI for the management of her asthma. Which of the following instructions should be given to the patient?
   1. Shake the inhaler before use
   2. Breathe slowly and fully before administration
   3. Administer by pressing the canister downward
   4. Hold your breath as long as possible

4. Buccal tablets are administered:
   1. under the tongue.
   2. between the upper lip and gum.
   3. by injection.
   4. through inhalation.

5. What steps should the nurse follow when administering a liquid cough syrup to a patient?
   1. Hold the medicine glass at eye level and pour the prescribed dose
   2. The measurement line should be even with the fluid level at the base of the meniscus
   3. Discard any excess
   4. Dilute all liquids with water

6. Which of the following drug administration routes is the safest and most convenient?
   1. Oral
   2. Topical
   3. Vaginal
   4. Nasal

7. Which of the following drug administration routes is through the epidermal layer of skin into the dermis?
   1. Oral
   2. Topical
   3. Inhalation
   4. Intravenous

8. Which of the following drug administration routes is rapid and across a large surface area?
   1. Oral
   2. Topical
   3. Inhalation
   4. Rectal

9. After administering medication in the enteral tube, how much water do you use to clear the tube?
   1. 20 to 30 ml
   2. 25 to 35 ml
   3. 5 to 15 ml
   4. 30 to 60 ml

ANSWERS 1. 4, 2. 3, 4, 3. 1, 2, 3, 4, 4. 2, 5. 1, 2, 3, 6. 1, 7. 2, 8. 3, 9. 1

Critical Thinking Exercise

Answers available online.

1. A patient with a bleeding ulcer has a nasogastric tube in place that is connected to low intermittent suction. There is an order for Carafate suspension (to coat the ulcer) per tube. What concerns do you have and what will you do?

Additional Resources

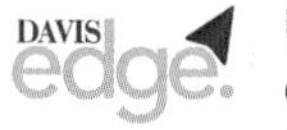

Use the scratch off code on the inside front cover of your book to access online quizzes that will help you to improve your scores on course exams and prepare for the NCLEX-PN®.

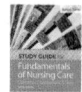

Study Guide

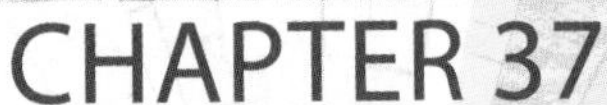

CHAPTER 37
Administering Intradermal, Subcutaneous, and Intramuscular Injections

KEY TERMS

Air-lock (AIR-LOK)
Ampule (AM-pyool)
First-pass metabolism (FERST-PASS muh-TAB-uh-lizm)
Gauge (GAYJ)
Insulin syringe (IN-su-lin si-RINJ)
Intradermal (IN-trah-DER-muhl)
Intramuscular (IN-trah-MUS-kyoo-lar)
Prefilled syringe (pree-FILD si-RINJ)
Subcutaneous (sub-kyoo-TAY-nee-us)
Tuberculin syringe (tyoo-BER-kyoo-lin si-RINJ)
Vial (VYE-al)
Z-track (ZEE-TRAK)

CHAPTER CONCEPTS

Safety

LEARNING OUTCOMES

1. Define various terms associated with intradermal, subcutaneous, and intramuscular injections.
2. Explain the significance of first-pass metabolism.
3. Describe the different types of syringes, including volume capacity and the units of measurement marked on each type.
4. Identify the different parts of a syringe and needle.
5. Describe the appropriate sites used for intradermal and subcutaneous injections.
6. Identify the anatomical landmarks and muscles used for intramuscular injections in adults and children.
7. Describe the volumes of medication that may be administered via the intradermal, subcutaneous, and intramuscular routes of injection.
8. Select appropriate needle gauge and length for the different routes of administration in the various injection sites for adults and children.
9. Describe proper injection technique for intradermal, subcutaneous, and intramuscular injections, including Z-track.
10. Specify parts of the syringe and needle that must be kept sterile during preparation and administration of an injection.
11. Identify appropriate safety measures related to administration of injections.
12. Relate possible complications associated with different types of injections.
13. Explain the importance of compatibility of medications.
14. Identify appropriate steps to employ as you draw up and combine two types of insulin in a syringe and then administer it via the subcutaneous route.
15. Correctly draw up medications from a vial and from an ampule.
16. Discuss diluents and any restrictions for use related to various age groups.
17. Identify medication classifications that require verification by more than one nurse prior to administration.
18. Discuss how the administration of insulin and Capitalize Lovenox varies from other subcutaneous injection techniques.
19. Discuss information found in the Connection features in this chapter.
20. Identify specific safety features.
21. Answer questions about the skills in this chapter.

SKILLS

37.1 Reconstituting and Withdrawing Medication From a Vial
37.2 Withdrawing Medication From an Ampule
37.3 Administering an Intradermal Injection
37.4 Combining and Administering Insulin Subcutaneously
37.5 Administering an Intramuscular Injection
37.6 Administering a Z-Track Injection

CRITICAL THINKING CONNECTION

Clinical Assignment

You will be caring for a 42-year-old male patient with poorly controlled diabetes who had a below-the-knee amputation 2 days ago. His medication orders include an injection of two types of insulin, NPH and regular insulin, every morning. In addition, he has meperidine ordered intramuscularly (IM) every 4 to 6 hours prn for incisional pain or phantom pain.

Critical Thinking Questions:

1. What laboratory values do you monitor prior to administering insulin?
2. How do you research how to administer insulin injections and how to mix two types of insulin in one syringe?
3. What is the purpose of administering insulin and rotating sites?
4. How do you administer an IM injection and select the appropriate site?
5. What size of needle would you use for the IM injection?

This is the chapter that most student nurses have been waiting for—how to administer an injection—because injections are one of the skills that people most commonly relate to nurses. In this chapter, you will learn how to be a safe practitioner while administering medications via the intradermal (ID), subcutaneous (subcut), and IM routes. This includes more than just the technique of the injection itself. ***Safety: A safe practitioner must know how to select the proper syringe and correct gauge and length of needle and must know the sites where different medications may be administered, the potential complications, which medications are compatible, and much more that you may not have thought about until now.***

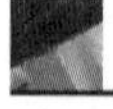

INJECTIONS

Injections are considered to be administered via the parenteral route, which means not through the gastrointestinal tract. The parenteral routes of medication administration include ID, subcut, IM, and IV; all of these will be covered in this chapter except the IV route. You will learn about the IV route in Chapter 38.

The advantages of administration of medications by injection include the following:

- Bypass of the gastrointestinal tract, thereby preventing gastrointestinal irritation
- Rapid onset time compared to the oral route
- Ease of administration to uncooperative or unconscious patients
- Better absorption of drugs that are poorly absorbed via the oral route

However, parenteral administration also has it disadvantages, including the following:

- Invasive and uncomfortable for the patient
- Expensive
- Requires additional supplies and equipment
- Requires qualified personnel to administer
- Carries a risk of infection and nerve injury

KNOWLEDGE CONNECTION

What are the parenteral routes of medication administration? What are the advantages of administering medication by injection? The disadvantages? Is it safe to delegate injections to unlicensed personnel?

Supplies and Equipment

Administration of medication per an injectable route requires various supplies and equipment, including a syringe, needle, alcohol prep pads, dry cotton ball or gauze pad (2 × 2 inch, 5 × 5 cm), needle disposal container, examination gloves, and bandage.

Syringes

A syringe is used to hold and introduce the medication into the needle, which will direct the medication into the body tissue. Medical syringes are typically disposable and made of plastic, while glass syringes are more prevalent in research settings. Syringes are available in numerous sizes, ranging from 0.3 to 60 mL, with the most common sizes being 1 mL and 3 mL. Each syringe has calibrations marked on the barrel in milliliters or units indicating the volume of medication to administer, depending on the type of syringe and the type of medication to be injected with the syringe (Fig. 37.1).

PARTS OF A SYRINGE. A syringe has three main parts: a barrel, a plunger with a flange on the end, and a tip that connects to the needle (Fig. 37.2).

• WORD • BUILDING •

intradermal: intra – within + derm – skin + al – related to
subcutaneous: sub – under + cuta – skin + neous – related to
calibration: calibr – quality or merit + ation – action

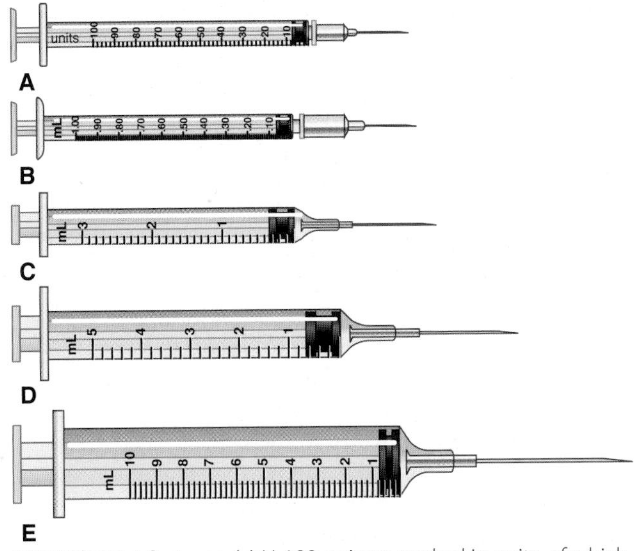

FIGURE 37.1 Syringes: (a) U-100 syringe marked in units, of which there are 100/mL; (b) 1-mL tuberculin syringe marked in 0.01 mL (1/100th of a milliliter) and minims (16 minims equals 1 mL); (c) 3-mL standard syringe marked in whole milliliters and 0.1 mL (1/10th of a milliliter); (d) 5-mL standard syringe marked in whole milliliters and 0.2 mL (2/10ths of a milliliter); (e) 10-mL standard syringe marked in whole milliliters and 0.2 mL (2/10ths of a milliliter) (from Wilkinson JM, Treas LS. *Fundamentals of Nursing: Theory, Concepts & Applications.* Vol. 2. 3rd ed. Philadelphia, PA: FA Davis; 2016).

Barrel

The barrel is the hollow cylindrical chamber that holds the medication. It has graduated unit-of-measurement marks that indicate the various volumes of medication the syringe can hold. One end of the barrel has a tip that connects to the needle. The other end of the barrel is open and has a plunger inserted into it.

Tips

A syringe may have one of two types of tips (Fig. 37.3):

- **Luer-Lok tip** has threaded grooves that screw onto the needle hub and lock it in place.
- **Slip-tip** has a smooth, slightly tapered tip that inserts into the needle hub, requiring a slight twist of the syringe or needle to securely snug the needle and syringe together.

Plunger

The plunger is a pistonlike rod that fits inside the barrel and slides up and down the barrel to either draw up medication

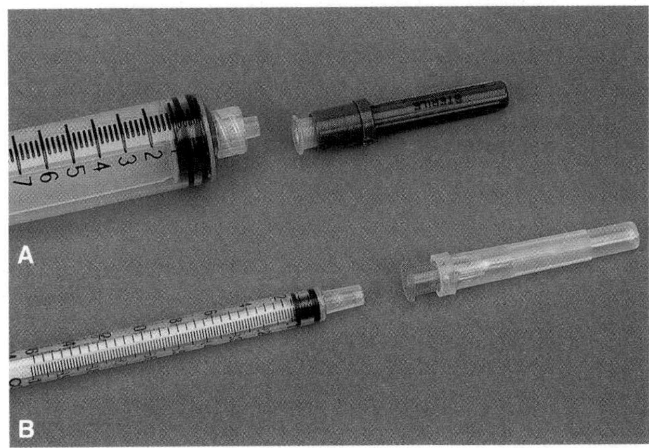

FIGURE 37.3 Syringe tips: (a) Luer-Lok tip that screws on; (b) Slip-tip that applies with a gentle push-and-twist motion (from Wilkinson JM, Treas LS. *Fundamentals of Nursing: Theory, Concepts & Applications.* Vol. 1. 3rd ed. Philadelphia, PA: FA Davis; 2016).

or push it out of the barrel. The end of the plunger that is inserted into the barrel is rubber tipped to provide traction against the barrel. On the other end of the plunger is a flange that allows you to grip the plunger to pull it back when drawing up medication (refer to Fig. 37.2).

SYRINGE TYPES. There are four major types of syringes, two of which are designed for administration of specific medications.

Regular Syringe. A standard syringe is most frequently used for IM or subcut injections. It is calibrated in milliliters (mL), and some also have minims (m) marked on them as well. Standard syringes are available in 1-, 3-, 5-, 10-, 20-, and 60-mL sizes. You will use the 1-, 3-, and 5-mL syringes for most injections.

Tuberculin Syringe. The **tuberculin (TB) syringe** is a smaller diameter syringe that holds a total volume of 1 mL and is calibrated in tenths and hundredths of a milliliter as well as sixteenths of a minim, making it an excellent choice for administration of the small and precise volumes of medication required by newborns and infants as well as for the TB skin test for which it was designed (Fig. 37.4).

Insulin Syringe. The **insulin syringe** is similar in size and shape to a TB syringe, but it is calibrated in units of insulin and used only for injecting insulin. ***Safety: It is no longer considered safe to abbreviate the word unit with "U." The Joint Commission has included it on the list of Do Not Use***

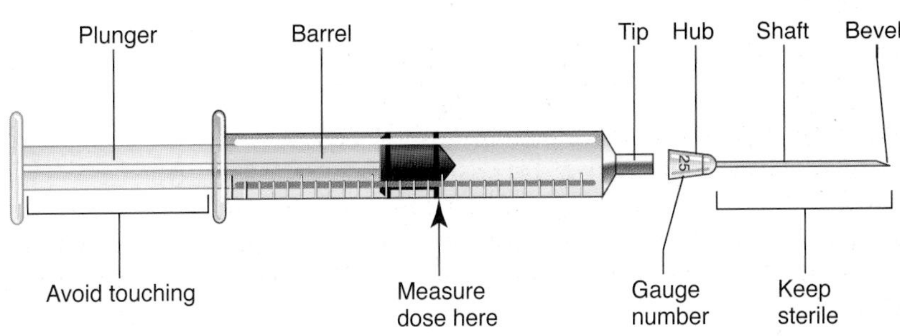

FIGURE 37.2 Parts of a syringe and safety needle (from Wilkinson JM, Treas LS. *Fundamentals of Nursing: Theory, Concepts & Applications.* Vol. 1. 3rd ed. Philadelphia, PA: FA Davis; 2016).

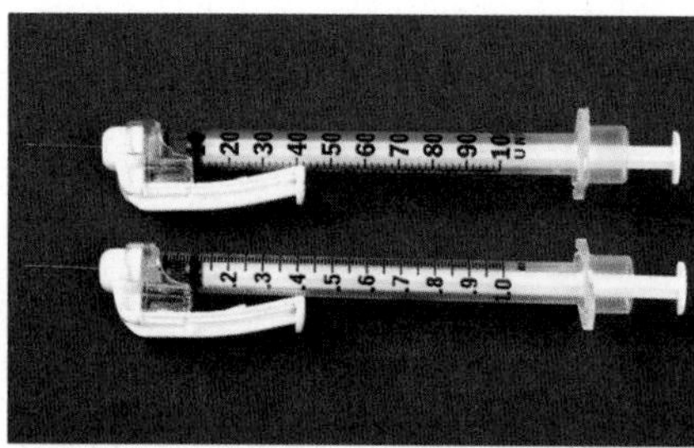

FIGURE 37.4 Top: Insulin syringe. Bottom: Tuberculin syringe (from Wilkinson JM, Treas LS. *Fundamentals of Nursing: Theory, Concepts & Applications.* Vol. 2. 3rd ed. Philadelphia, PA: FA Davis; 2011).

Abbreviations. The word "units" must always be spelled out. There are several sizes of insulin syringes that hold different total volumes of 0.3, 0.5, or 1 mL. A standard insulin syringe is 1 mL and holds up to 100 units of insulin. The smaller size that holds only 0.3 mL is best for children who need very small doses of insulin and for people with poor eyesight. The calibrations are printed in a larger font, making it easier for patients with impaired vision to see the numbers more accurately.

An insulin syringe usually has a tiny-gauge, short, permanently attached needle. The most common syringe size is marked for use with U-100 insulin, meaning the strength of the insulin is 100 units of insulin per 1-mL volume (see Fig. 37.4).

Prefilled Syringes. **Prefilled syringes** are single-dose, ready-to-use, disposable syringe cartridges, some with an attached needle and some to which you must attach a needle, that contain specific dosages of specific medications. The cartridge is loaded into a reusable plastic holder for administration. This drug-delivery device offers various advantages, including ease of use, convenience, and safety. Prefilled injection systems such as Carpuject® (Abbott) and Tubex® (Wyeth-Ayerst) are designed for safe and quick loading and unloading (Fig. 37.5).

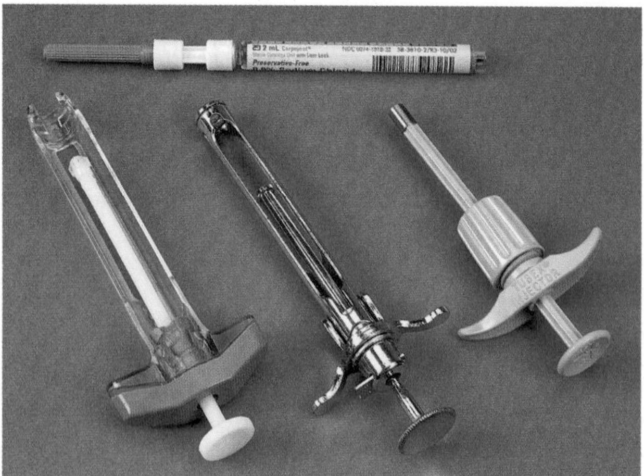

FIGURE 37.5 Left: Prefilled syringe unit dose cartridge with holder; Right: Disposable, prefilled, self-controlled system (from Wilkinson JM, Treas LS. *Fundamentals of Nursing: Theory, Concepts & Applications.* Vol. 1. 3rd ed. Philadelphia, PA: FA Davis; 2016).

After using the cartridge, unscrew it from its holder and drop it vertically into a disposal container. ***Safety: Do not recap the needle.***

Needles

The needle is a small, hollow, cylindrical tube with a sharp, beveled cutting-edge tip used to pierce the skin. It is usually made of steel or other metal. For administering injections, the needle must be attached to a syringe, which contains the medication.

PARTS OF A NEEDLE. A hypodermic needle consists of a plastic *hub* used to attach the needle to the syringe, the *bevel,* the *cannula* or *shaft,* and a *safety guard* to cover the used needle as soon as it is withdrawn from the patient's body (see the orange safety needle guard in Fig. 37.6). All facilities should have both needle and syringe safety devices or use one of the needleless systems developed to reduce contaminated needle sticks.

The bevel is the slanted tip of the needle, designed to facilitate needle insertion and prevent *coring* (punching out a circular piece of skin) when inserting the needle. ***Safety: The bevel should always face upward when piercing the skin.*** The

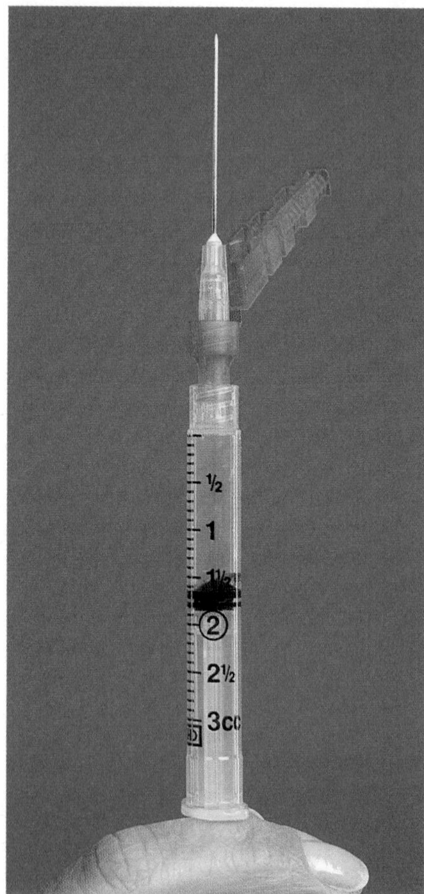

FIGURE 37.6 Standard syringe attached to a safety needle with orange guard, containing 1.7 mL of air (from Wilkinson JM, Treas LS. *Fundamentals of Nursing: Theory, Concepts & Applications.* Vol. 2. 3rd ed. Philadelphia, PA: FA Davis; 2016).

pointed tip entering the skin in front of the bevel limits the degree of tissue injury as the bevel allows for gradual increase in the size of the opening made in the skin. The shaft denotes needle length. ***Safety: Maintain the sterility of the entire needle. Do not touch any part of it.***

The needle has a plastic cap or cover that must be removed before use. ***Safety: To prevent accidental needle sticks with contaminated needles, never recap a used needle.*** Blood-borne pathogens can be transmitted from the patient to anyone stuck with the contaminated needle.

GAUGE. The **gauge** (G) of a needle refers to the diameter of the needle and is indicated by numbers, typically between 14 G (2.1 mm) and 30 G (0.3 mm). The *higher* the gauge number, the *smaller* the diameter of the needle. A 14-G (2.1-mm) needle is a very large-diameter needle, while a 30-G (0.3 mm) needle is very tiny. The choice of needle gauge depends on several factors:

- Viscosity of the medication
- Route of administration
- Size of patient and muscle mass

A smaller gauge, from 14 G (2.1 mm) to 20 G (0.9 mm), has a larger diameter and because of this is required for *viscous,* or thick, medications; larger gauges, from 21 G (0.8 mm) to 30 G (0.3 mm), have smaller diameters and are used for thin medications. Smaller-gauge needles generally cause less pain; however, larger-gauge needles, such as 29 G (0.34 mm) and 30 G (0.3 mm), are so tiny that they are easily bent. The size of the muscle targeted for an IM injection also affects the gauge somewhat. For example a thin, water-consistency medication might flow easily through a larger-gauge (but smaller-diameter) needle such as a 27 G (0.4 mm) or 29 G (0.34 mm). However, if the medication is to be injected IM into a 225-pound muscular male, a smaller-gauge (but larger-diameter) needle such as a 22 G (0.7 mm) would be required in order to be strong enough to pierce a large muscle, whereas a 27-G (0.4-mm) to 30-G (0.3-mm) needle would be appropriate to administer the same medication to a newborn with tiny muscles. Needle manufacturers may color-code needles according to gauge, although color coding is not universal and may vary between different manufacturers.

LENGTH. Needles come in different lengths, typically ranging from ¼ inch to 2 inches (0.64 to 5 cm). The length is measured from the tip of the bevel to the junction of the hub and shaft. The choice of length depends on the weight, amount of fat, and muscle development of the patient; the site of injection; and the route of administration. A subcut injection, which is injected into the layers of subcutaneous fat of an adult, is administered with a shorter needle, between ⅜ and ⅞ of an inch (0.9 to 2.2 cm) depending on the patient's size. For a subcut injection in an infant, you might need a ¼-inch (0.64-cm) needle. For a school-age child, a ⅝-inch (1.6-cm) needle would be a likely choice.

An IM injection for an adult, injected into the muscular layer below the subcutaneous layer, is administered in the body or largest portion of a muscle and requires a longer needle length, from 1 to 2 inches (2.5 to 5 cm). Children range in size from tiny newborns to adolescents who are similar in size to adults, so the range of needles used for IM injections varies significantly. A newborn might require a ⅜-inch (0.9-mm) needle, and a school-age child might require a ⅝- to 1-inch (1.6- to 2.5-cm) needle depending on the child's size.

Handling Syringes and Needles

Asepsis is a primary concern when handling syringes and needles. Always wash your hands before handling sterile injection supplies, and clean the work surface where you will be preparing the injection. Keep a facility-approved cleaning agent near the medication cart or counter where you routinely prepare medications so that it will be handy to use.

Get Ready

Begin by reviewing the health-care provider's order so that you know the type and volume of medication that you are to draw up and the route of administration. Assess your patient's age and size, the site you will use, and the amount of muscle mass or subcutaneous tissue at the site. Now you are prepared to select the appropriate syringe and the correct gauge and length of needle.

Gather all the supplies you will need before beginning the preparation of the injection. It will save you time and energy, make you more efficient and enable you to be more productive, make you appear more competent, and make it easier to maintain sterile technique required for proper preparation. If you have to stop what you are doing, set down supplies and equipment, and possibly leave the patient room or medication cart in order to get something you forgot, this has the potential to require extra handwashing, as well as repeated entering and exiting of the work site or patient room, and may force you to redirect your thoughts and focus, all of which reduce your organization and ability to be efficient and complete nursing care in a timely manner. It also forces the patient to wait, and it may even require you to use additional sterile supplies, which increases costs. Taking the few extra minutes to assess which supplies you will need to administer an injection will save you time over the whole shift.

Maintain Asepsis

Safety: It is important to maintain sterility of the appropriate parts of the syringes and needles you work with. As you prepare the syringe, peel the sterile package open and lay the package down with the syringe still resting in one side of the package until you are ready to attach the needle. ***Safety: Avoid taking the syringe out of the package and laying it on the bare countertop, where you risk contaminating the tip of the syringe.***

When handling a syringe, keep all parts that contact the medication or the patient sterile. This includes the syringe tip, the inside of the barrel, and the length of the plunger from the rubber tip inside the barrel to approximately 1 inch from the flange end. That keeps the portion of the plunger that comes in contact with the medication and goes in and out of the syringe barrel sterile. The outside of the barrel and the flange are the only parts that may be touched. It is not necessary to wear gloves for preparation of an injection, but always wear clean examination gloves for the actual administration of every injection to protect you from possible contact with body fluids and blood-borne pathogens.

The only part of a needle that may be touched is the plastic needle cap. The hub of the needle that attaches to the syringe must be kept sterile while preparing to attach it. Without touching the needle, peel the package open just far enough to expose the hub, fold the two package flaps down to the sides of the needle package, and hold them down with your nondominant fingers and thumb. With your dominant hand, pick up the sterile syringe from its wrapper, and if it has a cap on the syringe tip, aseptically remove it using both hands, one holding the syringe and one holding the cap, and then attach the needle hub to the syringe. ***Safety: Do not attempt to remove needle covers or syringe tip caps using a one-handed method. It is virtually impossible to push or flip the cover or cap off the needle or syringe without contaminating it with the thumb that is pushing it off. Never use your teeth to pull off a needle cover.***

To attach the needle to a Luer-Lok syringe, place the hub of the needle against the threaded connector of the syringe and gently twist clockwise. The same type of needle will attach to a slip-tip syringe with a gentle push and twist. The needle and syringe are then ready for use.

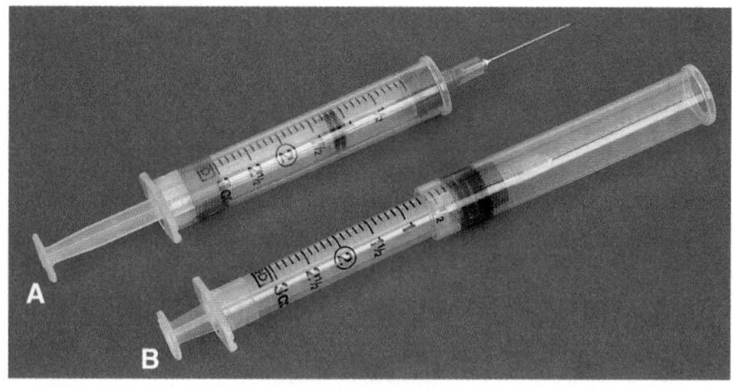

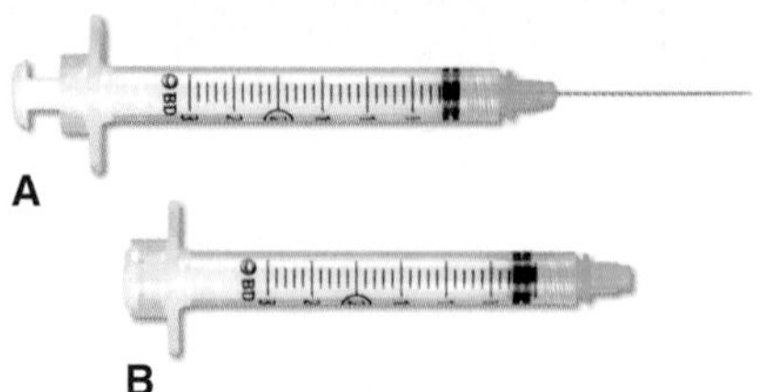

FIGURE 37.7 Top: (a) Before injection (safety device has not been activated); (b) After injection and activation of safety device. Bottom: (a) Needle before activation of retracting device; (b) After needle retraction (from Wilkinson JM, Treas LS. *Fundamentals of Nursing: Theory, Concepts & Applications.* Vol. 2. 3rd ed. Philadelphia, PA: FA Davis; 2016).

Preventing Needle-Stick Injuries

Percutaneous injuries, commonly referred to as *needle-stick injuries,* are a significant occupational hazard for nurses and other health-care workers. These injuries provide the perfect mode of transmission for blood-borne infectious diseases, including HIV, hepatitis B, and hepatitis C. Needle-stick injuries commonly occur when recapping contaminated needles. They also may result from improper needle disposal.

Safety: To prevent needle-stick injuries, never recap used needles. Do not bend, break, or cut needles before disposal. Be vigilant to activate the needle safety guard immediately after use, as soon as the needle tip leaves the patient's body as you withdraw the needle after administering an injection. (See Fig. 37.7 for an example of two additional types of needle safety devices.) ***Safety: Drop the syringe and needle as one unit into the sharps container, which is made of a hard plastic that is nonpervious, or puncture proof*** (Fig. 37.8). Sharps containers come in various sizes, ranging from a small, approximately 8-ounce size all the way up to a 1.5-gallon size, and usually they are red. Some are designed to set on a countertop or medication cart, while others are designed to mount on the room wall.

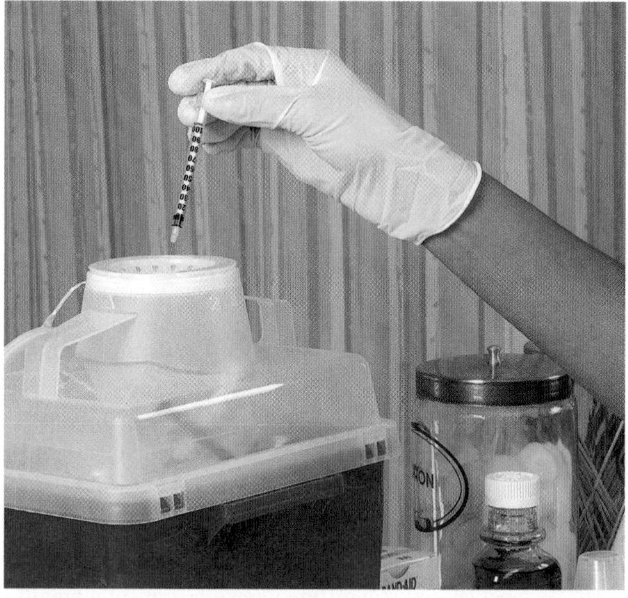

FIGURE 37.8 Always dispose of needles and glass vials/ampules in a sharps container made of puncture-proof plastic, usually red (from Wilkinson JM, Treas LS. *Fundamentals of Nursing: Theory, Concepts & Applications.* Vol. 1. 3rd ed. Philadelphia, PA: FA Davis; 2016).

Occupational safety guidelines published by the U.S. Centers for Disease Control and Prevention (CDC) and the Occupational Safety and Health Administration recommend against recapping any needles, both new and used, even when disposing of them. To maintain sterility of the needle and because carrying an uncovered needle while walking down the hallway is unsafe, it is sometimes necessary to recap a clean needle after drawing up a medication so that you may carry it to the patient's room. ***Safety: When recapping a clean needle, use the one-handed scoop technique.*** Lay the cap on a flat surface with the open end extending a short distance beyond the edge of the flat surface. Maintaining sterility, scoop the cap onto the tip of the syringe needle held in your dominant hand (Fig. 37.9A). The free hand

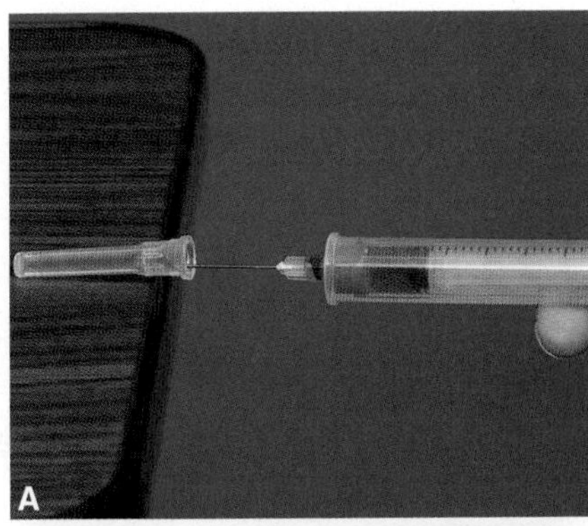

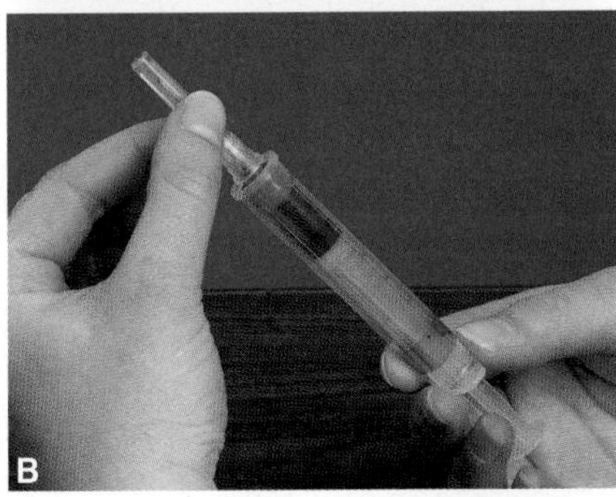

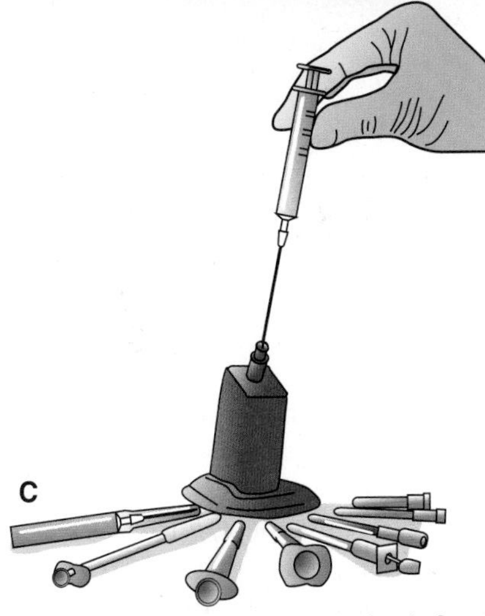

FIGURE 37.9 The one-handed "scoop" method of recapping sterile needles: (a) Without touching the sterile needle to the outside of the needle cap, scoop the cap onto the needle; (b) Use the other hand to "pull" the cap down over the needle until secure (do not place your finger on the end of the cap and "push" it on); (c) An alternative is a needle recapping device (a, b: from Wilkinson JM, Treas LS. *Fundamentals of Nursing: Theory, Concepts & Applications*. Vol. 2. 3rd ed. Philadelphia, PA: FA Davis; 2016).

should be kept away from the exposed needle. Once the cap has been scooped up onto the needle, you may use your nondominant hand to pull the cap farther onto the needle until it secures.

There is also an alternative method that works well for individuals whose hand might be shaking: First open a sterile package containing an alcohol pad, using care to touch only one corner of the alcohol pad to pull it out of the package. Lay the pad on the countertop and place the open end of the cap in the middle of the alcohol pad. Now scoop the cap onto the needle. The sterile alcohol pad provides an extra degree of sterility should you touch it on the way to the open end of the cap. ***Safety: Never push on the end of the cap because it is possible for a large needle to go through the end of the cap and into your finger. You should not use the two-handed method to recap even the sterile needle because this develops a habit that can be performed with contaminated needles without even thinking about it.*** There also are various recapping devices that can be purchased for one-handed recapping of sterile needles (see Fig. 37.9).

Ensure that proper needle disposal containers are conveniently located. This helps ensure proper needle disposal and may reduce the inclination to recap used needles before disposal. There should be one container in each patient room and on each medication cart or work counter where medications are prepared. ***Safety: Never place needles in the garbage or in a recycling bin to prevent accidental needle sticks of housekeeping employees and other department employees. It also decreases public access to disposed needles.***

If a needle-stick injury occurs, immediately wash the punctured area with soap and water, which encourages bleeding from the site. Follow facility protocol and seek medical attention. Most facilities require testing for blood-borne pathogens—from both the individual on whom the needle was used and the recipient of the contaminated needle stick. It is important to get the patient's consent for blood draws. The testing is normally done the same day of reporting and two to three more times at specified intervals. Documentation, usually an incident or variance occurrence form, is completed according to facility policy and protocol.

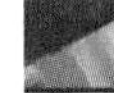

KNOWLEDGE CONNECTION

What are the parts of a syringe? What are the parts of a needle? How should you dispose of needles? How are needle-stick injuries prevented?

MEDICATIONS

You must be knowledgeable about all medications that you are preparing to administer, and administration by the injectable routes increases the importance of this knowledge because the medication will take effect faster than via many other delivery methods. The injectable routes can also result in an increased intensity of the drug's effect. In addition, an injected drug cannot be retrieved even immediately after administration, whereas orally administered drugs have limited potential for retrieval of part of or an entire dose by using gastric lavage or emetic medications to induce vomiting, and some topical medications can be at least partially removed with soap and water if caught quickly.

It will serve you well and make you a safer nurse to be vigilant in your research efforts regarding drugs to be administered per injection. The absolute minimum knowledge that you should acquire about each drug includes the following:

- Is the patient allergic to it?
- What is its classification?
- What does it do? How does it work?
- Why does this patient need this medication?
- Is the ordered dose within the safe dose parameters for this patient's age, size, and condition?
- Is the route appropriate for this particular drug? This patient?
- What assessments should you make prior to administering the medication? Afterward?
- How quick is the onset of drug action?
- For which side effects must you watch?
- Is there an antidote if one is needed?
- Is it compatible with other medications the patient is receiving?

Reconstitution and Drawing Up Medications

Injectable medications may come in the form of a liquid or a powder that needs to be dissolved in a liquid. The powder form is used for medications that are not stable for very long once they are in solution. The process of dissolving powdered drugs using a liquid or diluent such as sterile normal saline or sterile water is known as *reconstitution.* Some medication labels or inserts will provide more than one volume of diluent to use for the purpose of mixing different concentrations of the medication. ***Safety: It is always your responsibility to read the label and accompanying insert to determine the type and volume of diluent to use for reconstitution and the strength of the medication once it has been reconstituted.***

Vials

A **vial** is a glass or plastic container of medication with a rubber stopper that must be punctured with a needle for medication removal (Fig. 37.10). If the label or insert indicates that the rubber stopper is designed for use with needleless systems, a needleless piercing device may be used in place of a needle (Fig. 37.11). However, do not use blunt needles or needleless piercing devices on any vial stopper or IV tubing injection port unless it specifies that it is designed for use with needleless systems. ***Safety: Using nonsharps to pierce rubber stoppers that are not designed for such use allows the device to core the rubber. This means a round piece of the stopper is punched out and now is either in the medication or aspirated into the needle or syringe.***

MULTIPLE-DOSE VERSUS SINGLE-DOSE VIALS. Vials of parenteral solutions may be labeled as *single-dose* or *single-use* as well as *multiple-dose* or *multiple-use* vials. All multiple-dose vials contain bacteriostatic preservatives that reduce the risk of microorganism growth, while the single-dose vials do not. ***Safety: Avoid using single-dose vials more than once.*** Upon opening a multiple-dose vial, write the date, time, and your initials on the label. Some medications are good for only 24 hours; others vary in the length of time for which the drug may safely be used after opening.

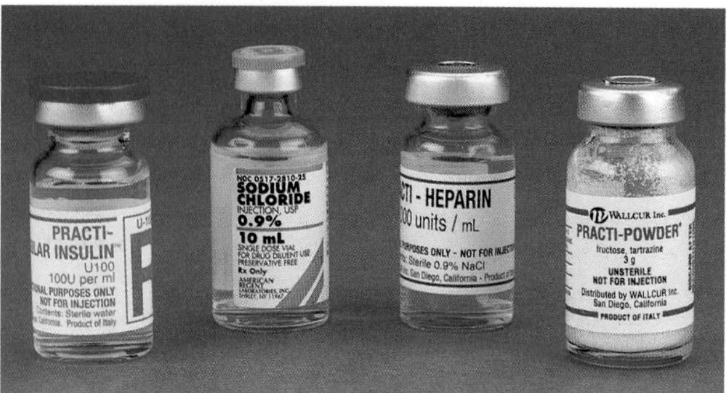

FIGURE 37.10 Medication vials (from Wilkinson JM, Treas LS. *Fundamentals of Nursing: Theory, Concepts & Applications.* Vol. 1. 3rd ed. Philadelphia, PA: FA Davis; 2016).

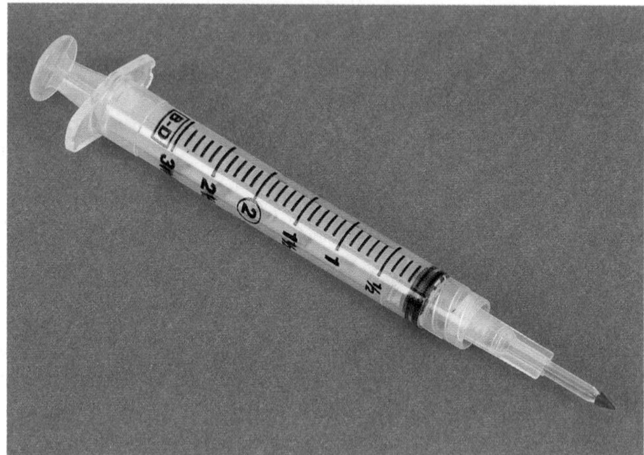

FIGURE 37.11 A syringe with a needleless piercing device (from Wilkinson JM, Treas LS. *Fundamentals of Nursing: Theory, Concepts & Applications.* Vol. 1. 3rd ed. Philadelphia, PA: FA Davis; 2016).

It is important to know that benzyl alcohol 0.9%, the bacteriostatic preservative used in multiple-dose vials of sterile water for injection and sodium chloride 0.9% for injection, is contraindicated for use in newborns. The warning is generally printed in red letters right on the label. Benzyl alcohol has been found to be toxic to neonates. Remember this when using multiple-dose vials.

WITHDRAWING MEDICATION FROM A VIAL. Wash your hands before handling medication and supplies. Remove the plastic cap from the top of the vial and then wipe the rubber stopper of the vial with an alcohol wipe. Using two hands, remove the needle cover from the needle attached to your syringe and lay the cover down or stand it in a needle-recapping device (refer to Fig. 37.9). Hold the syringe in your nondominant hand, and use your dominant hand to grasp the plunger, holding it only by the flange. Pull the plunger back, filling

• WORD • BUILDING •

diluent: dilu – wash away + ent – agent or action

bacteriostatic: bacterio – bacteria + static – stopping

the syringe reservoir with air equal to the amount of solution to be drawn up. For example, if you are to draw up 1.7 mL of medication, pull back on the plunger to fill the syringe reservoir with 1.7 mL of air.

With the needle, pierce the rubber stopper of the medication vial at a 90-degree angle, allowing the pointed tip (the long side of the bevel) to enter the stopper first. Keep the needle tip above the fluid level and slowly inject the air from the syringe into the air space above the medication in the vial (Fig. 37.12). This slightly pressurizes the vial so that the medication can be drawn out easily. ***Safety: Do not inject air directly into the medication; doing so may introduce bubbles that will take up some of the space in the syringe and prevent you from drawing an exact dose of medication.***

After instilling the air into the vial, leave the needle inserted into the vial; invert both the vial and the syringe and carefully draw up the appropriate volume of medication by slowly pulling the plunger back (Fig. 37.13). ***Safety: Be certain to maintain sterility of the entire needle and the plunger that enters into the syringe barrel.*** Draw up the exact amount and inspect the syringe carefully for bubbles. If bubbles are present, pull back on the plunger and fill the syringe with approximately 1 mL of extra medication; most bubbles will then go to the top of the syringe, where they can be expelled from the syringe. If not, gently tap the side of the syringe to release the bubbles so that they rise toward the needle (Fig. 37.14). Be certain to use care when tapping on the syringe; if you tap it too hard and do not have a secure hold on both the vial and the syringe, it is easy to bend the shaft of the needle. Slowly reinstill the air and any overfill of medication back into the vial. Withdraw the needle from vial. Skill 37.1 (page 846) provides more information on reconstituting and withdrawing medications from a vial.

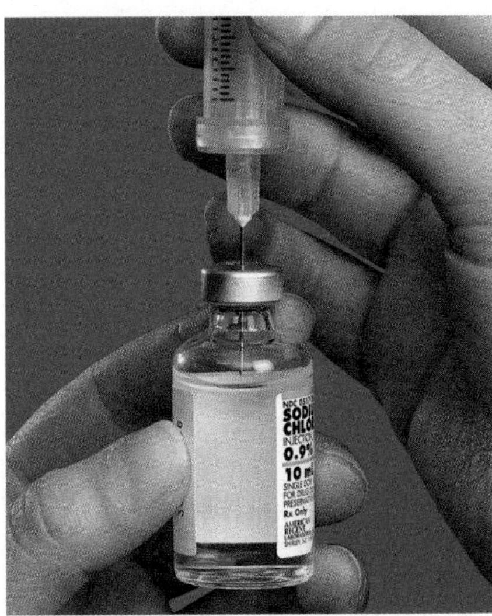

FIGURE 37.12 When instilling air into a vial, keep the needle tip above the fluid level (from Wilkinson JM, Treas LS. *Fundamentals of Nursing: Theory, Concepts & Applications*. Vol. 2. 2nd ed. Philadelphia, PA: FA Davis; 2016).

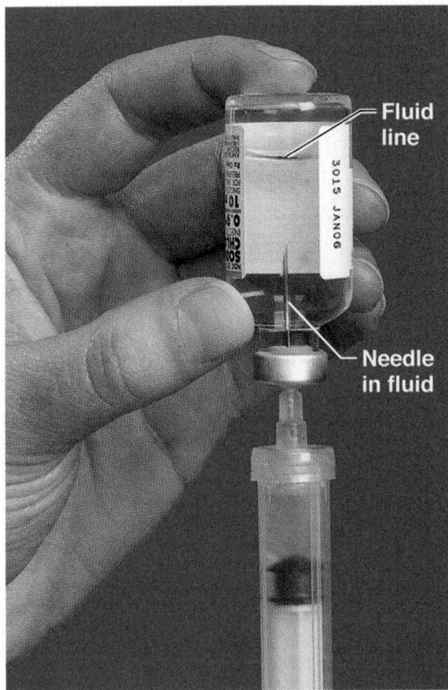

FIGURE 37.13 Invert the vial with the needle still inside the vial. Begin to pull back on the plunger to withdraw the desired volume of medication (from Wilkinson JM, Treas LS. *Fundamentals of Nursing: Theory, Concepts & Applications*. Vol. 2. 2nd ed. Philadelphia, PA: FA Davis; 2016).

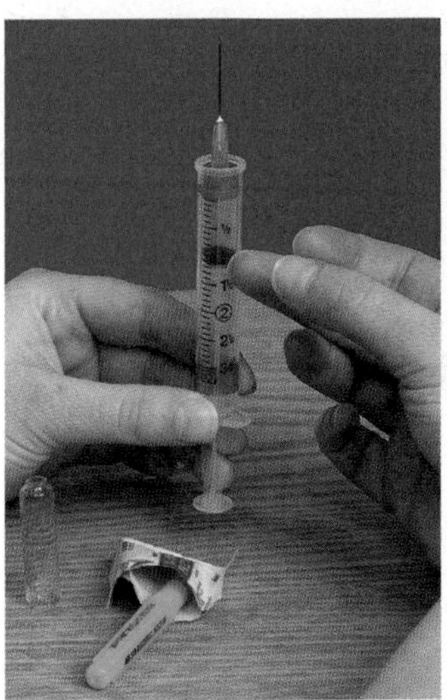

FIGURE 37.14 If unable to get air out of a syringe, gently tap on the side of the syringe to free the air bubble so that it will rise to the top of the syringe, where it can be expelled (from Wilkinson JM, Treas LS. *Fundamentals of Nursing: Theory, Concepts & Applications*. Vol. 2. 3rd ed. Philadelphia, PA: FA Davis; 2016).

Ampules

An **ampule** is a small, sealed glass drug container that must be broken to withdraw the medication. To prepare the ampule for withdrawal of medication, tap the top of the ampule to distribute the medication to the lower portion of the ampule. Wipe the neck of the ampule with an alcohol wipe to reduce bacterial contamination on the outside of the ampule. Use either a plastic device designed specifically for breaking an ampule or an alcohol wipe or gauze pad held between your fingers and the neck of the ampule that you intend to break off. Snap the neck of the ampule, breaking it away from your body to avoid injury (Fig. 37.15).

Safety: Attach a filter needle, which has a device for filtering debris such as glass shards from ampules or rubber cores from vials, to the syringe you will use to draw up medication. Invert or tilt the ampule to facilitate withdrawal of the medication. Maintaining sterility of the filter needle and the medication in the ampule, insert the filter needle you attached to the syringe into the ampule without touching the needle to the outside of the ampule (Figs. 37.16 and 37.17). Unless you accidently instill air into the inverted ampule, medication will

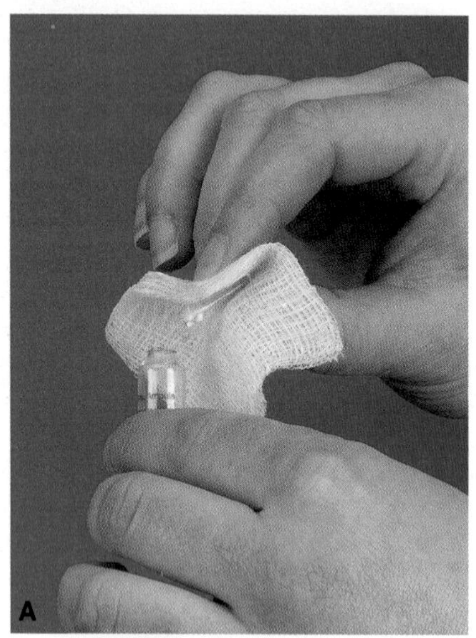

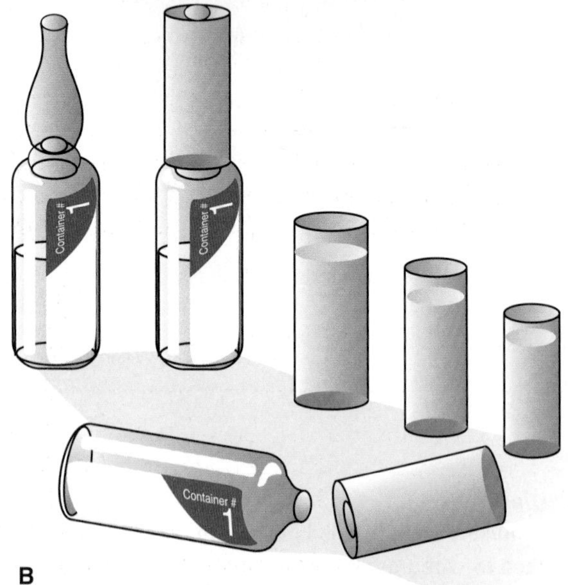

FIGURE 37.15 (a) Use gauze or an alcohol wipe to protect your fingers when breaking an ampule; (b) If available, break ampule necks with a special device designed for this purpose (a: from Wilkinson JM, Treas LS. *Fundamentals of Nursing: Theory, Concepts & Applications.* Vol. 2. 3rd ed. Philadelphia, PA: FA Davis; 2016).

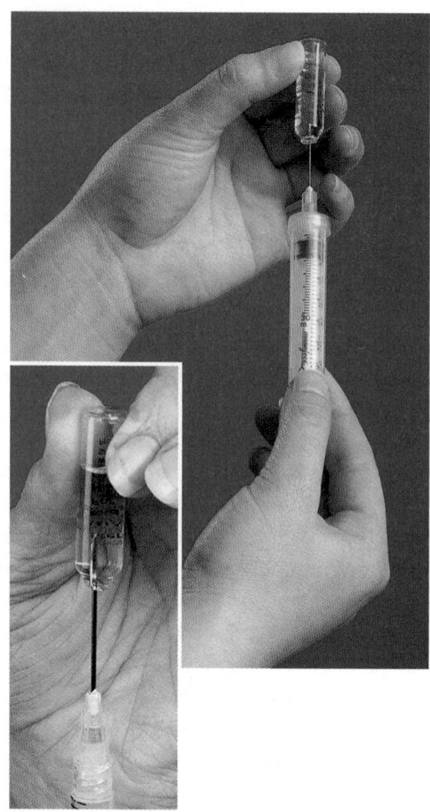

FIGURE 37.16 Invert the ampule and insert a sterile needle into the ampule, keeping the needle tip below the fluid level (from Wilkinson JM, Treas LS. *Fundamentals of Nursing: Theory, Concepts & Applications.* Vol. 2. 3rd ed. Philadelphia, PA: FA Davis; 2016).

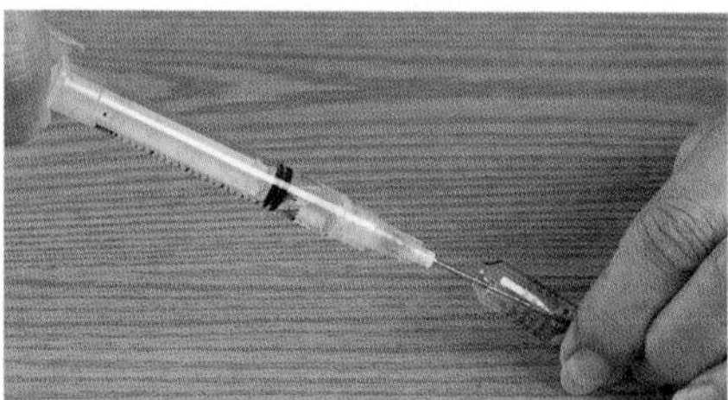

FIGURE 37.17 Tilting the ampule for medication removal (from Wilkinson JM, Treas LS. *Fundamentals of Nursing: Theory, Concepts & Applications.* Vol. 2. 2nd ed. Philadelphia, PA: FA Davis; 2016).

not leak out of the ampule even though it is upside down because of the surface tension of the fluid. Keeping the needle tip below the fluid level in the ampule, pull back on the syringe plunger until the appropriate volume of medication has been withdrawn, and then remove the filter needle from the ampule. ***Safety: You must change the filter needle after drawing up the medication and attach a new regular needle before administering the injection.***

If air is present in the syringe, tap the barrel of the syringe near the hub to move air toward the needle. Push carefully on the plunger to expel air or excess medication. Empty the unused portion of medication from the ampule. ***Safety: Remove the filter needle from the syringe prior to administration of medication. Injecting the medication back through the same***

filter needle and into the patient will also instill any glass shards that the filter might have caught. You must change the needle after withdrawing the medication from the ampule and then discard the ampule glass and filter needle in a puncture-resistant container to prevent accidental injury. Skill 37.2 (page 847) provides more information on withdrawing medication from an ampule.

Mixing Medications

Sometimes it may be appropriate to combine more than one drug in a syringe to avoid the discomfort of multiple injections. ***Safety: It is crucial to check the compatibility of medications before mixing and injecting them.***

Compatibility/Incompatibility of Medications

You must assess whether drugs are compatible with each other before you administer them together and especially before you mix them together in the same syringe. *Incompatibility* is an unwanted reaction that occurs between the drug and the solution, container, or another drug. There are physical, chemical, and therapeutic types of incompatibilities that can occur. Physical incompatibilities produce visible reactions such as color changes, precipitate formation, cloudiness, gas formation, or haze. A chemical incompatibility involves the degradation of the drug resulting from a chemical reaction. Therapeutic incompatibility occurs within the patient as the result of two concurrently administered drugs that interact. If there is a question about compatibility, review drug inserts and drug information texts and consult with a pharmacist.

Ready to Mix

Once compatibility is established, cleanse both tops of the two vials with separate alcohol pads. Attach a filter needle to the syringe to draw up medications. If one or both of the vials are multiple-dose vials, fill the syringe with the amount of air equal to the medication dose needed from the first medication (for textbook purposes, we will call the first one *vial A* and the second one *vial B*). Maintain the vial in an upright position and inject the air into vial A, but be careful not to touch the needle to the solution. This prevents medication from vial A from being transported on the needle and contaminating the medication in vial B when the needle is inserted. Remove the needle from vial A.

Then fill the syringe with the appropriate volume of air and inject the air into vial B. Without removing the needle from vial B, invert the vial and syringe and withdraw the required volume of medication into the syringe. Withdraw the needle from vial B and then reinsert it into vial A. Invert vial A carefully, and withdraw the required volume of medication, using caution to avoid drawing more than you need because you will be unable to inject any of it back into the vial now that the two medications are mixed. Replace the filter needle with an appropriate needle to be used for injection. The syringe then contains a mixture of medications from vials A and B.

The process is much easier when both vials are single-dose vials. Instill air in each vial and then withdraw medication from one vial and then the second vial. There is no need to protect the needle from contact with the first medication.

MIXING MEDICATIONS FROM PREFILLED SYRINGES. Medications from prefilled syringes may also be mixed. There are two ways to perform the task: both medications can be drawn into a separate syringe, or the second medication can be drawn into the prefilled cartridge if there is adequate room.

The first method is to draw the medication from the prefilled cartridge into a separate syringe. The end of the prefilled cartridge has a plastic adapter that may have its own attached needle, or it may be designed so that a needle can be attached to it (refer to Fig. 37.5). For this method, apply gentle pressure to the entire plastic adaptor, bending it sideways, and it will slide easily off the end of the prefilled cartridge, exposing a rubber stopper at the end of the cartridge.

Cleanse the stopper with an alcohol wipe and then pierce the stopper with a hypodermic needle attached to a syringe, withdrawing the medication from the cartridge into the syringe. If the second medication is in a single-dose vial, first clean the vial stopper with alcohol. Pull into the same syringe a volume of air equal to the volume of medication to be withdrawn from the second medication vial. Insert the syringe needle into the vial and instill the air. Now withdraw the correct volume of medication into the syringe with the first medication, where they mix.

To mix both medications in the cartridge, place the cartridge in the plastic holder, retain the amount of air in the cartridge that will need to be instilled into the second medicine vial, and expel any excess air over that amount from the cartridge. Wipe the vial stopper with an alcohol wipe, then invert the vial prior to piercing the vial stopper with the needle on the prefilled cartridge. Hold the syringe with the first medication in a vertical position, with the needle tip pointing up. This allows air in the syringe to rise toward the needle and settle on top of the medication so that it can be injected rather than the medication in the syringe. Instill the air from the cartridge and withdraw the appropriate volume of medication into the cartridge, where the two medications mix (Fig. 37.18).

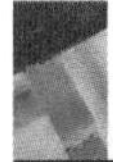

COMPARISON OF ROUTES OF ADMINISTRATION

Generally oral administration is the safest and most convenient route; however, it has the slowest onset of action of all the routes and provides a lower blood level than all other routes of administration. Before an oral medication can begin to work, it must first be absorbed from the gastrointestinal tract into the portal circulation that transports the medication to the liver. One of the liver's most important functions, due to its protective nature, is metabolizing and detoxifying potentially harmful agents in the blood. As the liver metabolizes the drug, it decreases the amount of

Anatomy and Physiology Connection

Anatomy of the Tissues You Inject

The skin is the largest organ of the body. The skin regulates body temperature, provides a physical barrier for protection, prevents excess water loss or absorption, and contains nerve endings for sensory perception. The skin is divided into two main layers: the epidermis, which is the outermost layer of skin, and the dermis, which is the connective tissue layer of the skin located below the epidermis. The dermis, which is composed of collagen, elastic tissue, and reticular fibers, is attached to an underlying hypodermis, commonly known as the *subcutaneous connective tissue.* The subcutaneous connective tissue stores adipose tissue and contains larger blood vessels and nerves. The muscular tissue layer is deeper yet, beneath the subcutaneous layer. The dermal layer, the subcutaneous layer, and the muscle layer are each composed of different types of cells and tissue. The drug manufacturers design medications to work best in specific tissues; rarely is a drug compatible with all three layers of tissue. There are numerous drugs that are caustic and damaging when injected into the improper tissue layers.

Because the skin that covers all the layers underneath is the primary or first line of defense against microorganism invasion, any break in the skin's integrity places the patient at risk for infection, which is why it is imperative that you use stringent sterile technique when withdrawing medications from containers and during administration of injections. If you consistently use good technique, you will not find yourself responsible for an abscess or other infection because of an improperly administered injection.

drug remaining in the blood after it leaves the liver to enter the systemic circulation, where it can perform its intended function. This process is known as **first-pass metabolism.** In other words, the drug is weakened during metabolism that occurs during the first pass through the liver. The routes of administration that escape first-pass metabolism include sublingual, buccal, and parenteral routes because they all provide absorption directly into the systemic circulation rather than into the portal circulation of the digestive tract. Parenteral drugs elicit rapid responses because they circumvent first-pass metabolism, but because they cannot be retrieved, parenterally administered drugs may present more risks.

The most common parenteral routes are classified as **intradermal, subcutaneous,** and **intramuscular.** An ID injection deposits the medication into the *epidermis,* or the outer layers of the skin, while a subcut injection is injected under the layers of the skin into the subcutaneous tissue layer. An IM injection is administered into the deep muscle tissue below the subcutaneous layer of tissue.

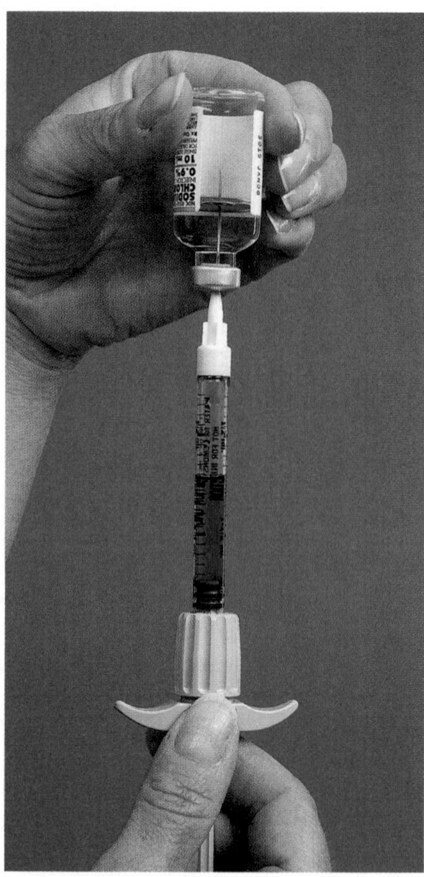

FIGURE 37.18 Hold the syringe vertical, needle tip upward. This allows the air inside the syringe to rise above the medication so that air can be instilled into the vial to maintain air pressure. Invert the vial before piercing the rubber stopper with the needle (from Wilkinson JM, Treas LS. *Fundamentals of Nursing: Theory, Concepts & Applications.* Vol. 2. 2nd ed. Philadelphia, PA: FA Davis; 2016).

Intradermal Injections

An ID injection is the injection of a small amount of fluid into the dermis, or true skin layer immediately below the epidermis (Fig. 37.19). It is commonly used as a diagnostic tool, such as testing for allergies or tuberculosis. (Box 37.1 provides a description of administering an ID tuberculin skin test.) The left or right ventral forearm is the site most frequently used for tuberculin testing, using a substance called tuberculin purified protein derivative (P.P.D.). The left or right ventral forearm, upper chest, and upper back over the scapulae are the sites used for allergy testing.

The length of the needle for an ID injection should be ¼ to ⅝ inch, with a very small-diameter needle between 25 and 30 G (1.27 to 1.58 cm). Position the needle bevel up and use a 15-degree angle for insertion of the needle. Instill the medication between the layers of the dermis to create a *bleb,* which looks somewhat like a small, raised, fluid-filled blister (Fig. 37.20). Avoid applying pressure or massaging the injection site. If a drop of blood or fluid leaks from the puncture

• WORD • BUILDING •

intramuscular: intra – within + muscul – muscle + ar – related to

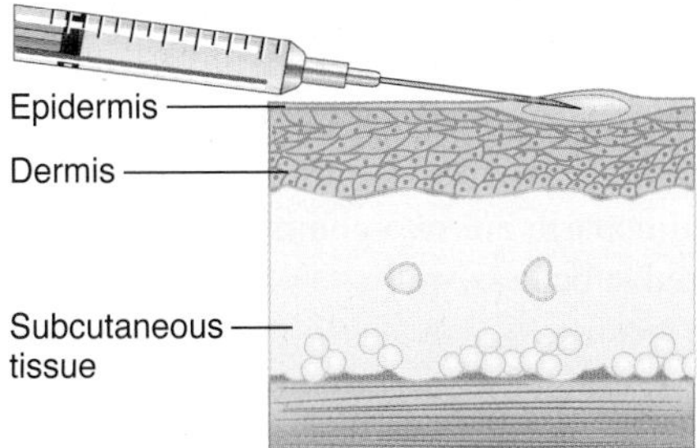

FIGURE 37.19 Intradermal injection delivers a small volume of medication into the dermal layer (from Wilkinson JM, Treas LS. *Fundamentals of Nursing: Theory, Concepts & Applications*. Vol. 2. 3rd ed. Philadelphia, PA: FA Davis; 2016).

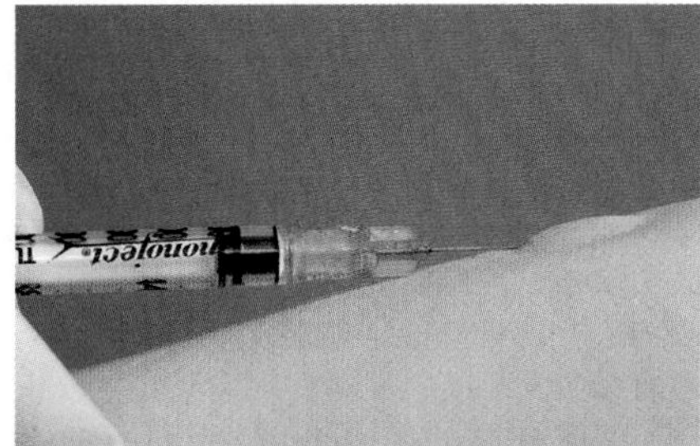

FIGURE 37.20 A small, discreet, pale, raised *bleb* should arise if you have the needle positioned correctly (from Wilkinson JM, Treas LS. *Fundamentals of Nursing: Theory, Concepts & Applications*. Vol. 2. 3rd ed. Philadelphia, PA: FA Davis; 2016).

Box 37.1

Tuberculin Skin Testing

A substance known as tuberculin purified protein derivative, commonly called P.P.D., is used to test an individual for the presence of tuberculosis. Inject a small volume (0.1 mL) intradermally on the ventral side of the left or right forearm. If the correct ID injection technique is used, a pale elevation of the skin, called a wheal, that is approximately 6 to 10 mm in diameter will result, looking somewhat like a tiny blister that absorbs within a few minutes. Use an ink pen to circle the wheal and write the date and time next to the circle. Advise the patient to have the site read between 48 to 72 hours later for interpretation.

The interpretation involves determining whether or not the site is indurated and, if so, the size of the induration. Induration is a palpable raised and hardened area where the P.P.D. was injected. If blisters are present, they also indicate a positive result. Any redness that may occur does not indicate a positive result. If induration or blistering is present, measure the size. Induration 2 mm or less in diameter is considered negative. In a healthy individual, 15 mm is considered a positive reading. In a health-care worker who has been exposed to TB, 10 mm is considered a positive reading. In some types of immunocompromised patients, even 5 mm may be considered a positive reading.

site after withdrawing the needle, gently touch the corner of the drop with a dry cotton ball or alcohol wipe to remove it, but do not apply pressure to the site.

Safety: Activate the needle guard immediately after removal of the needle from the skin. You must be vigilant about this safety mechanism while you are still learning and perfecting your technique for this to become an automatic habit. Skill 37.3 (page 848) provides more information on administering an ID injection.

KNOWLEDGE CONNECTION

What is a P.P.D. skin test for? What volume of drug is administered for a P.P.D. test? Describe the range of needle gauges and lengths that are used for ID injections. What is meant by first-pass metabolism? Why is it important? What is a bleb?

Subcutaneous Injections

A subcut injection deposits the medication into the subcutaneous layer below the skin and above the muscle layer (refer to Fig. 37.19). It contains fewer blood vessels than muscle, producing a slower absorption time compared to IM injections. ***Note: The Joint Commission has mandated that because previously used abbreviations for subcutaneous, including SC, SQ, and sub-q, increase the risk of medication errors, they should no longer be used. The only abbreviation that may be used is subcut.*** Sites for a subcut injection include the back of the upper arms, the abdomen (but stay a minimum of 2 inches away from the umbilicus), the anterior thighs, the area of the back just below the scapulae, and the upper buttocks (Fig. 37.21).

The subcut route is useful when slow and continuous absorption is required. The abdomen provides more rapid absorption than the other subcutaneous sites and is the preferred sites for insulin and Lovenox, an anticoagulant. To prevent irritation and tissue damage, the medication must be isotonic and must be the same pH as the tissue.

To administer an adult subcut injection, you will need a needle between ⅜ and ⅞ inch (0.95 to 2.22 cm) in length with

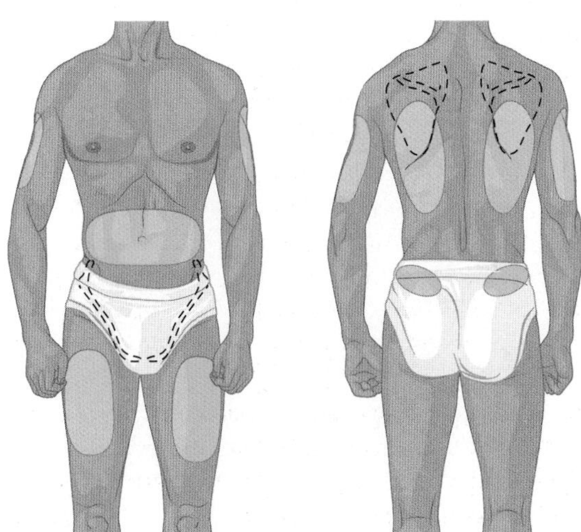

FIGURE 37.21 Subcutaneous injection sites (from Wilkinson JM, Treas LS. *Fundamentals of Nursing: Theory, Concepts & Applications*. Vol. 1. 3rd ed. Philadelphia, PA: FA Davis; 2016).

a diameter between 24 and 29 G. You will administer the injection at a 45-degree angle. However, the angle of needle insertion and the length of needle may vary somewhat based on the amount of fat and size of the patient. For example, if you are administering a subcut injection into the abdomen of an extremely obese adult male, you could use any needle length between ⅜ and ⅞ inch (0.95 and 2.22 cm) and could use a 45-degree angle or even a 90-degree angle, because the layer of subcutaneous tissue would be thick enough that any of these would deposit medication within the subcutaneous tissue layer. This would not be the case if you were administering a subcut injection in the abdomen of a petite, 101-pound, 22-year-old female. For this patient, you would need the shorter ⅜- or ⅝-inch (0.95- to 1.58-cm) needle length and would use a 45-degree angle. Anything longer would deposit medication into the muscular tissue.

According to most facility policies, the maximum volume for subcut injection is 1 to 2 mL. It is your responsibility to know your facility's policy. You will pinch or bunch up the skin and underlying fat layer into a fold between your finger and thumb, which helps to lift the subcutaneous layer off the muscle, helping to ensure that you inject only subcutaneous tissue rather than muscle (Fig. 37.22). As with all injection techniques, the insertion of the needle should be swift, piercing the skin and subcutaneous layer in one smooth motion. ***Note: Avoid inserting the needle only a short distance and then having to push the needle farther in to reach the proper depth, which results in additional discomfort for the patient.***

Do not aspirate before injecting medication as there are few large blood vessels in the subcutaneous tissues, making it difficult to hit a vessel. You will apply gentle pressure to the site after removing the needle and gently massage to distribute the medication into the tissue for better absorption unless you are administering insulin or heparin. ***Safety: Activate the needle safety device immediately after removal of the needle from the skin.*** You must be vigilant about this safety mechanism while you are still learning and perfecting your technique for this to become an automatic habit.

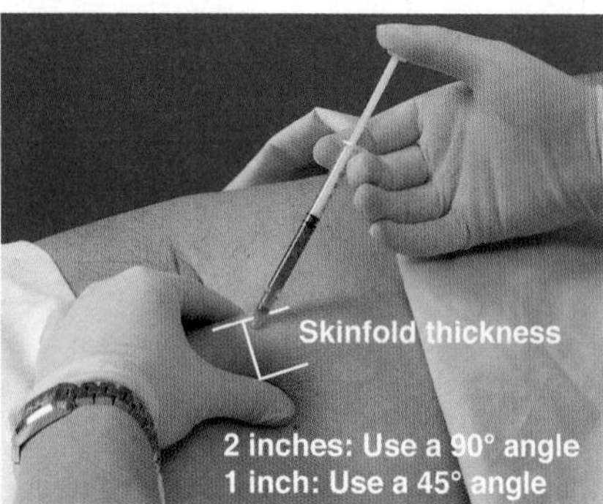

FIGURE 37.22 For subcutaneous injection, pull the skin taut as you pinch a large skinfold between your thumb and fingers, lifting the subcutaneous layer off the muscle (from Wilkinson JM, Treas LS. *Fundamentals of Nursing: Theory, Concepts & Applications.* Vol. 2. 2nd ed. Philadelphia, PA: FA Davis; 2016).

Safety: Do not massage the site after injection of insulin or heparin.

Insulin and Heparin

Insulin and heparin are two commonly used drugs that are administered subcut as well as IV. ***Safety: Both drugs, if administered incorrectly, can be life-threatening; therefore, you must follow specific safety steps that are not necessary for other medications*** (Table 37.1).

INSULIN. Insulin is a hormone that is necessary for transporting glucose from the blood into each individual cell of all the tissues in the human body. If insulin is not present to transport the glucose from the blood, the blood level of glucose elevates. Without glucose to utilize for energy production within the cells, all body processes and functions are impaired, which is what happens when an individual has diabetes mellitus: The pancreas does not produce adequate insulin to meet the body's needs.

Insulin types are designated according to their speed of action, including how long the interval is from administration of the insulin to the onset of its action, the timing of the insulin's strongest or peak action, and the duration of effect. Classifications generally are categorized as very rapid acting, rapid acting, intermediate acting, long acting, and very long acting. ***Safety: You will need to learn the onset, peak, and duration of the various insulins so that you can adequately assess patients for effectiveness of their insulin.*** It is particularly important when a patient receives several doses or two or more types of insulin each day. The peak and duration times of multiple insulins will overlap with onset and peak times of previously administered insulins, compounding the effects on the patient's blood glucose level, which places the patient at increased risk for dangerously low glucose levels, known as *hypoglycemia* or *insulin shock.*

A patient whose blood glucose is unstable may require finger stick blood sugar (FSBS) measurements several times per day to monitor glucose levels, followed by administration of insulin, the dosage of which is determined according to a *sliding scale* that is dependent on the FSBS results obtained at specified intervals (Table 37.2). Some more recent research recommends using an algorithm for insulin dosing instead of a sliding scale in order to deliver a more individualized insulin dose for the patient's needs.

You will also need to know the signs and symptoms of both hypoglycemia and hyperglycemia so that you can identify the problems quickly and prevent a delay in treatment (Table 37.3). ***Safety: It is important that you teach the patient with diabetes to wear a bracelet or necklace that states the patient has diabetes and uses insulin.*** The bracelet or necklace should be easily seen so that the patient having a hypoglycemic reaction can be immediately identified as having diabetes, helping to ensure appropriate care for the patient.

Insulin preparations are measured in units and require use of specific insulin syringes for administration. Now most insulin is concentrated at 100 units per milliliter

Table 37.1
Tips for Safe Insulin and Heparin Administration

Medication	*Tips for Safe Administration*
Insulin	• Monitor finger stick blood glucose or serum glucose levels. • Use a syringe matching the strength of the insulin. • Have a second and a third nurse verify that you have the correct type of insulin and the correct dosage drawn into the syringe. • Do not aspirate before injecting insulin. • Do not massage the site after removing the needle. • Monitor the patient for signs and symptoms of hypoglycemia and hyperglycemia.
Heparin	• Assess laboratory results—prothrombin time, international normalized ratio, and partial thromboplastin time—before administering. • After checking the heparin label against the medication administration record three times, check it again. • Have a second and a third nurse verify that you have the correct strength of heparin and the correct dosage drawn into the syringe. • Do not aspirate before instilling heparin. • Do not massage the site after withdrawing the needle. • Monitor the patient for bleeding gums, red blood cells in the urine, blood in the stools, and excessive bruising.

Table 37.2
Example of an Insulin Sliding Scale

FSBS Results	*Regular Insulin per Subcutaneous Route (number of units to administer)*
150–200 mg/dL	Give 2 units
201–250 mg/dL	Give 4 units
251–300 mg/dL	Give 6 units
301–350 mg/dL	Give 8 units
Greater than 350 mg/dL	Call health-care provider

(U-100). Always confirm that you have the corresponding U-100 syringe to use with U-100 insulin. Rapid-acting insulin and short-acting insulin are often combined with intermediate-acting insulins. Not all types of insulins can be mixed. ***Safety: Long-acting insulins, such as insulin glargine (Lantus), are never mixed with other insulins.*** Some combination products come premixed in a single vial, such as Novolin 70/30, which is 70% intermediate-acting insulin and 30% short-acting insulin.

KNOWLEDGE CONNECTION

What primary function of insulin makes it so important? What test result should you view prior to insulin administration?

Table 37.3
Signs and Symptoms of Hypoglycemia and Hyperglycemia

Condition	*Signs and Symptoms*	*Immediate Actions to Take*
Hypoglycemia	Pale, cool, clammy skin Tremors or palpitations Hunger or nausea Increased irritability Fatigue Difficulty concentrating Headache Dizziness or restlessness Drowsiness or lethargy	Assess finger stick blood sugar (FSBS). If below 90 mg/dL and the patient is able to swallow, give a small glass of orange juice or other simple carbohydrates, followed by a protein source and complex carbohydrates such as peanut butter on wheat bread, cheese and crackers, or a glass of milk and a sandwich, to maintain glucose level.

Continued

Table 37.3
Signs and Symptoms of Hypoglycemia and Hyperglycemia—cont'd

Condition	*Signs and Symptoms*	*Immediate Actions to Take*
Critically low hypoglycemia	Delirium Violent behavior Seizures Obtunded (diminished arousal/awareness) Coma Death	Assess FSBS. Patients may vary dramatically in how low the glucose must go before they exhibit these serious central nervous system signs and symptoms: Some will exhibit them at 40 mg/dL, while others may not until the blood glucose is down to 20 mg/dL. Treat these patients symptomatically. Notify the laboratory to draw a serum glucose level stat and then reassess the FSBS within 30 minutes and prn. Assess vital signs and apply oxygen. Initiate an IV line if not already infusing. Notify the health-care provider. Initiate standing orders until contact is established with the health-care provider; this generally includes IV administration of dextrose 50%. If the patient is having a seizure, ensure a patent airway, protect from injury, and administer antiepileptic medication according to health-care provider's orders.
Hyperglycemia	Hot, dry, flushed skin Thirst Fatigue or weakness Sleepiness Sweet or acetone odor to breath	Assess FSBS. If glucose is above 200 mg/dL and there are no health-care provider's orders specifying whether or not to administer insulin at this level of elevation, notify the health-care provider. Administer rapid-acting insulin according to health-care provider's orders. Reassess FSBS in 1 hour and prn.
Critically high hyperglycemia	Vagueness Mental confusion Hypotension Coma Death	Assess FSBS. As with extreme hypoglycemia, blood glucose may vary greatly from patient to patient: One may not exhibit these signs and symptoms even when glucose is 700 mg/dL or higher, while another may be already hypotensive or comatose at 500 mg/dL. Treat symptomatically as well as administering insulin to lower glucose. Notify the laboratory to draw a stat serum glucose. Reassess FSBS in 1 hour and prn. Assess vital signs and apply oxygen. Notify the health-care provider stat. Initiate an IV line if not already infusing. Administer rapid-acting insulin according to physician's orders.

Insulin should be kept refrigerated. However, before withdrawing it, gently roll the vial between both hands for approximately 1 minute to resuspend and warm the medication. Avoid shaking or vigorously agitating the insulin. When mixing insulins in the same syringe, the *clear* rapid-acting insulin must be withdrawn into the syringe first, followed by the *cloudy* intermediate-acting insulin. Just remember "clear before cloudy." Skill 37.4 (page 849) provides more information on combining and administering insulin subcutaneously.

The preferred injection site for insulin is the abdomen because it provides faster and more consistent absorption, but the back of the upper arms, the thighs, and the buttocks also may be used. ***Safety: Injection sites should be rotated to establish consistent blood insulin levels and reduce the risk of tissue damage, which will affect absorption.*** If a patient is able to self-administer insulin, teach the patient to use a clock method on the abdomen; giving the insulin at the position of 12 o'clock, then 1 o'clock, then 2 o'clock, and so forth.

Patients who require repeated insulin injections may develop *lipoatrophy,* the breakdown of subcutaneous fat at the site of repeated insulin injections, or *lipohypertrophy,* the buildup of subcutaneous fat at the site of repeated insulin injections. To prevent these complications, rotate injection sites around the abdomen, keeping them typically a fingerbreadth, or 1 inch, apart. ***Safety: Do not massage after injecting insulin because this may cause erratic absorption of the drug.***

Patient Teaching Connection

Insulin Self-Administration

It is important to help patients to be as independent as possible, including being adequately skilled to administer their own insulin. Part of your responsibility as a nurse will be to provide appropriate levels of patient education regarding this task. It helps to keep patient teaching as simple and straightforward as possible. The following steps provide simple but thorough instruction regarding self-administration of insulin.

- Wash your hands. (There is no need for the patient to wear gloves to self-administer.)
- Rotate injection sites with each dose to prevent tissue damage and increase absorption.
- Before drawing up the insulin suspension, gently roll and invert the bottle. Do not shake, because this can cause bubbles or foam to develop.
- Clean the rubber stopper of the vial with alcohol.
- Remove the needle cap without contaminating the needle.
- Inject a volume of air into the bottle equal to the volume of insulin you are going to remove.
- Then pull back on the plunger slowly until the syringe contains the desired number of units.
- Remove the needle from the bottle, maintaining sterility of the needle.
- Pinch the skin by squeezing a couple of inches of skin between your thumb and two fingers, pulling the skin and fat away from the underlying muscle.
- Cleanse the site with alcohol and allow to dry.
- With the needle bevel pointing upward, hold the syringe like a pencil in a vertical position, with the "eraser" end pointing toward the ceiling.
- Use a dartlike wrist action to make a swift puncture.
- Insert the needle at a 45-degree to 90-degree angle to the skinfold, depending on the length of the needle and the thickness of the subcutaneous tissue layer.
- Push the plunger to inject the insulin.
- Release your grip on the skinfold.
- Remove the needle from the skin and activate the safety mechanism immediately. Do not recap used needles.
- Do not massage the site or cover the skin with a gauze pad.
- Dispose of the needle and syringe in a puncture-proof container.

Basal and Bolus Insulin. Insulin can be administered with injections one or more times per day, or by pump, which delivers a small amount of short-acting insulin hourly throughout the day. This keeps the blood sugar levels within normal range between meals and overnight. Then when the diabetic using an insulin pump needs additional insulin, such as at mealtime, a bolus of short-acting insulin is administered via the pump to mimic the body's production of insulin. When a person eats, the body produces extra insulin to utilize the carbohydrates ingested. The bolus amounts can be programmed into the pump. The term *bolus* refers to an amount of medication given all at once. The term *basal* refers to the minimum requirements when the body is at rest and no additional demands are being made.

A relatively new approach to injecting insulin is called the basal/bolus system, or MDI (multiple daily injection) system. This system works somewhat like an insulin pump, but the insulin is injected rather than delivered by a pump. The basal/bolus system allows some diabetics to have more flexibility in their mealtimes and lifestyle. The person injects the prescribed amount of Lantus or Levemir long-acting insulin once or twice per day. Then, based on checking FSBS and the timing of meals, the person injects rapid-acting insulin such as Humalog or Novolog to keep their blood sugar stable after meals.

Diabetics with active lifestyles who find it difficult to eat meals at the same time every day may find the basal/bolus system preferable to injecting insulin and having to eat at a certain time or suffer a hypoglycemic reaction. However, this system requires multiple finger sticks (4 to 10 times per day) plus the injection of Lantus or Levemir, with additional rapid-acting insulin injections throughout the day (four to five injections each day). The use of an insulin pen may make this system easier to manage.

Research indicates better blood sugar control using this system because it more closely resembles the way the body delivers insulin to the bloodstream. It also makes the diabetic's lifestyle more flexible.

KNOWLEDGE CONNECTION

Explain the technique for preparing and administering a subcut injection of insulin. Which insulin cannot be mixed with any other type? If you must mix insulins, which type should you draw first, rapid acting or intermediate acting?

HEPARIN. Heparin is an anticoagulant drug that is administered to reduce and prevent formation of blood clots, which can cause cerebrovascular accidents and heart attacks, or myocardial infarctions. ***Safety: Heparin comes in various strengths, such as 1,000 units/mL, 5,000 units/mL, 10,000 units/mL, and 20,000 units/mL.*** Heparin can be life-threatening if an incorrect dosage is administered. ***Safety: It is paramount that you always have a second nurse verify the strength of heparin and the dosage you have drawn into the syringe.*** You should always monitor the laboratory results of the partial thromboplastin time, activated partial thromboplastin time, prothrombin time, and international normalized ratio prior to administration. Heparin can be administered subcutaneously or intravenously, delivered by direct IV injection or a continuous IV drip. ***Safety: Heparin should never be given IM. A continuous IV drip will require constant monitoring of the infusion rate.***

The abdomen is the preferred site for a subcut injection. ***Safety: Administer heparin slowly into the subcutaneous tissue and leave the needle in place for about 10 seconds before withdrawing it.*** Do not administer anywhere that has a scar or bruise. Do not rub or ice the site after injection as this can cause hemorrhage or bruising.

KNOWLEDGE CONNECTION

What needle gauges and lengths could you use for administering subcut injections? Which site is recommended for administration of subcut insulin? Why? What special instructions should you teach the patient learning to self-administer insulin? Explain the technique for administering a subcut injection of heparin. How many nurses should verify an insulin or heparin dose after drawing it into the syringe?

Laboratory and Diagnostic Connection

Prothrombin Time and Activated Partial Thromboplastin Time

The international normalized ratio (INR) and prothrombin time (PT) are used to assess the patient's system of blood clot formation. This test is also known as PT/INR. When a patient is taking an anticoagulant such as warfarin, rivaroxaban, or dabigatran, his or her blood is tested to be sure it is not becoming too anticoagulated. The PT time is measured in seconds, and the goal is for it to be 1 ½ to 2 ½ times the normal clotting time, which is 10 to 13 seconds. The INR is determined by dividing the patient's protime result by the normal patient average. The goal for INR is to have the patient's level between two to three.

The PT and the activated partial thromboplastin time (APTT) both assess the patient's own system of blood clot formation, evaluating clotting factors I, II, V, VIII, IX, X, XI, and XII. Recall that factor I is fibrinogen, and factor II is prothrombin. The only difference between these two tests is the activators that have been added to the reagent used to determine the PT. This results in a shorter clotting time using a more narrow normal range.

These tests are a measurement of the length of time that the body takes to complete the clotting process. Thus, a longer time result would indicate a slower clotting process, while a shorter time result would mean the blood is completing its intrinsic clotting process faster than it should, contributing to the formation of clots, which are a source of problems for the patient. Heparin interferes with the intrinsic clotting process by inactivating prothrombin for several hours after administration of drug. This prolongs the clotting process.

The goal of heparin therapy is to lengthen both the PT and APTT to 1 ½ to 2 ½ times the normal range. The normal ranges and the therapeutic ranges desired for patients on anticoagulant therapy with heparin are as follows:

- PT
  - Normal range: 60 to 70 seconds
  - Therapeutic range: 90 to 175 seconds
- APTT
  - Normal range: 30 to 40 seconds
  - Therapeutic range: 45 to 100 seconds

Intramuscular Injections

An IM injection is an injection directly into the largest portion of a muscle, called the *body* of the muscle. It is used for certain types of medications, particularly those that are rapid and long lasting, such as vaccines, and medication solutions that are irritating to the subcutaneous tissue.

Depending on the chemical properties of the drug, the medication may be absorbed either somewhat quickly or more gradually. Drugs in aqueous solution are rapidly absorbed. Drugs in oil or in other repository vehicles deliver a slow, constant absorption.

IM injections are administered in the larger muscles of the leg and hip, and smaller volume injections are administered in the deltoid of the upper arm. The maximum volume to inject intramuscularly is based on the site and the patient's muscle development:

- 2 to 3 mL for injecting a *large* ventrogluteal site (gluteus medius and gluteus minimus muscles) or a very large vastus lateralis muscle of the leg in an adult
- 1 to 2 mL for a ventrogluteal (gluteus minimus and medius muscles), vastus lateralis, or rectus femoris site in trim, average-size adults; older children with adequate muscle development; older adults; and thin patients
- 0.5 to 1 mL for small muscles in infants and small children
- 0.5 to 1 mL for the deltoid muscle in small children and up, through older adults

For average adults, the needle should be 1 to 1 ½ inches (2.5 to 3 cm) in length, with a gauge size between 20 and 22 G (1.1 to 0.7 mm). If a medication is thin, use the smallest size needle that can be used for the injection, but if the medication is thick and viscous, you may have to use a larger 20-G (1.1-mm) needle. On occasion a medication is so thick and viscous that even an 18-G (1.2-mm) needle may be required, such as with gamma globulin.

Administer IM injections at a 90-degree angle into the body of the target muscle. As with all injection techniques, the insertion of the needle should be swift, quickly piercing

• WORD • BUILDING •

anticoagulated: anti – against + coagulated – congealed

ventrogluteal: ventro – anterior + gluteal – related to the gluteus muscles

the skin and muscle in one smooth motion. ***Note: Avoid inserting the needle only a short distance and then having to push the needle farther in to reach the proper depth, which results in additional discomfort for the patient.***

The IM route is generally used for irritating or caustic drugs and allows for administration of larger volumes of medication. Skill 37.5 (page 850) provides more information on administering an IM injection.

Some nurses prefer to use an **air-lock** for the purpose of reducing irritation of the tissue along the path the needle made through the skin, subcutaneous layer, and muscle. The air-lock technique is quite simple. After drawing up the exact volume of medication, continue to aspirate 0.1 to 0.2 mL of air into the syringe. When inverting the syringe to make the skin puncture and instill the medication, be certain to position the syringe so that it is vertical, allowing the air to rise above the medication in the syringe, toward the plunger. This is necessary so that the air is not injected until after the medication, when it can help to lock the medication within the muscle (Fig. 37.23). The air clears any medication that remains in the needle, making it less irritating to the subcutaneous tissue during needle withdrawal. Medications such as interferon, iron dextran, and hydroxyzine hydrochloride (Vistaril) and vaccines such as diphtheria, tetanus toxoid, and pertussis may be administered using the air-lock technique.

After withdrawing the needle from the tissue after an IM injection, hold pressure on the site with a 2×2-inch gauze pad or cotton ball and massage the site to increase absorption. The exception is any IM injection administered using the Z-track method; do not massage a Z-track. ***Safety: Activate the needle safety device immediately after removal of the needle from the skin.***

Evidence-Based Practice

Deciding Whether or Not to Aspirate When Administering Intramuscular Immunizations and Vaccine Injections

Clinical Question

Do you aspirate for IM immunization and vaccine injections?

Evidence

It is common practice to aspirate for IM immunizations and vaccine injections prior to giving the injection. However, the CDC and Advisory Committee on Immunization Practices (ACIP) does not recommend aspirating for immunizations and vaccine injections. When giving an IM immunization or vaccine, the evidence shows the nurse is less likely to hit a neural or vascular structure. Research has expanded to include not aspirating any IM injections except dorsogluteal and certain medications.

Implications for Nursing Practice

The CDC and ACIP highlight the importance of not aspirating for IM and SC immunizations and vaccines in the healthcare setting. Also, evidence shows not to aspirate any IM injection except dorsal gluteal and certain medications.

Sources: Kroger AT, Sumaya CV, Pickering LK, et al. General Recommendations on Immunization: Recommendations of the Advisory Committee on Immunization Practices (ACIP). Cdc.gov. https://francais.cdc.gov/mmwr/preview/mmwrhtml/rr6002a1.htm?s_cid=rr6002a1_w. Accessed 9/12/18; National Center for Immunization and Respiratory Diseases. Vaccine Administration. Cdc. Gov. https://www.cdc.gov/vaccines/pubs/pinkbook/vac-admin.html. Accessed 9/12/18; Sisson, H. Aspirating During the Intramuscular Injection Procedure: A Systematic Literature Review. *Journal of Clinical Nursing*. 2015; *24*(17-18): 2368-2375. http://onlinelibrary.wiley.com/doi/10.1111/jocn.12824 /abstract

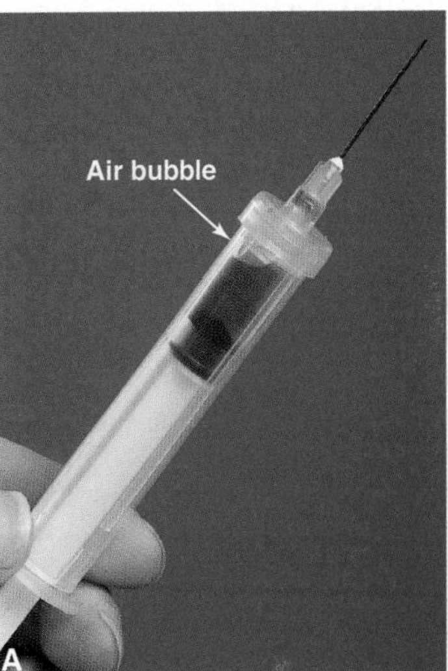

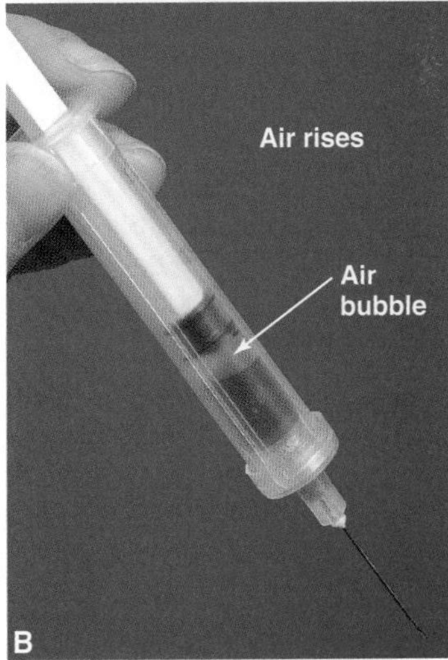

FIGURE 37.23 (a) Hold the syringe vertical so that air is not trapped on the side of the syringe: Air should rise to the top of the medication solution; (b) Once you invert the syringe to administer the injection, the air rises to the top, once more enabling it to enter the needle and patient after the medication has gone in (from Wilkinson JM, Treas LS. *Fundamentals of Nursing: Theory, Concepts & Applications.* Vol. 2. 2nd ed. Philadelphia, PA: FA Davis; 2016).

Preventing Complications of IM Injections

Complications from IM injection can arise from the needle puncture solution, incorrect technique, or the drug solution itself. To prevent infection of the injection site:

- Wash hands before you begin to prepare injections.
- Wash hands again after you enter the patient's room.
- Clean the injection site with alcohol or a facility-approved antiseptic. Use adequate friction and clean the site beginning in the center and wiping concentric circles outward until a 2-inch area is clean.
- Cover the puncture wound with a new bandage to allow the skin time to seal over.

Repetitive injections can cause bleeding, bruising, soreness, and muscle spasm. To prevent these complications:

- Make certain you review the patient's medical record and know whether the patient has any medical problems that might increase the risk of bleeding, such as hemophilia, anticoagulant therapy, or disease of the blood cell–producing tissue or if the patient takes supplements or herbs that increase bleeding. Box 37.2 provides a list of common vitamins and herbs that increase bleeding.
- Rotate sites faithfully and document them to provide the next nurse with accurate data.
- Use the smallest gauge needle appropriate for the medication, site, and patient size.
- Make the needle puncture swiftly and at the correct angle.

Box 37.2

Common Supplements That May Increase Bleeding

Even though supplements are easily obtained because they are considered over-the-counter drugs and do not require a prescription, this does not mean that they cannot cause dangerous problems. It is important to make the health-care provider aware of all herbs, supplements, and even nonprescription drugs such as antacids, aspirin, or acetaminophen products that a patient takes.* Most surgeons will stop the following herbal supplements prior to a scheduled surgery because of their effect of increasing bleeding:

- Cayenne
- Feverfew
- Ginkgo biloba
- Ginseng
- Omega-3 fatty acids
- St. John's wort
- Vitamins A and C
- Antiplatelet drugs

*Even though aspirin and acetaminophen are not herbal supplements, they are over-the-counter medications that most individuals feel free to take frequently, even on a daily basis. Both are known to have antiplatelet properties that increase bleeding and should be included on the patient's list of medications, herbs, and supplements if taken regularly.

- Apply a cotton ball, gauze pad, or alcohol wipe to the site immediately upon removal of the needle unless contraindicated, as for insulin and heparin.
- Apply a cool pack if bruising appears.

Z-TRACK. The **Z-track** method of IM injection prevents irritating and dark-colored medications, such as iron dextran, from leaking out of the injection site into sensitive tissues or subcutaneous tissues that may stain. It also helps to reduce the inflammation and discomfort that can be caused by the medication irritating the subcutaneous tissue. The technique achieves this by closing the needle track in the tissue, preventing seepage of medication. Medications such as haloperidol (Haldol) and hydroxyzine (Vistaril) typically are administered by this method.

Place the lateral aspect of your nondominant hand against the patient's skin next to the intended insertion site, and pull or displace the skin and subcutaneous layer between 1 and 2 inches (2.5 and 5 cm) to one side, holding the tissue back while you use your dominant hand to swiftly pierce the skin and tissue with the needle to enter the muscle (Fig. 37.24). Without moving your nondominant hand from its tissue-securing position, close the index finger and thumb of that hand against the syringe to stabilize the needle. Inject the medication over 10 to 15 seconds per milliliter of solution to reduce discomfort. Then wait 5 to 10 seconds to allow some of the medication to disperse away from the needle tip and track. Swiftly withdraw the needle as you immediately release the skin and tissue being held back by your nondominant hand. This effectively closes off the needle track pathway and seals the medication within the body of the muscle. You may place an alcohol pad or cotton ball on the injection site and cover it with a bandage, but do not massage it, which can force medication into the SC tissue. ***Safety: Activate the needle safety device immediately after removal of the needle from the***

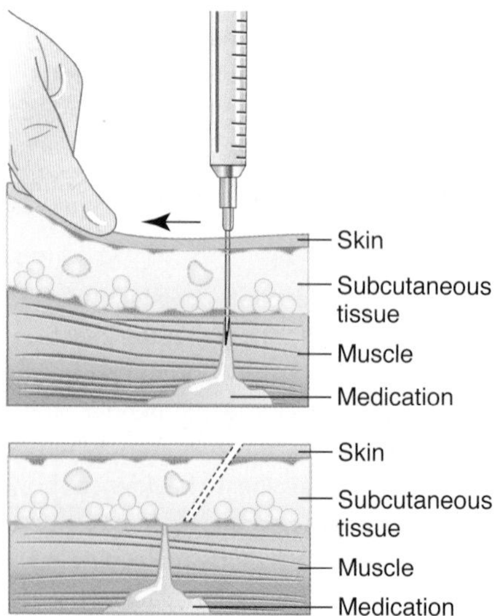

FIGURE 37.24 Z-track injection provides for closure of the needle track when you release the skin and tissue (from Wilkinson JM, Treas LS. *Fundamentals of Nursing: Theory, Concepts & Applications.* Vol. 2. 3rd ed. Philadelphia, PA: FA Davis; 2016).

skin. You must be vigilant regarding performance of this safety mechanism while you are learning and perfecting your technique so that it eventually becomes an automatic action that you do without having to consciously think about it. Skill 37.6 (page 851) provides more information on administering a Z-track injection.

Injection Site Identification

Correctly selecting the sites for IM injections requires you to know specific anatomical landmarks. Without this knowledge, you are at risk for causing discomfort, injury, and possibly permanent damage to the patient. Make it a priority to learn the correct anatomical landmarks and how to locate them for each IM injection site.

VENTROGLUTEAL. The safest and most comfortable IM injection site for all patients older than 7 months is the ventrogluteal site. In the past, this was not the site of choice. In fact, nurses who trained prior to the 1990s were not taught about this site. Most were taught to use the dorsogluteal site, which is no longer recommended because of the risk of damaging the extremely large sciatic nerve that extends across the buttock and travels down the posterior aspect of the leg (Fig. 37.25).

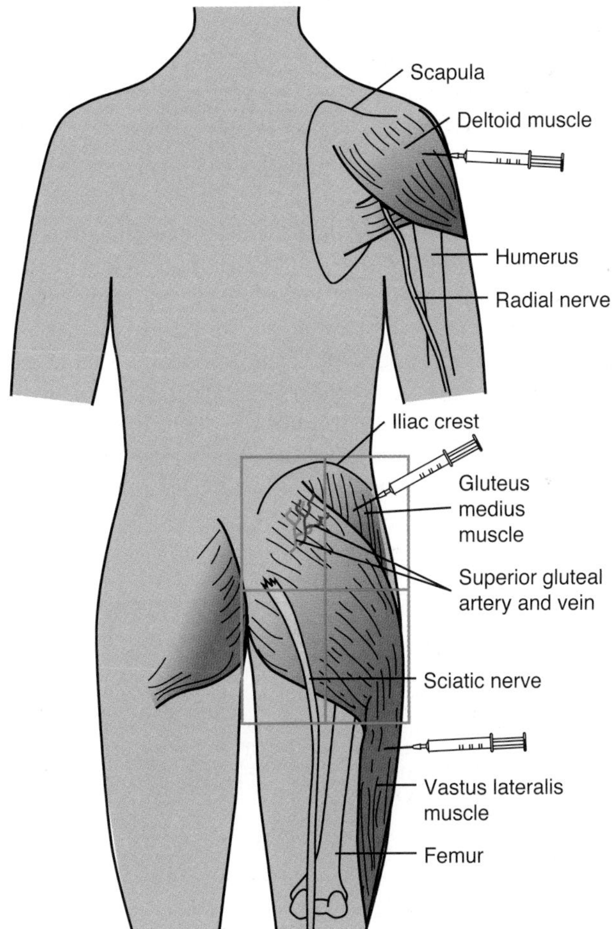

FIGURE 37.25 The injection site must be accurately determined to avoid injury to the sciatic nerve.

This is your chance to help make a positive change in nursing by learning to use the ventrogluteal site as the site of choice. The dorsogluteal site should *only* be used if all other sites are not accessible.

The ventrogluteal site is the safest for IM injections because it is not close to any major blood vessels or nerves and there is little subcutaneous tissue overlying the gluteus medius and gluteus minimus muscles. To locate this site, have the patient assume a side-lying position with the foot on the top leg inverted to relax the hip muscles. Use your right hand for an injection on the patient's left hip and your left hand for an injection on the patient's right hip. Place

Real-World Connection

Ventrogluteal Injection Site

The nursing instructor was taking weekly injections of vitamin B12 prescribed by her health-care provider. Rather than give them herself, she thought it would provide the practical nursing students opportunity to get some injection practice. So she announced to the clinical students in preconference that for the next few months a different student each week would get the opportunity to administer an IM injection to the instructor. Although somewhat good-naturedly reluctant to inject their instructor yet wanting to take advantage of the opportunity, each week students would draw straws to determine which student received the honor of "sticking" the instructor. The students were allowed to select the injection site, and the second week, a student selected the ventrogluteal site, a site in which the instructor had never received an injection. The instructor was slightly apprehensive regarding use of the site but agreed to allow the student to follow through with her selection. The student was nervous and shaking, but administered the IM injection into the ventrogluteal site using perfect technique. Not only was the instructor impressed with the total lack of discomfort, but she had not been able to identify when she was actually stuck because of the swiftness and perfect angle of insertion applied by the student. Through the following weeks, some students selected the vastus lateralis muscle and one other selected the dorsogluteal site, but the majority of the students followed suit and selected the ventrogluteal site for their turn at sticking the instructor.

Not only did the students receive the opportunity to administer an injection, but the instructor, who had never wanted to receive a ventrogluteal injection, was so impressed with the fact that she did not experience even minor discomfort from any of the injections at the site that she was determined to use the ventrogluteal site as her primary injection site from that day forward, as did some of the students. This goes to show that using good technique when administering ventrogluteal injections will lead to minimal or no discomfort to the patient.

the palm of your hand on the patient's greater trochanter with the index finger on the anterior superior iliac spine and your middle finger pointing toward the iliac crest. The "V" formed by your index and middle fingers marks your injection site. You should insert the needle in the center of the "V," slightly closer to the base of your two fingers (Fig. 37.26).

DELTOID. The most common site for injection of small volumes such as 0.5 or 1 mL is the deltoid muscle on the superior aspect of the upper arm. It is a smaller muscle than those of the other sites and is in close proximity to the brachial artery and radial nerve. Use the deltoid only for children with adequate muscle mass and adults. It is not suitable for newborns and small infants because of the lack of muscle development.

To select your site, locate the acromion process, place your little finger on the process and measure three fingerbreadths down. Inject into the fullest part of the deltoid (Fig. 37.27). Avoid going too low and posterior, where the radial nerve and artery are located. This site is appropriate for children ages 1 year to older adults. It is the most convenient to access of all the IM injection sites, and the patient may be sitting up or lying in bed for the injection.

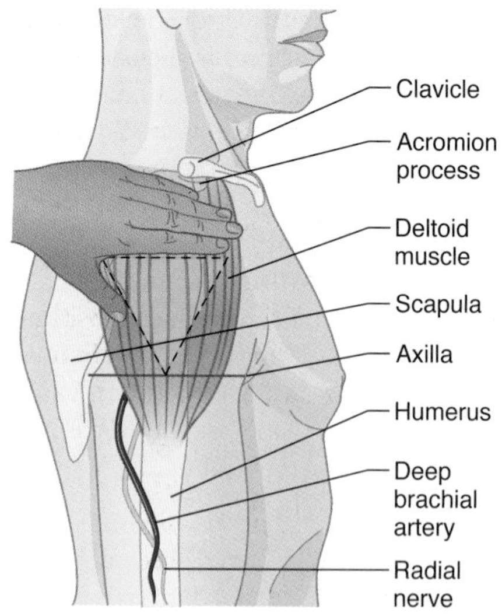

FIGURE 37.27 Locating the deltoid site (from Wilkinson JM, Treas LS. *Fundamentals of Nursing: Theory, Concepts & Applications.* Vol. 2. 3rd ed. Philadelphia, PA: FA Davis; 2016).

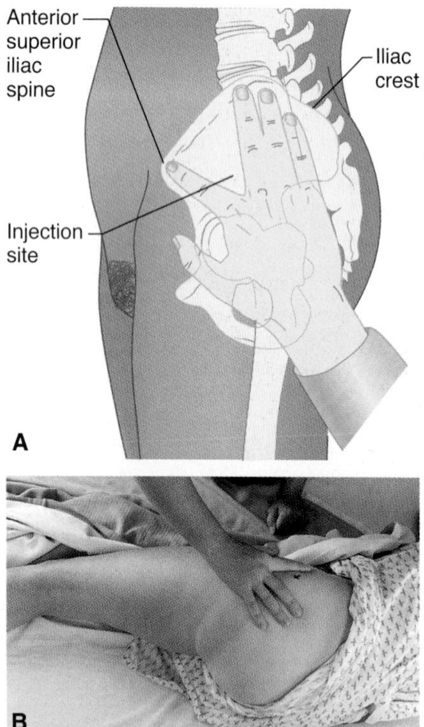

FIGURE 37.26 (a) Diagram marking the number one choice for IM injections: the ventrogluteal injection site; (b) Position the patient in a lateral side-lying position and place the palm of your hand over the greater trochanter. Point the index finger at the anterior superior iliac spine and the middle finger toward the iliac crest. The injection site is in the middle of the "V" form made by your fingers. If you are using the patient's left hip, you will use your right hand to make the "V." If you are using the patient's right hip, you will use your left hand to make the "V" (from Wilkinson JM, Treas LS. *Fundamentals of Nursing: Theory, Concepts & Applications.* Vol. 2. 3rd ed. Philadelphia, PA: FA Davis; 2016).

VASTUS LATERALIS. The vastus lateralis on the lateral aspect of the thigh is the second-choice site for injections greater than 1 mL if the ventrogluteal site cannot be accessed. It is the number one choice for newborns and infants who have not developed any of the gluteal muscles or the deltoid muscle. Absorption from this site is better than from other IM sites.

To locate this site, have the patient assume either a supine position or a sitting position on the side of a bed or in a chair. Divide the thigh into thirds: Place one of your hands across the thigh next to the femoral crease (or next to the head of the trochanter) and your other hand across the distal aspect of the upper leg, just above the patella. The midpoint between your hands is the middle third of the thigh. Inject into the fullest portion of the muscle, just a little lateral to the longitudinal midline of the upper leg (Fig. 37.28).

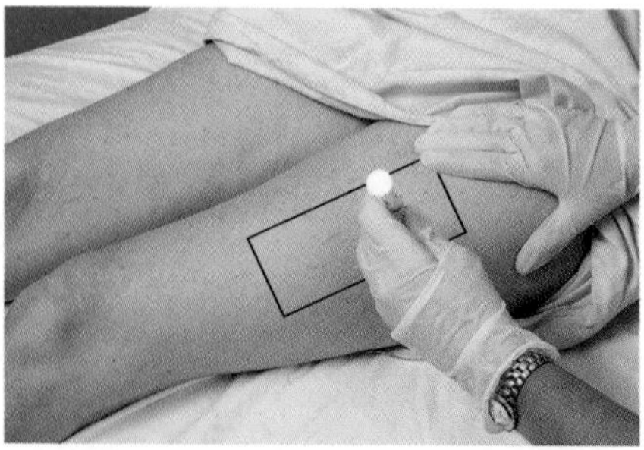

FIGURE 37.28 Administering an IM injection in the vastus lateralis muscle (from Wilkinson JM, Treas LS. *Fundamentals of Nursing: Theory, Concepts & Applications.* Vol. 2. 3rd ed. Philadelphia, PA: FA Davis; 2016).

RECTUS FEMORIS. The rectus femoris is located in the longitudinal midline of the anterior thigh, but it is the last choice of sites to use and is for use in adults only, whenever rapid absorption is desired and other sites are inaccessible. ***Safety: The rectus femoris site is not used in infants and children.*** Many patients who self-administer injections at home use this site for its convenience. The disadvantage is that it is sometimes painful. It is near the vastus lateralis site but lies more to the midline of the thigh. If you use this site, position the patient in the supine position and have the patient relax the thigh muscle as much as possible.

DORSOGLUTEAL. The dorsogluteal site, as was mentioned earlier, is no longer the site of choice for IM injections—and it is never used in infants and small children. In adults, it should be used only as a last resort because of its proximity to the sciatic nerve, which can suffer injury and sometimes permanent damage when stuck by an errant needle. To identify the landmarks for this site, have the patient assume a prone position with the toes turned inward to relax the hip muscles. Palpate the posterior superior iliac spine and the greater trochanter. Draw an imaginary line between the two landmarks. From the midpoint of this line, move approximately 1 inch above the line (toward the patient's head). This should place your finger in the upper, outer aspect of the buttock, where you are an adequate distance from the sciatic nerve (Fig. 37.29). Aspirate to ensure that the needle is not in a vessel. If blood returns into the syringe with aspiration, withdraw the needle, dispose of the medication-filled syringe in a sharps container, and draw up another dose of medication using a new syringe and needle. This site is the last choice in adults when better sites are inaccessible, and it is never a choice in infants and small children. For tips to decrease discomfort of injections, see Box 37.3.

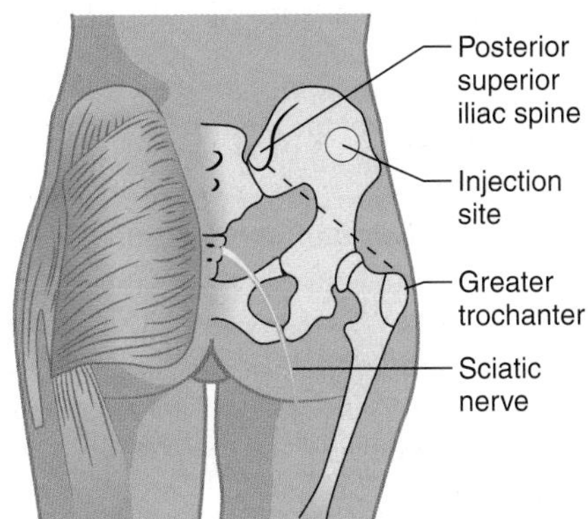

FIGURE 37.29 Locating the landmarks for the dorsogluteal site (from Wilkinson JM, Treas LS. *Fundamentals of Nursing: Theory, Concepts & Applications.* Vol. 2. 2nd ed. Philadelphia, PA: FA Davis; 2011).

Settings Connection: Medical Office

Injection Variations in Newborns, Infants, and Toddlers

- Sites: In newborns, infants, and toddlers, the vastus lateralis muscle on the anterolateral aspect of the upper leg is the muscle of choice for IM injections. The gluteus muscles of the hip do not develop until a child begins to walk, and even then they should not be used because of the proximity of the sciatic nerve in the tiny buttock. For school-age children through older adults, the thicker gluteal muscle at the ventrogluteal site, where there are fewer nerves and blood vessels, is rapidly becoming the number one choice of sites; the vastus lateralis or the deltoid muscle of the arm also may be used. The rectus femoris on the anterior thigh is no longer recommended in children of any age because of the increased discomfort of the site. However, the site is safe for IM injection in teenagers and adults if for some reason all other sites are deemed unsatisfactory.
- Needle size: For infants, use a 5/8-inch needle length in a 23- to 27-G needle. For children, older adults, or thin adults, use a ⅝- to 1-inch needle length in a 22- to 25-G needle. Always select the length of the needle based on the size of the muscle to be injected as well as the size of the patient.

KNOWLEDGE CONNECTION

Describe the technique for IM injection. Identify various needle lengths and gauges to use for IM injection. What is the maximum volume you may inject in the various muscles of each age group? How should a patient be positioned when administering an IM injection? Describe the Z-track method for injection.

Box 37.3
Tips to Decrease Injection Discomfort

Sometimes needles and the medications themselves can be the cause of discomfort during an injection. Your knowledge and injection technique will also impact the level of discomfort accompanying your injections. However, there are innumerable things you can do to improve your injection technique and make injections nearly "undetectable." There is nothing quite as rewarding after administering an injection as hearing the patient say, "You're already done? I didn't even feel the stick." This is the challenge you should set out to achieve. Try all of the following tips, and both you and your patients will be rewarded.

- Always use the smallest needle appropriate for the medication, site, and patient size.

Continued

Box 37.3 Tips to Decrease Injection Discomfort—cont'd

- Be accurate in identifying landmarks for all injection sites: Just 1 inch off the correct site can cause unnecessary discomfort and injury to tissues and nerves.
- Know your medications: Identify those that are caustic and irritating to tissues. Make certain the correct route is ordered for the specific medication.
- Avoid administering a greater volume of medication than should be given at the site or that is too great for the size of the muscle.
- Avoid preparing the injection within the patient's view; this increases anxiety and discomfort.
- After inserting the needle through a vial stopper to draw up medication, change the needle for a new one that has not been dulled by the stopper and does not have medication on it.
- Explain what you are about to do to the patient to gain his or her compliance in holding still and relaxing the muscle.
- If the patient is a child, explain according to child's level of growth and development. Do not lie and say it will not hurt. Be truthful, but offer hope by saying, "Try to hold real still and I'll try to be as easy as I can. It will sting for a minute and then it will be all over." Or you can say, "Hold onto your dolly real tight. I'll count to three, and then you and I will both say OUCH together. It will be over quickly."
- Distract the patient by engaging him or her in conversation.
- Assist the patient to assume the best position to relax the muscles of the site you select.
- Pull the skin over the site taut.
- Use the Z-track technique for all IM injections.
- Puncture the skin swiftly and to the proper depth to lessen the discomfort. Avoid shallow sticks where you then have to "push" the needle the rest of the way in.
- Stabilize the syringe and needle while injecting medication; do not allow any movement of the needle while it is within the tissues.
- Inject the medication slowly, no faster than 10 to 15 seconds per milliliter of medication.

Skill 37.1 Reconstituting and Withdrawing Medication From a Vial

Assessment Steps

1. Review the health-care provider's orders and the medication administration record (MAR) for the correct patient, medication, dose, route, indication, and time. ***This will ensure accuracy and currency of orders and prevent medication errors.***
2. Review a drug book for actions, required assessments, correct dosage, route, side effects, and expected results; review the drug insert for proper diluent, volume, and instructions for reconstitution. ***This will ensure proper reconstitution steps are followed and will maintain stability of the drug.***
3. Assess the patient's allergies ***to reduce risk of an allergic reaction.***
4. Select the correct medication vial, including medication name, dosage strength, dosage volume, dosage route and its appropriateness, and expiration, ***to reduce the risk of medication error.***
5. Assess the vial contents for cloudiness, color changes, or particulate matter ***to ensure quality of the medication.***

Planning Steps

1. Clean the workstation ***to reduce microorganisms*** before preparation of medication.
2. Gather needed supplies: appropriate syringes, needles, diluent, and alcohol pads. ***Being prepared saves time and energy. It also works to increase the patient's perception of your competence.***

Implementation Steps

1. Perform the Initial Implementation Steps located on the inside back cover.
2. Wash hands ***to prevent cross-contamination.***
3. *Safety: Perform at least three medication label comparisons to the MAR to reduce the risk of medication error.*
4. Remove the cap from the medication vial and the diluent vial for access to the contents. Clean the rubber stoppers of both vials with separate alcohol swabs, rubbing in a circular motion, ***to reduce microorganisms. Discard the swabs.***
5. Attach the needle or vial access device (VAD) to the syringe using aseptic technique ***to reduce the risk of contamination of the medication.***
6. Pull back on the syringe plunger to draw up an amount of air equal to the amount of diluent you plan to withdraw from the vial. ***This helps to maintain equal pressure inside the vial to ease removal of the medication.*** Handle only the flange and the most distal 1 inch of the plunger ***to avoid contaminating the portion of the plunger that will be reinserted into the sterile barrel with the medication.***
7. Inject air through the rubber stopper into the vial, keeping the tip of the needle or VAD above the fluid line ***to prevent injecting air into the solution.***
8. Draw up the specified volume of the specified diluent to ensure proper dissolving and concentration. *Safety: Note whether or not the diluent contains a bacteriostatic preservative, and correlate this with appropriateness for the patient's age.*
9. If using a multiple-dose vial, write the date, time, and your initials on the label ***so that staff will know when the vial was first opened.*** If using a single-dose vial, dispose of it once you are through with it.
10. Wipe the stopper of the medication vial again with an alcohol wipe ***to remove any contamination before puncturing the stopper again.***
11. Inject the diluent into the medication vial and mix until dissolved ***to prevent particulate matter.***
12. Calculate the volume to withdraw from the vial to equal the health-care provider's medication order, ***to reduce the risk of medication error.***

Skill 37.1 (continued)

13. Pull back on the syringe plunger to draw up an amount of air equal to the amount of medication you plan to withdraw from the vial. ***This helps to maintain equal pressure inside the vial to ease removal of the medication.*** Handle only the flange and the most distal 1 inch of the plunger ***to avoid contaminating the portion of the plunger that will be reinserted into the sterile barrel with the medication.***
14. On a flat surface, hold the vial in one hand. Inject air through the rubber stopper into the vial, keeping the tip of needle above the fluid line ***to prevent injecting air into the solution.*** *Safety: Avoid using needleless piercing devices to access regular rubber stoppers because they core the stopper. Obtain and attach a needleless vial adapter so that you can use a needleless piercing device, or use a safety needle to withdraw the medication from the vial.*
15. Invert the vial and move the needle tip below the fluid level ***to avoid drawing up air.*** Withdraw the ordered amount of medication. Keep the syringe at eye level ***to ensure accuracy.***
16. Check the syringe for air bubbles. If bubbles are present, tap the syringe to remove them.
17. Remove the needle or VAD from the vial, holding the barrel of the syringe securely and maintaining sterility of the needle. ***Activate the safety device to prevent needle stick.***
18. Change the needle ***to prevent injecting the patient with a dull needle.*** Before removing the needle from the tip of the syringe, pull back slightly on the plunger ***to move the medication away from the tip of the syringe and reduce the risk of contamination or loss of medication.*** Remove the needle and aseptically apply the new needle. Push the plunger gently ***to dispel air from the syringe.***
19. Drop the contaminated needle into the sharps container ***to reduce risk of needle sticks.***
20. Dispose of the vial or return it to the storage area if medication remains in a multiple-dose vial.

Evaluation Step

1. Recheck your calculations and ***evaluate if what you have drawn up is correct.***

Skill 37.2 Withdrawing Medication From an Ampule

Assessment Steps

1. Review the health-care provider's orders and the medication administration record (MAR) for the correct patient, medication, dose, route, indication, and time. ***This will ensure accuracy and currency of orders and reduce the risk of medication error.***
2. Review a drug book and the drug insert for drug information ***for accuracy.***
3. Assess the patient's allergies ***to reduce the risk of an allergic reaction.***
4. Select the correct ampule, including medication name, dosage strength, dosage volume, dosage route and its appropriateness, and expiration, ***to reduce the risk of medication error.***
5. Assess the ampule contents for cloudiness, color changes, or particulate matter ***to ensure quality of the medication.***

Planning Steps

1. Clean the workstation ***to reduce microorganisms*** before preparation of medication.
2. Gather needed supplies: appropriate syringes, needles, alcohol pads, and either a gauze pad or a commercial ampule-breaking device. ***Being prepared saves time and energy.***

Implementation Steps

1. Perform the Initial Implementation Steps located on the inside back cover.
2. Wash hands ***to prevent cross-contamination.***
3. *Safety: Perform at least three medication label comparisons to the MAR to reduce the risk of medication error.*
4. Attach the filter needle to the syringe. ***This filters out shards of glass that may have fallen into the medication when breaking the ampule.***
5. If the medication is stuck at the top of the ampule, use your fingertip to gently flick the neck of the ampule. ***This helps to ensure that an adequate volume of medication is available for withdrawal from the ampule.***
6. Holding the ampule below and away from your face, wrap a sterile gauze pad around the ampule neck ***to protect your fingers*** and snap the top off toward you ***so that the ampule breaks away from you, helping any shards of glass to fly away from you.***
7. Attach the filter needle to the syringe. ***This filters out shards of glass that may have fallen into the medication when breaking the ampule.***
8. Holding the ampule with your nondominant hand, invert it or tilt it slightly. Insert the filter needle below the level of the liquid without contaminating the needle by touching it to the outside of the ampule; draw up the medication into the syringe. ***This reduces contamination of the medication with glass shards.***
9. Pull back on the plunger, moving medication away from the end of the syringe ***to reduce the risk of contamination or loss of medication.*** Remove the filter needle and replace it aseptically with the injection needle ***so that filtered glass within the needle will not be injected into the patient.***
10. Dispose of the ampule and filter needle in an appropriate container ***to prevent needle sticks.***
11. Label the syringe with the drug name, dose, date, patient name, and time ***to reduce chance of error.***

Evaluation Step

1. Evaluate that the drug, dosage, route, and appropriate needle have been prepared.

Skill 37.3 Administering an Intradermal Injection

Assessment Steps

1. Review the health-care provider's orders and the medication administration record (MAR) for the correct patient, medication, dose, route, indication, and time. ***This will ensure accuracy and currency of orders and help to prevent medication errors.***
2. Review a drug book and the drug insert for drug information ***to ensure accuracy.***
3. Assess the patient's allergies ***to reduce the risk of an allergic reaction.***
4. Assess the site to be used for injection, noting cuts, bruises, or other wounds that might contraindicate site usage. ***Avoid injecting sites previously injected on the same day.***

Planning Step

1. Gather needed supplies: 1-mL syringe, 24- to 28-G needles for drawing up an ID administration, alcohol wipes, dry cotton ball, black ink pen, and examination gloves. ***Being prepared saves time and footwork.***

Implementation Steps

Before Going to the Patient's Room

1. Wash hands ***to prevent cross-contamination.***
2. *Safety: Perform two medication label comparisons to the MAR for right patient, right drug, right dose, right route, right indication, and right time to reduce risk of medication error.* Also check the expiration date of the medication.
3. Withdraw the medication from the ampule or vial, ***maintaining sterility of appropriate pieces of equipment and medication.*** Dispel any air from the syringe.
4. Recap the needle before walking to the patient's room ***to maintain sterility of the needle.*** Use the one-handed method of recapping or use a commercial recapping device ***to prevent needle stick.***

After Entering the Patient's Room

5. Perform the Initial Implementation Steps located on the inside back cover.
6. *Safety: Perform a third medication label comparison to the MAR for right patient, right drug, right dose, right route, right indication, and right time to reduce risk of medication error.*
7. Explain the procedure to the patient ***to reduce anxiety and increase cooperation.***
8. Wash hands again ***to prevent cross-contamination*** and apply clean examination gloves ***to reduce risk of contact with body fluids.***
9. Select a site on the left or right inner forearm, if injecting P.P.D. You can use the left or right inner forearm, upper chest, or upper back for other ID injections.
10. Cleanse the area with an alcohol swab by wiping with a circular motion and moving outward from the injection site ***to reduce microorganisms.*** Allow the skin to dry.
11. Remove the needle cap with your nondominant hand by pulling it straight off to prevent contamination of the needle.
12. Spread the skin taut over the injection site ***to ease piercing of the skin with the needle.***
13. Hold the syringe with the needle at a 5- to 15-degree angle to the patient's skin on the left or right inner forearm, bevel side up. Insert the needle into the skin to a maximum depth of ⅛ inch (3 mm). Apply a very GENTLE lift at the needle tip to ensure that you can see the bevel through the dermis, ***which indicates you are not too deep.***
14. Slowly inject the medication while holding the GENTLE lift on the bevel, so that a 1/4- to 1/5-inch (6- to 10-mm) ***wheal,*** or discreet pale raised area of skin, forms at the tip of the needle. If a wheal does not begin to appear, withdraw the needle *very slightly* and continue to inject until a wheal forms. ***This ensures deposition of medication where it belongs, in the dermal layer.***
15. Remove the needle quickly at the same angle it was inserted and release the skin. ***This prevents the medication from leaking out.*** Activate the safety device ***to reduce the risk of needle stick.***
16. Blot any remaining blood from the injection site with a 2×2 gauze.
17. Do not massage the area after removing the needle. ***Doing so may cause the medication to spread and alter its absorption.***
18. Discard the needle and syringe in the sharps container ***to prevent needle stick.***
19. If injecting P.P.D., circle the site and write the date, time, and your initials by the circle.
20. Instruct the patient that the P.P.D. results must be read once for interpretation between 48 to 72 hours. ***This helps to gain patient compliance.***
21. Follow the Ending Implementation Steps located on the inside back cover.
22. Document the injection and site in the MAR and nurse's notes ***for continuity of care.***

Evaluation Step

1. Immediately following the injection, observe the injection site ***for bleeding, swelling, or any signs of adverse reactions to the medication.***
2. Monitor the patient for at least 15 minutes after the injection ***for signs of adverse reactions.***

Sample Documentation

11/01/22 0840 Administered 0.1 mL P.P.D. ID injection in left inner forearm. 8-mm bleb obtained. No reaction noted. Instructed that test must be read for interpretation at 48 and again at 72 hrs. for valid results. Verbally acknowledged understanding. ________

________ *Nurse's signature and credentials*

Skill 37.4 Combining and Administering Insulin Subcutaneously

Assessment Steps

1. Assess finger stick blood sugar (FSBS) or check the last blood sugar reading for the patient ***to ensure that the glucose level is not too low to safely administer insulin.***
2. Assess the patient for signs and symptoms of hypoglycemia and hyperglycemia.
3. Review the health-care provider's order and compare with the medication administration record (MAR) ***for accuracy and currency and to reduce the risk of medication error.***
4. Review the type of insulin to be injected in a drug text or resource to verify onset time, peak action time, and duration of insulin effect ***to reduce risk of failure to identify critical overlap times of multiple doses.***
5. Assess time and site of the last insulin dose ***so that you will know when to anticipate overlapping of multiple doses of insulin, which can cause sudden drops in blood glucose.***

Planning Steps

1. Determine the injection site. Rotate sites. Plan to use the abdomen for better absorption. Use the "clock" method of rotation of sites on the abdomen. Avoid using the same injection site as a previous injection on the same day ***to reduce discomfort and excessive trauma to tissues.***
2. Clean the work area ***to reduce microorganisms.***
3. Gather needed supplies: correct two types of insulin (check expiration dates), insulin syringe to match insulin strength (such as U-100 regular), alcohol wipes, and gloves. ***This saves time and footwork.***

Implementation Steps

Before Going to the Patient's Room

1. Wash hands ***to prevent cross-contamination.***
2. *Safety: Perform two label comparisons of each type of insulin to the MAR for right patient, right drug, right dose, right route, right indication, and right time to reduce risk of medication error.* Also check the expiration date of the insulin.
3. For NPH insulin, gently roll the vial between the palms of your hands ***to warm and mix the insulin.*** Do not shake.
4. Remove the needle cap and draw up air into the syringe equal to the total units of insulin to be drawn up from both vials ***to maintain equal pressure.***
5. Clean the vial stoppers with a separate alcohol swab for each one ***to reduce microorganisms.***
6. If regular insulin and NPH insulin are to be mixed, the ***clear*** regular insulin should be drawn up first, after injecting air into both vials. ***This sequence of drawing prevents regular (fast-acting) from being contaminated with NPH (intermediate-acting) insulin.***
7. Insert the needle into the stopper of the NPH vial and instill the number of units of air equal to the units of insulin to be removed. Then aseptically remove the needle from the stopper ***to prevent contamination of the needle.***
8. Insert the needle into the stopper of the regular insulin vial and instill the remaining units of air to equal the units of insulin you plan to withdraw ***to maintain equal pressure.*** Do not remove the needle from the insulin vial.
9. Invert the vial with the needle still in the stopper. Carefully draw up the exact number of units of regular insulin ordered. Do not remove the needle from the insulin vial. *Safety: Take the MAR and written FSBS results along with the insulin to another staff nurse. Ask the nurse to tell you what you have.* The nurse should check the name on the MAR, name and type of insulin, and number of units drawn into the syringe; compare and verify that it is the amount indicated on the MAR for the patient's current blood sugar; and check the expiration date on the vial. The nurse should then initial the MAR ***as the second witness of the insulin dose.*** Depending on facility policy, you may be required to obtain a third nurse to witness the dose.
10. Withdraw the needle from the vial, taking care ***to maintain sterility and to not bend the needle.***
11. Wipe the NPH insulin vial stopper again with an alcohol pad ***to remove microorganisms.***
12. Insert the needle into the NPH insulin vial and invert the vial carefully ***to avoid bending the needle.***
13. Withdraw slowly the ***exact*** number of units of NPH insulin. It must be exact, ***because you are unable to reinstill any of it back into the vial as it is now mixed with regular insulin.*** Do not remove the needle from the vial ***so that you can obtain verification of the correct dosage.***
14. Again, take it to the second nurse to compare and verify that you have what the MAR and blood sugar indicates you should administer. Have the nurse initial the MAR as the second witness. ***This reduces chances of error.***
15. Remove the needle from the vial aseptically.
16. Recap the needle using the one-handed scoop method or a commercial recapping device ***to prevent needle stick.***
17. Take the insulin to the patient's room.

After Entering the Patient's Room

18. Perform the Initial Implementation Steps located on the inside back cover.
19. *Safety: Perform a third medication label comparison to the MAR for right patient, right drug, right dose, right route, right indication, and right time to reduce risk of medication error.*
20. Explain the procedure to the patient ***to reduce anxiety and increase cooperation.***
21. Wash hands again and apply clean gloves ***to protect the patient from cross-contamination and you from blood-borne pathogens.***
22. Check the patient's identity using two methods according to facility policy ***to reduce errors.***
23. Cleanse the skin site and allow to dry.
24. Pinch up a fold of skin and subcutaneous tissue, lifting it off the muscle layer ***to prevent accidental injection into the muscle.***
25. Using a dart action, insert the needle at the appropriate 45- or 90-degree angle, as determined by the size of the

(skill continues on page 850)

Skill 37.4 (continued)

patient and the length of the needle ***to ensure deposition of insulin into the subcutaneous layer.***

26. Do not aspirate. Inject the insulin and withdraw the needle using the same angle at which it was inserted.
27. Immediately activate the safety device ***to prevent needle stick.***
28. Do not wipe the site.
29. Drop the syringe with the needle into the sharps container ***to prevent needle stick.***
30. Follow the Ending Implementation Steps located on the inside back cover.
31. Document insulin administration and site on the MAR ***for continuity of care.***

Evaluation Steps

1. Immediately following the injection, observe the injection site ***for bleeding, swelling, or any signs of adverse reactions to the medication.***
2. Monitor for signs and symptoms of hypoglycemia.

Sample Documentation

11/01/22 0750 FSBS 245 mg/dL. Reg insulin 4 units with NPH 10 units administered subcutaneously directly left of umbilicus @ 3 o'clock position. Skin warm and dry. alert. oriented × 4 spheres. ________
________ Nurse's signature and credentials

Skill 37.5 Administering an Intramuscular Injection

Assessment Steps

1. Review the health-care provider's orders and the medication administration record (MAR) for the correct patient, medication, dose, route, indication, and time. ***This will ensure accuracy and currency of orders.***
2. Review the drug book and drug insert for drug information ***to increase safety of administration.***
3. Determine what assessments, if any, must be made prior to administration of the injection. If administering a prn medication, assess the length of the time interval since the last dose ***to ensure an adequate time between doses.***
4. Assess the patient's allergies ***to reduce chances of an allergic reaction.***
5. Determine the site of the last injection and where to inject this time, evaluating the patient's size and the length of needle to obtain ***to ensure medication is deposited in correct muscle layer.*** Avoid using the same injection site as used for a previous injection.
6. Ensure that the injection site area is not tender and is free of lumps.

Planning Steps

1. Clean your work surface ***to prevent contamination of sterile injection supplies.***
2. Select a needle of the smallest suitable gauge and length based on the patient's size and muscle mass ***to ensure the best IM deposition of the medication.*** Gather needed supplies: correct size syringe, two needles, alcohol wipes, gauze pad, and gloves. ***Being prepared saves time and effort.***

Implementation Steps

Before Going to the Patient's Room

1. Wash hands ***to prevent cross-contamination.***
2. *Safety: Perform two label comparisons to the MAR for right patient, right drug, right dose, right route, right indication, and right time to reduce risk of medication error.*
3. Use aseptic technique to aspirate an amount of air into the syringe equal to the volume of medication you plan to withdraw from the vial ***to maintain equal pressure in the vial.***
4. Wipe the vial stopper with an alcohol wipe ***to reduce microorganisms.***
5. Use aseptic technique to inject the air into the vial, keeping the needle tip above the medication level ***to prevent instilling air into the medication.***
6. With the needle still in the vial stopper, invert the vial and move the needle tip underneath the medication level ***to avoid withdrawing air*** while withdrawing medication from the vial.
7. Withdraw the appropriate dose, using care to remove any air from the syringe. Remove the needle from the medication vial.
8. Use the one-handed scoop method or a commercial cap holder to recap the needle. ***This reduces risk of needle sticks.***
9. Pull back on the plunger to move medication away from the tip of the syringe ***to avoid losing or contaminating medication.*** Then remove the needle and drop the needle in the sharps container.
10. Open a new needle of appropriate gauge and length and apply it to the syringe without contaminating it. ***This reduces the risk of contamination and provides the patient with a sharp needle that has not been dulled by going through stoppers.***
11. Take the medication to the patient's room.

After Entering the Patient's Room

12. Perform the Initial Implementation Steps located on the inside back cover.
13. *Safety: Perform a third medication label comparison to the MAR for right patient, right drug, right dose, right route, right indication, and right time to reduce risk of medication error.*
14. Explain the procedure to the patient ***to reduce anxiety and increase cooperation.***
15. Wash hands again and apply clean examination gloves ***to reduce cross-contamination and protect you from body fluids.***
16. Check the patient's identity using two methods as dictated by facility policy ***to reduce medication errors.***

Skill 37.5 (continued)

17. Position the patient comfortably ***to allow access to the target site.*** Use the ventrogluteal site as first choice in patients older than 7 months. Avoid using the dorsogluteal site unless it is the only choice ***to reduce the risk of damaging the sciatic nerve.***
18. Wipe the site with alcohol and allow to air dry ***to prevent burning.***
19. Pull the skin taut with your nondominant hand ***to ease piercing the skin with the needle.***
    Note: It is considered by some nurses to be best practice to administer all IM injections in sites other than the deltoid, using the Z-track method as an additional step to reduce discomfort of injections. It helps to prevent medication from ascending back up the needle track after removal of the needle. This is your choice. If you desire to use the Z-track method, see Skill 37.6.
20. Using your dominant hand, holding the needle so that the bevel is up, and using a 90-degree angle, swiftly pierce the skin and into the muscle with one smooth dartlike motion. ***This reduces the discomfort of needle insertion.***
21. Secure the syringe with your nondominant hand ***to prevent movement of the needle.***
22. Hold the syringe steady while injecting the medication slowly, no faster than 5 to 10 seconds per milliliter of medication, ***to prevent unnecessary discomfort by allowing the tissue to expand and the medication to disperse as the medication is injected.***
23. Swiftly withdraw the needle at the same angle you used to insert it, applying a gauze pad to the site with your nondominant hand as soon as the needle leaves the skin. Immediately activate the safety device ***to prevent needle stick.*** *Safety: If a sharps container is available at the bedside, drop the syringe and needle into it.*
24. Massage the area gently ***for better distribution and absorption.***
25. Follow the Ending Implementation Steps located on the inside back cover.
26. Document in the MAR and in nurses' notes if this is a new order, a one-time injection, or a prn injection.

Evaluation Steps

1. Immediately following the injection, observe the injection site ***for bleeding, swelling, or any signs of adverse reactions to the medication.***
2. If this is first dose of a new medication, monitor the patient for at least 15 minutes after the injection ***for signs of adverse reactions.***
3. Evaluate the effectiveness of the medication and document results.

Sample Documentation

11/01/22 1845 Third dose of Kefzol 500 mg IM given in right ventrogluteal site without complaining of discomfort.

———————— Nurse's signature and credentials

Skill 37.6 Administering a Z-Track Injection

Assessment Steps

1. Review the health-care provider's orders and the medication administration record (MAR) for the correct patient, medication, dose, route, indication, and time. ***This will ensure accuracy and currency of orders.***
2. Review the drug book and drug insert for drug information ***to increase safety of administration.***
3. Determine what assessments, if any, must be made prior to administration of the injection. If administering a prn medication, assess the length of the time interval since the last dose ***to ensure an adequate time between doses.***
4. Assess the patient's allergies ***to reduce chances of an allergic reaction.***
5. Determine the site of the last injection and where to inject this time, evaluating the patient's size and the length of needle to obtain, ***to ensure the medication is deposited in the correct muscle layer.*** Avoid using the same injection site as used for a previous injection.
6. Ensure that the injection site area is not tender and is free of lumps.

Planning Steps

1. Clean your work surface ***to prevent contamination of sterile injection supplies.***
2. Wash hands ***to prevent cross-contamination.***
3. Select a needle of the smallest suitable gauge and length based on the patient's size and muscle mass ***to ensure the best IM deposition of the medication.*** Gather needed supplies: correct size syringe, two needles, alcohol wipes, and gloves. ***Being prepared saves time and effort.***

Implementation Steps

Before Going to the Patient's Room

1. Wash hands ***to prevent cross-contamination.***
2. *Safety: Perform two label comparisons to the MAR for right patient, right drug, right dose, right route, right indication, and right time to reduce risk of medication error.*
3. Use aseptic technique to aspirate an amount of air into the syringe equal to the volume of medication you plan to withdraw from the vial ***to maintain equal pressure in the vial.***
4. Wipe the vial stopper with an alcohol wipe ***to reduce microorganisms.***
5. Use aseptic technique to inject air into the vial, keeping the needle tip above the medication level ***to prevent instilling air into the medication.***
6. With the needle still in the vial stopper, invert the vial, and move the needle tip underneath the medication level ***to avoid withdrawing air*** while withdrawing medication from the vial.

(skill continues on page 852)

Skill 37.6 (continued)

7. After withdrawing the correct volume of medication, draw up 0.2 to 0.5 mL of air into the syringe to use for an air-lock. ***This air-lock helps to prevent medication from re-ascending back up the needle track into the subcutaneous tissues, where it may be caustic.***
8. Remove the first needle and attach a second needle ***to prevent tracking the medication through the subcutaneous tissue.***
9. Recap the new needle using the one-handed method ***to reduce risk of needle sticks.***

After Entering the Patient's Room

10. Perform the Initial Implementation Steps located on the inside back cover.
11. *Safety: Perform a third medication label comparison to the MAR for right patient, right drug, right dose, right route, right indication, and right time to reduce risk of medication error.*
12. Explain the procedure to the patient ***to reduce anxiety and increase cooperation.***
13. Wash hands again and apply clean examination gloves ***to prevent cross-contamination and protect you from body fluids.***
14. Place the patient in the appropriate position ***to expose the targeted muscle.***
15. Use appropriate landmarks to select the injection site and ***reduce the risk of nerve injury.***
16. Cleanse the site with alcohol using concentric circles ***to remove microorganisms.***
17. Just prior to injection, use the lateral aspect of your nondominant hand to pull the skin and underlying subcutaneous tissue to the side, displacing it laterally by 1 to 1 ½ inches.
18. Using your dominant hand, hold the syringe with the needle bevel upward and swiftly pierce the skin, entering at a 90-degree angle, inserting the needle almost to the hub ***to ensure deposition of medication in the muscle layer.***
19. Without moving the needle, slowly inject the medication into the muscle, including instillation of the air-lock.
20. Wait for 5 to 10 seconds before withdrawing the needle. Withdraw the needle and then immediately release the skin and tissue being held by your nondominant hand. ***This allows the tissue to close the needle track at the muscle layer, preventing medication from entering the subcutaneous layer.*** Activate the needle guard as soon as the needle leaves the skin ***to reduce needle sticks.***
21. Blot any remaining blood from the injection site with a 2 × 2 gauze.
22. Do not massage the site. ***Massaging the site after a Z-track injection may allow medication to be dispersed above the muscle as the needle track is manipulated.***
23. Discard the needle and syringe in the sharps container ***to reduce needle sticks.***
24. Document the injection, technique used, and site in the MAR. Include any reactions to the injection.

Evaluation Steps

1. Immediately following the injection, observe the injection site ***for bleeding, swelling, discoloration, or any signs of adverse reactions to the medication.***
2. If this is the patient's first exposure to the medication, monitor the patient for at least 15 minutes after the injection ***for signs of adverse reactions.***

Sample Documentation

07/19/22 2115 Cyanocobalamin 100 mcg administered IM using Z-track technique in right vastus lateralis without reports of discomfort. ——————————
—————————— Nurse's signature and credentials

POST CONFERENCE

You share about your day with your classmates in post conference, allowing them to learn from your insights. Most of the injection procedure went well, especially when you were preparing the insulin. You were nervous, but you did remember to draw clear first and then cloudy insulin after you had injected the exact amount of air into each vial. You had difficulty recapping the needle to take it to the patient's room. You felt like you chased it all over the countertop. Your instructor helped you find a way to place it so that you did not do that the next time. Your IM injection was rather nerve wracking for you because the patient was in a great deal of pain after therapy when he asked for the meperidine. You were nervous and trying to hurry to get the pain relief to him. As a result, you accidentally touched the needle to your bare hand and had to change needles before you could give the medication. You identified the ventrogluteal site on his unaffected leg. You were so worried about hurting him with the injection, but he was just relieved to have the medication to relieve his pain. He assured you that any injection pain was quite minor to the pain he was experiencing in his amputated leg.

Key Points

- Parenteral routes include ID, between the layers of the skin; subcut, beneath the skin but above the muscle; and IM, in muscle tissue.
- A syringe has three main parts: a barrel, a plunger on one end, and a tip on the other.
- The syringe tip will have either a slip-tip or a Luer-Lok connection, which attaches to a hypodermic needle.
- Syringes are available in numerous sizes, typically ranging from 0.5 to 60 mL.
- There are standard syringes, TB syringes, and insulin syringes.
- There are three parts of a needle: the bevel, or slant at the tip of the needle; the hub, or attachment point of the needle to the syringe; and the shaft or barrel, the main body of the needle.
- Needle sizes are designated by length and gauge. Gauges range from 14 to 30. The smaller the diameter of the needle, the higher the gauge number. Needle lengths range from ¼ to 2 inches (0.64 to 5 cm).
- The viscosity of the medication, the route of injection, and the size of the patient help to determine the choice of needle gauge and length.
- Ampules contain single doses of medication in liquid form and require use of a filter needle to withdraw medication.
- Filter needles must always be changed after drawing up medication from a glass ampule and before administering the injection.
- A vial is a container for parenteral medication that has a metal-enclosed rubber stopper on top. It can be a single-dose or multiple-dose vial.
- The term *bolus* refers to an amount of medication given all at once. The term *basal* refers to the minimum requirements when the body is at rest and no additional demands are being made.
- The site of choice for administering an IM injection for all patients older than 7 months is the ventrogluteal site.
- The site of choice for newborns and infants younger than 7 months is the vastus lateralis. The rectus femoris is not used on infants or small children.
- The maximum volume that can be injected in the deltoid muscle is 1 to 2 mL in older children and adults and 0.5 to 1 mL in infants.
- The maximum volume that can be injected in the ventrogluteal site is 1 to 2 mL in infants and children, the elderly, and average-size adults.
- The maximum volume that can be injected into a very large individual's ventrogluteal site is 3 mL.
- Activate the safety device immediately after withdrawing the needle from the patient's skin.
- Dispose of needles in sharps containers immediately after use.
- Sterile needles should only be recapped using the one-handed method or a commercial recapping device.
- Never recap used needles.

Review Questions

Select the answer that is most appropriate for each of the following questions. Some questions may have more than one correct answer. Select all that apply.

1. A parenteral route of medication administration is one that bypasses which of the following?
   1. Stomach
   2. Kidneys
   3. Skin
   4. Heart
   5. Liver

2. Injection of a drug into the upper layers of the skin is known as which route of medication administration?
   1. Intra-articular
   2. Intradermal
   3. Subcutaneous
   4. Intramuscular

3. Which site of subcutaneous administration has the most rapid absorption of insulin?
   1. Vastus lateralis
   2. Dorsogluteal site
   3. Back of upper arm
   4. Abdomen
   5. Deltoid

4. Which of the following steps should the nurse perform when combining two types of insulin and administering them?
   1. Always withdraw intermediate-acting insulin first
   2. When mixing insulins, remember "clear before cloudy"
   3. Inject with 20-G, 1-inch needle
   4. Insert needle at a 45- or 90-degree angle
   5. Mix Lantus with regular insulin

5. A nurse needs to administer medication from an ampule. What of the following steps should the nurse take when drawing up this medication?
   1. Snap off the ampule neck using a sterile gauze pad
   2. Hold the ampule away from the body when breaking
   3. Tilt the ampule and place the injection needle into the liquid
   4. Avoid tapping the top of the bottle
   5. Use a filter needle to draw up medication

6. What gauge and length of needle would you select to administer an IM injection of a nonviscous medication in the ventrogluteal site of a 40-year-old male construction worker who is in good health and weighs 185 pounds?
   1. 25 G, 1 inch
   2. 18 G, 1 ½ inch
   3. 22 G, 1 ½ inch
   4. 24 G, 2 inch
   5. 20 G, ⅝ inch

7. You are about to administer a standard P.P.D. to a 31-year-old male. Which of the following needles and syringes would be appropriate to use?
   1. Tuberculin syringe with 27-G, ⅝-inch needle
   2. 1-mL syringe with 20-G, 1 ½–inch needle
   3. Insulin syringe with 25-G, ⅝-inch needle
   4. 3-mL syringe with 25-G, ½-inch needle
   5. 1-mL syringe with 18-G, 1-inch needle

8. In which of the following injections should you avoid aspirating before injecting the medication?
   1. IM injection of antibiotics
   2. ID tuberculosis test
   3. Subcut insulin
   4. IM pain medication
   5. Subcut anticoagulant

9. Select the correct anatomical landmarks for the ventrogluteal site.
   1. Iliac crest
   2. Greater trochanter
   3. Acromion process
   4. Coccyx
   5. Anterior superior iliac spine

10. A nurse is caring for a 65-year-old female with type 1 diabetes. The patient is receiving an insulin bolus for a glucose reading of 310 mg/dL. How will the nurse give the insulin bolus?
    1. Give the medication all at once
    2. Give the medication before meals
    3. Give the medication after meals
    4. Give the medication before and after meals and at bedtime

ANSWERS 1. 1, 5, 2. 2, 3. 4, 4. 2, 4, 5. 1, 2, 3, 5, 6. 3, 7. 1, 8. 2, 3, 5, 9. 1, 2, 5, 10. 1

Critical Thinking Exercises

Answers available online.

1. Describe the differences between the ID, IM, and subcut injection routes, including any choice/most advantageous muscles or sites or restricted sites. Be thorough.

2. You are preparing to administer an antibiotic injection to a newborn that must be reconstituted before use. The medication label states that sterile normal saline for injection, sterile water for injection, and sterile bacteriostatic water for injection are appropriate diluents that may be used for reconstituting the antibiotic. When you go to the medication cart to obtain the diluent, you see three unopened vials to choose from: sterile normal saline 0.9% (multiple-dose vial), sterile water for injection (multiple-dose vial), and sterile water (single-dose vial). Which of the three diluents cannot be used in this particular situation? Why not, if the label says both normal saline for injection and water for injection are acceptable diluents?

Additional Resources

Use the scratch off code on the inside front cover of your book to access online quizzes that will help you to improve your scores on course exams and prepare for the NCLEX-PN®.

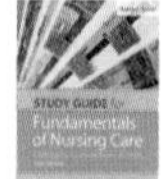

Study Guide

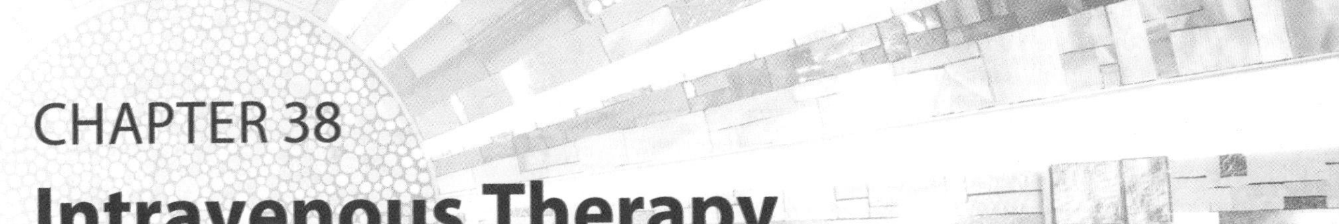

CHAPTER 38
Intravenous Therapy

KEY TERMS

Cannulation (KAN-yoo-LAY-shun)
Drug–drug interaction (DRUG-DRUG IN-ter-AK-shun)
Extravasation (eks-TRAV-uh-SAY-shun)
Flange (FLANJ)
Hypertonic IV solution (HYE-per-TON-ik FOR so-LOO-shun)
Hypotonic IV solution (HYE-poh-TON-ik FOR so-LOO-shun)
Hypovolemia (HYE-poh-voh-LEE-mee-ah)
Infiltration (IN-fil-TRAY-shun)
Isotonic IV solution (EY-soh-TON-ik FOR so-LOO-shun)
Nonvesicant (non-VESS-ik-ant)
Packed red blood cells (PAKT RED BLUHD SELLS)
Patent (PAT-ent)
Plasma (PLAZ-mah)
Precipitate (pree-SIP-ih-tayt)
Speed shock (SPEED SHOCK)
Thrombus (THROM-bus)
Vesicant (VESS-ik-ant)

CHAPTER CONCEPTS

Safety
Patient-Centered Care

LEARNING OUTCOMES

1. Define various terms associated with preparing, initiating, and maintaining peripheral IV therapy.
2. Identify the purposes and benefits of peripheral IV therapy.
3. List the common components of IV fluids, their uses, and special considerations for use.
4. Compare the effects of infusing hypotonic, isotonic, and hypertonic IV solutions.
5. Describe equipment used for peripheral IV therapy.
6. Discuss the importance of asepsis during IV therapy.
7. Relate possible complications of IV therapy, as well as their causes, prevention, and treatment.
8. Contrast IV therapy in children, adults, and older adults.
9. Explain how to prepare, initiate, and maintain a peripheral IV infusion.
10. Calculate an infusion rate for a gravity infusion and a pump infusion.
11. Discuss peripheral IV therapy nursing care.
12. Discuss the components and uses of various blood products.
13. Summarize how to prepare, initiate, and monitor infusion of blood and blood products.
14. Apply knowledge of IV therapy in specific scenarios.
15. Identify the purpose of each central venous access device.
16. Discuss information found in the Connection features in this chapter.
17. Identify specific safety features.
18. Answer questions about the skills in this chapter.

SKILLS

38.1 Administering IV Push Medication via PRN Lock or IV Line
38.2 Administering IV Piggyback Medication
38.3 Converting an IV Infusion to a PRN Lock
38.4 Calculating IV Infusion Rate
38.5 Adding Medications to a Primary IV Solution
38.6 Initiating Peripheral Venipuncture
38.7 Adding a New Bag of IV Solution to an Existing IV Line
38.8 Discontinuing an IV Infusion or PRN Lock
38.9 Preparing, Initiating, and Monitoring the Infusion of Blood and Blood Products

CRITICAL THINKING CONNECTION

Clinical Assignment

You will be caring for a 77-year-old male who was admitted to the hospital with nausea, vomiting, and dehydration. The cause of his symptoms is not yet determined. He is NPO and has an IV infusion of D5 1/2NS infusing at 60 mL per hour in his left forearm. According to his chart, it was difficult for the nurse to get the IV infusion started. When you go in to introduce yourself, he tells you that his arm is hurting and points to the IV site.

Critical Thinking Questions:

1. Your most immediate focus at this moment will be?
2. What will you do about the infusion and IV site problem?
3. Describe how you would determine the size and type of IV catheter to reinsert?
4. What fluids will you infuse and at what rate?

As you learned in Chapter 29, fluid is one of the body's most essential substances, second only to oxygen. During illness or recovery from injury, the body often is unable to tolerate medications, fluids, and nutrition by mouth, thus necessitating infusion of medications, fluids, electrolytes, and nutritional components by a route other than the usual route of the alimentary canal. Any other route of administering medications, including the intravenous, subcutaneous, or intramuscular route, is known as the parenteral route. This chapter is devoted to the *peripheral intravenous route,* which means to infuse directly into the vascular system by the way of a peripheral vein, as opposed to a larger central vein such as the subclavian or jugular. This chapter will introduce you to the entry-level knowledge and skills of peripheral IV therapy. Much skill and knowledge are required to prepare an infusion, initiate IV access, and maintain the infusion in a safe manner. Practice, and practice alone, will help you to develop stellar IV therapy skills and techniques.

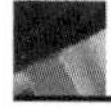

PURPOSES OF INTRAVENOUS THERAPY

Infusion of fluids intravenously may serve multiple purposes:

- Maintaining or providing daily body fluid and electrolytes because of inability to ingest fluids and nutrients by mouth
- Replacing abnormal or excessive loss of fluids and electrolytes
- Providing an avenue for IV administration of medications

Maintaining Fluids and Electrolytes

Whenever an individual refuses to drink adequate fluids or is unable to ingest fluids orally, whether it is because of nausea, inability to swallow, disease of the digestive tract, decreased level of consciousness, or NPO status for surgery, the body requires the necessary fluids be administered via a different route. Without maintenance of adequate fluid supply, the body can:

- Become dehydrated
- Develop imbalances between levels of fluid and electrolytes
- Develop impairment of cellular function, which impacts the functions of each body system
- In severe cases cease to function, resulting in death

Provision of maintenance fluids generally will include not only water, the primary need, but also electrolytes, glucose, and sometimes vitamins. The electrolytes are necessary to maintain homeostasis of fluids and electrolytes, which contribute to correct function of all body systems. Glucose is required for production of energy. It provides the calories, or fuel, that will be burned during all cellular functions. Glucose is also stored in the form of glycogen in the liver, to be converted back to glucose at a later time when energy needs require more fuel. Vitamins are required for various cellular functions such as growth of new tissue.

Replacing Fluid and Electrolyte Losses

There are numerous ways an individual can lose excessive amounts of fluids. Recall from Chapter 29 that fluids are normally lost on a daily basis through the kidneys, intestinal tract, skin, and lungs. Excessive losses in any of these areas, such as from high fever or working outside in extreme heat, require that the fluids be replaced to prevent dehydration. Diseases that cause excessive vomiting or diarrhea, require gastrointestinal suctioning, or simply prevent oral intake of fluids increase the fluid replacement needs. When the loss of water is accompanied by the loss of specific electrolytes, they also must be replaced. For example, gastric suctioning or vomiting can deplete sodium, chloride, potassium, and hydrochloric acid, resulting in hyponatremia, hypochloremia, hypokalemia, and metabolic alkalosis. Loss occurring with diarrhea includes loss of potassium, sodium, and bicarbonate. You may find it helpful to refer back to Chapter 29 regarding these imbalances.

Recall that when fluids and electrolytes are lost in balanced proportions from extracellular spaces, the decrease in blood volume is called **hypovolemia.** The direct loss of blood from the cardiovascular system, in the form of hemorrhage, is another avenue of fluid and electrolyte loss along with the other components of blood. *It is important to remember that inadequate fluid within the cardiovascular system makes it impossible to provide adequate circulation to the cells, tissues, and organs, all of which are required to sustain life.* Replacement of lost fluids and electrolytes should be based on actual fluid losses, increased metabolic needs, and laboratory results of serum electrolyte levels.

• WORD • BUILDING •

hypovolemia: hypo – deficient + vol – volume + em – blood + ia – condition

Infusion of Intravenous Medications

The administration of IV solutions provides an avenue through which we can ensure the rapid and direct delivery of medications to the blood in the intravascular space when they are needed. Administering medications via the IV route delivers an increased potency of medication compared to the intramuscular or subcutaneous injection route. Because of the increased drug potency and the immediacy of the drug's effects, the IV route of drug administration can be very dangerous if the person giving the drug does not have adequate knowledge of the drug's therapeutic effects, side effects, adverse reactions, and antidote, when appropriate.

Medications can be added to larger volumes of IV fluids, such as 500 or 1,000 mL, and infused continuously, or they can be added to smaller volume of fluids, ranging from 50 to 250 mL, for delivery at specified intervals. Figure 38.1 shows the different IV container volume sizes.

Continuous IV Infusion

When continuous IV infusion of a drug is desired, the healthcare provider orders the dosage of medication to be administered. The pharmacist or nurse performs the calculations to determine the amount of drug to add to a specific volume of IV solution in order to achieve the desired concentration. The volume of solution may vary from 250 to 1,000 mL. Now the infusion rate that will deliver the prescribed dosage must be calculated. ***Safety: All infusions of IV solution must be monitored closely to maintain the ordered rate of infusion, but it is doubly important if medication is added to the solution.***

IV Push

Some medications can be administered directly by a method known as *IV push,* which means the medication is injected directly into the vein using a needle and syringe. The IV push route of administration has two advantages: it produces an immediate therapeutic blood level and instantaneous effects of the drug. However, these same advantages serve as disadvantages as well. If the incorrect drug or dosage is administered, the unintentional blood level and effects of the wrong drug are immediate, sometimes harming the patient. It also is possible that the patient may suffer adverse reactions or be allergic to the drug. The immediacy of effects requires your vigilance in verifying that you are administering the right drug and dosage to the right patient at the right time, by the right route, and slowly according to the manufacturer's recommendations.

This route is commonly used in emergencies, surgery, and other situations in which immediate results are desired. If the patient has an intermittent infusion device, also known as a *PRN lock,* the medication can be administered IV push via the injection port without having the discomfort of another needle stick. Another way to administer IV push drugs is through the Y-injection port nearest the insertion site of a primary IV line with continuous infusion of IV fluids (Fig. 38.2).

Safety: The administration of IV push medication requires that the medication be compatible with the IV solution as well as any medications that have been added to the solution. Many facilities have policies in place requiring that all venous access devices (VADs) be flushed with 1 to 10 mL of sodium chloride, or normal saline (NS), prior to administration of IV push medications and again after the IV push medication regardless of compatibility or incompatibility. Other facilities may require NS flushes only if there is an incompatibility issue.

If the medication is not compatible, the flow must be stopped by pinching off the tubing just proximal to the injection port to be used. One to 10 mL of NS is injected through the injection port, followed by the medication. Then the medication is flushed out of the line with another 1 to 10 mL of NS before resuming infusion of the incompatible IV solution. Most facilities stock prefilled syringes of NS flush, which save you the time of gathering supplies and drawing NS up each time you need a flush (Fig. 38.3). However, because some facilities charge what seem like exorbitant prices for the prefilled syringe of NS, it does significantly raise the cost to the patient.

Many medications must be diluted in 1 to 10 mL of NS prior to IV push administration. By diluting the medication,

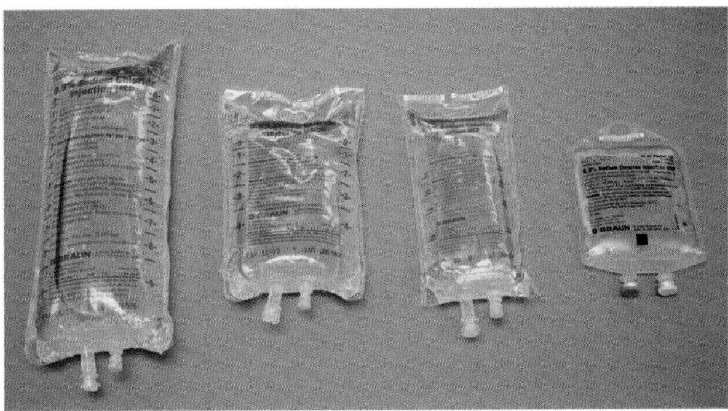

FIGURE 38.1 IV solutions come in a variety of bag sizes/volumes: 50 mL, 250 mL, 500 mL, and 1,000 mL.

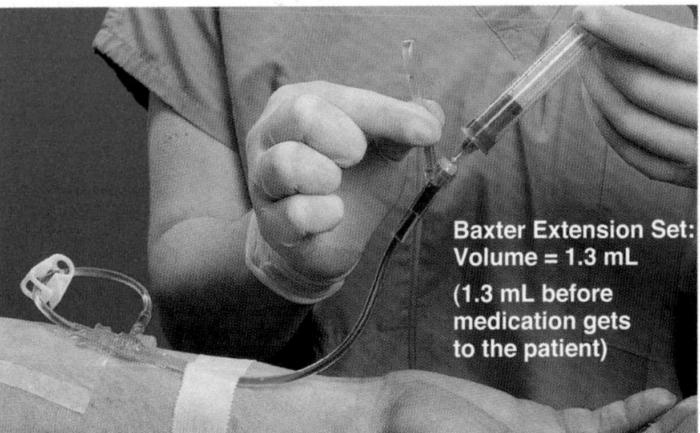

FIGURE 38.2 Administering IV push medication into the injection port closest to the insertion site of a continuously infusing IV. The nondominant hand pinches off the primary line between the Y-injection port and the IV bag to ensure that the medication infuses down-line toward the patient rather than up-line toward the IV solution bag (from Wilkinson JM, Treas LS. *Fundamentals of Nursing: Theory, Concepts & Applications*. Vol. 2. 3rd ed. Philadelphia, PA: FA Davis; 2016).

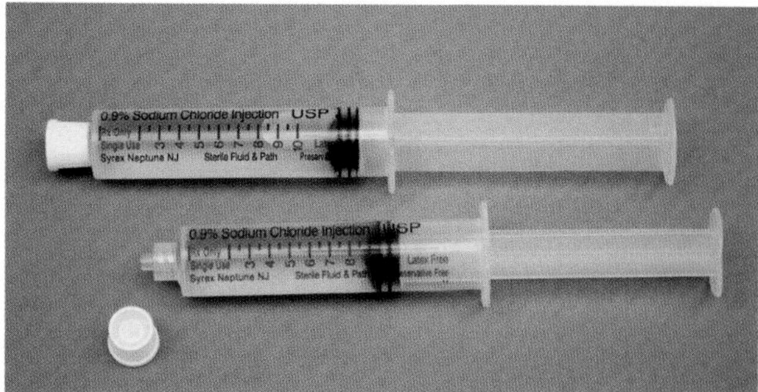

FIGURE 38.3 Prefilled syringes of normal saline with Luer-Lok tips and sterile caps; used to flush IV lines.

the level of vein irritation and patient discomfort are reduced. All IV push drugs must be administered over the manufacturer's recommended length of time. Some medications require an administration time of only 2 to 5 minutes; others require 7 to 10 minutes or more. ***Safety: It is your responsibility to research the length of time over which you should give a medication.*** This information can be found in the drug insert that comes with the drug or in a drug book, or it can be obtained from the pharmacist. Skill 38.1 (page 889) provides more information on administering IV push medications.

Some state boards of nursing, some nurse practice acts, and certain facilities place restrictions on who may administer IV push medications. Some designate that it is strictly the responsibility of the registered nurse (RN), while others allow both licensed practical/vocational nurses (LPN/LVNs) and RNs to perform this skill. Some facilities allow LPN/LVNs to administer IV push medications but restrict administration of certain categories, such as cardiac emergency drugs, to RNs. It is your responsibility to know your own state board of nursing's philosophy and Nurse Practice Act scope of practice, as well as your facility's policy regarding this issue.

IV Piggyback

A third method of administering medications intravenously is called IV piggyback (IVPB). The medication is added to a smaller volume of IV solution, usually a volume between 50 and 250 mL, of either 0.9% sodium chloride (NS) or dextrose 5% in water (D5W). The medication is then infused over a specified period of time between 15 and 90 minutes depending on the medication. A specially designed, shorter tubing connects the IVPB solution container to the most proximal Y-injection port located on the primary IV line, similar to *riding piggyback* on the primary line, thus the name. You will also hear it called *secondary tubing* as well as simply *piggyback tubing*. The terms are synonymous. The IVPB route is commonly used for administering medications that require intermittent infusion, such as every 4 hours or every 8 hours. Figure 38.4 identifies the parts of the primary and secondary IV tubing and shows how they work together. Skill 38.2 (page 891) provides more information on administering IVPB medications.

Some patients will no longer have a need for a continuously infusing IV solution but will still need the IV access

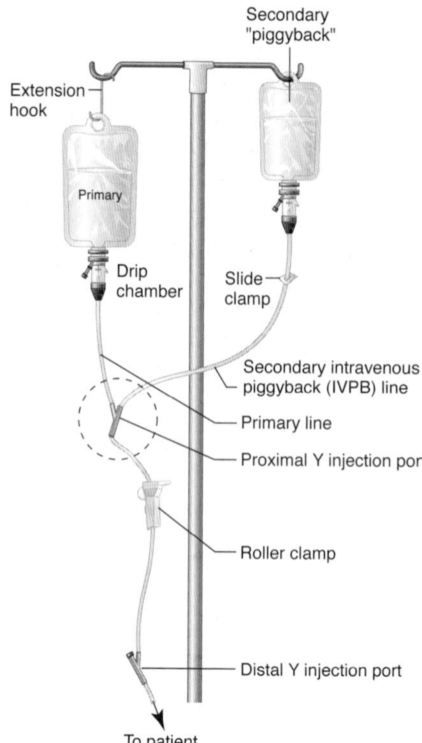

FIGURE 38.4 IVPB medication infusing into the most proximal (closest to bag) Y-injection port on the primary administration set (from Wilkinson JM, Treas LS: *Fundamentals of Nursing: Theory, Concepts & Applications*. Vol. 2. 3rd ed. Philadelphia, PA: FA Davis; 2016).

for administration of intermittent IVPB or IV push medications. In such a situation, the health-care provider may order to discontinue the IV fluids and convert to an intermittent infusion lock, termed a *PRN lock* or *saline lock*. The IV tubing is disconnected from the cannula in the vein and a PRN lock device is attached to the cannula. The PRN device is kept **patent** (open allowing fluids to pass through, or the opposite of clogged), with IV flushes of NS administered at least every 8 hours. Skill 38.3 (page 892) provides more information on converting an IV infusion to a PRN lock.

If a patient has a PRN lock rather than a continuous primary IV solution, the shorter secondary tubing would not be long enough to administer an IVPB because it would not reach from the IVPB solution bag on the IV pole to the PRN lock injection port secured to the patient's arm or hand. Therefore, instead of using a secondary piggyback tubing, it would be necessary to use a basic primary IV tubing so that it would be of adequate length.

KNOWLEDGE CONNECTION

What are three reasons for administration of IV fluids? Explain the difference in IV push and IVPB routes of administration. List four ways in which body fluids may be lost. What is the minimum time frame in which an IV push drug may be administered?

Compatibility Versus Incompatibility

Medications must be compatible with other drugs, additives, and IV solutions that are mixed or administered at the same time or immediately after each other. So many medications are available today that numerous medications can be incompatible and result in **drug–drug interactions.** This means the interaction between the two drugs causes a change in the activity or components of one or more of the drugs. Some drug reactions may even produce a product that is totally unsafe to administer. Certain incompatible drugs, when mixed, cause a precipitate to form. A **precipitate** forms when one of the agents in a solution separates from the solvent and becomes a solid, insoluble product. It may or may not be visible to the naked eye, but when you can see it, it may look cloudy, hazy, or like fine floating crystals. Never allow an infusion to continue if you see precipitates forming in the fluid.

Some incompatible drugs require use of separate tubing sets to administer each medication, while others only require a specified interval of time to elapse between administrations of the two incompatible medications. When incompatible drugs require separate tubing sets for each medication, you must label the tubing with the date and time hung, name of the drug, and your initials. Other medications might only require that you flush the intermittent infusion lock or the primary IV line with NS both before and after giving each medication. This prevents the two medications from ever coming in contact with each other.

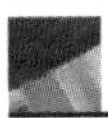

SAFE ADMINISTRATION OF IV DRUGS

Knowledge required to safely administer IV medications includes the following:

- Patient's medication allergies
- Patient's disease or condition
- Sterile technique
- Integrity of the IV access
- Effects of the drug
- Correct form of medication for IV use
- Correct dosage for specific patient's age or weight
- Type of diluent to use if needed
- Volume of dilution required
- Rate of safe administration
- Expected effects of the medication
- Possible drug–drug interactions
- Possible adverse reactions, including the most common and those that are life-threatening
- Appropriate nursing interventions to use if an adverse reaction occurs

> **KNOWLEDGE CONNECTION**
>
> Explain what drug incompatibility means. What does the term *precipitate* mean with regard to incompatibility? Identify at least 10 things you must know to safely administer IV medications.

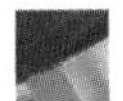

IV SOLUTIONS

IV fluids are comprised of water to which various percentages of components have been added. Common components found in different IV fluids include glucose, electrolytes, vitamins, and amino acids. The amounts of these solutes that are dissolved in the water determine the fluid's *tonicity* (the solute concentration of IV solutions and the effect that it will have on the blood volume, cell size, and energy production).

Tonicity serves to meet the individual needs of patients as they are treated at different stages of diseases and conditions, each of which may require differing volumes of water and solutes to provide or maintain homeostasis throughout the body. IV fluids are responsible for saving lives every day. ***Safety: The danger that you need to understand is that the administration of improper amounts of water and solutes or the wrong concentration of the two components can cause complications and possibly patient death.*** It is important that you learn the differences among isotonic, hypotonic, and hypertonic fluids and what occurs physiologically after infusion of these solutions into the patient.

Isotonic Solution

An **isotonic IV fluid** solution is fluid that contains an amount of solute that produces a concentration of dissolved particles equal to that of the intracellular and extracellular fluids of the human body. Because the concentration is equal, administration of the isotonic solution will not cause movement of water between the intravascular space, the interstitial space, and the intracellular space. In other words, there will be no movement of fluids across the semipermeable membranes of the blood vessels or cellular membranes as long as this ratio remains balanced (Fig. 38.5). Table 38.1 lists common isotonic fluids and their uses.

Hypotonic Solution

A **hypotonic** solution has a lower osmolarity than body fluids, which simply means there is less solute dissolved in the water, making the concentration of the dissolved particles less than that of the body fluids. Hypotonic solution infused into the intravascular space, or blood vessels, will cause shifting of body fluids out of the intravascular space and into the interstitial spaces, and then eventually into the intracellular spaces, rehydrating the cells (Fig. 38.6). (For further detail of this process, refer to the Anatomy and Physiology Connection: Maintaining Compartmental Fluid Balance.)

This process makes a hypotonic solution good for use in patients who need simple water replacement because of lack of fluid intake or loss of body water without loss of electrolytes, known as *hypertonic dehydration.* For a list of common hypotonic fluids and their uses, refer to Table 38.1.

• WORD • BUILDING •

hypotonic: hypo – deficient + tonic – muscle tone
hypertonic: hyper – excessive + tonic – muscle tone
osmolarity: osmol – standard unit of osmotic pressure + arity – degree or quality

Anatomy and Physiology Connection

Maintaining Compartmental Fluid Balance

The body strives to maintain a homeostatic balance of fluids and electrolytes at all times. One of the mechanisms by which this is accomplished is the movement of the solvent, or liquid, component of body fluid. The fluid shifts that occur with hypertonic or hypotonic solutions result due to changes in *solute,* or particle, concentration dissolved in the solvent. By administering a hypotonic solution (one with a lower solute concentration than that in the body fluids) into the blood vessels, the solute concentration of the blood is lowered and the concentration in the interstitial space outside the blood vessels is now higher than that in the blood. Because of this imbalance, water then moves from inside the blood vessels, across the semipermeable membrane of the vessel walls, and into the interstitial space in an attempt to balance the two levels of solute concentration. As this water moves into the interstitial space, the solute concentration in the fluid there is being diluted in an effort to equalize it to that of the fluid inside the blood vessels. As this process continues, the solute concentration of the fluid in the interstitial space now becomes less than that of the fluid within the cells. This imbalance causes water to move across the semipermeable cellular membrane from the interstitial space to the inside of the cells in an effort to maintain balance of the solute concentration of the interstitial and intracellular fluids. As water is moved from the interstitial spaces into the cells, the cells are rehydrated.

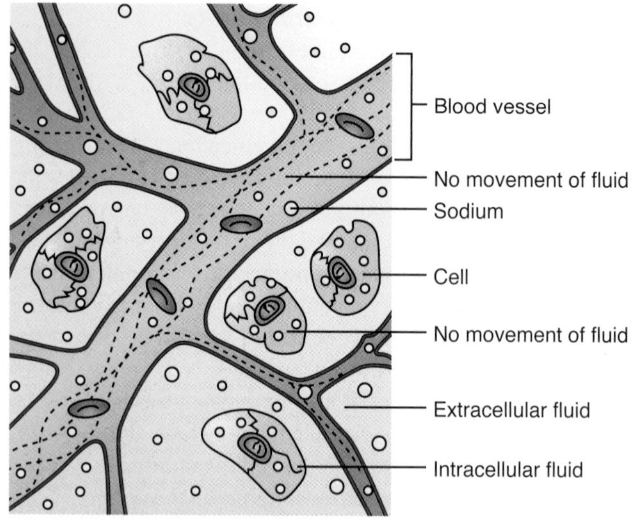

End result of infusing isotonic IV solution:

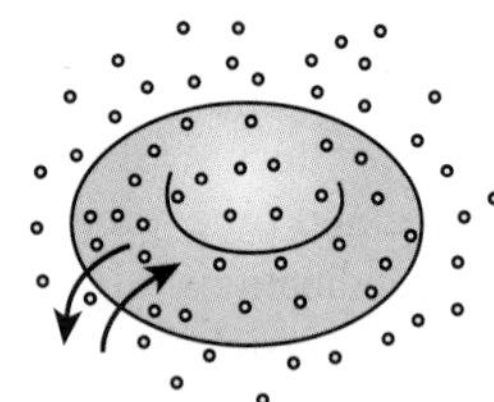

FIGURE 38.5 Fluid movement during infusion of isotonic IV solution. During infusion of isotonic IV solution, the body maintains balance as equal volumes of water cross back and forth continuously between the two extracellular spaces (blood inside the intravascular space and fluid in the interstitial spaces) and the intracellular spaces inside the cells. The end result is the balance shown inside and outside of a cell.

Table 38.1
Common IV Solutions and Their Uses

Solution	*Uses*	*Special Considerations*
Hypotonic		
Half-strength saline: may be written as ½NS or 0.45% NaCl	Water replacement Fluid and electrolyte replacement during gastric suction Hypertonic dehydration Depletion of Na^+ and Cl^-	Avoid use in patients with liver disease, head trauma, or burns Can cause cerebral edema ***Safety: Should not be used in patients with hypotension because it will further drop BP.***
One-third strength saline: may be written as ⅓NS or 0.33% NaCl	Free water replacement to aid kidneys in elimination of wastes	***Safety: Should not be used in patients with hypotension because it will further drop BP.***
Isotonic		
5% Dextrose in water: may be written as D5W	Provide some calories for energy Provide free water Reduce protein breakdown for energy	***Safety: Do not use in patients who are allergic to corn.*** Irritates veins, causing phlebitis

Table 38.1
Common IV Solutions and Their Uses—cont'd

Solution	*Uses*	*Special Considerations*
	Short-term treatment of dehydration, at controlled infusion rate To administer medications by intravenous piggyback (IVPB) route	Use cautiously in patients with renal and cardiac disease; can result in fluid overload ***Safety: Observe for early signs and symptoms of fluid overload.*** Continual infusion can result in electrolyte deficits *After dextrose is metabolized, it becomes hypotonic;* has been known to cause cerebral edema with continuous infusion ***Safety: Observe for early signs and symptoms of cerebral edema (increased intracranial pressure).*** Avoid using for resuscitation; can cause hyperglycemia Cannot be mixed with blood components; causes hemolysis
NS or sodium chloride: may be written as NS or 0.9% NaCl	Replacement of nutrients and electrolytes when no fluid shift is desired *Only* fluid used to initiate and discontinue blood transfusion Irrigant for IV access devices to prevent clotting Vascular expander	Can result in fluid volume excess; use cautiously in patients with congestive heart failure ***Safety: Observe for early signs and symptoms of fluid overload.*** Dilutes concentration of hemoglobin in the blood May lower potassium levels
Lactated Ringer's solution: may be written as LR	*Is most similar to electrolyte content of the blood* and is therefore used for fluid replacement in all types of dehydration and fluid volume deficits Electrolyte replacement in intravascular fluid	***Safety: Has some incompatibilities with medications. Check for compatibility before administering medication.*** Can result in fluid volume excess
Normosol-R: may be written as Normosol	Similar to LR	Can result in circulatory overload
5% Dextrose in 0.22% sodium chloride: may be written as D5 ¼NS	Supplies some calories Treat dehydration As a "fluid challenge" to assess kidney function	***Safety: Do not use in patients who are allergic to corn.*** Can result in circulatory overload Fluid challenge: give 8 mL/m^2 of body surface area for 45 minutes to determine if kidneys begin to function by making urine
Hypertonic		
5% Dextrose in 0.45% sodium chloride: may be written as D5 ½NS	Replace nutrients Treat dehydration	***Safety: Do not use in patients who are allergic to corn.*** Can result in circulatory overload
5% Dextrose with 0.9% normal saline: may be written as D5NS	Supplies calories Used to expand blood volume	***Safety: Do not use in patients who are allergic to corn.*** Can result in circulatory overload

Continued

Table 38.1
Common IV Solutions and Their Uses—cont'd

Solution	*Uses*	*Special Considerations*
10% to 50% Dextrose: may be written as D10W, D20W, D50W	Prefilled syringes of dextrose 50% in water are used to treat severe hypoglycemia, but dextrose 50% IV fluids are not used for continuous IV infusion	***Safety: Any IV fluid with dextrose concentration greater than 10% cannot be given through peripheral veins. It must be administered via central veins.*** ***Safety: Do not use in patients who are allergic to corn.***
3% to 5% Sodium chloride: may be written as 3% NaCl and 5% NaCl	To treat severe sodium depletion and water overload (not commonly used)	***Safety: Dangerous. Only small volumes are infused.*** Irritates veins Administer slowly May cause circulatory overload

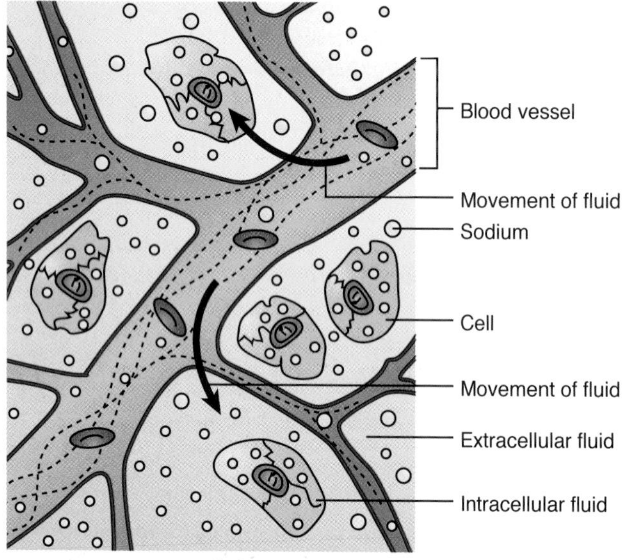

End result of excessive hypotonic IV solution:

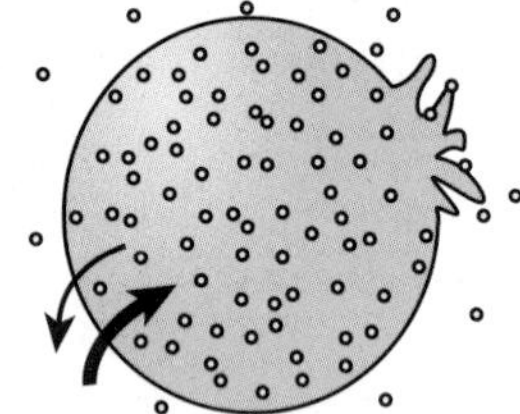

FIGURE 38.6 Fluid movement during infusion of hypotonic IV solution. The body tries to maintain balance when infusion of hypotonic IV solution dilutes the blood, making it less concentrated than the interstitial fluid. Osmosis pulls water from the blood to the interstitial spaces to dilute the more concentrated interstitial fluid. Once the interstitial fluid becomes less concentrated than the fluid inside the cells, osmosis will pull water from the interstitial spaces into the intracellular space inside the cells. If this is allowed to continue beyond the patient's specific needs, the cells will continue to fill with extra water, swelling until they eventually rupture and die, as seen in the diagram of a cell.

Recall from Chapter 29 that the movement of an excessive volume fluid from the vascular spaces into the interstitial spaces is known as third-spacing, which lowers both blood volume and blood pressure (BP) and causes edema. The increased volume of interstitial fluid dilutes the solute concentration, making the interstitial fluid hypotonic; excessive water then moves into the cells, causing them to swell and possibly rupture. ***Safety: Infusion of an excessive volume of hypotonic IV solutions can result in cerebral edema, increased intracranial pressure, overhydration and rupture of brain cells, and death of the patient.*** Box 38.1 lists early signs and symptoms of increased intracranial pressure.

Hypertonic Solution

If a fluid has a higher concentration of particles dissolved in it than the concentration in fluids of the body, it is known as **hypertonic** solution. Intravenous infusion of excessive hypertonic fluids causes water to be pulled from the interstitial space into the intravascular space in an attempt to balance the solute concentration on both sides of the semipermeable membrane, the vessel wall. This overloads the fluid volume within the vascular spaces, resulting in elevated BP. The fluid movement

Box 38.1
Early Signs of Increased Intracranial Pressure

It is best to detect increasing intracranial pressure before it has progressed to the point that the vital signs deteriorate. Be alert to the following earlier signs:

- Change in level of consciousness
- Confusion
- Disorientation
- Headache increasing in severity
- Pupillary changes
- Purposeless movements
- Restlessness

does not stop here, however. The solute concentration of the interstitial fluid will increase as the water is pulled out of it to move into the blood vessels. Now the solute concentration of the interstitial fluid becomes greater than that found within the cells. The water will then be pulled out of the cells and into the extracellular spaces in an attempt to balance the solute concentration on both sides of the semipermeable cell membrane (Fig. 38.7). This reduction in cellular fluid can result in shrinking of the cells. Cells in this condition will not function appropriately and even can die as a result. Table 38.1 lists common hypertonic solutions and their uses.

KNOWLEDGE CONNECTION

Compare isotonic, hypotonic, and hypertonic fluids. Explain which direction fluid movement occurs when hypertonic fluid is administered intravenously. Explain the same for hypotonic fluid.

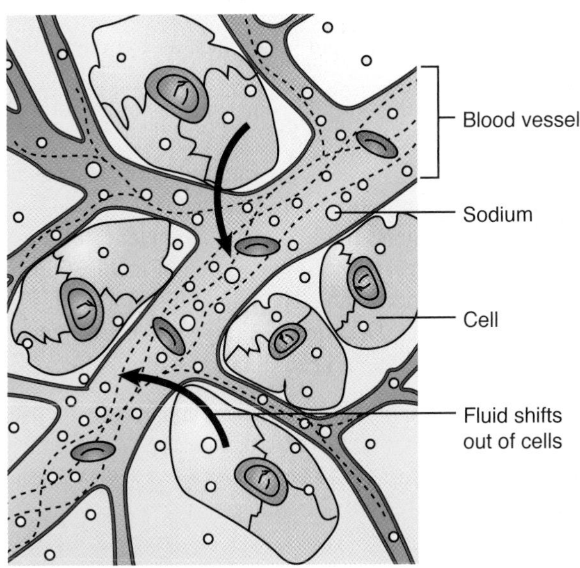

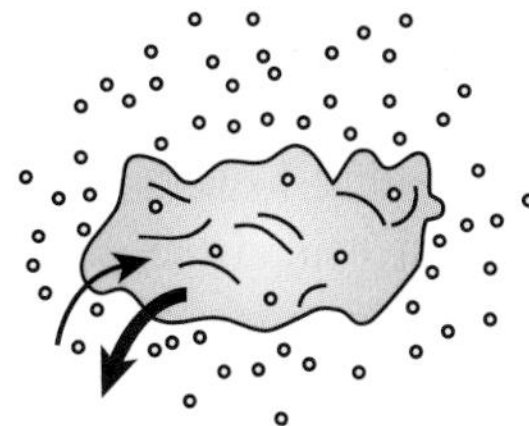

FIGURE 38.7 Fluid movement during infusion of hypertonic IV solution. The body tries to maintain balance when infusion of hypertonic IV solution raises the concentration of the blood. Then osmosis pulls the less concentrated interstitial fluid into the blood vessel to dilute the now more concentrated blood. This shifting causes the interstitial space to begin to dehydrate, increasing its concentration. This causes osmosis to pull the less concentrated intracellular fluid from inside the cells to the outside of the cells, where it can dilute the concentration of the interstitial fluid. The effect is cell shrinkage. If allowed to continue beyond the patient's level of need, the cells eventually will dehydrate, collapse, and lyse, ultimately destroying the cells, as seen in the diagram of a cell.

INTRAVENOUS EQUIPMENT

A wide variety of IV equipment is available for use, and advancing technology provides new and improved choices of equipment at an amazingly rapid rate. The equipment that you learn to use in development of your IV skills probably will not be in use 10 years from now. The equipment of basic IV therapy includes numerous varieties of the following components:

- **IV needle cannula or catheter:** a needle covered with a flexible plastic cannula that is used to access a peripheral vein and through which IV fluid can enter the vein. Once the plastic sheath has been advanced off the needle into the vein, the needle is removed (Fig. 38.8).
- **Winged butterfly:** a steel needle with plastic wings at the base of the needle, also known as a *scalp-vein needle* (Fig. 38.9). Used for shorter infusion times, usually less than 24 hours; for phlebotomy; and for when the longer, larger IV cannulas cannot be successfully inserted into a vein.

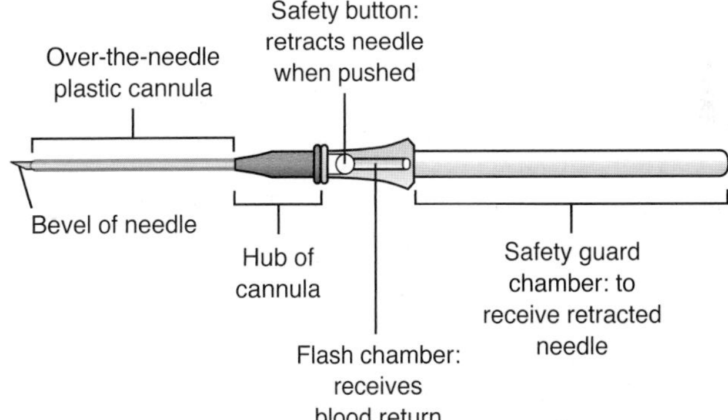

FIGURE 38.8 The parts of a safety IV needle with over-the-needle cannula: needle, bevel of needle, over-the-needle cannula, flashback chamber, hub, needle retraction button, and safety guard to receive retracted needle.

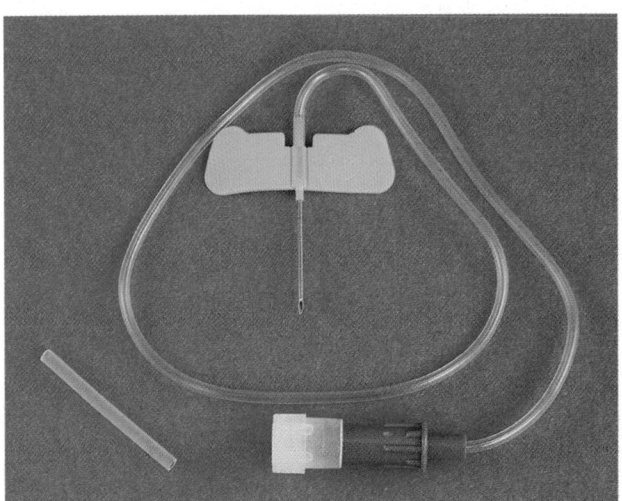

FIGURE 38.9 Winged butterfly device, also known as a scalp-vein needle (from Wilkinson JM, Treas LS. *Fundamentals of Nursing: Theory, Concepts & Applications*. Vol. 1. 3rd ed. Philadelphia, PA: FA Davis; 2016).

- **IV tubing:** tubing through which IV fluids may infuse from the IV bag to the patient.
- **IV infusion pump or controller:** an electronic or computerized pump/controller that is manually set to control the volume of solution to be infused and the rate of infusion.
- **Intermittent infusion IV access tubing or PRN locks:** devices that are designed to connect directly to the cannula and have an injection port on the opposite end through which medications can be intermittently infused without requiring a continuously infusing IV line (Fig. 38.10). The purpose of both PRN lock designs is to maintain venous access without continuously infusing fluids.
- **IV start kit:** a small kit containing generic supplies required to initiate an IV access device.

Intravenous Needle Cannula

The IV needle cannula comes in many different designs, lengths, and *gauges* (G), which means the diameter size of the inner bore of the hollow needle. The needle is covered by a plastic sheath called an *IV cannula* or *catheter*. The cannula is slightly shorter than the needle, allowing the bevel at the tip of the needle to extend just beyond the end of the cannula (refer to Fig. 38.8). Once the bevel of the needle, followed by the end of the cannula, has entered the vein, the cannula is carefully advanced off the end of the needle into the vein. Then the needle itself is removed. The process of advancing the IV cannula into the vein is known as **cannulation.**

IV cannulas have been found to be a better way to maintain IV access for a longer period of time than a regular steel needle. The plastic IV cannula does not irritate the vein as much as a steel needle. Neither does it become displaced by piercing through the other side of the vein as easily as a sharp steel needle.

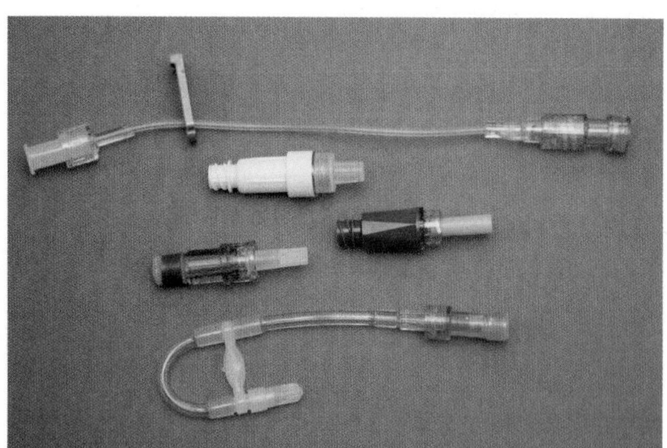

FIGURE 38.10 Various PRN lock injection port devices. Top: The "pigtail" PRN lock device has an injection port on one end of the PRN lock and on the other end a 4-inch extension tubing that ends in a Luer-Lok connection that screws directly onto the IV cannula hub; Middle: These three short PRN locks without attached extensions are about 1 inch (2.5 cm) in length and attach directly to the IV cannula hub; Bottom: This PRN device has an approximately 3-inch-long extension tubing that is shaped like the letter "J" and is hard and does not flex like the "pigtail."

The larger the gauge number, the smaller the diameter of the needle bore; the smaller the gauge number, the larger the diameter. The cannula sizes include even numbers from the tiniest 24 G (0.6 mm) to the very large 12 G (2.8 mm). They also come in different lengths from ½ to 2 inches (1.2 to 5 cm). The gauge and length to be used depend on the size of the vein to be accessed, the viscosity or thickness of the solution to be infused through the cannula, and the rate at which it is to be infused (Table 38.2). Larger-bore needles, such as 18 G (1.2 mm) to 20 G (0.9 mm), are used in the following situations:

- Administration of blood or blood product transfusions so that the viscous fluid can be rapidly infused
- When the risk of hemorrhage, fluctuation of vital signs, or shock exists, such as when a patient is scheduled for surgery
- When the patient has experienced some type of major trauma or disease and may need rapid infusion of fluids

Smaller-bore needles, such as 22 or 24 G, are indicated in the following situations:

- When the patient has small veins, such as a young child or older adult
- When the patient has fragile veins, such as older adults or those who have had repeated IV medications
- When IV access is needed only intermittently, such as to administer IV antibiotics every 6 hours
- When the purpose is simply to maintain patency of the access device in case IV administration of medications or fluids should be necessary. The rate of infusion in this situation is known as *TKO* (to keep [the vein] open), which is 20 to 30 mL per hour, according to facility policy.

The most commonly selected gauges and lengths for use in adult patients are 20 to 22 G (0.9 to 0.7 mm) and 1 to 1.5 inches (25 to 40 mm). Figure 38.11 presents a variety of IV cannula sizes.

Winged Butterfly

The winged butterfly is also known as a *scalp-vein needle*. It has two small plastic wings, one extending from each side at the base of a steel needle. Both wings fold upward to provide a place for you to grasp the device while initiating IV access. The two wings are designed to lie flush to the skin surface. Tiny, flexible tubing extending from behind the wings attaches

Table 38.2
IV Cannula Gauge Infusion Capability

IV Cannula Gauge	*Fluid Volume Capability*
20 G	Can infuse up to 3,900 mL/hr
22 G	Can infuse up to 2,200 mL/hr
24 G	Can infuse up to 1,400 mL/hr

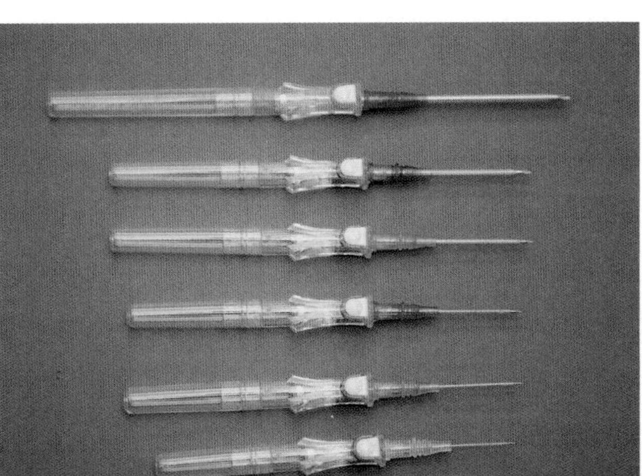

FIGURE 38.11 Various sizes of IV needles with over-the-needle cannulas: 14 G, 16 G, 18 G, 20 G, 22 G, and 24 G.

directly to the IV tubing. The winged butterfly sizes include the odd numbers from 19 to 29 G (1 to 0.3 mm) in diameter and from ⅜ to 1 inch (9.5 to 25 mm) in length (refer to Fig. 38.9).

Butterfly needles, though easy to insert and secure, infiltrate easier than a plastic over-the-needle cannula. The steel tip of the needle will more easily pierce the vein wall and allow seepage of solution into the interstitial tissues. Butterflies are mostly for short-term use, such as administration of single doses of IV push medication and *phlebotomy,* which is the drawing of blood samples. (Refer to Chapter 34 for further information related to phlebotomy.) Butterflies may be used to access scalp veins in newborns and infants up to 18 months of age for the infusion of IV fluids. The scalp veins are often selected in these infants due to the ease of securing the site on the head. Butterflies also may be used for patients in whom insertion of a typical IV cannula has been unsuccessful and IV therapy is required.

KNOWLEDGE CONNECTION

Describe what a cannula is. What sizes and lengths do they come in? Which is smaller, an 18-G (1.2-mm) or a 24-G (0.6-mm) cannula? Which VAD is commonly used to access a newborn's scalp veins?

Intravenous Tubing

IV tubing is flexible, small-diameter tubing that either delivers IV solutions and medication from the solution bag to the cannula in the patient's vein or provides an avenue to deliver solution from a second bag to the primary IV line of a different solution. IV tubing must have a sterile spike or piercing pin on one end to insert into the solution bag port. Extending just below the piercing pin is a **flange,** a hard plastic projection that provides a place for your fingers to push the piercing pin into the solution bag port without contaminating the sterile piercing pin. Immediately below the flange is a drip chamber that holds a small volume of the IV solution before it enters the IV tubing. The drip chamber is filled one-third to one-half full and is the site you will observe to determine that solution is flowing. If the IV fluid is being infused by gravity, you will observe the drip chamber to count the number of drops per minute. Some IV tubing has an in-line filter to remove any foreign particles that might be found in the IV solution. There will be clamps on the tubing to shut off solution flow and control the rate of flow. Different types of clamps you may see include a *slide clamp,* which simply allows solution to flow or stops the flow, and a *roller clamp,* which allows you to not only start or stop the solution flow but also to regulate the rate of infusion by rolling the clamp either tighter or looser. Some IV pump tubing has a cassette chamber that inserts into the pump mechanism. The opposite end of the tubing is the sterile end that inserts into the cannula hub. Both this end and the piercing pin are covered with caps when you take the tubing out of the package to help you in maintaining their sterility.

IV tubing comes in many different styles, and it would be impossible to discuss them all here. The following are the basic types that are commonly used:

- **Primary IV tubing administration set:** The long, main tubing that allows continuous flow of IV fluids. It may be designed to flow by gravity or to be used with a pump or controller.
  - **Primary IV administration set for infusion by gravity:** The primary tubing for gravity flow has one or more Y-injection ports and a roller clamp to control the infusion rate (refer to Fig. 38.4).
  - **Primary IV administration set for infusion by pump:** Each primary pump tubing is designed and dedicated solely for use with the specific pump indicated by the manufacturer. These sets are not interchangeable with different brands of IV pumps. Some have a small cassette chamber on them that inserts into the pump mechanism, and others do not.
- **Secondary medication (or IVPB) tubing administration set:** A shorter IV tubing, often termed *piggyback tubing,* that is used to administer medications at intervals. The tubing connects (piggybacks) to the most proximal Y-injection port of the primary IV tubing administration set (refer to Fig. 38.4).
- **Blood administration Y-set:** Tubing shaped like the letter "Y" (Fig. 38.12). Two piercing pins on two upper ends insert into the bag of blood product and the bag of NS used to accompany blood product infusions. The tail of the Y-set consists of a single tubing end that connects directly to the IV cannula in the patient's vein (Fig. 38.13).

Intravenous Tubing Extenders

There are various devices that may be used either to add length to the primary IV tubing or to connect the IV tubing directly to the IV cannula that is inserted into the vein.

- **Extension tubing** is a 6- to 24-inch length of tubing inserted between the patient's IV cannula and the primary IV tubing for the purpose of extending the length of tubing

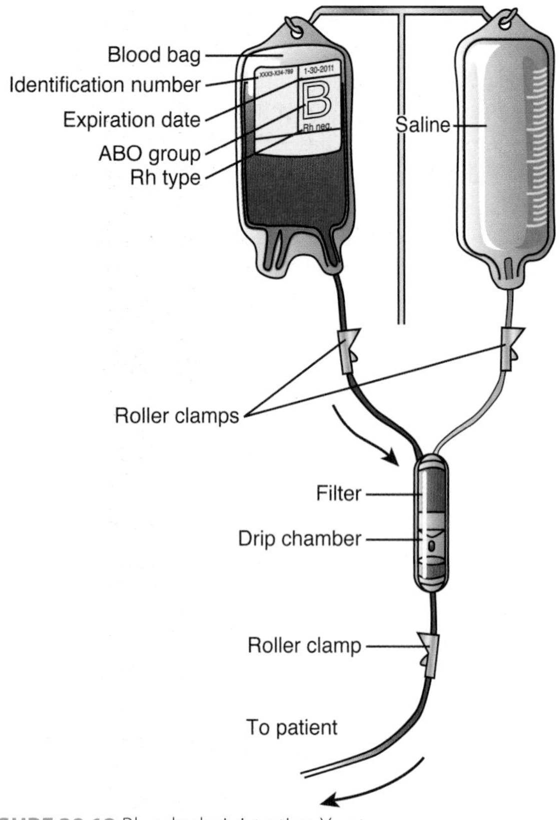

FIGURE 38.12 Blood administration Y-set.

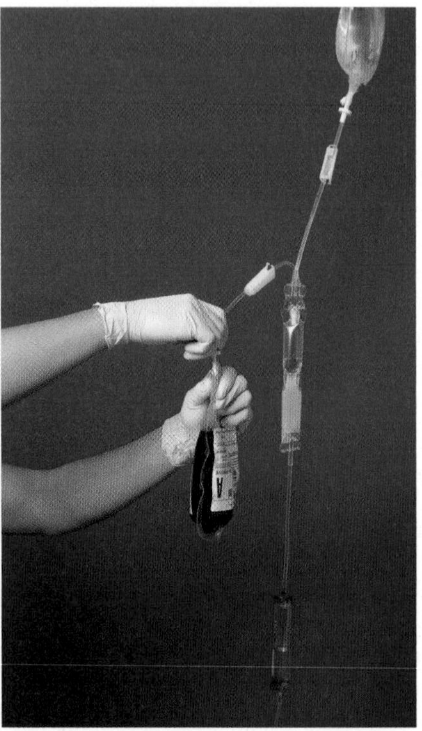

FIGURE 38.13 Blood administration Y-set primed with NS, showing insertion of the piercing pin into the unit of blood (from Wilkinson JM, Treas LS. *Fundamentals of Nursing: Theory, Concepts & Applications*. Vol. 2. 3rd ed. Philadelphia, PA: FA Davis; 2016).

to provide the patient with more mobility or to provide additional injection ports where medications can be injected directly into the patient's IV line.

- **Intermittent infusion lock or PRN lock** is a small device that attaches to the IV cannula inserted into the vein and provides an injection port on the end of it through which IV fluids or medications can be administered either continuously or at intervals (Box 38.2). Although technically not an IV tubing "extender," it may have a 1- to 4-inch length of tubing built into it (refer to Fig. 38.10).

KNOWLEDGE CONNECTION

What is the difference between a continuous IV infusion and a PRN lock? What does the term *patent* mean? What danger is inherent when using heparin to maintain patency of a PRN lock?

Real-World Connection

Reduced-Strength Heparin Versus Regular-Strength Heparin

A 7-month-old infant presented to the hospital's emergency room (ER) with *status epilepticus,* back-to-back seizures that would not stop. Over the course of several hours, the ER staff treated the infant with intermittent doses of IV anticonvulsant medication via an intermittent infusion lock. In between the doses of seizure medication, the nurse was to administer a dose of reduced-strength heparin, 10 units per 1 mL, to maintain the patency of the IV cannula. Later, after the infant had received at least seven doses of the anticoagulant, it was discovered that the nurse had mistakenly been administering full-strength heparin, at a concentration of 5,000 units per 1 mL, rather than the reduced-strength heparin designed for flushing intermittent infusion locks. Even though a dose of vitamin K was given as an antidote, the infant developed the signs of severe pallor, bleeding from the gums, and constant oozing from the intermittent infusion lock site. When the infant began to develop a decreased level of consciousness and vital signs became unstable, the infant was medi-flighted to a specialty children's hospital for intensive care. The problem? The accidental but massive overdose of anticoagulant had resulted in hemorrhaging within the brain. The infant did survive but suffered death of a sufficient number of brain cells, resulting in major neurological deficits and leaving the child in a vegetative state. The infant's mother filed a lawsuit against the first hospital and the nurses who made the mistake. What a horrible tragedy for the infant and the infant's loved ones. But the tragedy does not really end with the lawsuit. Imagine the burden of guilt that the nurses must live with, knowing that something as *basic* as *reading the label* could have prevented this immeasurable loss.

Box 38.2

Heparin Flushes

PRN locks are used to maintain venous access without continuously infusing fluids. To keep the vein *patent,* or open, the lock and IV cannula must be flushed intermittently with 1 to 10 mL NS, depending on health-care provider's orders and facility policy, usually once every 8 hours. Although it is now rare to see, you may see a health-care provider's order for heparin to flush a PRN lock. Flush-strength heparin is available in strengths from 10 units/mL to 100 units/mL. It is a very low-dose anticoagulant that was created solely for use in PRN locks. However, more concentrated strengths of heparin are used for anticoagulation therapy, and an excessive number of accidental overdoses occurred due to inadvertently flushing PRN locks with the higher concentrations of heparin intended only for anticoagulant use. Some of these overdoses resulted in serious hemorrhages and some in death. NS has been shown to be equally as effective at maintaining vein patency without the risk of overdose and is now used almost exclusively over flush-strength heparin. However, if you should receive an order for heparin to flush a PRN lock, remember the following safety guideline. ***Safety: When flushing a PRN lock with heparin, make certain to use the correct flush strength. Heparin also comes in much higher concentrations for treatment of life-threatening blood clots. It comes in 1,000 units/mL, 5,000 units/mL, 10,000 units/mL, and 20,000 units/mL*** (see the Real-World Connection box).

Each manufacturer produces various versions of each of these types of tubing, many to be used only with specific brands or models of IV pumps or infusers. You will need to familiarize yourself with the specific IV equipment and supplies used at the facility where you work.

Drop Factor

A characteristic that differs from one IV tubing to another is the *drop factor,* which represents the number of drops it takes for that specific tubing to equal 1 mL of volume of IV fluid (Fig. 38.14). The drop factor number may be found on the tubing package. If the drops produced by the tubing are large, it requires fewer drops to equal 1 mL of volume than it takes if the drops are smaller. The range of drop factors in IV tubing includes drop factors of 10, 15, 20, and 60, with 10 being the largest drop size and 60 being the smallest (Box 38.3). A drop factor of 10 simply means that it takes 10 of these *largest* drops to equal 1 mL of fluid. On the opposite end of the scale, a drop factor of 60 means that it takes 60 of these tiniest drops to equal 1 mL of fluid (Fig. 38.15).

The size of the fluid drop produced by the tubing is categorized as either a microdrop or a macrodrop. The tiny drops produced by tubing with a drop factor of 60 are known as *microdrops.* All the other drop factors produce larger drops and are known as *macrodrops.* The drop factor number is important because it is used in the formula to calculate IV infusion rates that you will be learning later in this chapter.

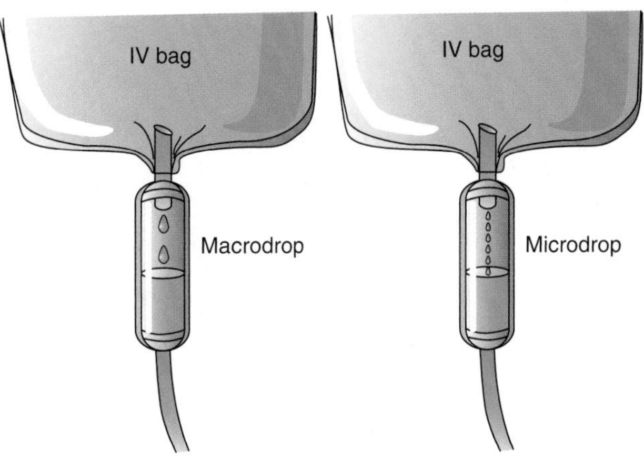

FIGURE 38.14 Drip chamber and number of drops equaling 1 mL.

Box 38.3

IV Tubing Drop Factors

The drop factor represents the number of drops that an IV tubing delivers to deliver 1 mL of fluid. The drop factor can be found on the tubing box.

- **Drop factor of 10:** 10 drops equals 1 mL
- **Drop factor of 15:** 15 drops equals 1 mL
- **Drop factor of 20:** 20 drops equals 1 mL
- **Drop factor of 60:** 60 drops equals 1 mL

KNOWLEDGE CONNECTION

Explain what is meant by *drop factor.* Where can you locate this information?

Needleless IV Systems and Safety Needles

In an attempt to reduce contaminated needle sticks among health-care workers, manufacturers have devised several needleless IV systems that do not require the use of sharp needles to inject medication into the tubing injection ports. The systems have incorporated the technology used in the manufacturing of medication vials that do not require the use of sharps to withdraw their contents. Numerous safety needles have been invented to make administration of intramuscular, subcutaneous, and intradermal injections safer as well.

The Occupational Safety and Health Administration has mandated that hospitals must use either safety needles, safety syringes, or needleless systems to decrease the risk of transmission of blood-borne pathogens such as HIV and hepatitis B via contaminated needle sticks. There are many such systems, each a little bit different than the other. Figure 38.16 presents an example of one type of safety syringe and how it works. It is your responsibility to be knowledgeable regarding the system that is used in your facility. Most of the current systems allow you to screw a Luer-Lok–tipped syringe directly to the injection port to inject medication into the IV line. Others require a needleless piercing device, or

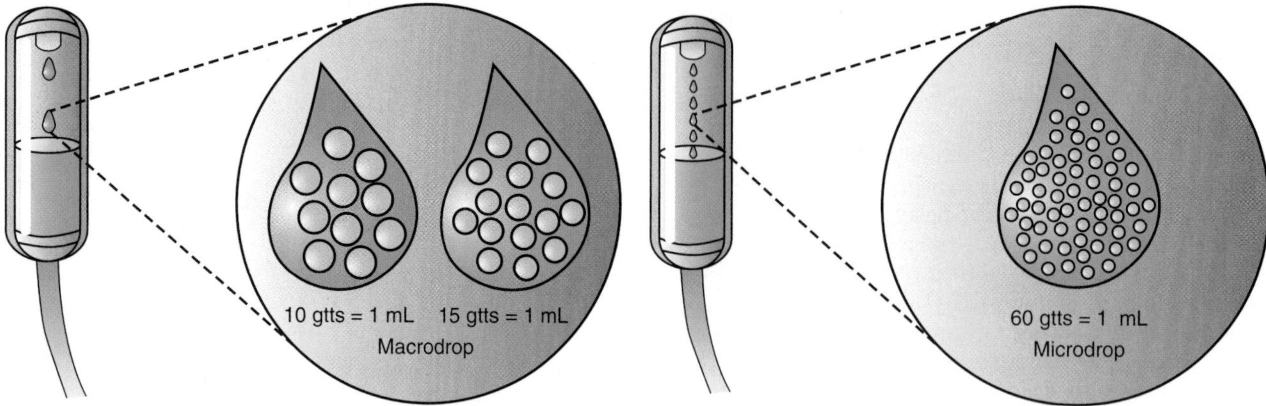

FIGURE 38.15 A tubing with a drop factor of 10: The drops are larger, and it takes 10 of these larger drops to equal 1 mL of fluid. On the opposite end of the scale is a tubing with a drop factor of 60: The drops are quite tiny, and it takes 60 of these tiniest drops to equal 1 mL of fluid.

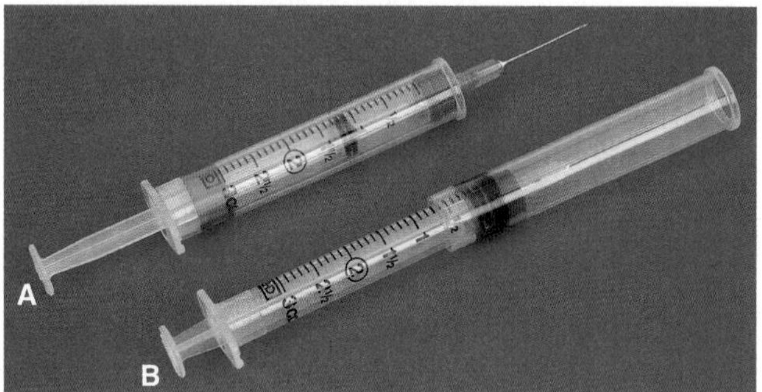

FIGURE 38.16 An example of one type of safety syringe (a) before and (b) after activation (from Wilkinson JM, Treas LS. *Fundamentals of Nursing: Theory, Concepts & Applications*. Vol. 2. 3rd ed. Philadelphia, PA: FA Davis; 2016).

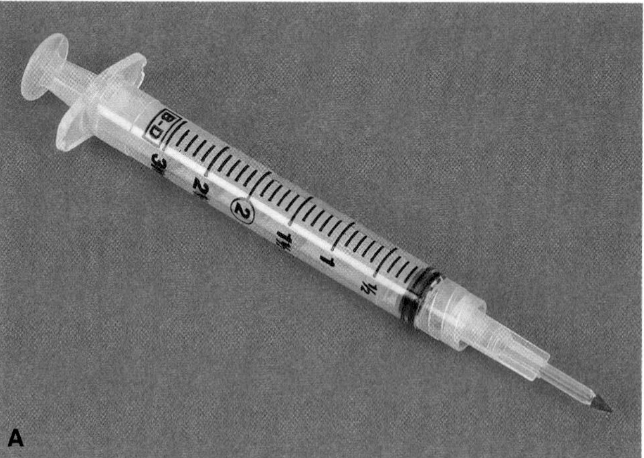

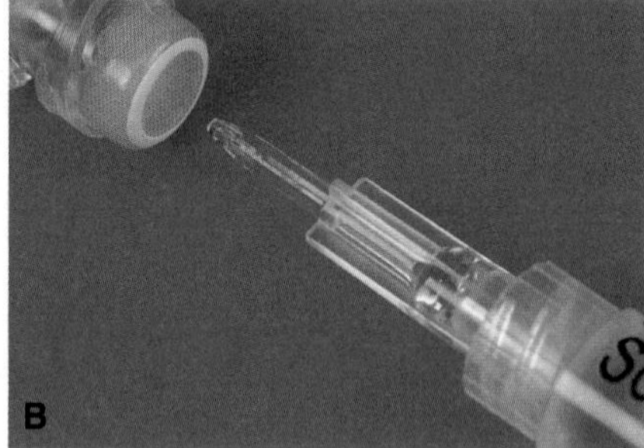

FIGURE 38.17 (a) Syringe with a needleless piercing device attached; (b) needleless piercing device which inserts into the needleless port designated by the white ring around the rubber port (from Wilkinson JM, Treas LS. *Fundamentals of Nursing: Theory, Concepts & Applications*. Vol. 2. 3rd ed. Philadelphia, PA: FA Davis; 2016).

blunt-tipped adapter, that inserts into the injection ports. Figure 38.17a shows a close-up of a syringe with an attached needleless piercing device.

IV tubing was also adapted to work with the safety needles and needleless systems. The rubber ports had to be designed so that blunt-tipped piercing devices could be inserted without destroying the rubber stopper, which would cause leakage and provide an open entry site for microorganism access. By gaining access to the once-sterile IV tubing, microorganisms had a direct route into the sterile cardiovascular system of the patient, resulting in sepsis and even death. Figure 38.17b shows an injection port with a white ring that indicates it is a needleless port designed to receive blunt-tipped piercing devices. Figure 38.18 shows a variety of needleless devices.

However, it is important to know that even though these safety needles and needleless systems are in place in most facilities, there are still some older styles of IV tubing and medication vials in use that do not accept these needleless piercing devices. ***Safety: Needleless blunt-tip adapters cannot be inserted into vials and injection ports of systems that are not designed to be needleless. To do so carries the potential of punching out a small core from the rubber stopper that falls into the solution and inside the IV tubing. This is known as "coring" and is not a safe practice. Most needleless systems are identified by a white or blue ring painted around the edge of the injection ports.***

Intravenous Infusion Pumps and Controllers

IV infusion pumps and controllers provide an immeasurable amount of protection against accidental infusion of too much fluid, as is possible when an IV solution is infused solely by

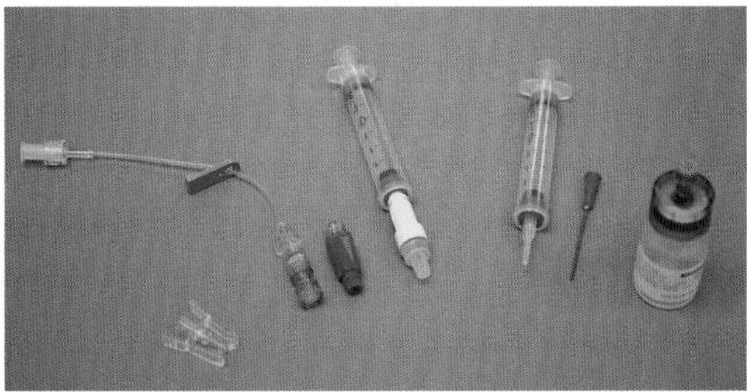

FIGURE 38.18 Various needleless supplies. From left to right: piercing device that secures with a clothespin-like clip; "pigtail" PRN lock; short PRN lock; safety syringe with attached piercing device inserted into a short PRN lock; safety syringe with attached piercing device ready for use; "blunt needle" piercing device; and vial converter cap, converting a regular vial to a needleless access vial.

gravity. When infusing by gravity, a 1,000-mL bag of IV solution conceivably could accidentally infuse the complete volume in an hour or less. This would present a very dangerous situation for the patient. Many patients would be unable to tolerate that much fluid instilled into their cardiovascular systems that quickly and could go into circulatory fluid overload and pulmonary edema. Elderly individuals and children are especially prone to fluid overload. You will learn more about this complication later in this chapter.

Each manufacturer produces an infusion pump that looks and works a little differently than other available products, but the premise is the same: They can be programmed to control the total volume of fluid to be infused and the rate of infusion and to coordinate primary fluid infusion with intermittent infusion of IVPB medications. Pumps provide accurate total volume infused over a particular period of time, such as an 8- or 12-hour shift (Fig. 38.19). They also have alarms to indicate when:

- The IV line is occluded
- Air is present in the line
- The IV bag is empty
- The preset volume of fluid has infused

It is easy to understand how infusion pumps increase the safety of IV therapy for the patient and save time for you, as well as providing an extra measure of safety for you.

KNOWLEDGE CONNECTION

How does use of an IV pump or controller provide a measure of safety for the patient?

Intravenous Start Kit

Many companies package the basic supplies that are used to initiate, or start, an IV access device (Fig. 38.20). These kits are designed exclusively for the health-care worker's convenience: It saves you the time of gathering the individual

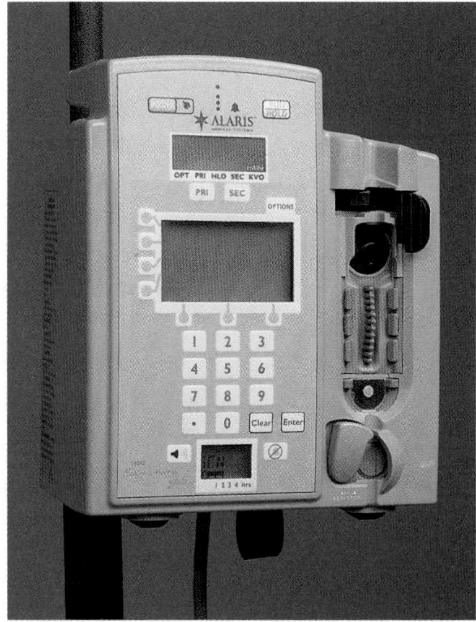

FIGURE 38.19 An example of an IV pump (from Wilkinson JM, Treas LS. *Fundamentals of Nursing: Theory, Concepts & Applications*. Vol. 2. 3rd ed. Philadelphia, PA: FA Davis; 2016).

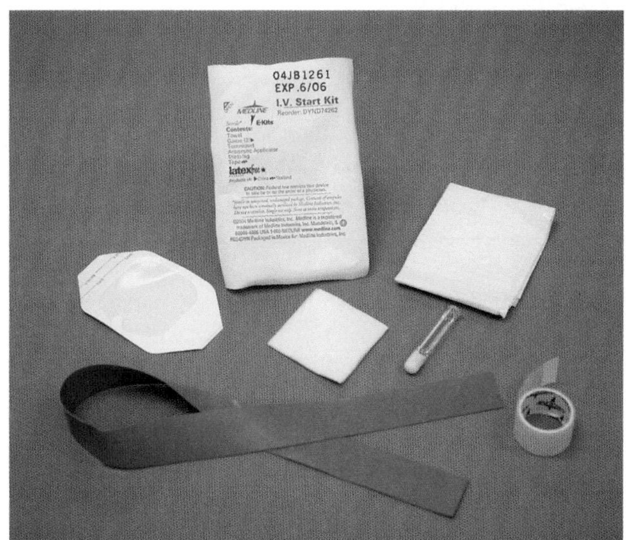

FIGURE 38.20 Typical contents of an IV start kit.

generic supplies that are required for virtually every IV access start. Usually included in these kits are the following items:

- **Tourniquet:** to block venous blood return while selecting a vein and making the initial stick
- **Antiseptic prep pad:** to cleanse the skin site to be punctured
- **Sterile 2×2-inch (5×5-cm) gauze pad:** to dry the puncture site before applying adhesive dressing
- **Sterile 2×3-inch (5×7.6-cm) transparent occlusive, semi-permeable adhesive dressing:** applied over the needle insertion site to reduce contamination by microorganisms
- **Label:** placed on the site dressing with date and initials to indicate when the IV access was started
- **Tape:** to secure the VAD

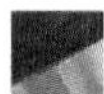

ASEPSIS AND INTRAVENOUS THERAPY

As you previously learned, the body's first line of defense against invasion by microscopic organisms is the skin. ***Safety: When this first line of defense is broken by piercing the skin with an IV cannula needle, you must use strict aseptic technique.*** Even with use of aseptic technique, the patient remains at risk for infection of the IV site. Infection at the site can progress to infection of the bloodstream, known as *sepsis,* which can be fatal. Even a local infection at the IV site, without progression to the bloodstream, can cause the following:

- Increase the patient's discomfort and anxiety; risk of **thrombus,** or blood clot, formation; and length of hospital stay and expense of hospitalization
- Decrease the patient's trust and rapport with health-care providers
- Increase the nurse's workload and liability

Therefore, use of asepsis during IV therapy cannot be adequately emphasized.

Handwashing

You must thoroughly wash your hands for at least 20 seconds immediately prior to handling any of the supplies you will be using for initiation of IV access or maintenance of IV therapy.

Gloves

Clean examination gloves are worn for any nursing care of IV therapy that places you at risk of contact with the patient's body fluids, including the following types of care:

- Initiating the IV access
- Changing the occlusive IV site dressing
- Touching a leaking IV site dressing
- Discontinuing an IV line
- Converting an IV infusion to a PRN lock
- Changing primary IV tubing
- Any care that requires you to come in contact with the insertion site or supplies used at the insertion site
- Any other nursing care of IV therapy that places you at risk of contact with patient body fluids

Supplies

Certain parts of IV supplies must be kept sterile at all times (Box 38.4). Once the IV access has been initiated, everything is connected, and fluids are infusing, you should have an enclosed sterile system from the inside of the solution bag through the tubing into the patient's vein. ***Safety: Any intrusion into the inside of this system requires that principles of strict asepsis be followed.*** This includes introduction of a needle, blunt-tipped adapter, or Luer-Lok syringe tip into either the solution bag or IV tubing at any injection port or connection.

The Infusion Nurses Society (INS) recommends that you change "continuously infusing" primary and secondary IV tubing at least every 72 hours and any time contamination of tubing is even suspected. If a facility's rate of IV-related infections increases using the 72-hour schedule, the INS recommends changing the continuous infusion tubing every 48 hours. INS also recommends that tubing used for "intermittent infusions," such as secondary tubing used for infusion of IVPB medication, be changed every 24 hours. The increased frequency of opening the sterile system to spike the next IVPB medication bag provides more opportunities for contamination, thus requiring more frequent changing. A bag of IV solution should never be allowed to infuse longer than 24 hours. It is common practice to dispose of any remaining solution and to hang a new sterile bag of solution every 24 hours.

A tourniquet must be used on only one patient before discarding it. Studies have shown that use of a tourniquet on multiple patients increases nosocomial infections.

Box 38.4

IV Supplies That Must Be Kept Sterile

Maintaining sterile technique during IV initiation is paramount. Because there are "specific parts" of each supply item that must be kept sterile, you will need to be able to identify them on sight while you are manipulating the supplies during IV initiation. You may find it helpful to locate the parts listed below on the actual items. If so, obtain (1) an IV needle with cannula, (2) a primary IV tubing, (3) a bag of IV solution, (4) a PRN lock, and (5) a transparent occlusive dressing. Identify the parts on each item that must be kept sterile:

- Entire length of the IV needle barrel and cannula or butterfly
- Opening to the hub of the IV cannula or butterfly that connects directly to the IV tubing end
- Open end of the IV tubing that connects into the IV cannula or needle hub
- IV tubing spike, or *piercing pin,* that enters the sterile IV solution bag
- IV solution bag insertion port into which the IV tubing spike enters
- IV solution being infused
- Adhesive side of the transparent occlusive dressing prior to application over the IV insertion site
- All direct connection points of tubing extensions or adapters

Patient's Skin

Safety: The skin site to be pierced with the IV cannula or needle must be thoroughly cleansed using the antiseptic agent specified in facility policy to reduce skin surface microorganisms. The following are the four solutions recommended by the INS:

1. 10% povidone-iodine
2. 2% tincture of iodine
3. 2% aqueous chlorhexidine gluconate
4. 70% isopropyl alcohol

• WORD • BUILDING •
nosocomial: nosocomi – hospital + al – related to

If povidone-iodine is to be used, assess the patient for allergy to iodine or shellfish. If the patient has no allergy, use alcohol to remove skin oils and then proceed with the iodine solution. Vigorously scrub the selected site for at least 20 seconds, beginning in the center and working outward in concentric circles until a 3-inch diameter circle has been cleansed. Avoid retouching the center of the cleansed area with the wipe that has touched the outer edges of the circle and the contaminated skin next to it. ***Safety: Touching the cleansed site with the gloved finger requires recleansing of the site prior to piercing the skin with a needle.*** Allow the solution to dry. If alcohol is the sole agent used, extend the scrub time to 30 seconds. Avoid using alcohol *after* povidone-iodine because it has been shown to negate the effect of the iodine.

KNOWLEDGE CONNECTION

Explain why asepsis is so important during IV initiation and maintenance therapy. Which parts of the IV catheter must be kept sterile? Which parts of the primary or main IV tubing must be kept sterile? For how long should you cleanse the skin site to be punctured?

CALCULATION OF INFUSION RATE

Many formulas have been devised to calculate the IV infusion rate. One formula that is simple to understand and that works for the calculation of both gravity infusion and infusion by pump is described in this chapter. However, before proceeding with the formula itself, there are a few things you must first understand:

1. You will hear several terms used to describe the rate at which an IV solution is to infuse into the patient. They include *infusion rate, flow rate, drop rate,* and *drip rate.*
2. These terms are not to be confused with the *drop factor.*
3. When infusing an IV solution by *gravity,* the drop factor is printed on the tubing container. It will be stated as a number of "*drops per mL.*" Do not confuse this factor with "drops per minute," which refers to the rate of infusion. The drop factor tells you how many drops that specific tubing must "drip" to equal 1 mL of fluid, or "*drops per mL.*"
4. When using a *pump* or *controller,* the *drop factor is always 60.* It does not matter which drop factor is printed on the tubing box because the machine is electronically designed to equal the drop factor of 60 since the pump is set in milliliters per hour (mL/hr) rather than drops per minute (gtts/min).
5. When the IV solution is to infuse via *gravity,* the infusion rate (or flow rate, drop rate, or drip rate) is measured by visually counting the number of *drops per minute.*
6. When the IV solution is to infuse via an IV *pump* or *controller,* the pump electronically measures the infusion rate in *milliliters per hour.*
7. The abbreviation for *drops* is *gtts.*

Until you have a working knowledge of calculating IV infusion rates, you should memorize these seven points. This will make using the following formula easier to learn.

Three numbers are required in order to use this formula:

1. Specified volume of fluid that is to infuse
2. Amount of time, in minutes, in which the specified volume of fluid is to infuse
3. Drop factor of the tubing/pump

The formula to calculate an IV infusion rate is:

$$\frac{\text{Volume} \times \text{drop factor}}{\text{Time}} = \text{rate of infusion},$$

where *Volume* is the volume of fluid to be infused, *Time* is the time (in minutes) in which the specified volume of fluid is to infuse, and the rate of infusion is measured in mL/hr if an IV pump is used or in gtts/min if gravity flow is used.

For this formula to work, you must make certain that *Volume* and *Time* are directly related. For example, if you are calculating the rate for the *Volume* of the entire bag, the *Time* must be the number of minutes, not hours, for the entire bag to infuse. If the entire bag of *1,000 mL* of fluid is to infuse in 2 hours; you would perform the calculation using *120 minutes* for *Time.* If the *1,000 mL* is to infuse in 4 hours, you would use *240 minutes* for *Time.* If the order is to run the *1,000 mL* bag for 8 hours, you would use *480 minutes* for *Time* in the formula.

However, if you are just calculating the rate of infusion for a 50-mL bag of IVPB antibiotic that must infuse within *1 hour,* you would use *50 mL* for *Volume* and *60 minutes* for *Time.* Remember, the *Volume* of fluid to infuse must correlate with the *Time* in which it is to infuse. Skill 38.4 (page 894) covers calculation of the IV infusion rate.

Most IVPB medications will be infused over a period of 15, 30, 45, 60, or 90 minutes. If the health-care provider and pharmacy both fail to provide you with the length of time for infusion of a specific medication, you can find this information in a drug book. It is your responsibility to know the appropriate length of time to infuse medication.

Practice

The only way to be able to correctly calculate IV infusion rates is to practice until you are competent and confident that you fully understand the formula and what each number represents, the actual working steps of the problem, and the application of the process to specific situations. Some sample problems are included in Table 38.3, in the workbook, and on the DavisPlus Web site.

KNOWLEDGE CONNECTION

If you are to infuse D5W 500 mL at 30 mL per hour to keep the vein open, at how many drops per minute would you set the gravity flow rate? You must administer the following IVPB antibiotic: ampicillin 500 mg in D5W 50 mL over 20 minutes. At how many drops per minute would you set the gravity flow rate? At how many milliliters per hour would you set an IV pump for this same IVPB?

Table 38.3
Sample Calculations of IV Infusion Rates

Infusion Order	*Calculations for* *Gravity Infusion (measured in gtts/min)*	*Pump Infusion (measured in mL/hr)*
Infuse Unasyn 500 mg in D5W 50 mL IVPB over 15 minutes (Tubing drop factor: 20)	$\frac{50 \text{ mL} \times 20}{15 \text{ min}}$ = 66.6 or 67 gtts/min	$\frac{50 \text{ mL} \times 60}{15 \text{ min}}$ = 200 mL/hr
Infuse vancomycin 1 g in NS 250 mL IVPB over 90 minutes (Tubing drop factor: 10)	$\frac{250 \text{ mL} \times 10}{90 \text{ min}}$ = 27.7 or 28 gtts/min	$\frac{250 \text{ mL} \times 60}{90 \text{ min}}$ = 166.7 or 168 mL/hr
Infuse gentamycin 80 mg in D5W 100 mL IVPB over 30 minutes (Tubing drop factor: 15)	$\frac{100 \text{ mL} \times 15}{30 \text{ min}}$ = 50 gtts/min	$\frac{100 \text{ mL} \times 60}{30 \text{ min}}$ = 200 mL/hr
Infuse IV LR 1,000 mL over 10 hours (Tubing drop factor: 15)	$\frac{1{,}000 \text{ mL} \times 15}{600 \text{ min}}$ = 25 gtts/min	$\frac{1{,}000 \text{ mL} \times 60}{600 \text{ min}}$ = 100 mL/hr
Please note that the above order would be the equivalent of infusing 100 mL in 1 hour. These numbers came from dividing the total volume (1,000 mL) by the number of hours (10) in which it all should infuse (1,000 ÷ 10), to get the number of mL that should infuse in 1 hour (1,000 ÷ 10 = 100 mL/hr). It allows you to work with smaller numbers than calculating the entire 1,000-mL bag.	$\frac{100 \text{ mL} \times 15}{60 \text{ min}}$ = 25 gtts/min	$\frac{100 \text{ mL} \times 60}{60 \text{ min}}$ = 100 mL/hr

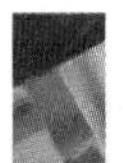

INITIATING PERIPHERAL VENIPUNCTURE

Before you initiate peripheral venipuncture, whether it is to infuse fluids or to place an intermittent infusion lock, review the facility's policy for the procedure and review the patient's medical record for several pieces of information.

Medical Record Review

Review the health-care provider's orders for verification of what is to be done. Review the patient's medical record to determine the patient's condition, including his or her medical diagnoses and reason for IV access, as well as the patient's age, mental cognition, and allergies.

Health-Care Provider's Order

Make certain that the health-care provider's order includes the date, time, type of solution, size of solution container, route, indication, and infusion rate. Note whether there is an order for additives such as vitamins or potassium chloride.

Patient's Medical Condition

You need to know not only the patient's current admission diagnosis but also his or her medical history. Does the patient have congestive heart failure or other cardiac problems? Does he or she have renal disease? Does the patient have any chronic respiratory problems? All of these affect the patient's ability to receive different types of fluids and rates of infusion. Is this patient stable or unstable? Is the patient at risk for hemorrhaging or going to surgery? Why does the patient need IV access? All of these things help to determine what gauge of IV intracatheter would be appropriate, what type of fluid is needed, and whether or not the patient can receive faster rates of infusion.

Patient's Age and Mental Cognition

How old is the patient? Is he or she an infant, child, teenager, adult, or older adult? Infants and children do not require the same fluid volumes as teenagers and adults. They are unable to tolerate a fast rate of infusion. Many older adults also are intolerant of faster rates of infusion. IV infusion of fluids in infants, small children, and elders must be controlled and observed even more frequently than in average adults for signs and symptoms of circulatory fluid overload. Younger children and confused patients have added risk because of their inability to call for a nurse when needed.

Allergies

Assess whether the patient is allergic to iodine, medications, latex, or tape. Nonlatex gloves and tourniquets are available for use with patients with latex allergies. A BP cuff can be used in place of a tourniquet in patients who are allergic to latex or rubber. Numerous types of tape are available for use when the patient is allergic to a particular type, including paper, silk, plastic, micropore, and old-fashioned adhesive tape. As you read earlier in this chapter, other types of antiseptic solutions are available for site preparation if the patient is allergic to iodine.

KNOWLEDGE CONNECTION

What assessment data should you collect prior to initiating an IV access? Why should you review the facility policy for a skill you are about to perform?

Preparing the Equipment

Identify your patient using two methods of identification. Introduce yourself and explain the procedure, answering any questions the patient might have. To assist you in determining which gauge of IV cannula to bring, assess the patient's veins for size and characteristics.

Safety: Wash your hands for at least 20 seconds. Obtain the correct volume container of the ordered IV solution. Check the label three times as you would any medication, checking the type of solution and the expiration date. Check the bag for leaks by squeezing the bag and inspecting for pinhole leaks. If there are any leaks in the bag, the solution is considered contaminated and should be discarded. Inspect the solution for clarity, ensuring there is no cloudiness or any floating particulates.

Calculate the rate of infusion, in mL/hr for pump infusion and in gtts/min for gravity infusion. Label the solution container, including the patient's name, room number, date, rate of infusion, time infusion is to start, and your initials. If an additive is ordered, fill out a red or other bright-colored medication label as dictated by facility policy and attach it to the solution container. Add the appropriate dose of additive to the solution. Skill 38.5 (page 895) provides more information on adding medications to a primary IV solution.

Obtain an infusion pump or controller if available and an IV pole. Following the instructions accompanying the pump or controller, set the pump button labeled "Primary VTBI" (volume to be infused) for the total volume of primary IV solution that is to be infused; also set the health-care provider ordered rate of infusion button that is labeled "Primary Rate." The rate will be measured and marked with "mL/Hr" as the unit of measurement. It is helpful to set the VTBI setting at a few milliliters less than the actual total volume in the bag. This will prevent the bag from running dry, which can allow air to enter the drip chamber and proximal end of the IV tubing. For example, if the solution bag holds 1,000 mL, set the pump VTBI setting around 940 or 950 mL. When the pump alarm signals that the VTBI has been infused, you will still have fluid left in the bag. You can then set a new VTBI at 30 or 40 mL, giving you adequate time to obtain the next bag of solution and hang it before the original bag runs dry.

Obtain the required tubing administration set that works with the pump or one designed for infusion by gravity flow if a pump is not available for use. Inspect the packaging of the sterile IV tubing administration set, ensuring that it is still intact and not expired. Remove the tubing from the package and close the roller clamp. Remove the cap from the solution container port. Aseptically insert the piercing pin of the tubing set into the port on the solution container. Read the instructions on the package for priming the tubing set because each set is designed to prime differently, especially those with a cassette feature that inserts into the pump mechanism. Prime the tubing according to instructions, ensuring that all air is removed from the tubing set. Replace the sterile cap on the end of the tubing. Do not insert the IV tubing into the IV pump until after cannulation has been verified by free flow of IV fluid in the drip chamber by gravity. You do not want it attached to the pump to force fluid into the vein until you are certain that the site is not going to swell.

Most nurses prefer to bring the two different sizes of IV cannulas or winged butterflies that would work for the patient's medical diagnosis, condition, and reason for IV access as well as the preview of vein size and characteristics. The final selection of cannula size and length will be made after you make further assessment at the bedside. Get a towel or waterproof pad to protect the bed. Gather an IV start kit or the individual supplies that would be contained in the kit.

KNOWLEDGE CONNECTION

What preparation does the container or bag of IV solution require? What should you assess before opening packages containing IV tubing administration sets? What data must you enter into an IV pump or controller prior to use?

Selecting a Vein

The most common veins used in peripheral IV therapy include the veins of the forearm. On the forearm, the cephalic, basilic, median cubital, median antebrachial, and accessory cephalic veins are the superficial veins commonly used (Fig. 38.21).

If there are no suitable veins on the forearm, the dorsal side of the hand may be used, but this is not the best choice because of the proximity of nerves and tendons. Cannulation of hand veins can limit the patient's use of the hand, so use of the nondominant hand is preferred over the dominant hand. If use of the hand veins becomes necessary, the basilic vein, metacarpal veins, and cephalic veins are used (Fig. 38.22).

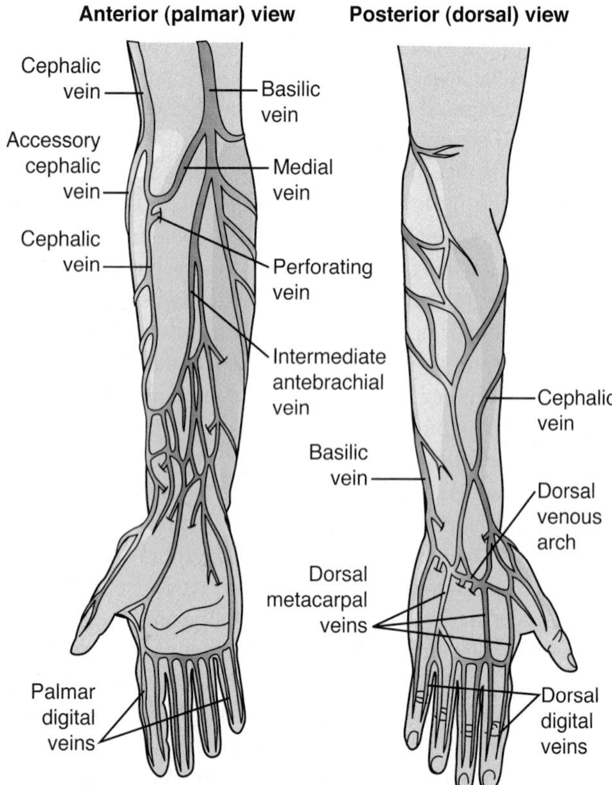

FIGURE 38.21 The superficial veins of the forearm.

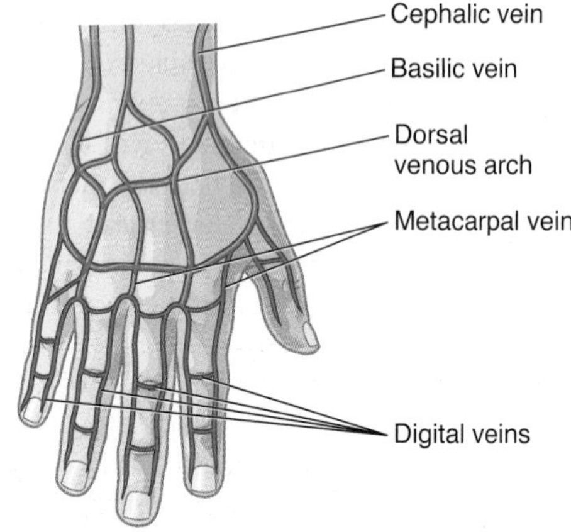

FIGURE 38.22 The superficial veins of dorsal aspect of hand (from Wilkinson JM, Treas LS. *Fundamentals of Nursing: Theory, Concepts & Applications*. Vol. 1. 3rd ed. Philadelphia, PA: FA Davis; 2016).

Leg veins are the farthest veins from the heart and are used only as a last resort, although sometimes they are the only veins accessible in infants or small children. It is not advisable to use the leg or foot veins in elders or anyone with peripheral vascular disease because of the decreased circulation to the extremities. A facility may have a policy requiring a health-care provider's order before an IV access can be initiated in a lower extremity.

Once a vein has been pierced and cannulated, the vein should not be accessed distally for IV restarts. An IV restarted distal to a previously used site has an increased chance of infiltration. A site proximal to the previous site should be used if another IV cannula must be inserted into the same vein. If the patient is apt to have IV therapy for several days, it is best to select the most distal vein that is suitable.

KNOWLEDGE CONNECTION

Locate and name the common forearm veins used for IV therapy on your arm and on another classmate's arm. If an IV restart becomes necessary, what are the limitations for selecting the next vein to cannulate?

Apply the tourniquet proximal to the elbow; inspect and palpate the veins. Make certain that the distal arterial pulse is still palpable after application of tourniquet. You only want to occlude the venous blood flow, not the arterial blood flow. Select a vein that is large enough to accommodate the gauge of IV cannula needed for the patient's condition. You also want to choose a vein that is stable and does not roll when you palpate it. Feel for bumps and observe for vein *bifurcations,* which are where veins separate into two branches. These are both indications of valves in the veins, whose purpose is to control the direction of blood flow back toward the heart. Inserting the IV needle into a valve may result in damage that can cause blood to pool distally from the damaged valve. Any time blood pools, there is an increased risk of thrombosis.

A good vein should feel slightly rounded, spongy, resilient or elastic, and bouncy, but not flat. It is always best to initiate an IV access in the patient's nondominant arm if at all possible. This allows the patient free use of the dominant hand. Do not use extremities on the same side as a mastectomy, paralysis, or a dialysis access device. Avoid selecting a vein site that:

- Extends over a flexible joint
- Feels sclerosed or hardened
- Is bruised, red, or edematous
- Lies adjacent to an infected area
- Has been recently used for IV therapy or is distal to a recent stick site
- Is too small for the IV cannula
- Has a bump or bifurcation indicating a valve
- Rolls

Once the vein has been selected, remove the tourniquet to allow return of blood flow while you set up your work site. There are several ways to increase the blood flow to the veins if further dilation is needed (Box 38.5). If the vein selected for IV initiation is located over a flexible joint because

• WORD • BUILDING •

sclerosed: skleros – hard

bifurcation: bi – two + furc – fork + ation – action

Box 38.5

Tips for Dilating Veins

At times the patient on whom you need to start an IV will not have a clearly visible or palpable vein. There are several simple techniques you may use to help stimulate vein dilation. In almost all situations except life-and-death emergencies, the few extra minutes that it may take you to perform one, or even all, of these techniques will serve you well. The majority of the time, being patient and working to stimulate the veins will provide you with a more appealing vein, increase your confidence, and reduce the number of attempts to cannulate the vein. However, the greatest and most important benefit belongs to the patient who will not be forced to endure more needle sticks than absolutely necessary. Try the following techniques:

- Use gravity by allowing the extremity to hang dependent off the side of the bed to a position lower than the heart for several minutes.
- Apply a BP cuff rather than a tourniquet.
- Have the patient squeeze a rolled-up washcloth or rubber ball, clasping and unclasping the fist several times.
- Apply moist, warm packs to the extremity for 10 to 15 minutes.
- Use an alcohol wipe and friction to rapidly wipe back-and-forth over the vein for several seconds.*
- Use the thumb and middle finger to gently flick the skin over the vein.*
- ***Note: Avoid slapping the patient's skin with your hand. It really stings and is uncomfortable.***

*These two methods of stimulation cause a release of histamine under the skin, which dilates the vein.

of the lack of other suitable sites, you will want to stabilize the joint after the IV access has been initiated. This is done by placing the patient's hand or arm on top of an arm board and wrapping it securely, but not so tightly as to impair venous return, with an Ace bandage, roller gauze, or Coban, a stretchable roller bandage that is secured when it sticks to itself (Fig. 38.23).

KNOWLEDGE CONNECTION

What are the characteristics of a *good* vein for IV therapy? Why should you avoid puncturing a vein where there is a known valve? Which vein sites should be avoided for IV therapy?

Performing Final Preparation of Supplies

After selecting the vein, place a towel underneath the patient's extremity to protect the bed from blood drips. It will save you a linen change. Open and arrange all your supplies on the towel so that each item is within easy reach. You want to avoid reaching or turning to pick up an item while you are holding the cannula, which cannot be bent or crimped. Inspect the cannula and needle bevel for intactness and burrs. Open several alcohol

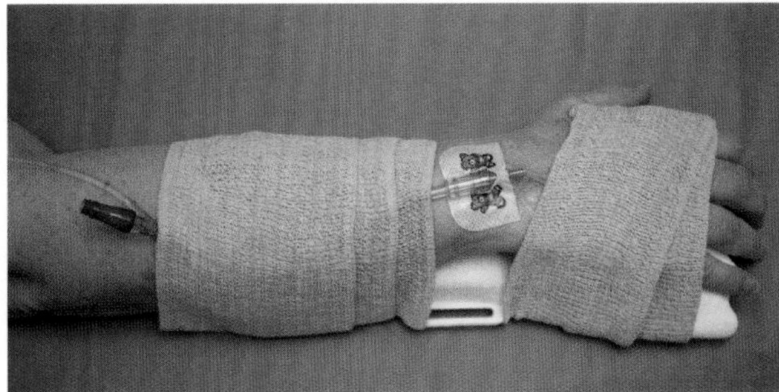

FIGURE 38.23 Hand with IV secured to arm board with Coban. IV site is beneath the wrap, so IV would be positional when wrist is bent.

wipes to use to clean the puncture site after cannulation of the vein and prior to applying the dressing. Place the capped sterile end of the IV tubing or PRN lock on the towel so that it can be easily reached when it is time to connect it to the cannula hub. Label the IV tubing set according to facility policy so that nurses will know when to change the tubing.

If you have not already applied clean examination gloves, do so at this point before proceeding. Position your body in linear alignment with the patient's arm. This is done by positioning the patient's arm in front of you so that, when you look straight ahead, you are looking linearly up the arm. In other words, you are lined up with the arm as if you are an extension of the hand. Avoid trying to start an IV access with your body perpendicular to the arm (standing to the side of the arm). Linear alignment allows you optimal visualization of the IV catheter needle and its relationship to the selected vein you are attempting to cannulate. Because you are lined up with the arm and vein, it also allows you to have a more accurate mental image of the exact location of the vein as it extends beyond your point of needle insertion.

Make a visual *marker* to help you know the exact location and path of the vein even when you cannot see the vein but can palpate it. This may help prevent the need to palpate the vein location again after you have already cleansed the site, thus contaminating the intended insertion site.

Prepare the sterile end of the primary IV tubing by making certain the cap over the sterile end has been slightly loosened so that you will be able to easily remove the cap once you have advanced the cannula into the vein. Place the tubing end, with the cap loose but still covering the sterile tip, within easy reach on your work surface, towel, or waterproof pad. This decreases the risk of inadvertently pulling the cannula out of the vein while reaching for the tubing to connect it to the cannula.

KNOWLEDGE CONNECTION

Why is positioning of your body in relationship to the patient's arm important? Explain the purpose of arranging all IV initiation supplies on the towel or protective pad work surface directly in front of you prior to attempting vein cannulation.

Cleaning the Site

Next, cleanse the site with the antimicrobial agent indicated by facility policy. Use the method of cleansing described earlier in the section on asepsis and IV therapy.

> **KNOWLEDGE CONNECTION**
>
> Describe the proper technique for cleansing the site chosen for venipuncture, including the length of time to spend scrubbing the site. Is it a problem to confirm the location of the vein by palpating the site with your gloved hand immediately prior to puncturing the skin? Explain your answer.

Performing Venipuncture and Cannulation

Without contaminating the cleansed site, apply the tourniquet 4 to 6 inches proximal to the selected site. (Refer to Chapter 34, Skill 34.1, page 766, for application instructions.) Place your nondominant hand distal to the intended puncture site. Use your thumb to pull the skin taut, which will stabilize the skin and underlying vein. This should help to prevent the vein from rolling. Make sure your hand pulling the skin taut is an adequate distance from the site to prevent contamination of your needle and cannula when you perform the venipuncture. If the selected site is the distal portion of the forearm, flex the patient's wrist to help pull the skin taut.

Safety: The needle must be inserted in the same direction that the venous blood flows, back toward the heart. Hold the flashback chamber of the needle in your dominant hand with the bevel up. Line the needle up linearly with the vein, as if the vein were an extension of the IV catheter needle. Inform the patient of the ensuing prick. Hold the needle at a 20- to 30-degree angle to perform the venipuncture. A very superficial or fragile vein may necessitate decreasing the angle to 15 degrees, while a deeper vein on an obese patient may require an increase in the needle's angle up to 45 degrees. Pierce the patient's skin and vein using one of following two methods: direct or indirect.

- **Direct method:** a one-step method that consists of puncturing the skin and the vein in one motion or movement of the needle. Useful for entry into rolling veins, fragile veins, and hand veins and when using smaller-gauge needles, such as 22 G (0.7 mm) or 24 G (0.6 mm).
- **Indirect method:** a two-step method. First, the skin is pierced parallel to the vein, and then the tip of the needle is angled toward the vein and gently inserted into the vein. Useful for entry into all veins.

Once the bevel of the needle enters the vein, you will see blood enter the flashback chamber, commonly known as a *flash* or *blood return.* Lower the angle of the needle, advance the needle and cannula as one unit just far enough to ensure that the entire bevel of the needle and the end of the over-the-needle cannula are inside the vein, and then stop. ***Safety: Never advance the full length of the needle while still inside the cannula as one unit into the vein.*** Use your nondominant thumb and index finger to carefully advance the over-the-needle cannula off the end of the needle into the vein lumen.

If the cannula remains in the vein as you advance it, you should observe a steady backflow of blood. While advancing the cannula off the needle, make certain your dominant hand holding the flashback chamber does not move. If you experience difficulty advancing the cannula all the way, sometimes it helps to "float" it in with IV solution. After advancing the cannula as far as it will go:

- Remove the needle
- Attach the IV tubing
- Open the roller clamp on the IV tubing
- Allow a slow infusion of solution
- Use your nondominant hand to reapply traction to the vein
- Use your dominant hand to attempt further advancement of the cannula into the vein

After you have advanced the full length of the cannula into the vein, use the nondominant hand to gently release the tourniquet. Then place the middle or ring finger of your nondominant hand on the vein proximal to the end of the cannula to block venous flow. Use your thumb and index finger to stabilize the needle hub against the patient's skin without contaminating the skin puncture or the sterile open end of the hub. Use your dominant hand to activate the needle retraction device or remove the needle manually from the inside of the cannula. Quickly pick up the end of the IV tubing or PRN lock, remove the cap from the sterile end, and insert the end into the needle hub without contaminating the tubing end or needle hub.

Safety: Never use your teeth to remove the cap from the sterile end of the tubing and avoid trying to remove the cap from the end of the tubing using only one hand. You are bound to contaminate the end of tubing. It is safer to make certain the cap is loosely attached to the tubing just before performing the venipuncture. Then when you pick up the tubing with your dominant hand, you can place the capped end between two of the fingers of your nondominant hand that is occluding the vein and securing the cannula hub. A gentle grasp of the cap by the two fingers will allow you to easily and gently pull the tubing end from the cap with your dominant hand and yet maintain its sterility. This requires good fine motor skills and practice. Initially, until you have become skilled using this or an equivalent technique, you may want to simply have a classmate or instructor present who can assist you by removing the cap from the sterile end of the tubing.

Encountering Difficulty

If your initial venipuncture does not produce a blood return into the flashback chamber indicating that you are in the vein, you will simply continue using the indirect method: The skin has been punctured, but you are not in the vein. Continue to use your dominant hand to hold the needle in place. Before moving the needle again, use the index finger of your nondominant hand to relocate the vein. Feel the skin just proximal to the insertion site. Without contaminating the insertion site, locate the end of the needle and its position in relation to the intended vein. When a needle is not in the vein, it has to be in one of four places: on top of the vein, to the right side of the vein, underneath the vein, or to the left side of the vein. It is important to know the needle's location and proximity to the vein before you make further attempt to enter the vein.

Lower or increase the needle's angle, according to the depth of the vein. Try again to enter the vein. If you are at the side of the vein, you will need to angle the needle *just slightly* toward the vein. If you are under the vein, you will need to *pull the needle back slightly* to reposition it for entry. ***Safety: If using an over-the-needle cannula, you must place the index finger of your dominant hand on the colored hub of the plastic needle while you gently pull the needle and cannula back as one unit. If you do not hold the cannula hub, the inner needle will pull back without the cannula. Once this occurs, you cannot reinsert the needle into the plastic cannula. Doing so could sever the tip of the cannula, creating a migrating embolism requiring emergency surgical removal of the severed cannula tip.*** After repositioning the needle, gently insert the needle into the vein, avoiding quick movements such as jabbing or stabbing because they can cause pain and damage nerves and veins.

You will want to limit the number of unsuccessful venipuncture attempts on a patient to no more than three times. Then it is best to ask another nurse to try to start the IV access. No one likes to "miss" the vein during venipuncture, but all of us will be unsuccessful at one time or another, even nurses who are highly skilled at venipuncture. Do not allow initial unsuccessful attempts to discourage you. Continue to take advantage of opportunities to perform venipuncture until you become confident and skilled. Skill 38.6 (page 896) provides more information on initiating peripheral venipuncture.

KNOWLEDGE CONNECTION

What degree of angle is commonly used to puncture the vein? If it is a fragile vein lying close to the surface, what degree of angle will serve you better? What area of the IV catheter needle do you hold while inserting it? How will you initially determine you have accessed the vein? Which part of the IV catheter and needle is advanced its full length into the vein lumen?

Determining Proper Cannulation

Once you have secured the IV cannula, flush the IV with 1 to 10 mL of 0.9% sodium chloride (NS) flush. Observe the venipuncture site for swelling as the fluid flows in. Site swelling is indicative of displacement of the IV cannula outside the vein. Immediately close the roller clamp and remove the cannula from the vein.

If the normal saline flush is hard to push, there is some type of problem with the cannulation. You may try pulling the cannula back just slightly, not even ⅛ inch. If it is just lying against a valve or the wall of the vein, this will allow it to free-flow. It is also wise to assess that all the clamps on the tubing are open and that there are no crimps in the tubing that might slow the fluid flow. Once you have verified free flow of fluid with no site swelling, you may proceed to secure the site.

Securing the IV Site

Secure the Luer-Lok by screwing it onto the cannula hub. Avoid screwing it tightly; the Luer-Lok connects securely without excessive tightening. Clean all blood from the connection and skin with alcohol wipes, using care not to bend the cannula where it attaches to its hub. Use the sterile 2×2-inch (5×5-cm) gauze pad to dry the skin. Peel the backing from and apply the transparent occlusive dressing over the site and the hub of the cannula. Do not cover the Luer-Lok connector on the IV tubing (Fig. 38.24). Doing so would necessitate removal of the primary sterile dressing just to change the IV tubing. (If your facility does not use transparent occlusive dressings, apply the type of sterile dressing dictated by facility policy.)

After applying the transparent occlusive dressing, apply several 3- to 4-inch (7.6- to 10-cm) pieces of tape to secure the Luer-Lok connection and the first 6 to 8 inches (15 to 20 cm) of the IV tubing to the patient's arm. Place a small label on the dressing indicating the date and time of venipuncture, gauge and length of needle, and your initials.

KNOWLEDGE CONNECTION

Why is it important to determine proper cannulation of the vein with gravity free flow of IV solution prior to inserting the tubing administration set into the pump? Why is it recommended to cover the puncture site with a sterile transparent occlusive dressing?

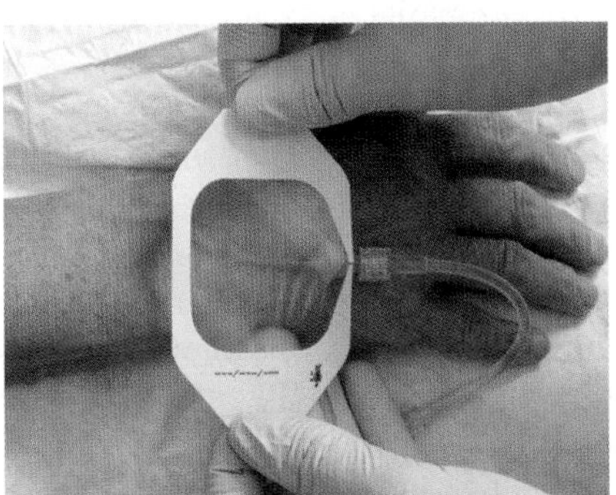

FIGURE 38.24 Applying transparent occlusive dressing to new IV site (from Wilkinson JM, Treas LS. *Fundamentals of Nursing: Theory, Concepts & Applications*. Vol. 2. 3rd ed. Philadelphia, PA: FA Davis; 2016).

Starting the IV Pump

Place the IV tubing in the IV pump according to the manufacturer's instructions. Open all tubing set clamps. Check that the volume to infuse and the rate of infusion both are correctly set. Start the pump and assess its proper function. Reassess the venipuncture site for swelling or leaking. Make certain the patient is feeling no discomfort at the site before you leave the room.

Setting Gravity Infusion Rate

If the solution is to infuse by gravity, hold your watch with a second hand next to the drip chamber on the IV tubing. Count the number of drops that fall during 1 minute. Does it match your calculations? Use the roller clamp to adjust the flow until you achieve the desired rate (Fig. 38.25).

Here is a time-saving hint: Divide by four the total number of drops per minute that you calculated prior to beginning the infusion. That will be the number of drops that should infuse per 15 seconds. Adjust the flow with the roller clamp and recount the drops until you obtain the desired number of drops per 15 seconds. Once you have regulated the drip rate for the 15 seconds, count the drops for an entire minute to ensure that the rate is correct. By counting the number of drops for 15 seconds, you will save 45 seconds every time you have to regulate the roller clamp. This generally will save you anywhere between 1 and 5 minutes; this may not sound like much time, but over the course of a shift, every 5 minutes you can save is better used somewhere else. Refer to the Calculation of Infusion Rate section earlier in this chapter for further assistance.

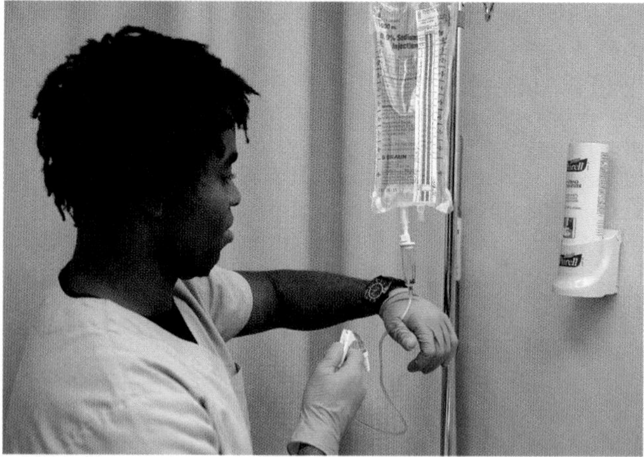

FIGURE 38.25 Counting the number of drops per minute to calculate a gravity flow infusion rate.

KNOWLEDGE CONNECTION

What is the formula for calculating the infusion rate? What unit of measurement is used for gravity flow infusion rates? An infusion controlled by a pump?

Monitoring Intravenous Infusions

You should monitor the rate of infusion and the condition of the IV site frequently. The site and surrounding tissue should be assessed for the signs and symptoms of infiltration (Box 38.6), phlebitis (Box 38.7), and infection. ***Safety: The accepted nursing standard for frequency of IV site assessment is to assess and document the condition of the site at least every 2 hours in an adult and every 1 hour in children, the elderly, and those patients who might be prone to circulatory fluid overload.*** Some experts even recommend assessment of the site every hour in adults. Your facility may have policies that differ from these standards. If the facility policy dictates assessment to be done at *shorter* intervals, you must perform it accordingly. However, if the facility policy dictates *longer* intervals, such as every 4 hours, you are ethically and legally held to the more frequent schedules. Refer to Figure 38.26 for an example of electronic documentation of IV site assessment.

Box 38.6
Signs and Symptoms of Infiltration

Assess adult IV sites at least every 2 hours, and more often if indicated, for the following signs and symptoms of infiltration. Assess IV sites every 60 minutes in infants, children, and older adults.

- Blanching or pallor of skin around site
- Complaint of tightness or discomfort around site
- Edema at site
- Lack of blood return upon lowering IV solution bag or aspirating with needle and syringe
- Site cool to touch
- Sluggish flow or lack of infusion
- Solution leakage at site
- Taut skin around site

Box 38.7
Signs and Symptoms of Phlebitis

Each time you assess the IV site for infiltration, also assess for the following signs and symptoms of phlebitis, or vein inflammation.

- Edema of site
- Erythema at site
- Increased warmth at site compared to surrounding area
- Reports of burning or discomfort at IV site or along vein track
- Sluggish infusion rate
- Vein feels like a hard cord when palpated

Monitor the volume of solution remaining in the primary bag so that you are prepared and have time to obtain the next ordered bag of solution before the hanging bag runs completely dry. Plan to prepare the next bag of solution when there is still a minimum of 50 to 100 mL of solution remaining. Skill 38.7 (page 900) provides more information on adding a new bag of IV solution to the existing IV line.

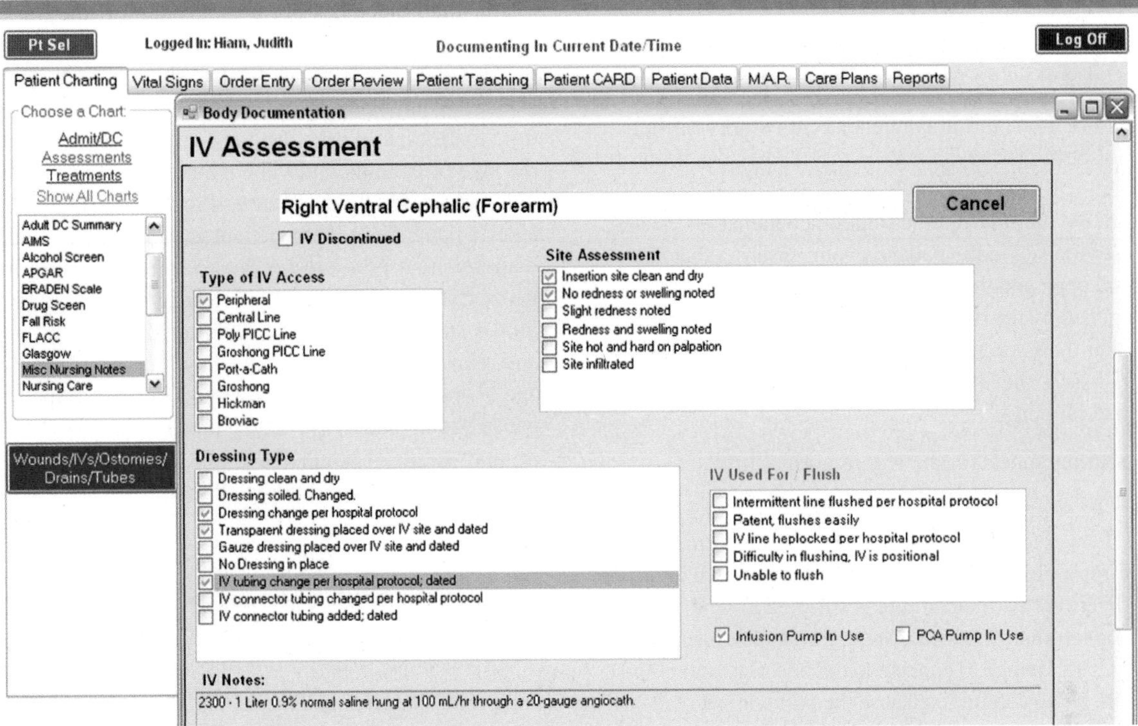

FIGURE 38.26 Example of electronic documentation of IV site assessment (from Wilkinson, Treas LS. *Fundamentals of Nursing.* Vol. 2. 3rd ed. Philadelphia, PA: FA Davis; 2016).

Documenting the Venipuncture

Document the venipuncture, including the date and time; gauge, length, and type of needle; site of placement; number of attempts it took; type of fluid and size of fluid container; whether it is flowing by gravity or pump; rate of infusion; site assessment; any difficulties experienced; and how the patient tolerated the procedure. (Refer to the sample documentation at the end of Skill 38.6.)

KNOWLEDGE CONNECTION

How frequently should you assess an IV site in a child? In an adult without risk of fluid overload?

Elder Care Connection

Performing Venipuncture in Elders

Venipuncture of elderly persons can present different challenges. Sometimes their skin is very thin, fragile, and even somewhat transparent. Their veins often are tiny, fragile, and sclerosed, making it easy to go completely through the vein with the needle. Here are some hints to make venipuncture of elders a little easier:

- Avoid use of a tourniquet if possible: Fragile veins often "blow" or rupture, causing a hematoma, when a tourniquet is used. If a tourniquet is needed, it is less uncomfortable and easier on their fragile skin to apply the tourniquet less tightly and over the sleeve of the patient's gown.
- Use a BP cuff in place of a tourniquet: Position it at least 6 inches proximal to the site of intended venipuncture. Pump it only 10 to 20 mm Hg higher than the diastolic pressure.
- Avoid excessive friction or prolonged tapping as methods to distend the vein: It is best to use the smallest gauge needle and cannula that is available, usually 22 G and 1 inch (0.7 mm × 25 mm) in length. Use no more than a 15-degree angle of the needle during venipuncture.
- Be selective when choosing tape to use on fragile skin: Silk or micropore tape usually will come off without tearing the fragile skin, as plastic and adhesive tape can do. Some nurses prefer paper tape for fragile skin, while others feel that if any moisture comes in contact with paper tape once applied to the skin, it becomes similar to glue.
- Be careful when removing tape: When removing any type of tape from fragile skin, use adhesive remover to loosen the adhesive. Then, after lifting the end of the piece of tape, *use your fingers to gently pull the skin from the tape* as opposed to *peeling the tape from the skin.* This helps to prevent skin tears.

Problem-Solving

If the IV solution stops infusing or the pump alarms *occlusion,* take the following steps:

- Make certain the solution container is not empty or that the pump setting for *volume to be infused* has not been completed.
- Inspect the IV tubing from the solution container all the way to the insertion site in the patient's vein, ensuring that all clamps are open and that the tubing has not been inadvertently pinched by the bed rails or by the patient lying on it.
- Ensure that there are no air bubbles in the tubing or pump cassette. Assess the site for signs and symptoms of infiltration and phlebitis.

If everything appears to be within normal limits:

- Remove the solution container from the pump and IV pole. Lower the bag below the level of the vein. Observe for a blood return in the cannula hub, which is an indication that the cannula is still in the vein.
- If no blood return is obtained, hang the container back on the IV pole. Use a syringe to connect to the injection port closest to the vein, being careful to cleanse the port with alcohol first. Pinch the tubing proximally to the port while aspirating with the syringe. Observe for a blood return. If no blood is returned, the cannula is no longer in the vein and must be removed. If there is a vacuum when you attempt to aspirate (if the syringe does not allow you to aspirate), most likely there is a blood clot obstructing the end of the cannula. The cannula should be discontinued and the IV restarted. ***Safety: Do not use NS to force flush or push the clot from the end of the cannula.*** The clot then becomes an embolism that can migrate to and occlude vessels in major organs, causing necrosis of tissue. You may see other nurses do this, but it is not acceptable and presents a clear danger to your patient.

Discontinuing an Intravenous Infusion

When you have a health-care provider's order to discontinue an IV infusion or PRN lock, or there is a problem that necessitates removal, turn off the IV pump. Then close the roller clamp, apply clean examination gloves, and gently remove the tape securing the tubing set to the arm. Use adhesive remover if needed.

While securing the cannula hub with your nondominant hand, lift each of the four transparent occlusive dressing edges toward the insertion site. Use caution to avoid crimping or bending the plastic cannula where it attaches to the hub. Once the transparent occlusive dressing is completely loosened from the patient's skin, use your nondominant hand to apply pressure with a sterile 2×2-inch (5×5-cm) gauze pad *proximal* to the end of the cannula that is still within the vein. ***Safety: Do not apply pressure over the cannula itself or you can dislodge the cannula from the hub and free it to migrate through the vascular system as an embolism.*** Allow your hand applying pressure on the vein to slide toward the puncture site as you carefully remove the cannula from the vein using your dominant hand.

While removing the cannula, maintain a pull that is parallel to the vein. Inspect the cannula to be sure that it is intact and that a small piece has not been broken off the tip. Once the cannula is completely out of the vein, apply firm pressure with the 2×2-inch (5×5-cm) gauze pad directly over the puncture site to prevent bleeding and bruising while allowing the blood time to clot. Hold pressure for 1 to 2 minutes, depending on the size of cannula and vein. The larger they are, the longer you may need to hold pressure. If the vein is fragile, as in some elderly patients, or if the patient is taking anticoagulant medications, hold pressure for 3 to 5 minutes before lifting the gauze to assess cessation of bleeding. While holding pressure on the site, cleanse the surrounding skin with alcohol wipes and allow to air dry. Once bleeding has ceased, apply a bandage or apply a piece of tape to hold a clean 2×2-inch (5×5-cm) gauze pad in place. Instruct the patient to remove the bandage or tape within 24 hours. Skill 38.8 (page 901) provides more information on discontinuing an IV infusion or PRN lock.

KNOWLEDGE CONNECTION

Explain the danger of forcing a blood clot from the end of the IV cannula so that the IV solution will drip again. What are the steps you should take in problem-solving a pump warning of *occlusion?* What is the risk of applying manual pressure against the cannula in the vein during removal? How long do you hold pressure on the site after removal of the cannula?

Supervision/Delegation Connection

IV Push and IVPB Medications

IV access initiation and administration of IV push and IVPB medications should not be delegated to CNAs or UAPs. These invasive skills should be performed by either a trained and certified LPN/LVN or an RN. It is helpful and provides a certain degree of protection for a nurse to have documented proof that he or she has received formal IV therapy training and testing. While some practical and vocational nursing schools include IV certification in their programs, others do not. Some state nurse practice acts prohibit the LPNs and LVNs from performing IV therapy.

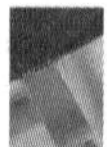

COMPLICATIONS OF PERIPHERAL INTRAVENOUS THERAPY

Due to the invasive nature of IV therapy, it has potential for numerous complications that can have serious or fatal consequences:

- **Infiltration:** leakage of nonvesicant IV fluid or medication into the tissue surrounding the IV insertion site;

• WORD • BUILDING •

nonvesicant: non – not + vesicant – blistering

nonvesicant means that it does not cause blistering and death of tissue

- **Extravasation:** leakage of vesicant IV fluid or medication into the tissue surrounding the IV insertion site; **vesicant** means that it causes blistering, necrosis, and sloughing of tissue
- **Phlebitis:** inflammation of the inner layer, or *intima,* of a vein
- **Thrombophlebitis:** inflammation of a vein in conjunction with the formation of a thrombus
- **Localized infection:** infection at the IV cannula insertion site
- **Septicemia:** life-threatening infection of the bloodstream
- **Severed cannula:** a piece of the IV cannula breaks off inside the vein
- **Air embolism:** obstruction of a blood vessel by an air bubble traveling through the circulatory system
- **Circulatory fluid overload:** excessive fluid volume within the cardiovascular system
- **Speed shock:** shock caused by rapid IV infusion of medication/solution

Infiltration

Infiltration can be caused by displacement of the IV cannula outside of the vein, either at the insertion site or by piercing through the other side of the vein, allowing nonvesicant fluid to leak from the vein into the surrounding tissues. Other causes of infiltration include puncturing the other side of the vein during venipuncture, excessive movement of the cannula inside the vein, or a too-rapid rate of infusion of IV fluid. Signs and symptoms of infiltration include the following:

- Edema around or dependent to the site; a good way to detect edema is to compare both arms
- Cool, pale, or taut skin around site
- Absence of or decreased blood return upon lowering the solution bag below the level of the insertion site or when aspirating with a syringe at an injection port close to the IV site
- IV fluid will not infuse at all or will only infuse at a slow rate, even when the tubing clamp is wide open
- Complaint of discomfort at the IV site or proximal to it
- Blanching around the insertion site or proximal to the end of the IV cannula

Prevention

Assess the IV site for edema, erythema and increased skin warmth, pallor and coolness of skin, leaking of IV solution, drainage, patency of site, and patient reports of discomfort at least every 1 hour in infants, children, older adults, and anyone who might be at risk for fluid volume overload. Keep the IV site well secured to reduce movement of the cannula.

Nursing Care

The IV infusion should be immediately discontinued and restarted as needed. The extremity should be elevated and positioned according to patient comfort. Warm or cool packs may be applied to the site according to facility policy.

Extravasation

Safety: Extravasation, the leakage of vesicant medications into the subcutaneous tissues, can have serious consequences. The initial indications of extravasation are the same as those for infiltration. An alert patient may complain of significant pain at or proximal to the IV site, or the site may exhibit erythema or edema.

The extent of tissue damage will be dependent on the specific type and concentration of medication, as well as the volume of vesicant fluid that has leaked into the tissues. There may be blistering and death of tissue. The necrotic tissue sloughs and can leave an extensive crater that will have to granulate and heal by second or third intention or be surgically covered with grafts. Extravasation can result in disfigurement, loss of function, and even amputation of the extremity. Box 38.8 provides a list of vesicant medications.

Prevention

Safety: When infusing vesicant medications, the dorsal hand should not be used for IV placement because it is more prone to tendon and nerve damage. Assess the IV site at least every 2 hours for adults and every 1 hour for infants, children, older adults, and anyone who might be at risk for fluid volume overload. Always assess IV site condition prior to administering IV medications. Be knowledgeable regarding all medications you administer intravenously so that you are aware of which ones are vesicants.

Nursing Care

As soon as extravasation is even suspected, stop the infusion, leave the cannula in place, estimate the volume of extravasated vesicant fluid, and notify the health-care provider immediately. Stat response and treatment must be carried out to reduce the amount of damage to tissues. The prescribed antidote is instilled into the tissues after aspirating any residual vesicant solution from the cannula. Elevate the affected extremity and apply either cold or heat packs according to the drug manufacturer's recommendations or facility policy. Document the situation in the patient's medical record. Depending on the extent of damage, long-term wound care, surgical débridement, skin grafts, cosmetic surgery, or amputation may be required.

Phlebitis and Thrombophlebitis

Inflammation of the intima of the vein without a blood clot is known as *phlebitis,* while inflammation in conjunction with a thrombus is termed *thrombophlebitis;* both cause burning, tenderness, or pain at the IV site. The skin at the site will become erythematous and feel warmer than the unaffected skin surrounding the phlebitis. Edema may or may not be present. The vein may feel hard or cordlike. The infusion rate may

• **WORD • BUILDING** •

extravasation: extra – outside of + vas – vessel + ation – action

thrombophlebitis: thrombo – blood clot + phleb – vein + itis – inflammation

Box 38.8

Vesicant Medications

When allowed to extravasate into surrounding tissues, a vesicant medication causes blistering. Some of the more commonly used vesicants are listed below by drug classification.

Antibiotics
Amphotericin B
Cefoxitin sodium (Mefoxin)
Erythromycin
Nafcillin
Tetracycline
Vancomycin

Anticonvulsants
Phenytoin
Valium

Antiemetics
Promethazine

Chemotherapy Drugs
Cisplatin
Streptozocin
Vincristine

Electrolytes
Calcium chloride and calcium gluconate
Potassium chloride

become sluggish. The presence of a thrombus adds the risk of it breaking away from the vein wall and becoming a moving embolus.

The following are factors that contribute to the development of phlebitis:

- Using a vein that is too small
- Using an IV cannula that is too large
- Failure to change the IV site at least every 72 hours
- Infusion of irritating or caustic medications
- Poorly secured IV site allowing excessive motion of the IV cannula inside the vein
- Contamination of insertion site during IV initiation
- Failure to use strict asepsis during IV therapy
- Failure to treat infiltration quickly

Prevention

When proactive steps are not taken to prevent it, phlebitis becomes a fairly common complication of peripheral IV therapy; thrombophlebitis does not occur as often. Be proactive and do not let any of the listed factors occur.

Nursing Care

There are numerous actions you should take to help prevent phlebitis. As previously noted, it is important to select the correct size of both IV cannula and vein. Maintain strict asepsis during IV initiation and IV maintenance. Secure the IV cannula hub to the extremity with tape to prevent movement or dislodgment. Also secure to the arm the first 6 to 8 inches (15 to 20 cm) of the IV tubing from where it connects into the IV cannula. Infuse concentrated or irritating drugs only through larger central venous lines whenever possible. Assess the IV site at least every 2 hours for signs and symptoms of infiltration and phlebitis. As soon as any are noted, take immediate action to remedy the problem.

If phlebitis develops, stop the flow of the IV fluid and discontinue the IV cannula. Elevate the affected arm on pillows. Apply warm moist packs to the site for 20 to 30 minutes every 2 hours until signs of phlebitis are gone. If there is purulent drainage from the puncture site or red streaks going up the arm, or if fever develops indicating infection, the site should be cultured. Antibiotics most likely will be required. If thrombophlebitis develops, administration of an anticoagulant may be necessary.

KNOWLEDGE CONNECTION

What signs and symptoms indicate infiltration? Phlebitis? Contrast infiltration to extravasation. Why is it important to know which drugs are vesicants? What nursing intervention should you perform after removal of a cannula because of phlebitis?

Localized Infection

Once a needle pierces the skin, the body's first line of defense against infection is breached. Even though the skin is cleansed and the needle is sterile, there still is a great risk of site infection. If microorganisms gain access to the site, infection sets in. Infection is manifested by erythema, edema, discomfort, purulent drainage, and fever.

Prevention

Prevention is key. ***Safety: Strict asepsis is required for all contact with any parts of the infusion system, during IV initiation, and throughout the span of the entire infusion.*** The following actions are included in prevention:

- Handwashing thoroughly for at least 20 seconds prior to contact with any aspect of the IV set-up
- Using alcohol-based hand cleanser after handwashing according to facility policy
- Visually examining IV solution containers for cloudiness of fluid, leaks, and expiration date
- Using the facility's approved antiseptic pads to thoroughly cleanse the skin prior to needle stick
- Maintaining strict asepsis of the IV needle, cannula, or winged butterfly
- Covering the site with a sterile dressing, preferably a clear adhesive dressing, which allows visual observation of the immediate site
- Firmly securing the IV cannula hub and IV tubing

- Assessing and documenting the condition of the IV site at least every 2 hours in adults and every 1 hour in children, elders, and patients prone to circulatory fluid overload
- Changing the IV site dressing if it becomes moist or soiled
- Removing the IV cannula at the first sign of inflammation or contamination
- Never allowing a solution container to hang longer than 24 hours
- Changing the IV site and IV tubing every 48 to 72 hours based on facility policy

Nursing Care

The initial step to assess inflammation is to perform a phlebitis score. The phlebitis score ranges from 0 to 4, 0 meaning no symptoms and 4 being the most severe. The initial treatment is the same as for phlebitis: Discontinue the IV cannula and apply warm packs to the site for 20 to 30 minutes every 2 hours until drainage and erythema have abated. *Applying a warm pack allows the fluid to be reabsorbed into the body.* The health-care provider probably will order antibiotics. Monitor the patient for further worsening of his or her condition.

Septicemia

Once a vein becomes inflamed and infected, it is possible for the microorganisms to travel through the bloodstream and cause system-wide infection, known as *septicemia.* Left untreated, septicemia quickly becomes life-threatening. More than one-fourth of septicemia cases due to IV therapy are fatal. Signs and symptoms include the following:

- High fever
- Chills and shivering
- Diaphoresis
- Nausea, vomiting, and diarrhea
- Tachycardia
- Tachypnea
- Hypotension
- Confusion
- Backache

Prevention

Assess for signs and symptoms of localized infection and discontinue the IV infusion upon detection. Notify the physician for new orders.

Nursing Care

The top priority once you suspect septicemia is to stop the IV flow and notify the physician stat. Discontinue the IV infusion and, according to facility policy or the physician orders, culture the cannula tip, tubing, and fluid. Restart a new IV infusion in the other extremity using a completely new setup, including cannula, tubing, and fluids. The physician will generally order blood cultures and IV antibiotics to be administered. It will be necessary to monitor the patient and vital signs closely for worsening of the patient's condition.

> **KNOWLEDGE CONNECTION**
>
> What are the signs and symptoms of local infection at the IV site? Of septicemia? What is the difference between the two diagnoses? List at least eight ways you can help prevent these infections.

Severed Cannula

The plastic IV cannula that is left in the vein after the steel needle is removed is extremely fragile and bends or crimps very easily. Crimping and flexing of the cannula increase the risk of the cannula separating from the hub or a piece of the cannula breaking off to become an embolus. An embolus can result in occlusion of vessels, including those of the heart and lungs, and can be fatal. Signs and symptoms include sudden sharp pain at the IV site, chest pain, cyanosis, tachypnea, tachycardia, and hypotension.

Prevention

Prevention is the best course of action. ***Safety: Take care to avoid bending the cannula during IV initiation and maintenance.*** Secure the site to minimize movement of the cannula. Avoid applying pressure directly over the cannula while removing an IV cannula from the vein. During IV initiation, use caution to prevent bending the cannula while you are connecting the tubing and securing the site. Avoid insertion of the IV cannula across a flexible joint.

Nursing Care

If a cannula does break away from the hub or a piece of the cannula breaks off inside the vein, immediately apply strong manual pressure on the vein several inches proximal to the insertion site. The goal is to prevent the cannula embolism from traveling from the periphery into the central circulation. Some facilities have policies dictating application of a tourniquet just proximal to the antecubital area. Notify the physician and radiology personnel stat. Start a new IV line in the opposite arm. Measure the remaining cannula length that you removed to determine the length of the severed cannula now acting as an embolism.

Air Embolism

An air embolism can occur if a large volume of air is introduced into the patient's vascular system. The occurrence of air embolism is rare in peripheral IV therapy, but the risk is there. It is more commonly seen with cannulation of central veins. The exact amount of air deemed to be fatal is not known, and a rapid rate of infusion of the air is as important as the amount of air infused. Signs and symptoms of air embolism are cyanosis, dyspnea, chest or shoulder pain, hypotension, tachycardia, and loss of consciousness.

Prevention

The first step in prevention of air embolism is to prime the IV tubing, PRN devices, and extensions before connecting them to the IV cannula. Remove all air from the syringe before injecting medication into the IV line. All tubing connections should have Luer-Lok tips if possible. If they do not have Luer-Lok connections, make certain the connections are snugly connected. Never allow the solution container to run dry; hang the next container of solution while there is still 30 to 50 mL of fluid remaining in the original container.

Nursing Care

If air should enter the IV line during infusion, stop the infusion, use a needle or blunt-tipped adapter attached to a syringe to pierce the injection port closest to the air in the tubing, and aspirate to remove all the air before restarting the flow of solution. If you suspect an air embolism, call for help to notify the physician and bring the crash cart. Place the patient on his or her left side in the Trendelenburg position. Once the air enters the right atrium of the heart, this position causes the air to rise to the top of the atrium, which reduces the chance of the air entering the pulmonary artery, traveling to the lungs and back to the left side of the heart, and then out into the systemic circulation. Apply supplemental oxygen and monitor vital signs until the physician arrives. Talk factually, firmly, and calmly to the patient to achieve compliance with your requests but to avoid frightening the patient more than necessary.

Circulatory Fluid Overload and Pulmonary Edema

Too much fluid infused into the cardiovascular system can result in fluid overload. Extreme fluid volume overload can result in pulmonary edema, where the excess fluid is forced into the pulmonary tissues. Patients with cardiovascular, renal, or respiratory disease, children, and elders are most susceptible to these complications. Fluid overload causes a rise in BP as the circulatory volume increases the pressure against the walls of the vasculature. Heart rate increases as the heart works harder to pump the increased fluid volume through the cardiovascular system. If the initial signs and symptoms are not detected and the infusion rate slows, hypertension, tachycardia, and tachypnea worsen. The patient begins to manifest signs of anxiety and restlessness, and moist breath sounds called *crackles* can be auscultated. The severity increases very quickly, and respirations become labored and gurgling. The patient becomes extremely dyspneic and cyanotic and starts coughing up pink frothy fluid. Box 38.9 presents other signs and symptoms of fluid overload.

The following are causes of fluid overload:

- Infusion of an excessive volume of fluid above the needs of the patient
- Too much sodium chloride for the needs of the patient
- An infusion rate that is too fast

An excessive infusion of isotonic fluid can result in overloading the circulatory system even though it does not cause third-space shifting. Infusion of hypertonic fluid, especially one with sodium chloride, when the patient does not need a hypertonic solution will pull excess fluid into the vascular spaces.

Once the overload has progressed to pulmonary edema, the patient's situation becomes critical. Without immediate treatment including, among other things, supplemental oxygen and IV diuretics, this patient will die.

Box 38.9

Signs and Symptoms of Circulatory Fluid Overload

It is important to detect circulatory fluid overload as early as possible. The patient may only exhibit one or two signs before the vital signs begin to change and the patient begins to rapidly decline. Each patient will be different. Be alert to the following signs in all patients receiving IV fluids and be ever vigilant in infants, children, older adults, and any patient with a diagnosis or medical history of diseases such as congestive heart failure.

- Anxiety without identifiable cause
- Cough
- Distention of neck veins
- Facial, hand, or foot edema
- Headache
- Increased BP
- Increased pulse rate
- Crackles in lungs
- Restlessness
- Shortness of breath

Prevention

It is better to prevent fluid overload than to try to treat it after it occurs. Using an infusion pump is the best way to control the rate of infusion. Always make certain that you are aware of the reason for infusion of the IV fluids as well as the patient's medical history so that you will be able to identify the potential for development of fluid overload and pulmonary edema. Monitor intake and output, auscultate breath sounds, and monitor vital signs for tachycardia, hypertension, and tachypnea. You must monitor the type and osmolality of fluid infusing as well as the infusion rate. *Do not be afraid to discuss the type of fluid or infusion rate with the physician if you are concerned that either one does not match the patient's needs.* Be respectful and tactful, but by all means talk to the physician about your concerns. The physician may very well appreciate it when you point out something that he or she may have overlooked. Remember that you are the patient's advocate. The best nurses are the ones who will seek answers and clarification of orders from physicians when they have a concern, doubt, or question regarding a patient's care. Be one.

Nursing Care

At the first sign or symptom of fluid overload, decrease the IV infusion rate and apply supplemental oxygen. Assess the vital signs and auscultate breath sounds after placing the patient in the high Fowler's position. Notify the physician immediately.

Speed Shock

When an IV solution or medication is infused rapidly, causing a harmfully elevated blood level, it can result in a condition known as speed shock. It is characterized by flushed skin, dizziness, headache, chest tightness, hypotension, irregular pulse, syncope or fainting, and cardiac arrest.

Prevention

The best care is prevention by monitoring the rate of infusion of the primary IV solution. Again, if you are concerned about the rapid rate of infusion, talk to the physician. Administer IVPB and IV push medications slowly and according to the manufacturer's recommendations. Make it a habit to use a drug reference book and look up the safe rate of administration. Use an IV pump when available, especially for medications, or use microdrip tubing (60 gtts/mL) administration sets if the solution is infused by gravity.

Nursing Care

If signs and symptoms of speed shock occur, stop the medication infusion and notify the physician. Call for assistance and the crash cart. Administer a medication antidote if there is one. Continually assess the patient's response to each intervention. Document the episode thoroughly afterward.

> **KNOWLEDGE CONNECTION**
> Explain why it is dangerous to reinsert the needle into the cannula once it has been pulled partially out. What should be your first intervention if the cannula is severed while it is in the patient's vein? List the signs and symptoms of circulatory fluid overload.

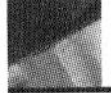

CENTRAL VENOUS ACCESS DEVICES

As a nurse, you may care for patients with central venous access devices, such as a peripherally inserted central venous catheter (PICC), a central venous catheter (also known as a *central line*), or an implanted venous access device (also known as an *implanted port*). Alternative vascular access devices are used when a peripherally inserted IV is not optimal. The venous catheter is used for short-term or long-term IV therapy, IV nutrition, and fluid replacement for 6 to 8 weeks. The vascular access devices are used in the hospital, in long-term care, and in home health, often to deliver chemotherapy. They may also be used for blood draws.

A single-lumen catheter is a long, thin catheter with one hub at the end. A multiple-lumen catheter is a long, thin catheter with multiple hubs at the end. The multiple-lumen allows for multiple types of IV therapy to be delivered at the same time. Complications with vascular access devices include bloodstream infections, pneumothorax, thrombosis, and misplacement.

Peripherally Inserted Central Venous Catheter

The PICC is advanced into a peripheral vein such as the basilic, brachial, or cephalic vein then advanced into the superior vena cava or right atrium (Fig. 38.27). In many hospitals, a PICC line is inserted by the peripheral venous access team (VAT) using sterile technique. The VAT consists of specially trained registered nurses. Before administering any IV therapy, an x-ray will be taken to verify placement. As the nurse, you may be asked to set up the sterile supplies needed for vascular access insertion at the bedside.

Central Venous Catheter

A nontunneled central venous catheter is inserted into a peripheral vein such as the femoral vein, jugular vein, or subclavian vein and is then advanced into the superior vena cava or right atrium (Figure 38.28). A nontunneled central venous catheter is used for short-term therapy. Ultrasound is used during the placement to allow the health-care provider to place the catheter in the correct location. A central venous catheter is used for IV therapy, nutrition, to obtain blood specimens for lab testing, to obtain central venous pressure readings, and to measure central venous oxygen saturation. The central venous catheter is inserted by a health-care provider using sterile technique.

Implanted Venous Access Device

An implanted port is surgically implanted under the skin below the collarbone and is usually placed in the right upper chest (Fig. 38.29). The port is connected to a catheter that is advanced through a large vein into the right atrium. Then the port itself is secured to the skin with sutures. The implanted port consists of one or two disk-shaped lumens under the

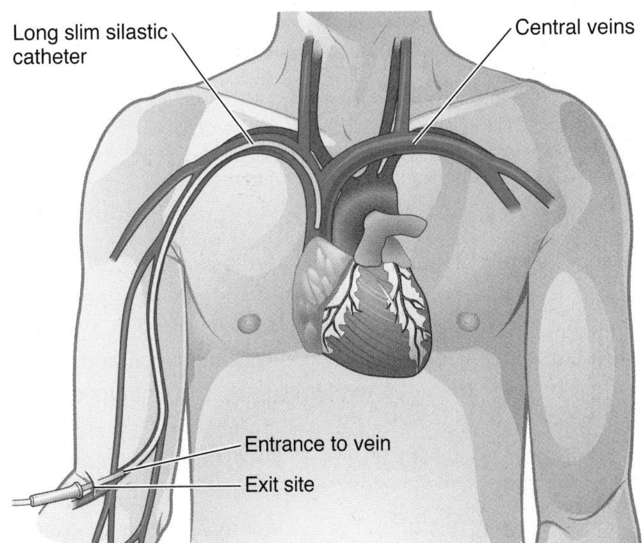

FIGURE 38.27 A PICC line is a long, soft, flexible catheter inserted through a vein in the arm and threaded into a central vessel (from Wilkinson JM, Treas LS. *Fundamentals of Nursing: Theory, Concepts & Applications*. Vol. 1. 3rd ed. Philadelphia, PA: FA Davis; 2016).

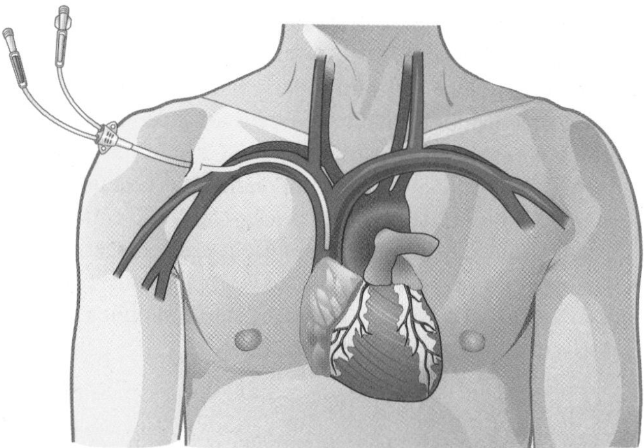

FIGURE 38.28 Nontunneled central venous catheters are inserted into the jugular; subclavian; and, occasionally, femoral veins (from Wilkinson JM, Treas LS. *Fundamentals of Nursing: Theory, Concepts & Applications*. Vol. 1. 3rd ed. Philadelphia, PA: FA Davis; 2016).

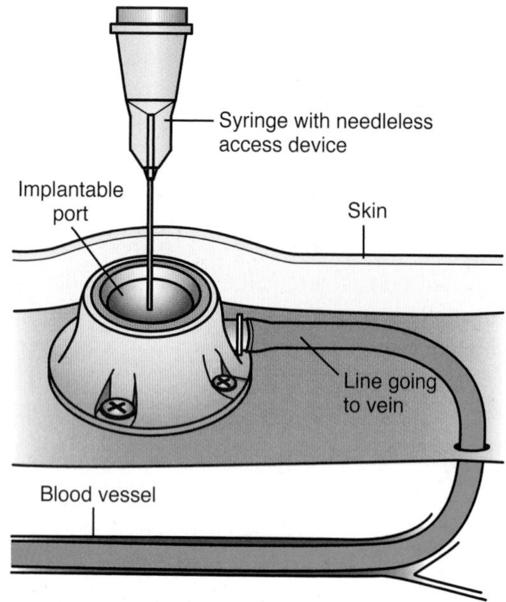

FIGURE 38.29 Central vascular access device, an implantable port (from Wilkinson JM, Treas LS. *Fundamentals of Nursing: Theory, Concepts & Applications*. Vol. 1. 3rd ed. Philadelphia, PA: FA Davis; 2016).

skin. The nurse will use a special needle called a *Huber* needle to access the port. Prior to doing so, it may be appropriate to place a local anesthetic cream to numb the skin over the port before the needle is inserted. The implanted port is inserted by a health-care provider using sterile technique.

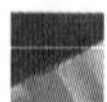

BLOOD AND BLOOD PRODUCTS

Blood has many functions, but it primarily serves as the transporter of oxygen and nutrients to body cells and transporter of waste substances removed from the cells. There are many variations of blood and blood products that may be transfused to meet various patient needs (Box 38.10).

Box 38.10

Examples of Blood Products and Their Uses

Research and technology have made it possible to isolate individual components and factors that compose the blood. It is no longer necessary to transfuse whole blood to every patient who only needs specific components. These are examples of specific blood components and possible situations in which they might be administered.

- **Albumin:** increase plasma volume
- **Cryoprecipitate:** replace coagulation factors I, VII, and XIII
- **Fresh-frozen plasma:** replace coagulation factors V and XI, drug reversal of warfarin (Coumadin)
- **Liquid plasma:** replace plasma proteins
- **PRBCs:** acute blood loss, hemoglobin less than 8 to 10 g/dL, symptomatic anemia
- **Platelets:** prevent/control bleeding related to low platelet count, acute leukemia, thrombocytopenia
- **Whole blood:** rarely used but restores blood volume along with all its components; mostly broken down for use of its individual components

Not all cultures and organized religions believe in or approve of transfusing blood or blood products. Some actually prohibit their members from receiving blood transfusions, an example of which is Jehovah's Witnesses.

Transfusion

A written physician's order is required for both the transfusion of blood or blood products and the pretransfusion laboratory tests. An informed consent for transfusion of blood or blood products also is required. The patient who is to receive transfusion of blood or blood products must have his or her own blood tested for its specific ABO type and Rh grouping. The blood of both the potential recipient and the blood donor are tested for compatibility and screened for antibodies. Known as *typing and crossmatching tests,* they are necessary to prevent antigen–antibody reactions during transfusion therapy. After the typing, crossmatching, and compatibility tests have been completed and verified by the laboratory or blood bank staff, a specific identification number is assigned to the blood product and is used for verification that it is the correct blood product for the specified patient.

Safety: Blood and blood products are not compatible with any IV solution other than 0.9% sodium chloride (NS). Therefore, no other IV solutions are used in conjunction with blood product infusion. Dextrose can cause hemolysis, meaning lysis or destruction of red blood cells. Even medications cannot be mixed with blood products. If infusion of IV medication is scheduled during the transfusion, a separate IV line should be established. The transfusion is initiated by

• WORD • BUILDING •

hemolysis: hemo – blood + lysis - dissolution

infusing NS, and completion of transfusion is followed by infusion of the same. The NS is also used to dilute packed red blood cells to a thinner consistency so that they can be infused. **Packed red blood cells** (PRBCs) are those that have been separated from **plasma,** the liquid portion of the blood.

Transfusion Reactions

Because transfusions have the potential for serious risks to the patient, you are responsible to be knowledgeable regarding safe administration, signs and symptoms of reactions, steps to prevent reactions, and interventions to treat reactions. There are at least a dozen types of transfusion reactions that create significant risks to the patient, but we will only address six primary types of reactions in this chapter:

- Acute hemolytic
- Bacterial
- Allergic
- Febrile
- Circulatory overload
- Anaphylactic reactions

Table 38.4 presents descriptions and treatments of these reactions.

> **KNOWLEDGE CONNECTION**
> Which IV solution must always be used to begin and end blood product transfusions? Contrast the signs and symptoms of an acute hemolytic reaction to those of an allergic reaction.

Supplies

Transfusions are generally administered with a special Y-shaped administration set, often referred to as a *Y-set.* Each of the two top branches of the Y-set end in piercing pins, one of which is used to spike the bag of blood product and the other to spike the bag of NS solution. The long tail of the Y-set contains an in-line filter and attaches to the cannula hub at the site of insertion into the patient's vein (refer to Figs. 38.12 and 38.13). Most commonly an 18-G (1.2-mm) or 20-G (0.9-mm) IV cannula is used to administer blood products. Infusing blood through a cannula that is too small is likely to lyse the blood cells.

Nursing Care Pretransfusion

Once blood products are ordered, inquire if the patient has ever received a blood transfusion before. Provide the appropriate level of patient teaching regarding the transfusion process. Discuss signs and symptoms that the patient should report to you if they are experienced during the transfusion, making certain that none of these signs and symptoms are present prior to initiating the transfusion so that they will not be misinterpreted as reactions to the transfusion.

Assess the patient's vital signs immediately before beginning the blood or blood product transfusion; this will serve as a baseline against which you can compare vital signs taken during the transfusion. If the patient's temperature is elevated, you should notify the physician before proceeding with initiation of the transfusion. The physician may order an antihistamine such as diphenhydramine hydrochloride to be administered prior to beginning a transfusion. During the transfusion, it is not uncommon for the patient to experience a low-grade fever, but you still will report it to the physician.

SAFETY MEASURES. Just prior to initiating a blood product transfusion, most facilities require that two nurses, usually RNs, double-check the physician's order, comparing it to the actual blood product to make certain that the correct blood components have been prepared for transfusion. The nurses are responsible for ensuring that the patient's name and identification number on the blood product container match those on the patient's identification band and those on the patient chart. Each unit of blood product will also have its own specific identification number assigned to it during typing and crossmatching. The nurses must verify that this identification number on the blood product container matches the number on the blood bank form. Once all data have been matched and verified, both nurses are required to sign the blood bank form. Most states require two RNs to initiate and monitor the first 15 minutes of a blood transfusion. LVN/LPNs can monitor the patient after the first 15 minutes of the blood transfusion. *Review the LVN/LPN scope of practice before administering blood products.* ***Safety: If any type of discrepancy exists, the transfusion should not be started and the blood product should be returned to the blood bank.***

PREPARING BLOOD PRODUCT FOR INFUSION. Wash your hands and apply clean examination gloves for preparation of blood products. Prepare the NS, blood administration set, and blood product container for use before going to the patient's room. Follow the manufacturer's instructions on the blood administration Y-set package for spiking NS and blood product containers, maintaining sterility of appropriate parts of the equipment. Label the tubing with the date and time. Prime the entire Y-set with the NS solution, including *back-priming* the branch of tubing that will be inserted into the blood product container. Skill 38.9 (page 901) provides more information on preparing, initiating, and monitoring the infusion of blood and blood products.

Nursing Care During Transfusion

To initiate the transfusion, start the flow of NS first and reassess patency of the IV site. Assess vital signs. Then close the clamp to the NS and begin infusion of the blood product at a rate of 50 mL per hour according to facility policy. ***Safety: Once the transfusion has been initiated, you will remain at the patient's bedside to monitor the patient for the first 15 minutes of the transfusion, which is the most likely***

Table 38.4
Transfusion Reactions

Reaction Type	*Description*	*Signs and Symptoms*	*Nursing Interventions*
Acute hemolytic	Very serious Related to ABO incompatibility Causes lysis (destruction) of blood cells Can result in shock and death	Chest pain Back pain Bleeding Vein burning ↑R rate, ↑ P rate, ↓ BP	**Stop transfusion stat** Call a code Apply oxygen Start new IV line Administer colloidal plasma expanders to BP Monitor vital signs
Febrile	Related to release of proteins by white blood cells during blood storage Transient fever	Nausea/vomiting ↑ Temp Chills Headache Chest pain	Stop transfusion Start NS Notify the health-care provider Administer antipyretics as ordered Monitor vital signs
Mild allergic	Related to sensitivity to proteins in transfusion	Flushed Urticaria Itching Watery eyes Shortness of breath Mild wheezes	Stop transfusion Start NS Notify the health-care provider Administer antihistamines as ordered Monitor vital signs
Anaphylaxis (severe allergic)	Very serious Life-threatening Previously developed antibodies related to sensitivity to proteins in transfusion Can result in shock and death	Wide-eyed appearance Anxiety Extensive urticaria ↓ BP Severe wheezing Cyanosis	**Stop transfusion stat** Start NS Notify the health-care provider Administer antihistamines and corticosteroids as ordered Start a new IV line Administer fluids to maintain BP Call code prn
Circulatory overload	Related to decreased cardiac output or transfusion rate too rapid, or patient was at risk for fluid excess	Wide-eyed appearance Anxiety Dyspnea Crackles Frothy sputum↑SpO_2 ↑BP, ↑ P rate, ↑ R rate	Stop transfusion Raise head of bed Apply O_2 Notify the health-care provider Administer diuretic as ordered Monitor vital signs
Bacterial contamination	Related to earlier contamination of blood product Can result in renal failure and shock	Very high fever Flushed ↓BP, then compensatory ↑BP	Stop transfusion Notify the health-care provider Administer steroids and antibiotics as ordered

time for reactions to occur. Assess the patient's responses and vital signs every 5 minutes during this first 15 minutes. Also, this is a good time to complete documentation that may not have been done yet regarding pretransfusion assessments, patient teaching, and initiation of the transfusion.

If there are no indications of a problem during the first 15 minutes, increase the flow rate to ensure that the transfusion will be completed within a 2- to 4-hour window. After 4 hours, the unit of blood is at risk for contamination because it is the perfect medium for bacterial growth. The only exception to this rate of infusion is during emergency volume replacement, which may be infused more rapidly. Assess the patient's vital signs every 30 minutes to 1 hour according to facility policy throughout the remainder of the transfusion, obtaining one last set after the completion of the transfusion.

If there are any signs or symptoms of reaction during the transfusion, immediately stop the infusion of blood and resume the infusion of NS to keep the vein open. Refer to Table 38.4 for specific nursing interventions for different types of reactions.

Nursing Care Posttransfusion

When the blood has completely infused, close that tubing clamp and reopen the one to the NS solution, allowing the NS to flush the line. If there is no need to infuse another unit of blood product or wait for laboratory results, the IV infusion usually is discontinued as soon as the NS has flushed the line. Again, this will be according to facility policy and the physician's orders. The physician will generally order a blood count to be done 12 to 24 hours posttransfusion to determine the effect on the blood cell counts.

KNOWLEDGE CONNECTION

What gauge of needles may be used for blood product transfusions? Why is it not adequate for one nurse to verify that identification data assigned to the unit of blood product correspond with data on the chart, patient ID band, and transfusion form?

Skill 38.1 Administering IV Push Medication via PRN Lock or IV Line

Assessment Steps

1. Review the health-care provider's order for IV push medication ***to improve accuracy and decrease the risk for error.***
2. Unless you are familiar with the medication, use a drug book to research its therapeutic action, purpose, compatibility with the primary IV solution, drug–drug interactions, dosage, route, side effects, and length of time to infuse. ***This reduces the risk of administration of inappropriate solution and allergic reactions and better prepares you to detect problems. It also increases your ability to detect side effects and potential problems and to evaluate whether or not the medication does what is intended, and it reduces the risk of errors.***
3. Review the patient's diagnoses, medical history, and allergies to medications ***to ensure that it is safe to administer this medication to the specific patient.***
4. Perform any pertinent physical assessments such as BP, apical pulse, urine output, or auscultation of breath sounds ***for comparison with values after medication administration.*** **Review pertinent laboratory results.** ***Some medications should not be given unless specific laboratory results are within designated parameters.***
5. Assess the patient's IV access. Is it a continuous infusion or a PRN lock, or does it connect to a Luer-Lok syringe or require a needle or blunt-tipped adapter? ***This allows you to know what type of adapters you need.***
6. Calculate the volume of medication you will draw up. Recheck your calculations ***to decrease the risk of error.*** There are specific medications that MUST be rechecked by another nurse, such as heparin and insulin before administration.

Planning Steps

1. Gather needed equipment and supplies: syringe, needle or blunt-tipped adapter if required, two NS flushes (prefilled syringe if available), alcohol wipes, correct form and dosage of ordered medication, and examination gloves. ***Being prepared saves you time and effort and helps you to appear more confident and competent in the patient's eyes.***
2. Inspect packages for intactness and expiration date ***to ensure continued sterility.***

Implementation Steps

Before Going to the Patient's Room

1. *Safety: Wash hands to prevent cross-contamination.*
2. *Safety: To prevent error, compare the medication label to the medication administration record (MAR) three times, checking the patient name, medication name, dosage, route, and time. IV administration is so critical if errors are made. Check the labels an extra time before going to the patient's room. Check allergies.*
3. Cleanse the medication stopper with alcohol ***to remove any microorganisms.***
4. Draw up the ordered dosage of medication.
5. *Safety: Recap the sterile needle using the scoop method you learned in Chapter 37. You should never carry an uncovered needle down the hallway.*

After Entering the Patient's Room

6. Follow the Initial Implementation Steps located on the inside back cover.
7. *Safety: To prevent error, compare the medication label to the MAR a third time, checking the patient name, medication name, dosage, route, and time.*
8. Explain to the patient what you are about to do. Provide any necessary patient teaching ***to reduce patient anxiety and increase compliance.***
9. *Safety: Wash hands again to prevent cross-contamination.*
10. Assess the patient's IV site for signs of infiltration and phlebitis. ***You must not infuse IV solution or medications into a site that shows possible indication of infiltration or phlebitis.***

If Injecting Into the IV Line of a Continuous Infusion of IV Solution

11. Locate the Y-injection port closest to the insertion site in the patient's extremity. Cleanse the port with an alcohol wipe or CHG-alcohol combination product to remove microorganisms.
12. Attach the Luer-Lok NS flush syringe to the Y-injection port (or insert a needle or blunt-tipped adapter into the Y-injection port) and aspirate for blood to confirm catheter placement in the vein (refer to Fig. 38.2). Inject NS as dictated previously and disconnect the syringe from the Y-injection port.

(skill continues on page 890)

Skill 38.1 (continued)

13. Making certain the medication syringe contains no air, attach the syringe to the Y-injection port after cleansing the port with an alcohol wipe to reduce the risk of air embolism. Gently aspirate for blood return. Slowly inject the medication, evenly distributing the volume over the designated time frame. For example, if you have 3 mL of medication to inject over 3 minutes, inject about 1 mL over the first minute, 1 mL over the second minute, and the last milliliter over the third minute.
    - To inject the medication, pinch off the primary IV tubing just proximal to the Y-injection port, stopping the flow of IV solution. While pinching off the IV tubing, inject a small portion of the medication and then release the IV tubing, allowing the IV solution to flow behind the medication.
    - When it is time to inject another small amount of the medication, again pinch off the primary IV tubing and inject the designated portion of the medication. Release the IV tubing in between injecting the medication.
    - Repeat this process over the designated period of time until all the medication has been instilled. Follow medication with 1 to 3 mL NS flush according to facility policy. *Safety: Never administer an IV push too quickly. Injecting IV push medication over the recommended time span helps to protect the patient from too great a response in too short a time span and helps to protect against speed shock* (refer to Fig. 38.2).
    - *Safety: Continually monitor the patient's skin around the injection site for edema to ensure that the medication is still infusing into the vein and is not infiltrating.*
    - ***Note: If the medication is incompatible with the primary IV solution, rather than trying to adequately flush the IV line with NS before and after administering the medication, it is best to inject the medication via another access device or directly into a different vein using a needle.***
14. After all medication is injected, remove the syringe or needle from the injection port.
15. Dispose of all contaminated supplies appropriately.
16. Remove and dispose of contaminated gloves. Wash hands to reduce microorganisms and risk of cross-contamination.
17. Follow the Ending Implementation Steps located on the inside back cover.
18. Document the administration of the medication in the nurses' notes only if it was a one-time order or a prn order. Otherwise, it is only documented on the MAR. Document any adverse or side effects exhibited as well as the effectiveness of the medication.

If Injecting Into a PRN Lock

11. Cleanse the PRN lock injection port with alcohol or CHG-alcohol combination product ***to reduce microorganisms.***
12. While maintaining sterility of the syringe tip, dispel air from the Luer-Lok syringe and attach the syringe with 1 to 3 mL NS to the Y-injection port of the PRN lock (or insert a needle or blunt-tipped adapter into the injection port). Open the slide clamp on the PRN lock ***to reduce the risk of air embolism and infection.***
13. Aspirate with the syringe ***to verify blood return*** into the PRN lock. If blood return is noted, flush the PRN lock with part of the NS flush solution. Use the amount of NS dictated by facility policy. It should be a minimum of 1 to 3 mL but may vary up to 10 mL.
14. After completing the flush, disconnect the NS flush syringe from the PRN lock injection port.
15. Wipe the injection port with an alcohol or CHG-alcohol combination product wipe ***to reduce microorganisms.***
16. Making certain there is no air in the medication syringe, connect the Luer-Lok of the syringe holding the medication to the injection port of the PRN lock (or insert the needle or blunt-tipped adapter that is attached to the syringe into the injection port). ***This helps to reduce the risk of air embolism.***
17. Slowly inject the medication, evenly distributing the volume over the designated time frame ***to reduce the risk of adverse reactions and speed shock.***

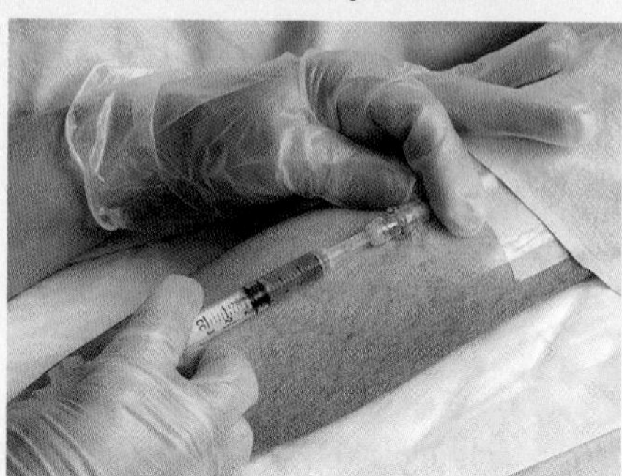

18. Once the medication is completely infused, disconnect the syringe from the injection port and repeat the NS flush as before.
19. Close the slide clamp on the PRN lock and remove the NS syringe or needle from the injection port.
20. Remove contaminated gloves and dispose of all contaminated supplies.
21. Wash hands ***to reduce cross-contamination.***
22. Follow the Ending Implementation Steps located on the inside back cover.
23. Document the administration of the medication in the nurses' notes only if it was a one-time order or a prn order. Otherwise, it is only documented on the MAR. Document any adverse or side effects exhibited as well as the effectiveness of the medication.

Evaluation Steps

1. *Safety: Make any assessments that should be made after administration of the medication, such as respiratory or pulse rate, to detect any untoward effects.*
2. Assess for effectiveness of the medication. ***This helps to determine if the medication needs to be changed.***
3. Assess the IV site one last time before leaving the patient's room ***to ensure that it is not becoming erythematous or edematous.***
4. Evaluate the adequacy and balance of patient's intake and output ***to detect possible signs of fluid imbalance.***

Sample Documentation

04/06/22 0415 Respirations 17 breathes per minute. Morphine Sulfate 6 mg diluted in NS 6 mL and administered slowly IV push over 5 minutes for C/O pain at a 6 on a scale of 0 to 10. States pain is down to a 2. Respirations 14 breathes per minute. ———

——— Nurse's signature and credentials

Skill 38.2 Administering IV Piggyback Medication

Assessment Steps

1. Review the health-care provider's order for IVPB medication and rate of infusion ***to clarify the order and reduce the risk of error.***
2. Unless you are familiar with the specific medication, use a drug book to research its therapeutic action, purpose, compatibility with primary IV solution and IVPB solution, possible drug–drug interactions, dosage, route, side effects, and length of time to infuse. This reduces the risk of administration of inappropriate solution and allergic reactions and better prepares you to detect problems. It also increases your ability to detect side effects and potential problems and to evaluate whether or not the medication does what is intended, and it reduces the risk of errors.
3. Review the patient's diagnoses, medical history, and allergies to medications to make certain it is safe to administer the medication.
4. Assess to determine whether short secondary or IVPB administration tubing is already hanging. Obtaining this information helps you to be properly prepared and have all the supplies that you will need to reduce the number of trips made to the supply room. It will save you time and energy. It also helps to raise the patient's perception of your competency.
5. Assess the patency of the IV line and assess the IV site for signs and symptoms of infiltration and phlebitis.

Planning Steps

IVPB Infusion Into Primary IV Line With Continual Infusion of IV Solution

1. Gather needed equipment and supplies: correct form and dosage of medication, solution (type and volume) in which to instill the medication if the IVPB medication is not premixed, medication label, IVPB secondary tubing administration set, alcohol wipes, and examination gloves. ***Being prepared increases your efficiency, saves time and footwork, and helps to increase the patient's perception of your competence.***
2. Calculate the recommended rate of infusion according to facility policy, a pharmacist, or a drug book: mL/hr for pump flow and gtts/min for gravity flow. ***This reduces the risk of error.***
3. Inspect packages for intactness and expiration dates ***to ensure sterility.***

Implementation Steps

Before Going to the Patient's Room

1. *Safety: Wash hands to prevent cross-contamination.*
2. *Safety: Compare the medication label to the medication administration record (MAR) twice, checking the patient name, medication name, dosage, route, and time, to prevent error.*
3. Inspect the IVPB tubing administration set package for intactness and expiration date ***to ensure continued sterility.***
4. Remove the tubing from the package and close the roller clamp. ***Closing the clamp reduces the risk of introducing air bubbles as the solution begins to flow.***
5. Locate the tubing port on the IVPB bag of medication and remove the rubber plug, maintaining the sterility of the port ***to reduce the risk of infection.***
6. Remove the cap from the tubing's piercing pin, maintaining the sterility of the pin ***to reduce the risk of infection.***
7. Placing your thumb and index finger behind the flange ***to reduce the risk of contaminating the sterile piercing pin,*** insert the pin into the tubing port on the IVPB medication bag. Use a twisting motion to aid insertion. *Safety: Use caution to prevent the piercing pin from piercing the sides of the port.*
8. If the injection ports on the patient's primary IV tubing are not compatible with the Luer-Lok ends on the IVPB tubing, attach a needle or blunt-tipped adapter to the end of the IVPB tubing before continuing. *Safety: Be careful to maintain sterility of the tubing end as well as both ends of the needle or blunt-tipped adapter.*
9. Squeeze the drip chamber on the IVPB tubing, filling it one-third to one-half full. ***This leaves adequate room in the drip chamber to observe the solution dripping.***
10. Remove the cap from the end of the IVPB tubing (or the attached needle or blunt-tipped adapter). Maintain sterility of the Luer-Lok end of IVPB tubing (or the attached needle or blunt-tipped adapter) ***to reduce the risk of infection.***
11. Open the roller clamp on the IVPB tubing, allowing only enough solution to run through the tubing to displace all air. *Safety: Avoid allowing excessive amount of solution to flow once all air has been removed from the tubing. The smaller volume in a piggyback, usually only 50 or 100 mL, necessitates that there be no excessive wastage of medication-containing fluid.*
12. Close the roller clamp ***to prevent premature dripping of solution*** and replace the sterile cap on the end of the IVPB tubing (or needle or blunt-tipped adapter) without contaminating it ***to reduce the risk of infection.***

After Entering the Patient's Room

13. Follow the Initial Implementation Steps located on the inside back cover.
14. *Safety: Compare the medication label to the MAR a third time, checking the patient name, medication name, dosage, route, and time, to prevent error.*
15. Explain to the patient what you are about to do. Provide any necessary patient teaching. ***This reduces patient anxiety and increases patient compliance.***
16. *Safety: Wash hands again to remove microorganisms.*
17. Reassess the patient's IV site for signs of infiltration and phlebitis.
18. Hang the IVPB medication bag on the IV pole. If infusing by pump, hang both bags at the same height. ***Note: If infusing by gravity rather than IV pump, use the extender wire to hang the primary IV solution bag lower than the IVPB medication bag. This allows the higher IVPB bag to infuse before the primary bag starts to run again.***
19. Locate the highest Y-injection port on the primary tubing. Cleanse the port with an alcohol wipe or CHG-alcohol combination product.
    Note: Some pump tubing has plastic cassettes that insert into the pumping mechanism of the controller or pump. The highest injection port may be located on the top of these cassettes.

(skill continues on page 892)

Skill 38.2 (continued)

20. Remove the cap from the end of the IVPB tubing (or needle or blunt-tipped adapter), maintaining the sterility of the end ***to prevent contamination and reduce the risk of infection.***
21. Cleanse the Y-injection port on the primary IV tubing with alcohol or CHG-alcohol combination product ***to remove microorganisms.*** Connect the IVPB tubing Luer-Lok adapter or blunt-tipped adapter to the primary tubing Y-injection port (refer to Fig. 38.4).

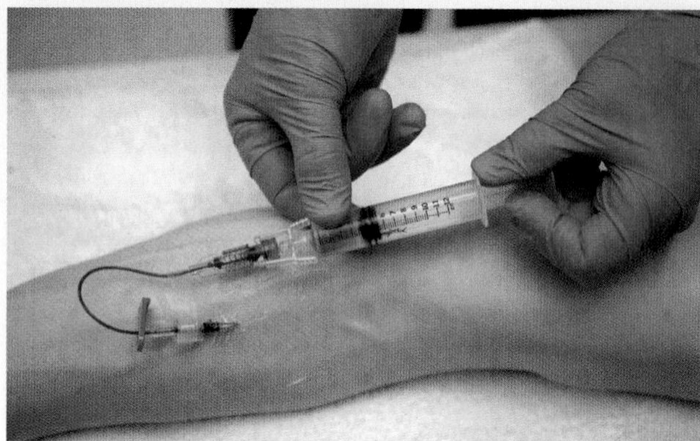

22. **If using an IV pump:** Program the settings for the IVPB: the ***secondary volume to be infused*** **and the** ***secondary rate of infusion.*** Open the clamp on the IVPB tubing and start the pump. Once the IVPB medication has entirely infused, the primary IV solution will resume its set rate of infusion.
    If using gravity flow: Open the roller clamp on the IVPB tubing and adjust the rate to the number of gtts/min that you previously calculated. Once the IVPB medication has completely infused, the lowered bag of primary IV solution will resume dripping at its previous rate of infusion.
23. Remove contaminated gloves and dispose of them properly.
24. Wash hands before leaving room ***to reduce risk of cross-contamination.***
25. Follow the Ending Implementation Steps located on the inside back cover.
26. Because routine medications are only documented on the MAR, the IVPB infusion itself is not documented in your nurses' notes. However, document the IV site assessment, any problems that develop, and the effectiveness of medication in the nurses' notes.

Sample Documentation

02/04/22 1205 Noted 1/2-in. edematous area just proximal to IV cannula during ampicillin IVPB infusion. Able to obtain blood return. C/O of IV site beginning to burn. IV DC'd. IV restarted in Left forearm with 22-G × 1-in. intracath with 1 attempt, no difficulty. IV infusing IVPB at 100 mL/hr. ——————— Nurse's signature and credentials

Skill 38.3 Converting an IV Infusion to a PRN Lock

Assessment Steps

1. Review the health-care provider's order for conversion to a PRN lock ***to reduce the risk of error.***
2. Assess whether the patient has IV tubing that connects directly to the cannula hub or has a PRN lock connecting the tubing to the cannula hub ***to determine the type of supplies you need.***
3. Assess the IV site for signs of infiltration or phlebitis.

Planning Steps

1. *Safety: Wash your hands to prevent cross-contamination.*

If Patient Has IV Tubing Connected Directly to the Cannula Hub

2. Gather needed equipment and supplies: PRN lock device, NS flush, needle or blunt-tipped adapter, alcohol wipes, and tape.
3. Inspect packages for intactness and expiration dates ***to ensure continued sterility.***
4. If the PRN lock device does not allow use of a Luer-Lok device, apply a needle or blunt-tipped adapter to the NS flush syringe. Maintain sterility of the tip of the NS flush syringe and the needle or blunt-tipped adapter ***to prevent contamination.***
5. Cleanse the injection port end of the new PRN lock device with alcohol or CHG-alcohol combination product ***to remove any microorganisms.***
6. Connect the sterile Luer-Lok tip of the syringe to the injection port, or insert the needle or blunt-tipped adapter into the injection port of the PRN lock, while maintaining sterility.
7. Prime the new PRN lock by injecting the NS into the lock until all air has been displaced with NS. ***This helps to prevent air embolisms.***

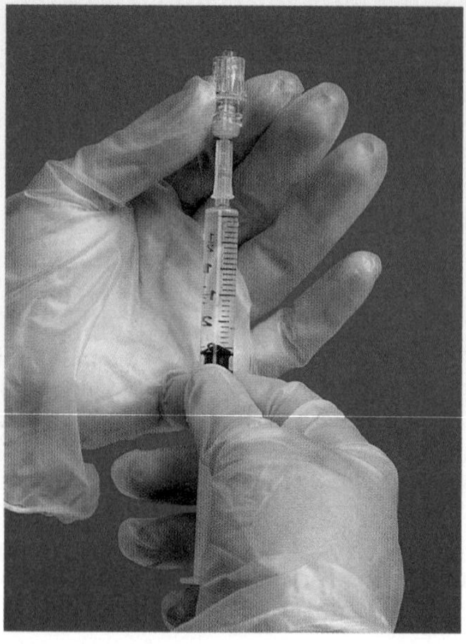

Skill 38.3 (continued)

8. Leave the syringe with the remaining NS attached to the PRN device so that ***it is ready to flush once connected to the cannula hub.***

Implementation Steps

1. Follow the Initial Implementation Steps located on the inside back cover.
2. Explain to the patient what you are about to do. Provide any necessary patient teaching ***to reduce patient anxiety and increase compliance.*** Place patient in a comfortable position and raise the bed to a working height.
3. *Safety: Once in the patient's room, wash hands again to prevent cross-contamination.*
4. Reassess the patient's IV site ***to ensure there are no signs of infiltration and phlebitis.***
5. Tear several 3- to 4-inch strips of tape to use for securing the PRN lock.
6. Stop the IV solution flow by turning off the IV pump or closing the tubing clamp if infusing by gravity flow.
7. ***To protect you from possible contact with patient body fluid,*** apply clean examination gloves.

If Patient Has IV Tubing Connected Directly to the Cannula Hub

8. Gently loosen the tape securing the IV tubing to the extremity and cannula hub, taking care not to lift the cannula hub away from the skin. *Safety: Lifting the hub bends the attached plastic cannula that is inserted into the vein, increasing the risk of a severed cannula. Pull the tape ends toward the cannula to decrease the risk of dislodging or bending the cannula.*
9. Once the tape is removed, place a sterile 2×2-inch (535-cm) gauze pad underneath the cannula hub connection to reduce the risk of contamination. Disconnect the IV tubing end from the cannula hub, maintaining the sterility of the cannula hub.

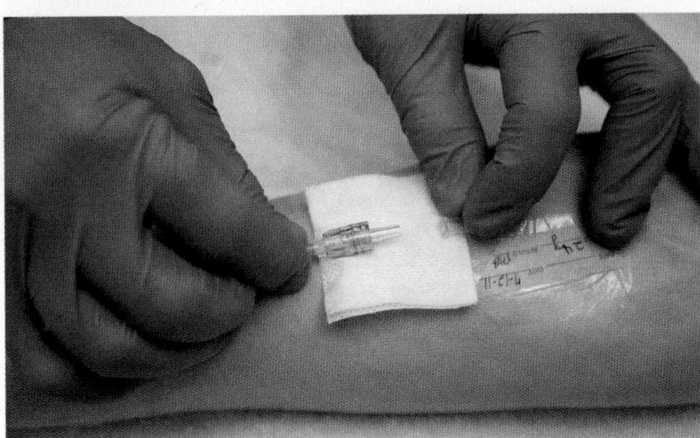

10. Remove the end cap from the connecting end of the new PRN lock device without contaminating the connecting end.
11. Insert the end of the PRN lock device into the sterile hub of the cannula in the patient's vein and scrub the PRN lock device with an alcohol wipe or CHG-alcohol combination product.
12. Screw the Luer-Lok connection device to the cannula hub ***to ensure that the PRN lock device will not be accidentally disconnected from the cannula hub.***

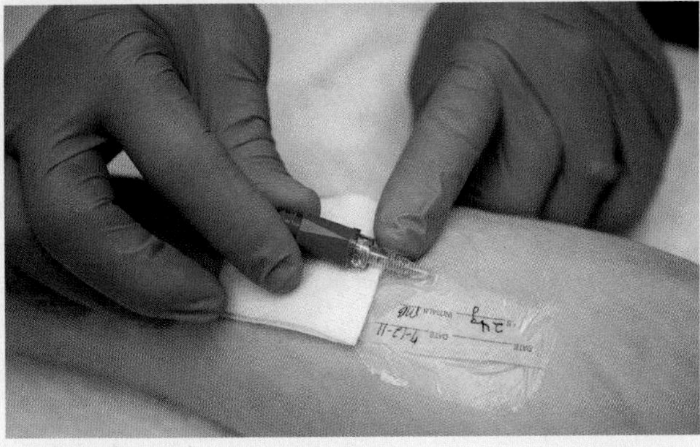

13. Secure the PRN lock device to the extremity with strips of tape ***to reduce the risk of displacement of the cannula from the vein and reduce irritation of the vein due to movement.***
14. Aspirate with the NS flush syringe and observe for a blood return from the cannula hub. ***Blood return indicates the cannula is still in the vein.***
15. Taking at least 1 minute, inject the remaining NS flush solution ***to clear blood out of the tip of the cannula to prevent clotting and obstruction of the cannula.***
16. Close the sliding clamp on the PRN lock device.
17. Disconnect the NS flush syringe from the cannula.
18. Remove contaminated gloves and dispose of all contaminated supplies.
19. Wash hands ***to prevent cross-contamination.***
20. Follow the Ending Implementation Steps located on the inside back cover.
21. Document the conversion from IV infusion to PRN lock.

If Patient Has a PRN Lock Device Connecting the Tubing to the Cannula Hub

8. Disconnect the IV tubing from the injection port of the PRN lock device.
9. Cleanse the injection port with an alcohol wipe or CHG-alcohol combination product ***to remove microorganisms.***
10. Connect the Luer-Lok tip of the NS flush syringe to the PRN lock device injection port or insert a needle or blunt-tipped adapter into the injection port of the PRN lock device.
11. Aspirate by pulling the syringe plunger back while observing for blood return ***to ensure placement of the cannula in the vein.*** If blood return is observed, flush the PRN lock device and cannula by injecting the NS flush slowly over at least 1 minute.
12. Close the slide clamp on the PRN device ***to prevent blood from backing up into the device, where it can clot.***
13. Disconnect the NS syringe.
14. Remove contaminated gloves and dispose of all contaminated supplies.
15. Wash hands ***to prevent cross-contamination.***

(skill continues on page 894)

Skill 38.3 (continued)

16. Follow the Ending Implementation Steps located on the inside back cover.
17. Document the conversion from IV infusion to PRN lock.

Evaluation Step

1. Reassess the site ***to ensure that there are no signs of infiltration before leaving the room.***

Sample Documentation

07/18/22 1520 IV converted to PRN saline lock. Site without edema or erythema. No C/O discomfort. ——— ——— Nurse's signature and credentials

Sample electronic documentation is below.

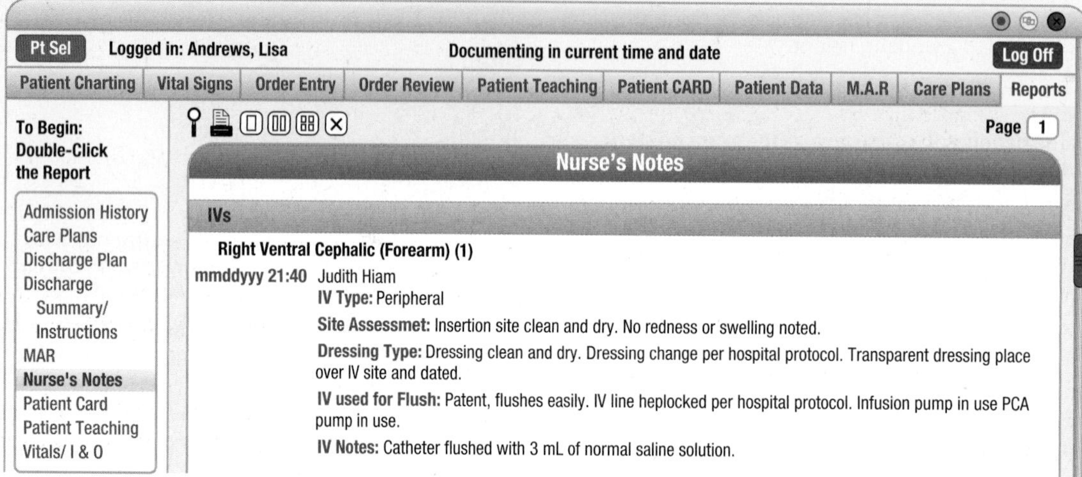

Skill 38.4 Calculating IV Infusion Rate

Assessment Steps

1. Review the health-care provider's order for size of IV solution bag and rate of infusion ***to reduce the risk of error.***
2. Assess whether you will infuse the IV solution by gravity flow or with an IV pump or controller.
3. Assess for the correct drop factor. If using gravity flow, check the tubing administration set box for the drop factor. If you are going to use a pump/controller, use 60 as the drop factor. ***This information is required to calculate the rate of infusion.***

Planning Steps

1. Plan to use this formula to calculate the infusion rate using the three pieces of data obtained during assessment:

$$\frac{\text{Volume} \times \text{drop factor}}{\text{Time}} = \text{rate of infusion,}$$

where *Volume* is the volume of fluid to be infused, *Time* is the time (in minutes) in which the specified volume of fluid is to infuse, and the rate of infusion is measured in mL/hr if an IV pump is used or in gtts/min if gravity flow is used.

2. Obtain the needed supplies: administration set package (for gravity flow), and calculator or pen and paper.

Implementation Steps

1. Multiply the volume of fluid you want to infuse times the drop factor.
2. Divide the total by the number of minutes in which you want this volume of fluid to infuse.
Note: Remember that, if you use the volume of the entire bag, you will have to use the total number of minutes in which you want to infuse the entire bag. If you use a lesser volume, such as the volume that is to infuse per hour, you must use only the number of minutes in 1 hour (60 minutes). If the volume is 50 mL and it must infuse in 20 minutes, then use these same two figures. The volume and time must be related to each other.

Evaluation Step

1. Evaluate your calculations and result, making certain you calculated the rate in gtts/min if it is to infuse by gravity flow and mL/hour if it is to infuse by pump.

Skill 38.5 Adding Medications to a Primary IV Solution

Assessment Steps

1. *Safety: Review the health-care provider's order to verify the type, route, and dosage of medication; type, size, and route of primary IV solution; and rate of infusion. This reduces the risk for error, reduces the risk of administration of inappropriate solution and allergic reactions, and better prepares you to detect problems.*
2. *Safety: Determine medication compatibility with primary IV solution and other drugs the patient is receiving. This prevents incompatibility errors.*
3. *Safety: Assess patient's allergies to make certain it is safe to administer the medication.*
4. Collect data regarding the medication's action, purpose, side effects, dosage, drug–drug interactions, and nursing implications. ***This provides you with the required knowledge to evaluate the appropriateness of the medication order and to be prepared to detect problems.***
5. If the patient already has the primary IV solution infusing, assess the IV site ***to rule out any signs and symptoms of infiltration and phlebitis.***

Planning Steps

1. Gather needed equipment and supplies: correct type and size of bag of IV solution; correct type, form, and dosage of medication; syringe large enough to draw up medication; 20- or 21-G (0.9- or 0.8-mm) needle; alcohol wipe; and orange or other bright-colored medication label. ***Being prepared saves you time and unnecessary footwork. Being prepared also helps you to appear more competent and confident, both of which are important to the patient's perception of and trust in you.***
2. Complete the "medication added" label, including the patient's name and room number; name, dosage, and rate of infusion of medication; date and time; and your initials.

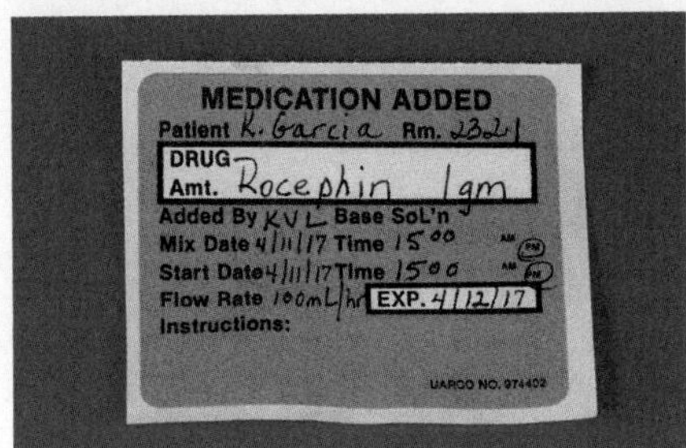

MEDICATION ADDED
Patient K. Garcia Rm. 2321
DRUG
Amt. Rocephin 1gm
Added By KVL Base SoL'n
Mix Date 4/11/17 Time 15⁰⁰ AM PM
Start Date 4/11/17 Time 15⁰⁰ AM PM
Flow Rate 100mL/hr EXP. 4/12/17
Instructions:
UARCO NO. 974402

3. Inspect packages for intactness and expiration dates ***to prevent use of unsafe supplies.***

Implementation Steps

1. Follow the Initial Implementation Steps located on the inside back cover.
2. *Safety: Check the medication label a minimum of three times to prevent medication error.*
3. *Safety: Use two methods of identifying the patient according to facility policy to reduce the risk of error.*
4. Explain to the patient what you are about to do. Provide any necessary patient teaching ***to reduce patient anxiety and increase compliance.***
5. *Safety: Wash hands to prevent cross-contamination.*
6. Using aseptic technique, attach the needle to the syringe. *Safety: The needle hub and the tip of the syringe must stay sterile to reduce the risk of infection.*
7. Cleanse the rubber stopper of the medication vial with an alcohol wipe or CHG-alcohol combination product ***to remove any microorganisms.*** If the medication requires dilution, add an appropriate volume of the proper diluent and mix well.
8. Using aseptic technique, instill an equal volume of air to displace the number of milliliters of medication you will remove from vial. *Safety: The cleansed rubber stopper on the vial and the needle must be kept sterile to reduce the risk of infection.*
9. Withdraw the correct volume/dosage of additive and remove the needle from the vial.
10. Locate the medication port on the IV solution bag. It normally does ***not*** have a cap or cover. Cleanse the port with an alcohol wipe or CHG-alcohol combination product ***to remove any microorganisms. Note: Do not confuse it with the port for the IV tubing, which has a rubber plug/cover over the end of it.***
11. Using aseptic technique, insert the needle through the medication port, using care to avoid puncturing the back side of the IV bag or port with the needle, ***which would require a new bag and tubing.*** *Safety: The cleansed port and needle must be kept sterile.*

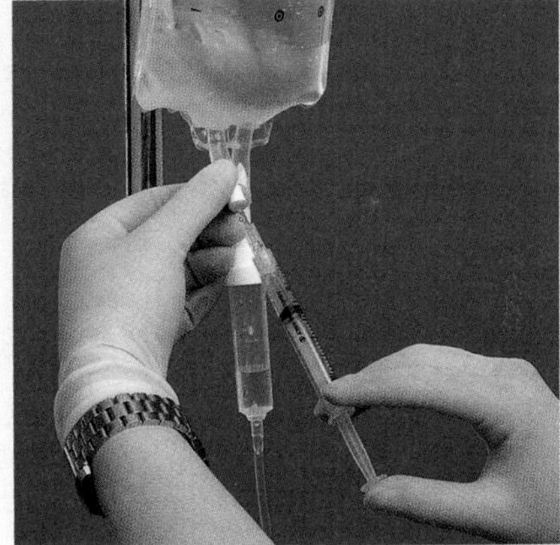

12. Instill the medication and remove the needle.
13. *Safety: Activate the needle safety mechanism and dispose of it in the sharps container.*
14. Gently invert the IV bag several times ***to distribute medication*** and hang it back on the IV pole.
15. Apply the label to the IV bag to which you will instill the medication ***to clarify what is infusing and help to reduce medication errors.***
16. Reassess the IV infusion rate ***to ensure it is still flowing at the ordered rate.***
17. Follow the Ending Implementation Steps located on the inside back cover.

(skill continues on page 896)

Skill 38.5 (continued)

Evaluation Steps

1. Evaluate for even distribution of medication and inspect for precipitation or clouding.
2. After the solution is infusing, again assess the patient's IV site ***to rule out any signs and symptoms of infiltration or phlebitis.*** Make certain the patient feels no discomfort.
3. Monitor for therapeutic effects, side effects, and adverse reactions ***to evaluate the effectiveness of the medication.***
4. Evaluate the adequacy and balance of the patient's intake and output ***to detect possible signs of fluid imbalance.***

Sample Documentation

12/31/22 1430 One vial potassium chloride added to hanging IV bag of D5W with approximately 900 mL left in bag. Infusing @ 125 mL/hr. IV site intact, clean, dry, without edema, erythema, or discomfort. ——————— Nurse's signature and credentials

Skill 38.6 Initiating Peripheral Venipuncture

Assessment Steps

1. Review the health-care provider's order for venipuncture, type and size of bag of IV solution, and rate of infusion. ***This provides you with the required knowledge to evaluate the appropriateness of the order and reduce errors.***
2. Review the patient's diagnoses; medical history; risk factors for circulatory fluid overload; reason for IV access; age; mental cognition; and any allergies to medications, solution, latex, iodine, and tape. ***This reduces the risk of administration of inappropriate solution and allergic reactions and better prepares you to detect problems.***
3. Assess whether the patient has ever had an IV before and determine what patient teaching needs to be done. ***Patient teaching reduces patient anxiety and increases patient compliance.***
4. Assess which side is the patient's dominant hand; assess the size and caliber of the veins in the nondominant extremity ***to determine the best site for IV initiation.***

Planning Steps

1. Gather needed equipment and supplies: IV pole, IV pump if available, correct type and size of bag of IV solution, correct primary IV tubing administration set that works with pump, extension tubing if desired, two sizes of IV needle catheter that will be suitable for the patient's needs, IV start kit or the components normally found in one (antiseptic wipe, tourniquet, sterile transparent occlusive dressing, roll of tape, sterile 2×2-inch gauze pad, and IV site label), labels for tubing and bag of solution, towel or waterproof pad, and clean examination gloves. ***Adequate preparation saves you time and footwork and helps you appear more confident and competent.***
2. *Safety: Check the solution label at least three times to avoid medication error.*
3. Calculate the rate of infusion in mL/hr for a pump or gtts/min for gravity, whichever applies. ***This reduces the risk of an incorrect administration rate.***
4. Inspect packages for intactness and expiration dates ***to ensure sterility and reduce the risk of infection.***

Implementation Steps

Before Going to the Patient's Room

1. *Safety: Wash hands to prevent cross-contamination.*
2. If a pump will be used, program or set the pump for the volume to infuse and rate of infusion.
3. Inspect the outer wrapper of the IV solution bag for intactness and moisture before removing the outer wrapper ***to detect leaking of solution, which would indicate a breach in sterility.***
4. Inspect the IV solution bag for the name or type of solution and expiration date. Inspect the solution for clarity. Make certain the fluid is clear, not cloudy, and contains no particulates. ***This helps to ensure the use of the correct solution and clarify whether it is safe for use.*** Squeeze the bag ***to observe for pinhole leaks.***
5. Apply a label to the bag of solution, including patient name, room number, date, time, and rate of infusion. ***This communicates the appropriate information to each nurse providing care to the patient.***

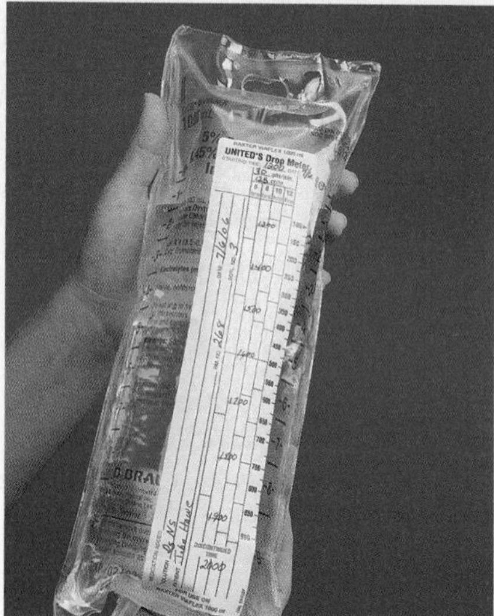

6. Verify that you have the correct primary IV tubing administration set for the type of pump being used or for gravity infusion. ***This increases efficiency and helps to control cost and waste of opening incorrect supplies.***
7. Open the package and remove the tubing administration set. Review the manufacturer's priming instructions if you are not familiar with this set ***to save time and increase competency.*** Close the roller clamp on the tubing ***to prevent premature dripping of solution into the administration set. This helps to reduce the risk of air bubbles while priming the tubing.***

Skill 38.6 (continued)

8. Locate the port on the IV bag of solution into which the tubing administration set piercing pin will be inserted. Remove the rubber plug or cover from the port. *Safety: Use caution to maintain sterility of the port.*
9. Remove the protective cap from the piercing pin, or spike, at the end of the tubing administration set. *Safety: Use care to maintain sterility of the piercing pin to reduce the risk of infection.*
10. Insert the piercing pin into the port of the IV bag without contaminating the piercing pin. Be certain to hold the port of the bag straight as you insert the piercing pin, ***to prevent piercing the side of the port with the piercing pin.***

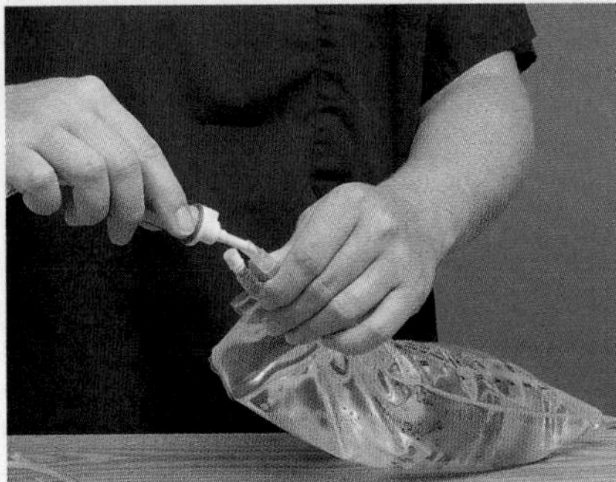

11. Squeeze the drip chamber on the tubing administration set and fill it approximately one-third to one-half full of solution. ***This leaves adequate room in the drip chamber to observe the solution dripping.***

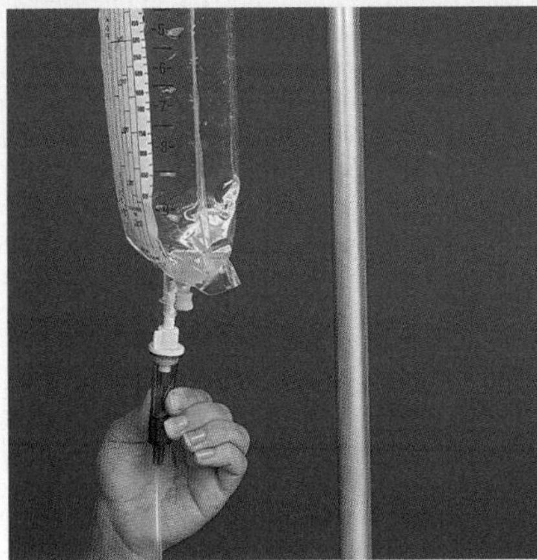

12. Hang the IV bag on an IV pole. Follow any special priming instructions from the manufacturer. Otherwise, remove the cap from the end of the tubing administration set, maintaining sterility of the tubing end. Next, prime the tubing by opening the roller clamp and allowing solution to run through the tubing set ***to displace all the air within the solution to reduce the risk of air embolism.*** Once all the air has been removed, close the roller clamp and recap the end of the tubing, maintaining sterility of the tubing end and the cap ***to reduce the risk of infection.***
13. Complete the label with the date and time started and date the tubing is due to be changed. Attach the label to the tubing. ***This communicates when the tubing should be changed to reduce the risk of infection.***
14. Drape the tubing over the top of the pole. *Safety: In order to prevent contamination, do not allow tubing to touch the floor.* If using a pump, do not insert the tubing into the pump mechanism until free flow of solution has ensured proper cannulation of the vein.

After Entering the Patient's Room

15. Follow the Initial Implementation Steps located on the inside back cover.
16. Explain to the patient what you are about to do. Provide any necessary patient teaching to reduce anxiety and increase patient compliance. Place patient in a comfortable position and raise the bed to a working height.
17. *Safety: Wash hands again to prevent cross-contamination.*
18. Place a towel or moisture-proof pad under the patient's nondominant arm. This saves you the extra work of changing soiled linens.

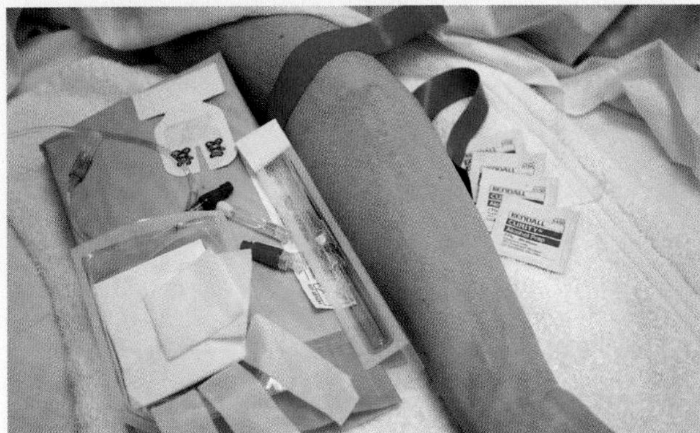

19. Apply a tourniquet and use recommended methods for dilating veins until adequate vein distention is obtained. This increases successful cannulation of the vein with fewer needle sticks for the patient.
20. Assess and palpate veins to select a vein.
21. Remove the tourniquet ***to allow venous circulation.***

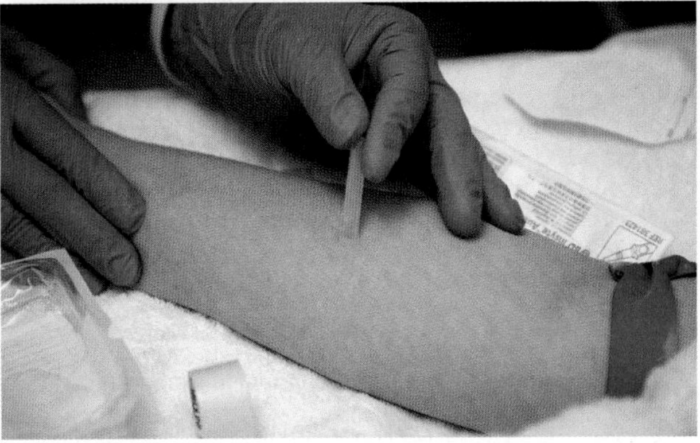

22. *Safety: Apply clean examination gloves to protect you from blood-borne pathogens.*

(skill continues on page 898)

Skill 38.6 (continued)

23. Select an appropriate IV catheter based on the vein.
24. Reapply the tourniquet 4 to 8 inches proximal to the venipuncture site without contaminating the cleansed site. The tail of the tourniquet should be tucked from the top side (proximal) rather than from below (distal). This results in both ends of the tourniquet coming out of the top side ***so that they do not contaminate the cleansed site.***
25. Cleanse the site with facility-preferred antiseptic wipe. Start in the center where you intend to perform the venipuncture. Using vigorous friction, cleanse in widening, concentric circles for at least 30 seconds. ***This removes microorganisms and reduces the risk of infection.***
26. Inform the patient of the impending prick ***to avoid surprising the patient, which can cause the patient to jump or move.*** Insert the needle through the skin and into the vein with one motion if possible, ***which reduces the discomfort of probing.***
27. Carefully remove the cap from the sterile IV needle cannula, maintaining sterility of the entire length of needle and cannula ***to reduce the risk of contamination and infection.***

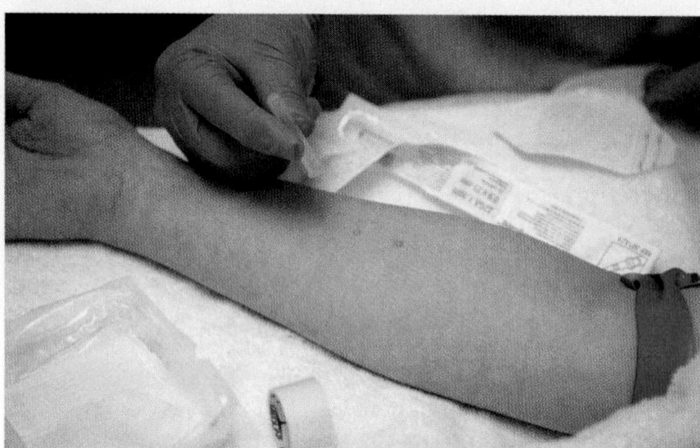

28. Place your nondominant hand ***several inches distal*** to the intended venipuncture site ***to reduce the risk of contaminating the IV cannula with your nondominant hand during initiation.*** Use the thumb on your nondominant hand to pull the skin taut ***to ease needle insertion through the skin and decrease patient discomfort.***
29. Hold the IV needle in your dominant hand with the bevel up. Use a 30- to 45-degree angle depending on the location and depth of the vein. If the vein is shallow and appears fragile, decrease the needle angle to 15 degrees. ***The bevel-up position eases needle insertion and reduces trauma to the vein, which decreases patient discomfort. Using too much angle will increase the risk of going through the vein.***
30. Upon obtaining blood return in the flashback chamber, advance the entire IV needle and cannula just far enough into the lumen of the vein to ensure that the end of the cannula is within the vein, usually less than ⅛ inch. *Safety: Do not insert the entire length of both the needle and cannula into the vein, which would increase the risk of the needle going through the vein.*
31. Once the bevel of the needle and the end of the cannula are inside the vein, use the aseptic technique to carefully advance the cannula over and off the end of the needle into the vein lumen.

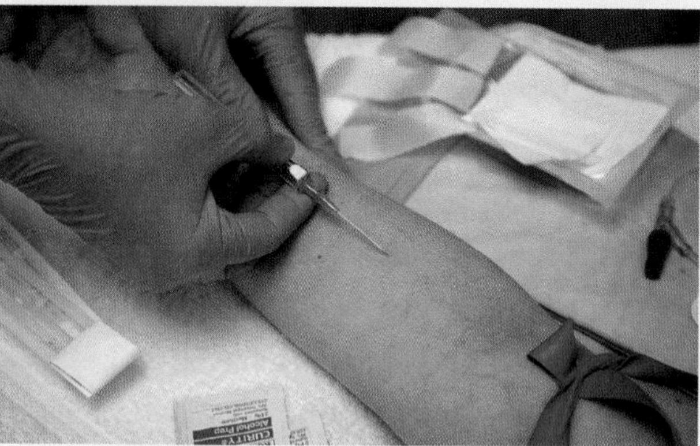

Avoid forcing the cannula, ***which can cause displacement of the cannula from the vein and damage to the vein walls.*** If resistance is met, gently apply traction to the vein or try to turn the cannula ever so slightly. If the cannula still does not advance with ease, it may be helpful to wait for further advancement of the cannula until you have connected the administration set tubing and slowly initiated flow of the solution. ***This sometimes helps to "float" the cannula into the vein.***

32. Once the cannula is fully inserted, use the thumb and index finger of your nondominant hand to secure the cannula hub. *Safety: Do not contaminate the open end of the hub.* Then use the middle or ring finger of your nondominant hand to apply pressure over the vein, beyond the end of the cannula, ***to prevent excessive bleeding during connection of the tubing.*** While your nondominant hand secures the cannula hub without contaminating it, use your dominant hand to carefully remove the needle from the cannula. Depending on the type and style of needle and cannula used, the needle may be removed from the cannula and vein by pressing the retracting button so that the needle retracts into the needle guard, or some other method may be used.
Some needle types require that you actually ***pull*** the needle from inside the cannula before the safety device will activate. Know your equipment and supplies and how they work prior to attempting IV initiation. Avoid "learning how to use" them at the bedside, ***which may increase patient anxiety and decrease the patient's perception of your competence.***

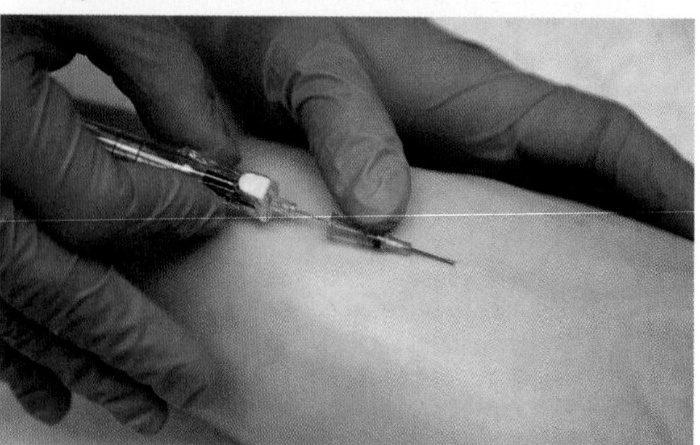

Skill 38.6 (continued)

33. Using aseptic technique, quickly remove the cap from the end of the IV tubing. With your nondominant hand, use a finger to apply pressure against the vein proximal to the cannula while securing the cannula hub with your thumb and index finger. With your dominant hand, aseptically insert the tubing end into the cannula hub, securing attachment by gently screwing on the Luer-Lok.

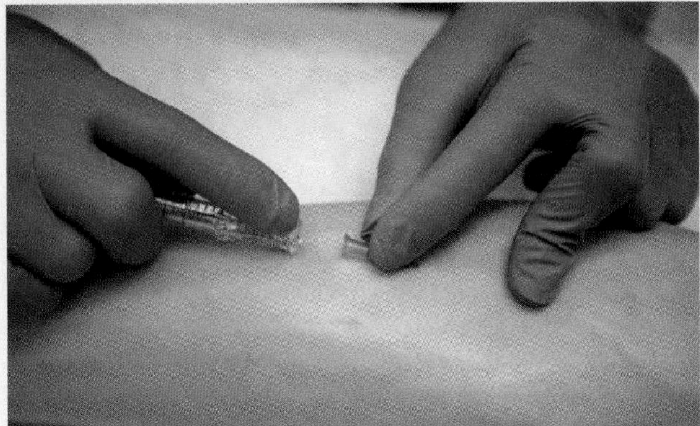

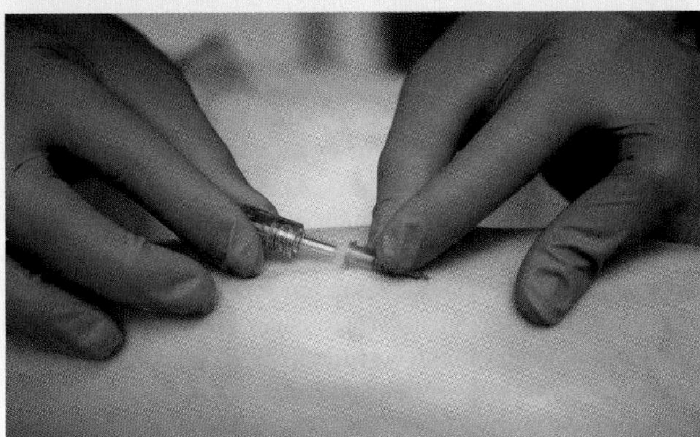

Safety: Avoid using a one-handed method of removing the cap from the tubing. It is virtually impossible to do without contaminating the sterile tubing end.

34. Do not apply a site dressing yet. Continue to hold the connection between the cannula hub and tubing securely against the patient's skin, preventing bending or crimping of the cannula. ***To ensure proper cannulation of the vein,*** open the roller clamp on the tubing and observe for free flow of solution. As solution is infused, make certain that there is no swelling at the site. Once free flow of solution is confirmed, partially close the roller clamp to prevent rapid infusion of solution while securing the site.
35. To secure the site, peel backing from a sterile transparent occlusive dressing and apply, covering the insertion site and the hub of the cannula only. ***This helps to secure the cannula and maintain the sterility of the puncture site, and it allows the tubing to be changed at the hub connection without having to remove the transparent occlusive dressing.***
36. Use strips of tape to secure the tubing to the extremity ***to reduce the risk of displacement of the cannula and infiltration.*** Avoid application of tape strips over the transparent occlusive dressing unless absolutely necessary. ***This allows tubing to be changed at the hub connection without having to remove the transparent occlusive dressing.***
37. Apply a small label with the date, time, cannula gauge, and your initials on the IV site. ***This communicates to staff when the IV should be changed to reduce the risk of phlebitis.***
38. Insert the tubing into the pump mechanism, set the volume to be infused (volume of bag) and rate of infusion (mL/hr), open the roller clamp all the way, and start the pump. This step will be different when using different manufacturer's IV pump models, so be certain to read the instructions prior to use.

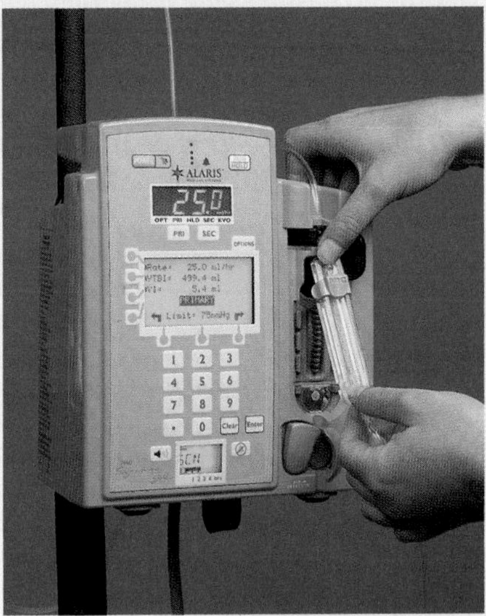

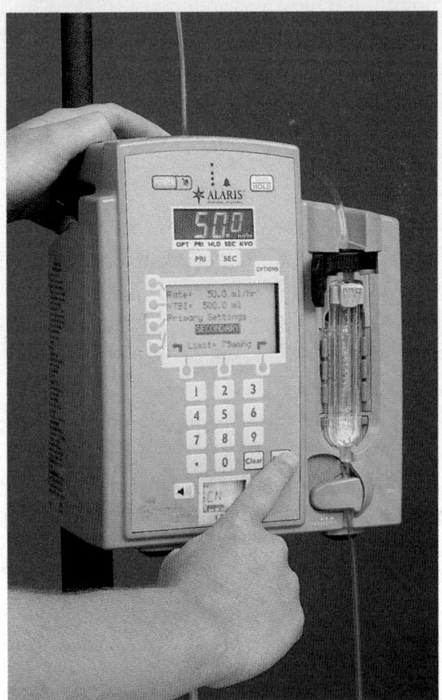

39. Dispose of used supplies and discard the needle in the sharps container ***to reduce the risk of contaminated needle sticks.***
40. Follow the Ending Implementation Steps located on the inside back cover.

(skill continues on page 900)

Skill 38.6 (continued)

Evaluation Steps

1. Observe the infusion site ***to make certain there is no swelling with infusion of the solution.*** Inquire of the patient regarding discomfort. ***Swelling and discomfort both are indicative of possible infiltration.***
2. Before leaving the room, reassess that the pump is working; the solution is flowing; and the site remains clean, dry, and without edema or erythema.
3. Evaluate the adequacy and balance of the patient's intake and output ***to detect possible signs of fluid imbalance.***

Sample Documentation

02/01/22 1915 IV initiated per health-care provider's orders, using aseptic technique, in Rt. forearm with 22-G × 1-in. intracath, one attempt, without difficulty. 1,000 mL D5W infusing per pump at 125 mL/hr. Site clean, dry, intact, and without erythema or edema. Voices no discomfort. ——————

—————— Nurse's signature and credentials

Skill 38.7 Adding a New Bag of IV Solution to an Existing IV Line

Assessment Steps

1. Review the health-care provider's order for type and volume of IV solution and rate of infusion ***to ensure correctness of the order.***
2. Review the patient's diagnoses, medical history, and allergies to medications ***to determine the appropriateness of the order.***
3. If the infusion rate is to be different from the rate at which the IV solution is now infusing, calculate the new rate in mL/hr for a pump or gtts/min for gravity flow.

Planning Steps

1. Obtain the ordered type and volume of solution and a new label for the bag. ***Being prepared saves time and effort.***
2. Inspect packages for intactness and expiration dates ***to ensure continued sterility.***
3. Fill out the label and apply to the bag ***for communication of contents to staff members.***

Implementation Steps

1. Follow the Initial Implementation Steps located on the inside back cover.
2. Explain to the patient what you are about to do. Provide any necessary patient teaching ***to decrease patient anxiety.***
3. *Safety: Wash hands to prevent cross-contamination.*
4. Assess the patient's IV site for signs of infiltration and phlebitis.
5. ***If using an IV pump or controller,*** press the button to stop the infusion. ***If infusing by gravity, clamp the tubing.***
6. Remove the rubber stopper covering the tubing port on the new IV solution bag, maintaining sterility.
7. Remove the IV solution bag from the IV pole and invert the bag (upside down) ***to prevent leakage of solution after removing the piercing pin.***
8. Remove the piercing pin, maintaining its sterility ***to lower the risk of infection.***
9. Insert the piercing pin into the tubing port on the new bag of IV solution, using care to maintain sterility of the piercing pin and the inside of the port.
10. Right the bag and hang it on the IV pole.
11. Squeeze the tubing drip chamber to fill the chamber one-third to one-half full. Do not overfill the chamber; leave room ***to observe dripping of the solution.*** If you accidently overfill, invert the bag and squeeze the drip chamber so that the extra fluid runs back into the bag.
12. ***If using an IV pump,*** set the volume to be infused and the rate of infusion on the pump. ***If infusing by gravity,*** count the drops falling in the drop chamber, setting the drop rate to the precalculated rate.
13. Place label with the time, date, and initials on the IV bag. ***This allows nurses to see when the IV bad was changed and by whom.***
14. Follow the Ending Implementation Steps located on the inside back cover.
15. If the new solution bag was added solely because the previous one had completely infused, document the bag of IV solution only on the medication administration record (MAR). If a new health-care provider's order prompted discontinuation of the infusing bag to hang a different new one, it should be documented in the nurses' notes as well as the MAR.

Evaluation Steps

1. Assess the IV site ***to ensure that there is no edema or erythema.***
2. Evaluate the adequacy and balance of the patient's intake and output ***to detect possible signs of fluid imbalance.***

Sample Documentation

06/25/22 0235 IV solution D5W discontinued and 1,000 mL NS hung & infusing at 80 mL/hr per health-care provider's order. IV site without erythema or edema. ——————

—————— Nurse's signature and credentials

Skill 38.8 Discontinuing an IV Infusion or PRN Lock

Assessment Step

1. Review the health-care provider's order to discontinue the IV infusion or PRN lock ***to reduce the risk of error.***

Planning Step

1. Gather needed supplies: alcohol wipes, sterile 2×2-inch (5×5-cm) gauze pad, bandage, and examination gloves. ***Being prepared saves you time and effort.***

Implementation Steps

1. Follow the Initial Implementation Steps located on the inside back cover.
2. Check the patient's identification using two methods according to facility policy.
3. Explain to the patient what you are about to do. Provide any necessary patient teaching. ***This reduces patient anxiety and increases patient compliance.***
4. *Safety: Wash hands to prevent cross-contamination.*
5. Apply clean examination gloves ***to protect you from bloodborne pathogens.***
6. Close the tubing clamp and turn the IV pump off if one is in use.
7. While securing the cannula hub with your gloved nondominant hand, use your gloved dominant hand to remove tape securing the tubing to the extremity, pulling the tape ends toward the IV site ***to avoid tearing skin at the puncture site.***
8. Continuing to secure the cannula hub, lift all four edges of the transparent occlusive dressing toward the insertion site until the transparent occlusive dressing is no longer secured to the patient's skin. ***This reduces the risk of crimping or breaking the cannula from the hub and decreases the risk of tearing the skin at the puncture site.***
9. Using your nondominant hand, apply gentle pressure to the vein immediately proximal to the inserted end of the cannula or needle, with a sterile ×2-inch (5×5-cm) gauze pad, *without* applying pressure over the cannula itself. ***Doing this proximally reduces the risk of accidental pressure on the cannula causing it to separate from its hub and become an embolism.*** As you use your dominant hand to gently remove the cannula from the vein, keeping the cannula parallel to the skin, slide the gauze pad in your nondominant hand toward the insertion site so that once the cannula tip is out of the vein, you can increase the pressure being applied to the insertion site to prevent formation of a hematoma. ***This helps to reduce the risk of hematoma at the site.***
10. Immediately inspect the tip of the cannula upon removal ***to ensure that the cannula tip is intact.***

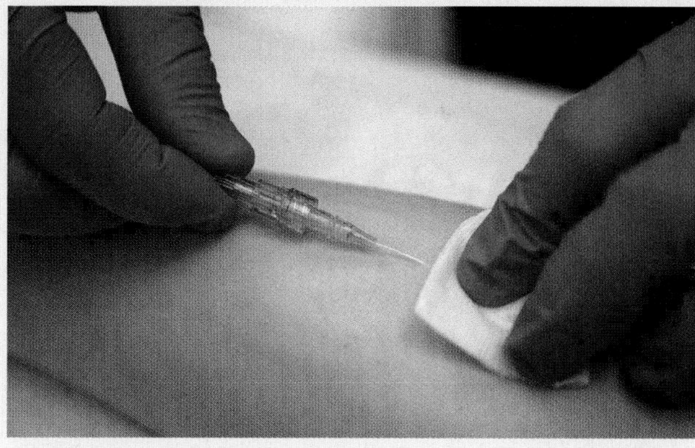

11. Hold pressure on the insertion site while cleansing the surrounding area of any blood using alcohol wipes. Maintain pressure to the site for 1 minute before lifting the gauze pad to inspect for cessation of bleeding. If the patient takes anticoagulants or bleeds easily, hold pressure for 3 to 5 minutes. ***This helps to reduce the risk of hematoma formation.***
12. Apply a bandage ***to reduce the risk of contamination with microorganisms.***
13. Remove and dispose of the contaminated gloves and cannula in proper biohazard bags.
14. Wash hands ***to prevent cross-contamination.***
15. Follow the Ending Implementation Steps located on the inside back cover.

Evaluation Steps

1. Evaluate to determine whether the tip of the cannula is intact as soon as it is withdrawn from the vein ***to ensure that the tip did not break off inside the vein, making it an embolism.***
2. Assess the site for bleeding or bruising.
3. Assess and record the total volume infused as noted on the IV pump on the intake and output record. Assess intake and output for imbalance.

Sample Documentation

08/27/22 1325 IV discontinued with intact 22-G cannula, according to health-care provider's order. No erythema, edema, or bruising noted at site. Total IV volume infused 635 mL. ————————————

———————— Nurse's signature and credentials

Skill 38.9 Preparing, Initiating, and Monitoring the Infusion of Blood and Blood Products

Assessment Steps

1. Verify that informed consent has been obtained. ***The patient's informed consent is required for administration of blood.***
2. Assess the patient's diagnoses and evaluate risk factors for fluid imbalance, urine output, and laboratory values.
3. Assess the patient's knowledge level regarding transfusion ***to determine teaching needs.***
4. Assess the patient's IV site ***to ensure there are no signs of infiltration or phlebitis.*** If there is *not* an IV access device already in place, initiate IV access using a 20-gauge or larger cannula depending on facility policy.

(skill continues on page 902)

Skill 38.9 (continued)

5. Assess the patient's history for blood transfusions and possible reactions.

Planning Steps

1. Perform any necessary patient teaching and explain signs and symptoms the patient should report during the transfusion. ***This helps to reduce patient anxiety and increase patient compliance.***
2. *Safety: Verify with a second nurse that the physician's order matches the blood components about to be infused, that the patient name and ID number on the unit of blood product container matches the one on the patient's ID band and the one on the transfusion record, that the unit of blood product identification number on the unit's label matches the one on the transfusion record, that the ABO blood type and Rh factor of the unit of blood matches that of the patient's, and finally that the blood's expiration date has not passed. Follow facility policy closely for this safety check. Document the date and time the infusion starts on the blood bank form and the MAR.*

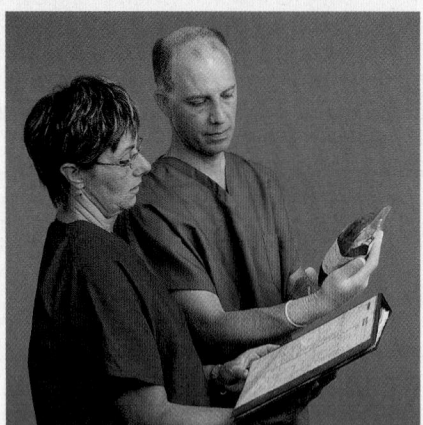

3. Gather needed equipment and supplies: blood administration Y-set, container of blood product that you have previously verified, container of 0.9% sodium chloride (NS) IV solution, alcohol wipes, tape, and clean examination gloves. ***Preparation saves you time and footwork.***

Implementation Steps

Before Going to the Patient's Room

1. *Safety: Wash hands and apply clean examination gloves to protect you from contact with blood-borne pathogens.*
2. Inspect the blood administration Y-set package for intactness and expiration dates ***to ensure continued sterility.*** Remove the Y-set from the package.
3. Close the clamps on both of the Y-shaped branches of the blood administration set ***to prevent premature dripping of solution.*** Label the tubing with date and time.
4. Remove the cap from one of the piercing pins and, ***to prevent contamination,*** aseptically spike the NS container port. *Safety: Use only 0.9% sodium chloride as companion to blood and blood products because of incompatibility of all other solutions.*
5. Prime the entire Y-set with the NS solution. ***Priming the Y-set removes air from the tubing.***
   - Begin by back-priming the branch of tubing that will insert into the blood product container. This is done by opening the clamp to the NS and priming the long tail of the tubing that will eventually connect to the patient's IV cannula.
   - Now close the main roller clamp on the long tail of the tubing and proceed with back-priming the second branch of the Y-set that is going to be inserted into the blood product container. Open the roller clamp on the second branch of the Y-set. This will allow NS to flow from the NS branch through the Y-set into the blood branch. As soon as all air in the blood branch of the Y-set has been replaced with NS, close the roller clamp.
   - Remove the cap from the piercing pin and aseptically spike the blood product container.
     - If the unit to be transfused is PRBCs, NS will need to be back-primed into the unit of PRBCs to dilute it to a consistency that will infuse through the Y-set and cannula. Open the roller clamp and allow NS to flow into the unit of PRBCs until the desired dilution is attained. Close the roller clamp.
     - After you close the roller clamp, it should remain closed while you initiate the flow of NS. The roller clamp on the blood product side of the Y-set is not to be opened again until you are ready to start the transfusion. ***The blood product is not infused until the NS has been initiated.***

After Entering the Patient's Room

6. Follow the Initial Implementation Steps located on the inside back cover.
7. Use two methods of identifying the patient according to facility policy ***to reduce the risk of error.***
8. Explain to the patient what you are about to do. Provide any necessary patient teaching. ***This reduces patient anxiety and increases patient compliance.***
9. *Safety: Wash hands to prevent cross-contamination.*
10. Aseptically connect the NS-primed Y-set to the IV cannula in the patient's vein.
11. Open only the clamp to the NS and set it to infuse at the TKO (to keep [the vein] open) rate or as dictated by facility policy.
12. Assess the patient's vital signs. Report any abnormal results to the physician ***prior to starting the blood transfusion.***
13. If vital signs are normal, close the NS roller clamp and open the blood roller clamp. Start the transfusion at a rate of 50 mL per hour for the first 15 minutes and according to facility policy. If there are no signs or symptoms of reaction, increase the rate of infusion. ***The initial slower rate of infusion limits the volume of blood infused should the patient have a reaction within the first 15 minutes.***
14. Remain with the patient for the first 15 minutes ***to assess for reactions.*** Assess vital signs again in 15 minutes, then 30 minutes, and then hourly until the infusion is complete. Monitor for signs and symptoms of reactions. If any are experienced, stop the transfusion immediately, open the roller clamp to begin infusion of NS, perform appropriate nursing interventions (refer back to Table 38.4), and notify the physician stat. Save the Y-set tubing, the unit of blood, and the bag of NS ***for return to the laboratory for testing.*** Leave the Y-set attached to the blood bag and NS. Also obtain a urine specimen from the patient and deliver it to the laboratory.
15. The transfusion will complete within a 2- to 4-hour window according to facility policy and patient's ability to tolerate rapid infusion of blood. Do not allow blood to hang longer than 4 hours.
16. Remove and dispose of contaminated gloves. Then wash hands ***to reduce microorganisms.***

Skill 38.9 (continued)

17. At completion of the blood transfusion, reapply clean gloves and close the blood clamp. Open the NS clamp and flush the line ***to ensure that the patient receives any blood product that might have remained in the line.***
18. Once the line has been flushed with NS, the IV site is maintained at TKO rate until it is determined that no further blood transfusion will be administered.
19. Some facilities require that the empty blood bag be returned to the laboratory even when there were no problems during transfusion.
20. After you have completed nursing care requiring contact with the blood bag and Y-set, remove and dispose of contaminated gloves.
21. Assess one final set of vital signs.
22. Wash hands ***to prevent cross-contamination.***
23. Follow the Ending Implementation Steps located on the inside back cover.
24. Document the transfusion procedure, including all assessment findings, any reactions experienced, vital signs, volume infused, time the transfusion was completed, and patient's condition posttransfusion.

Evaluation Steps

1. Evaluate the patient's tolerance of the transfusion throughout the entire infusion.

Sample Documentation

04/06/22 1730 Awake & alert. No C/O of pain, nausea, or discomfort. Skin pink, warm, & dry. IV Saline lock with 20-G cannula intact in left forearm, site without erythema or edema. Teaching done RE: blood transfusion procedure. States she has had numerous transfusions in the past and has no questions or concerns. Informed consent signed earlier and in the medical record. ——————— Nurse's signature and credentials

04/06/22 1755 Physician's order, plasma component, Pt. ID band, Type & Crossmatch results, Unit of plasma type, Rh factor, and ID number, plasma expiration date of 04/7/15, all checked by me and L. Cook, RN. Blood transfusion record completed and signed by Cook and Me. ——————— Nurse's signature and credentials

04/06/22 1757 I concur with the above entry. ——————— Nurse Cook's signature and credentials

04/06/22 1800 NS infusion initiated via 20-G cannula. BP 116/68, T - 98°F orally, AP - 73 reg & distinct, R - 19 reg & even. 1810 First unit, 250 mL of A + plasma, ID#329776105, began per gravity flow, infusing at 2 mL/min. ——————— Nurse's signature and credentials

04/06/22 1815 BP - 118/72, T - 98°F, P - 76, R - 21. No C/O voiced. ——————— Nurse's signature and credentials

04/06/22 1830 BP - 122/66, T - 98.2°F, P - 69, R - 22. No C/O voiced. ——————— Nurse's signature and credentials

04/06/22 1900 BP - 118/70, T - 98.2°F, P - 73, R - 20. No C/O voiced. Rate of plasma infusion increased to 125 mL/hr. ——————— Nurse's signature and credentials

04/06/22 2000 BP - 122/72, T - 98.4°F, P - 78, R - 21. No C/O voiced. IV site intact, no erythema or edema. Still infusing at 125 mL/hr. No S&S of reaction. ——————— Nurse's signature and credentials

04/06/22 2100 BP - 124/74, T - 98.4°F, P - 74, R - 22. No C/O voiced. IV site intact, no erythema or edema. Still at 125 mL/hr. No S&S of reaction. ——————— Nurse's signature and credentials

04/06/22 2200 Transfusion completed. NS started & infusing TKO. IV site intact, no erythema or edema. BP - 124/70, T - 98.4°F, P - 73, R - 22. ——————— Nurse's signature and credentials

POST CONFERENCE

Your experiences today were very valuable in helping you learn about IV therapy. You did have to discontinue your patient's current IV and start a new one. His veins were fragile, and you learned the value of not using a tourniquet the second time you attempted to initiate IV therapy. You were successful that time and were able to reestablish his IV fluids. Your patient began to have some complications of hypotonic solution infusion, which you recognized because you had studied your chapter carefully. You reported them immediately to your instructor, who then notified the charge nurse. The health-care provider decreased the rate of infusion and changed the IV fluid to normal saline to prevent further problems.

Key Points

- The purposes of IV therapy include providing daily body fluid and electrolytes, replacing abnormal loss of fluids and electrolytes, and providing IV administration of medications.
- Medications and IV solutions mixed or administered at the same time must be compatible.
- It is important for you to understand the differences between isotonic, hypotonic, and hypertonic fluids and when each is appropriate for use.
- Movement of excessive volumes of fluid from the vascular space into the interstitial spaces is known as third-space shifting, which lowers BP and causes edema and swelling of individual cells.
- Strict aseptic technique must be utilized during preparation of supplies, initiation of IV access, and maintenance of IV therapy.
- Never stick a patient more than three times before seeking the assistance of another nurse.
- Infusion rate is calculated by multiplying the volume times the drop factor and then dividing the total by the time in minutes. Gravity flow is measured by gtts/min. Pump flow is measured in mL/hr.
- Complications of IV therapy include infiltration, extravasation, phlebitis, thrombophlebitis, localized infection, septicemia, severed cannula, air embolism, circulatory fluid overload, and speed shock.
- The classic signs and symptoms of infiltration include edema; cool, pale, or taut skin; absence of blood return; sluggish flow or lack of infusion; site discomfort; and blanching of skin.
- Extravasation requires immediate intervention to reduce the amount of tissue damage.
- The best veins to consider for IV therapy are the cephalic vein, basilic vein, median cubital vein, and accessory cephalic vein.
- Blood products are compatible ONLY with 0.9% sodium chloride (NS).
- Informed consent is required for blood product transfusion.
- A type and crossmatch test must be performed prior to blood or blood component transfusion.
- Two nurses must check and confirm that the blood component matches the physician's order, the correct blood type and Rh factor, the patient name and ID number, that the blood unit ID number matches those on the transfusion record, and the blood's expiration date. Both nurses must sign the documentation.
- Vital signs must be monitored closely along with other signs and symptoms of reactions during blood product transfusion.
- Alternative vascular access devices are used when a peripherally inserted IV is not optimal.
- The PICC is advanced into a peripheral vein such as the basilic, brachial, or cephalic vein and then advanced into the superior vena cava or right atrium.

Review Questions

Select the answer that is most appropriate for each of the following questions. Some questions may have more than one correct answer. Select all that apply.

1. The minimum length of time that is safe for administration of IV push medication is:
   1. 1 hour.
   2. 30 seconds.
   3. 5 minutes.
   4. the amount of time designated by the medication manufacturer.
   5. 1 minute per 1 milligram.

2. The difference(s) between a primary IV administration set and a secondary IVPB administration set include(s) which of the following?
   1. The secondary IVPB administration set is used for administering IV push medication.
   2. The primary IV administration set always has a drop factor of 60.
   3. The primary IV administration set is longer than the secondary IVPB administration set.
   4. The secondary IVPB administration set has a drip chamber for visualizing the drip rate, while the primary administration set does not.
   5. There is no difference except the drop factor.

3. If set up correctly, through which of the following could you directly administer an intermittent infusion of medication?
   1. Secondary IVPB administration set
   2. PRN lock
   3. Primary IV administration set
   4. Y-set blood tubing

4. Which of the following strengths of heparin could you use for flushing a PRN lock?
   1. 1,000 units/mL
   2. 10 units/mL
   3. 5,000 units/mL
   4. 10,000 units/mL
   5. 100 units/mL

5. Which of the following preparations should be performed at the bedside?
   1. Mixing of IV medication
   2. Verification of health-care provider's IV order with MAR
   3. Site selection
   4. Priming primary IV administration set
   5. Calculation of infusion rate for gravity flow

6. If an IV order says to infuse 1,000 mL of fluid at the rate of 125 mL/hr, how many hours will it take to complete the infusion?
   1. 8 hours
   2. 6 hours
   3. 12 hours
   4. 10 hours
   5. 125 hours

7. Hypovolemia refers to a condition resulting from:
   1. dehydration caused by loss of intracellular and extracellular fluids.
   2. water losses that are greater than electrolyte losses.
   3. excessive loss of equal proportions of extracellular fluid and electrolytes.
   4. excessive loss of electrolytes in greater proportions than the loss of fluids.

8. What are the four IV tubing drop factors (drops equals 1 mL)?
   1. 10
   2. 15
   3. 35
   4. 20
   5. 60
   6. 5
   7. 50

9. What are the signs and symptoms of phlebitis?
   1. Site cool to touch
   2. Edema at the site
   3. Erythema at the site
   4. Blanching or pallor of skin around site
   5. Vein feels like a hard cord when palpated
   6. Solution leakage at site

10. Which veins are used during PICC placement?
    1. Basilic vein
    2. Jugular vein
    3. Carotid vein
    4. Brachial vein
    5. Cephalic vein

11. Which veins are used during central line placement?
    1. Brachial vein
    2. Cephalic vein
    3. Jugular vein
    4. Femoral vein
    5. Subclavian vein
    6. Basilic vein

ANSWERS 1. 4, 2. 5, 3. 1, 2, 3, 4. 2, 5. 3, 6. 1, 7. 3, 8. 1, 2, 4, 5, 9. 2, 3, 5, 10. 1, 4, 5, 11. 3, 4, 5

Critical Thinking Exercises

Answers available online.

1. Describe what you should do if your patient rings the call light and says, "My IV is not dripping anymore and the pump alarm is going off."

   For Questions 2–3: Calculate the rate of infusion or length of time it will take to complete the infusion for each of the following scenarios.

2. The health-care provider's order says to infuse 1,000 mL D5W at 125 mL/hr. You must infuse the solution by gravity because all the IV pumps are in use at this time. The drop factor on the primary administration set is 15 gtts/mL. How many gtts/min will you set the solution to infuse?

3. You know that the health-care provider has ordered dextrose 5% in 0.45% sodium chloride 1,000 mL to infuse over the next 10 hours. If you use an IV pump, at what rate will you set the pump?

Additional Resources

Use the scratch off code on the inside front cover of your book to access online quizzes that will help you to improve your scores on course exams and prepare for the NCLEX-PN®.

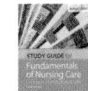

Study Guide

APPENDIX A
Photo and Illustration Credits for Unnumbered Figures

Except as noted, all photographs in this text are by Kris Piersall.

Unit 3

Chapter 13

Unnumbered Figures 13.1 through 13.4: Wilkinson JM, Treas LS. *Fundamentals of Nursing: Theory, Concepts & Applications.* Vol. 2. 3rd ed. Philadelphia, PA: FA Davis; 2016.

Chapter 14

Unnumbered Figures 14.1 through 14.10: Wilkinson JM, Treas LS. *Fundamentals of Nursing: Theory, Concepts & Applications.* Vol. 2. 3rd ed. Philadelphia, PA: FA Davis; 2016.

Chapter 15

Unnumbered Figures 15.8 through 15.13 and 15.16 through 15.31: Wilkinson JM, Treas LS. *Fundamentals of Nursing: Theory, Concepts & Applications.* Vol. 2. 3rd ed. Philadelphia, PA: FA Davis; 2016.

Chapter 16

Unnumbered Figures 16.2 through 16.5: © 2017 Hill-Rom Services, Inc. Reprinted with permission—All rights reserved.

Unnumbered Figures 16.21 and 16.25: Wilkinson JM, Treas LS. *Fundamentals of Nursing: Theory, Concepts & Applications.* Vol. 1. 3rd ed. Philadelphia, PA: FA Davis; 2016.

Unnumbered Figures 16.16 through 16.32: Wilkinson JM, Treas LS. *Fundamentals of Nursing: Theory, Concepts & Applications.* Vol. 2. 3rd ed. Philadelphia, PA: FA Davis; 2016.

Chapter 17

Unnumbered Figures 17.1 through 17.16, 17.19 through 17.21: Wilkinson JM, Treas LS. *Fundamentals of Nursing: Theory, Concepts & Applications.* Vol. 2. 3rd ed. Philadelphia, PA: FA Davis; 2016.

Unnumbered Figures 17.17 and 17.18: Dillon PM. *Nursing Health Assessment: A Critical Thinking Case Studies Approach.* 3rd ed. Philadelphia, PA: FA Davis; 2016.

Unnumbered Figures 17.20 through 17.22: Dillon PM. *Nursing Health Assessment: A Critical Thinking Case Studies Approach.* 3rd ed. Philadelphia, PA: FA Davis; 2016.

Chapter 21

Unnumbered Figures 21.1 through 21.10: Dillon PM. *Nursing Health Assessment: A Critical Thinking Case Studies Approach.* 3rd ed. Philadelphia, PA: FA Davis; 2016.

Chapter 22

Unnumbered Figures 22.3, 22.4, and 22.6: Wilkinson JM, Treas LS. *Fundamentals of Nursing: Theory, Concepts & Applications.* Vol. 2. 3rd ed. Philadelphia, PA: FA Davis; 2016.

Unit 4

Chapter 24

Unnumbered Figures 24.1 through 24.5: Wilkinson JM, Treas LS. *Fundamentals of Nursing: Theory, Concepts & Applications.* Vol. 2. 3rd ed. Philadelphia, PA: FA Davis; 2016.

Unnumbered Figure 24.6: Wilkinson JM, Treas LS. *Fundamentals of Nursing: Theory, Concepts & Applications.* Vol. 2. 2nd ed. Philadelphia, PA: FA Davis; 2011.

Chapter 25

Unnumbered Figure 25.1: Wilkinson JM, Treas LS. *Fundamentals of Nursing: Theory, Concepts & Applications.* Vol. 1. 3rd ed. Philadelphia, PA: FA Davis; 2016.

Chapter 26

Unnumbered Figures 26.1 through 26.3: Wilkinson JM, Treas LS. *Fundamentals of Nursing: Theory, Concepts & Applications.* Vol. 1. 3rd ed. Philadelphia, PA: FA Davis; 2016.

Unnumbered Figures 26.5 through 26.7, 26.13, 26.14, and 26.16 through 26.19: Wilkinson JM, Treas LS. *Fundamentals of Nursing: Theory, Concepts & Applications.* Vol. 2. 3rd ed. Philadelphia, PA: FA Davis; 2016.

Unnumbered Figures 26.15, and 26.20 through 26.25: Wilkinson JM, Treas LS. *Fundamentals of Nursing: Theory, Concepts & Applications.* Vol. 1. 3rd ed. Philadelphia, PA: FA Davis; 2016.

Chapter 27

Unnumbered Figures 27.2 and 27.3: Wilkinson JM, Treas LS. *Fundamentals of Nursing: Theory, Concepts & Applications.* Vol. 2. 3rd ed. Philadelphia, PA: FA Davis; 2016.

Chapter 28

Unnumbered Figures 28.1 through 28.23: Wilkinson JM, Treas LS. *Fundamentals of Nursing: Theory, Concepts & Applications.* Vol. 2. 3rd ed. Philadelphia, PA: FA Davis; 2016.

Chapter 29

Unnumbered Figures 29.1 and 29.2: Wilkinson JM, Treas LS. *Fundamentals of Nursing: Theory, Concepts & Applications.* Vol. 2. 3rd ed. Philadelphia, PA: FA Davis; 2016.

Chapter 30

Unnumbered Figures 30.1, 30.2, and 30.5 through 30.9: Wilkinson JM, Treas LS. *Fundamentals of Nursing: Theory, Concepts & Applications.* Vol. 2. 3rd ed. Philadelphia, PA: FA Davis; 2016.

Chapter 31

Unnumbered Figures 31.1 through 31.8: Wilkinson JM, Treas LS. *Fundamentals of Nursing: Theory, Concepts & Applications.* Vol. 2. 3rd ed. Philadelphia, PA: FA Davis; 2016.

Unnumbered Figures 31.10 and 31.11: Wilkinson JM, Treas LS. *Fundamentals of Nursing: Theory, Concepts & Applications.* Vol. 2. 3rd ed. Philadelphia, PA: FA Davis; 2016.

Chapter 34

Unnumbered Figure 34.6: Wilkinson JM, Treas LS. *Fundamentals of Nursing: Theory, Concepts & Applications.* Vol. 2. 3rd ed. Philadelphia, PA: FA Davis; 2016.

Unnumbered Figures 34.8 and 34.9: Wilkinson JM, Treas LS. *Fundamentals of Nursing: Theory, Concepts & Applications.* Vol. 2. 3rd ed. Philadelphia, PA: FA Davis; 2016.

Unit 5

Chapter 36

Unnumbered Figures 36.1 through 36.11: Wilkinson JM, Treas LS. *Fundamentals of Nursing: Theory, Concepts & Applications.* Vol. 2. 3rd ed. Philadelphia, PA: FA Davis; 2016.

Chapter 38

Unnumbered Figure 38.1: Wilkinson JM, Treas LS. *Fundamentals of Nursing: Theory, Concepts & Applications.* Vol. 2. 3rd ed. Philadelphia, PA: FA Davis; 2016.

Unnumbered Figure 38.3: Wilkinson JM, Treas LS. *Fundamentals of Nursing: Theory, Concepts & Applications.* Vol. 2. 3rd ed. Philadelphia, PA: FA Davis; 2016.

Unnumbered Figures 38.6 through 38.11: Wilkinson JM, Treas LS. *Fundamentals of Nursing: Theory, Concepts & Applications.* Vol. 2. 3rd ed. Philadelphia, PA: FA Davis; 2016.

Unnumbered Figures 38.19 and 38.20: Wilkinson JM, Treas LS. *Fundamentals of Nursing: Theory, Concepts & Applications.* Vol. 2. 3rd ed. Philadelphia, PA: FA Davis; 2016.

Unnumbered Figure 38.22: Wilkinson JM, Treas LS. *Fundamentals of Nursing: Theory, Concepts & Applications.* Vol. 2. 3rd ed. Philadelphia, PA: FA Davis; 2016.

Glossary

Abandonment: Leaving or walking away from patient assignments without replacement by another nurse.

Abrasion: A superficial open wound that generally heals well if kept clean.

Absorption: The process by which nutrients are taken from the end products of digestion into the villi (within the small intestine) that contain capillaries. This is the point where the majority of nutrients are absorbed into the bloodstream.

Accommodation response: A measure of the eye muscles' ability to focus on an image up close and in the distance.

Acidosis: An increase of acids.

Active listening: Techniques that use all the senses to interpret verbal and nonverbal messages. In this type of listening, attention is paid both to what the speaker is saying and also to what the speaker is not saying. The mind of the listener focuses on the interaction and detects feelings as well as the spoken words.

Activities of daily living (ADLs): Activities such as bathing, washing and styling hair, brushing and flossing teeth, dressing, and shaving.

Acupressure: A traditional Chinese therapy that is a blend of acupuncture and pressure.

Acupuncture: The ancient Chinese practice of inserting fine needles into carefully selected points located along meridians in the body.

Acute illness: An episode of illness that strikes suddenly and lasts for a limited time.

Acute pain: Pain that comes on suddenly and has a short duration (less than 6 months).

Adaptation: The ability to positively adjust to changes that occur in an individual's world.

Adjuvant: Something that assists or aids another treatment, therefore increasing the first treatment's effectiveness.

Admission process: The process of admitting a patient to a hospital during which the nurse begins establishing rapport and a trusting relationship with the patient.

Advance directive: Written documents that provide guidelines for making medical decisions in the event a person becomes incapacitated and is unable to make his or her wishes known. All states recognize two types of advance directives: power of attorney and a living will.

Adventitious breath sounds: Abnormal breath sounds, including crackles, rhonchi, wheezes, pleural friction rub, and stridor.

Adverse effect: An unexpected, unintended, and more severe or harmful effect than a side effect.

Advocate: To stand up for what is in the patient's best interest as opposed to what is in the best interest of the physician, hospital, or coworker. The nurse serves as the primary patient advocate.

Aerobic: A term used to describe organisms that grow and replicate in the presence of oxygen.

Afebrile: The state of being without fever.

Ageism: The practice of discrimination and prejudice against elders.

Age-related macular degeneration: The destruction of the area in the retina where the optic nerve attaches, leading to the loss of central vision.

Air-lock: An intramuscular injection of 0.1 to 0.2 mL of air that directly follows the medication from the syringe into the muscle. Its purpose is to clear irritating medications from the needle and needle track as the needle is withdrawn from the muscle through subcutaneous and dermal tissue layers.

Aldosterone: A hormone that regulates fluid and electrolyte balance by stimulating the kidneys to retain more sodium and excrete potassium.

Alkalosis: An increase in bases or alkaline substances.

Allergic reaction: A reaction that occurs when a patient's body reacts to a medication as a foreign invader to be destroyed.

Allopathic medicine: Traditional, conventional medicine that is practiced in the West.

Alternative therapy: Therapy used *instead* of conventional treatment.

Alzheimer's disease: A type of dementia that is strongly associated with aging and whose diagnosis is based on symptoms because a definitive diagnosis can only be made in autopsy of the brain.

Ambivalent: To have opposing feelings about someone or something.

Ambulate: To walk.

Ampule: A small, sealed glass drug container that must be broken to withdraw the medication.

Amputate: To remove a limb surgically.

Anabolism: The process by which the body uses components to build or reconstruct new components or tissue.

Anaerobic: A term used to describe organisms that can live and replicate without oxygen.

Analgesics: Pain medications.

Anaphylaxis: A life-threatening emergency due to an allergic reaction that involves swelling of the upper respiratory tract and that can result in occlusion of the airway.

Anastomoses: Junctions where veins join other veins and arteries join other arteries, providing alternate routes for blood flow if one pathway should become obstructed.

Anesthesia: The loss of sensation, with or without a loss of consciousness, accomplished by the administration of inhaled or injected medications.

Anorexia nervosa: An eating disorder marked by relentless self-starvation in an effort to reduce the body weight below normal. This disorder is characterized by an excessive leanness or wasting of the body, known as *emaciation*.

Antidiuretic hormone (ADH): A hormone released from the posterior pituitary that directs the kidney tubules to increase water reabsorption independently of solids, which helps to dilute the concentration of the blood.

Antiembolism hose: Often called an *AE hose* or *TED hose* (stands for *thromboembolic disorder*), they are a pair of strong support hose that are applied to compress the leg veins, assisting them to return blood back to the right side of the heart where it can be sent through the pulmonary artery to the lungs to be reoxygenated. This helps to prevent blood from pooling in the leg veins from inactivity and bedrest.

Antioxidants: Specific vitamins that help to deactivate free radicals before they can cause damage.

Anuria: The absence of urine or minimal urine production, which can be the result of a temporary illness or urinary tract obstruction or be a symptom of a serious underlying condition that must be diagnosed and treated.

Aphasia: An inability to speak or understand language.

Apnea: A period of no respirations.

Approximation: In wound infection, when the edges of a surgical incision meet and are aligned with one another.

Aquathermia pad: Also known as a *K-pad*, this device includes a small, electrically heated water storage tank and two tubes connected to a network of tubing within a disposable pad. It is used to safely apply heat to specific areas of the body.

Arteriography: Also known as *angiography*, this form of radiology requires that a contrast medium be instilled into designated arteries, which allows examination of the vessel to assess for abnormalities.

Ascites: A large collection of fluid within the peritoneal cavity.

Assault: Threatening a patient with harm or to show intent to touch him or her without permission.

Assisted care: A situation in which patients need some assistance with activities of daily living.

Associate degree nurse (ADN): A 2-year, entry-level educational program for registered nurses. Upon completion of all course work, a student takes the NCLEX-RN; upon successfully passing the examination, the graduate becomes a registered nurse and uses the title "RN" after her or his name.

Atelectasis: Severe pneumonia or lung collapse that causes a lack of or decreased excursion on one side of the chest.

Attachment: A type of emotional bonding, for example, mother–baby bonding.

Auditory learning: Learning by hearing and listening.

Auscultation: Listening to the sounds produced by the body.

Auscultatory gap: In some hypertensive patients, the period of silence between the first Korotkoff sound heard (the systolic blood pressure [BP]) and the next Korotkoff sound heard when it resumes at a number 30 to 40 mm Hg lower.

Autoclaving: A method of sterilization that delivers steam under pressure, with heat ranging from 250°F to 270°F, in order to sterilize instruments that will not be harmed by heat and water under pressure.

Baccalaureate degree nurse (BSN): A 4-year, entry-level educational program for registered nurses. Upon completion of all course work, the student takes the NCLEX-RN; upon successfully passing the examination, the graduate becomes a registered nurse and uses the title "RN" after her or his name. The focus of BSN nursing education puts more emphasis on management and leadership than ADN and diploma programs.

Barium enema: A type of test in which barium (a contrast medium) is instilled rectally for radiographic visualization of the large intestine in order to see its shape and any abnormalities that might be present. It is used to detect cancerous tumors, obstructions, polyps, inflammatory disease, or diverticula in the colon.

Base of support: The feet and lower legs, which give the body stability and balance. The wider one's base of support, the lower the center of gravity.

Bath blanket: A large lightweight flannel blanket used during a bath to prevent exposure.

Battery: Providing any type of medical care to a patient without his or her consent and/or agreement.

Bicarbonate: A main anion of extracellular fluid that is controlled by the kidneys. It is also present in lesser amounts in the intracellular fluid (ICF). Its normal range is 22 to 26 mEq/L.

Bier block: A common type of peripheral nerve block that is used as anesthesia. A tourniquet is placed around an extremity to decrease venous return while continuing to allow full arterial delivery of oxygenated blood to the site.

Biot's respirations: Respirations characterized by groups of several shallow breaths followed by variable-length periods of apnea.

Blood culture: The drawing of blood specimens to determine if organisms are present in the blood, and, if so, which specific organism is the culprit.

Blood urea nitrogen (BUN): A measure of urea nitrogen in the blood, which is a waste product normally eliminated from the body by the kidneys and excreted into the urine. The normal levels of BUN are 10 to 20 mg/dL in adults.

Body language: Nonverbal communication that reveals the attitude or mood through physical gestures, posture, or proximity.

Body mass index (BMI): A means of measuring obesity that uses a formula along with an individual's weight and height to calculate whether his or her level of fatness is within normal weight boundaries, underweight, overweight, or obese.

Body mechanics: The movement of muscles of the body for balance and leverage.

Boiling: A method of sterilization in which instruments and supplies are boiled in water for 10 minutes to kill non-spore-forming organisms; this method does not kill spores.

Bolus feedings: A type of intermittent tube feeding that is frequently used in which a physician-ordered volume of formula is administered at set intervals throughout the day.

Bone marrow aspiration: Under local anesthetic, a sample of marrow is removed from the sternum, tibia, or iliac crest by needle aspiration for evaluation of blood cell production. This test is performed to diagnose some serious anemias, thrombocytopenia, and cancerous tumors, and to stage Hodgkin's disease.

Bradycardia: A pulse that is less than 60 bpm.

Bradypnea: A respiratory rate below 12 respirations per minute.

Brand name: Also called the *trade name,* it is the name of a drug that usually is shorter and easier to remember than the drug's generic name. The brand name is owned by the pharmaceutical company, so it is sometimes referred to as the *proprietary name.*

Buccal route: A medication administration route in which medications are given between the cheek and the gum.

Buffer: A substance that can bind, or form an ionic bond, with a strong acid or base to prevent large changes in the pH of body fluids; a buffer binds with a strong acid to decrease acidity, or the buffer binds with a strong base to decrease alkalinity of the body.

Bulimia nervosa: Commonly referred to as *binge eating,* this eating disorder is accompanied by behavior to get rid of some of the calories that were ingested while bingeing, such as self- or medication-induced vomiting (known as *purging*), excessive exercise, fasting, or the overuse of laxatives.

Cannulation: The process of advancing the IV cannula into the vein.

Capitation: The payment system used by health maintenance organizations (HMOs).

Capsule: A gelatin shell that contains a powder or pellets of medication. It may be preferred over tablets because it is swallowed more easily.

Cardiopulmonary resuscitation (CPR): Actions to restart the heart or breathing of an unresponsive victim without a pulse or respirations.

Care plan: A documented plan for giving patient care that includes physician's orders, nursing diagnoses, and nursing orders.

Case management: The type of nursing care system that involves seeing each patient as an individual and each situation as unique. The goal of case management is to assist patients who are vulnerable, at risk, or cost intensive so that their care is coordinated, meets their specific needs, and is cost effective while still bringing them to optimum health.

Catabolism: The breaking down phase of metabolism. It breaks down complex substances into the simpler ones, sometimes releasing energy.

Cataract: A common visual disturbance in older adults that occurs when the lens of the eye becomes cloudy, or opaque, which causes visual blurring.

Cellulitis: Inflammation and infection of the skin and underlying tissue.

Center of gravity: The middle point of the body, below the umbilicus and above the pubis, around which the body's mass is distributed.

Centers for Disease Control and Prevention (CDC): A federal agency that helps protect the public by tracking outbreaks or occurrences of disease and by determining steps to take regarding treatment and containment of illness, immunizations, and future research.

Cephalocaudal: A pattern of growth that occurs in an orderly and predictable pattern, progressing from the head downward.

Cerebrovascular accident (CVA): Also known as *stroke* or *brain attack*, this condition is seen more often in older adults and may be caused by either a clot in a blood vessel or a bleeding blood vessel in the brain.

Chain of infection: A chain of events that occurs in order for infection to spread from one person to another.

Chair or bed monitor: A pressure-sensitive device that generates an alarm when the patient's weight is no longer sensed, indicating that the patient is attempting to get up.

Charting by exception: A type of charting in which only variances from "normal" in all activities of daily living, vital signs, and assessment findings are charted as entries. This method of charting is designed to drastically reduce time spent completing paperwork; however, opinions vary about its efficacy and safety.

Cheilitis/Chelosis: Inflammation of the lips.

Chemical disinfection: A method of sterilization used to kill pathogens on equipment and supplies that cannot be heated.

Chemical name: The name of the exact ingredients of the medication; it reads like a chemical formula.

Chest x-ray (CXR): A type of x-ray that allows one to see the bony structures of the thorax and also allows one to visualize the heart's position and size; the lungs, whether they are fully expanded or have collapsed lobes, and whether they are clear or congested; and densities that may indicate malignant tumors or tuberculosis.

Cheyne-Stokes respirations: A pattern of respirations that begin shallow, gradually increase in depth and frequency to a peak, and then begin to decrease in depth and frequency until they are slow and shallow; this is followed by a period of apnea lasting from 10 to 60 seconds.

Chiropractic: Manipulation of the spine to relieve pressure on the nerves.

Chronic illness: Illness that lasts for 6 months or longer and is characterized by intensifying or improving symptoms.

Chronic pain: Pain that lasts longer than 6 months.

Circadian rhythm: The body's 24-hour cyclical pattern, during which body metabolism and functions increase and decrease in rhythmic patterns.

Circulating nurse: A registered nurse who assists in the operating room (OR) by obtaining needed equipment and supplies. The circulating nurse is not "scrubbed in" on the case, so he or she may leave the operating suite to obtain needed items.

Circumoral cyanosis: Blueness (cyanosis) around the mouth.

Clear liquid diet: A type of diet ordered to provide hydration and calories in the form of simple carbohydrates that help meet some of the body's energy needs; most often used postoperatively or during recovery from gastrointestinal disease such as vomiting and diarrhea, when the gut must be introduced slowly to food. Examples of clear liquids include water, broth, and tea without milk.

Client-centered care: A type of care that empowers the patient to take control of and manage his or her care. It allows patients to achieve independence within the limits of their disability by permitting them to have a voice in their rehabilitation, schedule, goals, and method of attaining those goals.

Code team: A group of specially trained personnel designated to respond to codes throughout the hospital.

Cognitive development: How human beings learn.

Collaborative interventions: Nursing interventions that involve working with other health-care professionals in the hospital setting, such as therapists, social services workers, and dietitians.

Colonoscopy: Following patient sedation, the insertion of a flexible endoscope via the rectum into the colon and terminal ileum, allowing the physician to visualize the lining for abnormalities such as polyps, ulcerations, and tumors and to biopsy tissue as needed.

Colostomy: An opening in the bowel in the area of the large intestine used as an alternate form of bowel elimination.

Communication process: The exchange of information, feelings, needs, and preferences between two people.

Comorbidity: The presence of multiple, simultaneous diseases.

Complementary therapy: Therapy used *with* conventional treatment.

Complete blood cell count (CBC): The most common test ordered; it measures the number of leukocytes (white blood cells [WBCs]), erythrocytes (red blood cells [RBCs]), and thrombocytes/platelets (PLTs). It also differentiates the percentages of the five types of WBCs.

Complete metabolic panel: A specific grouping of blood chemistry tests in which 8 or 14 respective tests are done.

Complete proteins: A protein containing all of the essential amino acids.

Complex carbohydrates: Types of carbohydrates that are made up of starches and fiber (cellulose).

Computed tomography (CT): Also known as *computed axial tomography* or *CAT scanning,* CT is an x-ray procedure that takes many x-ray images of body parts from different angles. It then uses a computer to combine all the images to generate cross-sectional pictures and three-dimensional images of the internal organs and structures of the body.

Congruent: Two things that are in agreement. Congruent communication is one in which verbal and nonverbal languages effectively meet the goal of shared meaning in communication.

Connotative meaning: The emotional associations that can be attached to a word. Connotative language, whether used consciously or unconsciously, has the potential to shape a listener's attitude.

Conscious sedation: A type of sedation in which a patient is asleep but not totally unconscious.

Consensual reflex: Rapid, equal, and simultaneous constriction of the pupils that results from stimulation of the optic nerve by shining a light in either eye.

Constipation: A state of having less-frequent, hard, formed stools that are difficult to expel.

Contamination: The potential presence of pathogens on a sterile field or sterile object due to contact with an unsterile surface.

Continuous passive motion (CPM) machine: A machine designed to gently flex the patient's knee according to the number of degrees of flexion on the setting and then gently extend the knee.

Continuum: Related to health and wellness, a range that spans from severe illness to complete wellness.

Contractures: Shortening and tightening of the muscles because of disuse.

Contraindications: Situations that warrant *not* using something.

Controlled substances: Also known as *scheduled drugs,* these substances have greater capacity for addiction and abuse and are regulated by federal law.

Coping strategies: Positive or negative actions that people use to combat stress. Negative strategies cause harm to one's self or others, and positive strategies include those that are good for an individual's body, mind, and spirit.

Corrective surgery: A type of surgery done to repair an anatomical or congenital defect, such as repairing a cleft palate so that a child can nurse or eat normally.

Cosmetic surgery: A type of surgery performed to change or improve one's physical appearance.

Crackles: Discontinuous breath sounds usually heard during inspiration that may be either fine or coarse. Formerly called "rales."

Crepitus: Air in the subcutaneous tissues, in the chest wall, face, and neck.

Critical thinking: Using skillful reasoning and logical thought to determine the merits of a belief or action.

Cultural awareness: The knowledge of and sensitivity to a patient's cultural beliefs and values.

Cultural competence: The ability to interact well with individuals from different cultures and background. Culturally competent care occurs when the nurse provides care to the whole patient, incorporating within that care consideration of the patient's beliefs and values.

Cultural diversity: The differences between groups of people in a certain geographical area, such as a city, state, or country; a specific place, such as a church or factory; or a conceptual community, such as the medical community. It is a way of identifying the group through the differences found between groups of people.

Cultural sensitivity: Respect for an individual's specific cultural beliefs, values, and accepted patterns of communication.

Culture: The way of life that distinguishes a particular group of people from other groups. It is the whole of the learned behaviors of individuals within a specific group and includes things such as beliefs, values, art, music, laws, and customs.

Cutaneous pain: Pain that is more superficial or pertaining to the skin's surface and underlying subcutaneous tissue.

Cyanosis: A bluish color to the lips or skin that results from decreased oxygen levels in tissues.

Débridement: The surgical removal of the dead tissue.

Deep somatic pain: Also known as *osteogenic pain,* this type of pain is bone, ligament, tendon, and blood vessel pain. The pain may be diffuse and of longer duration than cutaneous pain.

Deep venous thrombosis: Blood clots in the lower leg.

Defecation: The process of bowel elimination.

Defining characteristics: The signs and symptoms exhibited by the patient.

Dehiscence: An uncommon but extremely serious complication of wound healing in which there is a partial or complete separation of the outer layers of a wound.

Dehydration: A loss of fluid only, which results in the increase of electrolyte concentrations in the remaining body fluid.

Dementia: A decrease in intellectual functioning that occurs over months or years and that eventually results in the inability to care for oneself.

Denotative meaning: The literal meaning of something, absent any interpretation.

Dependency phase: The phase of illness after which an individual has sought help and decides to follow the advice or recommended treatment or to seek help elsewhere. In this phase, a person relies on others for help in diagnosis and treatment. An individual with a chronic illness often remains in the dependency phase because complete recovery is not possible.

Dependent interventions: Interventions that require a health-care provider's order before they can be performed.

Desired effect: The reason a medication is prescribed or the purpose for which it is given.

Development: An increase in the complexity of skills performed by a person.

Diagnosis-related groups (DRGs): Classifications of illnesses and diseases that are used to determine the amount of money paid by Medicare to a hospital for the care of a patient with that particular illness or disease.

Dialysis: The process of using a machine to filter waste products and salts, and to remove excess fluid from the blood. This treatment may be temporary or long term, depending on the cause of the anuria.

Diarrhea: Loose or watery stools occurring three or more times a day.

Diastole: The time during which the ventricles are at rest.

Diastolic pressure: The measurement of the pressure exerted by the blood on the artery walls while the heart ventricles are not contracting, which is the lower of the two pressures.

Differential: The breakdown of the total WBC into percentages of the five types of white cells.

Diffusion: A process that allows a substance to flow over naturally from an area of higher concentration into an area of lower concentration.

Digestion: The process by which food is broken down in the gastrointestinal (GI) tract, releasing nutrients for the body to use. The process of digestion begins in the mouth, with saliva.

Diploma program nurse: A hospital-based nursing education program. Graduates of these programs also take the NCLEX-RN for licensure to become registered nurses.

Direct contact: The most common path of microorganism transmission; it spreads from one person directly to another, usually via the hands.

Direct patient care: Care performed when the nurse interacts directly with the patient; it includes activities such as bathing, teaching, listening, and administering medications.

Discharge instruction form: A form completed by the nurse when a physician writes a discharge order for a patient. It includes instructions for when the patient is to return to the physician's office for follow-up, medication directions, activity restrictions, dietary instructions, signs and symptoms that warrant notifying the physician, and treatment the patient is to continue at home.

Discharge planning: The process of planning for a patient's discharge; ideally, it should begin during the admission process in order to address the patient's needs for discharge.

Discharge process: The process of discharging a patient from his or her hospital stay. It includes the physician's discharge order, reconciliation of the patient's medications, providing discharge instructions to the patient, helping the patient to gather personal belongings, and assisting the patient to the car.

Discrimination: A type of unfair treatment of one or more persons or groups usually because of misguided and unfounded beliefs about the race, ethnicity, age, gender, or religion of the person or group.

Disinfectant: A cleaning agent that removes most pathogens.

Disinfection: The process of cleaning surgical supplies and equipment with solutions that kill pathogens.

Distention: The stretching out of intestinal walls that accommodates fecal material as it moves through the sigmoid colon into the rectum, eventually leading to the defecation reflex.

Documentation: The act of charting or making a written notation of all the things that are pertinent to each patient for whom a nurse provides care.

Do-not-attempt-resuscitation (DNAR) order: An order written by a patient's physician that specifies that no cardiopulmonary resuscitation (CPR) or other heroic efforts to restart the patient's heart and breathing are to be performed should the patient's heart and respirations cease.

Dorsiflexion: When lying in the supine position, the patient's ankles should be flexed approximately 90 degrees so that the toes point toward the ceiling.

Draw sheet: A type of sheet that is narrower than a flat sheet and has two narrow hems on each end. It is used to protect the bottom sheet from minor soiling and to help lift and turn heavier patients.

Drug-drug interaction: The interaction between two drugs that causes a change in the activity or components of one or more of the drugs. Some drug reactions may even produce a product that is totally unsafe to administer.

Dry-powder inhaler (DPI): A type of inhaler that does not contain a pressurized canister and does not spray out medication; instead, it relies on the force of the patient's own inhalation to dispense a dose of dry-powder medication.

Durable power of attorney: A legal court document that grants another individual the authority to make health-care decisions and act as proxy for the patient should the patient become disabled.

Dysphagia: Difficulty swallowing.

Dysphasia: Difficulty coordinating and organizing the words correctly in a sentence.

Dyspnea: Labored or difficult breathing.

Dysuria: Painful or difficult urination.

Echocardiogram: Ultrasonography of the heart, which is commonly used because it is noninvasive, quick, easy, and reliable. It can detect problems in heart wall motion, defective heart valves, the volume of blood that is pumped from the heart with each heartbeat, and enlargement of the heart wall muscles.

Edema: Swelling that occurs when excessive fluid leaves the vascular system and remains in the interstitial spaces.

Effleurage: The repetitive gentle, gliding stroking of one's fingertips over the surface of the skin, which is particularly effective during back massage to relax muscles or on the head to reduce tension headaches.

Electrocardiography (EKG): Also noted as *ECG*, this type of cardiac testing uses six electrodes that are applied to specific locations on the chest wall and four electrodes applied to the four extremities to graphically record the electrical activity through the heart's electrical conduction pathway. It detects any abnormalities by analyzing the heart's electrical activity from 12 different angles or views.

Electroencephalography (EEG): In this type of testing, electrodes are placed strategically on the scalp and record the electrical activity of the brain, known as *brain waves.* This study is beneficial in detecting epilepsy, diseases of the central nervous system, and tumors, and to confirm brain death.

Electrolyte: A salt, that when dissolved in water conducts electricity. It is present in blood, tissue fluids, and cells, and includes sodium, potassium, and chlorine.

Electronic Health Record (EHR): A computerized database that typically includes present and past medical and surgical information, laboratory, radiographic and drug information about a patient; most also contain billing and insurance information as well.

Elixir: A type of liquid medication that contains sweeteners or flavorings. It may also contain water and alcohol and is generally clear in appearance, although some may contain colorings.

Emancipated minor: An individual who has established his or her independence from parental control by court order, marriage, a history of living independently and being self-supporting, or service in the military.

Empathy: The ability to intellectually or emotionally understand the feelings of another person without actually experiencing or even agreeing with their situation, thoughts, feelings, distress, or pain.

Endorphins: Natural body chemicals produced by the brain in response to pleasant thoughts or feelings, exercise, laughter, sex, and massage.

Endotracheal tube: A firm but flexible plastic tube that may be inserted through the nose or the mouth.

Enteral nutrition: Nutrition that uses the GI tract as a delivery system and that involves tube feedings that usually replace all oral intake but may also be given as a supplement to oral ingestion of nutrients.

Enteric-coated: A type of tablet coating that does not dissolve until the medication reaches the intestines. This coating protects the stomach from ingredients in the medication that may be irritating, preventing nausea, vomiting, and ulcer formation.

Epidural anesthesia: The insertion of a small catheter into the epidural space of the spinal column to provide a continual administration of a stronger anesthetic agent. Some physicians utilize epidurals for postoperative pain control as well as during surgery.

Eructation: Belching.

Erythema: Redness.

Eschar: Hard, dry, dead tissue that has a leathery appearance.

Esophagogastroduodenoscopy (EGD): After a patient's mouth and throat is sprayed with a local anesthetic or mild sedation is administered, imaging that results from a flexible scope being inserted through the mouth, down the esophagus, through the stomach, and into the upper duodenum, which allows visualization of the lining of each. It is useful for detection and biopsy of polyps, ulcers, tumors, gastric reflux, and constrictions, as well as evaluation of chemical burns after ingestion of poisons.

Essential amino acids: One of the building blocks of protein, these types of amino acid are the most important because they must be obtained from food sources because the body is unable to produce them.

Ethics: The values that influence an individual's decisions and behavior.

Ethnicity: The categorization of a group of people by a distinctive trait, such as the line of genealogy or ancestry, race, or nationality.

Eupnea: Respirations in which the rate, depth, rhythm, pattern, and respiratory effort fall within normal parameters.

Euthanasia: Assisting a patient in suicide or knowingly administering an unsafe dosage of medication that will most likely kill the patient.

Evacuated tube: A plastic or glass tube used to draw a blood sample for laboratory testing that is closed with a colored rubber stopper or a rubber stopper surrounded by a colored plastic top, from which a certain amount of air has been evacuated.

Evidence-based practice (EBP): A problem-solving approach to delivering health care that uses the best evidence from nursing research studies and patient care data and also considers the patient's preferences and values.

Evisceration: The protrusion of abdominal contents through an opened abdominal wound.

Exacerbation: A period of chronic illness that is characterized by worsening symptoms.

Excoriation: Scrapes on the skin that may be due to scratching or that may occur during care.

Excursion: Equal chest expansion during respiration.

Exhalation: Also known as *expiration,* the process of releasing air from the lungs.

Expected outcomes: Statements of measurable action for the patient within a specific time frame and in response to nursing interventions.

Exploratory surgery: Surgery done to provide further data and determine a diagnosis for a problem.

External fixators: The wires, pins, tongs, and rods that may be used in skeletal traction.

Extracellular fluid (ECF): One-third of the body's fluid that is located in the compartments outside the cells.

Extravasation: Leakage of vesicant IV fluid or medication into the tissue surrounding the IV insertion site.

Extubation: The removal of an endotracheal tube after surgery.

Fall assessment rating scales: Forms that, when filled out, give a numerical rating for each patient's risk for falls. The higher the number, the greater the patient's risk.

Febrile: The state of having a fever.

Fecal incontinence: The loss of voluntary control of the rectal sphincters.

Feedback: A return message sent by the receiver of information that completes the communication process. It indicates that the original message has been received, processed, and comprehended.

Fight-or-flight response: An automatic response to a threat to an individual's well-being. The individual's brain engages the sympathetic nervous system, which stimulates the endocrine glands to pump cortisol, adrenaline, and other hormones into the bloodstream.

Filtration: The passage of fluid through a partial barrier that separates the fluid from certain particles that are too large to pass through the semipermeable membrane.

First-pass metabolism: When a medication is administered orally, it is absorbed into the portal circulation, going first to the liver where it is partially metabolized before leaving the liver to enter the systemic circulation where it can perform its function. Drugs that are administered buccally, sublingually, or parenterally go directly into the systemic circulation and escape the first-pass metabolism of the liver that occurs with oral drugs.

Flange: On the proximal end of an IV tubing just below the piercing pin, the hard plastic projection that provides a place for your fingers to push the piercing pin into the IV solution bag without contaminating the sterile piercing pin.

Flatus: Gas produced in the bowel.

Fluid volume deficit: An equal loss of both fluid and the electrolytes contained in that fluid; also known as *hypovolemia.*

Focus charting: A type of charting that is focused on the patient and patient concerns, problems, and strengths. Unlike PIE charting, there is not a constructed list of specific problems. It includes data, action, and response.

Fontanels: The spaces between the bones of the skull that are not yet fused together; sometimes called the *soft spots.*

Food intolerance: An adverse, nonallergic reaction to a food without activation of the immune response.

Footdrop: Permanent plantar flexion of the foot.

Fowler's position: Semi-sitting position with various degrees of head elevation with the knees slightly elevated.

Fracture: A break in a bone.

Full liquid diet: A diet that consists of all the liquids found in a clear liquid diet with the addition of all other opaque liquids and food items that become liquid at room temperature.

Gaseous disinfection: A method of sterilization that kills pathogens on supplies and equipment that are heat-sensitive or that must remain dry.

Gastric decompression: The process of reducing pressure within the stomach by emptying it of its contents, including ingested food and liquids, gastric juices, and gas.

Gauge (G): The diameter of needle, indicated by numbers, typically between 14 G (2.1 mm) and 30 G (0.3 mm). The *higher* the gauge number, the *smaller* the diameter of the needle.

General anesthesia: A type of sedation in which the patient is totally unconscious.

Generic name: Assigned by the U.S. Adopted Name Council (USANC), this is a drug name usually based, at least partially, on the chemical name but is more of a shorthand version.

Geri-chair: A recliner with side arms, a lap belt, and wheels for navigation through hallways that is used for residents who are unable to sit unassisted.

Glaucoma: An eye disease characterized by increased intraocular pressure that affects the optic nerve and can lead to blindness.

Glomerular filtration rate (GFR): Considered the most accurate test for evaluating kidney function, this test measures the volume of urine, in milliliters, that is filtered by the kidney within 1 minute; it involves a 24-hour collection of urine.

Glycosylated hemoglobin (A_{1c}): Also known as *glycated hemoglobin,* this test measures the hemoglobin that has become bound with glucose. It provides a method of calculating the average blood glucose for the previous 3-month period of time, giving a picture of how well controlled a patient's diabetes is.

Good Samaritan Law: A law that provides protection to the voluntary caregiver at sites of accidents and emergencies. It serves to provide protection to a citizen, nurse, or other nonemergency response health-care provider who chooses to stop and render aid to someone in an emergency situation, such as an automobile accident.

Granulation tissue: New, fragile tissue that grows and fills in a wound.

Grief: The mental and emotional distress and suffering that an individual experiences with death and loss; it is expressed in various ways by each individual.

Growth: The physical changes that occur in the size of human beings.

Guaiac test: A test used to determine the presence of occult blood in the bowel.

Guarding: The defense mechanism of tightening the abdominal muscles to prevent further compression of tender or inflamed areas.

Halitosis: Bad breath.

Hallucination: A false perception that has no relation to reality; an individual may believe that she or he sees, hears, or smells something that is not really present.

Health-care–associated infection (HAI): An infection that is acquired while the patient is being cared for in any health-care setting, including home health care and long-term care.

Health Insurance Portability and Accountability Act (HIPAA): Implemented by regulations of the U.S. Department of Health and Human Services in 1996, this federal law provides for confidential maintenance of protected patient health information.

Health literacy: The ability of individuals to understand basic health information and to use that information to make good decisions about their health.

Health maintenance organization (HMO): A cost containment program featuring a primary care physician (PCP) as the gatekeeper to eliminate unnecessary testing and procedures; this is a capitated system that requires the insured person to remain within the network.

Health Occupations Students of America (HOSA): A national organization specifically for students in health occupations educational programs. Membership is open to both high school and adult students, with separate chapters for each group.

Health promotion: The process of or actions related to ways of becoming or staying healthy.

Healthy People 2020: An initiative of the office of Disease Prevention and Health Promotions of the U.S. Department of Health and Human Services; it provides science-based health goals and objectives to prevent disease and improve national health. The goals and objectives are revised every 10 years.

Heimlich maneuver: An action to relieve choking by thrusting just below a person's xiphoid process.

Hematoma: A bruise.

Hematuria: The presence of blood in the urine, either visible or microscopic.

Hemoconcentration: A concentration of RBCs in the blood caused by a decrease in the volume of plasma allowed to flow.

Hemoglobin A_{1c} (Hb A_{1c}): A laboratory test that measures the amount of hemoglobin that has combined with glucose (known as glycated hemoglobin) in order to evaluate a patient's long-term glycemic control.

Hemolysis: Lysis or the destruction of red blood cells (RBCs).

Hemorrhage: Profuse bleeding.

Hemorrhagic stroke: A cerebrovascular accident (CVA) caused by a bleeding blood vessel that interrupts normal blood flow to an area of the brain, resulting in the death of brain tissue.

Hemostasis: The cessation of active bleeding.

Hemothorax: The presence of blood and draining in the pleural space, which pools in the lower portion of the cavity.

Holism: The relationships among all living things.

Holistic: A view of the physical, mental, social, and spiritual aspects of a person as parts of the integrated whole being.

Home health care: One or many types of health or medical services provided to patients in their homes because they are confined to their homes by an illness or disability.

Hospice: The National Hospice and Palliative Care Organization defines this type of care as "a medically-directed nurse-coordinated program providing a continuum of home and inpatient care for the terminally ill patient and family."

Hygiene: The practice of keeping oneself clean and well-groomed.

Hyperglycemia: An abnormally elevated blood glucose level.

Hypertension: High blood pressure; this term describes a systolic reading consistently above 130 or a diastolic reading consistently over 80.

Hypertension, primary: The rise in blood pressure that occurs as a result of the heart's having to work harder to pump blood through artery walls made less elastic due to arteriosclerosis; also known as *essential hypertension.*

Hypertension, secondary: Blood pressure that becomes elevated due to renal or endocrine disease.

Hypertonic solution: A solution that has a higher osmolarity, or lower concentration of particles dissolved in it than the concentration in fluids of the body.

Hypoglycemia: An abnormally low blood glucose level.

Hypotension: Low blood pressure; this term describes a blood pressure reading that suddenly falls 20 to 30 mm Hg below an individual's normal blood pressure or one that falls below the low normal of 100/60 mm Hg.

Hypothermia: A condition in which an individual's core temperature drops below 95°F (35°C).

Hypotonic solution: A solution that has a lower osmolarity, or lower concentration of particles dissolved in it than the concentration in fluids of the body.

Hypovolemia: A decrease in blood volume that results when fluids and electrolytes are lost in balanced proportions from extracellular spaces.

Hypoxemia: The dropping of oxygen levels in the blood below the normal range.

Hypoxia: As a result of hypoxemia, a state in which the blood cannot take adequate amounts of oxygen to the tissues during internal respiration.

Ileostomy: An opening in the bowel in the area of the small intestine used as an alternate form of bowel elimination.

Illusion: A misinterpretation of sensory stimuli, such as seeing one thing but believing it is another thing; an individual experiencing an illusion is often disoriented to time and place.

Impaction: The blockage of the movement of contents through the intestines by a bulk mass of very hard stool; it occurs as a result of constipation.

Incentive spirometer: A device with one or more chambers and a mouthpiece that patients use to take frequent deep breaths.

Incident report: Also known as an *unusual occurrence report* or *variance report,* this report is to be completed in the event of an unusual occurrence or an accident. It should include what happened, who was involved, who witnessed the event, and the treatment that was provided.

Incomplete proteins: A protein lacking one or more of the essential amino acids.

Incontinence: An inability to control the passing of urine.

Independent interventions: Nursing interventions that are provided without consultation with anyone else; a physician's order is not required to perform them.

Indications: A condition or situation for which a specific treatment or medication is considered therapeutic.

Indirect contact: A path of microorganism transmission in which microorganisms leave one person (the reservoir) and contaminate an object (the mode of transmission), which is then used on another patient (the susceptible host). The second patient becomes ill due to contact with the same microorganism.

Indirect patient care: Care that is performed when the nurse provides assistance in a setting other than with the patient. Examples include documenting care, participating in care conferences, talking with the health-care provider, and receiving new orders.

Indwelling catheter: Also known as a *double-lumen catheter* or *Foley catheter,* a device used to empty the bladder, usually for a few days and on a continuous basis.

Infiltration: The leakage of nonvesicant IV fluid or medication into the tissue surrounding the IV insertion site.

Informed consent: Written permission by a patient that allows medical treatment or surgical procedures. It requires the patient (or a legal representative if the patient is a minor or is unconscious) to have knowledge and understanding of the procedure or process to be performed, along with its accompanying risks and possible outcomes.

Inhalation: Also known as *inspiration,* the process of taking air into the lungs.

Inpatient: A patient who stays overnight or longer in a health-care facility, such as an acute medical or mental health-care hospital, a skilled nursing facility in a nursing home or hospital, a long-term acute care hospital, a long-term chronic care facility such as a nursing home or assisted living facility, or a rehabilitation facility.

Insulin syringe: A syringe that is calibrated in units of insulin and used only for injecting insulin; it is similar in size and shape to a TB syringe.

Integrative health care: The use of Western medicine and complementary and alternative medicine (CAM) in a coordinated way.

Interpreter: An individual who translates communication for another person.

Interstitial space: The space surrounding and between cells, which holds fluid known as either *tissue fluid* or *interstitial fluid.*

Intracellular fluid (ICF): Two-thirds of the body's fluids that is located inside the individual cells.

Intractable pain: Pain that cannot be relieved, is incurable, or is resistant to treatment.

Intradermal (ID): A type of medication route that deposits the medication into the *epidermis,* or the outer layers of the skin.

Intramuscular (IM): A type of medication route in which medicine is administered into the deep muscle tissue below the subcutaneous layer of tissue.

Intravascular space: A space that includes the blood vessels and the heart and that holds the plasma.

Intravenous pyelogram: This test uses an iodine-based contrast dye that is injected intravenously in order to take x-rays of the kidney parenchyma, pelvis, calyces, ureters, and bladder. This test evaluates renal structure and function, and aids in detecting kidney stones, obstruction, tumors, urinary tract disease, and trauma.

Intubation: The insertion of an endotracheal tube into the patient's trachea to maintain an open airway and administer oxygen and, for surgery, an inhalant anesthesia.

Ionizing radiation: A method of sterilization that kills pathogens on sutures, some plastics, and biological materials that cannot be boiled or autoclaved.

Ischemia: Reduced blood flow to an area.

Ischemic stroke: A cerebrovascular accident (CVA) caused by a blood clot that interrupts normal blood flow to an area of the brain, resulting in the death of brain tissue.

Isotonic IV solution: A solution that contains an amount of solute that produces a concentration of dissolved particles equal to that of the intracellular and extracellular fluids of the human body.

Jaundice: A yellowing of the eyes or skin resulting from excessive blood levels of bilirubin.

Jejunostomy tube (J-tube): A long-term feeding tube inserted into the jejunum.

Joint replacement: Surgery to remove damaged articular bone surfaces and replace them with metal and plastic surfaces.

Kardex: A type of flip chart with a page for each patient on the unit or floor that contains a summary of care required by the patient; it requires continual updating and maintenance by nursing staff.

Kayexalate enema: A type of enema administered for the purpose of lowering a very high potassium level.

Kinesthetic learning: Learning by touching and doing.

KUB: A flat-plate x-ray, also known as *KUB* (which stands for kidneys, ureters, and bladder), is an x-ray of the abdomen that shows the abdominal organs' structures and their position. This type of x-ray is often the initial diagnostic tool utilized when an abdominal organ disease is suspected.

Laceration: An open wound made by the accidental cutting or tearing of tissue.

Laparoscopic surgery: A type of surgery in which the scope is inserted into the surgical area through three or four tiny incisions between 1/2 and 3/4 inch (1.27 to 1.85 cm) in length. It reduces the risk of infection, decreases postoperative pain, and shortens recovery time.

Lateral position: Lying on the right or left side to relieve pressure on the back and on the sacral and coccygeal areas.

Learning: The act of acquiring knowledge or skills.

Leaving AMA: A situation in which a patient becomes unhappy with his or her care, decides against treatment, or for any other reason simply decides to leave the hospital before the physician authorizes a discharge; known as *leaving against medical advice.*

Left shift: The elevation of slightly immature neutrophils, called *bands,* which generally indicates bacterial infection.

Leg monitor: A type of chair monitor; it attaches to the patient's leg like a large bandage and generates an alarm when the leg is in a dependent position, indicating that the patient is attempting to stand.

Lesion: A localized, open area of diseased skin.

Lethargy: Drowsiness or mental sluggishness.

Leukoplakia: White patches on the tongue or oral mucosa that can be precancerous lesions.

Lice: Tiny parasites that live on the skin and scalp.

Licensed practical/vocational nurse (LPN/LVN): The most basic of all the entry-level options for nurses.

Living will: A written document prepared by a mentally competent patient that indicates that procedures and measures the patient does or does not want should an end-of-life condition or disability occur.

Local anesthesia: A type of sedation in which a very small area of tissue is blocked from sensory perception by injection of a local anesthetic numbing agent such as lidocaine.

Localized infection: An infection in one area of the body.

Logroll: Turning a patient's body as one unit after the patient has had spinal surgery or a spinal injury.

Lumbar puncture: The insertion of a spinal needle to obtain a cerebrospinal fluid (CSF) sample to culture for organisms and to measure the CSF pressure. This test is used to diagnose meningitis, subarachnoid hemorrhage, tumors, and other infections of the central nervous system.

Lymphostasis: Lack of movement of lymph fluid due to the surgical removal of lymph tissue.

Maceration: Softened skin due to continuous exposure to moisture.

Magnetic resonance imaging (MRI): A form of radiology that uses a magnetic scanner to detect the magnetic properties of atoms, usually hydrogen, while radiofrequency energy produces images of body tissues. It produces "slices" of the site being imaged, allowing the examiner to view organs and tissues at all depths.

Malignant hyperthermia: A rapid and severe rise in body temperature that occurs while the patient is under a general anesthesia; it is caused by an inherited genetic trait.

Malpractice: A situation in which a nurse's actions fail to meet professional standards of care and injure a patient.

Managed care: Per Myllahy and Jensen, this type of care is "a system of health-care delivery aimed at managing the cost and quality of access to health care."

Massage therapy: The application of stroking, pressure, friction, and kneading muscles and other soft tissue to relax muscles and decrease stress.

Mass casualty event (MCE): A public health or medical emergency involving thousands of victims.

Mechanical soft diet: The diet of choice for patients with acute or chronic difficulties with chewing, such as those with jaw problems, missing teeth, poorly fitting dentures, or severe weakness or fatigue. This diet includes all of the items from the full liquid diet plus the addition of soft foods such as scrambled eggs and cottage cheese.

Medicaid: A federal–state program in which the federal government helps states pay for the health care of those with an income below the poverty level as well as certain other individuals.

Medical asepsis: Practices performed to prevent the spread of infection; sometimes referred to as using *clean technique.*

Medicare: The federal government's health insurance program for people older than 65 years of age or those with certain disabilities or conditions.

Medication administration record (MAR): Record of medications, the times they are to be given, and documentation that they have been given. May be a paper MAR or for electronic health records, it is an e-MAR.

Medication reconciliation: One of the most important discharge responsibilities of the nurse. In this process, the nurse reconciles prescription and over-the-counter medications the patient was taking at home with the physician's orders while the individual was a patient in the facility. This safety measure was adopted in an effort to decrease medication omissions and duplications and potential drug interactions.

Melena: Small amounts of blood that come from higher in the digestive tract, such as the stomach, that have been partially digested and that have a distinctive "old blood" odor and a black, tarry appearance.

Menarche: The beginning of menstrual periods.

Meridians: Energy pathways in the body.

Metabolism: The chemical and physical processes required to build and maintain body tissues.

Metered-dose inhaler (MDI): Pressurized medication dispensers that spray a premeasured amount of drug into the lungs. They are the most efficient way to get medications into the airways.

Methicillin-resistant *Staphylococcus aureus* (MRSA): A resistant strain of *Staphylococcus aureus* that can live on the skin of healthy individuals without causing illness but which can cause serious illness when a wound is infected with it.

Microorganisms: Minuscule living bodies that cannot be seen without a microscope.

Mitered corner: A slanted corner that is created to anchor the linens more firmly than if the linens were only tucked at the foot of the mattress.

Moral development: The ability to think at higher levels and develop a value system that differentiates right from wrong.

Mottling: A purplish blotching of the skin that indicates that circulation has slowed greatly.

Mucosal route: A medication route in which medicine is absorbed through the mucosa, such as medications applied through the rectum, vagina, eye, or ear, and inhaled into the lungs and bronchi.

Myocardial infarction: Heart attack.

Narcotic: A medication made with opium and opium derivatives that control and relieve pain. Narcotics are controlled substances and may be formulated for oral, topical, injectable, and IV administration.

Narrative charting: A type of charting that details the patient's experiences during a hospital stay. It is written in chronological order and relates the patient's health status from admission and through all changes in condition, up to and including his or her discharge status.

Nasogastric (NG) tube: A feeding tube inserted through the nose, down the esophagus, and into the stomach.

National Association of Licensed Practical Nurses (NALPN): The professional organization for licensed practical/vocational nurses. Established in 1949 by Lillian Custer, it is available only to those with an LPN or LVN license, although student affiliation is allowed.

NCLEX-PN: The licensing examination taken by students completing their LPN/LVN educational program; it stands for the *National Council Licensure Examination for Practical Nursing.*

NCLEX-RN: The licensing examination taken by students completing their ADN educational program; it stands for the *National Council Licensure Examination for Registered Nursing.* Upon successfully passing the examination, the graduates become registered nurses and use the title "RN" after their names.

Nebulizer: A medication delivery system that contains an air compressor and a mask or handheld mouthpiece.

Necrotic: The death of cells or tissue.

Negligence: A patient injury that occurs because the nurse fails to meet his or her responsibility to the patient.

Neuropathic pain: The burning, stabbing, or sometimes deep ache that occurs when there is nerve compression caused by pressure from tumors, lymphedema, or compression fractures of the spine.

Nitrogen balance: An equal amount of nitrogen ingested in the form of protein with the level of nitrogen that is utilized by the body, with excesses removed from the body by the kidneys.

Nits: The eggs of lice.

Nociceptors: Nerve pain receptors.

Nocturia: Waking often during the night to urinate.

Nonessential amino acids: One of the building blocks of protein, this type is produced by the liver and thus is not essential for inclusion in our diet.

Nonverbal communication: Communication that is conveyed by body language. It is less conscious and more indirect than verbal communication and therefore often conveys more of what a person feels, thinks, and means than what is stated in words.

Nonvesicant: Something that does not cause blistering and the death of tissue.

Normal flora and fauna: Microorganisms that live in and on the body; they perform needed functions to protect the body from harmful pathogens as well as help break down and digest food.

NPO: An acronym that stands for "nothing per os," or nothing by mouth. It signifies that a patient is restricted from the oral intake of food or fluid, including water. It is frequently ordered before surgery, invasive procedures, and certain diagnostic studies in order to reduce the risk of aspiration.

Nurse Practice Act (NPA): In every state, the law that governs nurses' actions. This law is written to specifically address each level of nursing.

Nursing diagnosis: The formulation of a patient assessment through analysis of the information gathered. The nursing diagnosis is related to the needs or problems the patient is experiencing and is completely different than medical diagnoses.

Nursing drug guide: A guide that includes generic drugs listed in alphabetical order with information about the classification, brand names, absorption, indications for use, dosages, contraindications, cautions, interactions, nursing interventions, and patient teaching.

Nursing goal: The overall direction in which one must progress in order to improve a problem.

Nursing process: A decision-making framework used by all nurses to determine the needs of their patients and to decide how to care for them.

Objective data: Things that are observable through the senses of hearing, sight, smell, and touch.

Occult blood: Blood in the stool that is hidden or not visible.

Ocular prosthesis: Artificial eye.

Oliguria: Urinary output of less than 30 mL/hr, which can be caused by decreased fluid intake, dehydration, illness, urinary obstruction, renal failure, hemorrhage, or severe loss of body fluids.

Ophthalmoscope: A lighted instrument used to assess and examine the internal structures of the eyes.

Oral glucose tolerance test: A test that is used to diagnose diabetes mellitus or hypoglycemia. The patient drinks concentrated glucose syrup to stimulate pancreatic production of insulin, and blood and urine samples are collected at five to six intervals over a 3- to 6-hour span to evaluate glucose levels.

Oral route: Medication taken through the mouth, either by swallowing or by *sublingual* (under the tongue) or buccal (between cheek and gums) placement.

Orthopnea: A condition in which an individual finds it too hard to breathe unless he or she is positioned in an upright position, such as sitting or standing.

Orthopneic position: Sitting upright with the head of the bed elevated 90 degrees or sitting on the side of the bed with one's feet flat on the floor; in this position, the individual leans slightly forward with arms raised and elbows flexed, supported on an over-bed table.

Orthostatic hypotension: Also known as *postural hypotension,* this is a decrease in blood pressure that occurs when a patient changes from a reclining or flat position to an upright position, such as sitting or standing; it is common after a person has been restricted to bedrest.

Osmosis: The process in which water moves through a semipermeable membrane from the side where the fluid is lowest in solute concentration to the side where the fluid is highest in solute concentration.

Osteoarthritis: A disorder that causes degeneration and inflammation of joints over time.

Otoscope: A lighted instrument used to assess/examine the inside of the nose, the tympanic membranes, and the ear canals.

Outpatient: A patient who is provided care in many settings and typically in one day and then is allowed to return home. Outpatient care is preferred when possible to decrease costs while still providing quality care.

Over-the-counter (OTC) medications: Medications available without a prescription; also referred to as *nonprescription medications.* They may be purchased by the consumer for use at recommended dosages.

Packed red blood cells (PRBCs): Red blood cells that have been separated from plasma.

Palliative care: Comfort care that is physician directed and that is performed to alleviate uncomfortable symptoms such as pain, nausea, and vomiting but is not intended to cure the patient's disease.

Palliative surgery: Surgery that alleviates symptoms and provides comfort but does not necessarily cure the disease or heal the injury.

Pallor: Paleness of the skin.

Palpation: To examine by touch or feel.

Paracentesis: A test performed to drain ascites, which is the accumulation of fluid in the abdominal cavity.

Parenteral nutrition: A type of feeding administered directly into the bloodstream via a central venous catheter, bypassing the GI tract; it provides complete nutrition, including amino acids, dextrose, emulsified fats, vitamins, minerals, and trace elements. It is used for patients with one or more problems that are complicated by malnutrition and low protein levels.

Parenteral route: A medication route in which medicine is given beneath the skin. It includes all injections, such as *intradermal* (between the layers of the skin), *subcutaneous* (beneath the skin), *intramuscular* (within muscle layers), and *intravenous* (into the vein).

Paresthesia: Numbness or decreased sensation.

Parietal pleura: The portion of the pleura that lines the chest cavity.

Partial parenteral nutrition (PPN): A type of feeding administered through a peripherally inserted central catheter (PICC) inserted into a smaller peripheral vein.

Patent: Something, such as a PRN device, that is open.

Pathogens: Microorganisms that cause infection in humans.

Patient-controlled analgesia (PCA): Drugs that are administered, within preset boundaries, by the patient, who controls the frequency and administration of his or her pain medication. It uses a computerized IV infusion device consisting of a pump, a large syringe containing the analgesic, IV tubing, and a push button the patient presses for delivery of the analgesic.

Percussion: Striking body parts with the tips of the fingers to elicit sounds that can help locate and determine the size of structures beneath the surface, to identify whether the structure is solid or hollow, and to detect areas containing air or fluid.

Percutaneous endoscopic gastrostomy (PEG) tube: A long-term feeding tube inserted into the stomach through the skin and abdominal wall.

Peristalsis: Rhythmic, wavelike movements that begin in the esophagus and continue to the rectum to propel a bolus of food through the GI tract.

Permeable: Having pores or openings that allow for the passage of substances.

PERRLA: An acronym used in documentation that stands for *pupils equal* and *round* and *reactive to light* and *accommodation.* It is used to document a patient's pupils that are bilaterally brisk and equally reactive to light and accommodation.

Petechiae: Pinpoint areas of hemorrhage.

pH: A measure that is used to determine the acid-base balance; it stands for *parts hydrogen.* The pH ranges from 0 to 14.

Phagocytosis: The process by which certain white blood cells surround, engulf, and digest offending microorganisms and debris in cells and exudate, which helps to prevent infection.

Phantom limb pain: A type of neuropathic pain that feels as though it is coming from an extremity that has been *amputated,* meaning that it has been surgically or traumatically removed.

Phlebitis: Inflammation of a vein.

Phlebotomy: The practice of drawing blood samples.

Physical development: The physical size and functioning of a person. Influences on physical development include genetics, nutrition, and function of the endocrine and central nervous systems.

Physical therapist: A health-care team member responsible for assessing musculoskeletal deficiencies and developing the plan of care to strengthen muscles and restore mobility.

***Physician's Desk Reference* (PDR):** A comprehensive book that contains the same detailed information about a large number of medications that is found in drug package inserts. It is found at the nurses' station in hospitals or on electronic devices and is used by health-care providers to prescribe medications, as well as by nurses to research medications.

PIE charting: A type of charting styles that is shorter and documents fewer data than the SOAPIER charting style. It only addresses the patient's problems; therefore, the concept of treating the patient holistically is lost. It stands for ***p***roblem, ***i***nterventions, and ***e***valuation.

Plantar flexion: The downward pointing of the foot.

Plasma: The liquid portion of the blood.

Pleural effusion: Fluid in the chest cavity.

Pneumothorax: A serious condition in which air enters the pleural space through a hole, infiltrating an area of negative pressure.

Point-of-service (POS) plan: Similar to an HMO in that a primary care physician still serves as a gatekeeper, this type of plan is not capitated. Insured people can seek care from physicians who are both in and out of the network. The patient pays a part of the bill (usually 20% to 30%) and the insurance company pays the remainder.

Polyuria: Increased urinary output of greater than 3,000 mL/day, which can be caused by excessive fluid intake, consumption of alcohol, or use of certain medications, such as diuretics ("water pills").

Position of function: Placement of the extremities in an alignment to maintain the potential for their use and movement.

Postanesthesia care unit (PACU): A nursing area in which the immediate priority is to maintain a patent airway and verify respiratory and cardiac function.

Postmortem care: Care provided after an individual's death.

Precedent: Legal decisions put forth by courts by which similar future cases will be judged.

Precipitate: A substance that forms when one of the agents in a solution separates from the solvent and becomes a solid, insoluble product.

Preferred provider organization (PPO): A group of health-care providers who contract with a health insurance company to provide services to a specific group of patients on a discounted basis.

Prefilled syringe: A single-dose, ready-to-use, disposable syringe cartridge, sometimes with an attached needle and sometimes where you must attach a needle, that contains specific dosages of specific medications. The cartridge is loaded into a reusable plastic holder for administration. This drug-delivery device offers various advantages, including ease of use, convenience, and safety.

Prejudice: A determination or judgment about a person or group based on irrational suspicion or hatred of a particular group, race, or religion.

Prescription medication: A medication available with a written direction from a health-care provider with prescriptive authority. This includes physicians; nurse practitioners; and, in some situations, physician assistants, depending on state laws.

Pressure injury: A wound that results from pressure and friction.

Primary care nursing: A type of nursing care in which one nurse is responsible for all aspects of the care for his or her assigned patients. In this type of nursing, the nurse carries a great deal of responsibility, but a secondary nurse is assigned care for the patients when the primary nurse is off duty.

Primary care physician (PCP): A physician who is paid a set amount per member per month to manage the health care of those members. This PCP is considered the gatekeeper to health services for the individual enrolled in an HMO.

Primary data: Information provided by the patient.

Primary infection: An initial infection caused by one pathogen only.

Prodromal phase: The phase of illness just before the onset of symptoms in which an individual doesn't feel well and experiences generalized body aches and fatigue.

Prone position: Lying on one's stomach with the head turned to the side.

Prostaglandins: Chemicals that can stimulate the nerve pain receptors and that are released during injury and damage to tissue. These chemicals are hormones that act in the immediate area to initiate inflammation by sensitizing local pain receptors.

Prosthesis: An artificial limb, such as an arm or a leg.

Proxemics: The distance, or personal space, that people place between themselves and others.

Proximodistal: Growth that occurs from the center of the body outward.

Psychosocial development: Development that occurs throughout a human being's life in distinct stages. Each stage requires that specific tasks be mastered.

Ptosis: Drooping of the eyelids.

Puberty: The onset of the development of sexual characteristics and functions; it occurs between the ages of 11 and 14 years.

Pulse deficit: A state in which the radial pulse is slower than the apical pulse.

Pulse pressure: The measurement of the difference between the systolic and diastolic pressures, which is found by subtracting the smaller number, the diastolic, from the larger number, the systolic. A normal range is between 30 and 50 mm Hg.

Pureed diet: A type of diet that is processed in a blender/food processor. Any food item can be included, but its consistency must be changed.

Purulent: Containing pus.

Quality and Safety Education for Nurses (QSEN): Established in 2005, this project focuses on the knowledge, skills, and attitudes (KSAs) needed by nurses to continually improve the quality and safety of patient care. It includes prelicensure KSAs for nursing students and graduate KSAs.

Radiating pain: Pain that begins at a specific site and shoots out from or extends to a larger area beyond the site of origin.

Rapport: The creation of mutual trust and understanding.

Rebound phenomenon: Leaving heat packs in place longer than 45 minutes can cause constriction of vessels instead of dilation, worsening the original condition rather than improving it.

Recovery phase: The final phase of illness. During this phase, the individual slowly resumes independence and regains his or her health.

Rectal route: A medication administration route in which medications are inserted directly into the rectum. This route may be used when nausea or vomiting is present or when the patient cannot take anything by mouth.

Referral: The act, by a primary care physician, of providing a patient with a referral to a specialist. It provides a way of controlling access to more costly care and potentially redundant testing.

Referred pain: Pain felt in an area other than where the pain was produced.

Reflexes: Automatic responses by the central nervous system.

Regional anesthesia: A type of sedation in which specific nerves and the region innervated by the nerves, such as a finger, an arm, or the lower half of the body, are blocked from sensory perception by injection of a local anesthetic numbing agent such as lidocaine.

Regression: A return to earlier behaviors.

Rehabilitation: Often referred to as *rehab,* it is a level of care in which the patient can receive intense physical, occupational, and speech therapy services. The rehabilitation facility may be part of a hospital or it may be a free-standing facility.

Reinforce: To repeat.

Religion: The formal structured system of beliefs, values, rituals, and practices of a person or group, usually based on the teachings of a god or other spiritual leader.

Remission: A period of chronic illness that is characterized by either minimal symptoms or a complete absence of symptoms.

Renal calculi: Commonly referred to as *kidney stones,* these can occur anywhere in the renal system from the kidneys to the urethra.

Rescue breathing: Breathing for the patient in case of respiratory arrest when the pulse is still palpable.

Resident: The preferred term used to refer to an individual within a long-term care facility who resides in the facility.

Residual urine: Urine that remains in the bladder after the patient voids, which can be caused by bladder outlet obstruction or problems with the detrusor muscle's contractility.

Respiratory route: A medication administration route in which medications are dispersed in fine droplets and inhaled into the lungs and bronchial airways, usually through the use of inhalers or nebulizers.

Respite: Arrangements for the provision of care in order that the family members may have a time to get away, rest, and rejuvenate without the strain and worry of continual caregiving.

Restorative sleep: Sleep that allows an individual to awaken feeling rested, refreshed, rejuvenated, and energized, ready to meet new challenges.

Restraint alternatives: Less-restrictive ways than standard restraints that help the patient remember not to get up and try to walk, or to alert nursing staff that the patient is attempting to do so.

Restraints: Vests, jackets, or bands with connected straps that are tied to the bed, chair, or wheelchair to keep a patient in one place.

Retractions: Abnormal movements in which a patient's chest wall appears depressed, or sunken in, between the ribs or under the xiphoid process when the patient inhales. These movements indicate acute respiratory problems that need attention.

Rhonchi: Abnormal breath sounds, such as snoring, rattling, gurgling, squeaking, and low-pitched wheezes, caused by either secretions or partial occlusion of the airways. They are deeper and more rumbling sounds than crackles and usually are heard during expiration.

Right shift: The elevation of lymphocytes, which is a typical indicator of viral infection.

Risk factors: Physiological, psychological, or genetic elements that contribute to the development of an illness or disease.

Role reversal: A situation in which children who are accustomed to being cared for suddenly become the caregivers for their parents.

Safety data sheet (SDS): An organized, written summary identifying hazardous materials in the work environment and how to handle, store, contain, counteract, and dispose of them. It was formerly known as the *material safety data sheet.*

Sanguineous: Resembling blood.

Sclerosed: Veins that feel hard and ropey; they should not be used for venipuncture.

Scope of practice: The limitations and allowances of what a nurse can do.

Scrub nurse: The person who assists the physician throughout surgery by handing instruments, holding retractors, and performing other tasks that require sterile garb. This person, who may be a surgical technologist or a licensed practical nurse, does scrub in on the case.

Seborrhea: An overproduction of sebum.

Secondary data: Information obtained from family members, friends, and the patient's chart.

Secondary infection: An infection caused by a second, different pathogen than the pathogen of the primary infection.

Seeking help phase: The phase of illness in which an individual seeks help from a medical professional. In some cultures, an individual may seek help from a healer or other alternative practitioner.

Self-care: A situation in which patients are able to perform activities of daily living without assistance.

Semi-Fowler's position: A position in which the head of the bed is elevated 45 degrees.

Separation anxiety: Anxiety that develops from an individual's separation from familiar surroundings and significant others.

Septicemia: An infection in the blood.

Sequential compression devices (SCDs): Compression sleeve pads designed to wrap around the legs and capable of having air pumped into and out of them. These devices result in intermittent compression of the legs, aiding venous return of blood to the heart.

Serosanguineous: Having a pink appearance.

Serous: Having a somewhat clear to slightly yellow color.

Shared meaning: A goal of communication in which mutual understanding of the meaning of a message between two people is established.

Shearing: A situation in which the skin layer is pulled across muscle and bone in one direction while the skin slides over another surface, such as a bed sheet, in the opposite direction.

Side effect: An unintended but not always unexpected outcome of taking a medication.

Signs: Evidence of illness or injury that are objective and measurable.

Simple carbohydrates: Also known as *simple sugars,* this type of carbohydrate is chemically made up of one or two sugar molecules that are absorbed rapidly.

Sims' position: Lying on the back with the arms at the sides.

Sinus tract: A channel or tunnel that develops between two cavities or between an infected cavity and the surface of the skin.

Siphon enema: A sterile water enema used in a postsurgical patient to remove gas from the bowel.

Skeletal traction: A type of traction in which pins, screws, or tongs are surgically inserted into the bone.

Skin traction: A type of traction in which the limb is wrapped with an elastic bandage or fitted with a Velcro wrap to which a frame is attached.

SOAPIER charting: One of the lengthier documentation formats that typically is used in progress notes and the nurse's notes. It includes ***s***ubjective data; ***o***bjective data; ***a***ssessment data; a ***p***lan; an ***i***ntervention; an ***e***valuation; and, as needed, a ***r***evision.

Solar lentigines: Numerous spots of yellowish-brown discoloration caused by years of sun exposure; often evident in elderly patients.

Solution: A type of liquid medication that contains a dissolved substance.

Sordes: Dried mucus or food caked on the lips and teeth that can be treated with good oral hygiene.

Special mouth care: Oral care for patients whose conditions result in a need for more frequent care and who require assistance for this care.

Specific gravity: The result of comparing the weight of a substance with an equal amount of water. The normal specific gravity for urine is 1.001 to 1.029.

Speed shock: Shock caused by the rapid IV infusion of medication/solution.

Sphygmomanometer: The aneroid or electronic pressure manometer, or gauge, that is used to measure blood pressure.

Spica: A cast that encases the hips and one or both legs.

Spiritual care: Care that includes an understanding of the differences between spirituality and religion, and an understanding of one's own spirituality, beliefs, and values related to providing spiritual care to a patient.

Spiritual development: The development of faith that develops from a process of developing trust.

Spirituality: A way of being that includes an individual's spirit and the relationship of the spirit to the body, mind, and environment, including the patient's relationship to others.

Sprain: An injury to a joint that results in damage to muscles and ligaments. Severe sprains may cause ligaments to be completely torn.

Sputum: Mucus within the lungs.

Standard precautions: A group of safety measures performed to prevent the transmission of pathogens found in the blood and body fluids.

Standards of care: Standards of performance or clinical guidelines that represent the level of skill and nursing care that another nurse in the same area of the country, with the same educational level, would perform in the same situation.

Steatorrhea: Stool that contains an abnormally high amount of undigested fat: appears fluffy, floats on water, and has a foul odor.

Stereotyping: Having or creating preconceived ideas and fixed impressions about a person or group that may lead to prejudice and possible mistreatment. The preconceived ideas may be based solely on the person's physical characteristics.

Sterile conscience: Always being aware of potential or certain contamination of the sterile field or sterile objects and taking appropriate steps to correct the situation, such as replacing the contaminated object or reassembling the sterile field with new supplies.

Sterile field: An area that is free from all microorganisms where additional sterile items can be placed until they are ready for use.

Sterile technique: A method used to prevent contamination during invasive procedures or procedures that involve entering body cavities.

Sterilization: The process of using steam under pressure, gas, or radiation, to kill all pathogens and their spores on surgical supplies and equipment.

Stoma: The mouth of an opening in the bowel that is used as an alternate form of bowel elimination.

Straight catheter: A type of catheter used to empty the bladder of a patient who is unable to fully empty his or her bladder; also known as a *single-lumen catheter.*

Stress: A nonspecific response of the body to any demand made on it.

Stress incontinence: An inability to control the passing of urine that occurs with increased abdominal pressure, causing urine to leak out of the bladder; it is seen more in women than in men.

Stridor: An audible, high-pitched crowing sound that results from partial obstruction of the airways.

Stump: The remaining portion of a limb after amputation.

Subcutaneous (subcut): A type of medication route in which medication is injected under the layers of the skin into the subcutaneous tissue layer.

Subjective data: Information that is known only to the patient and the patient's family members.

Sublingual route: A medication administration route in which medications are given under the tongue.

Substance P: A chemical that can stimulate the nerve pain receptors and that is released during injury and damage to tissue. This chemical plays a role in eliciting localized tissue reactions similar to inflammation.

Supine position: Lying on one's back.

Surgical asepsis: A method that requires the use of sterile supplies and equipment that have been treated to kill all pathogens and spores.

Suspension: A type of liquid medication that contains fine particles of medication mixed with, but not dissolved in, a liquid. When the mixture sits, the particles will drift to the bottom of the liquid.

Sustained-release: Also called *controlled-release, delayed-release, extended-release,* or *modified-release tablets,* this is a type of tablet designed to slow absorption of the drug. This type of medication is absorbed slowly over time for a continuous effect.

Symptomatic phase: The phase of illness in which observable symptoms develop.

Symptoms: Evidence of illness or injury verbalized by the patient that is subjective and not directly measurable.

Syncope: Fainting.

Syrup: A type of liquid medication that consists of a concentrated aqueous preparation of sugars, with or without flavoring agents, and medicinal substances.

Systemic infection: The spread of infection from one organ to other organs via the bloodstream.

Systolic pressure: The measurement of the force exerted by the blood against the walls of arteries during contraction of the heart ventricles, which is when the pressure is highest.

Tablet: Powdered ingredients compressed into various sizes and shapes that are the most common form of oral medication.

Tachycardia: A pulse that is greater than 100 bpm.

Tachypnea: A respiratory rate that exceeds 20 respirations per minute.

Teachable moments: The time during which learning is easiest.

Team nursing: A team that consists of nurses and certified nursing assistants (CNAs) or unlicensed assistive personnel (UAPs) to provide care for a group of patients.

Tenesmus: Bowel cramping that is identified by increased rectal pressure and a feeling of the need to defecate.

Tension pneumothorax: A life-threatening type of pneumothorax in which air is trapped in the pleural cavity surrounding the lungs, which not only compresses and collapses the lungs but also causes pressure on the heart and major blood vessels and causes them to shift within the thorax.

Tepid: Cool but not cold.

Terminal cleaning: Following a patient's discharge, disinfection of the bed, furniture, bathroom, sink, and floor in order to prepare the room for the next patient.

The Joint Commission: The organization responsible for evaluating and accrediting health-care organizations and programs in the United States.

Therapeutic communication: Patient-centered communication in which the goal is to promote a greater understanding of a patient's needs, concerns, and feelings.

Therapeutic level: The amount of medication in the blood that it takes to reach the desired effects on the target organ or organs.

Third-party payer: A party that pays the bills of a beneficiary cared for by a physician or hospital; when a bill is sent to an insurance company, the insurance company is referred to as a *third party* or a *third-party payer.*

Third-spacing: A shift in fluids to areas where they can no longer contribute to fluid and electrolyte balance between ICF and ECF. The fluids are still within the body but are unavailable for normal use.

Thoracentesis: In this test, under local anesthetic, a needle is inserted through the chest wall into the pleural space to remove excess fluid for diagnostic purposes or to decrease respiratory distress due to excess fluid due to lung disease or cancer.

Thrombus: A blood clot.

Tinea capitus: A fungal infection that can affect any part of the body and can be spread from one person to another.

Topical route: A medication route in which medicine is applied to the skin; includes creams, ointments, lotions, and transdermal patches.

Tortuous: Veins that have many twists and turns.

Total care: A situation in which patients are able to do very little or nothing for themselves.

Total parenteral nutrition (TPN): A type of feeding administered through a central venous catheter (CVC) placed in a larger central vein.

Tourniquet: A rubber strap that can be snugly wrapped around a limb to occlude the venous return of blood toward the heart.

Toxicity: A state of having too much of a medication in the body.

Tracheostomy: An incision into the trachea that is held open with a tube to promote breathing.

Transcultural nursing: Care that crosses cultural boundaries or combines the elements of more than one culture.

Transdermal route: A medication administration route in which a drug is applied to the skin using a patch. The drug is absorbed through the skin into the bloodstream for a systemic effect.

Transfer: The movement of a patient from one place to another in a way that is safe both for the patient and for health-care personnel.

Transfer summary form: Documentation of the patient's condition and the reason for transfer and a comprehensive list of the patient's medications.

Transient ischemic attack: A temporary decrease in the blood supply to the brain, lasting a few minutes to a few hours, that causes sudden symptoms of dizziness, visual changes, weakness, numbness in one or more limbs, and difficulty swallowing; sometimes referred to as a "ministroke."

Transmission-based precautions: Precautions used to prevent the spread of known infection to patients or health-care staff. They are used when a patient has a communicable illness that can be spread through contact, through respiratory droplets, or through the air.

Trochanter roll: A rolled towel or cylindrical device placed snugly against the lateral aspect of the patient's thigh to prevent the leg from rotating outward.

Tuberculin (TB) syringe: A smaller-diameter syringe that holds a total volume of 1 mL and is calibrated in tenths and hundredths of a milliliter as well as sixteenths of a minim, making it an excellent choice for the administration of the small and precise volumes of medication required by newborns and infants as well as for the TB skin test for which it was designed.

Turgor: Skin elasticity, which is an indicator of hydration level in all ages of patients except elders. The skin of elderly patients loses its elasticity and is not a reliable assessment tool for hydration.

Ultrasonography: The use of ultrasound waves to produce images of organs and tissues that can be recorded and printed. It is painless and easy to use and can show motion of the organ.

Urge incontinence: Also known as *overactive bladder,* this type of incontinence is an inability to keep urine in the bladder long enough to get to the restroom.

Urinary diversion: The elimination of urine by an alternative route rather than traveling through the bladder, which may be established when there has been trauma to the bladder or the bladder has been removed as a result of bladder cancer.

Urinary retention: The inability to empty the bladder at all, or the inability to completely empty the bladder, which can be acute or chronic.

Urinary tract infection (UTI): An infection caused by the presence of pathogens within the urinary tract.

Vaginal route: A medication administration route used to provide medicine that comes in the form of suppositories, creams, aerosol foams, or tablets inserted into the vagina to dissolve there.

Validate: To ensure the correctness of something.

Value: An individual's belief of something's worth.

Vasoconstriction: Narrowing of the veins and capillaries.

Vasodilation: An increase in the size of the cavity or opening inside the vessel.

Vectors: Organisms, such as ticks and mites, that are carriers of microorganisms.

Venography: A form of radiology that requires a contrast medium be instilled into designated veins, which allows examination of the vessel to assess for abnormalities.

Venous return: Blood return from the extremities back to the heart.

Verbal communication: A conscious use of words, either spoken or written. This type of communication is more direct than nonverbal communication and is often used to give or receive specific information.

Vesicant: Something that causes blistering, necrosis, and sloughing of tissue.

Vessel lumen: The cavity or space inside a blood vessel.

Vial: A glass or plastic container of medication with a rubber stopper that must be punctured with a needle for medication removal.

Visceral pain: Sometimes known as *soft tissue pain,* this pain is experienced from stimulation of deep internal pain receptors.

Visceral pleura: The portion of the pleura that lines the lungs.

Visual learning: Learning by seeing, reading, and watching.

Void: To urinate.

Wellness strategies: Actions designed to promote healthy practices.

Wheezes: Abnormal breath sounds that are continuous melodious, musical, or whistling sounds. They are caused by constriction of the airways, and can be inspiratory or expiratory.

Yoga: A mind-body intervention that is used to decrease the negative effects of stress through the use of breathing exercises, physical postures, and meditation.

Z-track: A method of intramuscular injection that prevents irritating and dark-colored medications from leaking out of the injection site into sensitive tissues or subcutaneous tissues that may stain. It also helps to reduce the inflammation and discomfort that can be caused by the medication irritating the subcutaneous tissue.

Index

Note: Page numbers followed by b indicate boxes, page numbers followed by f indicate figures, page numbers followed by t indicate tables.

B

C

D

E

I

J

K

N

O

P

S

W

X

Y

Z